WK 585

This book is due for return on or before the last date shown below.

0 8 AUG 2006

DIAGNOSIS AND MANAGEMENT OF PITUITARY TUMORS

DIAGNOSIS AND MANAGEMENT OF
PITUITARY TUMORS

Edited by

KAMAL THAPAR, MD, PHD

*Division of Neurosurgery, Department of Surgery,
University Health Network, University of Toronto,
Toronto, Ontario, Canada*

KALMAN KOVACS, MD, PHD

*Department of Pathology and Laboratory Medicine
St. Michael's Hospital, Toronto, Ontario, Canada*

BERND W. SCHEITHAUER, MD

*Department of Pathology
Mayo Clinic, Rochester, MN*

RICARDO V. LLOYD, MD, PHD

*Department of Pathology
Mayo Clinic, Rochester, MN*

Foreword by

Michael O. Thorner, MB, BS, DSC

*Professor and Chair, Department of Internal Medicine
University of Virginia Medical School
Charlottesville, VA*

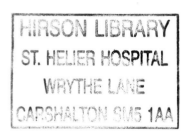
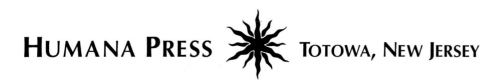

HUMANA PRESS ☀ TOTOWA, NEW JERSEY

Library of Congress Cataloging-in-Publication Data

Diagnosis and management of pituitary tumors / edited by Kamal Thapar ...[et al.]
     p. ; cm.
   Includes bibliographical references and index.
   ISBN 0-89603-403-8 (alk. paper)
   1. Pituitary gland--Tumors. I. Thapar, Kamal
   [DNLM: 1. Pituitary Neoplasms--diagnosis. 2. Pituitary Neoplasms--therapy. WK 585 D5355 2001]
RC280.P5 D49 2001
616.99'247--dc21
                     99-58333

To my beloved Hazel, whose love and encouragement sustain me; to our little daughters, Molly, Olivia, and Isabelle, who give my life purpose; and to my mentors, Kalman Kovacs, Edward Laws Jr., Bernd Scheithauer, and James Rutka, who have passed on to me their passion for science and discovery, and upon whose shoulders I continue to stand.

KAMAL THAPAR

To Eva, my wife and longtime companion in the exciting journey exploring the mysteries of pituitary tumors.

KALMAN KOVACS

To Chuckie and our children, Hans and Monika—more stimulation and inspiration than I could imagine.

BERND W. SCHEITHAUER

Sincere thanks to Debbie Lloyd and Vincent Lloyd for their continuous support during this project.

RICARDO V. LLOYD

Foreword

Diagnosis and Management of Pituitary Tumors is ambitious and is probably the most comprehensive text ever put together on this topic. The editors have selected leaders in the field to address the topic in an extremely thorough and inclusive manner—including historical, anatomical, physiological, epidemiological, pathophysiological, experimental, and pathological considerations—before turning to clinical considerations, both in terms of a general overview, neuroophthalmologic evaluation, imaging, surgery, medical therapy, and radiotherapy. Eminent clinicians, surgeons, pathologists, radiologists, and radiation oncologists cover in detail prolactinomas, somatotroph adenomas, corticotroph adenomas, thyrotroph adenomas, nonfunctioning tumors, pituitary tumors in children, as well as invasive adenomas and pituitary carcinomas, and lesions exclusive of pituitary adenomas that occur in the sellar region. The work finishes with a chapter on future perspectives for pituitary tumors. The authors have been carefully selected to provide authority for up-to-date reviews and the book provides not only back-ground information, but also specific and detailed information dealing with all aspects of pituitary tumors.

Diagnosis and Management of Pituitary Tumors meets a hitherto unfulfilled need for the collection of authoritative information on pituitary tumors. This volume is essential reading and an essential reference source for everyone dealing with pituitary tumor patients, including internists, endocrinologists, neurosurgeons, neuroradiologists, radiotherapists, as well as pathologists. The editors and the publisher are to be commended on undertaking this timely project, which is certain to be extremely useful and successful.

Michael O. Thorner, MB, BS, DSC
Henry B. Mulholland Professor
of Internal Medicine
Chair, Department of Internal Medicine
University of Virginia Health Sciences Center
Charlottesville, VA

Preface

Pituitary tumors represent a unique form of neoplasm. Both in concept and in practice, they differ fundamentally from virtually all other intracranial neoplasms. The most obvious difference relates to the dual nature of the clinical problem they pose, featuring endocrine concerns on the one hand, complicated by neurooncologic issues on the other. Thus, the diagnostic and therapeutic imperatives that surround pituitary tumors are correspondingly unique in calling upon the coordinated expertise of the clinical endocrinologist, neuroradiologist, neurosurgeon, pathologist, and radiation therapist. Indeed, the excellent long-term outcomes now enjoyed by many patients with pituitary tumors are directly attributable to this multidisciplinary approach and bears testament to the many innovations over the past two decades. These include new methods in endocrine diagnosis, high resolution imaging, receptor mediated pharmacotherapy, microsurgical technique, the development of a precise and physiologically meaningful classification of pituitary tumors, and improved methods of radiation delivery.

Whereas pituitary tumors are the subject of several current textbooks of endocrinology, neurosurgery, pathology, and radiology, their treatment in these contexts tends to represent a unidimensional view of the disease, one understandably skewed to a specialty-specific readership. This contrasts with the actual way in which pituitary tumors are clinically managed, an approach wherein optimal outcomes result from thoughtful, interactive decision-making by knowledgeable physicians of various disciplines. It is of this spirit of multidisciplinary cooperation that this text was born.

Our objective was to produce a comprehensive and up-to-date reference work encompassing all aspects of pituitary tumors, including consideration of basic science and molecular biology, their endocrine, radiologic, and pathologic diagnosis, and, lastly, issues of surgical, medical, and radiotherapeutic management. Thus, we hoped to transcend conventional boundaries and biases of the specialty-specific approach. Given the enormous and ever-increasing literature on the subject, our task of distilling it into a single volume was made possible only by enlisting the contributions of renowned clinicians, surgeons, pathologists, and scientists well known to the medical literature. The result, a collaborative multidisciplinary effort, should well serve the interests of all who deal with pituitary tumors.

We are indebted to a number of individuals whose support and encouragement sustained this project from beginning to end. In particular, we acknowledge the guidance and advice provided by our longtime colleague, Dr. Eva Horvath. We are also appreciative of the support provided by Mr. and Mrs. Steven Jarislowsky, Mr. and Mrs. Francis Wittern, and Mr. and Mrs. James Wooters; The Ellis Levitt I Welfare Fund; the Physicians Services Incorporated of Ontario; the Lloyd Carr Harris Foundation; Ms. Ann-Marie Creszenci, Office of Postgraduate Medical Education, University of Toronto; Dr. Charles Tator, Former Chairman, Division of Neurosurgery, University of Toronto; Dr. Avrum Gotlieb, Chairman, Department of Laboratory Medicine and Pathobiology, University of Toronto; Dr. Bernadette Garvey, Chief of Laboratory Medicine, St. Michael's Hospital; Dr. Robert Bear, St. Michael's Hospital, Toronto.

The publication of this book would not have been possible without the enthusiastic support and contributions of Mr. Thomas Lanigan and Mr. John Morgan, Humana Press. We are very much indebted to them. We are also grateful to Ms. Andrea Maher, who typeset the entire book, including some copious revisions that kept it up to date.

Kamal Thapar
Kalman Kovacs
Bernd W. Scheithauer
Ricardo V. Lloyd

Contents

FOREWORD   vii

PREFACE   ix

CONTRIBUTORS   xiii

COLOR PLATES   xv

1   Pituitary Adenomas:
Historic Considerations   1
*Raymond V. Randall, Bernd W. Scheithauer,
and Kalman Kovacs*

2   Anatomy of the Pituitary Gland
and Sellar Region   13
Albert L. Rhoton, Jr.

3   Hypothalamic–Pituitary Physiology
and Regulation   41
*Miklos I. Goth, Gabor B. Makara,
and Ida Gerendai*

4   Epidemiology of Pituitary Tumors   57
Shozo Yamada

5   Pathogenesis and Molecular Biology
of Pituitary Tumors   71
Ilan Shimon and Shlomo Melmed

6   Experimental Models
of Pituitary Tumorigenesis   81
Lucia Stefaneanu

7   Pathology of Pituitary Adenomas
and Pituitary Hyperplasia   91
*Bernd W. Scheithauer, Eva Horvath,
Ricardo V. Lloyd, and Kalman Kovacs*

8   Molecular Pathology of Pituitary Tumors   155
Ricardo V. Lloyd

9   Diagnosis, Management, and Prognosis
of Pituitary Tumors:
General Considerations   165
Mary Lee Vance

10   Neuro-Ophthalmologic Evaluation
of Pituitary Tumors   173
Shirley I. Stiver and James A. Sharpe

11   Imaging of Pituitary Tumors   201
Derek Emery and Walter Kucharczyk

12   Positron Emission Tomography
in Sellar Tumors: *In Vivo Metabolic,
Receptor, and Enzyme Characterization*   219
Carin Muhr

13   Pituitary Surgery   225
Kamal Thapar and Edward R. Laws, Jr.

14   Medical Therapy of Pituitary Tumors   247
Mark E. Molitch

15   Radiation Therapy of Pituitary Tumors:
Including Stereotactic Radiosurgery   269
B. Dawn Moose and Edward G. Shaw

16   Prolactinomas   279
Charles F. Abboud and Michael J. Ebersold

17   Somatotroph Adenomas:
Acromegaly and Gigantism   295
Hans-Jürgen Quabbe and Ursula Plöckinger

18   Corticotroph Adenomas: *Cushing's Disease
and Nelson's Syndrome*   317
*Joan C. Lo, J. Blake Tyrrell,
and Charles B. Wilson*

19   Thyrotroph Adenomas   333
Michael Buchfelder and Rudolf Fahlbusch

20   Clinically Nonfunctioning
Pituitary Adenomas   343
William F. Young, Jr.

21   Pituitary Tumors in Children   353
Nalin Gupta and James T. Rutka

22   Invasive Pituitary Adenoma
and Pituitary Carcinoma   369
Peter J. Pernicone and Bernd W. Scheithauer

23   Sellar Tumors Other Than Adenomas   387
*Paul E. McKeever, Mila Blaivas,
and Stephen S. Gebarski*

24   Tumor-like Lesions of the Sellar Region   449
Wolfgang Saeger

25   Pituitary Tumors: *Future Perspectives*   461
*Gregory M. Miller, Xun Zhang,
and Anne Klibanski*

Index   467

Contributors

CHARLES F. ABBOUD, MD, *Departments of Internal Medicine and Endocrinology, Mayo Clinic, Rochester, MN*

MILA BLAIVAS, MD, PHD, *Department of Pathology, University of Michigan Medical School, Ann Arbor, MI*

MICHAEL BUCHFELDER, MD, *Department of Neurosurgery, University of Erlangen-Nürnberg, Erlangen, Germany*

MICHAEL J. EBERSOLD, MD, *Department of Neurological Surgery, Mayo Clinic, Rochester, MN*

DEREK EMERY, MD, FRCP (C), *Department of Radiology and Diagnostic Imaging, University of Alberta, Edmonton, Alberta, Canada*

RUDOLF FAHLBUSCH, MD, *Department of Neurosurgery, University of Erlangen-Nürnberg, Erlangen, Germany*

STEPHEN S. GEBARSKI, MD, *Department of Pathology, University of Michigan Medical School, Ann Arbor, MI*

IDA GERENDAI, MD, DSCI, *Department of Human Morphology and Developmental Biology, Semmelweis University of Medicine, Budapest, Hungary*

MIKLOS I. GOTH, MD, PHD, *Faculty of Health Sciences, Semmelweis University, Budapest, Hungary*

NALIN GUPTA, MD, PHD, FRCSC, *Department of Neurological Surgery, University of California at San Francisco, San Francisco, CA*

EVA HORVATH, PHD, *Division of Pathology, Department of Laboratory Medicine, St. Michael's Hospital, Toronto, Ontario, Canada*

KALMAN KOVACS, MD, PHD, DSC, FRCP (C), FCAP, FRC (PATH), *Division of Pathology, Department of Laboratory Medicine, St. Michael's Hospital, Toronto, Ontario, Canada*

ANNE KLIBANSKI, MD, *Neuroendocrine Unit, Harvard Medical School, Massachusetts General Hospital, Boston MA*

WALTER KUCHARCZYK, MD, FRCP (C), *Professor and Chairman, Department of Medical Imaging, University of Toronto, Toronto, Ontario*

EDWARD R. LAWS, JR., MD, FACS, *Professor of Neurological Surgery and Medicine, University of Virginia School of Medicine, Charlottesville, VA*

RICARDO V. LLOYD, MD, PHD, *Department of Laboratory Medicine and Pathology, Mayo Clinic, Rochester, MN*

JOAN C. LO, MD, *Division of Endocrinology, University of California at San Francisco, San Francisco, CA*

GABOR B. MAKARA, MD, DSCI, *Institute of Experimental Medicine, Hungarian Academy of Sciences, Budapest, Hungary*

PAUL E. MCKEEVER, MD, PHD, *Section of Neuropathology, University of Michigan Medical School, Ann Arbor, MI*

SHLOMO MELMED, MD, *Cedars-Sinai Research Institute, Cedars-Sinai Medical Center, UCLA School of Medicine, Los Angeles, CA*

GREGORY M. MILLER, PHD, *Neuroendocrine Unit, Department of Medicine, Massachusetts General Hospital and Harvard Medical School, Boston, MA*

MARK E. MOLITCH, MD, *Center for Endocrinology, Metabolism, and Molecular Medicine, Northwestern University Medical School, Chicago, IL*

B. DAWN MOOSE, MD, *Department of Radiation Oncology, Wake Forest University School of Medicine, Winston-Salem, NC*

CARIN MUHR, MD, PHD, *Department of Neurology, University of Uppsala, University Hospital, Uppsala, Sweden*

PETER J. PERNICONE, MD, *Department of Pathology, Florida Hospital Medical Center, Orlando, FL*

URSULA PLÖCKINGER, MD, *Department of Hepatology and Gastroenterology, Division of Neuroendocrinology and Metabolism, Charité, Campus Virchow-Klinikum, Humboldt Universität zu Berlin, Berlin, Germany*

HANS-JÜRGEN QUABBE, MD, *Professor Emeritus, Department of Endocrinology, Klinik Steglitz, Freie Universität, Berlin, Germany*

RAYMOND V. RANDALL, MD, MS (MED), FACP, *Emeritus, Division of Endocrinology and Internal Medicine, Department of Medicine, Mayo Clinic, Rochester, MN*

ALBERT L. RHOTON, JR., MD, *Department of Neurological Surgery, University of Florida College of Medicine, Gainesville, FL*

JAMES T. RUTKA, MD, PHD, FRCSC, FACS, *Professor and Chairman, Division of Neurosurgery, The Hospital for Sick Children and the University of Toronto, Toronto, Ontario, Canada*

WOLFGANG SAEGER, MD, *Department of Pathology of the Marienkrankenhaus, University of Hamburg, Hamburg, Germany*

BERND W. SCHEITHAUER, MD, *Professor of Pathology, Mayo Medical School; Consultant, Mayo Clinic, Rochester, MN*

JAMES A. SHARPE, MD, *Department of Neurology and Neuro-Ophthalmology Clinic, The Toronto Hospital, Western Division, Toronto, Ontario, Canada*

EDWARD G. SHAW, MD, *Professor and Chair, Department of Radiation Oncology, Wake Forest University School of Medicine, Winston-Salem, NC*

ILAN SHIMON, MD, *Division of Endocrinology, Sheba Medical Center, Tel-Aviv University, Tel-Aviv, Israel*

LUCIA STEFANEANU, PHD, *Division of Pathology, Department of Laboratory Medicine, St. Michael's Hospital, Toronto, Ontario, Canada*

SHIRLEY I. STIVER, MD, PHD, *Division of Surgery, Beth Israel Deaconess Medical Center, Harvard Medical School, Boston, MA*

KAMAL THAPAR, MD, PHD, FRCSC, *Division of Neurosurgery, Department of Surgery, University Health Network (Toronto Western Division), and the University of Toronto, Toronto, Ontario, Canada*

MICHAEL O. THORNER, MB, BS, DSC, *Henry B. Mulholland Professor of Internal Medicine and Chair, Department of Internal Medicine, University of Viriginal Medical School, University of Virginia Health Sciences Center, Charlottesville, VA*

J. BLAKE TYRRELL, MD, *Division of Endocrinology, University of California at San Francisco, San Francisco, CA*

MARY LEE VANCE, MD, *Departments of Medicine and Neurological Surgery, Division of Endocrinology and Metabolism, University of Virginia, Charlottesville, VA*

CHARLES B. WILSON, MD, *Department of Neurological Surgery, University of California at San Francisco, San Francisco, CA*

SHOZO YAMADA, MD, PHD, *Department of Neurosurgery, Toranomon Hospital, Tokyo, Japan*

WILLIAM F. YOUNG, JR., MD, *Divisions of Endocrinology and Metabolism and Hypertension, Mayo Clinic, Rochester, MN*

XUN ZHANG, PHD, *Neuroendocrine Unit, Massachusetts General Hospital, Boston, MA*

Color Plates

Color Plates appear after p. 176, containing:

Figure 8-2 (See discussion on p. 156.) ISH applications in the pituitary. **(A)** Detection of PRL mRNA in normal pituitary with a ^{35}S-labeled oligonucleotide probe (×250); **(B)** the sense control probe is negative (×250); **(C)** incidental PRL adenoma detected by ISH with a digoxigenin-labeled oligonucleotide probe in an autopsy pituitary (×200); **(D)** an ACTH adenoma expressing pro-opiomelanocortin detected with a digoxigenin-labeled oligonucleotide probe (×300).

Figure 8-5 (See discussion on pp. 159, 160.) Comparison of *in situ* RT-PCR and ISH to detect PRL mRNA in GH$_3$ cells grown in serum-free media with low PRL mRNA levels. **(A)** *In situ* RT-PCR detects a strong signal for PRL by the indirect method in all of the tumor cells (×250). **(B)** There is a weak and focal hybridization signal for PRL mRNA detected by ISH in the same population of GH$_3$ cells (×250).

Figure 10-13 (See discussion on pp. 181, 184.) Fundoscopic image demonstrating band or bowtie atrophy in a patient with temporal hemanopia and acuity 20/20 in the ipsilateral eye and no light perception in the contralateral eye.

Figure 10-14 (See discussion on pp. 184, 185 and full caption on p. 185.) Cross-section mount of optic nerve stained for myelin, illustrating band atrophy of nerve fibers from the nasal retina.

Additional color illustrations may be found in Chapter 12:

Figure 12-1 (See complete caption on p. 220.) PET images comparing ^{11}C-L-methionine with ^{18}F-fluorodeoxyglucose.

Figure 12-2 (See complete caption on p. 220.) PET image demonstrating the effect of bromocriptine.

Figure 12-3 (See complete caption on p. 221.) PET images with ^{11}C-L-raclopride in patient with a prolactinoma.

Figure 12-4 (See complete aption on p. 221.) PET image of patient with a microprolactinoma.

Figure 12-6 (See complete caption on p. 222.) PET image demonstrating effect of cabergoline treatment.

Figure 12-7 (See complete caption on p. 222.) PET image demonstrating effect of Sandostatin treatment.

Figure 12-8 (See complete aption on p. 223.) PET image demonstrating differentiation of meningioma.

1 Pituitary Adenomas

Historic Considerations

RAYMOND V. RANDALL, MD, MS, BERND W. SCHEITHAUER, MD,
AND KALMAN KOVACS, MD, PHD, DSC

INTRODUCTION: HISTORIC CONSIDERATIONS

Pierre Marie's report on acromegaly in 1886 opened an era of interest in pituitary tumors and renewed inquiry into the function of the pituitary gland *(1)*. Prior to that time, abnormalities of the pituitary had been infrequently recorded. Landolt wrote that Plater in 1641 described a 24-yr-old man with progressive loss of vision, convulsions, and weakness *(2)*. Postmortem examination revealed a pituitary tumor the size of a hen's egg. Rolleston in his book, *The Endocrine Organs in Health and Disease (3)*, noted that Bonet in 1679 and Wepfer in 1681 reported enlargement of the pituitary, Vieussens in 1705 documented enlargement of the pituitary with blindness, and Gray and Ward in 1849 each reported a tumor of the pituitary to the Pathological Society of London. Ward's patient, a young woman who had experienced progressive loss of vision, was at postmortem found to have a large pituitary tumor also involving the infundibulum and pressing on the optic nerves *(4)*. Gray's patient was a 30-yr-old woman with headaches and confusion. At postmortem examination, her pituitary was "large," as was the sella, which contained pus, and communicated with the pharynx *(5)*. Earlier, in 1823, Ward published his findings in a 38-yr-old male who for 3 yr had failing vision and, in the last days of life, had become nearly blind. At postmortem examination, a tumor of the pituitary compressed the optic and olfactory nerves *(6)*. The same year, 1823, Rayer reported two patients with progressive loss of vision, headaches, apathy, and somnolence. At postmortem examination, each had a tumor of the pituitary *(7)*. Rayer also added from the literature, the findings on three patients with enlargement of the pituitary. One, a report from 1705, Vieussens' case cited above, stated that the patient had a tumor the size of a hen's egg and atrophy of the optic and olfactory nerves. Mohr, in 1840, described the case of a 57-yr-old woman with a 6-yr history of memory disturbances and vertigo, and decreased vision for 3 yr *(8)*. For several weeks prior to death following seizures, she had extremely severe headaches and weakness of her right extremities. At postmortem examination, she was enormously obese, had hydrocephalus, and an enlarged sella with a

goose egg-sized tumor of the pituitary, which impinged on the crus cerebri and displaced the optic chiasm.

Prior to Marie's report in 1886, little was known about the function of the pituitary. Rolleston wrote that Galen (130–200 AD) recognized the presence of the pituitary, and Vesalius (1514–1564) thought the brain excreted waste material through the infundibulum to the pituitary, where it was eliminated as phlegm into the nasopharynx *(3)*. Rolleston also related that over the centuries, other hypotheses regarding the function of the pituitary had been set forth. These included drainage of moisture from the brain, separation of phlegmatic serum from the blood and its passage into the nostrils, collection of cerebrospinal fluid and its passage into the circulation, and finally the production of fluid for nourishment of the brain. Neurologic function was also postulated. Medvi, in *A History of Endocrinology*, stated that Gall (1758–1828), as well as Carus (1789–1869) and Burdach (1801-1876) believed that the pituitary was either a large ganglion or the upper end of the spinal cord *(9)*. As late as 1845, Chater, apparently unaware of previous thoughts on the subject, wrote that the pituitary should be considered to be the "first or true cerebral ganglion of the sympathetic" *(10)*.

THE PIERRE MARIE ERA

Marie's 1886 article introduced the term *acromegaly*, described two patients (designated cases I and II in his paper) with the abnormality, and reviewed five previously published reports of patients (designated cases III–VII) who seemed to have similar findings *(1)*. The oldest observation mentioned by Marie (Figure 1) had been made over 100 years earlier—this, the 1772 report of Saucerotte, remains the first known description of a patient with acromegaly. There are two interesting aspects in Marie's report. Patient VII, a man of 36 yr, had died under the care of a Doctor Henrot, and at autopsy was found to have a pituitary tumor the size of a hen's egg. No significance was ascribed to the tumor. Two other patients (cases V and VI) were brothers and, as Marie wrote in a publication 4 yr later in 1890, did not have acromegaly *(11)*. In retrospect, they most likely had either familial pachydermoperistosis, a condition also called hereditary hypertrophic osteoarthropathy, or were afflicted with hypertrophic pulmonary osteoarthropathy (Marie-Bamberger's disease).

From: *Diagnosis and Management of Pituitary Tumors* (K. Thapar, K. Kovacs, B. W. Scheithauer, and R. V. Lloyd, eds.), ©Humana Press Inc., Totowa, NJ.

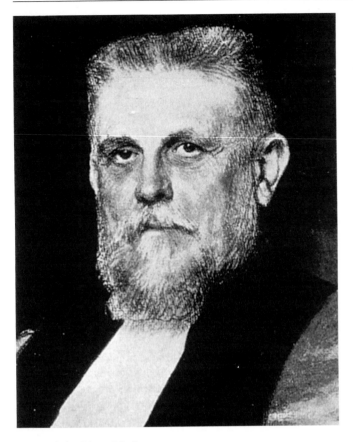

Figure 1-1 Pierre Marie.

In his 1890 publication, Marie also stated that he considered enlargement of the pituitary to be part of acromegaly, and that vision was often affected, blindness occurring in advanced disease owing to compression of the optic nerves by the enlarged pituitary. One year thereafter, The New Sydenham Society of London published *Essays on Acromegaly* by Marie and Souza-Leite *(12)*. The latter, a student of Marie had previously published a thesis on acromegaly. The New Sydenham report, a compilation of 48 cases, consists of a translation of Marie's 1886 paper with its 2 original cases and the 5 drawn from other sources, 32 cases from the literature added by Souza-Leite to his thesis, and another 9 cases that had appeared after the writing of the thesis. At the time of the publication of the report, the cause of acromegaly was not known, but enlargement of the pituitary was again recognized as part of the syndrome.

SPECULATIONS ON THE CAUSE OF ACROMEGALY

Following Marie's initial 1886 publication, there was widespread reporting of new cases of acromegaly and a continued searching of the older medical literature to uncover reports of patients who, in retrospect, seemed to have had the condition. There also arose an interest in gigantism. This is understandable, because some giants had features similar to those of acromegaly, and examination of the skulls of giants, in medical museums, invariably showed enlargement of the pituitary fossa. In 1889, Furnivall reviewed the literature, finding 48 autopsied patients with acromegaly, and added one of his own *(13)*. In all 49 cases, there was an abnormality of the pituitary and, in all but two instances, the gland was considered enlarged. The author mentioned that there were several theories regarding the cause of

acromegaly, but did not elaborate. In any event, the pituitary was not considered to be at fault. Two years later, Hutchinson published a series of four papers entitled *The Pituitary as a Factor in Acromegaly and Giantism (14)*. After taking into account the number of cases reported more than once, he stated that there were approx 218 reported cases of acromegaly and 7 of gigantism. To the latter, he added the case reports of six additional giants plus observations he had made on several more. Noting that previous authors had recorded the presence of acromegalic features in some giants, he suggested that acromegaly and gigantism were related conditions. Hutchinson arrived at several conclusions:

1. The body has "a sort of 'growth centre' or proportional regulator of the entire appendicular skeleton."
2. Acromegaly is an overgrowth that expresses itself after adult stature has been reached, whereas gigantism is the same condition manifesting itself before adult stature has been attained.
3. In the preponderance of cases of both conditions, there is hypertrophy of the pituitary.

For years after Marie's original 1886 report and well into the first decade of the present century, there persisted a contention and a lack of consensus regarding the cause of acromegaly. It is of note, however, that as early as 1887, only 1 yr after Marie's original report, Minkowski reported a patient with acromegaly and, despite a lack of anatomic information about the patient's pituitary, postulated that the condition was related to this gland *(15)*. Lewis, in a paper of 1905 *(16)*, and Cushing in his 1912 monograph entitled *The Pituitary Body and Its Disorders (17)*, reviewed the prevailing opinions regarding the cause of acromegaly. These can be summarized as follows. Marie, noting that his first two patients had premature menopause and that other patients had decreased sex drive with disease progression, originally thought the condition was due to a general or gonadal dystrophy caused by hypophyseal dysfunction, a view championed by several others. However, others looked on the condition as being the result of hypertrophy or hyperplasia of the anterior pituitary. Alternatively, other authors thought that the increase in pituitary size was merely one accompaniment of the widespread organ enlargement that characterized acromegaly. Still others concluded that acromegaly had no relation to abnormalities of the pituitary. Indeed, some looked on the findings in acromegaly to be the result of a nutritional disorder that also caused enlargement of the hypophysis. Changes in the nervous system, decreased function of the thyroid, enlargement of the thymus, and atavistic reversion to anthropoid ancestors were among other theories. Marie, in a 1911 communication to Cushing, stated that after going from one hypothesis to another, he had no definite position on this question. He went on to say that perhaps the important thing was less the quantity of function of the hypophysis than modification and alteration of its secretion *(17)*.

There were several reasons why the concept that a tumor of the pituitary was the underlying cause of acromegaly was slow to be accepted. These included:

1. The fact that involvement of the pituitary by other lesions, such tuberculosis, syphilis, aneurysm, and nonpituitary tumors of the sellar region could also cause headaches and visual disturbances, but without acromegaly.
2. Fröhlich's widely quoted 1901 report of a male patient with a presumed tumor of the pituitary, but without acromegaly *(18)*.

3. There were occasional reports of patients with acromegaly, but without an enlarged sella.

Thirty-eight years later, Fröhlich stated that he originally thought the problem with his patient lay in the pituitary, but then realized that it was in the hypothalamus (19). The occurrence of acromegaly without sellar enlargement was addressed by Lewis in his 1905 report of a patient with acromegaly who died of cerebral embolism with secondary hemorrhage (16). This case is of particular interest, since although the patient's sella was normal in size and the pituitary was grossly unremarkable, microscopic examination showed it to be almost completely composed of what was called "hyperplasia of the chromophile cells." Lewis was of the opinion that excess function of the glandular elements of the anterior lobe of the pituitary was responsible for the acromegaly.

OTHER DEVELOPMENTS

Although many original reports relating to the pituitary, including those of the early 20th century, dealt with acromegaly and/or gigantism, there were other clinically important developments of historic interest. In an 1893 publication, Boyce and Beadles, stated that among 3000 autopsy patients of the Colney Hatch Lunatic Asylum, there were 20 with intracranial growths, excluding cysts, abscesses, and aneurysms (20). Among these, six were said to be hypophyseal tumors. One was "the size of a walnut," but no further information was given. In another patient, the pituitary was cystic, but, again, without further elaboration. The third patient was blind and had findings compatible with anterior pituitary failure; a cyst was found "resting upon the sella," but no pituitary gland was found. The fourth patient died in 1884, 2 yr before Marie's report on acromegaly, and, in retrospect, had classic findings of acromegaly. At postmortem examination, there was a cystic pituitary tumor the size of a "hen's egg." The fifth patient had carcinoma of the breast and what seemed to be a metastasis to the pituitary. The last patient's lesion was called a dermoid cyst. The authors did an extensive review of the literature on various lesions, including tumors of the pituitary and sellar region. They described the signs and symptoms related to these abnormalities in such detail that little, other than associated endocrine and radiologic findings associated with such lesions, have subsequently been added. In an interesting footnote, the authors wrote, "In going over the descriptions of recent cases of acromegaly one certainly gains the impression that in the vast majority of them there is enlargement of the hypophysis."

In 1900, Babinski reported the case of a 17-yr-old female patient with retarded sexual development, moderate obesity, headaches, and bilateral papilledema (21). At postmortem examination there was a large tumor, diagnosed as an "epithelioma," adherent to the pituitary gland. Since it involved the pituitary, the author found it interesting that the tumor had not resulted in acromegaly or gigantism, and stated it would have been instructive to know to what extent the pituitary had been altered by the tumor. Knowing that lesions of the pituitary in adults altered gonadal function, suppressed menses, and caused atrophy of the uterus, Babinski stated it was reasonable to believe that a similar lesion could, as seemed to be the case in his patient, arrest genital development in a child.

PROLIFERATION OF LITERATURE ON ACROMEGALY AND THE PITUITARY

The explosion of literature relating to acromegaly and to the pituitary that took place following Marie's paper of 1886 can best be appreciated by referring to the *Index-Catalogue of the Library of the Surgeon-General's Office, United States*. When the first list of publications dealing with the pituitary appeared in 1890, there were only 24. Interestingly, Marie's 1886 paper on acromegaly was not among them. When the first list of publications on acromegaly appeared in 1896, it included 13 monographs, among which were The New Sydenham Society's *Essays on Acromegaly* by Marie and Souza-Leite, Souza-Leite's thesis on acromegaly, and articles by 142 authors, including Marie, many of whom had written more than one article on the subject. The list of publications on the pituitary again appeared in 1908, and there were 66 authors or pairs of authors. When the topic of acromegaly next appeared in the *Index-Catalogue* in 1918, the list of publications was over 7 pages long, and that of the pituitary in 1929, over 16 pages.

EARLY HISTOPATHOLOGIC FINDINGS

In 1724, Santorini recognized the unique nature of what he termed the "glandula pituitaria," and expressed from it a milky fluid, which he called "glandula pituitaria potior (9). Bell, in his book *The Pituitary* (22), credits Hannover for noting, in 1844, that the human anterior pituitary is composed of more than one type of cell. According to Lewis (16), it was Flesch in 1884 and Dostoiewsky in 1886 who described the cells of the anterior pituitary as being chromophobic or chromophilic, and Schonemann in 1902 who divided chromophilic cells as being cyanophilic or eosinophilic based upon their appearance in hematoxylin and eosin preparations. Benda, in 1900, noted that eosinophilic cells in the anterior pituitary contained varying numbers of granules and felt that those cells containing the most granules were the maximally active cells (23). In the same paper, he noted that a pituitary tumor associated with acromegaly contained eosinophilic cells. Subsequently, he and his colleagues reported the presence of eosinophilic cells in two pituitary tumors from acromegalic patients (24).

DIAGNOSTIC AND THERAPEUTIC RADIOLOGY

In 1895, Wilhelm C. Roentgen discovered X-rays, and their application to medical diagnosis and therapy soon followed. Oppenheim, in 1901, was the first to report the use of roentgenograms in the diagnosis of a pituitary tumor (25). In 1907, Gramegna used X-rays to treat a 45-yr-old woman with classic acromegaly and roentgenographically demonstrated sellar enlargement (26). She had experienced amenorrhea since age 32, headaches, and visual impairment. The therapeutic X-rays were directed through the mouth to the region of the sella. Though the patient's headaches ceased and vision improved, a relapse prompted another course of X-ray therapy. She again had a brief regression of symptoms followed by recurrence. Another course of X-ray therapy was of no benefit. Gramegna published his findings 2 yr later, in 1909, the same year that Béclère (27) published his experience in treating a 16-yr-old giantess with headaches, partial loss of vision, genital infantilism, adiposity, and sellar enlargement. Béclère stated that the X-rays were given "through four or five different areas on the fronto-temporal area." It had been planned to follow radiation therapy by surgery, but since her headaches ceased and vision improved in one eye, surgery was no longer considered. Emmanuel wrote that Béclère subsequently reported the patient to be alive and well 13 yr after treatment (28).

Radiation therapy of pituitary adenomas has undergone many changes since X-rays were first used to treat such a tumor in 1907. Various forms of radiation have subsequently been employed: orthovoltage X-rays; ^{60}Co (cobalt); intrasellar implantation of radioactive isotopes, including ^{90}Y (yttrium), ^{190}Au (gold), and, rarely, ^{222}Rn (radon); cyclotron-generated heavy particle radiation; stereotactic radiosurgery using cyclotron radiation; and linear accelerator, which is the radiation therapy most widely used at present. Over the past few years, a number of medical centers use the "Gamma Knife," stereotactic radiation with ^{60}Co through multiple ports, as initial treatment for selected pituitary tumors.

Radiation therapy for the treatment of pituitary adenomas is not without its drawbacks. As time goes on after treatment, some patients develop progressive anterior pituitary failure (29). Another problem is the subsequent development of benign or malignant intracranial tumors within the radiation field. Such patients had typically undergone both surgery and radiation therapy. Waltz and Brownell reported two cases of sarcoma and found 10 similar cases in the literature (30). Brada and colleagues reported the occurrence of tumors in 5 of 334 patients whose pituitary tumor was treated with surgery and radiation therapy (31). They estimated that the cumulative risk of developing a second brain tumor was 1.3% over the first 10 yr and 1.9% over the first 20 yr. Similar findings were reported by Tsang and coworkers (32). Among 305 patients with a pituitary tumor who had received radiation therapy, most often in conjunction with operation, four developed a glioma. They estimated the cumulative risk to be 1.7% at 10 yr and 2.7% at 15 yr.

As therapeutic radiology evolved over the years, so did diagnostic radiology, especially in recent years. For decades, standard techniques included lateral and posteroanterior roentgenographic views of the sella and adjacent areas, iv injection of contrast medium to highlight adenomas, and pneumoencephalography to identify both upward extension of adenomas and sellar enlargement owing to empty sella syndrome. Injection of intrathecal contrast medium was also used to assess suprasellar extension of adenomas and the presence of an empty sella. The introduction of computed tomography (CT) in 1973, as well as subsequent generations of improved scanners, significantly advanced the diagnosis of pituitary adenomas. In the recent years, magnetic resonance imaging (MRI) with and without contrast medium has effectively replaced CT.

PITUITARY SURGERY

In 1893, Caton and Paul reported the first operation for a pituitary tumor, the procedure being performed by Paul (33). The patient was 33 yr old in 1891 when she presented with advanced acromegaly and severe headaches. Two years later, she developed visual changes. Paul removed a portion of the right temporal bone to decrease intracranial pressure, thereby successfully relieving the headaches. The patient was not considered a candidate for resection of a presumed pituitary tumor. She died 3 mo later and at autopsy had a "tangerine orange" sized, hemorrhagic tumor, which was called a sarcoma. The surgical procedure used by Paul had been suggested by Horsley. In an address to the British Medical Association published in 1906, Horsley stated that he had operated on 10 patients with pituitary tumor (34). Unfortunately, he gave no details, except for brief mention of a patient with an inoperable "cystic adenosarcoma," which he had approached by the transfrontal route in 1889, 4 yr before Caton and Paul's publication. On the basis of this report, Horsley has occasionally been given credit for performing the first surgery on a pituitary tumor, but apparently he never published the details of any of his 10 operations. Over the next decade, there were numerous reports of

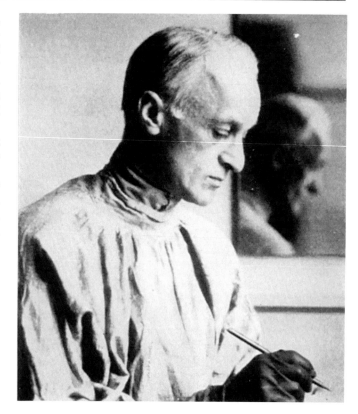

Figure 1-2 Harvey Cushing.

operations on pituitary tumors. They employed various surgical approaches, primarily transfrontal and transsphenoidal with various routes being used to approach the sphenoid sinus. Bell, in his 1919 monograph *The Pituitary*, had a full chapter devoted to descriptions of the various surgical procedures in use at the time (22).

In 1902, when Cushing (Figure 2) started to operate on lesions in and around the pituitary, he used subtemporal decompression to relieve pressure symptoms (17). In 1909, he began to remove pituitary tumors rather than simply doing a decompressing procedure. Cushing did his first transsphenoidal operation via resection of the anterior wall of the frontal sinus and nose. The following year, he began using a sublabial incision and submucosal resection of the septum to reach the sphenoid sinus and enter the pituitary fossa. Many neurosurgeons of the time, notably Hirsch (35), used this or a similar approach to the sphenoid sinus and pituitary fossa. A principal disadvantage of the sphenoidal approach was the occurrence of infection and meningitis, often complicating a postoperative cerebrospinal fluid leak. Furthermore, the approach did not permit the resection of large tumors. Consequently, Cushing abandoned the transsphenoidal method and turned to a transcranial approach for tumors in the pituitary, a procedure used by most neurosurgeons of his time.

From the 1930s through the 1970s, most operations for pituitary tumors were by way of the transcranial route. Nonetheless, the transsphenoidal approach continued to be used by Hirsch in Vienna and Dott in Edinburgh. The latter had worked with Cushing and taught the technique to Guiot of Paris. In turn, Guiot taught the transsphenoidal procedure to Hardy of Montreal, who refined the operation by using the operating microscope and intraoperative fluoroscopy. Hardy also advocated both the selective removal of pituitary microadenomas (adenomas <10 mm in diameter), leaving normal pituitary tissue in place, as well as the transsphenoidal approach for the removal of larger adenomas, again sparing normal pituitary tissue when possible. Hardy's technique of transsphenoidal surgery has been widely adopted, and the result has been a general shift away from radiation therapy for the initial treatment of pituitary adenomas. Instead, radiation therapy is used primarily in instances where surgery is unsuccessful in eradicating the tumor. A combination of transsphenoidal and transcranial surgery is used when an adenoma cannot be satisfactorily removed by either approach alone.

ROLE OF THE PITUITARY IN ACROMEGALY

As previously stated, there continued to be a quandary regarding the relationship between the pituitary tumors of acromegalic patients and the syndrome of acromegaly, and this was not settled until after surgeons began to operate on pituitary adenomas in patients with acromegaly. This question was resolved independently by Hochenegg (36) and by Cushing (37) after Schloffer in 1906 suggested that partial resection of the pituitary might alleviate the condition (38). In 1908, Hochenegg removed a pituitary tumor from a 30-yr-old woman with acromegaly, headaches, and visual disturbances. Immediately thereafter, the headaches disappeared, and visual improvement was noted. Within days, the patient noted her hands were smaller. At 1 mo, the same was true of her feet and facial features. One year later, Cushing undertook the partial resection of a pituitary tumor of a 38-yr-old man with typical acromegalic features and headaches. Following the procedure, the patient's headaches disappeared and his soft tissue changes regressed. Cushing believed that the results were in keeping with the fact that the tumor was responsible for the acromegaly, which he looked on as a state of hyperpituitarism. Based on the studies he and others had done on the effects of total and subtotal resection of the anterior pituitary in dogs, Cushing stressed that the pituitary was essential to life, and care should be taken to leave all or a portion of the anterior lobe in place when removing tumors of the pituitary and sellar region (39).

As previously noted, Cushing's monograph, *The Pituitary Body and Its Disorders*, appeared in 1912, a major landmark in the history of pituitary adenomas (17). Much of the text was devoted to a detailed review of the medical and surgical histories of 50 of his patients, most of whom had undergone one or more operations for a pituitary tumor. The role of chromophobic tumors in causing varying degrees of anterior pituitary failure was well documented. Likewise, pituitary tumors were convincingly shown to be the cause of acromegaly. Although a few of Cushing's 50 patients were treated with radiation therapy, in the closing pages of his text, he was not optimistic about the role of X-rays in treating pituitary tumors. It must be remembered, however, that the reports of Gramegna and Béclère regarding the use of radiation therapy appeared only 3 yr prior to the publication of Cushing's monograph and 7 yr after he had operated on the first of the patients in his series. Subsequently, many of Cushing's patients with pituitary tumors underwent radiation therapy at some stage of their treatment.

CUSHING'S DISEASE

In 1932, Cushing published his paper on pituitary basophilism, now better known as Cushing's disease (40). The first patient in this report was also patient XLV in his monograph of 1912, at which time the case was placed in the category of so-called polyglandular syndrome. Without sufficient evidence to implicate

the pituitary as the cause, he considered these patients to have evidence of a "ductless gland disorder." In the 1932 paper, in addition to the above-mentioned patient, Cushing added another of his patients (patient 11) and 10 from the literature. All had similar findings, which he again designated "polyglandular syndrome." Most came to autopsy at which time three had a basophilic adenoma of the pituitary, two had an undifferentiated pituitary adenoma, one had an "adenomatous-like structure" in the anterior lobe of the pituitary, and two had a "normal" pituitary. Two patients, one among the three with a basophilic adenoma, had adrenal cortical hyperplasia. One patient of the two patients with an undifferentiated pituitary adenoma had a small adrenal adenoma. Cushing astutely concluded, "if further study should prove that adrenal tumors in the absence of any demonstrable change in the pituitary body may cause a polyglandular syndrome it may well enough be assumed that when the same features characterize the syndrome of a basophilic adenoma, they in all probability are secondarily ascribable to a hypersecretory influence of adrenal cortex."

As noted above, patient 11 in the 1932 paper was one of Cushing's patients. Since the patient was too debilitated by his disease to undergo an exploration of the pituitary, he underwent radiation therapy to the pituitary region. The patient dramatically improved. A number of patients with Cushing's disease, especially children, have subsequently benefited from the effects of radiation therapy. Despite Cushing's correct belief that the "polyglandular syndrome" was inherently a pituitary disease, the issue of whether Cushing's disease was primarily a disorder of the pituitary or of the adrenal glands remained unsettled for several decades. Thus, many patients with this disorder were treated by bilateral subtotal or total adrenalectomy, rather than by an operation on the pituitary. A number of patients who had adrenal surgery subsequently developed an aggressive pituitary adenoma or pituitary carcinoma with generalized hyperpigmentation (Nelson's syndrome) (41,42).

SUBCLINICAL PITUITARY ADENOMAS

An interesting and provocative paper on pituitary adenomas appeared in 1936. Costello examined the pituitary glands of 1000 patients who came to autopsy (43). Ranging in age from 2 to 86 yr, they had no recognizable evidence of endocrine disease. On serial sections of the pituitaries, he found adenomas in 225 pituitaries. One (0.4%) had three adenomas, 41 (18%) had two, and the remaining 183 (81.6%) had a single adenoma. Histologically, the adenomas fell into one of several tinctorial groups: 52.8% were chromophobic, 27.2 % were basophilic, 7.5 % were eosinophilic cells, and 12.5% consisted of two or three cell types. Since this study was performed long before the introduction of immunostaining techniques, it is not known what hormones these adenomas contained. Nonetheless, the study demonstrates that many normal persons harbor one or more pituitary adenomas. It remains unknown whether, in some instances, these adenomas grow and/ or become hormonally active to produce clinical symptoms.

The presence of subclinical adenomas is not unique to the pituitary, for they occur in other endocrine glands, notably the thyroid and adrenals. Mortensen and coworkers examined 821 thyroid glands removed at autopsy (44). All thyroid glands had been found to be normal on palpation prior to death. One or more thyroid nodules were found in 406 thyroids (49.5 %). Russi and coworkers reported the findings of 131 instances of adrenocortical adenomas in 9000 autopsies (1.45%) (45). Since the autopsies were performed by many different persons, they surmised that many small adenomas may have been overlooked. Spain and Weinsaft found solitary adrenocortical adenomas in 29 of 100 consecutive postmortem examinations of elderly women (46). Interestingly, in 100 consecutive autopsies of elderly males, they found only two solitary adenomas.

Almost a half-century after Costello's publication, in 1983 McComb and coworkers published their study of 107 subclinical pituitary adenomas using conventional and immunohistochemical techniques (47). The 107 adenomas were found within 100 pituitaries obtained at unselected autopsies from patients dying of various diseases. None had evidence of pituitary hypersecretion, though a few patients had treated diabetes mellitus or hypothyroidism, and some had received long-term corticosteroids. Applying Costello's histologic classification, 4 of the 107 adenomas were acidophilic, 4 were basophilic, and the remainder were chromophobic. By immunohistochemical studies, 54 adenomas (50.5%) were considered null-cell adenomas, since they were nonreactive for any anterior pituitary hormones. Forty-five adenomas (42.1%) contained prolactin (PRL). Of the remaining eight adenomas, four contained adrenocorticotropic hormone (ACTH), two contained both PRL and growth hormone (GH), and the remaining two, thyroid-stimulating hormone (TSH) or luteinizing hormone (LH). These findings stand in contrast to those, in the same study, of 606 symptomatic pituitary adenomas removed at operation. Among these, 152 (25.1%) were null-cell adenomas, 176 (29.0%) contained PRL, 56 (9.2%) PRL and GH, 98 (16.2%) GH, 3 (0.5%) TSH, and 20 (3.3%) follicle-stimulating hormone (FSH) and LH. Of ACTH adenomas, 51 (8.4%) were functioning, whereas 36 (8.0%) were silent ACTH adenomas. Finally, 14 tumors (2.3%) were plurihormonal adenomas. The reason for the differences in the distribution of the various kinds of pituitary adenomas in the group of subclinical tumors compared to those surgically removed is not clear.

KERNOHAN AND SAYRE'S ATLAS

In 1956, Kernohan and Sayre published their monograph *Tumors of the Pituitary Gland and Infundibulum*, one of a series of Atlases of Tumor Pathology published under the auspices of the Armed Forces Institutes of Pathology (48). Based on 5000 intracranial tumors operated at Mayo Clinic and available for study to the authors, 605 (12%) were pituitary adenomas. Among these tumors were 565 chromophobic adenomas, 40 eosinophilic tumors, but there were no basophilic examples. During the period of time that these intracranial tumors were collected, patients with acromegaly at the Mayo Clinic were treated by irradiation, unless they had visual field and/or oculomotor changes. On the other hand, patients with Cushing's disease were treated with bilateral, subtotal or total adrenalectomy. Thus, the low number of eosinophilic tumors and the absence of basophilic tumors in this series were not representative of the actual proportion of patients with these pituitary adenomas seen at their institution.

The atlas of Kernohan and Sayre became the standard for the classification and nomenclature of pituitary tumors and remained so for many years. Since it was published before the advent of immunoassays and immunostains for pituitary adenomas, it was not appreciated that many chromophobic pituitary adenomas were in fact hormonally active. Even the existence of prolactin-secreting adenomas was not suspected, although, in retrospect, the following reports hinted at the existence of such tumors. Krestin, in 1932, reported two patients with persistent lactation and amenorrhea

with roentgenographic evidence of sellar enlargement; the pathology of the underlying lesions was unknown (49). In 1954, Forbes and colleagues, including Albright, described 15 nonacromegalic women with persistent lactation and amenorrhea or irregular menses (50). Eight had roentgenographic evidence of an enlarged sella; of these, three had a chromophobe adenoma on biopsy. The term, Forbes-Albright syndrome was subsequently used to designate persons with persistent lactation and a pituitary tumor. Two other syndromes of persistent lactation and amenorrhea were recognized prior to 1954. The term, Chiari-Frommel syndrome was applied to postpuerperal women with amenorrhea and persistent lactation (51), and the term Del Castillo syndrome was applied to those without a preceding pregnancy who had amenorrhea and galactorrhea (52). As expected, many patients with these disorders were subsequently found to harbor a prolactin-secreting pituitary adenoma.

TESTS FOR HORMONES OF THE ANTERIOR PITUITARY

As various hormones of the anterior pituitary were identified and isolated, bioassays and in vitro assays were devised to measure them. These assays were primarily used in animal studies and in the preparation of biologic standards. With some exceptions, they were not applicable to routine clinical use in humans, and it was not until the introduction of radioimmunoassays that measurements of the various pituitary hormones became readily available in both laboratory and clinical settings. It is of historic interest that we briefly mention several of the more notable assays gleaned from the extensive literature that preceded the radioimmunoassay method.

GROWTH HORMONE   Cushing, in a talk to the American Medical association in 1909, suggested, as had others, that the anterior pituitary elaborated a growth-promoting substance (39). It was not until 1933 that Evans, a former student of Cushing, and coworkers, described a test for the potency of growth hormone in pituitary extracts based on the gain in body weight of rats following the injection of these extracts (53). Later, Evans and his group used stimulation in growth of the rat tibial epiphyses as a bioassay of GH (54). In a clinical application of this effect on epiphyses, Sullivan and coworkers found that the costochondral junctions in patients with active acromegaly failed to close normally in early adulthood (55).

GONADOTROPINS   During their work on purification of LH (previously termed "metakentrin"), Greep et al. developed an assay for measuring LH based on increase in weight of the anterior lobe of the prostate of hypophysectomized, immature male rats (56). This assay proved to be superior to previous assays based on an increase in weight of the seminal vesicles of immature rats, be they intact or hypophysectomized.

Over the years, many methods for measuring FSH, once called "thylakentrin," were devised. These included increase in uterine weight or ovarian weight in immature, female rats; production of follicles in the ovaries of hypophysectomized, female rats; and increase in testicular weight in hypophysectomized, male rats. It was also known that human chorionic gonadotropin (HCG) augmented the action of FSH on the ovary. Applying this information, Steelman and Pohley used large doses of HCG to make intact, immature rats hypersensitive to FSH. They found, within a specific range, the relationship between administered FSH and ovarian weight was linear giving a simple, reliable assay (57). They also showed specificity for FSH by demonstrating that luteinizing hormone, thyrotropin, prolactin, adrenocorticotropic hormone, and growth hormone did not interfere with the assay.

The only practical way to study pituitary gonadotropins in humans was to measure the amount of these hormones excreted in the urine, usually in a 24- or 48-h specimen. The many assays developed usually involved concentrating and extracting gonadotropins from the urine, and injecting the preparation into mice or rats and measuring increase in weight of the ovaries or uterus, or noting vaginal histology, ovarian hyperemia, or size of the vaginal opening. None of these procedures distinguished between LH and FSH, but measured the aggregate of both. Although most laboratories could handle only a small number of assays, Albert devised a method to start processing sixteen 24- or 48-h urine specimens each day using as an end point the increase in ovarian weight of hypophysectomized, immature rats *(58)*. His method was used extensively for investigative as well as clinical evaluation of patients.

PROLACTIN It was the 18th century surgeon and naturalist John Hunter who described the secretion of "milk" from the crop glands of both female and male pigeons to feed their young. It was not until the present century that many investigators recognized the presence of a substance in the anterior pituitary that stimulated the growth of mammary glands and secretion of milk. By 1933, growth hormone as well as hormones stimulating the gonads, thyroid, and adrenals were recognized, but had not been isolated and purified. Therefore, it was not known whether the mammary-stimulating and milk-secreting substance of the anterior pituitary was an entity or an action of one or more of the other hormones. This question was settled by Riddle and coworkers, who isolated a substance from beef, sheep, and hog anterior pituitaries, which stimulated milk secretion, and which they named, prolactin *(59)*. In the same publication, they described a quantitative assay for prolactin based on promoting weight gain of the crop glands of immature pigeons and doves. This method of measuring prolactin enjoyed widespread use. Another widely used assay for the lactogenic factor was the injection of anterior pituitary extracts into rabbits made pseudopregnant by the administration of chorionic gonadotropin and measuring lactation. However, there was doubt whether the anterior pituitary factor that initiated lactation in mammals was identical to that which stimulated the crop gland of pigeons. Bergman et al. in a series of experiments using both rabbits and pigeons and lactogenic extracts of the anterior pituitary relatively free of other hormones of the anterior pituitary showed the lactating factor to act equally well in both species *(60)*.

ADRENOCORTICOTROPIC HORMONE Aware that ACTH reduces the ascorbic acid content of adrenal glands, Sayers and coworkers developed a sensitive assay of ACTH activity *(61)*. Since ACTH produces varying depletion of adrenal ascorbic acid in intact rats, they successfully used the effects of a highly purified preparation of ACTH on hypophysectomized rats as a reference standard when measuring ACTH activity in various biologic materials.

THYROTROPIN A number of attempts were made to measure thyrotropin in blood or serum, but most gave poor results when known amounts of thyrotropin were added to the blood or serum being assayed. However, the more reliable method of McKenzie was used clinically. He employed mice injected with I^{131} and suppressed their endogenous thyrotropin by injecting thyroxine followed by the administration of powdered thyroid in their diet *(62)*. Known amounts of thyrotropin were injected into the mice and the increase in blood I^{131} was measured, thus establish-

ing a response curve. Thyrotropin in the sera of patients was recovered by starch block electrophoresis and injected into test animals. With this technique, McKenzie measured thyrotropin activity in the serum from a patient with nonacromegaly and in six patients with myxedema.

RADIOIMMUNOASSAYS AND IMMUNOHISTOCHEMICAL STUDIES

Undoubtedly, the most significant advances in understanding the secretory function of the pituitary gland and in facilitating the diagnosis of pituitary adenomas followed Yalow and Berson's 1959 introduction of radioimmunoassay for the measurement of insulin concentrations in biologic fluids *(63)*. The technique led to the almost simultaneous development of radioimmunoassays for measuring human growth hormone (GH) by Berson's group *(64)* and others *(65,66)*. Subsequently, a number of investigators developed methods of measuring the other pituitary hormones, namely TSH, PRL, FSH, LH, ACTH, and alpha-subunit, the common subunit of the glycoprotein hormones, TSH, FSH, and LH. Clinicians were now able to measure the serum or plasma levels of hormones being secreted by the normal pituitary as well as by pituitary adenomas. Such measurements provide useful information, not only about the secretory products of a pituitary adenoma, but about possible compromise of the pituitary's own hormone secretion owing to the effects of the tumor. It also became possible to evaluate the efficacy of treatment of hormone-secreting pituitary adenomas, be it by surgery, radiation, medication, or a combination of these modalities, as well as to detect the early recurrence of such tumors. In addition, assays for measuring hypothalamic hormones, such as gonadotropin-releasing hormone (GnRH), corticotropin-releasing hormone (CRH), growth hormone-releasing hormone (GRH), and somatostatin (growth hormone-inhibiting hormone, GHIH) have been developed.

While immunoassays for pituitary hormones were being developed and applied to the diagnosis of pituitary adenomas, histopathologic methods for their study were also changing. It was evident that tinctorial methods, which divided pituitary adenomas into acidophilic, basophilic, and chromophobic groups, were inadequate for differentiating functioning from nonfunctioning adenomas, despite the availability of a fairly large number of staining techniques. Furthermore, in many instances, the results of these stains did not correlate with the endocrine function of the adenomas. For instance, chromophobic adenomas had for decades been looked on as nonfunctioning, causing symptoms only by compression or invasion of adjacent structures or by compromising the function of the normal pituitary. It was McCormick and Halmi who showed that the cells of chromophobic adenomas did indeed contain granules, the implication being that they were hormone-producing *(67)*. This reinforced the finding that in some instances, total or partial removal of a chromophobic adenoma alleviated endocrine syndromes owing to excessive secretion of one or more pituitary hormones.

Subsequently, the medical application of electron microscopy confirmed the secretory nature of adenohypophyseal cells. In addition, it permitted their classification into five basic types, including somatotropes, corticotropes, lactotropes, thyrotropes, and gonadotropes. With experience, it became possible to distinguish one cell type from another and to correlate their fine structural features with histochemical findings. Special fixation of fresh tissues is required for optimal electron microscopic studies. Given the difficulty inherent in obtaining fresh normal human pituitary tissues for study, much of the early ultrastructural work was performed on animal pituitaries. Unfortunately, findings based on animal studies often do not correlate well with human data.

The localization of the various anterior pituitary hormones in specific pituitary cells has added enormously to our knowledge of the structure and function of normal as well as neoplastic anterior pituitary cells. Initially, cellular location of the various hormones was achieved by immunofluorescence methods, the hormone antibodies being labeled with variously colored fluorescent compounds. Demonstrating more than one hormone in a given cell or in cells of different types was difficult, since the fluorescent compounds in early use tended to wash out when a second fluorescent antibody was applied to a previously stained tissue. To circumvent this problem, Nakane and Pierce used antibodies labeled with horseradish peroxidase to localize tissue antigens (68). In 1968, Nakane studied rat pituitary tissues using rabbit antisera against several human hormones, including chorionic gonadotropin, somatotropin, and thyrotropin, peroxidase-labeled sheep antirabbit γ-globulin, and three colored compounds, one for each of the three hormonal antisera (69). He found that each of the antisera labeled only one cell type, that some cells were not labeled, and none exhibited more than one label. The author concluded he had demonstrated the presence of individual thyrotropin, growth hormone, and luteinizing hormone-producing cells, the rationale for the latter being that antisera to chorionic gonadotropin crossreacts with luteinizing hormone. He also demonstrated that the immunoperoxidase method was applicable to paraffin-embedded tissues, did not require such special equipment as a darkfield fluorescence microscope, and that immunoperoxidase labeling was permanent.

KOVACS AND HORVATH'S ATLAS

The immunoperoxidase method has been successfully applied in the study of human pituitary disorders, including adenomas as well as a broad spectrum of medical diseases. Combining histochemical and immunoperoxidase techniques with ultrastructural studies of normal and adenomatous pituitary tissues, Kovacs and Horvath of St. Michaels Hospital, Toronto, placed pituitary pathology on a firm footing. Their efforts culminated in the 1986 publication of *Tumors of the Pituitary Gland*, a monograph in the second series of Atlas of Tumor Pathology published by the Armed Forces Institutes of Pathology (70). Like the 1956 monograph of Kernohan and Sayre, this new contribution became the standard reference for the classification of pituitary tumors. The Kovacs and Horvath classification, based on electron microscopy and immunohistology, consists of 14 tumor types. Concise descriptions of the characteristics of these various adenomas are presented in Chapter 7 of this volume. The multimodality approach to formulating the classification made clear the futility of using standard hematoxylin-eosin stains to categorize pituitary tumors, e.g., growth hormone cell, prolactin cell, mixed growth hormone and prolactin cell adenomas, as well as acidophil stem-cell adenomas may be either acidophilic or chromophobic, whereas functioning corticotroph cell, silent corticotroph cell, thyrotroph cell, and gonadotroph cell adenomas may be either basophilic or chromophobic. Kovacs and Horvath also emphasized that although some adenomas can be very aggressive and invasive of surrounding tissues, routine histopathologic findings are of no prognostic significance in so far as the clinical course of the patient is concerned. Aggressive behavior was, however, associated with several combinations of immunohistochemical and ultrastructural findings (71–74).

The Kovacs and Horvath classification with minor additions remains current and is the basis of the present World Health Organization Classification of Adenohypophysial Neoplasms (75).

MEDICAL TREATMENT OF PITUITARY ADENOMAS

Medical therapy of pituitary adenomas, a relatively recent development, is covered in Chapter 14, but some historic aspects are germane to our review. Consequently, developments in the treatment of patients with acromegaly and those with prolactinoma, those showing the best response to medical therapy, are briefly discussed.

ACROMEGALY　　Based on reports that L-DOPA stimulated growth hormone release in patients with Parkinson's disease and normal persons, Liuzzi and coworkers studied the effects of L-DOPA on eight patients with acromegaly (76). To their surprise, all patients responded with a transient fall in values for GH, with normal values being reached in two patients. Later they administered a longer acting dopamine agonist, 2-Br-α-ergocryptine (bromocriptine) to seven acromegalic patients and found a comparable, but longer-acting effect (77). Another dopamine agonist, pergolide, has similar effects, but in smaller doses and with slightly longer suppression of GH. Recently, a more potent, longer-acting dopamine agonist, cabergoline, has been successful in shrinking the pituitary macroadenomas (tumors > 10 mm in diameter) in five of seven patients with acromegaly (78).

Since the aforementioned drugs are ineffective in many patients with acromegaly, Hall and coworkers administered somatostatin (GH-release-inhibiting hormone) in the form of a synthetic tetradecapeptide to six normal persons and three acromegalic patients (79). In all instances, the medication inhibited the release of GH after insulin-induced hypoglycemia. Currently, octreotide acetate, a synthetic octapeptide form of somatostatin, is used in some patients with acromegaly, but a shortcoming is the need to administer it subcutaneously every 8 h. Lanreotide, a slow-release form of octreotide, has been shown to be effective in suppressing growth hormone when given intramuscularly every 2–4 wk (80–82).

PROLACTINOMA　　There have been rare reports of patients with galactorrhea responding favorably to treatment with clomophene, estrogens, or oral contraceptives, but more frequently, estrogens and contraceptives have been implicated as the causal agent. Drawing on the knowledge that 2-Br-α-ergocryptine, a dopamine agonist, inhibited prolactin secretion and lactation in animals, Lutterbeck and coworkers used this medication to suppress nonpuerperal galactorrhea in three women (83). Their findings were subsequently confirmed by del Pozo et al. (84) and Besser et al. (85). Pergolide, with its longer effect at a lower dose, has also proven effective, as has bromocriptine LAR, a long-acting form of bromocriptine. The latter has been reported to cause a macroprolactinoma to disappear and not reappear 3 yr after the medication was discontinued (86). Cabergoline, the most recently introduced dopamine agonist, has the advantage of being effective when given orally twice a week.

PITUITARY CARCINOMA

Over the years, a vexing problem has been the diagnosis of pituitary carcinoma. Reports of patients with anterior pituitary tumors published at the end of the 19th century and early part of the 20th century frequently stated that such lesions were malignant. In Furnivall's 1898 review of 49 reported cases of patients with acromegaly who had come to autopsy, a diagnosis of sarcoma of the pituitary was made in 11 instances, of sarcoma or lymphadenoma in one, of spindle-celled sarcoma in one, and of glioma or sarcoma in yet another *(13)*. Prior to the Kernohan era, what we now term pituitary adenomas were considered grade 1 adenocarcinoma in the files of the Mayo Clinic Tissue Registry. In retrospect, such diagnoses of malignancy are understandable. It has long been recognized that pituitary adenomas may expand the sella, elevate the sellar diaphragm, and show suprasellar extension with compression of the optic chiasm and brain tissues. In most instances, they do so without actual invasion of these structures. On the other hand, a significant proportion of pituitary adenomas infiltrate and destroy sellar bone, some with resultant cavernous sinus invasion. In addition, adenomas occasionally exhibit nuclear atypia, cellular pleomorphism, nucleolar enlargement, and occasional mitotic figures. Nonetheless, a diagnosis of malignancy cannot be made on such operative, radiographic, or histologic findings. By convention, it is the presence of metastases that is the *sine qua non* of pituitary carcinoma. Metastases may involve either the cerebrospinal axis or may be systemic, often affecting the skeleton or viscera, such as the liver. Pituitary carcinoma is exquisitely rare. Mountcastle and coworkers reported an acromegalic male with a GH-producing carcinoma of the pituitary with metastases to both the cerebrospinal space and cervical lymph nodes *(87)*. Immunostains demonstrated GH in the metastases. They reviewed 36 reported cases of pituitary carcinoma and found that almost half (44%) had syndromes of hormonal secretion. More recently, Pernicone and coworkers reported 15 cases of carcinoma of the pituitary *(88)*. Of these, seven tumors produced PRL, seven were ACTH-secreting (four with Nelson's syndrome), and one was ostensibly a nonsecreting null-cell tumor. Their study included a review of 53 published cases, including 16 PRL-producing tumors, and 15 ACTH, 5 GH, 1 TSH-producing, as well as 13 nonfunctioning tumors. The authors found that among their 15 cases, the tumors often showed increased mitotic activity, p53 protein overexpression, and elevated MIB-1 and PCNA proliferation indices. Values of these parameters in metastases often exceeded those in primary tumors. Since the prognosis of patients with carcinoma of the pituitary is so poor, with only one-third of the patients surviving 1 yr after the demonstration of metastases, the authors suggested that these parameters might serve to identify adenomas of uncertain malignant potential, lesions that if earmarked for close surveillance and aggressive therapy, might be prevented from metastasizing. Comparative studies of mitotic activity *(73)*, MIB-1-labeling indices *(71)*, and p53 expression by adenomas *(72)*, invasive adenomas, and pituitary carcinomas support the utility of this approach, one adopted in the new World Health Organization Classification of Adenohypophysial Neoplasms *(75)*.

HYPOTHALAMIC GANGLIOCYTOMAS

An interesting finding has been the demonstration of hypothalamic neuropeptides in gangliocytomas, sometimes called hamartomas or choristomas, which have been associated with pituitary tumors and endocrine syndromes in most instances. Asa and colleagues reported six such patients *(89)*. Five had acromegaly and, in addition to a pituitary adenoma with GH-containing cells, there were hypothalamic gangliocytoma cells containing human pancreatic tumor GH-releasing factor (hptGRF). The gangliocytoma cells also contained glucagon, somatostatin in four instances, and gonadotropin-releasing factor in two instances. The sixth patient also had a pituitary adenoma containing GH, but did not have clinical evidence of acromegaly. The gangliocytoma cells, in addition to containing hptGRF, also contained somatostatin and gluca-

gon. Why the patient did not have acromegaly is not clear. The tumor may not have been present long enough for acromegalic findings to develop, or release of somatostatin may have offset excess hptGRF, if indeed, the gangliocytoma cells were actually releasing these neuropeptides.

Hypothalamic gangliocytomas have also been found with other endocrine syndromes associated with pituitary adenomas. Kovacs' group demonstrated corticotropin-releasing factor in the neurons of a hypothalamic gangliocytoma associated with corticotrop cell hyperplasia and Cushing's disease reported by Lapresle and others *(90)*. Bracco et al. have reported a similar situation in a patient with an intasellar gangliocytoma and Cushing's disease *(91)*. Judge and coworkers had a patient with precocious puberty and a hypothalamic hamartoma containing gonadotropin-releasing factor *(92)*. It would be of interest to know if other tumors in and around the hypothalamic area, pinealomas for example, might contain neuropeptides and cause endocrine syndromes, such as precocious puberty.

THE FUTURE: NEW METHODS FOR THE STUDY OF PITUITARY DISEASE

With the introduction of a variety of molecular techniques during the last two decades, new knowledge has rapidly accumulated, the result being considerable progress in pituitary pathology. This has been particularly noticeable in regard to adenohypophyseal tumors. For example, immunoelectron microscopy using double-immunogold labeling has made it possible to demonstrate the presence of two hormones at the ultrastructural level and to answer the question of whether two hormones reside in the same or different cells, or even the same secretory granules *(93,94)*. *In situ* hybridization, which uses radioactive or nonradioactive probes, has permitted the localization of mRNAs, thus indicating gene expression *(95–97)*. This sensitive method can visualize not only hormone mRNAs, but also ones for receptors, growth factors, and oncogenes. New methods permitting the demonstration of cytogenetic and molecular genetic abnormalities are shedding light on the process of tumor development and progression. Fluorescence *in situ* hybridization provides opportunities to investigate chromosomal abnormalities *(98,99)*. The polymerase chain reaction, by amplifying genes, can detect a large number of molecular abnormalities *(100,101)*. A veritable gold mine is the introduction of transgenic animal models, which, like no other method, facilitate our understanding of the pathophysiology and pathomorphology of disease. Transgenic animals can either express foreign genes in excess or, as in the case of "knockout mice," the total lack of a gene, thus making it possible to examine the consequences of increased or decreased gene function *(102,103)*. Methods have also been developed to study the process of hormone secretion. These include the reverse hemolytic plaque assay, which permits the demonstration of hormone release by a single cell *(104,105)*. Sophisticated in vitro studies using pituitary tumor cells or cell lines also shed light on the mechanisms underlying "endocrine activity," for example, the regulation of hormone secretion *(106–108)*. Finally, newly discovered cell proliferation markers have already begun to explain the biologic behavior of pituitary tumors by quantifying their growth rate, correlating with conventional measures of aggressiveness, and shedding light on structure–function correlations. Such markers exceed in sensitivity the time-honored and still useful method of quantifying mitotic activity. The application of p53 protein immunohistochemical analysis was previously discussed.

CURRENT STATUS

Despite the many advances in our understanding of the varied presentations, clinical course, and pathology of pituitary adenomas, we are still left with the identical questions that have perplexed physicians throughout the last two centuries. Why do pituitary adenomas occur, and how can they be prevented or cured?

ACKNOWLEDGMENTS

We express our thanks to Mr. and Mrs. Ellis I. Levitt, Mr. and Mrs. F. A. Wittern, Jr., Mr. and Mrs. James L. Wooters, Mr. S. and Mrs. G. Jarislowski, and the Lloyd-Carr-Harris Foundation, Ontario, Canada for their generous support of some of the work in the text.

REFERENCES

1. Marie P. Sur deux cas d'acromégalie. Hypertrophie singulière non congénitale des extrémetiés supérieures, inférieures et céphalique. Rev Med 1886;6:297–333.
2. Landolt AM. History of pituitary surgery: transcranial approach. In: Landolt AM, Vance ML, Reilly PL, ed. Pituitary Adenomas. Churchill Livingston, New York, 1996, pp. 283–294.
3. Rolleston HD. The Endocrine Organs in Health and Disease. Oxford University Press, Oxford, UK, 1936.
4. Ward N. Tumour of the infundibulum. Trans Pathol Soc Lond 1848-50;ii:19.
5. Gray H. Ulceration of the sella turcica and softening of the brain. Trans Pathol Soc Lond 1846-50;ii:19-20.
6. Ward J. Case of amaurosis produced by enlargement of the pituitary gland. Lond Med Repository Rev 1823;20:217,218.
7. Rayer PFO. Observations sur les maladies de l'appendice sud-sphenoidal (glande pituitaire) du cerveau. Arch Gén Méd 1823;3:350–367.
8. Mohr B. Hypertrophie (markschwammige Entartung?) der Hypophysis cerebri und dadruch bedinger Druch auf die Hirngrundfläche, insbesondere auf die Schnerven, das Chiasma derselben und den linkseitgen Hirnschenkel. Wschr Ges Heilk 1840;6:565–571.
9. Medvei VC. A History of Endocrinology. MTP, Lancaster, UK, 1982.
10. Chater G. On the pituitary gland. Provincial Med Surg J 1845;390,391.
11. Marie P. Acromegaly. Brain 1890;xii:59–81.
12. Marie P, Souza-Leite. Essays on Acromegaly. The New Sydenham Society, London, 1891.
13. Furnivall P. Pathological report on a case of acromegaly, with an analysis of the results of forty-nine post-mortem examinations on cases of acromegaly. Trans Pathol Soc Lond 1898;xlix:204–223.
14. Hutchinson W. The pituitary gland as a factor in acromegaly and giantism. New York Med J 1898;lxvii:341–344, 450–453; 1900; lxxii:89–100, 133–145.
15. Minkowski O. Ueber einen Fall von Akromegalie. Berl Klin Wchnsch 1887;xxiv:371–374.
16. Lewis DD. Hyperplasia of the chromophile cells of the hypophysis as the cause of acromegaly, with report of a case. Bull Johns Hopkins Hosp 1905;XVI:157–164.
17. Cushing H. The Pituitary Body and Its Disorders. J.B. Lippincott Company, Philadelphia, 1912.
18. Fröhlich A. Ein Fall von Tumor der Hypophysis cerebri ohne Akromegalie. Wien klin Rdsch. 1901;15:883–886, 906–908.
19. Fröhlich A. In: Fulton JF, Ranson SW, Frantz AM, ed. The Hypothalamus and Central Levels of Autonomic Function, Proceedings of the Association for Research in Nervous and Mental Disease, vol. XX. Williams & Wilkins, Baltimore, 1940, 722,723.
20. Boyce R, Beadles CF. A further contribution to the study of the pathology of the hypophysis cerebri. J Pathol Bacteriol Edinburgh 1893;1:359–383.
21. Babinski MJ. Tumeur du corps pituitaire sans acromégalie et avec arrêt de développement des organes génitaux. Revue Neurologique 1900;viii:531–533.
22. Bell WB. The Pituitary. William Wood, New York, 1919.
23. Benda C. Beiträge zur normalen und pathologischen histologie der menschlichen Hypophysis cerebri. Berl klin Wschr 1900; xxxvii:1205–1210.
24. von Fraenkel A, Stadelmann E, Benda C. Zwei Fälle von Akromegalie. Deut Med Wschr 1901;27:536–539.
25. Oppenheim H. Arch fur Psychiat 1901;xxxiv:303,304.
26. Gramegna A. Un cas d'acromégalie traité par la radiothérapie. Rev Neurol 1909;xvii:15–17.
27. Béclère A. The radio-therapeutic treatment of tumours of the hypophysis, gigantism, and acromegaly. Arch Roentgen Ray 1909-10; 14:142–150.
28. Emmanuel IG. Symposium on pituitary tumors. (3) Historical aspects of radiotherapy, present treatment technique and results. Clin Radiol 1966;17:154–160.
29. Littley MD, Shalet SM, Beardwell CG, Ahmed SR, Applegate G, Sutton ML. Hypopituitarism following external radiotherapy for pituitary tumours in adults. Quart J Med 1989;70:145–160.
30. Waltz TA, Brownell B. Sarcoma: A possible late result of effective radiation therapy for pituitary adenoma. Report of two cases. J Neurosurg 1966;24:901–907.
31. Brada M, Ford D, Ashley S, Bliss JM, Crowley S, Mason M, et al. Risk of second brain tumour after conservative surgery and radiotherapy for pituitary adenoma. BMJ 1992;304:1343–1346.
32. Tsang RW, Laperriere NJ, Simpson WJ, Brierley J, Panzarella T, Smyth HS. Glioma arising after radiation therapy for pituitary adenoma. A report of four patients and estimation of risk. Cancer 1993;72:2227–2233.
33. Caton R, Paul FT. Notes of a case of acromegaly treated by operation. Br Med J 1893;ii:1421–1423.
34. Horsley V. On the technique of operations on the central nervous system. Br Med J 1906;2:411–423.
35. Hirsch O. Endonasal method of removal of hypophyseal tumors. With report of two successful cases. JAMA 1910;LV:772–774.
36. Hochenegg J. The operative cure of acromegaly by removal of a hypophyseal tumor. Ann Surg 1908;58:781–783.
37. Cushing H. Partial hypophysectomy for acromegaly. With remarks on the function of the hypophysis. Ann Surg 1909;1:1002–1017.
38. Schloffer H. Zur frage der Operationen an der Hypophyse. Beitr klin Chir 1906;1:767–817.
39. Cushing H. The hypophysis cerebri. Clinical aspects of hyperpituitarism and of hypopituitarism. JAMA 1909;LIII:249–255.
40. Cushing H. The basophil adenomas of the pituitary body and their clinical manifestations (pituitary basophilism). Bull Johns Hopkins Hosp 1932;L:137–195.
41. Nelson DH, Meakin JW, Dealy JB Jr, Matson DD, Emerson K Jr, Thorn GW. ACTH-producing tumor of the pituitary gland. N Engl J Med 1958;259:161–164.
42. Salassa RM, Kearns TP, Kernohan JW, Sprague RG, MacCarty CS. Pituitary tumors in patients with Cushing's syndrome. J Clin Endocrinol Metab 1959;19:1523–1539.
43. Costello RT. Subclinical adenoma of the pituitary gland. Am J Pathol 1936;12:205–216.
44. Mortensen JD, Woolner LB, Bennett WA. Gross and microscopic findings in clinically normal thyroid glands. J Clin Endocrinol Metab 1955;15:1270–1280.
45. Russi S, Blumenthal HT, Gray SH. Small adenomas of the adrenal cortex in hypertension and diabetes. Arch Intern Med 1945;76:284–291.
46. Spain DM, Weinsaft P. Solid adrenal cortical adenoma in elderly female. Arch Pathol 1964;78:231–233.
47. McComb DJ, Ryan N, Horvath E, Kovacs K. Subclinical adenomas of the human pituitary. New light on old problems. Arch Pathol Lab Med 1983;107:488–491.
48. Kernohan JW, Sayre GP. Tumors of the Pituitary Gland and Infundibulum. Atlas of Tumor Pathology. Armed Forces Institute of Pathology, Washington, DC, 1956.
49. Krestin D. Spontaneous lactation associated with enlargement of the pituitary: with report of two cases. Lancet 1932;1:928–930.
50. Forbes AP, Henneman PH, Griswold GC, Albright F. Syndrome characterized by galactorrhea, amenorrhea and low urinary FSH:

comparison with acromegaly and normal lactation. J Clin Endocrinol Metab 1954;14:265–271.

51. Chiari JBVL, Braun C, Spaeth J. Klinik der Geburtshilfe und Gynakologie. F. Enke, Erlangen, 1855.

52. Del Castillo EB, Lanari A. Syndrome caracterizado por crecimiento exagerado, amenorea y galactorrea. Semana Med 1933;1:1905–1911.

53. Marx W, Simpson ME, Evans HM. Bioassay of the growth hormone of the anterior pituitary. Endocrinology 1942;30:1–10.

54. Greenspan FS, Li CH, Simpson ME, Evans HM. Bioassay of the hypophyseal growth hormone: the tibia test. Endocrinology 1949;45:455–463.

55. Sullivan CR, Jones DR, Bahn RC, Randall RV. Biopsy of the costochondral junction in acromegaly. Proc Staff Meet Mayo Clin 1963;38:81–86.

56. Greep RO, van Dyke HB, Chow BF. Use of anterior lobe of prostate gland in the assay of metakentrin. Proc Soc Exp Biol Med 1941; 46:644–649.

57. Steelman SL, Pohley FM. Assay of the follicle stimulating hormone based on the augmentation with human chorionic gonadotropin. Endocrinology 1953;53:604–616.

58. Albert A. Human urinary gonadotropin. In: Pincus G, ed. Recent Progress in Hormone Research, vol 12. Proceedings of the Laurentian Hormone Conference, 1953. Academic, New York, 1956, pp. 227–293.

59. Riddle O, Bates RW, Dykshorn SW. The preparation, identification and assay of prolactin—a hormone of the anterior pituitary. Am J Physiol 1933;105:191–216.

60. Bergman AJ, Meites J, Turner CW. A comparison of methods of assay of the lactogenic hormone. Endocrinology 1940;26:716–722.

61. Sayers MA, Sayers G, Woodbury LA. The assay of adrenocorticotropic hormone by the adrenal ascorbic acid-depletion method. Endocrinology 1948;42:379–393.

62. McKenzie JM. The bioassay of thyrotropin in serum. Endocrinology 1958;63:372–382.

63. Yalow RS, Berson SA. Assay of plasma insulin in human subjects by immunological methods. Nature 1959;184:1648,1649.

64. Glick SM, Roth J, Yalow RS, Berson SA. Immunoassay of human growth hormone in plasma. Nature 1963;199:784–787.

65. Utiger RD, Parker ML, Daughaday WH. Human serum growth hormone: measurements of concentration and turnover with a radioimmunoassay. J Clin Invest 1961;40:1086.

66. Hunter WM, Greenwood FC. A radio-immuno-electrophoretic assay for human growth hormone. Acta Endocr Suppl 1962;67:59.

67. McCormick WF, Halmi NS. Absence of chromophobe adenomas from a large series of pituitary tumors. Arch Pathol 1971; 92:231–238.

68. Nakane PK, Pierce GB Jr. Enzyme-labeled antibodies for the light and electron microscopic localization of tissue antigens. J Cell Biol 1967;33:307–318.

69. Nakane PK. Simultaneous localization of multiple tissue antigens using the peroxidase-labeled antibody method: a study on pituitary glands of the rat. J Histochem Cytochem 1968;16:557–560.

70. Kovacs K, Horvath E. Tumors of the Pituitary Gland. Atlas of Tumor Pathology. Armed Forces Institute of Pathology, Washington, DC, 1986.

71. Thapar K, Kovacs K, Scheithauer BW, Stefaneanu L, Horvath E, Pernicone PJ, et al. Proliferative activity and invasiveness among pituitary adenomas and carcinomas: an analysis using the MIB-1 antibody. Neurosurgery 1996;38:99–107.

72. Thapar K, Scheithauer BW, Kovacs K, Pernicone PJ, Laws ER Jr. P53 expression in pituitary adenomas and carcinomas: correlation with invasiveness and tumor growth fractions. Neurosurgery 1996;38:765–771.

73. Thapar K, Yamada Y, Scheithauer BW, Kovacs K, Yamada S, Stefaneanu L. Assessment of mitotic activity in pituitary adenomas and carcinomas. Endocrin Pathol 1996;7:215–221.

74. Cattreroni G, Becker MHG, Key G, Duchrow M, Schluter C, Galle J, et al. Monoclonal antibodies against recombinant parts of the Ki-67 antigen (MIB-1 and MIB-3) detect proliferating cells in microwave processed formalin-fixed paraffin sections. J Pathol 1992;168: 357–363.

75. Kovacs K, Scheithauer BW, Horvath E, Lloyd RV. The World Health Organization Classification of Adenohypophysial Neoplasms. A proposed five-tier scheme. Cancer 1996;78:502–510.

76. Liuzzi A, Chiodini PG, Botalla L, Cremascoli G, Silvestrini F. Inhibitory effect of L-dopa on GH release in acromegalic patients. J. Clin Endocrinol Metab 1972;35:941–943.

77. Liuzzi A, Chiodini PG, Botalla L, Cremascoli G, Müller EE, Silvestrini F. Decreased plasma growth hormone (GH) levels in acromegalics following CB154 (2-Br-α-ergocriptine) administration. J Clin Endocrinol Metab 1974;38:910–912.

78. Howlett TA, Robertson IJA, Liddicoat A. Acromegaly: shrinkage of macroadenomas with cabergoline. Program & Abstracts 79th Meet. Endocrin Soc 1997:448.

79. Hall R, Besser GM, Schally AV, Coy DH, Evered D, Goldie DJ, Kastin AJ, McNeilly AS, Mortimer CH, Phenekos C, Tunbridge WMG, Weightman D. Action of growth-hormone-release inhibitory hormone in healthy men and in acromegaly. Lancet 1973; 2:581–584.

80. Lancranjan I and the Sandostatin LAR group. Efficacy, tolerability and safety of Somatostatin LAR in acromegalic patients: results of a multicentre study in 151 patients. Program & Abstracts 79th Meet. Endocrin Soc 1997;78.

81. Pedroncelli A, Lancranjan I, Montini M, Mazzocchi N, Gianola D, Pagani MD, Albani G, Gherardi F, Bruns Ch, Ørskov H, Pagani G. Long-lasting experience with Sandostatin LAR in the management of acromegaly. Program & Abstracts 79th Meet. Endocrin Soc 1997;448.

82. Aubert V, Leclere J, Klein M, Simonetta C and the french SMSC 300 E 00 acromegaly study group. Effect of Sandostatin LAR in 38 acromegalic patients: results at 6 months. Program & Abstracts 79th Meet. Endocrin Soc 1997;452.

83. Lutterbeck PM, Pryor JS, Varga L, Wenner R. Treatment of nonpuerperal galactorrhea with an ergot alkaloid. Brit Med J 1971; 3:228,229.

84. del Pozo E, Brun del Re R, Varga L, Friesen H. The inhibition of prolactin secretion in man by CB-154 (2-Br-α-ergocryptine). J Clin Endocrinol Metab 1972;35:768–771.

85. Besser GM, Parke L, Edwards CRW, Forsyth IA, McNeilly AS. Galactorrhoea: successful treatment with reduction of plasma prolactin levels by Brom-ergocryptine. Brit Med J 1972;3: 669–672.

86. Jamrozik SI, Thalamas CM, James-Deidier A, Rochiccioli P, Trémoulet M, Manelfe C, et al. 7-year follow-up in a teenage patient treated with Parlodel-LAR and GH for macroprolactinoma and growth retardation. Program and Abstracts 79th Meeting. Endocrin Soc 1997, p. 140.

87. Mountcastle RB, Roof BS, Mayfield RK, Mordes DB, Sagel J, Biggs PJ, et al. Case report: Pituitary adenocarcinoma in an acromegalic patient: response to bromocriptine and pituitary testing: a review of the literature on 36 cases of pituitary carcinoma. Am J Med Sci 1989;298:109–118.

88. Pernicone PJ, Scheithauer BW, Sebo TJ, Kovacs KT, Horvath E, Young WF Jr, et al. Pituitary carcinoma A clinco-pathologic study of 15 cases. Cancer 1997;79:804–812.

89. Asa SL, Scheithauer BW, Bilbao JM, Horvath E, Ryan N, Kovacs K, et al. A case for hypothalamic acromegaly: a clinicopathologic study of six patients with hypothalamic gangliocytomas producing growth hormone-releasing factor. J Clin Endocrinol Metab 1984; 58:796–803.

90. Lapresle J, Racadot J, Said G. Myasthenie, thymone et tumeur hypophysaire associant une prolifereration adenomateuse heterogene et un ganglio-neurome de la selle turcique. J Neurol Sci 1976; 28:249–254.

91. Bracco L, Archambeaud-Mouveroux F, Teissier MP, Labrousse F, Vidal J, Treves R, et al. Combined intra-sellar gangliocytoma and Cushing's disease. Program and Abstracts 79th Meeting. Endocrin Soc 1997, p. 457.

92. Judge DM, Kulin HE, Page R, Santen R, Trapukdi S. Hypothalamic hamartoma. A source of luteinizing hormone-releasing factor in precocious puberty. N Engl J Med 1977;296:7–10.

93. Bendayan M: Protein A-gold electron microscopic immunocytochemistry: methods, applications and limitations. J Electron Microsc Technol 1984;1:243–270.

94. Felix IA, Horvath E, Kovacs K, Smyth HS, Killinger DW, Vale W. Mammosomatotroph adenoma of the pituitary associated with gigantism and hyperprolactinemia. A morphologic study including immunoelectron microscopy. Acta Neuropathol 1986;71:76–82.

95. Stefaneanu L, Kovacs K, Horvath E, Lloyd RV. In situ hybridization study of pro-opiomelanocortin (POMC) gene expression in human pituitary corticotrophs and their adenomas. Virchows Arch Pathol Anat 1991;419:107–113.

96. Komminoth P. Digoxigenin as an alternative probe labeling for in situ hybridization. Diagn Mol Pathol 1992;1:142–150.

97. Stefaneanu L, Kovacs K, Horvath E, Lloyd RV, Buchfelder M, Fahlbusch R, et al. In situ hybridization study of estrogen receptor messenger ribonucleic acid in human adenohypophysial cells and pituitary adenomas. J Clin Endocrinol Metab 1994;78:83–88.

98. Kontogeorgos G, Kovacs K. FISHing chromosomes in endocrinology. Endocrine 1996;5:235–240.

99. Kontogeorgos G, Kaprano S. Interphase analysis of chromosome 11 in human pituitary somatotroph adenomas by direct fluorescence in situ hybridization. Endocr Pathol 1996;7:203–206.

100. Eidne KA. The polymerase chain reaction and its uses in endocrinology. Trends Endocrinol Metab 1991;2:169–175.

101. Jin L, Qian X, Lloyd RV. Comparison of mRNA expression detected by in situ PCR and in situ hybridization in endocrine cells. Cell Vision 1995;2:314–321.

102. Stefaneanu L, Kovacs K. Transgenic models of pituitary diseases (review). Microsc Res Technique 1997;39:194–204.

103. Stefaneanu L, Kovacs K, Horvath E, Asa SL, Losinski N, Billestrup N, et al. Adenohypophysial changes in mice transgenic for human growth hormone-releasing factor: a histological, immunocytochemical and electron microscopic investigation. Endocrinology 1989;125:2710–2718.

104. Yamada S, Asa SL, Kovacs K, Muller P, Smyth HS. Analysis of hormone secretion by clinically non-functioning human pituitary adenomas using the reverse hemolytic plaque assay. J Clin Endocrinol Metab 1989;68:73–80.

105. Neil JD, Frawley LS. Detection of hormone release from individual cells in mixed populations using a reverse hemolytic plaque assay. Endocrinology 1983;112:1135–1137.

106. Kohler PO, Bridson WE, Rayford PL, Kohler SE. Hormone productions by human pituitary adenomas in culture. Metabolism 1969; 18:782–788.

107. Adams EF, Brajkovich IE, Machiter K. Hormone secretion of dispersed cell cultures of human pituitary adenomas: effects of theophylline, thyrotropin-releasing hormone, somatostatin and 2-bromo-alpha-ergocriptine. J Clin Endocrinol Metab 1979;49:120–126.

108. Bethea CL, Weiner RI. Human prolactin secreting adenoma cells maintained on extracellular matrix. Endocrinol 1981;108:357–360.

2 Anatomy of the Pituitary Gland and Sellar Region

ALBERT L. RHOTON, JR., MD

INTRODUCTION

This chapter is divided into two sections. The first section deals with the relationships in the cranial base that are important in performing the various transcranial and subcranial approaches to the sellar region. The second section deals with the neural, arterial, and venous relationships in suprasellar and third ventricular regions that are important in planning surgery for pituitary adenomas.

SELLAR REGION

SPHENOID BONE   The sphenoid bone is located in the center of the cranial base (Figures 1 and 2) *(1–4)*. The intimate contact of the body of the sphenoid bone with the nasal cavity below and the pituitary gland above has led to the transsphenoidal route being the operative approach of choice for most pituitary adenomas. Some part of it is also exposed in the transcranial approaches to the sellar region.

The neural relationships of the sphenoid bone are among the most complex of any bone: the olfactory tracts, gyrus rectus, and posterior part of the frontal lobe rest against the smooth upper surface of the lesser wing; the pons and mesencephalon lie posterior to the clival portion; the optic chiasm lies posterior to the chiasmatic sulcus; and the second through sixth cranial nerves are intimately related to the sphenoid bone. All exit the skull through the optic canal, superior orbital fissure, foramen rotundum, or foramen ovale, all foramina located in the sphenoid bone.

The sphenoid bone has many important arterial and venous relationships: the carotid arteries groove each side of the sphenoid bone and often form a serpiginous prominence in the lateral wall of the sphenoid sinus; the basilar artery rests against its posterior surface; the circle of Willis is located above its central portion; and the middle cerebral artery courses parallel to the sphenoid ridge of the lesser wing. The cavernous sinuses rest against the sphenoid bone, and intercavernous venous connections line the walls of the pituitary fossa and dorsum sellae.

In the anterior view the sphenoid bone resembles a bat with wings outstretched (Figures 1 and 2). It has a central portion called the body; the lesser wings, which spread outward from the superolateral part of the body; the two greater wings, which spread upward from the lower part of the body; and the superior orbital fissure, which is situated between the greater and lesser wings. The vomer, the pterygoid processes, and the medial and lateral pterygoid plates are directed downward from the body. The body of the sphenoid bone is more or less cubical and contains the sphenoid sinus. The superior orbital fissure, through which the oculomotor, trochlear, and abducens nerves and the ophthalmic division of the trigeminal nerve pass, is formed on its inferior and lateral margins by the greater wing and on its superior margin by the lesser wing. The inferior surface of the lesser wing forms the posterior part of the roof of each orbit, and the exposed surface of the greater wing forms a large part of the lateral wall of the orbit. The optic canals are situated above and are separated from the superomedial margin of the superior orbital fissure by the optic strut, a bridge of bone that extends from the lower margin of the base of the anterior clinoid process to the body of the sphenoid. The sphenoid ostia open from the nasal cavity into the sinus.

In the superior view, the pituitary fossa occupies the central part of the body and is bounded anteriorly by the tuberculum sellae and posteriorly by the dorsum sellae (Figure 1). The chiasmatic groove, a shallow depression between the optic foramina, is boundered posteriorly by the tuberculum sellae and anteriorly by the planum sphenoidale. The frontal lobes and the olfactory tracts rest against the smooth upper surface of the lesser wing and the planum sphenoidale. The posterior margin of the lesser wing forms a free edge called the sphenoid ridge, which projects into the Sylvian fissure to separate the frontal and temporal lobes. The anterior clinoid processes are located at the medial end of the lesser wings, the middle clinoid processes are lateral to the tuberculum sellae, and the posterior clinoid processes are situated at the superolateral margin of the dorsum sellae. The dorsum sellae is continuous with the clivus. The upper part of the clivus is formed by the sphenoid bone and the lower part by the occipital bone. The carotid sulcus extends along the lateral surface of the body of the sphenoid.

The superior aspect of each greater wing is concave upward and is filled by the tip of each temporal lobe. The foramen rotundum, through which the maxillary division of the trigeminal nerve passes, is located at the junction of the body and greater wing. The foramen ovale transmits the mandibular division of the trigeminal nerve, and the foramen spinosum transmits the middle meningeal artery. When viewed from inferiorly, the vomer, a separate bone,

From: *Diagnosis and Management of Pituitary Tumors* (K. Thapar, K. Kovacs, B. W. Scheithauer, and R. V. Lloyd, eds.), ©Humana Press Inc., Totowa, NJ.

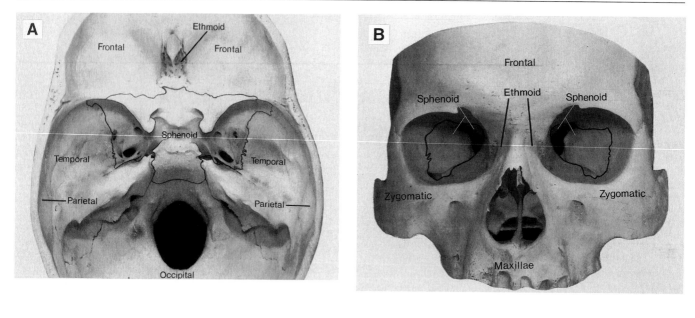

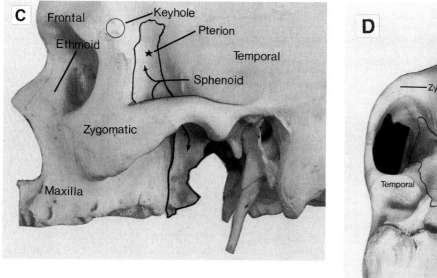

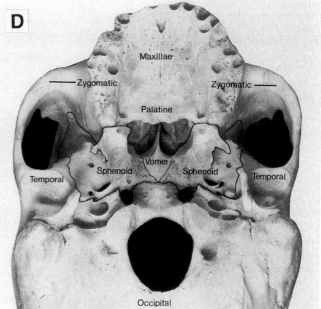

Figure 2-1 Osseous relationships of the sphenoid bone. The sphenoid bone is outlined in each view. (**A**) Superior view. (**B**) Anterior view. (**C**) Lateral view. (**D**) Inferior view (2).

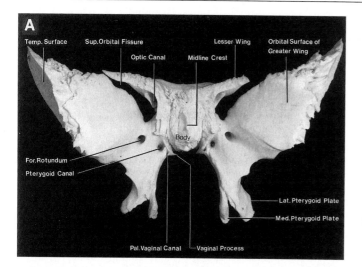

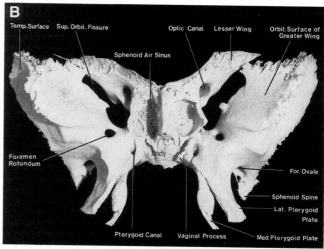

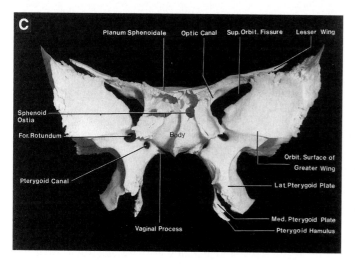

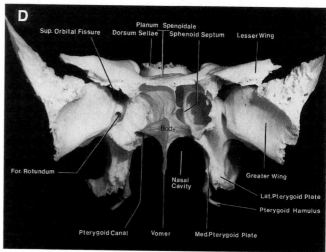

Figure 2-2   Sphenoid bone. Anterior views. **(A)** Conchal-type sphenoid bone. **(B)** Bone with presellar type sphenoid sinus. **(C)** Bone with sellar type sphenoid sinus and well-defined sphenoid ostia. **(D)** Bone with sellar type sphenoid sinus with poorly defined sphenoid ostia and obliquely oriented sphenoidal septae *(2)*.

frequently remains attached to the anterior half of the body of the sphenoid, and its most anterior portion separates the sphenoid ostia.

The pterion and the "keyhole" are two important anatomical landmarks in the region of the greater wing in the lateral view (Figure 1). The pterion is located over the upper part of the greater wing. The "keyhole" is located just behind the junction of the temporal line and the zygomatic process of the frontal bone several centimeters anterior to the pterion. A burr hole placed over the pterion will be located at the lateral end of the sphenoid ridge. A burr hole placed at the keyhole will expose the orbit at its lower margin and dura over the frontal lobe at its upper margin.

SPHENOID SINUS   The sphenoid sinus is subject to considerable variation in size and shape and to variation in the degree of pneumatization (Figure 2) *(5–7)*. It is present as minute cavities at birth, but its main development takes place after puberty. In early life, it extends backward into the presellar area, and subsequently expands into the area below and behind the sella turcica, reaching its full size during adolescence. As the sinus enlarges, it may partially encircle the optic canals. When the sinus is exceptionally large, it extends into the roots of the pterygoid processes or greater

wing of the sphenoid bone, and may even extend into the basilar part of the occipital bone. As age advances, the sinus frequently undergoes further enlargement associated with absorption of its bony walls. Occasionally there are gaps in its bone with the mucous membrane lying directly against the dura mater.

There are three types of sphenoid sinus in the adult: conchal, presellar, and sellar types, depending on the extent to which the sphenoid bone is pneumatized (Figure 2). In the conchal type, the area below the sella is a solid block of bone without an air cavity. In the presellar type of sphenoid sinus, the air cavity does not penetrate beyond a vertical plane parallel to the anterior sellar wall. The sellar type of sphenoid sinus is the most common, and here the air cavity extends into the body of sphenoid below the sella and as far posteriorly as the clivus. In our previous study in adult cadavers, this sinus was of a presellar type in 24% and of the sellar type in 75% *(8)*. In the conchal type, which is infrequent in the adult, the thickness of bone separating the sella from the sphenoid sinus is at least 10 mm.

The septae within the sphenoid sinus vary greatly in size, shape, thickness, location, completeness, and relation to the sellar floor

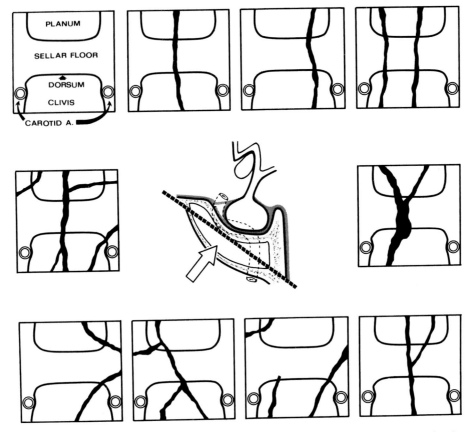

Figure 2-3 Septa in the sphenoid sinus. The heavy broken line on the central diagram shows the plane of the section of each specimen from which the drawings were taken, and the large arrow shows the direction of view. The planum is above, the dorsum and clivus are below, and the sella is in an intermediate position on each diagram. The heavy dark lines on the drawings show the location of the septae in the sphenoid sinus. A wide variety of septae separate the sinus into cavities that vary in size and shape, seldom being symmetrical from side to side *(8)*.

(Figure 3). The cavities within the sinus are seldom symmetrical from side to side and are often subdivided by irregular minor septae. The septae are often located off the midline as they cross the floor of the sella. In our previous study, a single major septum separated the sinus into two large cavities in only 68% of specimens, and even in these cases, the septae were often located off the midline or were deflected to one side *(8)*. The most common type of sphenoid sinus has multiple small cavities in the large paired sinuses. The smaller cavities are separated by septae oriented in all directions. CT or MRI of the sella provide the definition of the relationship of the septae to the floor of the sella needed for transsphenoidal surgery. Major septae may be found as far as 8 mm off the midline *(8)*.

The carotid artery frequently produces a serpiginous prominence into the sinus wall below the floor and along the anterior margin of the sella (Figures 4–6) *(8,9)*. Usually, the optic canals protrude into the superolateral portion of the sinus, and the second division of the trigeminal nerve protrudes into the inferolateral part. A diverticulum of the sinus, called the opticocarotid recess, often projects laterally between the optic canal and the carotid prominence.

Removing the mucosa and bone from the lateral wall of the sinus exposes the dura mater covering the medial surface of the cavernous sinus and optic canals (Figures 4–6). Opening this dura exposes the carotid arteries and optic and trigeminal nerves within the sinus. The abducent nerve is located between the lateral side of the carotid artery and the medial side of the first trigeminal division. The second and third trigeminal divisions are seen in the

lower margin of the opening through the lateral wall of sphenoid sinus. In half of the cases, the optic and trigeminal nerves and the carotid arteries have areas where bone 0.5 mm or less in thickness separates them from the mucosa of the sphenoid sinus, and in a few cases, the bone separating these structures from the sinus is absent *(8,9)*. The absence of such bony protection within the walls of the sinus may explain some of the cases of cranial nerve deficits and carotid artery injury after transsphenoidal operations *(11)*. The bone is often thinner over the carotid arteries than over the anterior margin of the pituitary gland.

DIAPHRAGMA SELLAE The diaphragma sellae forms the roof of the sella turcica. It covers the pituitary gland, except for a small central opening in its center, which transmits the pituitary stalk (Figures 7 and 8). The diaphragma is more rectangular than circular, tends to be convex or concave rather than flat, and is thinner around the infundibulum and somewhat thicker at the periphery. It frequently is a thin, tenuous structure that would not be an adequate barrier for protecting the suprasellar structures during transsphenoidal operation. In a prior anatomic study, Renn and Rhoton *(8)* found that the diaphragma was at least as thick as one layer of dura in 38% and in these would furnish an adequate barrier during transsphenoidal hypophysectomy. In the remaining 62%, the diaphragma was extremely thin over some portion of the pituitary gland. It was concave when viewed from above in 54% of the specimens, convex in 4%, and flat in 42%.

The opening in its center is large when compared to the size of the pituitary stalk. The diaphragmal opening is 5 mm or greater in

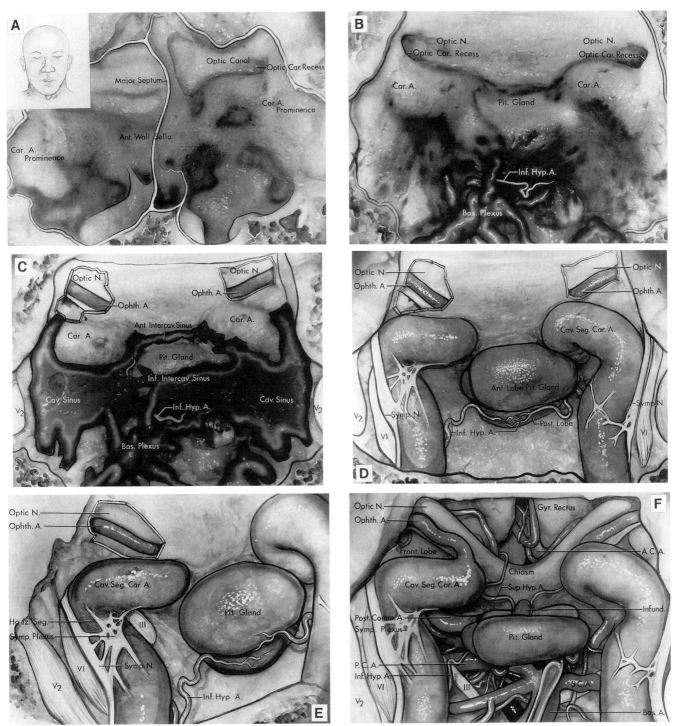

Figure 2-4 Transnasal view of sphenoid sinus and sellar region. **(A)** Orientation is as shown in the insert. Anterior view into a sphenoid sinus (Sphenoid Sinus) with the mucosa removed. The structures in the exposure include the major sphenoidal septum, anterior sellar wall (Ant. Wall Sella), and the bony prominences over the carotid artery (Car. A. Prominence) and optic canal. The opticocarotid recess (Optic Car. Recess) is located between the carotid artery and the optic nerve. **(B)** The bone in the walls of the sphenoid sinus has been removed. The pituitary gland (Pit. Gland), carotid artery (Car. A.), and optic nerve (Optic N.) are seen through the dura. The basilar venous plexus (Bas. Plexus), which forms the largest connection between the cavernous sinuses, is situated on the clivus behind the dorsum sellae. The inferior hypophyseal artery (Inf. Hyp. A.) courses inside the dura covering the posterior lobe of the pituitary gland. **(C)** The dura covering the medial and lower walls of the cavernous sinuses (Cav. Sinus) has been removed. Anterior (Ant. Intercav. Sinus) and inferior intercavernous sinuses (Inf. Intercav. Sinus) connect the paired cavernous sinuses. The dura in the floor of the optic canals has been opened to expose the ophthalmic arteries (Ophth. A.) and the optic nerves. The maxillary trigeminal division (V_2) courses in the lateral edge of the exposure. **(D)** The dark latex in the venous spaces has been removed to expose the cavernous segment of the carotid arteries (Cav. Seg. Car. A.), anterior (Ant. Lobe) and posterior (Post. Lobe) lobes of the pituitary gland, and the sympathetic (Symp. N.) and abducent (VI) nerves. **(E)** Oblique view of the cavernous segment of the right carotid artery. The oculomotor nerve (III) passes above the horizontal segment (Horiz. Seg.). The sympathetic plexus (Symp. Plexus) encircles the carotid artery. **(F)** The dura has been removed to expose the intradural structures in the region of the cavernous sinuses. Structures in the exposure include the gyrus rectus (Gyr. Rectus), pituitary stalk (Infund.), and superior hypophyseal (Sup. Hyp. A.), posterior communicating (Post. Comm. A.), anterior cerebral (A.C.A.), posterior cerebral (P.C.A.), basilar (Bas. A.), and superior cerebellar arteries (S.C.A.) *(10)*.

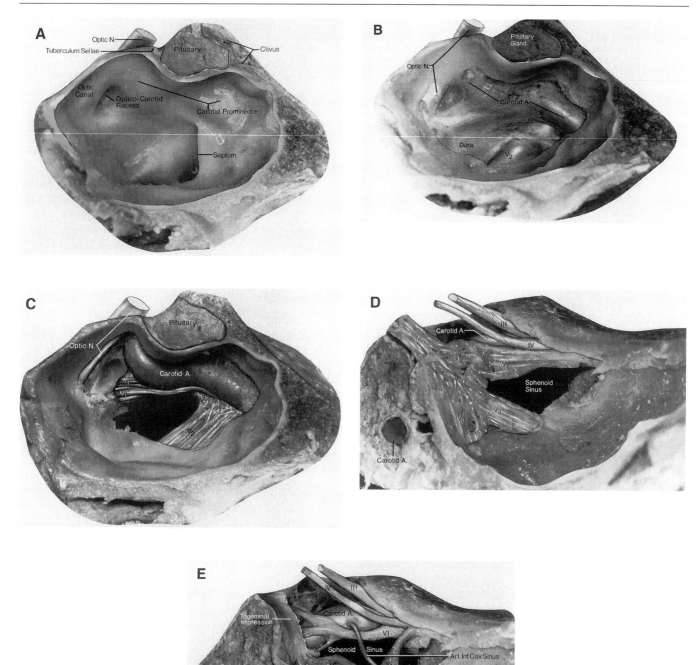

Figure 2-5 Stepwise dissection of the lateral wall of the right half of a sellar-type sphenoid sinus. **(A)** The opticocarotid recess separates the carotid prominence and optic canal. The optic nerve (Optic N.) is exposed proximal to the optic canal. The septum in the posterior part of the sinus is incomplete. **(B)** The sinus mucosa and thin bone forming the sinus wall have been removed to expose dura mater covering the carotid artery (Carotid A.), the second trigeminal division (V_2) just distal to the trigeminal ganglion, and the optic nerve. **(C)** The dura has been opened to expose the carotid artery, the optic nerve in the optic canal, the second trigeminal division below the carotid artery, and the abducens nerve (VI) between the first trigeminal division (V_1) and the carotid artery. **(D)** Lateral view of the specimen showing the cavernous sinus. The carotid artery courses medial to the oculomotor (III), and trochlear (IV) nerves and the ophthalmic division (V_1) of the trigeminal nerve. The petrous portion of the carotid artery is seen in cross-section behind the third (V_3) trigeminal division. **(E)** The trigeminal nerve has been reflected forward to expose the carotid artery, the trigeminal impression, the artery of the inferior cavernous sinus (Art. Inf. Cav. Sinus), and the abducens nerve, which splits into three bundles as it passes around the carotid artery *(6)*.

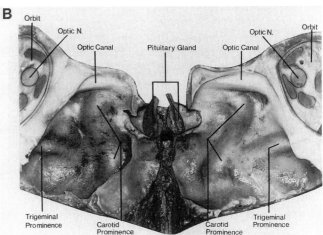

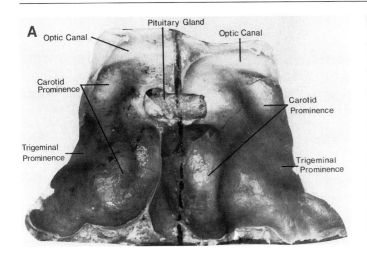

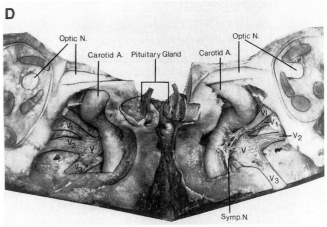

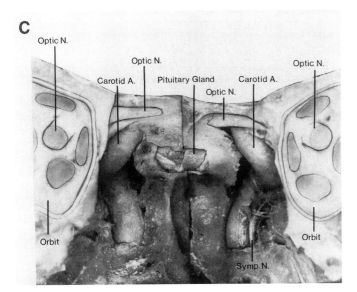

Figure 2-6 (**A**) Anterior views of a sellar-type sphenoid sinus. The anterior wall of the sella has been removed to expose the pituitary gland. The specimen was split at the midline. The air cavity is wider below than above, as is typical in a well-pneumatized sinus. The optic canals are above. The prominences over the carotid arteries form serpiginous bulges in the lateral walls of the sinus. The trigeminal prominences are situated below the carotid prominences. (**B**) The specimen is opened slightly to provide a better view of the carotid and trigeminal prominences in the lateral wall of the sinus. (**C**) The mucosa, dura, and bone in the lateral wall of the sinus have been removed to expose the intracavernous segment of the carotid artery. Sympathetic nerves (Symp. N.) ascend on the carotid arteries. The orbital contents appear laterally. (**D**) The halves of the specimen have been spread to show the abducens nerve (VI) and the ophthalmic (V_1), maxillary (V_2), and mandibular (V_3) divisions of the trigeminal nerve (V) *(6)*.

A

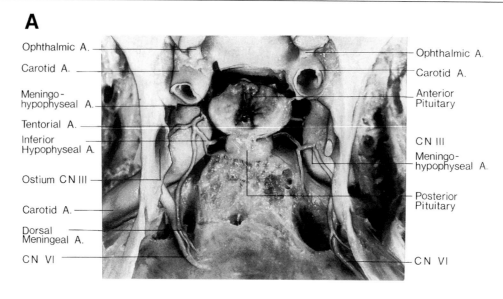

Ophthalmic A.
Carotid A.
Meningo-
hypophyseal A.
Tentorial A.
Inferior
Hypophyseal A.
Ostium CN III
Carotid A.
Dorsal
Meningeal A.
CN VI

Ophthalmic A.
Carotid A.
Anterior
Pituitary
CN III
Meningo-
hypophyseal A.
Posterior
Pituitary
CN VI

B

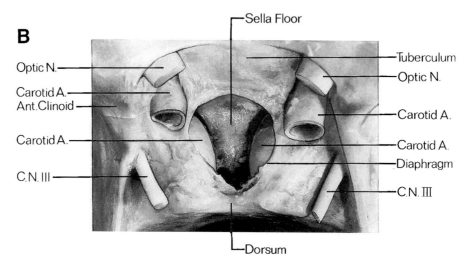

Sella Floor
Optic N.
Carotid A.
Ant.Clinoid
Carotid A.
C.N. III
Tuberculum
Optic N.
Carotid A.
Carotid A.
Diaphragm
C.N. III
Dorsum

Figure 2-7 *(continued on next page)* Superior views of the sellar region. **(A)** The ophthalmic artery arises below the optic nerve. The dorsum was removed to expose the posterior lobe of the pituitary. The meningohypophyseal trunk arises from the carotid artery and gives rise to the inferior hypophyseal, tentorial, and dorsal meningeal arteries. The sixth cranial nerve (CN VI) receives a branch from the dorsal meningeal artery. The oculomotor nerve (CN III) passes through a dural ostium in the roof of the cavernous sinus. **(B)** Carotid arteries bulge into the pituitary fossa.

56%, and in these cases, it would not form a barrier during transsphenoidal pituitary surgery. The opening was round in 54% of the cases, and elliptical with the short diameter of the ellipse oriented in an anteroposterior direction in 46%. A deficiency of the diaphragma sellae is assumed to be a precondition to formation of an empty sella. An outpouching of the arachnoid protrudes through the central opening in the diaphragma into the sella turcica in about half of the patients. This outpouching represents a potential source of postoperative cerebrospinal fluid leakage *(11)*.

PITUITARY GLAND   When exposed from above by opening the diaphragma, the superior surface of the posterior lobe of the pituitary gland is lighter in color than the anterior lobe. The anterior lobe wraps around the lower part of the pituitary stalk to form the pars tuberalis (Figures 9 and 10) *(2,14)*. The posterior lobe is more densely adherent to the sellar wall than the anterior lobe. The gland's width is equal to or greater than either its depth or its length in most patients. Its inferior surface usually conforms to the shape of the sellar floor, but its lateral and superior margins vary in

shape, because these walls are composed of soft tissue rather than bone. If there is a large opening in the diaphragma, the gland tends to be concave superiorly in the area around the stalk. The superior surface may become triangular as a result of being compressed laterally and posteriorly by the carotid arteries (Figure 7). Since the anterior lobe is separated from the posterior lobe, there is a tendency for the pars tuberalis to be retained with the posterior lobe. Intermediate lobe cysts are frequently encountered during separation of the anterior and posterior lobes.

PITUITARY GLAND AND CAROTID ARTERY   The distance separating the medial margin of the carotid artery and the lateral surface of the pituitary gland usually varies from 1 to 3 mm; however, in some cases, the artery will protrude through the medial wall of the cavernous sinus to indent the gland (Figure 7) *(5,8,12)*. Heavy arterial bleeding during transsphenoidal surgery has been reported to be caused by carotid artery injury, but may also be caused by a tear in an arterial branch of the carotid artery (e.g., the inferior hypophyseal artery) or by avulsion of a small capsular branch from the carotid artery *(11)*.

C

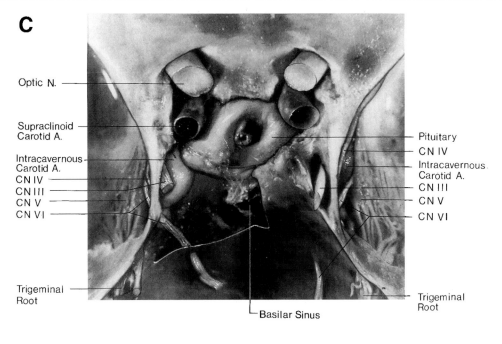

Optic N.

Supraclinoid Carotid A.

Intracavernous Carotid A.
CN IV
CN III
CN V
CN VI

Pituitary
CN IV
Intracavernous Carotid A.
CN III
CN V
CN VI

Trigeminal Root

Trigeminal Root

Basilar Sinus

D

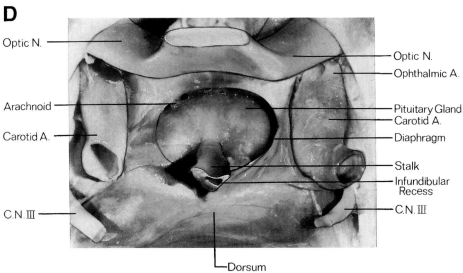

Optic N.

Arachnoid

Carotid A.

C.N. III

Optic N.
Ophthalmic A.

Pituitary Gland
Carotid A.
Diaphragm

Stalk
Infundibular Recess

C.N. III

Dorsum

Figure 2-7 Superior views of the sellar region. (**C**) The carotid arteries indent the lateral margins of the pituitary gland, and a tongue of pituitary gland extends over the top of the arteries. (**D**) The optic chiasm has been reflected forward. A congenitally absent diaphragma exposes the superior surface of the gland. A and C are from *(12)*; B and C are from *(8)*.

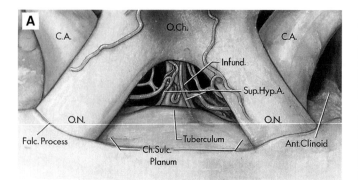

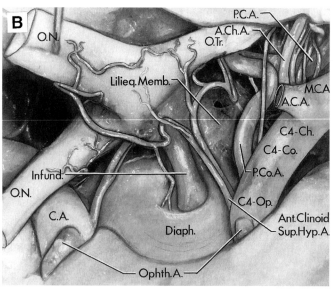

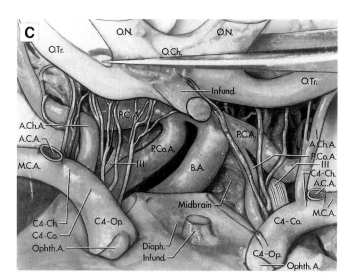

Figure 2-8 *(continued on next page)* Relationships in the sellar and suprasellar areas. **(A)** Anterior view. The optic nerves (O.N.) enter the optic canals medial to the anterior clinoid processes (Ant. Clinoid). The infundibulum (Infund.) is exposed below the optic chiasm (O.Ch.) and behind the planum sphenoidale, chiasmatic sulcus (Ch. Sulc.) and tuberculum sellae. The superior hypophyseal arteries (Sup. Hyp. A.) pass from the carotid artery (C.A.) to the infundibulum. The falciform process (Falc. Process) is a fold of dura mater that passes above the optic nerve proximal to the optic foramen. **(B)** The optic nerves have been divided and elevated to show the perforating branches of the carotid arteries. The supraclinoid portion of the carotid artery is divided into three segments based on the origin of its major branches: the ophthalmic segment (C4-Op.) extends from the origin of the ophthalmic artery (Ophth. A.) to the origin of the posterior communicating artery (P.Co.A.), the communicating segment (C4-Co.) extends from the origin of the posterior communicating artery to the origin of the anterior choroidal artery (A.Ch.A.), and the choroidal segment (C4-Ch.) extends from the origin of the anterior choroidal artery to the bifurcation of the carotid artery into the anterior (A.C.A.) and middle cerebral arteries (M.C.A.). The perforating branches arising from the ophthalmic segment pass to the optic nerve, chiasm, infundibulum, and floor of the third ventricle. The perforating branches arising from the communicating segment pass to the optic tract and the floor of the third ventricle. The perforating branches arising from the choroidal segment pass upward and enter the brain through the anterior perforated substance (Ant. Perf. Subst.). The diaphragma sellae (Diaph.) surrounds the infundibulum above the pituitary gland. Liliequist's membrane (Lilieq. Memb.) is situated between the infundibulum and posterior cerebral arteries (P.C.A.). **(C)** The optic nerves, anterior cerebral arteries, and infundibulum have been divided and the optic nerves and chiasm elevated to expose the diaphragma sellae, basilar artery (B.A.), and oculomotor nerves (III). The perforating branches of the carotid artery supply the infundibulum, optic chiasm and tracts, and the floor of the third ventricle.

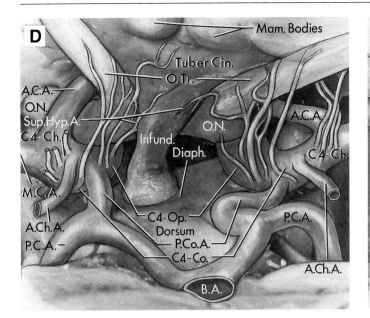

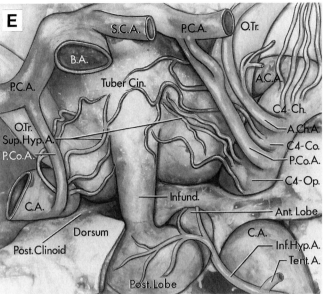

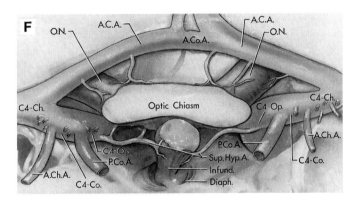

Figure 2-8 Relationships in the sellar and suprasellar areas. **(D)** Posterior view. The basilar artery and brainstem have been divided and the floor of the third ventricle elevated to provide this posterior view of the arteries in the suprasellar area. The tuber cinereum (Tuber Cin.) and mamillary bodies (Mam. Bodies) are exposed between the optic tracts. **(E)** The right half of the dorsum and the right posterior clinoid process (Post. Clinoid) have been removed to expose the anterior (Ant. Lobe) and posterior (Post. Lobe) lobes of the pituitary gland. The basilar, posterior cerebral and superior cerebellar arteries (S.C.A.) have been elevated to expose the pituitary stalk and floor of the third ventricle. The inferior hypophyseal (Inf. Hyp. A.) and the tentorial arteries (Tent. A.) arise from the carotid artery. **(F)** Posterior view of the anterior part of the circle of Willis. The optic chiasm has been divided posterior to its junction with the optic nerves and anterior to where the infundibulum arises from the floor of the third ventricle. The superior hypophyseal arteries pass to the infundibulum and send branches to the lower surface of the optic chiasm. The anterior cerebral arteries send branches to the upper surface of the optic chiasm. The anterior communicating artery (A.Co.A.) is situated above the optic chiasm *(13)*.

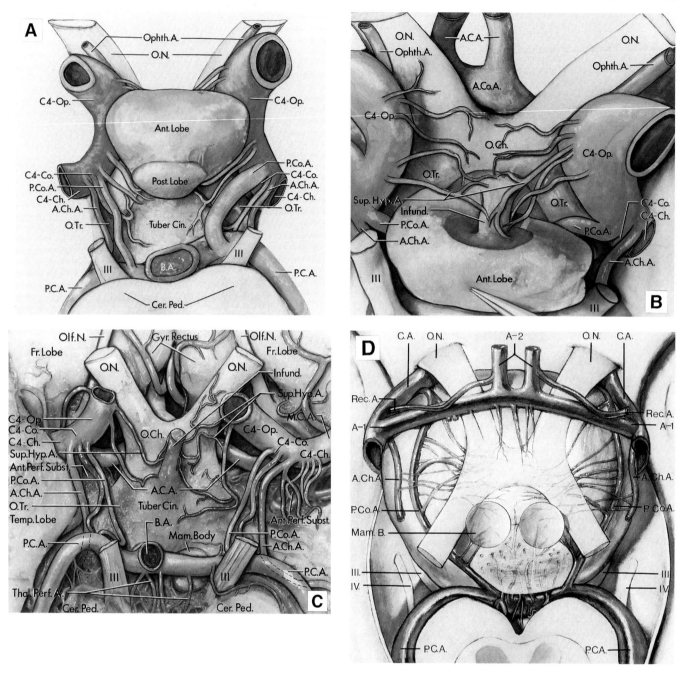

Figure 2-9 Relationships in the sellar and suprasellar areas. **(A)** Inferior view. The supraclinoid portion of the carotid artery is divided into three segments based on the site of origin of its major branches: the ophthalmic segment (C4-Op.) extends from the origin of the ophthalmic artery (Ophth. A.) to the origin of the posterior communicating artery (P.Co.A.); the communicating segment (C4-Co.) extends from the origin of the posterior communicating artery to the origin of the anterior choroidal artery (A.Ch.A.); and the choroidal segment (C4-Ch.) extends from the origin of the anterior choroidal artery to the bifurcation of the carotid artery. The optic nerves (O.N.) are above the ophthalmic arteries. The optic chiasm and optic tracts (O.Tr.) are above the anterior (Ant. Lobe) and posterior (Post. Lobe) lobes of the pituitary gland. The tuber cinereum (Tuber Cin.) is anterior to the apex of the basilar artery (B.A.). The posterior cerebral arteries (P.C.A.) pass around the cerebral peduncles (Cer. Ped.) above the oculomotor nerves (III). The perforating branches arising from the ophthalmic segment pass to the anterior lobe, optic nerve, and chiasm, and to the anterior part of the tuber cinereum. A single perforating branch arises from the communicating segment on each side and passes upward to the optic tract and the floor of the third ventricle. **(B)** The pituitary gland has been reflected backward to show the superior hypophyseal arteries (Sup. Hyp. A.) passing from the ophthalmic segments to the infundibulum (Infund.). The anterior cerebral (A.C.A.) and the anterior communicating (A.Co.A.) arteries pass above the optic chiasm (O.Ch.). **(C)** The superior hypophyseal arteries pass to the infundibulum of the hypophysis. The communicating segment sends one perforating branch on each side to the optic tracts and the region around the mamillary bodies (Mam. Body). The choroidal segment sends its perforating branches into the anterior perforated substance (Ant. Perf. Subst.). The thalamoperforating arteries (Thal. Perf. A.) arise from the basilar artery. Other structures in the exposure include the temporal (Temp. Lobe), and frontal lobes (Fr. Lobe), gyrus rectus (Gyr. Rectus), and olfactory nerves (Olf. N.). **(D)** Superior view of multiple arteries stretched around the suprasellar extension of a pituitary adenoma. The anterior cerebral arteries send branches to the superior surface of the optic nerves and chiasm. The posterior communicating, internal carotid, and posterior cerebral arteries send branches into the area below and behind the chiasm. The recurrent arteries (Rec. A.) arise just distal to the anterior communicating artery. The trochlear nerve (IV) is also exposed *(13).*

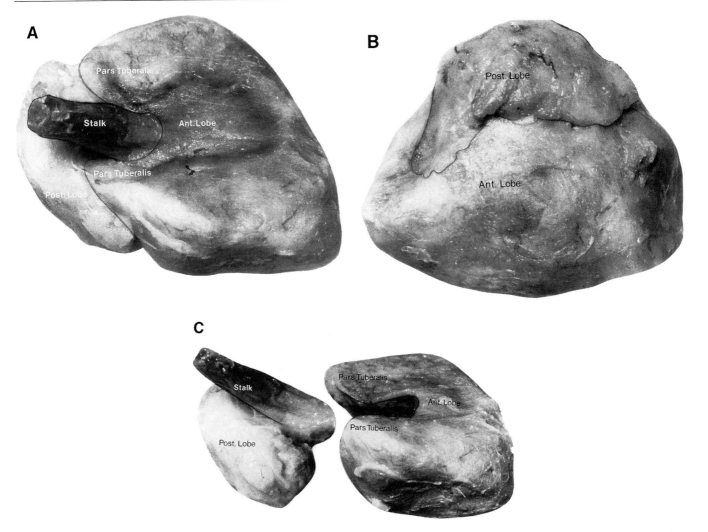

Figure 2-10 **(A)** Pituitary gland: superolateral view. The posterior lobe is a lighter color and has a different consistency, being less firm than the anterior lobe. The pars tuberalis partially encircles the stalk. The gland is concave around the stalk. **(B)** Pituitary gland: inferior view. Note the cleavage plane between the anterior and posterior lobes. **(C)** The anterior and posterior lobes have been separated. The pars tuberalis partially encircles the stalk *(2)*.

If the carotid arteries indent the lateral surfaces of the gland, the gland does lose its rounded shape and conforms to the wall of the artery, often developing protrusions above or below the artery. Intrasellar tumors are subjected to the same forces, which prevent them from being spherical, and the increased pressure within the tumor increases the degree to which the tumor insinuates into surrounding crevices and tissue planes. Separation of these extensions from the main mass of gland or tumor may explain cases in which the tumor and elevated pituitary hormone levels persist or recur after adenoma removal.

INTRACAVERNOUS VENOUS CONNECTIONS Venous sinuses may be found in the margins of the diaphragma and around the gland *(8)*. The intercavernous connections within the sella are named on the basis of their relationship to the pituitary gland; the anterior intercavernous sinuses pass anterior to the hypophysis, and the posterior intercavernous sinuses pass behind the gland (Figures 11 and 12). Actually, these intercavernous connections can occur at any site along the anterior, inferior, or posterior surface of the gland. The anterior sinus is usually larger than the posterior sinus, but either or both may be absent. If the anterior and posterior connections coexist, the whole structure constitutes the

"circular sinus." Entering an anterior intercavernous connection that extends downward in front of the gland during transsphenoidal operation may produce brisk bleeding. However, this usually stops with temporary compression of the channel or with light coagulation, which serves to glue the walls of the channel together.

A large intercavernous venous connection called the basilar sinus often passes posterior to the dorsum sellae and upper clivus (Figures 11 and 12). The basilar sinus connects the posterior aspect of both cavernous sinuses, and is usually the largest and most constant intercavernous connection across the midline. The superior and inferior petrosal sinuses join the basilar sinus. The abducent nerve often enters the posterior part of the cavernous sinus by passing through the basilar sinus.

CAVERNOUS SINUS The cavernous sinus surrounds the horizontal portion of the carotid artery and a segment of the abducent nerve (Figures 5, 7, and 13). The oculomotor and trochlear nerves, and the ophthalmic division of the trigeminal nerve are found in the roof and lateral wall of the sinus *(10,12,15,16)*. The lateral wall of the cavernous sinus extends from the superior orbital fissure in front to the apex of the petrous portion of the temporal bone behind. The oculomotor nerve enters the roof of the sinus

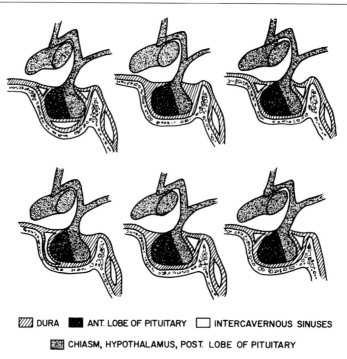

DURA   ANT. LOBE OF PITUITARY   INTERCAVERNOUS SINUSES

CHIASM, HYPOTHALAMUS, POST. LOBE OF PITUITARY

Figure 2-11   Six sagittal sections of the sellar region showing variations in the intercavernous venous connections within the dura. The variations shown include combinations of anterior, posterior, and inferior intercavernous connections and the frequent presence of a basilar sinus posterior to the dorsum. Either the anterior (lower center) or posterior (lower left) intercavernous connections or both (top center) may be absent. The anterior intercavernous sinus may extend along the whole anterior margin of the gland (lower left). The basilar sinus may be absent (lower right) *(8)*.

lateral to the dorsum sellae. The trochlear nerve enters the roof of the sinus posterolateral to the third nerve, and both nerves enter the dura mater immediately below and medial to the free edge of the tentorium. The ophthalmic division enters the low part of the lateral wall of the sinus and runs obliquely upward to pass through the superior orbital fissure. The abducent nerve enters the posterior wall of the sinus by passing through the dura lining the upper clivus and courses forward between the carotid artery medially and the ophthalmic division laterally. It frequently splits into multiple rootlets in its course lateral to the carotid artery.

The branches of the intracavernous portion of the carotid artery are the meningohypophyseal trunk, the artery of the inferior cavernous sinus, and McConnell's capsular arteries (Figure 7A). The ophthalmic artery may also take origin from the carotid artery within the sinus in few cases *(8,10)*. The most proximal branch of the intracavernous carotid artery, the meningohypophyseal trunk, usually arises below the level of the dorsum sellae near the apex of the curve between the petrous and intracavernous segments of the artery. The three branches of the meningohypophyseal artery are the tentorial artery (of Bernasconi-Cassinari), which courses toward the tentorium; the inferior hypophyseal artery, which courses medially to supply the posterior part of the capsule of the pituitary gland; and the dorsal meningeal artery, which perforates the dura of the posterior wall of the sinus to supply the region of the clivus and the sixth nerve (Figures 4 and 7).

The artery of the inferior cavernous sinus, which is also called the inferolateral trunk, originates from the lateral side of the horizontal segment of the carotid artery distal to the origin of the meningohypophyseal trunk (Figure 5E) *(10,12)*. It passes above the abducent nerve and downward medially to the first trigeminal division to supply the dura of the lateral wall of the sinus. In a few

cases, it arises from the meningohypophyseal trunk. McConnell's capsular arteries, if present, arise from the medial side of the carotid artery and pass to the capsule of the gland, distal to the point of origin of the artery of the inferior cavernous sinus.

SUPRASELLAR AND THIRD VENTRICULAR REGION

This section deals with neural, arterial, and venous relationships in the suprasellar and third ventricular regions that are important in planning surgery for pituitary adenomas.

NEURAL RELATIONSHIPS   The third ventricle is located in the center of the head, above the sella turcica, pituitary gland, and midbrain, between the cerebral hemispheres, thalami, and the walls of the hypothalamus, and below the corpus callosum and the body of the lateral ventricle (Figure 14). It is intimately related to the circle of Willis and deep venous system of the brain. Manipulation of the walls of the third ventricle may cause hypothalamic dysfunction as manifested by disturbances of consciousness, temperature control, respiration, and hypophyseal secretion, visual loss owing to damage of the optic chiasm and tracts, and memory loss owing to injury to the columns of the fornix in the walls of the third ventricle *(14,17,18)*. The third ventricle is a narrow, funnel-shaped, unilocular, midline cavity. It has a floor, a roof, and an anterior, posterior, and two lateral walls.

FLOOR   The floor extends from the optic chiasm anteriorly to the orifice of the aqueduct of Sylvius posteriorly (Figures 14–16). The anterior half of the floor is formed by diencephalic structures, and the posterior half is formed by mesencephalic structures.

When viewed from inferiorly, the structures forming the floor from anterior to posterior include the optic chiasm, infundibulum of the hypothalamus, tuber cinereum, mamillary bodies, posterior perforated substance, and (most posteriorly), the part of the teg-

A

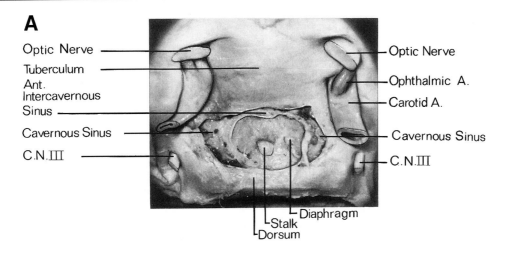

Optic Nerve

Tuberculum

Ant.
Intercavernous
Sinus

Cavernous Sinus

C.N. III

Optic Nerve

Ophthalmic A.

Carotid A.

Cavernous Sinus

C.N. III

Diaphragm
Stalk
Dorsum

B

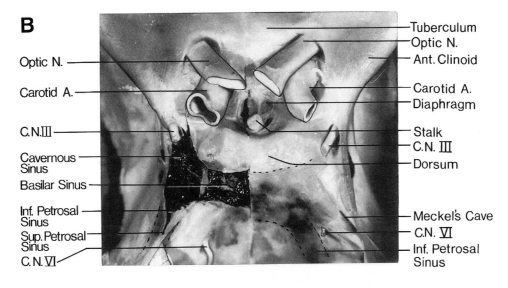

Optic N.

Carotid A.

C.N. III

Cavernous
Sinus

Basilar Sinus

Inf. Petrosal
Sinus

Sup. Petrosal
Sinus

C.N. VI

Tuberculum
Optic N.
Ant. Clinoid

Carotid A.
Diaphragm

Stalk
C.N. III
Dorsum

Meckel's Cave
C.N. VI
Inf. Petrosal
Sinus

C

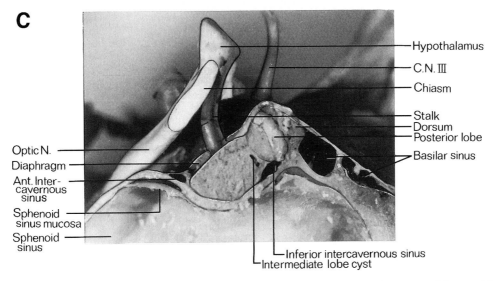

Optic N.
Diaphragm
Ant. Inter-
cavernous
sinus

Sphenoid
sinus mucosa

Sphenoid
sinus

Hypothalamus
C.N. III
Chiasm

Stalk
Dorsum
Posterior lobe

Basilar sinus

Inferior intercavernous sinus
Intermediate lobe cyst

Figure 2-12 Intercavernous venous connections. **(A)** The ophthalmic artery arises from the superior aspect of the carotid artery and courses laterally beneath the optic nerve to the optic foramen. The dura over the cavernous and anterior intercavernous sinuses has been opened to show the venous connection across the midline. **(B)** The basilar sinus connects the posterior portion of the two cavernous sinuses. The dura over the posterior aspect of the left cavernous sinus and the left half of the basilar sinus has been removed. The course of the basilar, inferior petrosal, and superior petrosal sinuses within the dura is shown by the dotted lines. **(C)** Midsagittal section of the sellar region. The anterior and inferior intercavernous sinuses are small. The basilar sinus, dorsal to the clivus and joining the posterior aspect of the two cavernous sinuses, is the largest connection across the midline *(8)*.

A

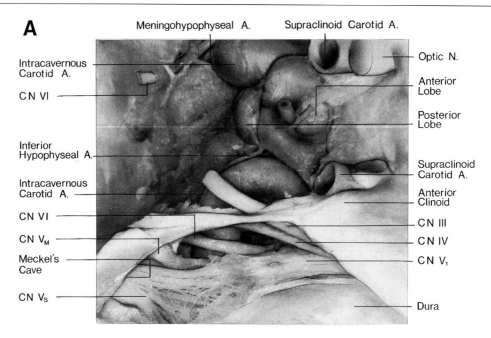

Meningohypophyseal A.   Supraclinoid Carotid A.

Intracavernous Carotid A.

CN VI

Optic N.

Anterior Lobe

Posterior Lobe

Inferior Hypophyseal A.

Intracavernous Carotid A.

CN VI

CN V$_M$

Meckel's Cave

CN V$_S$

Supraclinoid Carotid A.

Anterior Clinoid

CN III

CN IV

CN V$_1$

Dura

B

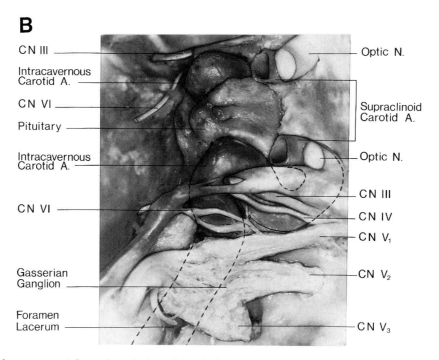

CN III

Intracavernous Carotid A.

CN VI

Pituitary

Intracavernous Carotid A.

CN VI

Gasserian Ganglion

Foramen Lacerum

Optic N.

Supraclinoid Carotid A.

Optic N.

CN III

CN IV

CN V$_1$

CN V$_2$

CN V$_3$

Figure 2-13 *(continued on next page)* Superolateral view of the pituitary gland and right cavernous sinus. **(A)** The lateral dural wall of the cavernous sinus has been removed. A tortuous carotid artery bulges superiorly, pushing the interclinoid ligament and roof of the cavernous sinus upward, and indenting the lateral margin of the pituitary gland. The inferior hypophyseal artery passes to the pituitary gland. The third (CN III) and fourth cranial nerves (CN IV) course in the upper part of the cavernous sinus. The sixth cranial nerve (CN VI) passes above the trigeminal sensory (CN V$_s$) and motor (CN V$_m$) roots, and medial to the first division (CN V$_1$). **(B)** Further dural removal exposes the trigeminal root and its second (CN V$_2$) and third (CN V$_3$) divisions below the cavernous sinus. The trigeminal root has been displaced laterally to show a second rootlet of the sixth cranial nerve lateral to the carotid artery.

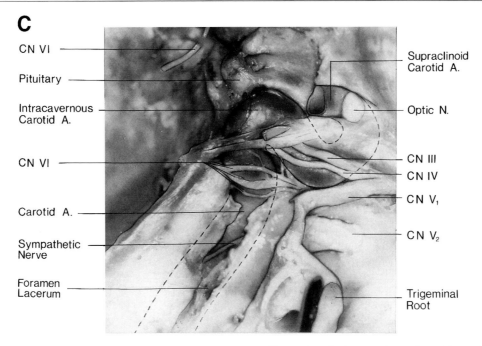

CN VI

Pituitary

Intracavernous
Carotid A.

CN VI

Carotid A.

Sympathetic
Nerve

Foramen
Lacerum

Supraclinoid
Carotid A.

Optic N.

CN III

CN IV

CN V₁

CN V₂

Trigeminal
Root

Figure 2-13   Superolateral view of the pituitary gland and right cavernous sinus. **(C)** The trigeminal root has been reflected forward, exposing the carotid artery in the foramen lacerum. A sympathetic nerve bundle courses on the carotid artery in the foramen lacerum. Three rootlets of the sixth cranial nerve pass around the carotid artery. The carotid artery is outlined in the areas where it is out of view in the temporal bone and cavernous sinus *(12)*.

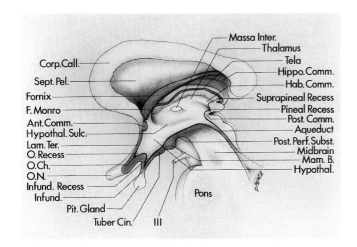

Corp. Call.

Sept. Pel.

Fornix

F. Monro

Ant. Comm.

Hypothal. Sulc.

Lam. Ter.

O. Recess

O. Ch.

O.N.

Infund. Recess

Infund.

Pit. Gland

Tuber Cin.   III

Massa Inter.

Thalamus

Tela

Hippo. Comm.

Hab. Comm.

Suprapineal Recess

Pineal Recess

Post. Comm.

Aqueduct

Post. Perf. Subst.

Midbrain

Mam. B.

Hypothal.

Pons

Figure 2-14   Midsagittal section of the third ventricle. The floor extends from the optic chiasm (O.Ch.) to the aqueduct of Sylvius and includes the lower surface of the optic chiasm, infundibulum (Infund.), infundibular recess (Infund. Recess), pituitary gland (Pit. Gland), tuber cinereum (Tuber Cin.), mamillary bodies (Mam. B.), posterior perforated substance (Post. Perf. Subst.), and the part of the midbrain anterior to the aqueduct. The anterior wall extends from the optic chiasm to the foramen of Monro (F. Monro) and includes the upper surface of the optic chiasm, optic recess (O. Recess), lamina terminalis (Lam. Ter.), anterior commissure (Ant. Comm.), and foramen of Monro. The roof extends from the foramen of Monro to the suprapineal recess and is formed by the fornix and the layers of the tela choroidea (Tela), between which course the internal cerebral veins and the medial posterior choroidal arteries. The hippocampal commissure (Hippo. Comm.), corpus callosum (Corp. Call.), and septum pellucidum (Sept. Pel.) are above the roof. The posterior wall extends from the suprapineal recess to the aqueduct and includes the habenular commissure (Hab. Comm.), pineal gland, pineal recess, and posterior commissure (Post. Comm.). The oculomotor nerve (III) exits from the midbrain. The hypothalamic sulcus (Hypothal. Sulc.) forms a groove between the thalamic and hypothalamic (Hypothal.) surfaces of the third ventricle *(17)*.

mentum of the midbrain located above the medial aspect of the cerebral peduncles. The optic chiasm is located at the junction of the floor and the anterior wall. The lower surface of the chiasm forms the anterior part of the floor, and the superior surface forms the lower part of the anterior wall. The optic tracts arise from the posterolateral margin of the chiasm and course obliquely away from the floor toward the lateral margin of the midbrain. The infundibulum, tuber cinereum, mamillary bodies, and posterior perforated substance are located in the space limited anteriorly and laterally by the optic chiasm and tracts, and posteriorly by the cerebral peduncles.

The infundibulum of the hypothalamus is a hollow, funnel-shaped structure located between the optic chiasm and the tuber cinereum. The pituitary gland (hypophysis) is attached to the infundibulum, and the axons in the infundibulum extend to the posterior lobe of the hypophysis. The tuber cinereum is a prominent mass of hypothalamic gray matter located anterior to the mamillary bodies. The tuber cinereum merges anteriorly into the infundibulum. The tuber cinereum, around the base of the infundibulum, is raised to form a prominence called the median eminence. The mamillary bodies form paired, round prominences posterior to the tuber cinereum. The posterior perforated substance is a depressed, punctuated area of gray matter located in the interval between the mamillary bodies anteriorly and the medial surface of the cerebral peduncles posteriorly. The posterior part of the floor extends posterior and superior to the medial part of the cerebral peduncles and superior to the tegmentum of the midbrain.

When viewed from above and inside the third ventricle, the optic chiasm forms a prominence at the anterior margin of the floor (Figures 15 and 16). The infundibular recess extends into the infundibulum behind the optic chiasm. The mamillary bodies form paired prominences on the inner surface of the floor posterior to the infundibular recess. The part of the floor between the mamillary bodies and the aqueduct of Sylvius has a smooth sur-

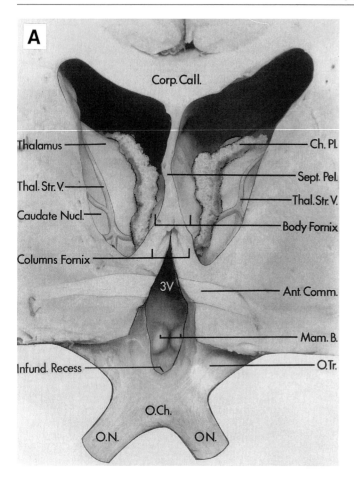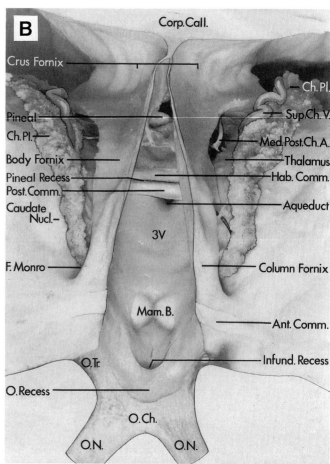

Figure 2-15 Anterosuperior views of the third ventricle. **(A)** The anterior part of the cerebral hemispheres and part of the anterior wall of the third ventricle have been removed. The optic chiasm (O. Ch.) and nerves (O. N.) are at the lower margin of the anterior wall. The optic tracts (O. Tr.) extend laterally below the floor of third ventricle (3V). The infundibular recess (Infund. Recess) extends downward posterior to the optic chiasm and anterior to the mamillary bodies (Mam. B.). The midportion of the anterior commissure (Ant. Comm.) has been removed to expose the columns of the fornix anterior to the foramina of Monro. The body and columns of the fornix join anterior to the foramina of Monro. The choroid plexus (Ch. Pl.) is attached along the cleft between the thalamus and fornix on each side. The thalamostriate veins (Thal. Str. V.) course between the caudate nucleus (Caudate Nucl.) and the thalamus. Other structures in the exposure include the septum pellucidum (Sept. Pel.) and corpus callosum (Corp. Call.). **(B)** The septum pellucidum and the medial part of the body of the fornix have been removed to expose the foramen of Monro (F. Monro) and the full length of the floor of the third ventricle. The floor extends from the optic chiasm to the aqueduct of Sylvius. The habenular commissure (Hab. Comm.) forms the upper margin of the stalk of the pineal gland, and the posterior commissure (Post. Comm.) forms the lower part of the stalk. The optic recess (O. Recess) extends anterior to the upper one-half of the optic chiasm between the chiasm and the lamina terminalis, which has been removed. Other structures in the exposure include the medial posterior choroidal arteries (Med. Post. Ch. A.) and superior choroidal veins (Sup. Ch. V.) *(17)*.

face, which is concave from side to side. This smooth surface lies above the posterior perforated substance anteriorly and the medial part of the cerebral peduncles and the tegmentum of the midbrain posteriorly.

ANTERIOR WALL The anterior wall of the third ventricle extends from the foramen of Monro above to the optic chiasm below (Figures 14–16). Only the lower two-thirds of the anterior surface is seen on the external surface of the brain; the upper one-third is hidden posterior to the rostrum of the corpus callosum. The part of the anterior wall visible on the surface is formed by the optic chiasm and the lamina terminalis. The lamina terminalis is a thin sheet of gray matter and pia mater that attaches to the upper surface of the chiasm and stretches upward to fill the interval between the optic chiasm and the rostrum of the corpus callosum.

When viewed from within, the boundaries of the anterior wall from superiorly to inferiorly are formed by the columns of the

fornix, foramen of Monro, anterior commissure, lamina terminalis, optic recess, and optic chiasm. The opening of the foramen of Monro into each lateral ventricle is located at the junction of the roof and the anterior wall of the third ventricle (Figures 14 and 17). The foramen is a duct-like canal that opens between the fornix and the thalamus into each lateral ventricle, and extends inferiorly below the fornix into the third ventricle as a single channel. The foramen of Monro is bounded anteriorly by the junction of the body and the columns of the fornix, and posteriorly by the anterior pole of the thalamus.

POSTERIOR WALL The posterior wall of the third ventricle extends from the suprapineal recess above to the aqueduct of Sylvius below (Figures 14–17). When viewed from anteriorly within the third ventricle, it consists, from above to below, of the suprapineal recess, the habenular commissure, the pineal body and its recess, the posterior commissure, and the aqueduct of Sylvius.

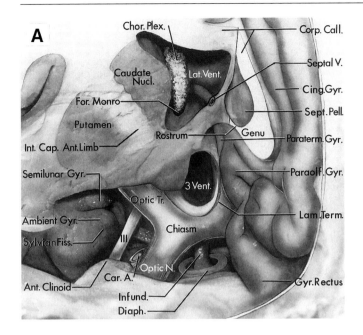

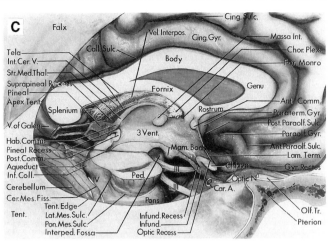

Figure 2-16 Suprasellar and third ventricular regions. Stepwise dissection. **(A)** Anterior-superior view. The anterior part of the frontal lobe has been removed to expose the anterior incisural space and suprasellar region. The section of the frontal lobe passes adjacent to the septum pellucidum (Sept. Pell.) and through the rostrum and genu of the corpus callosum (Corp. Call.), frontal horn of the lateral ventricle (Lat. Vent.), and the anterior limb of the internal capsule (Int. Cap. Ant. Limb). The anterior incisural space is located anterior to the midbrain and extends upward around the optic chiasm, lamina terminalis (Lam. Term.), and anterior part of the third ventricle (3 Vent.). The optic tract (Optic Tr.) extends posteriorly above the oculomotor nerve (III). The infundibulum (Infund.) of the pituitary gland passes through the diaphragma sellae (Diaph.). Choroid plexus (Chor. Plex.) extends through the foramen of Monro (For. Monro). Other structures in the exposure include the carotid artery (Car. A.), caudate nucleus (Caudate Nucl.), optic nerve (Optic N.), septal vein (Septal V.), cingulate (Cing. Gyr.), paraterminal (Paraterm. Gyr.), paraolfactory (Paraolf. Gyr.), semilunar (Semilunar Gyr.) and ambient gyri (Ambient Gyr.), gyrus rectus (Gyr. Rectus), sylvian fissure (Sylvian Fiss.), and anterior clinoid process (Ant. Clinoid). **(B)** The transverse section has been extended behind the foramen of Monro to include part of the cerebral peduncle (Ped.). The posterior part of the right optic nerve and the right half of the optic chiasm have been removed to expose the posterior part of the anterior incisural space. The thalamus and internal capsule are located directly above the cerebral peduncle. Other structures in the exposure include the olfactory tract (Olf. Tr.), substantia nigra (Subst. Nigra), red nucleus (Red Nucl.), parahippocampal gyrus (Parahippo. Gyr.), tentorial edge (Tent. Edge), temporal horn (Temp. Horn), globus pallidus (Globus Pall.), collateral (Coll. Sulc.), callosal (Call. Sulc.) and anterior hippocampal sulci (Ant. Hippo. Sulc.), anterior commissure (Ant. Comm.), mamillary bodies (Mam. Body), massa intermedia (Massa Int.), and choroidal fissure (Chor. Fiss.). **(C)** The right cerebral hemisphere has been removed to expose all of the third ventricle. The optic recess extends inferiorly between the optic chiasm and the lamina terminalis, and the infundibular recess (Infund. Recess) extends into the infundibulum behind the chiasm. The layer of tela choroidea that forms the upper wall of the velum interpositum (Vel. Interpos.) is adherent to the lower margin of the body and crus of the fornix. The layer of tela choroidea that forms the lower wall of the velum interpositum is attached anteriorly to the striae medullaris thalami (Str. Med. Thal.) and posteriorly to the superior margin of the pineal body. The striae medullaris thalami extend forward from the habenular commissure (Hab. Comm.) along the superomedial margin of the thalamus. Other structures in the exposure include the interpeduncular fossa (Interped. Fossa), tentorial apex (Apex Tent.), internal cerebral vein (Int. Cer. V.), lateral mesencephalic (Lat. Mes. Sulc.) and pontomesencephalic sulci (Pont. Mes. Sulc.), posterior commissure (Post. Comm.), vein of Galen (V. of Galen), trochlear nerve (IV), inferior colliculus (Inf. Coll.), cerebellomesencephalic fissure (Cer. Mes. Fiss.), and the anterior (Ant. Paraolf. Sulc.) and posterior paraolfactory sulci (Post. Paraolf. Sulc.) *(19)*.

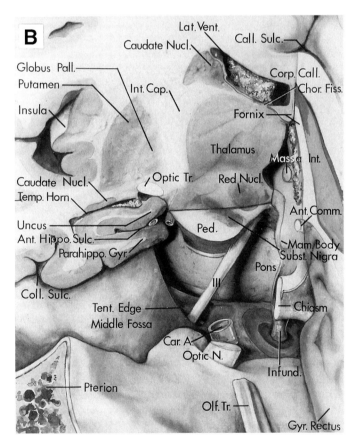

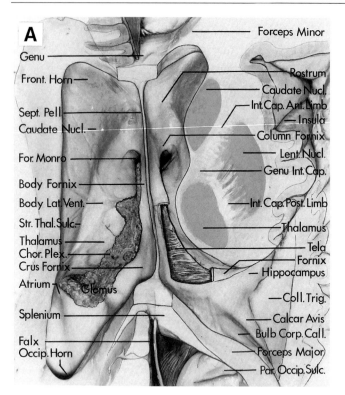

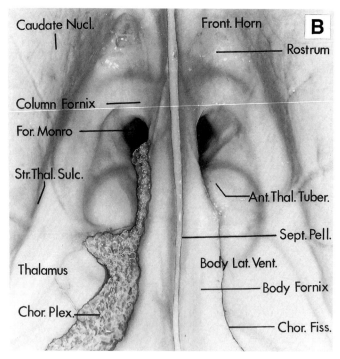

Figure 2-17 *(continued on next page)* Neural relationships. **(A)** Superior view. The upper part of the cerebral hemispheres have been removed to expose the lateral ventricles and roof of the third ventricle. The upper part of the roof of the third ventricle is formed by the body and crus of the fornix. The columns of the fornix pass anterior and superior to the foramen of Monro (For. Monro). Part of the fornix has been removed on the right side to expose the tela choroidea (Tela) in the roof of the third ventricle. The choroid plexus (Chor. Plex) has been removed on the right side. The anterior limb of the internal capsule (Int. Cap. Ant. Limb) is located between the head of the caudate nucleus (Caudate Nucl.) and the lentiform nuclei (Lent. Nucl.). The posterior limb of the internal capsule (Int. Cap. Post. Limb) is located between the thalamus and the lentiform nucleus. The genu of the internal capsule (Genu Int. Cap.) touches the lateral wall of the ventricle between the caudate nucleus and the thalamus. Other structures in the exposure include the frontal horn (Front. Horn), body (Body Lat. Vent.), and occipital horn (Occip. Horn) of the lateral ventricle, septum pellucidum (Sept. Pell.), parietooccipital (Par. Occip. Sulc.), and striothalamic sulci (Str. Thal. Sulc.), bulb of the corpus callosum (Bulb Corp. Call.), and collateral trigone (Coll. Trig.). **(B)** Enlarged view of the region of the foramen of Monro. The choroid plexus has been removed from its attachment along the choroidal fissure (Chor. Fiss.) on the right side. The anterior thalamic tubercle (Ant. Thal. Tuber.), which overlies the anterior nucleus of the thalamus, bulges upward at the posterior margin of the foramen of Monro. The columns of the fornix pass anterior and superior to the foramen of Monro.

ROOF   The roof of the third ventricle forms a gentle upward arch, extending from the foramen of Monro anteriorly to the suprapineal recess posteriorly (Figures 14, 16, and 17). It is infrequent that pituitary adenomas are approached through the roof of the third ventricle. However, other tumors involving the third ventricle are approached from above. The roof has four layers: one neural layer formed by the fornix, two thin membranous layers of tela choroidea, and a layer of blood vessels between the two sheets of tela choroidea (Figures 16 and 17).

The upper, or neural, layer is formed by the fornix. The upper layer of the anterior part of the roof of the third ventricle is formed by the body of the fornix, and the posterior part of the roof is formed by the crura and the hippocampal commissure. The body of the fornix splits into two columns at the anterior margin of the opening of each foramen of Monro into the lateral ventricle. The columns descend in the lateral walls of the third ventricle and terminate in the mamillary bodies.

The tela choroidea forms two of the three layers in the roof below the layer formed by the fornix (Figures 16 and 17). The tela choroidea consists of two thin, semiopaque membranes derived from pia mater, which are interconnected by loosely organized trabecu-

lae. The final layer in the roof is a vascular layer located between the two layers of tela choroidea. The vascular layer consists of the medial posterior choroidal arteries and their branches and the internal cerebral veins and their tributaries. Parallel strands of choroid plexus project downward on each side of the midline from the inferior layer of tela choroidea into the superior part of the third ventricle.

The velum interpositum is the space between the two layers of tela choroidea in the roof of the third ventricle. The upper layer of the tela choroidea is attached to the lower surface of the fornix and the hippocampal commissure (Figures 16 and 17). The lower wall is attached to the teniae thalami, small ridges on the free edge of a fiber tract, the striae medullaris thalami, which extends along the superomedial border of the thalamus from the foramen of Monro to the habenular commissure. The posterior part of the lower wall is attached to the superior surface of the pineal body. The internal cerebral veins arise in the anterior part of the velum interpositum, just behind the foramen of Monro, and they exit the velum interpositum above the pineal body to enter the quadrigeminal cistern and join the great vein. The velum interpositum is usually a closed space that tapers to a narrow apex just behind the foramen

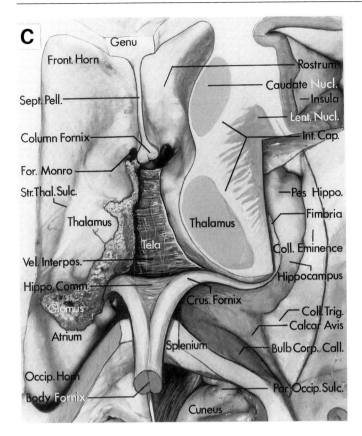
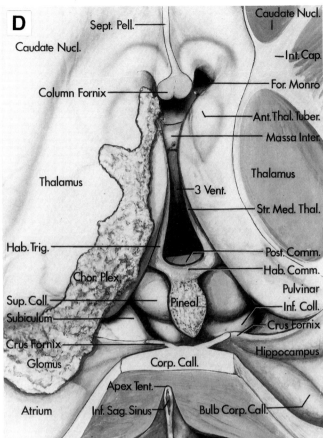

Figure 2-17 Neural relationships. **(C)** The fornix has been divided at the junction of its body and the columns above the foramen of Monro, and reflected backward to expose the velum interpositum (Vel. Interpos.) located between the layers of tela choroidea in the roof of the third ventricle. Other structures in the exposure include the pes hippocampus (Pes Hipp.), collateral eminence (Coll. Eminence), and hippocampal commissure (Hipp. Comm.). **(D)** The body and anterior part of the crura of the fornix have been removed to expose the third ventricle (3 Vent.). The massa intermedia (Massa Inter.) extends into the anterior part of the third ventricle, and the habenular (Hab. Comm.) and posterior commissures (Post. Comm.) cross the posterior part of the third ventricle. The layer of tela choroidea, which form the upper wall of the velum interpositum, is attached to the lower margin of the fornix and the layer that forms the lower wall is attached to the striae medullaris thalami (Str. Med. Thal.). Other structures in the exposure include the habenular trigones (Hab. Trig.), superior (Sup. Coll.) and inferior colliculi (Inf. Coll.), inferior sagittal sinus (Inf. Sag. Sinus), and tentorial apex (Apex. Tent.) *(20)*.

of Monro, but it may infrequently have an opening situated between splenium and the pineal body that communicates with the quadrigeminal cistern to form the cisterna velum interpositum.

LATERAL WALL The lateral walls are not visible on the external surface of the brain, but are hidden between the cerebral hemispheres (Figures 14 and 16). They are formed by the hypothalamus inferiorly and the thalamus superiorly. The lateral walls have an outline like the lateral silhouette of a bird's head with an open beak. The head is formed by the oval medial surface of the thalamus; the open beaks, which project anteriorly and inferiorly, are represented by the recesses in the hypothalamus: the pointed upper beak is formed by the optic recess, and the lower beak is formed by the infundibular recess. The hypothalamic and thalamic surfaces are separated by the hypothalamic sulcus, a groove that is often ill-defined and extends from the foramen of Monro to the aqueduct of Sylvius. The superior limit of the thalamic surfaces of the third ventricle is marked by narrow, raised ridges, known as the striae medullaris thalami. These striae extend forward from the habenulae along the superomedial surface of the thalamus at the site of the attachment of the lower layer of the tela choroidea.

The massa intermedia projects into the upper one-half of the third ventricle and often connects the opposing surfaces of the thalamus. The massa intermedia was present in 76% of the brains examined and was located 2.5–6.0 mm (average, 3.9 mm) posterior to the foramen of Monro *(17)*. The columns of the fornix form distinct prominences in the lateral walls of the third ventricle just below the foramen of Monro, but inferiorly they sink below the surface.

SUPRASELLAR CISTERNS AND TENTORIAL INCISURA
The suprasellar region is commonly approached through the cisterns surrounding the anterior part of the tentorial incisura *(19)*. The incisura is a triangular space situated between the free edges of the tentorium. The upper part of the brainstem formed by the midbrain sits in the center of the incisura. The area between the midbrain and the free edges is divided into:

1. An anterior incisural space located in front of the midbrain.
2. Paired middle incisural spaces situated lateral to the midbrain.
3. A posterior incisural space located behind the midbrain (Figure 16C).

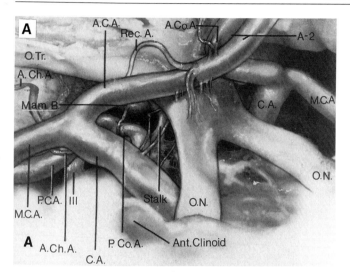
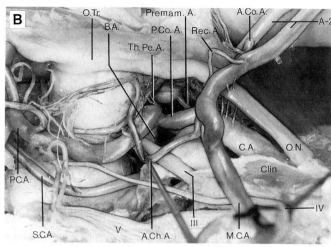

Figure 2-18 Right anterior and lateral views of the suprasellar area. (**A**) Right anterolateral view. The anterior clinoid process (Ant. Clinoid) and carotid artery (C.A.) are lateral to the optic nerve (O.N.). Perforating arteries pass from the carotid artery to terminate in the optic chiasm (O.Ch.) and tract (O.Tr.) and the hypothalamus anterior to the mamillary body (Mam. B.). The posterior communicating artery (P.Co.A.) courses medial to the carotid artery. The anterior choroidal artery (A.Ch.A.) arises from the carotid and passes above the posterior cerebral artery (P.C.A.). The third nerve (III) passes below the posterior cerebral artery. The recurrent artery (Rec. A.) arises from the anterior cerebral artery (A.C.A.) proximal to the anterior communicating artery (A.Co.A.). Other structures in the exposure include the middle cerebral (M.C.A.) and distal segment of the anterior cerebral arteries (A-2). (**B**) Right lateral view with the temporal lobe removed. The anterior clinoid process (Clin.) is lateral to the carotid artery. The premamillary artery (Premam. A.) arises from the posterior communicating artery, and the thalamoperforating arteries (Th. Pe. A.) arise from the posterior cerebral artery. The third and fourth (IV) cranial nerves course between the posterior cerebral and superior cerebellar arteries (S.C.A.). Other structures in the exposure include the trigeminal nerve (IV) and basilar artery (B.A.) *(21).*

Pituitary adenomas commonly involve the anterior incisural space.

The anterior incisural space corresponds roughly to the suprasellar area. From the front of the midbrain, it extends obliquely forward and upward around the optic chiasm to the subcallosal area. It opens laterally into the sylvian fissure and posteriorly between the uncus and the brainstem into the middle incisural space (Figure 16).

The part of the anterior incisural space located below the optic chiasm has posterior and posterolateral walls. The posterior wall is formed by the cerebral peduncles. The posterolateral wall is formed by the anterior one-third of the uncus, which hangs over the free edge above the oculomotor nerve. The infundibulum of the pituitary gland crosses the anterior incisural space to reach the opening in the diaphragma sellae. The part of the anterior incisural space situated above the optic chiasm is limited superiorly by the rostrum of the corpus callosum, posteriorly by the lamina terminalis, and laterally by the part of the medial surfaces of the frontal lobes located below the rostrum.

The anterior incisural space opens laterally into the part of the sylvian fissure situated below the anterior perforated substance. The anterior limb of the internal capsule, the head of the caudate nucleus, and the anterior part of the lentiform nucleus are located above the anterior perforated substance. The interpeduncular cistern, which sits in the posterior part of the anterior incisural space between the cerebral peduncles and the dorsum sellae, communicates anteriorly with the chiasmatic cistern, which is located below the optic chiasm. The interpeduncular and chiasmatic cisterns are separated by Liliequist's membrane, an arachnoidal sheet extending from the dorsum sellae to the anterior edge of the mamillary bodies. The chiasmatic cistern communicates around the optic chiasm with the cisterna laminae terminalis, which lies anterior to the lamina terminalis.

CRANIAL NERVES The optic and oculomotor nerves and the posterior part of the olfactory tracts pass through the suprasellar region and anterior incisural space (Figures 16 and 18). Each olfactory tract runs posteriorly and splits just above the anterior clinoid process to form the medial and lateral olfactory striae, which course along the anterior margin of the anterior perforated substance.

The optic nerves and chiasm and the anterior part of the optic tracts cross the anterior incisural space. The optic nerves emerge from the optic canals medial to the attachment of the free edges to the anterior clinoid processes and are directed posterior, superior, and medial toward the optic chiasm. From the chiasm, the optic tracts continue in a posterolateral direction around the cerebral peduncles to enter the middle incisural spaces. The optic nerve proximal to its entrance into the optic canal is covered by a reflected leaf of dura mater, the falciform process, which extends medially from the anterior clinoid process across the top of the optic nerve *(8).* The length of nerve covered by dura only at the intracranial end of the optic canal may vary from <1 mm to as great as 1 cm. Coagulation of the dura above the optic nerve just proximal to the optic canal on the assumption that bone separates the dura mater from the nerve could lead to nerve injury. Compression of the optic nerve against the sharp edge of the falciform process may result in a visual field deficit even if the compressing lesion does not damage the nerve enough to cause visual loss. Normally the optic nerve is separated medially from the sphenoid sinus by a thin layer of bone, but in a few cases, this bone is absent and the optic nerves may protrude directly into the sphenoid sinus, separated from the sinus by only mucosa and the dural sheath of the nerve *(6,8).*

OPTIC CHIASM The relationship of the chiasm to the sella is an important determinant of the ease with which the pituitary fossa can be exposed by the transfrontal surgical route (Figure 19).

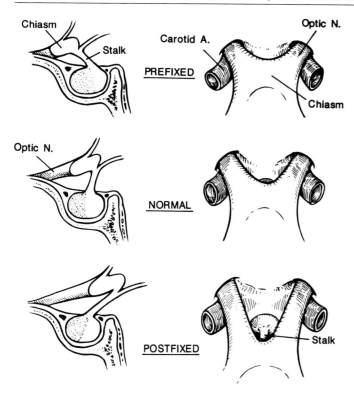

Figure 2-19 Sagittal sections and superior views of the sellar region showing the optic nerve (Optic N.) and chiasm, and carotid artery (Carotid A.). The prefixed chiasm is located above the tuberculum. The normal chiasm is located above the diaphragma. The postfixed chiasm is situated above the dorsum.

The normal chiasm overlies the diaphragma sellae and the pituitary gland, the prefixed chiasm overlies the tuberculum sellae, and the postfixed chiasm overlies the dorsum sellae. In approx 70% of cases, the chiasm is in the normal position. Of the remaining 30%, about half are "prefixed" and half "postfixed" *(8)*.

A prominent tuberculum sellae may restrict access to the sellae even in the presence of a normal chiasm. The tuberculum may vary from being almost flat to protruding upward as much as 3 mm, and it may project posteriorly to the margin of a normal chiasm *(8)*.

A prefixed chiasm, a normal chiasm with a small area between the tuberculum and the chiasm, and a superior protruding tuberculum sellae do not limit exposure by the transsphenoidal approach, but they limit the access to the suprasellar area provided by the transcranial approach. There are several methods of gaining access to the suprasellar area when these variants are present. One is to expose the sphenoid sinus from above by opening through the tuberculum and planum sphenoidale, thus converting the approach to a transfrontal-transsphenoidal exposure. If the chiasm is prefixed and the tumor is seen through a thin, stretched anterior wall of the third ventricle, the lamina terminalis may be opened to expose the tumor, but this exposure is infrequently used for pituitary adenomas. If the space between the carotid artery and the optic nerve has been enlarged (e.g., by a lateral or parasellar extension of tumor), the tumor may be removed through this space *(14,18)*.

An understanding of the relationship of the carotid artery, optic nerve, and anterior clinoid process is fundamental to all surgical approaches to the sellar and parasellar areas (Figure 18). The carotid artery and the optic nerve are medial to the anterior clinoid process. The artery exits the cavernous sinus beneath and slightly lateral to the optic nerve. The optic nerve pursues a posteromedial course toward the chiasm, and the carotid artery pursues a posterolateral course toward its bifurcation into the anterior and middle cerebral arteries.

ARTERIAL RELATIONSHIPS The arterial relationships in the suprasellar area are among the most complex in the head because this area contains all the components of the circle of Willis (Figures 8, 9, and 18). Numerous arteries, including the internal carotid and basilar arteries and the circle of Willis and its branches, may be stretched around tumors in this area: the posterior part of the circle of Willis and the apex of the basilar artery are located in the anterior incisural space below the floor of the third ventricle; the anterior part of the circle of Willis and the anterior cerebral and anterior communicating arteries are intimately related to the anterior wall of the third ventricle; both the anterior and posterior cerebral arteries send branches into the roof of the third ventricle; the internal carotid, anterior choroidal, anterior and posterior cerebral, and anterior and posterior communicating arteries give rise to perforating branches that reach the walls of the third ventricle and anterior incisural space; and all the arterial components of the circle of Willis and the adjacent segments of the carotid and basilar arteries, as well as their perforating branches may be stretched around suprasellar extensions of pituitary tumors *(13,21–24)*. Arterial lesions at the anterior part of the circle of Willis are more likely to result in disturbances in memory and personality, and those at the posterior part of the circle are more likely to result in disorders of the level of consciousness and are frequently combined with disorders of extraocular motion *(21,24)*.

INTERNAL CAROTID ARTERY The internal carotid artery exits the cavernous sinus along the medial surface of the anterior clinoid process to reach the anterior incisural space (Figures 8, 9, and 18). After entering this space, it courses posterior, superior, and lateral to reach the site of its bifurcation below the anterior perforated substance. It is first below and then lateral to the optic nerve and chiasm. It sends perforating branches to the optic nerve, chiasm, and tract, and to the floor of the third ventricle. These branches pass across the interval between the internal carotid artery and the optic nerve, and may serve as an obstacle to the operative approaches directed through the triangular space between the internal carotid artery, the optic nerve, and the anterior cerebral artery. The internal carotid artery also gives off the superior hypophyseal artery, which runs medially below the floor of the third ventricle to reach the tuber cinereum and joins its mate of the opposite side to form a ring around the infundibulum (Figures 8 and 9) *(13)*.

The supraclinoid (C_4) portion of the internal carotid artery is divided into three segments based on the origin of its major branches: the ophthalmic segment extends from the origin of the ophthalmic artery to the origin of the posterior communicating artery; the communicating segment extends from the origin of the posterior communicating artery to the origin of the anterior choroidal artery; and the choroidal segment extends from the origin of the anterior choroidal artery to the bifurcation (Figures 8 and 9) *(13)*. Each segment gives off a series of perforating branches with a relatively constant site of termination. The branches arising from the ophthalmic segment pass to the optic nerve and chiasm, infundibulum, and the floor of the third ventricle. The branches arising from the communicating segment pass to the optic tract and the floor of the third ventricle. The branches arising from the choroidal segment pass upward and enter the brain through the anterior perforated substance.

OPHTHALMIC ARTERY The ophthalmic artery is the first branch of the internal carotid artery above the cavernous sinus (Figures 8 and 9). It arises and enters the optic canal below the optic nerve. Its origin and proximal segment may be visible below the optic nerve without retracting the nerve, although elevation of the optic nerve away from the carotid artery is usually required to see the segment proximal to the optic foramen. The artery arises from the supraclinoid segment of the carotid artery in most cases, but it may also arise within the cavernous sinus or be absent in a few cases (8,10,12).

POSTERIOR COMMUNICATING ARTERY The posterior communicating artery arises from the posterior wall of the internal carotid artery and courses posteromedially below the optic tracts and the floor of the third ventricle to join the posterior cerebral artery (Figures 8, 9, and 18). Its branches penetrate the floor between the optic chiasm and the cerebral peduncle, and reach the thalamus, hypothalamus, subthalamus, and internal capsule. Its posterior course varies depending on whether the artery provides the major supply to the distal posterior cerebral artery. If it is normal, with the posterior cerebral artery arising predominately from the basilar artery, it is directed posteromedially above the oculomotor nerve toward the interpeduncular fossa (21,25). If the posterior cerebral artery has a fetal-type configuration in which it arises from the carotid artery, the posterior communicating artery is directed posterolaterally below the optic tract. The oculomotor nerve pierces the dura mater of the roof of the cavernous sinus 2–7 mm (average 5 mm) posterior to the initial supraclinoid segment of the carotid artery (2,12).

ANTERIOR CHOROIDAL ARTERY The anterior choroidal artery arises from the posterior surface of the internal carotid artery 0.1–3.0 mm above the origin of the posterior communicating artery (Figures 8, 9, and 18). It is directed posterolaterally below the optic tract between the uncus and cerebral peduncle. It passes through the choroidal fissure behind the uncus to supply the choroid plexus in the temporal horn. It sends branches into the optic tract and posterior part of the floor that reach the optic radiations, globus pallidus, internal capsule, midbrain, and thalamus (9,26).

ANTERIOR CEREBRAL AND ANTERIOR COMMUNICATING ARTERIES The anterior cerebral artery arises from the internal carotid artery below the anterior perforated substance and courses anteromedially above the optic nerve and chiasm to reach the interhemispheric fissure, where it is joined to the opposite anterior cerebral artery by the anterior communicating artery (Figures 8, 9, 18, 20, and 21) (24,27). The junction of the anterior communicating artery with the right and left A_1 segments is usually above the chiasm rather than above the optic nerves. In our studies, 70% were above the chiasm and 30% were in a prefixed position above the optic nerves (3,8). The shorter A_1 segments are stretched tightly over the chiasm, and the larger ones pass anteriorly over the nerves. Displacement of the chiasm against these arteries may result in visual loss before that caused by direct compression of the visual pathways by the tumor. The arteries with a more forward course are often tortuous and elongated, and some may course forward and rest on the tuberculum sellae or planum sphenoidale. The anterior cerebral artery ascends in front of the lamina terminalis and the anterior wall of the third ventricle, and passes around the corpus callosum.

The anterior cerebral and anterior communicating arteries give rise to perforating branches that terminate in the whole anterior wall of the third ventricle and reach the adjacent parts of the hypothalamus, fornix, septum pellucidum, and striatum (Figures 8, 20, and 21) (24,27). A precallosal artery may originate from the anterior cerebral or the anterior communicating artery, run upward across the lamina terminalis, and send branches into the anterior wall of the third ventricle (Figure 20).

The recurrent branch of the anterior cerebral artery, which is referred to as the recurrent artery of Heubner, is encountered frequently in approaches to the anterior part of the third ventricle (Figures 18, 20, and 21). It arises from the anterior cerebral artery in the region of the anterior communicating artery, courses laterally above the bifurcation of the internal carotid artery, and enters the anterior perforated substance (24,28). The recurrent artery courses anterior to the A_1 segment of the anterior cerebral artery and would be seen when elevating the frontal lobe before visualizing the A_1 segment in about two-thirds of cases. Of the remaining one-third, most coursed superior to A_1. Some of its branches reach the anterior limb and genu of the internal capsule.

POSTERIOR CEREBRAL ARTERY The bifurcation of the basilar artery into the posterior cerebral arteries is located in the posterior part of the suprasellar area below the posterior half of the floor of the third ventricle (Figures 8, 9, and 18) (21,25). A high basilar bifurcation may indent the floor. The posterior cerebral artery courses laterally around the cerebral peduncle, above the oculomotor nerve, and passes between the uncus and the cerebral peduncle to reach the quadrigeminal cistern. Its branches reach the floor, roof, and posterior, and lateral walls of the third ventricle.

The thalamoperforating arteries are a pair of larger perforating branches that arise from the posterior cerebral artery in the sellar region (Figures 9 and 18). The thalamoperforating arteries arise from the proximal part of the posterior cerebral arteries and the posterior part of the posterior communicating arteries, and enter the brain through the posterior part of the floor and the lateral walls. Infarction in the distribution of the thalamoperforating branches of the posterior cerebral artery may cause coma and death after the removal of a suprasellar tumor.

The medial posterior choroidal arteries also arise from the proximal portions of the posterior cerebral arteries in the suprasellar area and course around the midbrain to reach the quadrigeminal cistern (Figure 15) (9,26). They turn forward at the side of the pineal body to reach the velum interpositum, and supply the choroid plexus in the roof of the third ventricle and the body of the lateral ventricle.

VENOUS RELATIONSHIPS The deep cerebral venous system is intimately related to the walls of the third ventricle (Figure 22) (19,20). However, the veins do not pose a formidable obstacle to operative approaches to the suprasellar area and anterior third ventricle as they do in the region of the posterior third ventricle, because the veins in the suprasellar region are small.

The suprasellar area is drained, almost totally, by tributaries of the basal vein (19,20). The basal veins are formed by the union of veins draining the suprasellar area, and proceed posteriorly between the midbrain and the temporal lobes to empty into the internal cerebral or great vein (Figure 22). The veins joining below the anterior perforated substance to form the basal vein include the olfactory vein, which runs posteriorly in the olfactory sulcus; the fronto-orbital vein, which courses along the orbital surface of the frontal lobe; the deep middle cerebral vein, which receives the veins from the insula and passes medially across the limen insulae; the uncal veins, which course medially from the uncus; and the anterior cerebral vein, which descends on the lamina terminalis and

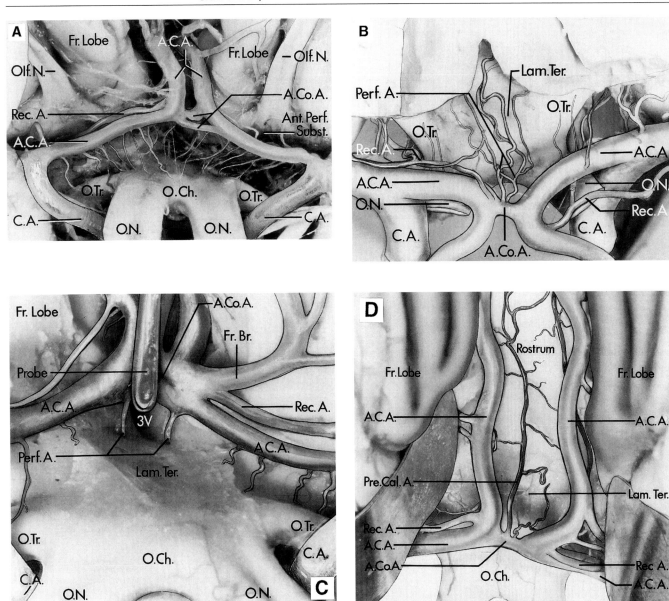

Figure 2-20   Arteries of the anterior wall of the third ventricle. Anterior views. **(A)** The anterior cerebral arteries give rise to perforating branches that enter the upper surface of the optic chiasm (O.Ch.). The recurrent arteries (Rec. A.) arise from the anterior cerebral arteries (A.C.A.) near the level of the anterior communicating artery (A.Co.A.). Other structures in the exposure include the optic nerves (O.N.) and tracts (O.Tr.), frontal lobes (Fr. Lobe), anterior perforated substance (Ant. Perf. Subst.), and olfactory nerves (Olf.N.). **(B)** The anterior communicating artery gives rise to a series of perforating arteries (Perf. A.) that enter the region of the lamina terminalis (Lam. Ter.). **(C)** A probe elevates the anterior communicating artery to expose two perforating arteries that pass through the lamina terminalis to reach the walls of the third ventricle (3V). The left recurrent artery arises in a common trunk with a branch to the frontal lobe (Fr. Br.). **(D)** A precallosal artery (Pre. Cal. A.) arises from the anterior communicating artery and passes upward on the lamina terminalis to reach the rostrum of the corpus callosum *(17)*.

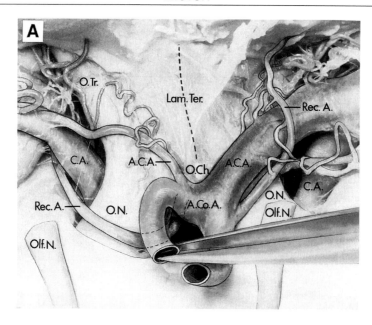

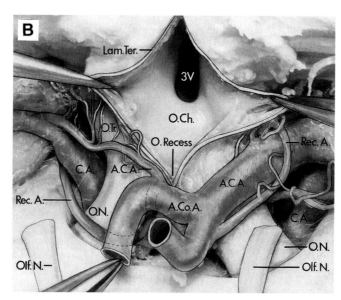

Figure 2-21 Anterior cerebral arteries and the lamina terminalis. **(A)** The anterior cerebral (A.C.A.), recurrent (Rec. A.), and anterior communicating arteries (A.Co.A.) have been retracted to expose the lamina terminalis (Lam. Ter.). Other structures in the exposure include the optic nerves (O.N.), chiasm (O.Ch.), and tracts (O.Tr.) and olfactory nerves (Olf. N.). The right anterior cerebral artery is hypoplastic. **(B)** The lamina terminalis has been opened along the dotted line shown in A to expose the cavity of the third ventricle (3V). The optic recess (O. Recess) extends downward between the lamina terminalis and the superior surface of the optic chiasm *(17)*.

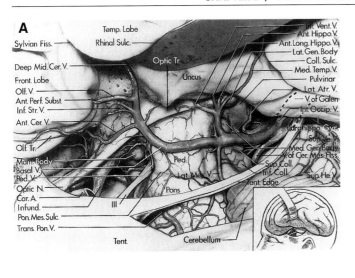

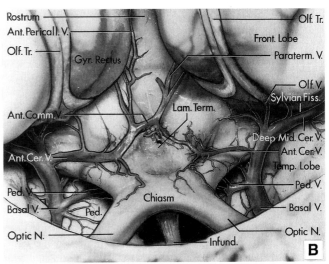

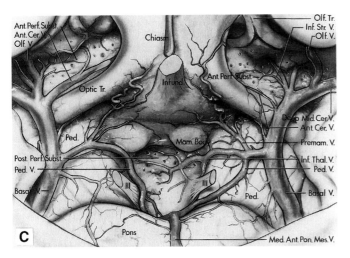

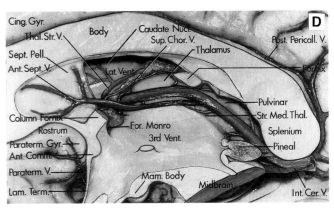

Figure 2-22 Veins in the suprasellar region. **(A)** Lateral view. Left side. The veins draining the suprasellar area converge on the anterior end of the basal vein (Basal V.). The temporal (Temp. Lobe) and frontal lobes (Front. Lobe) have been elevated, as shown in the insert. The basal vein arises below the anterior perforated substance (Ant. Perf. Subst.), passes around the cerebral peduncle (Ped.), and joins the vein of Galen (V. of Galen; dashed lines). The veins joining the anterior end of the basal vein include the olfactory veins (Olf. V.), which pass along the olfactory tract (Olf. Tr.); the inferior striate veins (Inf. Str. V.), which descend through the anterior perforated substance; the deep middle cerebral veins (Deep Mid. Cer. V.), which pass medially from the sylvian fissure (Sylvian Fiss.); and the anterior cerebral veins (Ant. Cer. V.), which pass across the optic chiasm. Other veins in the exposure include the peduncular (Ped. V.), lateral mesencephalic (Lat. Mes. V.), inferior ventricular (Inf. Vent. V.), anterior hippocampal (Ant. Hippo. V.), anterior longitudinal hippocampal (Ant. Long. Hippo. V.), medial temporal (Med. Temp. V.), lateral atrial (Lat. Atr. V.), internal occipital (Int. Occip. V.), transverse pontine (Trans. Pont.), superior vermian (Sup. Ve. V.) and superior hemispheric veins (Sup. He. V.), and the vein of the cerebellomesencephalic fissure (V. of Cer. Mes. Fiss.). Other structures in the exposure include the optic nerve (Optic N.) and tract (Optic. Tr.), carotid artery (Car. A.), lateral geniculate body (Lat. Gen. Body), infundibulum (Infund.), mamillary bodies (Mam. Body), tentorium (Tent.), tentorial edge (Tent. Edge), oculomotor nerve (III), parahippocampal (Parahippo. Gyr.), collateral (Coll. Sulc.), rhinal (Rhinal Sulc.) and pontomesencephalic sulci (Pon. Mes. Sulc.), lateral geniculate body (Lat. Gen. Body), and superior (Sup. Coll.) and inferior colliculi (Inf. Coll.). **(B)** Anterior view with the frontal lobe elevated. The anterior, deep middle cerebral, and olfactory veins join to form the basal vein. The anterior communicating (Ant. Comm. V.), paraterminal (Paraterm. V.), and anterior pericallosal veins (Ant. Pericall. V.) join the anterior cerebral veins in the region of the lamina terminalis (Lam. Ter.). The gyrus rectus (Gyr. Rectus) is also exposed. **(C)** Inferior view of the veins draining the floor of the third ventricle. The basal vein has its origin in the area below the anterior perforated substance. The peduncular veins cross the cerebral peduncle to join the basal veins. The premamillary veins (Premam. V.) drain the area around the infundibulum, and the inferior thalamic veins (Inf. Thal. V.) drain the region of the mamillary bodies and posterior perforated substance (Post. Perf. Subst.). The median anterior pontomesencephalic vein (Med. Pon. Mes. V.) courses in the midline on the midbrain and pons. **(D)** Midsagittal section showing the veins in the roof of the third ventricle (3rd Vent.). The brainstem has been sectioned at the level of the midbrain. Part of the septum pellucidum (Sept. Pell.) and body of the fornix has been removed to expose the right lateral ventricle (Lat. Vent.). The internal cerebral veins (Int. Cer. V.) course in the roof of the third ventricle. The thalamostriate (Thal. Str. V.), anterior septal (Ant. Sept. V.), posterior pericallosal (Post. Pericall. V.), and superior choroidal veins (Sup. Chor. V.) empty into the internal cerebral vein. Other structures in the exposure include the anterior commissure (Ant. Comm.), caudate nucleus (Caudate Nucl.), stria medullaris thalami (Str. Med. Thal.), paraterminal gyrus (Paraterm. Gyr.) and vein (Paraterm. V.), cingulate gyrus (Cing. Gyr.), and body of the corpus callosum (Body) *(20)*.

crosses the optic chiasm to reach the basal vein. The paired anterior cerebral veins are joined across the midline above the optic chiasm by the anterior communicating vein and receive the paraterminal veins from the paraterminal and parolfactory gyri and the anterior pericallosal veins from the rostrum and genu of the corpus callosum (Figure 22).

The veins on the surface of the brainstem that form the posterior wall of the anterior incisural space are divided into transversely and vertically oriented groups *(19,20)*. The transverse veins are the peduncular vein, which passes horizontally around the anterior surface of the cerebral peduncle and terminates in the basal vein, and the vein of the pontomesencephalic sulcus, which courses below the peduncular vein in the pontomesencephalic sulcus. The vertically oriented veins on the posterior wall of the anterior incisural space are the median anterior pontomesencephalic vein, which courses in the midline and connects the peduncular veins above with the pontine veins below, and the lateral anterior pontomesencephalic veins, which course on the anterolateral surface of the cerebral peduncle and the pons and join the basal vein superiorly and the vein of the pontomesencephalic sulcus below.

The internal cerebral veins course in the roof of the third ventricle and are only infrequently involved in pituitary adenomas (Figure 22). They originate just behind the foramen of Monro and course posteriorly within the velum interpositum. They join above or posterior to the pineal body to form the great vein.

REFERENCES

1. Pait TG, Zeal A, Harris FS, Paullus WS, Rhoton AL Jr. Microsurgical anatomy and dissection of the temporal bone. Surg Neurol 1977;8:363–391.
2. Rhoton AL Jr, Hardy DG, Chambers SM. Microsurgical anatomy and dissection of the sphenoid bone, cavernous sinus and sellar region. Surg Neurol 1979;12:63–104.
3. Rhoton AL Jr, Harris FS, Renn WH. Microsurgical anatomy of the sellar region and cavernous sinus. Clin Neurosurg 1977;24:54–85.
4. Rhoton AL Jr, Maniscalco J. Microsurgery of the sellar region. Neuroophthalmology 1977;9:106–127.
5. Bergland RM, Ray BS, Torack RM. Anatomical variations in the pituitary gland and adjacent structures in 225 human autopsy cases. J Neurosurg 1968;28:93–99.
6. Fujii K, Chambers SM, Rhoton AL Jr. Neurovascular relationships of the sphenoid sinus: A microsurgical study. J Neurosurg 1978; 50:31–39.
7. Hardy J. Transsphenoidal hypophysectomy. J Neurosurg 1971; 34:582–594.
8. Renn WH, Rhoton AL Jr. Microsurgical anatomy of the sellar region. J Neurosurg 1975;43:288–298.
9. Fujii K, Lenkey C, Rhoton AL Jr. Microsurgical anatomy of the choroidal arteries: Lateral and third ventricles. J Neurosurg 1980;52:165–188.
10. Inoue T, Rhoton AL Jr, Theele D, Barry ME. Surgical approaches to the cavernous sinus: A microsurgical study. Neurosurgery 1990;26:903–932.
11. Laws ER, Kern EB. Complications of transsphenoidal surgery. Clin Neurosurg 1976;23:401–416.
12. Harris FS, Rhoton AL Jr. Anatomy of the cavernous sinus: A microsurgical study. J Neurosurg 1976;45:169–180.
13. Gibo H, Lenkey C, Rhoton AL Jr. Microsurgical anatomy of the supraclinoid portion of the internal carotid artery. J Neurosurg 1981;55:560–574.
14. Rhoton AL Jr. Microsurgical anatomy of the region of the third ventricle. In: Apuzzo M, ed. Surgery of the Third Ventricle. Williams & Wilkins, Baltimore, 1987, pp. 92–166.
15. Gudmundsson K, Rhoton AL Jr, Rushton JG. Detailed anatomy of the intracranial portion of the trigeminal nerve. J Neurosurg 1971;35:592–600.
16. Parkinson D. Transcavernous repair of carotid cavernous fistula: A case report. J Neurosurg 1967;26:420–424.
17. Yamamoto I, Rhoton AL Jr, Peace DA. Microsurgery of the third ventricle: Part 1. Microsurgical anatomy. Neurosurgery 1981; 8:334–356.
18. Rhoton AL Jr, Yamamoto I, Peace DA. Microsurgery of the third ventricle: Part 2. Operative approaches. Neurosurgery 1981;8: 357–373.
19. Ono M, Ono M, Rhoton AL Jr, Barry M. Microsurgical anatomy of the region of the tentorial incisura. J Neurosurg 1984;60:365–399.
20. Ono M, Rhoton AL Jr, Peace DA, Rodriguez R. Microsurgical anatomy of the deep venous system of the brain. Neurosurgery 1984;15:621–657.
21. Saeki N, Rhoton AL Jr. Microsurgical anatomy of the upper basilar artery and the posterior circle of Willis. J Neurosurg 1977;46: 563–577.
22. Gibo H, Carver CC, Rhoton AL Jr, Lenkey C, Mitchell RJ. Microsurgical anatomy of the middle cerebral artery. J Neurosurg 1981;54:151–169.
23. Hardy DG, Peace DA, Rhoton AL Jr. Microsurgical anatomy of the superior cerebellar artery. Neurosurgery 1980;6:10–28.
24. Perlmutter D, Rhoton AL Jr. Microsurgical anatomy of the anterior cerebral-anterior communicating-recurrent artery complex. J Neurosurg 1976;45:259–271.
25. Zeal AA, Rhoton AL Jr. Microsurgical anatomy of the posterior cerebral artery. J Neurosurg 1978;48:534–551.
26. Rhoton AL Jr, Fujii K, Fradd B. Microsurgical anatomy of the anterior choroidal artery. Surg Neurol 1979;12:171–187.
27. Perlmutter D, Rhoton AL Jr. Microsurgical anatomy of the distal anterior cerebral artery. J Neurosurg 1978;49:204–228.
28. Rosner SS, Rhoton AL Jr, Ono M, Barry M. Microsurgical anatomy of the anterior perforating arteries. J Neurosurg 1984;61:468–485.

3 Hypothalamic–Pituitary Physiology and Regulation

Miklos I. Goth, MD, PhD, Gabor B. Makara, MD, DSci, and Ida Gerendai, MD, DSci

INTRODUCTION

This chapter briefly reviews the functional anatomy of the hypothalamohypophysial system, including the regulation of the major hypophysial hormones. The hypothalamohypophysial system is a major controller of integrated bodily functions, working alongside with other hormonal systems, as well as with the immune and the nervous systems. This system transmits brain signals to the various peripheral endocrine systems including the adrenals, gonads, and thyroid, which ultimately control gene expression in target tissues through peripheral hormones. Other pituitary cells transmit brain control using hormones acting on target cell surface receptors, such as prolactin, the growth hormone (GH)–insulin-like growth factor-I (IGF-I) axis, or vasopressin (VP).

In this system, we also find examples of local autocrine or paracrine events, medium- to long-range hormonal action via the blood conduit, and interplay of neuronal and hormonal signals, as in the neurohypophysis and the median eminence, where neuronal signals directly induce and modulate hormone secretion. Regulatory circuits of the endocrine axes include control systems with feedback elements, stimulatory and inhibitory neural control, and oscillatory and pulsatile secretory behavior.

HYPOTHALAMOHYPOPHYSIAL SYSTEM: OVERVIEW

NEUROSECRETION   One of the principal phenomena of the hypothalamohypophysial system is neurosecretion. In the late 1930, Ernst and Berta Scharrer observed that neurons of the supraoptic nucleus contain granules. These cells were called neurosecretory neurons, and the mechanism of synthesis and release of the substances in the granules were called neurosecretion. Since that time, the idea of neurosecretion has been extended. Now, it is generally accepted that endocrine functions in mammals are controlled by hypothalamic (HT) neurosecretory cells (also named neuroendocrine cells) producing specific neuropeptides, which are released into the portal vessels or into the general circulation. Therefore, these neurons are capable of transforming neural activity into hormonal signal. Recently, neurosecretion has been considered a more general event. Neurons producing peptides, and not

From: *Diagnosis and Management of Pituitary Tumors* (K. Thapar, K. Kovacs, B. W. Scheithauer, and R. V. Lloyd, eds.), ©Humana Press Inc., Totowa, NJ.

involved in the control of endocrine functions, are also considered to be neurosecretory cells which have all the morphological and functional properties (including electrophysiological characteristics) of the neurons. However, unlike other neurons, peptide synthesis and formation of membrane-bound secretory granules take place in the perikaryon (in the rough-surfaced endoplasmic reticulum and the Golgi complex, respectively). The neurohormone as part of the neurosecretory vesicle is transported to the nerve terminals by axonal flow, where it is stored until released by electrical stimulus. Neurosecretory cells receive neural input from other neurons, and, in addition, possess receptors that enable them to respond also to bloodborne, hormonal signals.

From the structural and functional point of view, the hypothalamohypophysial system can be divided into two systems: the hypothalamoneurohypophysial and the hypothalamoadenohypophysial system (1).

The hypothalamoneurohypophysial system (Figure 1) is composed of two HT cell groups, the supraoptic and paraventricular nucleus (magnocellular part), and of one main part of the pituitary (PIT) gland, i.e., neurohypophysis, which includes the neural lobe, the hypothalamohypophysial tract (neural stalk), and the median eminence (a special structure on the base of the HT, in the region of the tuber cinereum, through which neural fibers from the HT pass). The two cell groups of the HT contain large neurons whose unmyelinated axons run through the median eminence, then descend the neurohypophysial stalk (forming the hypothalamohypophysial tract) to the neural lobe. The hormones, oxytocin (OT), and VP, produced by the HT magnocellular neurons, travel in the axons to the neurohypophysis, where they are temporarily stored and released into the systemic circulation upon relevant physiological stimuli.

The hypothalamoadenohypophysial system is made up of the adenohypophysis and of neurons controlling its function (Figure 2). The adenohypophysis (2) can be divided into three parts: the pars distalis (anterior lobe), pars intermedia (intermediate lobe), and the pars tuberalis. The pars distalis makes up 80% of the adenohypophysis. The pars tuberalis is the upward extension of the anterior lobe. Because the pars tuberalis lies around the hypothalamohypophysial tract, these two structures form the hypophysial stalk. The pars intermedia (zona intermedia) is rudimentary in adult humans, but is well-developed in the human fetus and in some adult mammals. The classical hormones secreted by the adenohypophysis are the two gonadotropic hormones, luteinizing

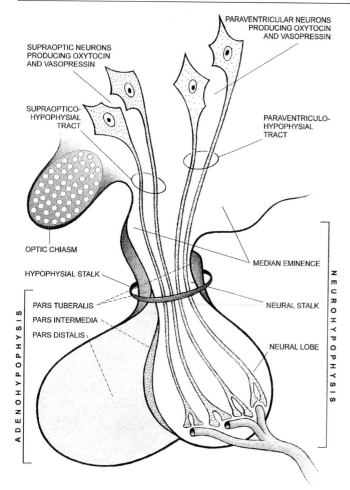

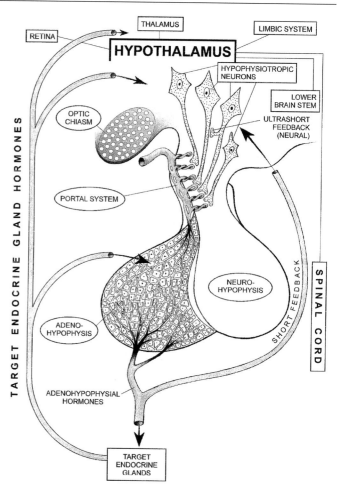

Figure 3-1 Schematic illustration of the organization of the hypophysis and the hypothalamoneurohypophysial system.

Figure 3-2 Schematic drawing of the hypothalamoadenohypophysial system and the main humoral and neural regulatory pathways.

hormone (LH) and follicle-stimulating hormone (FSH); the thyrotropin (TSH), the corticotropin (ACTH); the GH; and prolactin (PRL). The adenohypophysial hormone secretion is regulated by two primary and one additional intrapituitary local control mechanisms.

The neural control is exerted by HT neurons producing the HT-releasing and -inhibiting (hypophysiotropic) hormones and terminating in the median eminence, as well as neural inputs to the hypophysiotropic neurons. The chemically characterized hypophysiotropic neurohormones are gonadotropin-releasing hormone (GnRH), thyrotropin-releasing hormone (TRH), corticotropin-releasing hormone (CRH), growth hormone-releasing hormone (GHRH), somatostatin (SMS; somatotropin release-inhibiting hormone), and PRL-release-inhibiting hormone (PIF). Neurons of the arcuate nucleus also synthesize dopamine, which inhibits PRL release and is considered to be PIF, or at least one PIF. The axons of these nerve cells, terminating in the median eminence, release dopamine into the capillary loops; therefore, dopamine is transported to the adenohypophysis via the portal vessels.

The neurohormones synthesized by the hypophysiotropic cells are transported to nerve terminals in the median eminence, from where they are released into the portal vessels, which are in close topographical relation to the median eminence. The neurohormones reaching the adenohypophysial cells by vascular route activate specific hormone receptors, which in turn induce or inhibit

the synthesis and release of the corresponding adenohypophysial hormone.

The other chief mechanism controlling hormone secretion of the adenohypophysis is the feedback action of circulating hormones on the hypothalamoadenohypophysial system. All hypophysial hormones, either directly or indirectly through target hormones (gonadal, adrenal steroids, or thyroid hormones [THs]), exert regulatory actions on cerebral and hypophysial structures, which control the secretion of these hormones. This regulatory mechanism is called feedback control. Changes in the serum concentration of hormones secreted by the target endocrine glands alter the activity of the hypothalamohypophysial system. The phenomenon of negative feedback control is based on observations that indicated that increased serum concentration of a target gland hormone inhibits, and decreased hormone level stimulates, the secretion of the corresponding hypothalamohypophysial axis (long-loop feedback). The site of action of this hormone effect is both on the HT and on the adenohypophysis. In general, it seems that an increased level of peripheral endocrine gland hormone affects the secretion of the adenohypophysial hormone, acting most directly on the trop-hormone-synthesizing cell; the decrease in serum concentration exerts feedback action through the HT, altering primarily the secretion of the HT neurohormone, rather than acting directly on the pituitary. A special type of hormonal feedback is the positive feedback action of female sexual steroids on gonadotropins (positive estrogen feedback). This form of regulation is essential for the cyclic changes of gonadotrop secretion (further details in subheading, Control of Gonadotropin Secretion in Females). Circulating hormones, especially corticoids and sexual steroids, exert regulatory actions on cerebral structures other than the hypothalamohypophysial system.

Recently, a third, fine-tuning control mechanism has been recognized, based on the local (autocrine/paracrine) actions of different biologically active substances produced in and near the cells to be regulated. Local control is based on cell-to-cell communication through messenger molecules present in the microenvironment. Local regulatory factors in the PIT include different peptides, growth factors, and cytokines.

ENDOCRINE RHYTHMS Hormone secretion is not constant, but shows cyclic changes. Most cyclic changes are intrinsically driven by the biological clock. The suprachiasmatic nucleus is considered the pacemaker of circadian rhythms. The neurons of this cell group have the intrinsic capacity for spontaneous rhythms. The suprachiasmatic nucleus has rich neuronal connections with different HT nuclei and extra-HT structures, such as the retina and the pineal gland (discussed in subheading, Connections of HT). Certain hormone rhythms are influenced by light–dark period and sleep–awakeness status.

The endocrine rhythms can be classified according to the length of the cycle/period. Infradian rhythms include annual and seasonal rhythms and cycles longer than 1 d. In human physiology, annual and seasonal rhythms are of no importance, but, in certain species, such as in seasonally breeding animals, reproductive functions are closely associated to seasons. The infradian rhythm has a great significance in human reproductive processes. The activity of the hypothalamohypophysial–ovarian axis and the cyclic changes of the endometrium have a period of approx 28 d. Hormone secretion also shows patterns of 1 d (diurnal rhythm) and approx 1 d (circadian rhythm). Each adenohypophysial hormone secretion has a circadian rhythm with peak values characteristic to the given hormone. One early sign of HT dysfunction can be the loss of diurnal rhythm. Within the circadian rhythm there are rhythms of minutes or hours: ultradian or pulsatile rhythm. The pulsatile pattern of GnRH–gonadotrop hormone system is a prerequisite of reproduction. Pulsatile secretion of GH is also of physiological significance.

FUNCTIONAL ANATOMY OF ENDOCRINE HT

CONNECTIONS OF HT The HT is the ventral part of the diencephalon. In humans, the weight of the HT is approx 4 g; therefore, it makes up only 0.3% of the total brain. Despite its small volume, the HT has a functional significance that is out of proportion to its size.

The majority of the HT is surrounded by other cerebral areas, and only its small, basal portion, extending in rostrocaudal direction between the optic chiasm and the interpeduncular fossa, can be exposed to view. On the ventral surface are located the mamillary bodies. The area between the optic chiasm and the mamillary bodies is the tuber cinereum. The medial wall of the HT, together with the thalamus located above, form the lateral wall of the third ventricle *(3)*.

The HT (Figure 3) can be divided, in mediolateral extension, into three longitudinal areas: the periventricular area, a narrow region adjacent to the third ventricle; the medial HT; and the lateral HT. The border between the latter two areas is the fornix. The periventricular and medial areas are rich in neurons; the lateral

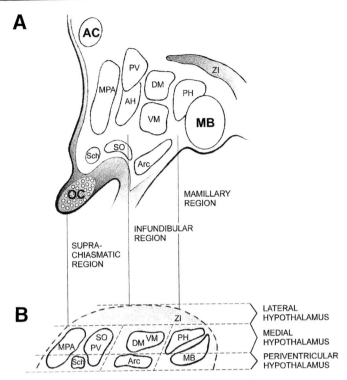

Figure 3-3 Schematic illustration of the regions and nuclei of the HT in the midsagittal (**A**) and in the horizontal (**B**) plane. AC, anterior commissure; AH, anterior HT nucleus; Arc, arcuate nucleus; DM, dorsomedial nucleus; MB, mamillary body; MPA, medial preoptic area; OC, optic chiasm; PH, posterior hypothalamus; PV, paraventricular nucleus; SCh, suprachiasmatic nucleus; VM, ventromedial nucleus; ZI, zona incerta.

area of the HT contains only few nerve cells, and therefore, is composed mostly of fibers. The majority of the fibers in the lateral HT area belongs to the medial forebrain bundle, which runs longitudinally in the rostrocaudal direction.

Rostrocaudally, the HT can also be divided into three parts, according to the main gross anatomical structures located below these areas: the suprachiasmatic, the infundibular, and the mamillary areas.

The suprachiasmatic zone contains the suprachiasmatic, the supraoptic, paraventricular, and the anterior HT nuclei. Anterior to the suprachiasmatic region, just behind the lamina terminalis, is the preoptic area, which belongs to the telencephalon. Just above the optic chiasm, i.e., in the medial rostral area of the HT is located the suprachiasmatic nucleus. This cell group contains small, densely packed neurons. Since the axons of these neurons do not project to the median eminence, the nucleus is not directly involved in the control of adenohypophysial hormone secretion. However, because of the afferent connections of the nucleus with the retina, and the reciprocal neural connections with hypophysiotropic neurons, this cell group plays an important integrative role in the control of daily and pulsatile hormone rhythms. The supraoptic nucleus, a cell group composed mostly of large neurons, is located above the optic tract. Dorsal to this cell group on the two sides of the third ventricle is the paraventricular nucleus, which is composed of two portions, the magnocellular and parvocellular parts.

In the medial basal part of the HT is located the arcuate seu infundibular nucleus, an arch-shaped cell group that surrounds the third ventricle. Dorsolateral to the arcuate nucleus is the ventromedial nucleus, and, dorsal to it can be found the dorsomedial nucleus. The periventricular nucleus occupies a narrow region close to the third ventricle.

The mamillary region includes the mamillary bodies and a not well-defined cell group, the posterior nucleus. These two nuclei do not project to the median eminence. However, the mamillary bodies, because of their rich connection with the thalamus, cerebral cortex, and limbic system, make the HT an integral part of these cerebral structures.

The axons of the arcuate, ventromedial, dorsomedial, and periventricular neurons, as well as fibers from the parvicellular part of the paraventricular nucleus, and a small portion of the supraoptic neurons, project to the superficial zone of the median eminence. Because the HT hormones are produced by neurons of the aforementioned cell groups, these HT nuclei are those that play a determining role in the control of adenohypophysial hormone secretion (hypophysiotropic neurons). In addition, the preoptic area also contains hormone-producing nerve cells with axons terminating in the median eminence.

The hypophysiotropic neurons also synthesize bioactive substances other than the HT-releasing and release-inhibiting hormones. Among others, opioid peptides (enkephalin, endorphins, dynorphin), vasoactive peptides (neurotensin, bradykinin, atrial natriuretic peptide, angiotensin II), and gastrointestinal peptides (vasoactive intestinal peptide, PIT adenylate-cyclase activating polypeptide, cholecystokinin, tachykinin, galanin, neuropeptide Y) are also produced in hypophysiotropic neurons. A given hypophysiotropic neuron might synthesize hormones that are different both in chemical nature and physiological function. Furthermore, synthesis of hypophysial hormones could also be demonstrated in extra-HT cerebral areas and also in nonneural tissues, in well-defined cell types of different viscera.

HT neurons producing hypophysiotropic hormones, besides their function as controlling hormone secretion, may act in the central nervous system as neurotransmitters or neuromodulators. The neuroanatomical basis of such functions is the intensive projection of hypophysiotropic neurons to other parts of the endocrine HT and extra-HT structures, such as the limbic system and autonomic nuclei.

The activity of the endocrine HT is under the integrated control of neural inputs to the hypophysiotropic neurons and the feedback action of peripheral and hypophysial hormones, exerted either on hypophysiotropic neurons or on extra-HT cerebral structures that possess specific hormone receptors. The HT receives information from diverse sources, in order to serve as a main integrator of the endocrine system. The majority of these pathways are reciprocal, i.e., they contain fibers both to and from the HT. The most extensive connections of the HT are with limbic structures, such as the amygdala, septum, and hippocampus.

The amygdala and the HT (especially the preoptic area and anterior nucleus) are interconnected by the stria terminalis and the ventral amygdalofugal bundles. The latter pathway contains fibers also from the olfactory system. The fornix, originating from the hippocampus, is the largest bundle to the HT. The majority of fibers terminate in the mamillary body or originate from it. However, a portion of the fibers, before reaching the column of the fornix, leaves the pathway and terminates in the septal region and in the preoptic area.

The well-defined pathway between the HT (mamillary body) and the anterior thalamic nucleus is the mamillothalamic tract.

Because the anterior thalamic nucleus is interconnected with the cingulate gyrus, the mamillothalamic tract provides a communication between the HT and the limbic cortex. There is a rich neural connection of great functional significance between the HT and brainstem nuclei, such as the central gray matter, locus ceruleus, other noradrenergic cell groups, raphe nuclei, nucleus of the solitary tract, and reticular formation.

Neurons of the paraventricular nucleus send descending fibers also to the preganglionic sympathetic neurons of thoracolumbar spinal cord segments. There is a direct neural pathway between the retina and the HT suprachiasmatic nucleus. Information from the olfactory system arrives at the HT via limbic structures. However, the HT is not directly linked to the main sensory systems (lemniscus pathways), because of connections of the HT with brainstem nuclei, and thalamic and cortical structures; secondary, tertiary sensory impulses are also conveyed to the HT. Recent studies have revealed multisynaptic, reciprocal neural connections between the peripheral endocrine glands and the HT.

Neural afferents terminating on hypophysiotropic neurons from several brain regions contain different neurotransmitters, amino acids, and neuropeptides, which may exert a regulatory action on the synthesis and release of hypophysiotropic hormones. The classical neurotransmitters, noradrenaline, adrenaline, serotonin, acetylcholine, and γ-amino-butyric acid (GABA), have been proven to influence the secretion of HT releasing and inhibiting hormones (*see* ref. *1*).

The HT does not contain neurons synthesizing noradrenaline. These neurons are located in different cell groups of the brainstem. The biggest of them is the locus ceruleus. Noradrenergic fibers from these cell groups, similar to other ascending bundles, travel in the medial forebrain bundle, then form synaptic contact either with hypophysiotropic neurons or nerve fibers in the median eminence. Noradrenaline plays a significant role in the control of HT neurohormones, such as GnRH or CRH. Adrenaline is also synthesized in extra-HT cell groups. These neurons are located in the brainstem. The adrenergic afferents to the HT exert an important regulatory action on structures involved in the control of GH secretion. The origin of cholinergic fibers innervating hypophysiotropic neurons is not established. Acetylcholine is an important regulatory factor of CRH, VP, and GHRH/somatostatin secretion.

Both the excitatory amino acids (glutamate, aspartate, glycine), and the inhibitory amino acid, GABA, are used by neurons in different HT nuclei. The amino acids binding to their receptors on the hypophysiotropic cells are able to stimulate or inhibit the secretion of the neurohormones. As mentioned, the HT neurons also synthesize several peptide hormones (opioid peptides, vasoactive intestinal peptide (VIP), substance P, galanine, and so on). These peptides and the gaseous neurotransmitter, nitric oxide, can also influence the activity of hypophysiotropic neurons.

Besides the rich neural connection of the HT with extra-HT structures, neuromorphological data have provided evidence for the existence of the extensive synaptic connections between HT nuclei. These studies have also revealed abundant intranuclear connections. Furthermore, axon collaterals of a given neurohormone-producing neuron form synaptic contact with the perikaryon where the axon originates.

BLOOD SUPPLY OF HYPOPHYSIS: PORTAL SYSTEM

Secretion of hormones by the adenohypophysis is under the control of the HT by a vascular route (*4*). Both hypophysial arteries

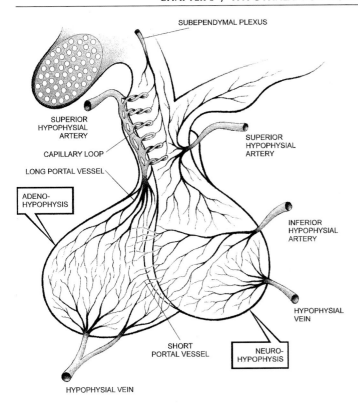

Figure 3-4   Schematic illustration of the blood supply of the HT.

(the superior and inferior hypophysial artery) originate from the internal carotid artery at the base of the brain (Figure 4). The superior hypophysial artery soon divides into precapillary arteries, forming a dense plexus and numerous loops in the median eminence. The plexus is remarkably dense in the contact zone between the median eminence and the pars tuberalis (Mantelplexus). From this plexus, capillary loops penetrate into the median eminence and the infundibular stem. The blood from the Mantelplexus and the capillary loops drains into the portal vessels located on the ventral surface of the PIT stalk: long portal vessels. Blood from a lesser portion of the capillary loops flows to the subependymal plexus of the third ventricle. The short portal vessels supplying the distal portion of the stalk and the neurohypophysis contribute also to the blood supply of the adenohypophysial tissue, providing a vascular communication between the adeno- and the neurohypophysis. The capillaries are drained by veins that enter the adenohypophysis, where they empty into the sinusoids. Approximately 80–90% of the blood to the adenohypophysis derives from the long portal vessels. The HT neurohormones are released from the nerve terminals in the median eminence into the portal vessels. The concentration of HT neurohormones in these vessels greatly exceeds that found in the systemic circulation. The majority of the portal blood from the median eminence flows toward the hypophysis, but, a small portion of it is supposed to flow in the opposite direction, i.e., toward the HT.

HYPOTHALAMONEUROHYPOPHYSIAL SYSTEM

The hypothalamoneurohypophysial system includes the magnocellular nuclei of the HT (supraoptic nucleus and the magnocellular part, and some neurons of the parvicellular neurons of the paraventricular nucleus), the median eminence, the supraopticohypophysial and paraventriculohypophysial tract (neural

stalk), and the neural lobe of the hypophysis. Some of the fibers originating from the supraoptic and paraventricular nuclei, however, do not terminate in the neural lobe, but in the median eminence; hence, these neurons are involved in the control of adenohypophysial hormone secretion. The neural lobe develops embryologically from the ventral part of the diencephalon; histologically, it is made up of thin, unmyelinated axons and terminals originating from the aforementioned HT nuclei, as well as of glial cells, also called pituicytes. The two neurohypophysial hormones (vasopressin [VP] and oxytocin [OT]) are synthesized in the HT and transported along the neural stalk, to the neural lobe. They are stored in neurosecretory granules (diameter 100–200 nm) of the axon terminals. Appropriate physiological stimuli induce the release of these hormones into sinusoids, which are lined by fenestrated endothelium (5).

As mentioned above, VP and OT are synthesized in cell bodies of both the supraoptic and paraventricular nuclei. However, individual neurons of these nuclei produce only one of the neurohypophyseal hormones. VP-ergic neurons co-express CRH, tyrosine hydroxylase (rate-limiting enzyme of catecholamine synthesis), VIP, angiotensin II, dynorphin, galanin, enkephalin, cholecystokinin, and TRH. OT-ergic neurons co-express many of the above peptides. The co-localization of VP and CRH in paraventricular neurons is of great physiological significance, since these two hormones play the major role in induction of ACTH release.

A subpopulation of VP-ergic and OT-ergic neurons project also to areas other than the neural lobe, namely, to the brainstem and the spinal cord. These HT neurons are presumably involved in cardiovascular control. Both the supraoptic and paraventricular nuclei are rich in different incoming fibers. Brain areas outside the blood–brain barrier, such as the organum vasculosum of the lamina terminalis and the subfornical organ, are interconnected with these magnocellular HT nuclei. The magnocellular nuclei receive important neural afferentation also from catecholaminergic cell groups of the brainstem and the nucleus of the solitary tract.

CHEMICAL STRUCTURE, SYNTHESIS, AND RECEPTOR OF VP AND OT   Chemical Structure   Both VP and OT are nonapeptides (composed of nine amino acids) and have a Cys–Cys bridge in position 1–6. Both are synthesized as a part of a larger precursor molecule. The prohormones for VP and OT share an extensive homology, consistent with the view that the two neurohypophysial peptides originate from the same gene located on chromosome 20. Both VP and OT are associated with the carrier protein, neurophysin, characteristic to each hormone (OT is associated with neurophysin I, VP with neurophysin II). Neurophysin, a 10-kDa peptide, is synthesized from the same precursor molecule as the neurohormones. The precursor molecules, packaged into secretory granules, travel by the axonal flow to the axon terminals, where they are released; in the secretory granules, VP and OT are processed by proteolytic processing to their bioactive forms. The hormones released into the general circulation are free arginine–vasopressin (VP) and OT.

VP and OT receptors belong to the family of G-protein-coupled receptors. VP receptors can be subdivided into two classes: the VP_1- and the VP_2-type receptors. Activation of VP_1 receptors induces increase in intracellular calcium via stimulation of phosphoinositol turnover. Two types of VP_1 receptors have been identified: the VP_{1a} and VP_{1b} or V_3 receptors. VP_{1a} receptors have been demonstrated in the central nervous system, smooth muscle cells of blood vessels, in the liver, adrenal cortex, uterus, and platelets. VP_{1b} receptors have different localization: They are present in the anterior pituitary, and are involved in the control of ACTH release. In contrast to VP_1 receptors, activation of VP_2 receptors of the kidney results in stimulation of adenylate cyclase.

OT (only one type is known) are present on smooth muscle cells and endometrial cells of the uterus, and in the mammary gland. Besides the presence of OT in those female reproductive organs, receptors for OT have been identified in the central nervous system, and in the PIT, kidney, testis, and thymus.

PHYSIOLOGICAL ACTION OF VP The chief physiological actions of VP are antidiuretic effect (water reabsorption) at the level of the distal convoluted tubules and medullary collecting ducts of the kidney (VP_2 receptor-mediated action); vasomotor effect resulting from contraction of vascular smooth muscle cells (VP_{1a} receptors are involved); regulatory action of blood pressure in concert with other peptide hormones (VP_{1a}-receptor-mediated effect); and hypophysiotropic effect (like CRH, VP-ergic fibers terminating in the median eminence release the hormone into the portal vessels, stimulating ACTH release).

VP release is controlled by neural and hormonal factors acting on VP-synthesizing neurons. Among the neurogen regulators is acetylcholine, which stimulates VP release. The effect is mediated through nicotinergic receptors. In contrast, adrenergic signal to VP neurons, through β-adrenergic receptors, suppresses hormone secretion. Angiotensin II induces VP release and thirst. Atrial natriuretic peptide inhibits VP release and prevents the stimulatory action of angiotensin II and hypertonic saline effect on VP release. Opioid peptides and morphine are well-known factors for inducing antidiuresis, by inhibiting VP release. Nitric oxide and cytokines have recently been reported to be additional regulatory factors of VP release. The involvement of glucocorticoid hormones in VP secretion is indicated by the observation that adrenocortical insufficiency leads to activation of VP-neurons and increase in serum VP concentration.

The chief physiological stimulus of VP secretion is alteration of plasma osmolarity and fall in blood volume. Hypotension, nausea, emotional stress, pain, and hypothermia also affect VP release. Increase in blood osmolarity results in VP release, and waterload inhibits hormone secretion. In other words, plasma osmolarity and VP release represent the two components of a control system based on negative feedback. Changes in plasma osmolarity are sensed by osmoreceptors present in special structures: the circumventricular organs located around the third ventricle. Osmoreceptors have been identified also in the periphery, in the hepatoportal blood vessels. Activation of these receptors induces stimulation of vagus fibers, which carry the signal to brainstem neurons innervating HT VP-ergic neurons. Osmoreceptors are very sensitive and respond to changes in osmolarity as small as 1%.

Receptors for blood volume control, called baroreceptors, capable of sensing changes in blood volume, are located in the left atrium, the carotid sinus, and the aorta. Activation of baroreceptors is followed by stimulation of nerve afferents projecting to brainstem nuclei. From these cell groups, multisynaptic pathways originate, which terminate on VP-producing HT neurons.

VP plays a regulatory role also in other bodily systems. VP acting on platelets, induces increased platelet aggregation. VP as a neurotransmitter, is involved in cognitive processes and aggressive behavior. In fever, VP acts as an antipyretic agent; the hormone is capable of decreasing body temperature.

PHYSIOLOGICAL ACTION OF OT The chief physiological actions of OT include milk ejection and uterine contraction.

During lactation, OT induces contraction of myoepithelial cells surrounding mamillary acini, which results in ejection of milk into the excretory ducts, and thence into the nipple. This process is initiated by mechanical stimulation of the breast, mostly the nipple or nearby areas. Stimulation of these mechanoreceptors induces a neuroendocrine reflex. The components of this reflex arc are mechanoreceptors in the nipple area; sensory fibers originating from this region (conducting neural impulses through the spinal cord, brainstem, and midbrain to the HT); supraoptic and paraventricular neurons producing OT (which, upon stimulus, generate high-frequency, synchronized discharges); the neuroendocrine component of the reflex: release of OT from nerve terminals of the neural lobe into the circulation; and the activation of OT receptors of the breast, which leads to milk ejection. Also, in the nonlactating state, mechanical stimulation of the nipple area or of the vagina results in OT release. In addition, estrogen, plasma hyperosmolarity, mild stress, and hemorrhage also act as stimulators of OT release.

The other important physiological role of OT is the stimulation of uterine smooth muscle contraction. The contractility response of uterine smooth muscle cells to OT is modulated by sexual steroids: Estrogen enhances, while progesterone decreases, the response. During delivery, there is a marked increase of OT secretion. Movement of the embryo in the birth canal activates mechanoreceptors located in the pelvic wall. The stimulus is transformed into neural signal, which is conducted by multisynaptic pathways (including ascending afferent fibers and different cell groups in the brainstem) to the OT-ergic neurons. The excitation of these nerve cells results in release of OT sufficient for delivery.

As far as the neural control of OT release is concerned, the hormone release is stimulated by acetylcholine; adrenalin, through β-adrenergic receptors, inhibits OT release. The stress-induced inhibition of OT release is also mediated by β-adrenergic receptors. Inhibin B, synthesized in brainstem neurons as a neurotransmitter/neuromodulator, is also involved in the control of OT release. Estrogen induces gene expression of OT and also regulates tissue- and stage-specific regulation of OT receptors. Prior to parturition, uterine OT receptors are highly upregulated and rapidly downregulated after delivery. At the beginning of lactation, the mammary gland OT receptors slowly rise in number and remain highly expressed throughout lactation.

HYPOTHALAMOADENOHYPOPHYSIAL SYSTEMS

GONADOTROP HORMONES **Chemical Structure, Synthesis, and Hormone Receptors** *Chemical Structure* The gonadotrop hormones, LH and FSH, together with TSH, belong to the hypophysial glycoprotein hormone family. The fourth member of the family, the choriogonadotropin (CG), is the product of the placenta. These hormones are composed of two noncovalently linked subunit chains, termed α- and β-subunits. The α-subunit is common to all these hormones. The β-subunit gives to each hormone its biological and structural specificity. The β-chain of choriogonadotropin shows 85% homology with the β-chain of LH. Free α-subunit is present in the serum. In the human, the mol wt of the α-subunit is approx 20–22 kDa, and it contains 92 amino acids. The β-subunit of both LH and FSH contains 115 amino acids and has two side chains.

Synthesis The two subunits are encoded by separate genes (6), present on different chromosomes (in the human, the α-subunit gene is located on chromosome 6, the LH β gene is found on chromosome 19, and the FSH β gene is present on chromosome 11).

Gonadotrop Hormone Receptors LH receptor is found in testicular Leydig cells and ovarian theca, granulosa, and interstitial cells. The FSH receptor is localized to Sertoli cells of the testis and granulosa cells of the ovary. Both receptors play a pivotal role in reproduction. The gonadotropin receptors belong to the family of G-protein-coupled receptors characterized functionally by their interaction with guanine nucleotide-binding proteins, and structurally by their seven hydrophobic, α-helical transmembrane domains.

Action and Secretion of Gonadotrop Hormones The term "gonadotrop hormones" derive from their role in controlling ovarian functions. FSH stimulates follicular growth, and, together with LH, follicular steroidogenesis *(7)*. LH is the ovulatory hormone, and stimulates formation and steroid secretion of the corpus luteum. In the male, FSH is responsible for the initiation and maintenance of spermatogenesis, acting mostly on Sertoli cells; LH stimulates Leydig cell steroidogenesis.

Both gonadotropins are secreted in a pulsatile manner. Pulsatile LH release is characterized by a marked increase in serum LH concentration, which occurs over a period of about 5 min, as the result of a preceding GnRH pulse. In humans, FSH pulses are usually synchronized with LH pulses. Each pulse of GnRH is accompanied by a pulse of both LH and FSH.

Regulation of Gonadotrop Hormone Secretion Secretion of gonadotrop hormones is primarily under the control of HT GnRH, which is released in a pulsatile manner into the hypophysial portal circulation. Gonadotropin secretion is also regulated by the feedback action of gonadal hormones (steroids, peptides). The activity of GnRH neurons is determined by several neural impulses.

GnRH Synthesis, Localization, and Ontogenesis of GnRH Neurons and Receptors Only a single GnRH has thus far been identified and synthesized. The neurohormone, a decapeptide, causes the release of both PIT gonadotropins.

Synthesis GnRH, like other neuropeptides, is synthesized as part of a large prohormone, and cleaved enzymatically in GnRH-expressing cells.

Localization of GnRH Neurons The majority of GnRH neurons are present in two HT areas: in the region of the preoptic, supraoptic, and septal areas, and in the mediobasal part of the tuber cinereum, especially in the arcuate (infundibular) and in the premamillary nuclei *(8)*. In humans, GnRH neurons are located mostly in the infundibular region, and only a few GnRH cell bodies are present in the preoptic area. Besides the HT, GnRH-expressing nerve cells can be detected in the olfactory bulb, the induseum griseum, and in the hippocampus.

Ontogenesis of GnRH Neurons Unlike other hypophysiotropic neurons, GnRH neurons are differentiated outside the brain, in the medial olfactory placodal epithelium of the developing nose. The GnRH neurons then migrate across the nasal septum and the cribriform plate, enter the forebrain with the nervus terminalis, an accessory nerve that is part of the olfactory system, and project from the nose to the septal–preoptic area and the HT. Along this route, GnRH neurons reach their final destination in the preoptic area and the infundibular region of the HT with projections to the median eminence. In the targeting process, neural and glial elements, as well as specific cell adhesion molecules, pave the migratory route. The common origin of the GnRH neurons from the olfactoric neuroepithelium explains the human disorder hypogonadotropic hypogonadism with hyposmia.

GnRH Receptor This receptor is a member of the seven-transmembrane-domain class, characteristic of G-protein-linked receptors. The action of GnRH starts with binding to the specific surface receptor on LH and FSH cells, which leads to activation of a specific G protein, stimulation of phospholipase activity in the cell membrane, modulation of inositol-1,4,5-triphosphate (IP$_3$) and diacylglycerol signal, and cytoplasmic calcium response.

GnRH receptors are located also in different brain areas, such as the septal region, HT ventromedial nucleus, amygdala, and hippocampus, where GnRH exerts a variety of effects, including modulation of sexual behavior.

Action and Secretion of GnRH *Action of GnRH* GnRH stimulates the secretion of both LH and FSH. The relative amounts of LH and FSH vary; under most circumstances, and particularly at low dosage, more LH than FSH is released. The rate at which GnRH pulses are administered, influences the patterns of LH and FSH secretion: Fast frequencies increase the secretion of both gonadotropins; slower frequencies stimulate FSH relative to LH; constant exposure to GnRH suppresses secretion of both gonadotropins. Whether a separate follicle-stimulating, hormone-releasing hormone exists remains controversial.

Secretion of GnRH, and GnRH Pulse Generator Activity Secretion of GnRH shows a pulsatile pattern. This pulsatile release pattern is essential for maintaining normal gonadotropin secretion, it is an obligatory factor of reproductive functions. The neurons, which release the decapeptide in the pulsatile manner, are collectively referred to as the GnRH pulse generator. The GnRH pulse frequencies vary according to sex, age, and physiological conditions. The pulsatile type of GnRH secretion first appears in late intrauterine life, followed by a period until early puberty, when the secretion is nonpulsatile or the pulsatility is markedly reduced. In the prepubertal period, nocturnal episodes of GnRH pulsatility are present. After this transitional period, the pulsatile pattern characteristic to adults develops. The GnRH pulse generator is located in the mediobasal part of the HT, in the arcuate nucleus. Recent in vitro data suggest that GnRH neurons have the intrinsic capacity to release the neurohormone in a pulsatile fashion *(29)*. It is not known which factor(s) synchronize the GnRH neurons located, in many cases, far from each other.

The pulsatile pattern of GnRH release is of great clinical importance. In both men and women with various forms of HT hypogonadotropic hypogonadism (inappropriate or insufficient GnRH secretion), pulsatile administration of GnRH can restore normal gonadotropin secretion. In adults, the pulsatile release of GnRH is characterized by a period of 90 min between the peak values. This time period is optimal for inducing maximal stimulation of gonadotrop hormone secretion. The activity of the GnRH pulse generator is influenced both by neural and hormonal factors.

GnRH secretion can be stimulated by neurotransmitters of different chemical structure *(9)*. Among these are norepinephrine (acting on β-adrenergic receptors), neuropeptide Y, galanine, glutamic acid, nitric oxide, transforming growth factor-α, and prostaglandins. In certain conditions, any of the above substances are able to induce GnRH release; pharmacological blockade of any of these transmitters can prevent the preovulatory GnRH surge. Inhibiting neural factors of GnRH secretion are the opioid peptides, which exert a tonic suppressive effect on the activity of the GnRH neurons. It is well known that stress has an inhibitory effect on gonadotrop secretion that results from the inhibitory action of CRH, VP, and cytokines on GnRH neurons. If the neural control of GnRH secretion is altered, first the amplitude of the GnRH pulses diminishes, then, in severe conditions, the pulsatile pattern completely disappears. Severe stress in the prepubertal period can result in delayed puberty. PRL is also known to suppress GnRH secretion, hyperprolactinemia causes amenorrhea.

Control of Gonadotropin Secretion in Males   Increased circulating testosterone exerts negative feedback on LH secretion. High serum testosterone level leads to decrease in LH pulse frequency and diminished pulse amplitude. Presumably, the action of the steroid is exerted both at HT level, by suppressing GnRH pulses, and on the gonadotrops, by decreasing the sensitivity of LH cells to respond to GnRH. Feedback control of FSH is exerted by inhibin and testosterone. FSH binding to plasma membrane of Sertoli cells stimulates synthesis and release of inhibin, which, in turn, acting on gonadotrops, suppresses FSH release, both in the absence or presence of GnRH. Testosterone reduces GnRH pulses, and therefore inhibits FSH release. FSH does not affect testosterone secretion, but the steroid is able to mediate negative feedback on FSH cells.

Control of Gonadotropin Secretion in Females   Because of the cyclic character of gonadotrop hormone secretion in females, the control system is more complex than that in males, and, in females, secretion of gonadotropins is closely associated with cyclic morphological and functional changes of the ovary *(10)*. The development of ovarian follicles is mostly under the control of FSH. Follicular growth includes proliferation of granulosa cells and differentiation of connective tissue cells around the follicle to form theca interna. In this phase of the ovarian cycle (follicular phase), FSH also induces synthesis of aromatase in granulosa cells. In response to LH, theca interna cells synthesize androstendione and, to a lesser extent, testosterone. These steroid hormones diffuse to the granulosa cells, where they are aromatized to estrogen. The increasing concentration of estrogen in the follicular fluid is essential for the maturation of the follicle. In the last portion of the follicular phase, the secretion pattern of estrogen becomes episodic, and the hormone exerts negative feedback on LH and FSH release, acting both in the brain and the PIT.

The granulosa cells of the maturing follicle secrete increasing amounts of estrogen into the blood. The continuously elevating level of estrogen eventually causes the disappearance of negative feedback. In the preovulatory period, serum estrogen concentration reaches a critical level that leads to a sharp increase of serum LH level (LH surge), i.e., in this particular condition, estrogen exerts a positive feedback on LH release. For the induction of LH surge, a constant (lasting at least 36 h), extremely high (approx 150 pg/mL) serum estrogen concentration is required. It seems that, at the beginning of the LH surge, the still moderately increased LH results in enhanced progesterone secretion. For the induction of LH surge, markedly increased estrogen and moderately elevated serum progesterone concentrations are essential. Concomitant with LH surge, there is an increase also in serum FSH concentration (FSH surge). It is supposed that the site of action of estrogen positive feedback is the anterior PIT (GnRH neurons lack estrogen receptors). During preovulatory LH surge, gonadotrop cells exhibit increased responsiveness to GnRH. In addition, there is a marked increase in the amount of newly synthesized LH that is readily releasable. After ovulation, the remaining granulosa and theca interna cells of the ruptured follicle transform into corpus luteum (luteal phase of the ovarian cycle). These morphological changes are controlled by LH (FSH level is low in this phase). Moreover, LH is also involved in altering steroid secretion of these cells (instead of estrogen, corpus luteum cells secrete progesterone). If

pregnancy does not occur, corpus luteum stops to synthesize progesterone; therefore, the progesterone-induced suppression of GnRH pulses and gonadotropin release ceases. This neurohormonal milieu is optimal for inducing neuronal and hormonal processes that lead to the initiation of the follicular phase of a new cycle.

In addition to estrogen and progesterone, nonsteroidal ovarian signal is also involved in the feedback control of gonadotropins. As in males, inhibin (secreted by granulosa cells in response to FSH) suppresses both GnRH-dependent and GnRH-independent FSH release. In females, however, the negative feedback effect of inhibin on FSH secretion is less remarkable than in males.

TSH   TSH is a glycoprotein, synthesized and secreted by the thyrotropes, which are mostly concentrated in the anteromedial portion of the PIT gland. Thyrotropes account for about 5% of anterior PIT cells. TSH is composed from an α-subunit of about 20 kDa, which is common to LH, FSH, and CG, and the specific β-subunit of about 18 kDa, a 112-amino-acid protein. The human PIT contains 100–150 μg TSH; the secretion rate of TSH in healthy humans is 50–200 μg/d. Full glycosylation of TSH is required for complete biologic activity. The plasma half-life of TSH is about 30 min.

TSH is responsible for normal thyroid function, and regulates both synthesis and secretion of thyroid hormones. The binding of TSH to its receptors in the thyroid cell membrane results in an increase in the size and vascularity of the gland, and an increase of the follicular epithelium and decrease in amount of colloid. The consequences are augmented iodide transport, thyroglobulin synthesis, iodothyrosine and iodothyronine production, thyroglobulin proteolysis, T_3 and T_4 secretion.

The secretion of TSH is regulated by negative feedback by thyroid hormone and open-loop neural control by HT hypophyseotropic factors, and is also modified by other factors, in order to guarantee appropriate thyroid stimulation.

HT Control   The dominant stimulatory role of the HT in the control of TSH synthesis and release is mediated by TRH, which was the first HT hormone to be isolated and structurally characterized. TRH is a small, weakly basic tripeptide, pyroGlu-His-Pro-NH2, derived from posttranslational cleavage of a larger precursor molecule containing multiple copies of the peptide. It is inactivated by a peptidase, the TRH-degrading ectoenzyme. TRH is necessary for the secretion of TSH with full biological activity. Stimulatory effects of TRH are initiated by binding of the peptide to specific receptors on the plasma membrane of the thyrotrope. These receptors belong to the family of seven-transmembrane-domain, G-protein-coupled receptors *(11)*. In normal subjects given TRH intravenously, serum TSH concentrations increase within 2–5 min, are maximal at 20–30 min, and return to basal levels by 2–3 h. In addition to stimulating TSH release, TRH also stimulates TSH synthesis by promoting transcription and translation of the TSH-subunit genes *(12)*.

The stimulatory effect of TRH is counterbalanced by the direct PIT inhibition of TSH synthesis and secretion by THs. The inhibition of circulating THs is exerted primarily on the thyrotropes, but also, to a lesser extent, on the TRH-producing neurons of the HT. In this process, local intra-PIT conversion of T_4 to T_3 is particularly important: the thyrotrope has a potent intracellular type II deiodinase. More than half of pituitary T_3 is derived from the local conversion of T_4 to T_3 by type II deiodinase, and the reminder is derived from the circulation. T_4 in the blood gains access to TRH-secreting neurons in HT by way of the cerebrospinal fluid, in which T_4 is also converted to T_3 by type II deiodinase. T_3 interacts with subtypes of the cytosolic/nuclear TH receptors, $TR\alpha1$, $TR\beta1$, and $TR\beta2$, in the PIT and in the paraventricular nucleus (13).

The major action of THs, after binding to specific nuclear receptors, is to regulate gene expression. Transcription of both the α- and β-subunits is suppressed by TH, although the effect on β-subunit is greater. In addition to the direct inhibitory actions of THs on TSH-subunit gene expression and TSH release, THs also modulate the expression of the TRH-receptor gene (14). Feedback control of the PIT by TH is remarkably accurate. The administration of small doses of T_3 and T_4 inhibits TSH response to TRH, and tiny decreases in plasma TH levels are sufficient to sensitize the PIT to TRH. TH action, mediated by intranuclear receptors, requires several hours.

The level of TRH mRNA in the paraventricular nuclei is also increased in hypothyroidism, and is reduced by TH treatment. The paraventricular nuclei are target for the action of THs in the control of TRH gene expression and release (15,16). Although THs mediate the feedback regulation of TSH secretion, it has been suggested that TRH determines its set point (16).

Important secondary modulators of TSH secretion are SMS and dopamine, both of which inhibit the function of the thyrotropes. SMS administration reduces the elevated serum TSH response to TRH, abolishes the nocturnal elevation in TSH secretion, and prevents TSH release after administration of dopamine antagonist drugs. Dopamine has an acute inhibitory effect on TSH secretion, and also decreases the levels of α-subunit and TSH-β-subunit mRNAs and gene transcription. Dopamine-induced decreases in TSH secretion result from direct action on the PIT or median eminence, which is mediated by the D_2 class of dopamine receptor. In addition to its effects on the release of TSH, dopamine also inhibits the release of α-subunit and TSH-β-subunit.

In contrast to dopamine, adrenergic activation stimulates TSH release. Endogenous adrenergic pathways have a modest stimulatory role in TSH control in humans. The catecholaminergic control of TSH secretion appears to act as a fine-tuning mechanism, rather than being of primary importance.

In addition to TRH action and feedback control by circulating TH levels, TSH secretion is also influenced by cold exposure and stress.

Circadian Rhythm   Plasma TSH in humans is characterized by a circadian periodicity, with a maximum between 9 PM and 5 AM and a minimum between 4 PM and 7 PM. Smaller ultradian TSH peaks take place every 90–180 min, probably because of bursts of TRH release from the HT, and are physiologically important in controlling the synthesis and glycosylation of TSH.

Exposure of infants to cold at the time of delivery causes an increase in blood TSH levels. Serum TSH levels are higher in the winter than in the summer in individuals in cold climates. However, it is uncertain whether changes in environmental or body temperature in adults influence TSH secretion. Stress also inhibits TSH release. The cytokines, (interleukin-1β (IL-1β), IL-6, and tumor necrosis factor-α inhibit TSH release (17).

ACTH   Adrenocorticotropin (ACTH) is a major stimulus of the various zones of the adrenal cortex, which secretes glucocorticoids, mineralocorticoids, and adrenal androgens. It is a 39-amino-acid peptide derived from the large multifunctional precursor protein, pro-opiomelanocortin (POMC), which is expressed in the corticotropic cells of the anterior PIT gland, in the intermediate lobe cells, and in a few neuronal cell groups in the brain, peripheral chromaffin cells, and selected immune cells.

In the anterior pituitary, the corticotropic cells comprise about 6–10% of the cells, in an uneven distribution. Enzymatic cleavage of the POMC at dibasic amino acids in the corticotropes yields ACTH, together with lipotropin, β-endorphin, some α-melanotropic stimulating hormone, and various other peptides encoded in the precursor protein. In the anterior PIT the major secretory product is ACTH and β-endorphin. ACTH is packaged in small to medium-sized (150–400 nm) granules, which are relatively few in number in the cytoplasm, and line the periphery of the ovoid or angular-shaped corticotrope cells.

HT Control   Brain control of the corticotrope cells is via CRH and VP, released in relatively high concentrations by the hypophysiotropic neurons of the HT paraventricular nucleus into the portal circulation (18). CRH and VP act through specific membrane receptors: the CRH-R1 and the V_3 receptors (V_{1b} in the rat) localized in the membrane of the corticotropic cells.

Second messengers for these receptors differ: CRH-R1 is linked via G proteins to adenylate cyclase, and, on stimulation, generates marked increases of cyclic adenosine monophosphate (cAMP); V_3 receptors activate phospholipase C to release IP_3 and calcium from intracellular stores, and activate protein kinase C through diacylglycerol. The two HT hormones markedly potentiate each other's actions, and together are more potent than each one alone. Because only CRH-induced actions are sensitive to rapid glucocorticoid inhibition, the coordinated secretion of the two neurohormones may play a role in the adaptation of chronic stress, in which high glucocorticoid secretion is maintained, despite the potent feedback action.

HT control is by CRH/VP-containing neurons located in the parvocellular region of the HT paraventricular nucleus, which project to the median eminence and the PIT stalk. Co-expression of CRH and VP is common, even in baseline conditions.

Feedback Control: Long Loop via Glucocorticoids and Short Loop via ACTH   Glucocorticoids inhibit ACTH secretion acting at the PIT and the brain. Removal of the adrenal gland or pharmacological interference with the synthesis of the cortisol strongly stimulates ACTH secretion via increased CRH and VP secretion into the portal circulation.

Glucocorticoids inhibit the CRH-stimulated secretion of ACTH acting at the level of the corticotrops. On sustained action, they decrease POMC mRNA levels and cellular content of ACTH. Glucocorticoids also act at the paraventricular CRH/VP-containing neurons, in which both CRH/VP mRNA levels and peptide content are decreased. The brain region richest in glucocorticoid receptors is the hippocampus. The neurons of the hippocampus project to the HT, and have an inhibitory influence on the activity of the hypothalamoPIT–adrenocortical system. Glucocorticoid inhibitory action is both at the nuclear level on gene expression, and on neuronal cell membrane, rapidly influencing neuronal behavior.

ACTH can also influence its own secretion via direct action on the HT, called short-loop feedback. It is believed to result at least in part from the vascular connections via the stalk, which may bring some secretions of the PIT back to the median eminence.

Actions   ACTH is the major stimulus to the zona fasciculata of the adrenal gland, in which both the structure of the tissue and its secretory activity are dependent on the effect of ACTH on its membrane receptors. Membrane receptors of ACTH are coupled to G proteins and markedly stimulate adenylate cyclase. The elevation of cAMP activates protein kinase A, which in turn phosphorylates various regulatory proteins. ACTH action is both very fast and lasting. The initial action occurs within minutes, and elevation of glucocorticoids in adrenal venous blood can be demonstrated within seconds of ACTH administration. In addition to the rapid secretory effects, ACTH also has trophic effects on the adrenal cortex: stimulation of expression of various stroidogenetic enzymes and maintenance of mitochondrial structure.

Neural Control of Basal Secretory Activity and Stress-Induced Changes *Circadian Rhythm* Basal activity of the system is highest at the beginning of the active cycle (morning in humans, evening in rodents), and lowest a few hours after the beginning of sleep. Secretion, even under basal conditions, is pulsatile, with a relatively uneven occurrence and varying pulse height. Feedback inhibition of a superimposed stimulus is strong during the rising phase of the corticoid pulses, compared to a stimulus occurring during the interpulse intervals.

Stress External, stressful stimuli strongly influence the activity of the hypothalamoPIT–adrenocortical system. Several stressors stimulate the system. Sudden emotional stimuli or failure of psychological coping in pressure situations markedly activate the system. Acute or chronic physical stressors, such as pain, tissue damage, infection, inflammatory mediators, toxins, and circulatory shock, all result in ACTH release and consequent increase of glucocorticoid blood levels. The set point of the glucocorticoid regulation is apparently reset during chronic stress, because hyperactivity of ACTH secretion is maintained, despite elevated glucocorticoid levels. An apparent change in glucocorticoid feedback occurs in a substantial proportion of depressive patients, who have elevated glucocorticoid levels throughout the day, with a diurnal rhythm.

Growth Hormone GH is synthetized and secreted by somatotropes in the anterior PIT gland. Most PIT GH (70–80%) is a nonglycosylated, single-chain, 191-amino-acid, 22-kDa protein with two intramolecular disulfide bonds, and 6–8% is a 20-kDa form. The somatotrope cells make up about 50% of the hormone-producing cells of the anterior PIT. The human adenohypophysis contains 5–10 mg GH, which circulates in several forms, including a 22-kDa form, a 20-kDa form, and acidic forms.

GH receptor is a single-chain protein with a unique transmembrane domain *(19)*. In humans, the GH receptor is composed of 620 amino acids. Soluble GH-binding proteins, identical to extracellular domains of full-length receptors, have been isolated from human plasma. GH receptors belong to class 1 of the cytokine receptor superfamily. Each GH molecule has two binding sites for the GH receptor. The binding of the hormone to the extracellular portion of the receptor induces dimerization of two identical α-receptor molecules by one hormone molecule, and forms a complex containing one GH molecule and two GH receptors.

The principal GH-binding protein binds 22-kDa GH with high affinity and limited binding capacity. Of 22-kDa GH, 40–50% and 20–30% of 20-kDa GH are complexed with the binding proteins, and the high-affinity binding protein accounts for 85% of this binding. The exact biologic significance of the binding proteins is unknown. The high-affinity binding proteins may compete with receptor for the binding of GH, and thus impair GH action; alternatively, the binding proteins may enhance the biologic activity of GH. Binding is decreased in Laron dwarfism and pygmies, and during prolonged fasting.

The effects of GH on cell metabolism are mediated either directly, through the GH receptor, or indirectly, through the GH-regulated production of IGFs. The GH–IGF-I axis is a highly complex system, involving GH, IGF-I and -II, six high-affinity and four lower-affinity IGF-binding proteins (IGFBPs).

IGFs are single-chain peptides that exhibit sequence homology with human proinsulin, synthetized primarily by the liver, but are also produced locally by most tissues, in which they act in an autocrine or paracrine manner. IGF-I is important for both fetal and postnatal growth. IGF-II is one of the major fetal growth factors. Serum concentrations of IGF-I are usually parallel with the 24-h mean serum concentrations of GH. Both IGFs activate the IGF-I receptor, which mediates the anabolic actions of both IGF-I and IGF-II. The interaction of GH with its hepatic receptor stimulates expression of the IGF-I gene and the release of the IGF-I peptide.

IGFs are bound to IGFBPs in the plasma. The IGFBPs constitute a family of six structurally related proteins that bind IGF peptides with high affinity. They share an overall protein sequence identity of approx 50%. Besides the classical six IGFBPs, the low-affinity IGF binders are the IGFBP-related protein-1, -2, -3, and -4, which are members of the IGFBP superfamily *(20)*. Under most conditions, the IGFBPs appear to inhibit IGF action, by competing with IGF receptors for binding IGF peptides. IGFBPs are carrier proteins, which extend the serum half-life of the IGF peptides, modulate IGF action, and regulate their bioavailability. IGFBP-3 binds more than 95% of the IGF in serum. The IGF–IGFBP-3 dimer forms a complex with another protein subunit, the acid-labile subunit, and, in this ternary complex, the IGFs have a serum half-life of many hours. Once released from the complex, the IGFs leave the circulation and enter the target tissues, with the aid of other IGFBPs. GH increases the serum concentrations of both the acid-labile subunit and IGFBP-3.

Actions of GH GH is essential for normal postnatal growth and development. GH is an anabolic hormone that has an important role in the regulation of protein synthesis, stimulating the uptake and retention of amino acids by muscle and liver *(21)*. GH enhances positive nitrogen balance, and decreases urea production. GH is a powerful lipolytic hormone that increases the oxidation of fats as a source of calories, mobilizes free fatty acids from fat stores, and redistributes body fat. GH has a direct effect on fat cells, stimulating their differentiation from precursor and increasing their number. GH is secreted when plasma glucose falls too low, i.e., when glucose utilization is greater than supply, by decreasing the use of glucose by peripheral tissues. Both continuous GH exposure and pharmacologic GH doses produce alterations in carbohydrate metabolism, cause insulin resistance and glucose intolerance, and produce fasting hyperglycemia and hyperinsulinemia. GH induction of insulin resistance at postreceptor site may be the mechanism for these effects. The site of insulin resistance being the liver. GH promotes growth and mineralization of the bone. GH stimulates the division of chondrocytes at the epiphyseal plates. These effects are mediated, at least indirectly, through the local production of IGF-I. After closure of the epiphyseal plates, GH still has an important role in bone metabolism and the maintenance of bone mineral density throughout life. GH has an important role in regulation of body water, particularly extracellular fluid, and it promotes the retention of both sodium and water.

HT Control The pulsatile secretion of GH by the somatotropes (Figure 5) is controlled by at least two antagonistic HT peptides:

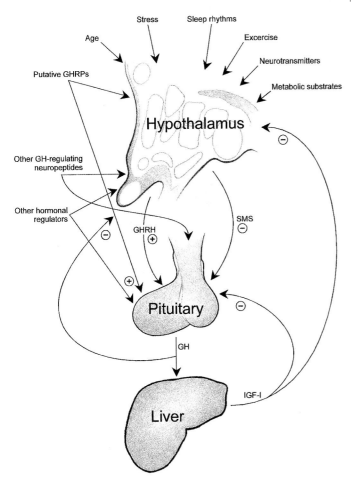

Figure 3-5 Neuroendocrine control of GH and IGF-I secretion. GH, growth hormone; GHRH, GH-releasing hormone; GHRP, GH-releasing peptide; IGF-I, insulin-like growth factor-I; SMS, somatostatin. The PIT somatotrope cell expresses receptors for GHRH, GHRP, and SMS. Metabolic substrates, e.g., amino acids, glucose, fatty acids. Neurotransmitters, such as acetylcholine, catecholamines, GABA, histamine, serotonin. Other GH-regulating neuropeptides, e.g., galanin, neuropeptide Y, opioid peptides. Other hormonal regulators, e.g., glucocorticoids, gonadal sex hormones, thyroid hormones.

GHRH, which stimulates GH release, and SMS, which inhibits GH release. Three biologically active molecular forms of GHRH occur in the human HT: GHRH 10-44-NH2, GHRH-1-40-OH, and GHRH 1-37-OH. The two larger forms are equipotent, and the smaller one is less active.

The GHRH peptide binds to its specific receptors on the membranes of the somatotropes. The human receptors for GHRH have been cloned, and they are a member of the seven-transmembrane-domain, G-protein-linked receptor superfamily *(22)*. GHRH stimulates both GH synthesis (by increasing the transcription rate of the GH gene) and GH release. GHRH activates cAMP by binding to a stimulatory G protein. GHRH increases the amplitude of GH pulses, but does not affect pulse frequency (the neural networks that generate spontaneous GH pulses are not affected by GHRH).

Growth-hormone-releasing Peptides (GHRPs) Several peptide analogs of metenkephalin stimulate rhythmic secretion of GH. The first was the GH-releasing hexapeptide, hexarelin (GHRP-6, His-DTrp-Ala-Trp-DPhe-Lys-NH2) *(23)*. Nonpeptidic

analogs of GHRP-6 (for instance, MK-0677, L-692429, L-692429, L-692585) have also been developed. These compounds, active when administered by intranasal and oral routes, are more effective in vivo than in vitro, and are more effective in the presence of GHRH; they are almost ineffective in the absence of GHRH. The analogs do not bind to the GHRH receptor *(24)*, and do not act by suppressing SMS secretion or by activating adenylate cyclase in the PIT. GHRPs potentiate the stimulatory effects of GHRH and inhibit SMS action on GH release. GHRPs and their nonpeptidyl analogs are referred collectively as GH secretagogues. Demonstration of GHRP receptor in the PIT and HT *(25)* suggests the existence of an endogenous GHRP that may be involved in the physiological regulation of GH secretion. These analogs act through a mechanism different from that of GHRH. The natural ligand for this receptor remains to be identified.

SMS is expressed, in the brain and in the periphery, in two principal forms: SMS-14 and SMS-28. SMS-14 is identical with the terminal 14 amino acids of SMS-28. One SMS gene is present in the human, and tissue-specific processing determines whether the 14- or 28-amino-acid form will be expressed. Somatostatin-14 is the predominant form in the brain (including the HT); SMS-28 is the major form in the gastrointestinal tract, especially in the colon.

In the PIT, SMS inhibits secretion of GH and TSH. As a PIT regulator, SMS is a true neurohormone. In addition, it exerts inhibitory effects on virtually all endocrine and exocrine secretions of the pancreas, gut, and gallbladder.

SMS binds to a family of specific receptors and inhibits adenylyl cyclase via G-protein-coupled receptors, with additional actions to reduce net calcium influx. SMS determines the timing and amplitude of GH pulses, and inhibits GH release, but has no effect on GH biosynthesis. Five SMS receptor subtypes (SSTR1–5), containing seven transmembrane domains, have been cloned and characterized *(26)*. There is a good correlation between SMS binding to SSTR2 and inhibition of GH release. When cells are exposed to both SMS and GHRH, SMS exerts the dominant effect.

Feedback control of GH release is mediated by GH itself, and by its nearly ubiquitous tissue mediator, IGF-I. Direct GH effects on the HT act by short-loop feedback; those involving IGF-I are long-loop systems. Control of GH secretion thus includes two closed-loop systems (GH and IGF-I) and one open-loop regulatory system (neural).

In the HT, both GH and IGF-I increase the secretion of SMS and inhibit the release of GHRH. In the PIT IGF-I (but not GH) inhibits the stimulatory effect of GHRH. In conditions in which circulating levels of IGF-I are low, such as Laron dwarfism (the result of a defect in the GH receptor), blood GH concentrations are elevated.

So-called autofeedback can be demonstrated in normal subjects, because GH injection reduces the subsequent GH secretory response to a GHRH stimulus. GH autonegative feedback stimulates SMS release from the HT. The GH receptor plays a primary role in mediating physiological GH autonegative feedback.

Neural Control Both GHRH and SMS are regulated by cerebral neurotransmitters and neuropeptides (Table 1). The GH regulatory system receives impulses from dopaminergic, noradrenergic, adrenergic, serotoninergic, histaminergic, and cholinergic fibers. Dopamine stimulates GHRH secretion by direct action on

Table 1
Factors Influencing Normal GH Secretion in Humans

Stimulation	Inhibition
Acetylcholine agonist	Acetylcholine antagonists
α_2-adrenergic agonists (clonidine)	Aging
α-MSH	α-adrenergic antagonists
Amino acids (arginine, leucine, lysine)	β_2-adrenergic agonists
Arginine vasopressin	Calcitonin
β-adrenergic antagonists (propranolol)	Chlorpromazine
β-endorphin	Elevated GH level
Decrease in blood glucose level	Emotional deprivation
Dopamine agonists	Endotoxin
Enkephalin analogues	GABA (stimulated)
Exercise	High cortisol level
Fasting	High IGF-I level
Fall in free fatty acid level	Hypothyroidism
GABA (basal)	Increase in blood glucose level
Galanin	Increase in free fatty acid level
GH-releasing peptides	Obesity
GHRH	Opioid receptor antagonists (naloxone)
Glucagon	Serotonin antagonists
Gonadal steroids[a]	Sleep (rapid eye movement)
Histamine	Somatostatin
Inflammatory cytokines	
Interleukins (IL-1, IL-2, IL-6)	
Leptin (inversely correlated with GH)	
Levodopa	
Low IGF-I level	
Neuropeptide Y?	
Neurotensin	
Opiates	
Physiological cortisol levels	
Serotonin	
Sleep (stage III and IV)	
Stress[b]	
Substance P	
Thyroid hormone	
TRH[c]	
VIP	

[a]Estrogen (amplitude), progesterone, testosterone.
[b]Physical, psychological, acute, chronic.
[c]In certain conditions, e.g., in acromegaly.

neuronal dopamine receptors, and by stimulation of α-adrenergic receptors.

Acetylcholine seems to be an important regulator of GH secretion. Blockade of acetylcholinergic muscarinic receptors reduces or abolishes GH secretory responses to different stimuli. In contrast, drugs that potentiate cholinergic transmission increase basal GH levels and enhance GH response to GHRH in normal individuals. Neurotransmitters may be specific for different physiological stimuli of GH secretion. For example, sleep-induced GH release is mediated by serotoninergic, and possibly by cholinergic, fibers. Probably both paracrine and neuroendocrine effects are mediated by VIP and galanin, which are intrinsic to the PIT, in stimulating GH release. Central TRH pathways generally inhibit GH secretion, however, in some conditions, such as acromegaly, TRH acts on the PIT to stimulate GH secretion.

Circadian Rhythm   GH is secreted in a pulsatile manner, with a marked diurnal rhythm. The amount of GH secreted can be altered by changing the frequency or amplitude of individual pulses. Under basal conditions, GH levels are low most of the time, with an ultradian rhythm of secretion of about 13 pulses/24 h. The amplitude of GH secretory bursts is maximal during the night. The most consistent period of GH secretion coincides with the onset of the first slow-wave sleep, usually within the first 60 min of sleep. GH levels are highest during slow-wave sleep (stages III and IV), and lowest during rapid eye movement sleep. Probably decreased HT SMS secretion initiates GH secretory bursts. Slow-wave sleep may be associated with low levels of HT SMS secretion; rapid eye movement sleep may be associated with high levels.

Secretion of GH is also modified by age, sex, metabolic status, external stimuli, hormonal factors, stress, and by certain neurotransmitters (Table 1). Levels of GH are maximal during adolescence and decline gradually with age. Serum GH concentrations rise twofold in the late follicular phase of the normal menstrual cycle. Premenopausal women have higher GH secretion than do young men. GH release is greater in women than men for arginine and hypoglycemia. The gender difference in pulsatile GH release arises from higher GH-secretory burst mass present in women.

Serum IGF-I levels in hypopituitary women are less responsive to exogenous GH.

Obesity also impairs spontaneous and induced GH secretion. The predominant effect appears to be the reduction in the amplitude of the GH secretory bursts. The metabolic clearance rate of GH is also accelerated in obesity. The diminished GH secretion in obesity may result from high levels of SMS. Gonadal steroids, particularly estradiol, are important in the regulation of GH secretion. GH secretory responses to a number of stimuli are augmented by treatment with estrogens. Oral glucose acts rapidly to suppress GH release by increasing HT SMS release.

Glucocorticoids are both inhibitors and stimulators of regulated GH secretion. Physiological amounts of glucocorticoids probably play an important long-term role in maintaining basal somatotrope secretory reserve in humans. GH secretion is inhibited in patients with Cushing's syndrome, and in patients receiving high-dose, long-term glucocorticoid treatment.

PRL Human PRL consists of 199 amino acids, and has three intramolecular disulfide bonds. 16% of amino acids of PRL are homologous with those of GH. PRL circulates in blood predominantly in a monomeric form (little PRL, 23 kDa), but also exists in dimeric (big PRL, 48–56 kDa) and polymeric (>100 kDa) forms. The larger forms have reduced receptor-binding affinity and biologic activity. Lactotrope cells have a wide distribution throughout the pars distalis of the PIT. The number of lactotrope cells in this region varies from 12 to 28%. Adult human PIT contains about 0.1 mg PRL. The normal serum PRL level is less than 15 ng/mL. Women tend to have slightly higher levels than men, probably because of estrogen stimulation of PRL secretion.

Several PRL-related proteins are also produced in many mammalian tissues, including the brain, uterus, placenta, and cells of the immune system. The physiological functions of extrahypophysial PRL-related proteins are not entirely known.

PRL acts through PRL receptors in multiple tissues, including breast, ovary, prostate, testis, and liver. In humans, these receptors are stimulated by both GH and PRL, since the PRL and GH receptors share sequence homology.

The main site of PRL action is the mammary gland. PRL plays a decisive role in preparation and maintenance of mammary gland milk production. During pregnancy, the breast undergoes considerable development through an interaction of several hormones. Estrogen, progesterone, PRL, and placental mammotropic hormones, including GH and probably insulin, cortisol, and TH are also involved in breast development. Lactation is inhibited during pregnancy by the high levels of estrogen and progesterone. Lactation begins when the maternal breast is subjected to sudden withdrawal of the estrogen and progesterone, then continues at a relatively high, although declining, PRL level, and at low estrogen and progesterone concentrations.

Physiological and pathologic hyperprolactinemia are associated with suppression of the HT–PIT–gonadal axis, probably because of the PRL-mediated inhibition of pulsatile secretion of GnRH, which results in impaired gonadotropin release and inhibition of gonadal function. PRL acts also at sites other than the breast, but the physiological function of these actions is poorly understood. PRL has a role in response to stress, normal immune function, osmoregulation, and angiogenesis.

Secretion of PRL like other anterior PIT hormones, is regulated by neural influences from the HT and hormonal feedback. Secre-

tagogues that affect PRL secretion bind to specific cell-surface receptors.

HT Control There are two major mechanisms by which the HT can influence PRL secretion from the PIT gland: inhibition by PIFs and stimulation by PRL-releasing factors (PRFs) (Table 2). PIT PRL secretion is under tonic and predominant inhibition exercised by the medial-basal HT. Thus, in contrast to the secretion of other PIT hormones, the secretion of PRL is increased in the absence of HT influences. The tonic suppression is mediated by regulatory hormones synthetized by tuberoinfundibular neurons. Theoretically, HT neuronal activity can enhance PRL release from the PIT gland by inhibition of a PIF and/or by stimulation of a PRF.

Dopamine, the most important PIF, is the best-established HT hypophysiotropic inhibitor of PRL secretion, and is produced by neurons in the arcuate–periventricular nucleus of the HT. This HT dopaminergic system can functionally be divided into two different parts: tuberoinfundibular and tuberohypophyseal dopaminergic neurons. PRL tonically and permanently inhibits and suppresses the secretory function of mammotropes, and DNA synthesis and cell division. PIT stalk interruption leads to increased levels of PRL. The inhibition is mediated by the interaction of dopamine with receptors of the D_2-subtype on PIT lactotrope membranes. This interaction activates an inhibitory G protein, leading to decreased adenylate cyclase activity. These actions are responsible for the therapeutic effect of dopamine agonists, such as bromocriptine in hyperprolactinemic states.

Plasma levels of PRL increase after adrenalectomy, and this can be reversed by administration of corticosteroids. Similarly, the synthetic glucocorticoid, dexamethasone, decreases PRL release (27).

Although tonic suppression of PRL release by dopamine is the dominant effect of the HT on PRL secretion, a number of stimuli promote PRL release. The genuine physiological significance of the several putative PRFs in humans is unknown.

TRH has been considered a physiologically relevant PRF of HT origin. Exogenous TRH stimulates PRL release with the same dose–response characteristics as for TSH release. TRH has high-affinity membrane receptors on mammotropes, and can stimulate PRL release only when dopaminergic input has previously been reduced or is absent.

VIP is a known stimulator of PRL release: It is produced in the anterior lobe, and is present in mammotropes. It has been concluded that the ability of mammotropes to release PRL spontaneously at a high rate may partly be the result of the tonic positive feedback of VIP as an autocrine factor. Another candidate for PRF is the peptide-histidine-isoleucine-27 (PHI-27), which is structurally homologous with VIP, and is synthetized as part of the VIP prohormone. PHI is co-localized with CRH in paraventricular neurons.

PRL synthesis is also regulated by effects of estrogen on PRL gene expression, so that serum PRL levels are higher in normal premenopausal women than in men. Similarly, PRL levels rise during menarche and during pregnancy. Ovarectomy reduces, and estrogen, alone or in combination with progesterone, increases PRL secretion. These effects are mediated by influencing HT dopaminergic neurons, by directly affecting mammotropes, and/or by indirectly releasing an unidentified mammotrope recruitment factor from the intermediate lobe. α-MSH is also considered as a paracrine PRF.

Table 2
Factors and Conditions that Change PRL Secretion in Primates and Humans

Stimulation	*Inhibition*
Acetylcholine	Dopamine
α-MSH	γ-Aminobutyric acid
Angiotensin	Glucocorticoids
Bombesin	Sleep cycle
Bradykinin	Epidermal growth factor
Central serotoninergic pathways	
Cholecystokinin	
Dopamine[a]	
Endorphinergic pathways	
Estrogen	
Exercise	
Exogenous opioids	
Fibroblast growth factor	
Gastrin	
Mating	
Melatonin	
Neurotensin	
Orgasm in women	
Oxytocin	
PACAP[b]	
Peptide-histidine-isoleucine-27	
Sleep cycle	
Stimulation of the nipple in women	
Stress (emotional and physical)	
Substance P	
Suckling	
TRH	
Uncharacterized neurointermediate lobe factor(s)	
Vasoactive intestinal peptide	

[a]Under certain conditions.
[b]Pituitary-adenylate-cyclase-activating polypeptide.

Suckling provides an essential stimulus for the release of PRL, and is one of the most important physiological regulators of PRL secretion. Within a few minutes of nipple stimulation, PRL rises and remains elevated for 10–20 min. It is generally accepted that the other two parts of the PIT gland, the neural lobe and the intermediate lobe, have a significant influence on PRL secretion (28). Suckling-induced PRL release in the rat is mediated in part by the neurointermediate lobe. However, the significance of the neurointermediate lobe for PRL regulation in humans is not clear, because this structure is rudimentary in primates and in humans.

Within the PIT, paracrine interactions with mammotropes have been demonstrated for three cell types: the gonadotropes, folliculostellate cells, and the corticotropes. It seems unlikely that such paracrine interactions are important in the acute release of PRL, but rather they may be involved in gradual or chronic changes in PRL secretion.

PRL exhibits a circadian rhythm with peak values in the early morning hours and lowest values at midday. Values are not closely correlated with other hormonal circadian rhythms. Nursing mothers retain the nocturnal PRL surge, which begins from a higher basal level. In healthy subjects, there are approx 14 pulses of PRL secretion per day. Enhanced PRL secretion during the night results from increased pulse amplitude.

Feedback is exerted by PRL itself at the level of the HT. Negative feedback control of PRL secretion is mediated through PRL receptors, located on the tuberoinfundibular dopamine-secreting neurons of the arcuate nucleus. Activation of the receptors increases the output and turnover of dopamine.

REFERENCES

1. Reichlin S. Neuroendocrinology. In: Wilson JD, ed. Williams Textbook of Endocrinology, vol. 1, 9th ed. W. B. Saunders, Philadelphia, 1998, pp. 165–249.
2. Thorner MO, Vance ML, Laws ER Jr, Horvath E, Kovacs K. The Anterior pituitary. In: Wilson JD, ed. Williams Textbook of Endocrinology, vol. 1, 9th ed. W. B. Saunders, Philadelphia, 1998, pp. 249–341.
3. Chadwich DJ, Marsch J, eds. Functional Anatomy of the Neuroendocrine Hypothalamus. Wiley, Chichester, West Sussex, UK, 1992.
4. Halász B. Hypothalamo-anterior pituitary system and pituitary portal vessels. In: Imura H, ed. The Pituitary Gland, 2nd ed. Raven, New York, 1994, pp. 1–28.
5. Ishikawa S, Okada K, Saito T. Vasopressin secretion in health and disease. In: Imura H, ed. The Pituitary Gland, 2nd ed. Raven, New York, 1994, pp. 331–350.
6. Nagaya T, Jameson JL. Structural features of the glycoprotein hormone genes and their encoded proteins. In: Imura H, ed. The Pituitary Gland, 2nd ed. Raven, New York, 1994, pp. 63–89.
7. Blake CA. Control of gonadotropin secretion. In: Knobil E, Neill JD, eds. Encyclopedia of Reproduction, vol. 2. Ep-L Academic, San Diego, 1998, pp. 528–551.
8. Silverman A-J, Line I, Witkin JW. Gonadotropin-releasing hormone (GnRH) neuronal systems: immunocytochemistry and in situ hybridization. In: Knobil E, Neill JD, eds. The Physiology of Reproduction, vol. 1, 2nd ed. Raven, New York, 1993, pp. 1683–1710.

9. Kordon C, Drouva SV, de la Escalera GM, Weiner RI. Role of classic and peptide neuromediators in the neuroendocrine regulation of luteinizing hormone and prolactin. In: Knobil E, Neill JD, eds. The Physiology of Reproduction, vol 1, 2nd ed. Raven, New York, 1993, pp. 1621–1682.

10. Hotchkiss J, Knobil E. Menstrual cycle and its neuroendocrine control. In: Knobil E, Neill JD, eds. The Physiology of Reproduction, vol 2. 2nd ed. Raven, New York, 1993, pp. 711–750.

11. Persani L. Hypothalamic thyrotropin-releasing hormone and thyrotropin biological activity. Thyroid 1998;8:941–946.

12. Duthie SM, Taylor PI, Anderson I, Cook J, Eidne KA. Cloning and functional characterization of the human TRH receptor. Mol Cell Endocrinol 1993;95:R11–R15.

13. Lechan RM, Qi Y, Jackson IM, Mahdavi V. Identification of thyroid hormone receptor isoforms in thyrotropin-releasing hormone neurons of the hypothalamic paraventricular nucleus. Endocrinology 1994;135:92–100.

14. Yamada M, Monden T, Satoh T, Iizuka M, Murakami M, Irruchijima T, Mori M. Differential regulation of thyrotropin-releasing hormone receptor mRNA levels by thyroid hormone in vivo and in vitro (GH3 cells). Biochem Biophys Res Comm 1992;184:367–372.

15. Kakucska I, Rand W, Lechan RM. Thyrotropin-releasing hormone gene expression in the hypothalamic paraventricular nucleus is dependent upon feedback regulation by both triiodothyronine and thyroxine. Endocrinology 1992;130:2845–2850.

16. Greer MA, Sato M, Wang X, Greer SE, McAdams S. Evidence that the major physiological role of TRH in the hypothalamic paraventricular nuclei may be to regulate the set-point for thyroid hormone negative feedback on the pituitary thyrotroph. Neuroendocrinology 1993;57:569–575.

17. Van Haasteren GAC, Van Der Meer MJM, Hermus ARMM, Linkels E, Klootwijk W, Kaptein E, et al. Different effects of continuous infusion of interleukin-1 and interleukin-6 on the hypothalamic-hypophysial thyroid axis. Endocrinology 1994;135:1336–1345.

18. Antoni FA. Vasopressinergic control of pituitary adrenocorticotropin secretion comes of age. Front Neuroendocrinol. 1993;14:76–122.

19. Goffin V, Kelly PA. Prolactin and growth hormone receptors. Clin Endocrinol 1996;45:247–255.

20. Baxter RC, Binoux MA, Clemmons DR, Conover CA, Drop SLS, Holly JMP, et al. Recommendations for nomenclature of the insulin-like growth factor binding protein superfamily. Endocrinology 1998;139:4036

21. Umpleby AM, Russell-Jones DL. The hormonal control of protein metabolism. Bailliere Clin Endoc 1996;10:551–570.

22. Gaylinn D, Harrison JK, Zysk JR, Lyons CE Jr, Lynch KR, Thorner MO. Molecular cloning and expression of a human anterior pituitary receptor for growth hormone-releasing hormone. Mol Endocrinol 1993;7:77–84.

23. Bowers CY. GH releasing peptides. Structure and kinetics. J Pediatr Endocrinol 1993;38:87–91.

24. Goth M, Lyons CE, Canny BJ, Thorner MO. Pituitary adenylate cyclase activating polypeptide, growth hormone (GH)-releasing peptide and GH-releasing hormone stimulate GH release through distinct pituitary receptors. Endocrinology 1992;130:939–944.

25. Howard AD, Feighner SD, Cully DF, Arena JP, Liberator PA, Rosenblum CI, et al. Receptor in pituitary and hypothalamus that functions in growth hormone release. Science 1996;273:974–977.

26. Patel YC, Greenwood MT, Panetta R, Demchyshun L, Niznik H, Sirkant CB. Somatostatin receptor family. Life Sci 1995;57:1249–1265.

27. Goth M, Kovacs L, Szabocs I, Nagy GM. Effect of dexamethasone (DEX) on prolactin secretion in rats and human. Fourth International Congress of Neuroendocrinology. October 12–16, 1998, Kitakyushu, Japan. Abstracts No. P016.

28. Liu JW, Ben-Jonathan N. Prolactin-releasing activity of neurohypophysial hormones: structure-function relationship. Endocrinology 1994;134:114–118.

29. Wetsel WC, Valença MM, Merchenthaler I, Liposits Z, López FJ, Weiner RI, Mellon PL, Negro-Vilar A. Intrinsic pulsatile secretory activity of immortalized luteinizing hormone-releasing hormone-secreting neurons. Proc Natl Acad Sci USA 1992;89:4149–4153.

4 Epidemiology of Pituitary Tumors

Shozo Yamada, MD, PhD

INTRODUCTION

Pituitary adenomas are benign tumors consisting of and arising from adenohypophyseal cells. Although endocrinological and morphological investigations on pituitary adenomas have yielded substantial data in the last decade, epidemiological studies have been limited *(1–3)*. This chapter will review current knowledge of the epidemiological characteristics of pituitary adenoma.

INCIDENCE AND PREVALENCE OF PITUITARY ADENOMA

The true incidence of pituitary adenoma is difficult to establish with certainty. The incidence and prevalence of tumors in a given population usually depend on several factors, such as the level of interest and activity in pituitary surgery, the diagnostic methods, the indications for surgical intervention, the admitting policies of physicians, and the pathological classification used. All these factors differ among the periods studied and between countries, or even among hospitals. Therefore, such influences must always be kept in mind when assessing differences between periods, institutions, and countries.

There are data from several countries or investigators regarding the frequency of pituitary adenoma as a proportion of all primary brain tumors *(4–36)* (Table 1). The frequency of pituitary adenoma varies widely between 3.4 and 23.2% *(4–36)*. On the whole, it accounts for 12.1% (14,078/115,897) of primary brain tumors. These differences in the incidence of pituitary adenoma may not reflect real international variation, since several possible factors may account for discrepancies in reported frequencies. For example, there may be differences in diagnostic technology, and in the interest of physicians between different countries and periods. Moreover, granuloma and nonneoplastic cystic, or vascular, lesions have been included in some reports, and even craniopharyngiomas were also classified as pituitary adenomas by some investigators. These lesions, as well as metastatic brain tumors, are excluded from Tables 1 and 2 as far as possible. Moreover, some reports are based on surgical materials, whereas others include tumors only diagnosed at autopsy or by neuroimaging studies. Thus, the number of cases without histological verification may also be a source of bias. These factors are indicated in Tables 1 and 2.

From: *Diagnosis and Management of Pituitary Tumors* (K. Thapar, K. Kovacs, B. W. Scheithauer, and R. V. Lloyd, eds.), ©Humana Press Inc., Totowa, NJ.

It has been reported that approx 2500 new cases of pituitary adenoma are diagnosed annually in the US *(37)*. Epidemiological data on the incidence rates in the general population are available for a few countries, especially developed Western countries *(2,4–8,10,11,14,15,29,38–40)* (Table 2). Ambrosi and Faglia estimated that the total prevalence was 19.9/100,000 inhabitants and the total incidence was 1.55 patients/100,000 at the end of 1986 in Milan, Italy *(2)*, whereas Lovaste et al. investigated brain tumors in another Italian district (the province of Trento) and reported that the incidence of pituitary adenoma in the 20- to 44-yr-old age group (including childbearing women) was 1.3 for men and 2.1/100,000/yr for women *(15)*. In other reports, the age-adjusted prevalence ranges from 4.8 to 8.9/100,000 *(1,9,33)*, whereas the age-adjusted incidence of pituitary adenoma/100,000 population was estimated as 0.8 in Carlisle, England *(39)*, 0.7 in Israel *(16)*, and 0.6 in Iceland *(14)* based on clinical or autopsy cases, but it was 0.9 (national survey, US) based only on cases diagnosed prior to death *(10)*. In recent reports, the average annual age- and sex-adjusted incidence of pituitary adenoma was 2.8/100,000 from 1950 to 1989 (symptomatic cases: 2.4; asymptomatic cases: 0.4) in Rochester, MN and 1.8 from 1989 to 1994 in Kumamoto prefecture, Japan *(11,29)*. These differences in the reported incidence of pituitary adenoma are probably mainly artifactual, and owing to differences in period as well as variations in the definitions and the diagnostic methods used. In addition, the higher incidence in England and Wales may be because the data were based on hospital discharges for pituitary disease, which could include some other pituitary lesions as well as patients readmitted with recurrence *(40)*.

In contrast, there is little epidemiological information about the incidence of each type of adenoma. Batrinos et al. found 117 prolactinomas (4.2%) in 4199 women aged 14–43 yr *(41)*, whereas Japanese investigators reported hyperprolactinemia in 14 men and 26 women among 10,640 inhabitants aged 20–60 yr, with prolactinoma being detected in 3 and 2 of the 14 men and 26 women, respectively *(42)*. Regarding acromegaly, the prevalence was reported to be 5.3/100,000 in 1968 and 6.3 in 1984, but the mean annual incidence was 0.3 (over 12 yr) and 0.4 (over 25 yr)/100,000 population in the Newcastle region and in Northern Ireland, respectively *(43,44)*. This rate would be equivalent to about 200 new cases per year in the UK. Similarly, the prevalence at the end of 1989 was reported as 6.0 and 6.9/100,000 and the average annual incidence was 0.3 and 0.3/100,000 in Vizcaya, Spain *(45)* and in Goteborg and the surrounding counties in Sweden *(46)*, respectively. However, the prevalence and incidence of Cushing's disease are not accurately known. A recent epidemiological study

Table 1
Pituitary Adenomas as a Proportion of Primary Intracranial Tumors[a]

Country and author, ref. no.	Time period	% of Adenoma		No. of tumor adenoma/total	Source of data	Histological confirmation	Diagnosed before death
US-Connecticut, Schoenberg et al. (4)	1935–1964		9.5%	241/2538	Connecticut Tumor Registry	100%	100%
US-Rochester, MN, Percy et al. (5)	1935–1968		9.8%	17/174	Mayo Clinic records	93%	64%
US-Rochester, MN, Kurland (6)	1945–1954		20.6%	7/34	Mayo Clinic records	85%	Both
US-Rochester, MN, Annegers et al. (7)	1935–1977		13.0% (17.2%)[b]	29/223	Mayo Clinic records	72%	86%
US-Washington, DC, Heshman et al. (8)	1960–1969	White Black	5.4% 17.9%	41/766 84/469	Records and registries of 26 hospitals	95%	Both
US-Washington. DC, Fan et al. (9)	1958–1970	White Black	7.9% 18.6%	646/8264 113/606	AFIP	100%	Both
US National survey, Walker et al. (10)	1973–1974		14.4%	1970/13720	Records of 166 cooperating hospitals (include other pituitary lesions)	74%	100%
US-Rochester, MN. Radhakrishnan et al. (11)	1950–1989		16.2%	55/339	Mayo Clinic records	>95%	63%
Canada-Newfoundland, Maroun and Jacob (12)	1966–1969		3.4%	3/88	Hospitals' records (cyst and bony tumors are excluded)	100%	Both
Denmark-Faroe Islands, Joensen (13)	1962–1975		9.6%	5/52	Records and registries of three hospitals	Almost all	100%
Iceland, Gudmundsson (14)	1954–1963		6.5%	12/186	All hospitals and state records	98%	Both
Italy-Trento, Lovaste et al. (15)	1977–1984		15.3%	46/301	All cases were collected in the province of Trento	72%	Both
Israel, Leibowitz et al. (16)	1961–1965		7.2%	69/958	National Tumor registry in the Ministry of Health (unspecified cases are excluded)	69%	Both
India-Madras, Ramamurthi (17)	During 22 yr		15.9%	176/1106	Madras Center (vascular tumors and tuberculoma are excluded)	58%	100%
India-Bombay, Dastur et al. (18)	1953–1966		7.1%	67/948	Mainly three hospitals in Bombay	100%	88%
Ceylon-Colombo, Weinman (19)	1962–1971		7.0%	42/597	Single neurosurgical center	100%	100%
Thailand, Shuangshoti and Panyathanya (20)	1956–1973		4.9%	42/857	Records of several hospitals	100%	91%
Hong Kong, Wen and Cheung (21)	1968–1972		8.9%	20/224	Restricted to chinese patients in Hong Kong	100%	100%
China, Cheng (22)	1950–1976		11.8%	1410/11951	Records of 10 hospitals	No data	Both
China, Wen-qing et al. (23)	During 20 yr		10.2%	2137/20931	Combined 12 series	100%	Most
Taiwan, Shn (24)	1951–1973		8.6%	92/1074	Records of 4 hospitals	Most	100%
Taiwan, Kepes et al. (25)	1975–1982		17.3%	167/966	Records of 2 hospitals	100%	100%

Study (Ref)	Years	Cases	Percentage			Source
Taiwan-South part, Hwang and Howng (26)	1983–1992	107/462	23.2%	100%	100%	Kaohsiung Medical college Hospital records
Brasil, Lana-Peixoto et al. (27)	1938–1979	21/294	7.1%	100%	57%	Hospital records
Japan, Sano (28)	1969–1983	4503/28424	15.8%	Most	100%	The Committee of Brain Tumor Registry of Japan
Japan-Kumamoto, Kuratsu and Ushio (29)	1989–1994	204/1117	18.2%	79%	100%	Records of 27 hospitals
Personal series						
Cushing (US) (30)	1932	360/1893	20.0%			
Courville (US) (31)	1945	34/410	8.3%			
Olivecrona (Sweden) (32)	1952	368/3805	9.7%			
Razdlovsky (USSR) (33)	1954	75/669	11.2%			
Grant (US) (34)	1956	206/2088	9.9%			
Zimmerman (US) (35)	1969	229/3603	6.4%			
Zülch (West Germany) (36)	1986	480/5760	8.3%			
Total		14078/115897	12.1%			

[a]Metastatic brain tumors, granulomas, skull bone tumors, or nonneoplastic cysts are excluded whenever it may be possible. Percentage of histological confirmation or diagnosed cases before death means such cases/total primary brain tumors examined. Ref: reference.

[b]Only cases diagnosed before death.

Table 2
Average Annual Incidence Rates per 100,000 Population for Pituitary Adenomas[a]

Country and author, ref. no.	Time period	Source of Data	Incidence rate			Notes
			Male	T	Female	
US-Rochester, MN, Kurland (6)	1945–1954	Mayo Clinic records		1.5		
US-Rochester, MN, Percy et al. (5)	1935–1968	Mayo Clinic records	2.9	8.9	0.5	(Prevalence)
US-Olmsted County, MN, Annegers et al. (38)	1935–1977	Mayo Clinic records	2.8	1.1	1.1	(Craniopharyngiomas were included)
			0.5 (0.5)[b]		0.7 (0.7)[b]	(15–44 yr) } 1935–1969 yr
			2.8 (–4.6)		0.4 (0.7)	(<45 yr) }
			0 (0)		7.1 (7.1)	(15–44 yr) } 1970–1977 yr
			2.8 (4.1)		1.1 (1.1)	(<45 yr) }
US-Washington, DC, Heshman et al. (8)	1960–1967	Records and registries of 26 hospitals		0.4		
			0.23		0.22	(White)
			1.02		0.76	(Black)
US-Connecticut, Schoenberg et al. (4)	1935–1964	Connecticut Tumor Registry	0.43		0.46	(Craniopharyngiomas were included)
				0.16		(1935–44 yr)
				0.36		(1945–54 yr)
				0.71		(1955–64 yr)
US-Rochester, MN, Annegers et al. (7)	1935–1977	Mayo Clinic records	1.5 (2.1)[b]	1.7	1.7 (1.7)[b]	
				1.1		(1935–49 yr)
				0.9		(1950–64 yr)
				2.0		(1965–77 yr)
				0.9		
US-National survey, Walker et al. (10)	1973, 1974	Records of 166 cooperating hospitals				
US-Rochester, MN, Radhakrishman et al. (11)	1950–1989	Mayo Clinic records	2.4	2.8[b]		
			0.73	1.05		(1950–69 yr)
			3.55	4.02		(1970–89 yr)
Iceland, Gudmundsson (14)	1954–1963	All hospitals and state records		0.6		(Included autopsy cases)
				4.8		(Prevalence)
Israel, Leibowitz et al. (16)	1961–1965	National Tumor registry in the Ministry of Health		0.7		(Asia-born)
				0.6		(African-born)
				0.4		(Europe-born)
				0.6		(Israel-born)
				0.8		
Italy-Trento, Lovaste et al. (15)	1977–1984	Province of Trento	1.0		1.6	(Included autopsy)
			1.3		2.1	(20–44 yr)
Italy-Lombardian region, Ambrosi and Faglia (2)	1967–1986	Lombardian region		1.55		(Prevalence)
England-Carlisle, Brewis et al. (39)	1955–1961			19.9		(Prevalence)
				0.8		
England and Wales, Robinson et al. (40)	1957–1976	Hospital in-patient enquiry		5.6		(Prevalence)
			3.0		4.4	(15–44 yr) } 1957–1970 yr
			5.1		7.7	(45–64 yr) }
			3.3		7.2	(15–44 yr) } 1971–1976 yr
			5.1		7.5	(45–64 yr) }
Japan-Kumamoto, Kuratsu and Ushio (29)	1989–1994	27 Hospital records	1.5	1.8	2.2	

[a]T: total incidence rate, (prevalence): prevalence rate, yr: year.
[b]Includes the asymptomatic cases that were diagnosed by autopsy or neuroimaging examinations.

carried out in Vizcaya, Spain estimated that the total prevalence between 1975 and 1992 was 3.9/100,000 and the average annual incidence over the preceding 18 yr was 0.24/100,000 *(47)*.

TIME TRENDS

The study of time trends in the incidence of disease is important, since a true increase would have important implications with regard to environmental carcinogenesis and public health. Several investigators have reported that the frequency of primary brain tumors has increased substantially during the past two decades *(48,49)*. Some investigators have attributed this increase to the introduction of computed tomography (CT) in the 1970s and magnetic resonance imaging (MRI) in the 1980s, as well as improved medical care for the elderly *(50,51)*. Radhakrishnan et al. reanalyzed the incidence of primary brain tumors diagnosed in Rochester, MN over the 40 yr between 1950 and 1990, and recently concluded that the reported increase in primary brain tumors was an artifact resulting from improvements in diagnostic technology and medical practice, because they found no significant increase in the incidence of symptomatic primary brain tumors between 1950 and 1969 (9.5/100,000/yr) and 1970 and 1989 (12.5/100,000/yr), whereas there was a marked increase over the last two decades in tumors diagnosed incidentally by neuroimaging studies *(11)*.

There have been several reports on the time trends in the incidence of pituitary adenoma. Annegers et al. reported a rapid increase in the number of pituitary adenomas in women of childbearing age after 1970 in Olmsted County, MN: the mean annual incidence of 7.1/100,000 women aged 15–44 yr during 1970–1977 represented an impressive increase compared to the level of 0.7/100,000 in the population with the same age and sex during 1935–1969, whereas no such changes in incidence were found among males and older women *(38)*. They attributed the 10-fold increase in Minnesota since 1970 to improved diagnosis of these tumors in women suffering from galactorrhea, amenorrhea, and infertility owing to introduction of the measurement of serum prolactin (PRL) by radioimmunoassay (RIA) in the 1970s and advances in diagnostic radiology *(38,52)*. However, no such trend was detected in England and Wales when hospital discharge rates for pituitary tumors and related diseases were analyzed in women aged 15–44 yr from 1966–1967 to 1974–1976 *(40)*. In addition, Radhakrishnan et al. reported that the incidence of symptomatic pituitary adenoma increased significantly between 1950 and 1969 (0.73/100,000/yr) and 1970–1989 (3.55/100,000/yr) (*p* = 0.04), especially in the age group of 64 yr and younger, although the incidence of other symptomatic tumors showed no significant change *(11)*. They speculated that the increase in the incidence of pituitary adenoma among women of childbearing age may be owing to the increasing use of endocrinological and neuroradiological studies leading to the discovery of these tumors, accompanied by a great improvement of surgical treatment during the last two decades. A similar impressive increase in the incidence of pituitary tumors has been reported in Italy, where there was an upward trend from 1967 to 1982, followed thereafter by a slight decline *(2)*. In addition, they found a steeper slope for prolactinomas in the observed population after introduction of the RIA for PRL in 1974, whereas the trends for growth hormone (GH) cell adenoma and nonfunctioning adenoma were constant. They speculated that the increase may have been owing to the recognition of prolactinoma, the improvement of endocrinological and radiological techniques, or the greater attention of doctors to pituitary disease, with the decrease in new cases after 1982 being attributed to the expansion of knowledge and

interest in endocrinology causing referral of patients to other non-specialist hospitals and universities *(2)*. Such a tendency is also found in other reports comparing the incidence before and after 1970, since the average incidence was 0.77 (range: 0.1–1.5) *(4,6,7,14,16)* before 1970, whereas it was 1.57 (range: 0.9–2.0) after this date *(7,10,30)*. The total number of pituitary tumors and the incidence among primary brain tumors also both increased from the mid1970s to 1979 and then remained stable in Japan, according to data based on surgical material *(29)*. In contrast, the annual incidence of acromegaly, as mentioned already, shows no difference before 1971 (0.3) *(43)* and afterward (0.4) *(44)* (0.3) *(45)*. Moreover, the annual number of new cases of acromegaly between 1955 and 1985 varied from 2 to 10 in Northern Ireland, but there was no significant difference before and after 1970 *(46)*. Therefore, an increase in the incidence or frequency of pituitary adenomas may not be owing to epidemiological factors, but to the recognition of prolactinoma and to diagnostic improvement, although these data did not always include patients with prolactinoma treated by medication alone.

AGE AND GENDER DISTRIBUTION

The age distribution of pituitary tumors has been reported by a number of authors. There is a significant age difference between women and men, and the number of patients younger than 20 yr and older than 71 yr is very low in any series *(2,28,53,54)*. The peak incidence in both sexes occurs in the third decade *(2,53)*, the fourth decade *(18,23,26,28,54)*: 57.3% (Canada) *(54)*, 66.5% (US) *(53)*, 66.8% (Japan) *(28)*, and 72.5% (Italy) *(2)* of pituitary adenomas was found between the third and the fifth decades. With respect to the average annual sex- and age-specific incidence of pituitary adenoma, Leibowitz et al. reported two blunt incidence peaks in the fifth and seventh decades *(16)*. In contrast, Kuratsu and Ushio reported two peaks in women, one during the childbearing years (third decade) and the other in the seventh decade, whereas the rate increased with age in males *(29)*.

A male predominance of pituitary adenoma with a male:female ratio ranging from 1.1 to 5.8 was found before 1970, whereas a female preponderance was observed more recently, with a female:male ratio ranging between 1.23 and 2.05 *(2,5–8,10,11, 14–17,19,21,23,25,26,28,29,38)* (Table 3). This recent female preponderance may be mainly owing to the marked female preponderance of PRL cell adenoma. In addition, the much higher female:male ratio reported by Ambrosi and Faglia in Italy may be because they also included patients treated by medication alone as opposed to other reports based solely on surgical material *(2)*. Few authors studied the age and sex distribution according to the type of adenoma. In addition, it is quite difficult to compare these data among different studies, because each author used a different classification of pituitary adenoma. However, several common trends were revealed by these reports *(2,28,53,54)*. In general, functioning tumors were more common at a younger age, whereas nonfunctioning tumors were more common at an older age *(53,55,56)*. PRL cell adenomas were found in young women, with a peak incidence in the third decade of life and were the most common adenoma from the third to fourth decades. After the fifth decade, however, PRL cell adenomas decreased in all series and showed an equal frequency in both sexes or even became more common in men. In addition, Ambrosi and Faglia reported that the female:male ratio was very high for microprolactinoma (19.84), but it was almost 1 for macroprolactinoma *(2)*. Another type of

Table 3
Male:Female Ratio of Reported Cases or of Incidence Rate of Pituitary Adenomas

Author, ref. no.	Time period	No. of cases	Male/female ratio
Gudmundsson (14)	1954–1963	12	2.0
Leibowitz et al. (16)	1961–1965	69	1.2
Weinman (19)	1962–1971	42	3.7
Wen and Cheung (21)	1968–1972	20	1.2
Ramamurthi (17)	During 22 yr	176	2.2
Walker et al. (10)	1973,1974	1970	0.6
Wen-qing et al. (23)	During 20 yr	2137	1.4
Radhakrishnan et al. (11)	1950–1989	55	0.4
Kepes et al. (25)	1975–1982	167	1.4
Hwang and Howng (26)	1983–1992	107	0.8
Sano (28)	1969–1983	4503	0.8
Ambrosi and Faglia (2)	1967–1986	2137	0.5

Country, ref. no.	Time period	Male/female ratio of incidence rate, include autopsy cases		
US-Rochester, MN (6)	1945–1954	5.8		
US-Rochester, MN (5)	1935–1968	2.5		
US-Rochester, MN (7)	1935–1977	0.9	(1.2)	
US-Olmsted County, MN (38)	1935–1969	0.7	(0.7)	(15–44 yr)
		7	(6.6)	(<45 yr)
	1970–1977	All female		(15–44 yr)
		2.5	(3.7)	(<45 yr)
US-Washington, DC (8)	1960–1967	1.1	(white)	
		1.3	(black)	
Italy-Trento (15)	1977–1984	0.6		
		0.6	(20–44 yr)	
Japan-Kumamoto (29)	1989–1994	0.7		

functioning adenoma, GH cell adenoma, shows the peak occurrence in the fifth decade with no sex predominance. However, some reports have described a female preponderance of acromegaly with a sex ratio of 1.8–2.0:1 (45,57). In addition, pure GH cell adenomas can be classified into densely granulated and sparsely granulated types (55). The latter has been reported in Japan to be more common in younger females, but no such tendency was observed in Canada (54,57). Corticotropic (ACTH) cell adenomas are also a disease found in women, with a female:male ratio of 3–8:1. The peak occurrence of this tumor is in the fourth decade owing to a female preponderance in the same age group. However, other authors have reported a much higher female predominance (15:1) and a higher frequency in the sixth decade, with no explanation of such discrepancies (47). In contrast, the occurrence in men remains almost constant throughout life. The peak occurrence of nonfunctioning pituitary adenoma was in the fifth or seventh decade without a sex preponderance in Japan, or with a male predominance (29). The much older peak incidence of nonfunctioning adenoma reported by Terada et al. may be because they only classified null-cell adenoma and oncocytoma as nonfunctioning adenoma (54). Clinically nonfunctioning adenomas are histologically heterogeneous and include null-cell adenomas or oncocytomas and silent adenomas (55). The former is more common in men over 50 yr old, whereas silent types of nonfunctioning adenomas are more common in younger females (56). In addition, the peak incidence of oncocytoma is one decade older than that of null-cell adenoma (56). These data may reflect the finding of Mindermamm and Wilson that nonfunctioning adenomas before the fourth decade were more common in women (53).

INCIDENCE OF VARIOUS TYPES OF PITUITARY ADENOMA

Comparison of the incidence of various types of pituitary adenoma among studies is quite difficult because of the different tumor classifications that were employed, ranging from clinical data or staining properties alone to immunohistochemical data or electron microscopic features plus immunohistochemistry. Based on clinical endocrine activity, the most frequent type of pituitary adenoma is prolactinoma, accounting for 50.1% of 2252 patients in Italy and 39.0% of 2230 surgical cases in San Francisco, followed by nonfunctioning adenoma (23.1 or 27.4%), GH cell adenoma (21.4 or 16.4%), ACTH cell adenoma (4.7 or 16.3%), and thyroid-stimulating hormone (TSH) and follicle-stimulating hormone (FSH)/luteinizing hormone (LH) cell adenoma (0.4–0.2 and 0.9%, respectively) (2,53). The lower incidence of prolactinoma among surgical cases may be owing to the absence of patients treated by medication alone. The same trends in the incidence of various types of adenoma are found in surgical cases in Japan: prolactinoma, 33.6%; nonfunctioning adenoma, 30.3%; GH cell adenoma, 20.1%; ACTH cell adenoma, 8.6%; and other functioning adenomas, 1.4% (28). These data suggest no racial predilection in the incidence of various types of adenoma. When adenomas are classified based on immunohistochemical and/or ultrastructural examination of surgical material, the incidence is quite difficult to compare among studies, because each investigator has used his or her own classification and investigation of a more widely accepted new classification is still ongoing (58–61). When we compared two studies that used the Kovacs and Horvath classification (55,62), both seemed to show no great differences and

Table 4
Incidence of Pituitary Adenomas Based on Histopathological Findings

	Terada et al. (54)		Kameya (59)	
	No. of cases	Incidence, %	No. of cases	Incidence, %
GH cell adenoma	85	13.1	31	13.7
Densely granulated	36	5.6	20	9.3
Sparsely granulated	49	7.6	10	4.4
PRL cell adenoma	178	27.5	43	18.9
Densely granulated	172	26.6	41	18.1
Sparsely granulated	6	0.9	2	0.8
GH and PRL cell adenoma	40	6.2	41	18.1
ACTH cell adenoma	84	13.0	9	4.0
TSH cell adenoma	6	0.9	3	1.3
Gonadotroph cell adenoma	64	9.9	25	11.0
Nonfunctioning adenoma	168	26.0	69	30.4
Null-cell adenoma	57	8.8	42	18.5
Oncocytoma	84	13.0	22	9.7
Silent adenoma	27	4.2	5	2.2
Unclassified plurihormonal adenoma	19	2.9	6	2.6
Unclassified adenoma	3	0.5		
Total	647	100	227	100

reflected the incidence as classified by the clinical endocrine activity *(54,59)* (Table 4). However, densely granulated and sparsely granulated GH cell adenomas show an almost equal incidence in North America *(54)*, whereas densely granulated adenomas are reported to be about twice as common as sparsely granulated adenomas in Japan *(57,59)*. It is still unclear whether this difference is significant and why it exists, but it might be because of some genetic factor. Recent studies on GH cell adenomas have suggested that a somatic mutation of G_s protein is found in a subset of these tumors and plays an important role in tumorigenesis. Such mutations have been reported in 40 and 36% of GH cell adenomas in the US and Italy, respectively *(63,64)*. In contrast, there is a significantly lower incidence of G_s protein mutation in Japan (<10%) *(65,66)*.

AUTOPSY MATERIALS

Pituitary adenomas that have existed without any apparent or recognized clinical symptoms are rather common at autopsy. Despite Erdheim and Stumme's report of an incidence of 8.5% in the autopsy pituitary glands *(67)*, these adenomas were considered rare until the early 1930s, when Susman and Costello reported adenomas in 8.5 and 22.5%, respectively, of pituitary glands examined at autopsy *(68,69)*. These adenomas incidentally found at autopsy were termed "subclinical adenomas" by Costello, since the majority (irrespective of type) were entirely benign, caused no recognizable symptoms, and could be demonstrated only by rather detailed examination of the pituitary gland. There have been several subsequent reports on the occurrence of incidental pituitary adenoma at autopsy (Table 5) *(67–85)*, and the incidence has ranged widely between a high of 27, 24, and 22.5% *(69,78,79)* and a low of 1.5, 2.7, and 3.2% *(72,81,85)*. Overall, 1301 adenomas were incidentally found in 13,792 examined pituitaries (9.4%). The main factors affecting the incidence are the definition of pituitary adenoma used by the investigators and how many sections of the pituitary gland are studied. For example, Hardy and Uei et al. reported the lowest frequencies (2.7 and 3.2%, respectively), but only used a single-section technique to study the pituitary *(72,85)*, whereas Burrow et al. and Costello reported a higher incidence and

sectioned the pituitary at 1- and 1.5-mm intervals *(69,79)*. Therefore, the single-cut technique probably missed many small adenomas. However, Muhr et al. reported the lowest frequency of 1.5%, although multiple sections were studied *(81)*. Similarly, the incidence of multiple adenoma at autopsy also varies, ranging from 0 to 25% *(69,71,74,76–81,84,85)*. Overall, multiple adenomas were found in 32 out of 323 patients with pituitary adenoma detected incidentally at autopsy (9.9%). This percentage is much higher than that reported for surgical cases (0.37%) *(86)*. The reason for this great differences in the frequency of multiple adenoma between surgical and autopsy materials remains unknown at present.

The age- and sex-related occurrence of pituitary adenoma at autopsy is also different from that in surgical cases. Incidental adenomas are found at autopsy in patients of all ages from 2 to 98 yr old. The highest incidence is variously noted in the fifth *(80,87)*, sixth *(69,77,85,87)*, seventh *(78,80)*, and eighth and higher *(80)* decades of life. In contrast, Burrow et al. reported that pituitary adenoma occurred in all age groups and that the age distribution of patients with adenoma did not differ from that of the whole autopsy population *(79)*. Moreover, Uei et al. reported that the incidence of adenoma was significantly lower under the age of 30 in both sexes *(85)*. The male:female ratio varies from 1.0 to 2.0, suggesting a slight male predominance *(69,71,76,80,81,85)*. The size of the adenomas found at autopsy also varies, but the vast majority are microadenomas <5 mm in diameter, and only three tumors more than 10 mm in greatest diameter have been reported *(74,77,85)*. This suggests that most of the adenomas found at autopsy are slowly growing tumors with no mass effect on the surrounding tissues and have a relatively benign course. These incidental microadenomas are mainly localized in antero-lateral wing of the pituitary *(77,80,85,87)*. Immunohistochemical studies have disclosed that PRL cell adenoma and nonfunctioning adenoma (null-cell adenoma and oncocytoma) are the most common types of the pituitary adenoma found at autopsy (PRL: 21–42%, nonfunctioning: 18–63%) *(76,79,80,85,87)*. Burrow et al. calculated that more than 1 in 10 persons in the general population dies with a prolactinoma *(79)*. McComb et al. studied 107 adenomas

Table 5
Frequency of Pituitary Adenomas Found at Autopsy[a]

Author, ref. no.	Year	No. of autopsies	No. of sections	Adenomas			The highest age incidence, range	M:F ratio	Multiple adenoma		Staining property	Immunohistochemistry
				No.	MA	Percent			No.	Percent		
Erdheim and Stumme (67)	1909	118		10		8.5						
Susman (68)	1933	260	Routine necropsy	22		8.5					C:26%, E:32%, B:42%	
Close (70)	1934	280	Single or 6–12 sections	39		14.0					C:95%, E:5%	
Costello (69)	1936	1000	1 to 1.5-mm intervals	225	0	22.5	6th (2–86 yr)	1.1	Several		C:53%, E:8.0%, B:27%, M:12%	
Sommers (71)	1959	400	Single	26	0	6.5		1.0	2	7.7		
Hardy (72)	1969	1000	Single section	27	0	2.7						
McCormick and Halmi (73)	1971	1600	Three sections	145	0	9.1					C: 0%, E: 59%, B: 18%, M: 16%	
Haugen (74)	1973	170 (All males and ≤40 yr)	Two sections	33	1	19.4			3	9.1		
Landolt (75)	1980	100	Two sections	13	0	13.0						
Kovacs et al. (76)	1980	152 (All ≥80 yr)	One or two sections	20	0	13.0		2.0	2	10.0	C: 100%	PRL: 53% GH + PRL: 6% others: 6% immunonegative
Parent et al. (77)	1981	500	Three sections	42	1	8.5	6th (6–85 yr)		3	7.1	Mainly chromo-phobic	
Mosca et al. (78)	1980	100	1-mm intervals	24	0	24.0	7th (28–98 yr)		0			
Burrow et al. (79)	1981	120	1-mm intervals	32	0	27.0	Even distribution (16–86 yr)		8	25.0		PRL: 41%
Teramoto et al. (80)	1981	1000	Three sections	58	0	5.8	5th and 7th	1.2	3	5.2	C: 95%, E: 5%, B: 0%	PRL: 30% GH: 7% Non: 63%
Muhr et al. (81)	1981	205	400-μ intervals	3	0	1.5		1.5	0			
Chambers et al. (82)	1982	100		14	0	14.0						
Schwesinger and Warzok (83)	1982	5100	Five sections	482	0	9.5						
Kontogeorgos et al. (84)	1991	470	Single up to 12 sections	49		10.2			4	8.2		
Uei et al. (85)	1994	1117	Single	36	1	3.2	6th (16–80 yr)	1.6	7	19.0	C: 68%, E: 18%, B: 14%	GH: 18% PRL: 21%

[a]MA: Number of macroadenoma. M:F ratio: male:female ratio, C: chromophobic, E: eosinophilic, B: basophilic, M: mixed.

found at autopsy, and stated that null-cell adenoma (51%) and PRL cell adenoma (42%) were the two most common types (87). In addition, there is no sex preponderance in the incidence of prolactinoma at autopsy unlike the female predominance in surgical patients (79,87). This may suggest that the initiating events for PRL cell adenoma are the same in both sexes, but the promoting factors (e.g., estrogen) are more active in women, resulting in clinical manifestation of this adenoma in the female sex. It has been reported that estrogen can enhance tumor growth-promoting factors in pituitary cell lines (88). In contrast, it is not surprising that other types of functioning adenoma secreting GH, TSH, or ACTH are rare, because these tumors are generally associated with clinically apparent endocrinopathy, and thus are diagnosed early and removed surgically. Kovacs et al. reported on a series of 152 unselected autopsy patients more than 80 yr old, and found that 9 of 17 cases examined by the immunoperoxidase technique were immunopositive for PRL (76). These findings suggest that the most common adenoma in autopsy pituitaries, the occurrence of which is not limited by age or sex, is the PRL cell adenoma. Some investigators have reported that incidental microadenomas are more frequent at autopsy in patients with cancer of the pancreas, rectum, or bronchus (68), patients with prostate carcinomas (74), or patients with hypertension or diabetes mellitus (77), whereas no correlation was found in most reports between the adenoma and the clinical findings, underlying disease, other endocrine disease, duration of illness, treatment, or cause of death.

In contrast, the frequency of incidental pituitary adenoma in normal persons is unknown. Hall et al. recently studied 100 normal volunteers (70 women and 30 men aged 18–60 yr) using high-resolution MRI before and after gadolium-diethylenetriaminepentaacetic acid (Gd-DTPA) administration, and concluded that 10 (7 women and 3 men) had suspected pituitary adenomas ranging from 3 to 6 mm in greatest diameter (89). Interestingly, this value (10%) corresponds well with that (9.3%) of incidental adenoma in autopsy series.

These epidemiological studies show a very high frequency of subclinical adenomas (9.4%) compared with clinically overt adenomas, suggesting that pituitary adenomas are generally benign, slow-growing, and that they rarely become symptomatic. An alternative interpretation is that the initiating events for pituitary tumorigenesis are quite common, whereas the factors promoting tumor growth are rarer. However, the true factors explaining discrepancy between these findings remain unknown.

PITUITARY ADENOMAS IN CHILDHOOD

Pituitary adenoma is very rare in childhood, and Gold reported that the average annual incidence was 0.1/million in Denmark from 1935 to 1959, accounting for 1.1% of all childhood intracranial tumors (1). This figure is comparable with other series reporting an incidence of 1.2% among all supratentorial tumors (90) and 0.1–1.6% among all intracranial tumors in children (22,28,91). It has also been reported that children represent 2.3–3.6% of all individuals with pituitary adenoma treated by transsphenoidal surgery (92–95). These data suggest that the incidence of pediatric pituitary adenoma does not differ between countries.

Pituitary adenomas in pediatric patients generally become symptomatic in childhood, but the majority of operations are undertaken during the adolescent years (95). However, several cases of ACTH cell adenoma and one case of GH cell adenoma in infancy have been reported (96–99). In childhood, ACTH and PRL cell adenomas are the most common types, especially before puberty for ACTH cell tumors and during or after puberty for PRL

cell tumors, whereas nonfunctioning adenomas (including silent gonadotroph cell adenomas) are extremely rare (92,94,95,100). This is opposite to the situation in adults among whom nonfunctioning adenomas predominate. In addition, as in adults, TSH cell adenomas seem to be extremely rare in children (100). In contrast, GH cell adenomas are reported to have the most even distribution in the various age groups and account for about 10% of surgically treated pituitary adenomas in patients under 20 yr of age (100). Regarding sex, a preponderance of females has been described, which may largely reflect the relative contributions of the two major types of adenomas, PRL and ACTH cell tumors (92,95). However, an equal sex predilection of childhood ACTH cell adenoma has been reported, unlike the female preponderance of this tumor in adults (101,102). In addition, when compared with adults, pituitary adenoma (Cushing's disease) is a less common cause of Cushing's syndrome in children (accounting for about 50%), especially younger children (102). Also, when compared with children having other adenoma types, multiple pituitary adenoma seems to occur more frequently (4.7%) in children with ACTH cell adenoma (100).

Histological examination suggests that a high proportion of the tumors have plurihormonal immunopositivity (95). Scheithauer et al. found in their review of plurihormonal adenomas that 10% of them were operated on during childhood or adolescence (103). Moreover, a predominance of macroadenomas (macro:micro, 1.4:1) has been noted (94), especially among PRL cell adenomas (92). Some authors have also suggested that childhood pituitary adenomas were more likely to be locally invasive or aggressive than those in adults (104,105), whereas others have not found such evidence (94,106).

PATHOGENESIS OF PITUITARY ADENOMAS

Accumulating evidence indicates that the development of pituitary adenoma is a multistep and multietiology process consisting of an initiation phase and a subsequent promotion phase. In addition, recent advances in molecular biology have confirmed that most pituitary adenomas are monoclonal in origin, which favors a somatic mutation contributing to tumorigenesis (107–109). Nevertheless, initiating mutations have only been discovered in a minority of these tumors, e.g., somatic mutations in the α-chain of the GTP-binding protein G_s have been reported in some GH cell adenomas (63,64). Somatic mutations of G_s protein into a putative oncogene termed "gsp (G_s protein)" via point mutation at two critical sites (arginine 201 and glycine 227) lead to constitutive activation of G_s by inhibiting GTP hydrolysis and stabilizing α in the active GTP-bond form. This G_s protein in adenoma cells provides a continuous signal for endocrine activity and cell proliferation without the need for promoting factors (63,64). However, G_s protein is usually restricted to GH cell adenomas (110) and is rarely found in other types of adenomas (111). They are found in 35–40% of Caucasians (112,113) and 40% of Koreans with acromegaly (114), whereas there is a significantly lower incidence (<10%) in Japan (65,66). In contrast, mutations of another candidate oncogene involving ras, protein kinase C (PKC), and c-erbB2 (neu) are rare or absent in pituitary adenomas (115), although ras mutations may play a role in invasive or malignant transformation of pituitary adenomas (116). Recently, a novel pituitary tumor transforming gene (PTTG) has been isolated by differential-display polymerase chain reaction using mRNA derived from rat pituitary tumor cells and normal pituitary tissue (117). Overexpression of PTTG mRNA was found in most pituitary adenomas, suggesting that PTTG is an early molecular requirement for pituitary tumor formation *(118)*.

Inactivation of suppressor genes is another possible cause of tumorigenesis. Familial pituitary adenomas are well known to be associated with multiple endocrine neoplasia type 1 (MEN 1). MEN 1-susceptibility locus was mapped to chromosome llql3 by a genetic linkage study *(119)* and, after a decade of intensive search, the *MEN1* gene was identified by positional cloning and its 610- amino acid predicted protein was termed "menin" *(120)*. In MEN 1, germ-line mutations in the *MEN1* gene have been found in most familial and sporadic patients with *MEN1 (121,122)*. The author and his colleagues reported specific loss of heterozygosity (LOH) on chromosome llql3 in brothers with familial acrogigantism *(123)*, but no germ-line mutation of *MEN1* gene was detected in three pedigrees of familial pituitary adenoma without *MEN1 (122)*, suggesting that a suppressor gene on chromosome llql3 other than *MEN1* gene may be etiological for familial pituitary adenoma without *MEN1*. Similarly, LOH on chromosome 11 was reported in sporadic pituitary adenomas *(110)*, but no mutations of *MEN1* gene were found in these tumors *(124)*, suggesting that an additional suppressor gene at this locus may be more commonly involved in the pathogenesis of sporadic pituitary adenomas. Moreover, extensive studies of other suppressor genes, including the *Rb* gene *(125)*, p53 *(126)*, cyclindependent kinase (CDK) inhibitors *(127)*, and purine-binding factor nm23 *(128)*, have confirmed inactivation in the few exceptional cases but not in most adenomas. Thus, these data suggest that most pituitary adenomas originate from a single cell that undergoes spontaneous or acquired somatic change (initiation) and grow by subsequent clonal expansion (promotion) related to intrinsic mutation or to extrinsic promoting factors, but there have been no common somatic mutations found in the majority of these tumors.

Factors causing an excess of hypothalamic releasing hormones or the lack of inhibitory hormones could play a role in promoting tumors. Moreover, intratumoral hypothalamic-releasing hormones and several growth factors can act as self-maintaining promoting agents by paracrine and/or autocrine mechanisms *(129–131)*. However, it still remains uncertain whether such chronic hyperstimulation itself can cause somatic mutation or can facilitate spontaneous mutation. Animal experiments have indicated that estrogen, oral contraceptives, thyroidectomy, and gonadectomy can all induce pituitary adenomas *(1)*. Moreover, a recent study using GH releasing hormone (GHRH) transgenic mice indicated true pituitary adenoma formation from GH cell hyperplasia *(132)*. However, pituitary adenomas do not usually arise in a setting of endocrinological imbalance, although GH cell adenoma associated with a parasellar neuronal tumor producing GHRH has been reported *(133)*. Epidemiological studies have also indicated neither an increased risk of pituitary adenoma *(134,135)*, nor tumor enlargement in women on oral contraceptives *(136)*. Similarly, there is no definite evidence that radiation or chemical carcinogens, both reviewed well by Gold *(1)*, play a role in the development of pituitary adenoma in human, although both can induce this tumor in experimental animals. Finally, there is no evidence that viruses are involved in pituitary tumorigenesis, despite the rare detection of virus-like particles in human pituitary adenomas *(137)*.

REFERENCES

1. Gold EB. Epidemiology of pituitary adenomas. Epidemiol Rev 1981;3:163–183.
2. Ambrosi B, Faglia G. Epidemiology of pituitary tumors. In: Faglia G, Beck-Peccoz P, Ambrosi B, Travaglini P, Spada A, eds. Pituitary Adenomas: New Trends in Basic and Clinical Research. Elsevier Science Publishers, Amsterdam, The Netherlands, 1991, pp. 159–168.
3. Faglia G. Epidemiology and pathogenesis of pituitary adenomas. Acta Endocrinol 1993;129(Suppl):1–5.
4. Schoenberg BS, Christine BW, Whisnant JP. The descriptive epidemiology of primary intracranial neoplasms: Connecticut experience. Am J Epidemiol 1976;104:499–510.
5. Percy AK, Elveback LR, Okazaki H, Kurland LT. Neoplasms of the central nervous system. Neurology 1972;22:40–48.
6. Kurland LT. The frequency of intracranial and intraspinal neoplasms in the resident population of Rochester, Minnesota. J Neurosurg 1958;15:627–641.
7. Annegers JF, Schoenberg BS, Okazaki H, Kurland LT. Epidemiologic study of primary intracranial neoplasms. Arch Neurol 1981;38:217–219.
8. Heshman MY, Kovi J, Simpson C, Kennedy J, Fan KJ. Neoplasms of the central nervous system. Incidence and population selectivity in the Washington DC, Metropolitan area. Cancer 1976;38: 2135–2142.
9. Fan K-J, Kovi J, Earle KM. The ethnic distribution of primary central nervous system tumors: AFIP, 1958 to 1970. J Neuropath Exp Neurol 1977;36:41–49.
10. Walker AE, Robins M, Weinfeld FD. Epidemiology of brain tumors: the national survey of intracranial neoplasms. Neurology 1985; 35:219–226.
11. Radhakrishnan K, Mokri B, Parisi JE, O'Fallon WM, Sunku J, Kurland LT. The trends in incidence of primary brain tumors in the population of Rochester, Minnesota. Ann Neurol 1995;37:67–73.
12. Maroun FB, Jacob JC. The frequency of intracranial neoplasms in Newfoundland. Can J Public Health 1973;64:53–57.
13. Joensen P. Incidence of primary intracranial neoplasms in an isolated population (The faroese) during the period 1962-1975. Acta Neurol Scand 1981;64:74–78.
14. Gudmundsson KR. A survey of tumors of the central nervous system in Iceland during the 10-year period 1954-1963. Acta Neurol Scand 1970;46:538–552.
15. Lovaste MG, Ferrari G, Rossi G. Epidemiology of primary intracranial neoplasms. Experiment in the province of Trento (Italy), 1977-1984. Neuroepidemiology 1986;5:220–232.
16. Leibowitz U, Yablonski M, Alter M. Tumors of the nervous system. J Chron Dis 1971;23:707–721.
17. Ramamurthi B. Intracranial tumors in India: incidence and variations. Int Surg 1973;58:542–547.
18. Dastur DK, Lalitha VS, Prabhakar V. Pathological analysis of intracranial space-occupying lesions in 1000 cases including children. Part 1. age, sex and pattern; and tuberculomas. J Neurol Sci 1968;6:575–592.
19. Weinman DF. Incidence and behavior pattern of intracranial tumors in Ceylon. Int Surg 1973;58:548–554.
20. Shuangshoti S, Panyathanya R. Neural neoplasms in Thailand: a study of 2897 cases. Neurology 1974;24:1127–1134.
21. Wen HL, Cheung SYC. Incidence of tumors in the nervous system in Hong Kong. Int Surg 1973;58:555–556.
22. Cheng MK. Brain tumors in the People's Republic of China: a statistical review. Neurosurgery 1982;10:16–21.
23. Wen-qing H, Shi-ju Z, Qing-sheng T, Jian-qing H, Yu-xia L, Qingzhong X, et al. Statistical analysis of central nervous system tumors in China. J Neurosurg 1982;56:555–564.
24. Shih C-J. Intracranial tumors in Taiwan. A cooperative survey of 1,200 cases with special reference to intracranial tumors in children. J Formosan Med Assoc 1977;76:301–310.
25. Kepes JJ, Chen WYK, Pang LC, Kepes M. Tumors of the central nervous system in Taiwan, Republic of China. Surg Neurol 1884;22:149–156.
26. Hwang SL, Howng SL. An analysis of brain tumors in south Taiwan. Kaohsiung J Med Sci 1992;8:656–664.
27. Lana-Peixoto MA, Pittella JEH, Arouca EMG. Tumores primarios intracranianos. ARQ (San Paulo) 1981;39:13–24.

28. Sano K. Incidence of primary tumors (1969–1983) In: Brain Tumor Registry of Japan. Neurologia Medico Chirurgica, 37. Special Issue, 1992, pp. 391–441.

29. Kuratsu J, Ushio Y. Epidemiological study of primary intracranial tumors: a regional survey in Kumamoto Prefecture in the southern part of Japan. J Neurosurg 1996;84:946–950.

30. Cushing HW. Intracranial Tumours. Notes upon a Series of Two Thousand Verified Cases with Surgical Mortality Percentages Pertaining Thereto. Charles C. Thomas, Springfield, IL, 1932, p. 150.

31. Courville BC. Pathology of the Central Nervous System, 2nd ed. Pacific Press, Palo Alto, CA, 1945, p. 351.

32. Olivecrona H. The cerebellar angioreticulomas. J Neurosurg 1952;9:317–330.

33. Razdlovsky EY. Tumors of the Brain. Izdatelstvo Meditsina, Moscow, 1954, pp. 12–13, 206–207.

34. Grant FC. A study of the results of surgical treatment in 2,326 consecutive patients with brain tumor. J Neurosurg 1956;13:479–488.

35. Zimmerman HM. Brain tumors: their incidence and classification in man and their experimental production. Ann NY Acad Sci 1969;159:337–359.

36. Zülch KJ. Brain tumors. Their Biology and Pathology, 3rd ed. Springer-Verlag, Berlin, 1986.

37. Christy NP. Diagnosis and treatment of pituitary tumors. In: Beeson PB, McDermott W, eds. Textbook of Medicine, 14th ed. WB Saunders, Philadelphia, 1975, pp. 1687–1689.

38. Annegers JF, Coulam CB, Abboud CF, Laws ER Jr, Kurland LT. Pituitary adenomas in Olmsted country, Minnesota, 1935–1977. Mayo Clin Proc 1978;53:641–643.

39. Brewis M, Poskanzer DC, Rolland C, Miller H. Neurological disease in an English city. Acta Neurol Scand 1966;42(Suppl):21–23, 41–46.

40. Robinson N, Beral V, Ashley JS. Incidence of pituitary adenoma in women. Lancet 1979;22:630.

41. Batrinos ML, Panitsa FC, Tsiganou E, Liapi C. Incidence and characteristics of microprolactinomas (3–5 mm) in 4199 women assayed for prolactin. Horm Metab Res 1992;24:384–391.

42. Katayanagi N, Miyachi Y. Statistical survey of prolactin producing tumor in Japan. Nippon Rinsho 51(Suppl):33–38, 1993 (in Japanese).

43. Alexander L, Appleton D, Hall R, Ross WM, Wilkinson R. Epidemiology of acromegaly in The Newcastle region. Clin Endocrinol 1980;12:71–79.

44. Ritchie CM, Atkinson AB, Kennedy AL, Lyons AR, Gordon DS, Fannin T, et al. Ascertainment and natural history of treated acromegaly in Northern Ireland. Ulster Med J 1990;59:55–62.

45. Etxabe J, Gaztambide S, Latorre P, Vazquez JA. Acromegaly: an epidemiological study. J Endocrinol Invest 1993;16:181–187.

46. Bengtsson BA, Eden S, Ernest I, Oden A, Sjogren B. Epidemiology and long-term survival in acromegaly. A study of 166 cases diagnosed between 1995 and 1984. Acta Med Scand 1988;223:327–335.

47. Etxabe J, Vazquez JA. Morbidity and mortality in Cushing's disease: an epidemiological approach. Clin Endocrinol 1994;40:479–484.

48. Greig NH, Ries LG, Yancik R, Rapoport SI. Increasing annual incidence of primary malignant brain tumors in the elderly. J Natl Cancer Inst 1990;82:1621–1624.

49. Davis DL, Ahlbom A, Hoel D, Percy C. Is brain cancer mortality increasing in industrial countries? Am J Ind Med 1991;19:421–431.

50. Doll R, Peto R. The causes of cancer: quantitative estimates of avoidable risks of cancer in the United States today. J Natl Cancer Inst 1981;66:1191–1308.

51. Helseth A. The incidence of primary central nervous system neoplasms before and after computerized tomography availability. J Neurosurg 1995;83:999–1003.

52. Collins WF. Adenomas of the pituitary gland-an epidemic? Surg Clin North Am 1980;60:1201–1206.

53. Mindermann T, Wilson CB. Age-related and gender-related occurrence of pituitary adenomas. Clin Endocrinol 1994;41:359–364.

54. Terada T, Kovacs K, Stefaneanu L, Horvath E. Incidence, pathology, and recurrence of pituitary adenomas: study of 647 unselected surgical cases. Endocrinol Pathol 1995;6:301–310.

55. Horvath E, Kovacs K. The adenohypophysis. In: Kovacs K, Asa SL, eds. Functioning Endocrine Pathology, vol. 1. Blackwell, Boston, 1990, pp. 245–281.

56. Yamada S, Aiba T, Horvath E, Kovacs K. Morphological study of clinically nonsecreting pituitary adenomas in patients under 40 years of age. J Neurosurg 1991;75:902–905.

57. Yamada S, Aiba T, Sano T, Kovacs K, Shishiba Y, Sawano S, Takada K. Growth hormone-producing pituitary adenomas: correlations between clinical characteristics and morphology. Neurosurgery 1993;33:20–27.

58. Trouillas J, Girod C. Adenomes hypophysaires: histologie et cytologie. Encyclopedie Medico-Chirurgicale (Paris) 10-023-A-10, 1994, pp. 1–15.

59. Kameya T. Classification of pituitary adenomas: proposal of a new classification by surgical pathologist. Horumon To Rhinsho 44(Suppl):26–29, 1996 (in Japanese).

60. Osamura RY, Sanno N, Teramoto A. Clinical and cytofunctional classification of pituitary adenomas: proposal of a new classification [Editorial]. Endocrinol Pathol 1995;6:253–256.

61. Kovacs K, Scheithauer BW, Horvath E, Lloyd RV. The WHO classification of adenohypophysial neoplasms: a proposed five-tier scheme. Cancer 1996;78:502–510.

62. Kovacs K, Horvath E. Tumors of the pituitary gland. In: Atlas of Tumor Pathology. Fascicle 21, 2nd ser. Armed Forces Institute of Pathology, Washington, DC, 1986.

63. Vallar L, Spada A, Giannattasio G. Altered Gs and adenylate cyclase activity in human GH secreting pituitary tumors. Nature 1987;330:566–567.

64. Landis CA, Masters SB, Spada, A, Pace AM, Bourne HR, Vallar L. GTPase inhibiting mutations activate the alpha chain of Gs and stimulate adenyl cyclase in human pituitary tumors. Nature 1989;340:692–696.

65. Yoshimoto K, Iwahana H, Fukuda A, Sano T, Itakura M. Rare mutations of the Gs alpha subunit gene in human endocrine tumors. Cancer 1993;72:1386–1393.

66. Hosoi E, Yokogoshi Y, Hosoi E, Horie H, Sano T, Yamada S, et al. Analysis of the Gs α gene in growth hormone-secreting pituitary adenomas by the polymerase chain reaction-direct sequencing method using paraffin-embedded tissues. Acta Endocrinol 1993;129:301–306.

67. Erdheim J, Stumme E. Uber die Schwangelschaftsveranderung der Hypophyse. Beitr Pathol Anat 1909;46:1–132.

68. Susman W. Pituitary adenomas. Br Med J 1933;2:1215.

69. Costello RT. Subclinical adenoma of the pituitary gland. Am J Pathol 1936;12:205–215.

70. Close HG. The incidences of adenomas of the pituitary body in some types of new growth. Lancet 1934;1:732–734.

71. Sommers SC. Pituitary cell relations to body states. Lab Invest 1958;8:588–621.

72. Hardy J. Transsphenoidal microsurgery of the normal and pathological pituitary. Clin Neurosurg 1969;16:185–217.

73. McCormick WF, Halmi NS. Absence of chromophobe adenomas from a large series of pituitary tumors. Arch Pathol 1971;92:231–238.

74. Haugen OA. Pituitary adenomas and the histology of the prostate in elderly men. Acta Pathol Microbiol Scand, Section A 1973;81:425–434.

75. Landolt AM. Biology of pituitary microadenomas. In: Faglia G, Giovanelli MA, MacLeod RM, eds. Pituitary Microadenomas. Academic, New York, 1980, pp. 107–122.

76. Kovacs K, Ryan N, Horvath E, Singer W, Ezrin C. Pituitary adenomas in old age. J Gerontol 1980;35:16–22.

77. Parent AD, Bebin J, Smith RR. Incidental pituitary adenomas. J Neurosurg 1981;54:228–231.

78. Mosca L, Solcia E, Capella C, Buffa R. Pituitary adenomas: surgical versus post mortem findings today. Proc Serono Symp 1980;29:137–142.

79. Burrow GN, Wortzman G, Rewcastle NB, Holgatw RC, Kovacs K. Microadenomas of the pituitary and abnormal sellar tomograms in an unselected autopsy series. N Engl J Med 1981;304:156–158.

80. Teramoto A, Tamura A, Hori T, Sano K, Hirakawa K, Osamura Y, et al. Subclinical pituitary microadenoma. No To Shinkei 1981; 33:625–632 (in Japanese with English abstract).

81. Muhr C, Bergstrom K, Grimelius L, Larsson SG. A parallel study of the roentgen anatomy of the sella turcica and the histopathology of the pituitary gland in 205 autopsy specimens. Neuroradiology 1981;21:55–65.

82. Chambers EF, Turski PA, LaMasters D, Newton TH. Regions of low density in the contrast-enhanced pituitary gland: normal and pathologic processes. Radiology 1982;144:109–113.

83. Schwesinger G, Warzok R. Hyperplasien und adenome der hypophyse im unselektierten sektionsgut. Zentralbl Allg Pathol 1982;126:495–498.

84. Kontogeorgos G, Kovacs K, Horvath E, Scheithauer BW. Multiple adenomas of the human pituitary. A retrospective autopsy study with clinical implications. J Neurosurg 1991;74:243–247.

85. Uei Y, Kanzaki M, Yabana T. Incidental adenomas of the human pituitary gland. Endocr Pathol 1994;5:90–99.

86. Kontogeorgos G, Scheithauer BW, Horvath E, Kovacs K, Lloid RV, Smyth HS, et al. Double adenomas of the pituitary: a clinicopathological study of 11 tumors. Neurosurgery 1992;31:840–849.

87. McComb DJ, Ryan N, Horvath E, Kovacs K. Subclinical adenomas of the human pituitary. Arch Pathol Lab Med 1983;107:488–491.

88. Lloyd RV, Lin L, Fields K, Kulig E. Effects of estrogens on pituitary cell and pituitary tumor growth. Pathol Res Pract 1991;187:584–586.

89. Hall WA, Luciano MG, Doppman JL, Patronas NJ, Oldfield EH. Pituitary magnetic resonance imaging in normal human volunteers: occult adenomas in the general population. Ann Intern Med 1994;120:817–820.

90. Hoffman HJ. Pituitary adenomas. In: American Association of Neurological Surgeons: Pediatric Neurosurgery: Surgery of the Developing Nervous System. Grune & Stratton, New York, 1982, pp. 493–499.

91. Matson DD. Neurosurgery of Infancy and Childhood, 2nd ed. Charles C. Thomas, Springfield, IL, 1969, pp. 403–409.

92. Haddad SF, VanGilder JC, Menezes AH. Pediatric pituitary tumors. Neurosurgery 1991;29:509–514.

93. Ludeche DK, Herrmann HD, Schulte FJ. Special problems with neurosurgical treatment of hormone-secreting pituitary adenomas in children. Prog Exp Tumor Res 1987;30:362–370.

94. Kane LA, Leinung MC, Scheithauer BW, Bergstralh EJ, Laws ER Jr, Groover RV, et al. Pituitary adenomas in childhood and adolescence. J Clin Endocrinol Metab 1994;79:1135–1140.

95. Partington MD, Davis DH, Laws ER Jr, Scheithauer BW. Pituitary adenomas in childhood and adolescence. J Neurosurg 1994;80:209–216.

96. Levy SR, Wynne CV Jr, Lorentz WB Jr. Cushing's syndrome in infancy secondary to pituitary adenoma. Am J Dis Child 1982;136:605–607.

97. Sumner TE, Volberg FM. Cushing's syndrome in infancy due to pituitary adenoma. Pediatr Radiol 1982;12:81–83.

98. Stegner H, Ludecke DK, Kadrnka-Lovrencic M, Stahnke N, Willig RP. Cushing's disease due to an unusually large adenoma of the pituitary gland in infancy. Eur J Pediatr 1985;143:221–223.

99. Blumberg DL, Skiar CA, David R, Rothenberg S, Bell J. Acromegaly in an infant. Pediatrics 1989;83:998–1002.

100. Mindermann T, Wilson CB. Pituitary adenomas in childhood and adolescence. J Pediatr Endocrinol Metab 1995;8:79–83.

101. Styne DM, Grumbach MM, Kaplan SL, Wilson CB, Conte FA. Treatment of Cushing's disease in childhood and adolescence by transsphenoidal microadenomectomy. N Engl J Med 1984;310:889–893.

102. Thomas CG, Smith AT, Griffiths JM, Askin FB. Hyperadrenalism in childhood and adolescence. Ann Surg 1984;199:538–548.

103. Scheithauer BW, Horvath E, Kovacs K, Laws ER Jr, Randall RV, Ryan N. Plurihormonal pituitary adenomas. Semin Diagn Pathol 1986;3:69–82.

104. Martins AN, Hayes GJ, Kempe LG. Invasive pituitary adenomas. J Neurosurg 1965;22:268–276.

105. Ortiz-Suarez H, Erickson DL. Pituitary adenomas of adolescents. J Neurosurg 1975;43:437–439.

106. Richmond IL, Wilson CB. Pituitary adenomas in childhood and adolescence. J Neurosurg 1978;49:163–168.

107. Herman V, Fagin J, Consky R, Kovacs K, Melmed S. Clonal origin of pituitary adenomas. J Clin Endocrinol Metab 1990;71:1427–1433.

108. Schulte H, Oldfild EH, Allolio B, Katz DA, Merkman RA, Unnissa A. Clonal composition of pituitary adenomas in patients with Cushing's disease: Determination by X-chromosome inactivation analysis. J Clin Endocrinol Metab 1991;73:1302–1308.

109. Alexander JM, Biller BMK, Bikkal H, Zervas N, Arnold A, Klibanski A. Clinical nonfunctioning pituitary tumors are monoclonal in origin. J Clin Invest 1990;86:336–340.

110. Boggild MD, Jenkinson S, Pistorello M, Boscard M, Scanarini M, McTernan P, et al. Molecular genetic studies of sporadic pituitary adenomas. J Clin Endocrinol Metab 1994;78:387–392.

111. Tordjman K, Stern N, Ouaknine G, Yossiphov Y, Razon N, Nordenskjold M, et al. Activating mutations of the Gs alpha gene in nonfunctioning pituitary tumors. J Clin Endocrinol Metab 1993;77:765–769.

112. Landis CA, Harsh G, Lyons J, Davis RL, McCormick F, Bourne HR. Clinical characteristics of acromegalic patients whose pituitary tumors contain mutant Gs protein. J Clin Endocrinol Metab 1990;71:1416–1420.

113. Spada A, Arosio M, Bochicchio D, Bassoni N, Vallar L, Bassetti M, et al. Clinical, biochemical, and morphological correlates in patients bearing growth hormone-secreting pituitary tumors with or without constitutively active adenyl cyclase. J Clin Endocrinol Metab 1990;71:1421–1426.

114. Yang I, Park S, Ryu M, Woo J, Kim S, Kim J, et al. Characteristics of gsp positive growth hormone-secreting pituitary tumors in Korean acromegalic patients. Eur J Endocrinol 1996;137:720–726.

115. Asa SL, Ezzat S. The cytogenesis and pathogenesis of pituitary adenomas. Endocr Rev 1998;19:798–827.

116. Cai WY, Alexander JM, Hedley-Whyte ET, Scheithauer BW, Jameson JL, Zervas NT, et al. Ras mutations in human prolactinomas and pituitary carcinomas. J Clin Endocrinol Metab 1994;78:89–93.

117. Pei L, Melmed S. Isolation and characterization of a pituitary tumor-transforming gene (PTTG). Mol Endocrinol 1997;11:433–441.

118. Melmed S. Pathogenesis of pituitary tumor, in Advances in the management of pituitary tumors. Endocrinol Metab Clin North Am 1999;28:1–12.

119. Larsson C, Skogseid B, Oberg K, Nakamura Y, Nordenskjold MC. Multiple endocrine neoplasia type 1 gene maps to chromosome 11 and is lost in insulinoma. Nature 1988;332:85–89.

120. Chandrasekharappa SC, Guru SC, Manickam P, Olufemi SE, Collins FS, Emmert-Buck MR, et al. Positional cloning of the gene for multiple endocrine neoplasia-type 1. Science 1997;276:404–407.

121. Agarwal SK, Kester MB, Debelenko LV, Heppner C, Emmert-Buck MR, Skarulis MC, et al. Germline mutation of the MEN1 gene in familial multiple endocrine neoplasia type 1 and related states. Hum Mol Genet 1997;6:1169–1175.

122. Tanaka C, Yoshimoto K, Yamada S, Nishioka H, Ii S, Moritani M, et al. Absence of germ-line mutations of the multiple endocrine neoplasia type 1 (MEN1) gene in familial pituitary adenoma in contrast to MEN1 in Japanese. J Clin Endocrinol Metab 1998;83:960–965.

123. Yamada S, Yoshimoto K, Sano T, Takada K, Itakura M, Usui M, et al. Inactivation of the tumor suppressor gene 11q13 in brothers with familial acrogigantism without multiple endocrine neoplasia type 1. J Clin Endocrinol Metab 1997;82:239–242.

124. Tanaka C, Kimura T, Yang P, Moritani M, Yamada S, Sano T, et al. Analysis of loss of heterozygosity on chromosome 11 and infrequent inactivation of the MEN1 gene in sporadic pituitary adenomas. J Clin Endocrinol Metab 1998;83:2631–2634.

125. Zhu J, Leon SP, Beggs AH, Busque L, Gilliland DG, Black PM. Human pituitary adenomas show no loss of heterozygosity at the retinoblastoma gene locus. J Clin Endocrinol Metab 1994;78:922–927.

126. Levy A, Hall L, Yeundall WA, Lightman SL. p53 gene mutations in pituitary adenomas: rare events. Clin Endocrinol 1994;41:809–814.

127. Tanaka C, Yoshimoto K, Yang P, Kimura T, Yamada S, Moritani M, et al. Infrequent mutations of p27kipl gene and trisomy 12 in a subset of human pituitary adenomas. J Clin Endocrinol Metab 1997;82:3141–3147.

128. Takino H, Herman V, Weiss M, Melmed S. Purine-binding factor (nm23) gene expression in pituitary tumors: marker of adenoma invasiveness. J Clin Endocrinol Metab 1995;80:1733–1738.

129. Levy A, Lightman S. Growth hormone-releasing hormone transcripts in human pituitary adenomas. J Clin Endocrinol Metab 1992;74:1474–1476.

130. Webster J, Ham J, Bevan JS, ten-Horn CD, Scanlon MF. Preliminary characterization of growth factors secreted by human pituitary tumors. J Clin Endocrinol Metab 1991;72:687–692.

131. Jones TH, Justices S, Price A, Chapman K. Interleukin-6 secreting human pituitary adenomas in vitro. J Clin Endocrinol Metab 1991;73:207–209.

132. Stefaneanu L, Kovacs K, Norvath E, Asa SL, Losinski NE, Price J, et al. Adenohypophyseal changes in mice transgenic for human growth hormone-releasing factors: A histological and immunocytochemical, and electron microscopic investigation. Endocrinology 1989;125:2710–2718.

133. Asa SL, Scheithauer BM, Bilbao JM, Horvath E, Ryan N, Kovacs K, et al. A case for hypothalamic acromegaly: a clinicopathological study of six patients with hypothalamic gangliocytomas producing growth hormone releasing factor. J Clin Endocrinol Metab 1984;58:796–803.

134. Wingrave SJ, Kay CR, Vessey MP. Oral contraceptives and pituitary adenomas. Br Med J 1980;1:685–686.

135. Shy KK, McTiernan AM, Daling JR, Weiss NS. Oral contraceptive use and the occurrence of pituitary prolactinoma. JAMA 1983;249:2204–2207.

136. Corenblum B, Donovan L. The safety of physiological estrogen plus progestin replacement therapy and with oral contraceptive therapy in women with pathological hyperprolactinemia. Fertil Steril 1993;59:671–673.

137. Kovacs K, Horvath E, Kerenyi NA. Intracisternal virus-like particles in a human pituitary adenoma. Z Krebsforsch 1976;85:111–115.

5 Pathogenesis and Molecular Biology of Pituitary Tumors

ILAN SHIMON, MD, AND SHLOMO MELMED, MD

INTRODUCTION

Pituitary tumors are mostly benign adenomas arising from adenohypophyseal cells. These monoclonal tumors may either express and secrete hormones autonomously, leading to clinical hormone-excess syndromes, such as acromegaly and Cushing's disease, or may be functionally silent and initially diagnosed as a sellar mass. Although mechanisms for pituitary mitogenesis and tumor proliferation and progression are still unclear, in recent years new information on the role of intrinsic pituitary genetic defects, growth factors, and hypothalamic and peripheral factors in pituitary tumorigenesis have been reported. In addition, the linkage between neoplastic cell transformation and unrestrained pituitary hormone secretion that characterizes these tumors may be associated with their pathogenesis.

HYPOTHALAMIC ROLE IN PITUITARY TUMORIGENESIS

Normal pituitary function is under predominant hypothalamic control, mediated by the effects of several hypothalamic releasing and inhibiting hormones. Peripheral hormones, including thyroid hormone, sex steroids, corticosteroids, and insulin-like growth factor-1 (IGF-1) also regulate the transcription of their respective pituitary trophic hormones. In addition to regulating pituitary hormone gene expression and secretion, it has been suggested that hypothalamic hormones may have a specific role in the pathogenesis of pituitary cell mitogenesis.

The role of growth hormone-releasing hormone (GHRH) in control of somatotroph proliferation has been demonstrated in both clinical and experimental studies. Ectopic GHRH-secreting tumors (bronchial carcinoids, pancreatic islet-cell tumors or small-cell lung carcinomas) and eutopic hypothalamic GHRH-secreting tumors (hamartomas, gangliocytomas) result in growth hormone (GH) hypersecretion, acromegaly, somatotroph hyperplasia, and occasionally somatotroph adenoma formation (1,2). However, the majority of these patients do not develop true adenomas. In vitro, GHRH stimulates proliferation of rat somatotrophs (3). In transgenic mice expressing a human GHRH transgene, the pituitary size increases dramatically owing to somatotroph hyperpla-

sia (4,5), and mice than older 12 mo of age develop mammo-somatotrophs adenomas (6). In contrast to the results of GHRH, corticotropin-releasing hormone (CRH) does not appear to be mitogenic. In Cushing's syndrome caused by ectopic CRH oversecretion from prostate carcinoma (7) or an intrasellar gangliocytoma (8), no corticotroph adenoma was identified despite the persistence of corticotroph hyperplasia. Transgenic mice overexpressing the CRH transgene develop Cushing-like syndrome, but do not demonstrate significant changes in pituitary weight or corticotroph adenoma formation (9). Thus, clinical and animal evidence indicates that CRH oversecretion probably does not induce corticotroph adenomas in vivo.

The inhibitory hypothalamic hormones also have a potential role in regulating pituitary tumor growth. Administration of dopamine agonists to prolactinomas (10) and somatostatin analogs to GH-secreting adenomas (11) suppresses hormone secretion, but also results in tumor size reduction.

It is highly unlikely that the hypothalamic hormones alone play a significant role in the proximal initiation of pituitary tumorigenesis. Histologic studies of pituitary adenomas show that tumor edges are clearly demonstrated and are not surrounded by hyperplastic pituitary tissue. This consistent observation supports the assumption that hypothalamic stimulation is not the key player in pituitary tumor pathogenesis. In addition, hormonal secretion by the adenoma is usually independent of physiologic hypothalamic control, and the surgical resection of small well-defined adenomas usually results in definitive cure of hypersecretion states. These observations imply that these tumors are derived from monoclonal expansion of a single transformed cell (see below) as the result of an intrinsic cellular defect, rather than the result of excessive polyclonal pituicyte proliferation owing to hypothalamic stimulation. However, hypothalamic factors may participate in promoting growth of the already transformed pituitary cell, which usually is maintained over many years (or decades).

CLONALITY OF PITUITARY ADENOMAS

Using X-chromosomal inactivation analysis, the monoclonal origin of GH-, prolactin- (PRL) (12), and adrenocorticotropin- (ACTH) secreting adenomas (12–14), and nonfunctioning pituitary tumors (12,15) was confirmed in female patients heterozygous for variant alleles of the X-linked genes hypoxanthine phosphoribosyltransferase (HPRT), and phosphoglycerate kinase (PGK). In contrast, normal pituitary (12) and corticotroph hyper-

From: *Diagnosis and Management of Pituitary Tumors* (K. Thapar, K. Kovacs, B. W. Scheithauer, and R. V. Lloyd, eds.), ©Humana Press Inc., Totowa, NJ.

Table 1
G Proteins in Pituitary Tumors

Tumor	gsp mutation	Other alterations
GH cell adenoma	[a]arginine (201) → cysteine, histidine	[a]Elevated activated CREB
	[a]glutamine (227) → arginine, leucine	[a]Elevated WT G$_s$α
Nonfunctioning adenoma	[a]arginine (201) → cysteine	gip2 mutations:
	[a]glutamine (227) → arginine, leucine	[b]glutamine (205) → arginine
McCune-Albright	[a]arginine (201) → cysteine, histidine	

[a]Elevated cAMP.
[b]Suppressed cAMP.
WT = wide-type.

plastic tissue *(14)* were found to be polyclonal. Thus, these observations suggest that an intrinsic somatic pituitary cell mutation gives rise to clonal expansion of a single cell and ultimate adenoma formation, which may be either secreting or nonsecreting. The monoclonal origin of adenomas makes it highly unlikely that hypothalamic effects alone initiate the process of pituitary transformation.

ACTIVATING gsp MUTATIONS

The G-proteins are a group of guanosine triphosphate (GTP) binding proteins coupled to a superfamily of polypeptide receptors with seven membrane-spanning domains *(16)*, and involved in transmembrane signal transduction. The G-proteins are heterotrimers composed of three distinct subunits: α, β, and γ. The α-subunit differs from one G-protein to another to define functional specificity of the different G-proteins. The G-protein mediates stimulation or suppression of different effector enzymes, including adenylyl cyclase, guanylyl cyclase, phospholipases, and ion channels. At least 20 different α-subunits have been cloned to date, and those of the α$_s$ class have been defined as adenylyl cyclase activators. Gain of function and loss of function mutations in G-proteins and G-protein-coupled receptors have been identified in several endocrine syndromes with altered signal transduction *(17)*.

A subset of human GH-secreting adenomas has been described with constitutively active G-protein α-subunit (G$_s$α), persistent activation of adenylyl cyclase, and high levels of intracellular cAMP *(18)*. These tumors harbor somatic heterozygous activating point mutations of the G$_s$α gene involving either arginine 201 (replaced by cysteine or histidine) or glutamine 227 (replaced with arginine or leucine) (Table 1) *(19,20)*. These residues are critically involved in GDP/GTP binding, and mutations there constitutively activate the G$_s$α protein by inhibiting its intrinsic GTPase activity, and convert it into an oncogene (gsp). As GHRH signaling is mediated by cAMP, this G-protein activation bypasses the somatotroph normal requirement for GHRH ligand-mediated receptor activation, increases cAMP levels, activates protein kinase A (PKA), which in turn phosphorylates the cAMP response element binding protein (CREB), and leads to sustained constitutive GH hypersecretion and cell proliferation *(21)*. Activating gsp mutations are present in up to 40% *(22–24)* of GH-secreting adenomas, and compared with nonmutant tumors the gsp-bearing adenomas are smaller, have mildly lower GH levels and enhanced intratumoral cAMP, do not respond briskly to GHRH, and are extremely sensitive to the inhibitory effect of somatostatin *(22,23)*. Interestingly, gsp mutations are rare (5%) in GH-secreting pituitary adenomas in Japan *(25)*. Similar early postzygotic somatic mutations in codon 201 of the G$_s$α were identified in various tissues of patients with McCune-Albright syndrome, including GH-producing pituitary adenomas *(26,27)* (Table 1). The mosaic distribution of mutant alleles of G$_s$α gene may cause the involved tissues to exhibit increased cellular proliferation and abnormal differentiation.

In contrast to GH-cell adenomas, these gsp-activating mutations are rarely present in nonfunctioning pituitary tumors (Table 2), and are absent in prolactinomas *(28,29)* and in TSH-producing adenomas *(30)*. Interestingly, several nonfunctioning adenomas also harbor gip2 mutations at codon 205 of the Gi2α protein, replacing glutamine with arginine *(29)*, but resulting in adenylyl cyclase inhibition and cAMP suppression (Table 1).

cAMP RESPONSE ELEMENT BINDING PROTEIN (CREB)

Most of the transcriptional effects of cAMP are mediated by the CREB. Transgenic mice overexpressing an inactive mutant of CREB in the anterior pituitary exhibit a dwarf phenotype and somatotroph hypoplasia *(31)*. Thus, the phosphorylated and, therefore, activated CREB may serve as the biochemical intermediate in the mechanism by which cAMP stimulates somatotroph proliferation. Recently, all 15 human GH-secreting pituitary adenomas studied were found to contain elevated levels of activated CREB, compared with nonfunctioning pituitary tumors *(32)*. Only four of these GH tumors contained a mutant gsp oncogene, but two additional secreting adenomas overexpressed wild-type G$_s$α protein that may promote CREB phosphorylation and somatotroph proliferation.

PROTEIN KINASE C (PKC)

Protein kinase C (PKC) is a calcium- and phospholipid-dependent protein kinase that participates in the signal transduction of several growth factors and hormones, thus regulating cell proliferation and survival. PKC activity and protein expression are increased in human secreting and nonsecreting pituitary adenomas as compared to normal human and rat pituitaries *(33)*. Recently, increased expression of the PKC α-isoform was demonstrated in both secreting and nonsecreting pituitary adenomas *(34)*. In addition, an identical point mutation in codon 294 of αPKC (aspartic acid replaced by glycine) was detected in all four invasive tumors studied, but not in the noninvasive tumors *(34)*. Thus, the structurally altered αPKC in invasive adenomas may be a hallmark for tumor growth.

Ras ONCOGENES

The *ras* family consists of three homologous functional genes, H-*ras*, K-*ras*, and N-*ras* *(35)* that encode 21-kDa (p21) proteins,

Table 2
Known Genetic Mutations and Alterations in Pituitary Tumor Cell Types

Tumor	Mutation/alteration	Incidence	References
GH cell adenoma	gsp mutations	35–40%	Landis et al. (19,22)
			Spada et al. (23)
			Boggild et al. (24)
	Activated CREB	100%	Bertherat et al. (32)
	Truncated GHRH-R	33%	Hashimoto et al. (86)
PRL cell adenoma	hst oncogene	4/4	Gonsky et al. (106)
	hst/FGF-4 protein	36%	Shimon et al. (107)
	Overexpressed PTTG	100%	Zhang et al. (99)
ACTH cell adenoma	p53 protein	50%	Buckley et al. (68)
Nonfunctioning adenoma	gsp mutation	7–9%	Tordjman et al. (28)
			Williamson et al. (29)
	11q13 allelic loss	20%	Boggild et al. (24)
Invasive adenoma	α-PKC mutation	4/4	Alvaro et al. (34)
	13q14 allelic loss	100%	Pei et al. (64)
	Reduced nm23 protein		Takino et al. (71)
Carcinoma	13q14 allelic loss	100%	Pei et al. (64)
	H-ras mutations	60%	Pei et al. (43)
MEN 1 associated adenoma	MEN-1 mutations	90–100%	Chandrasekharappa et al. (53)
			Agarwal et al. (55)
	Circulating FGF-2	40%	Zimering et al. (100–102)
McCune-Albright	gsp mutation		Weinstein et al. (26)

which possess GTPase activity, are involved in growth control, and have significant sequence homology with G-proteins (36). These characteristics suggest that ras proteins have an important role in signal transduction across the cell membrane. Missense mutations in *ras* genes convert them into active oncogenes. Most of these mutations occur at codons 12, 13, and 61. *Ras* mutations are commonly identified in human colon, lung, bladder, pancreas, breast and kidney carcinomas, and other solid and hematologic malignancies (37). They are the most frequently detected oncogenes in human neoplasms, and it is estimated that from 10 to 40% of human tumors arise from cells with abnormal forms or elevated levels of p21 (38).

In contrast, *ras* mutations are rare in pituitary adenomas. Karga et al. (39) studied 19 pituitary tumors, and identified a mutation in codon 12 of H-*ras* in one highly invasive prolactinoma. Herman et al. (40) did not find *ras* gene mutations in 22 GH cell adenomas and 22 nonfunctioning pituitary tumors. No evidence of oncogene amplification or rearrangement at the *ras* locus was found by Boggild et al. (24) in 88 pituitary adenomas, including secreting (GH-, PRL-, and ACTH-), and nonsecreting tumors, and by Cai et al in 78 prolactinomas and pituitary carcinomas (41). H-*ras* point mutations were identified in three distant pituitary carcinoma metastases, but not in their respective primary carcinomas, nor in other six invasive adenomas (42). Thus, activation of *ras* oncogene does not appear to be a critical event for initiation of pituitary adenomas, but may be important in the rare pituitary metastases formation or growth.

NUCLEAR ONCOGENES

c-*myc*, c-*myb*, and c-*fos* proto-oncogenes play an important role in regulation of cell proliferation and differentiation. Their encoded nuclear proteins are involved in transcription of other genes, including specific hormone genes (43). Woloschak studied mRNA expression of c-*myc* and c-*myb* in 30 pituitary tumors, and found c-*myc* mRNA elevation in nine tumors, whereas c-*myb*

mRNA expression was unchanged (44). However, c-*myc* protein immunoreactivity was rarely found (45), and c-*myc* gene amplification or rearrangements are uncommon in pituitary adenomas (24). The oncogenic effect of the nuclear phosphoprotein, c-*fos*, is sporadic (44), and c-*fos* activation is probably not a common feature of pituitary tumors. Therefore, the current evidence indicates that these nuclear proto-oncogenes are not involved in pituitary tumorigenesis.

PITUITARY TUMOR-TRANSFORMING GENE (PTTG)

Recently, a pituitary tumor-transforming gene (PTTG) was isolated from experimental rat pituitary tumors (43). The human homologues of PTTG comprise several separate PTTG genes. PTTG is located on chromosome 5q33 and is abundantly expressed in most human pituitary tumors (44), as well as in non-pituitary neoplasms. Pituitary PTTG expression is induced by estrogens and it stimulates bFGF production (45). The role of PTTG in the early transformation of pituitary cells through hyperplasia to frank adenoma formation has been demonstrated in experimental rat prolactinomas (45).

TUMOR SUPPRESSOR GENES

In contrast to the dominant proto-oncogenes, which initiate neoplasia when converted to oncogenes, tumor suppressor genes that normally suppress cell proliferation when present as two normal alleles, induce tumor cell growth as the result of functional loss of both alleles (46). Thus, tumorigenesis is generated by two recessive genetic changes (two-hit mutation theory), where the first event (first hit) may be a somatic mutation in the tumor itself, or germline mutation that is dominantly inherited, and the second genetic event (second hit) is usually loss of tumor heterozygosity (LOH), a deletion of the tumor suppressor gene and its flanking sequences. This somatic event, revealed by a comparison of leukocyte and tumor alleles, renders the cell hemizygous for the original allelic mutation, and leads to inactivation of the suppressor gene and to unrestrained tumor growth.

MEN-1 Gene   Multiple endocrine neoplasia type 1 (MEN-1) is an autosomal dominant disorder characterized by the combined occurrence of parathyroid, pancreatic islet, and anterior pituitary tumors. The MEN-1 gene was mapped to chromosome 11q13 (47,48). LOH of the MEN-1 locus on the pericentromeric region of the long arm of chromosome 11 has been demonstrated in the majority of parathyroid tumors removed from MEN-1 patients (49–51), in 25% of sporadic parathyroid adenomas (51), and in pancreatic islet tumors (47,52). These findings indicate that inactivation of a tumor suppressor gene on chromosome 11 is pathogenetically related to these MEN-1 associated endocrine tumors. Allelic losses for chromosome 11q markers were determined in both MEN-1 associated and sporadic pituitary adenomas (52). However, most sporadic pituitary tumors studied (40,51) did not demonstrate LOH of 11q13 loci.

Recently, the gene for MEN-1 has been cloned and characterized (53,54). The MEN-1 gene contains 10 exons and encodes a predicted 610-amino acid protein product, termed menin. Mutational analysis of the gene-coding sequence in unrelated MEN-1 families revealed different heterozygous mutations, including missense, nonsense, insertional and deletional frameshifts alterations in almost all cases (53–55), most of which predict a premature truncation of the menin protein. Thus, this confirms that MEN-1 is suppressor gene according to Knudson's two-hit theory, where the first hit are the germ-line MEN-1 mutations, and the second hit is a somatic deletion of the second MEN-1 allele on chromosome 11q13, resulting in LOH. MEN-1 gene mutations were also identified in most cases of sporadic MEN-1 syndrome (55,56), but not in cases of familial pituitary adenomas (56). In contrast to MEN-1 syndrome, patients with sporadic pituitary adenomas, both secreting and nonfunctional, usually do not demonstrate pathogenic changes, neither germ-line nor somatic, in the coding sequence of MEN-1 gene, even in tumors with LOH of 11q13 (57,58), and only two cases of sporadic pituitary adenomas (of 94 tumors studied) had specific MEN-1 mutations (57,58). Thus, MEN-1 gene mutations do not play a role in pituitary tumorigenesis in most sporadic adenomas.

RETINOBLASTOMA GENE   The retinoblastoma (Rb) gene is a tumor suppressor gene located at chromosome 13q14 that was first characterized because of its association with human retinoblastomas. Inactivation of both Rb alleles by somatic mutations leads to sporadic retinoblastomas (59), and LOH on chromosome 13q is associated with other types of tumors, including breast cancer, bladder, esophageal, renal cell, and prostate carcinoma. Subjects with germline mutations in one Rb allele develop the hereditary form of retinoblastoma at an early age. The Rb protein regulates the cell cycle, and is important for cell survival and differentiation. This protein is missing from retinoblastoma cells, and reintroducing a nonmutant Rb gene into these cells suppresses tumor formation.

Studies using transgenic disruptions of the Rb gene in mice revealed that embryos homozygous for the disrupted Rb gene die within days 14–15 of gestation (60). Mice heterozygous for the Rb mutation do not develop retinoblastomas, but have a high frequency (approx 90%) of pituitary tumors associated with LOH at the Rb locus (60). These tumors originate from the intermediate lobe of the pituitary, and are classified histologically as adenocarcinomas. However, no Rb allelic deletions were detected in benign

pituitary adenomas studied by four different groups (61–64). Pei et al. (64) showed LOH in proximity to the Rb locus in 13 malignant or highly invasive pituitary tumors, and in their respective metastases. Immunohistochemical studies, however, revealed the presence of Rb protein in tumors with chromosome 13 allelic loss (64). In another study of 24 benign pituitary tumors, no Rb mutations in exons 20–24 of the Rb gene were found, and the expression of Rb protein was confirmed (65). Thus, inactivation of Rb suppressor gene does not appear to play a role in pathogenesis of benign human pituitary adenomas. Another tumor suppressor gene located on chromosome 13 adjacent to the Rb locus may be involved in the development of invasive pituitary adenomas and carcinomas.

p53 GENE   The p53 suppressor gene encodes a sequence-specific DNA binding protein that stimulates expression of downstream genes, which negatively control cell proliferation. p53 is located on chromosome 17p13.1, and is the most common gene mutated and/or deleted in human neoplasia, associated with 50% of cancer types. Characteristically, one allele of the p53 is lost, and the remaining allele is mutated and results in a mutant p53 protein. This altered protein fails to suppress transformation and contributes to the development of malignancy. The wild-type p53 protein cannot be detected by immunohistochemistry owing to its short half-life, but the mutated protein is more stable and can be detected by specific antibodies.

p53 mutations were not detected using cycle sequencing of exons 5–8 (where the p53 mutations usually occur) in 22 nonsecreting and 22 GH-secreting pituitary adenomas (40), or in 29 adenomas (including all major types) (66) or in 4 pituitary carcinomas and their respective metastases (42). In addition, immunohistochemical analysis of p53 protein in 40 pituitary adenomas also detected no alteration of this protein (67). However, Buckley et al. (68) detected p53 protein accumulation by immunohistochemistry of sporadic pituitary adenomas in 16% of invasive tumors, but in only ACTH-producing and nonfunctional tumors, and in 50% of noninvasive ACTH-secreting tumors.

Interestingly, transgenic mice homozygous or heterozygous for p53 mutations develop lymphomas and sarcomas, but not pituitary tumors (69). However, mice heterozygous for both p53 and Rb mutations develop pituitary tumors, as well as lymphomas and sarcomas (69). These observations suggest that p53 probably has no role in pituitary adenoma formation. Its suggested involvement in Cushing's adenoma pathogenesis, and the progression of some nonfunctional tumors toward invasiveness still requires elucidation.

nm23   The purine binding factor (nm23) gene was identified as a tumor suppressor gene on the basis of reduced expression in highly metastatic cancer, including breast, hepatic, and colorectal carcinomas (70), compared with its abundant expression in low metastatic potential tumors. Recently, nm23 RNA expression was studied in 22 pituitary tumors, and the H2 isoform expression was significantly reduced in invasive adenomas, and correlated inversely with cavernous sinus invasion (71). nm23 H2 protein immunoreactivity was also reduced in invasive tumors (71). However, nm23 gene mutations were not detected in those aggressive tumors.

CYCLIN-DEPENDENT KINASE (CDK) INHIBITORS

The cyclin-dependent kinase (CDK) complexes play a central role in the regulation of cell-cycle progression. The Rb protein is one of their putative substrates, and phosphorylation of the protein by CDK4 inactivates its ability to control cell cycle (72). p16, the specific inhibitor of CDK4, was identified as a tumor suppressor gene that is inactivated in several human tumor-derived cell lines and functions in a feedback regulatory loop with the Rb protein. Inverse correlation between p16 and Rb is present in several tumor types, where wild-type p16 protein accumulates in cells with altered Rb, and p16 is absent in tumor cells expressing wild-type Rb. In a recent study of 25 human pituitary tumors, p16 mRNA levels were low, and p16 gene product was undetectable in all tumors studied (73). This decreased expression was not associated with p16 mutation or gene loss (73), ant it is unclear whether altered p16 expression in pituitary tumors has direct effects on cell-cycle control that results in tumorigenesis.

p27 is another negative regulator of the kinase activity of the cyclin–CDK complexes. It may have a critical role in regulation of entry into and exit from the mitotic cycle. p27 gene disruption in transgenic mice resulted in larger knockout mice (without GH or IGF-1 increase), multiple-organ hyperplasia, hyperplasia of the intermediate lobe of the pituitary, and a high incidence (almost 100%) of benign pituitary tumors that involved the entire intermediate lobe (74–76). Interestingly, only deletions of p27 and Rb (60) in mutant mice cause pars intermedia tumors, and both do so with almost 100% penetrance. This similarity in the unusual pattern of tumor development may be a consequence of the interaction of p27 and Rb proteins in a common regulatory pathway.

Pit-1

Pit-1 (also known as GHF-1), a 33-kDa nuclear protein, is a member of the POU homeodomain family of transcription factors. This factor is specifically expressed in normal somatotrophs, lactotrophs, and thyrotrophs, and is critical for GH, PRL, and TSH-β gene transcription. Children with mutations in the Pit-1 gene present with a syndrome of congenital hypothyroidism, dwarfism, and prolactin deficiency (77). In dwarf mouse strains with naturally occurring mutations or deletions of Pit-1 gene, somatotrophs, lactotrophs, and thyrotrophs failed to proliferate, and GH, PRL, and TSH-β were absent (78). In addition to the activation of the three hormone genes, Pit-1 may be involved in cell proliferation and survival of these three pituitary cell types. The GHRH receptor expression failure in Pit-1-defective dwarf mice (79) suggests that Pit-1 may control somatotroph proliferation through transcriptional regulation of the GHRH receptor.

Several studies have been performed to determine the distribution of Pit-1 in different human pituitary adenoma types. Asa et al. (80) demonstrated, not surprisingly, selective expression of Pit-1 mRNA and protein in somatotroph, mammosomatotroph, lactotroph, and thyrotroph adenomas, but not in corticotroph, gonadotroph, or null-cell tumors. Similar patterns of Pit-1 expression in specific adenoma types has also been reported by others (81–83). Thus, the presence of Pit-1 in GH-, PRL- and TSH-producing adenomas is not specific to neoplastic adenohypophyseal tissue, but is consistent with Pit-1 distribution and transcript size in the normal pituitary. This is somewhat expected, since Pit-1 is essential for the expression of these three hormones. However, several other groups have also localized Pit-1 transcripts and protein in some nonsecreting adenomas (84), indicating that these tumors may possibly arise from an uncommitted precursor cell expressing Pit-1. No mutations in the Pit-1 cDNA cloned from pituitary adenomas were identified in one study (82), but two

mutations have been reported by Delhase in the sequence of Pit-1 derived from a GH-secreting ademoma (83). However, their biological significance was not determined. Pit-1β isoform expression in normal and adenomatous tissues was similar to Pit-1 pattern of distribution (82). In summary, therefore, the evidence to date indicates that altered Pit-1 gene expression is probably not involved in pituitary adenoma pathogenesis.

RELEASING AND INHIBITING HORMONE RECEPTORS

Under physiologic conditions, hypothalamic GHRH stimulates pituitary somatotroph GH secretion, and somatostatin and IGF-1 inhibit GH release. GHRH receptor also acts as a critical molecule for the proliferation and differentiation of somatotrophs, and a missense mutation in the *little (lit)* mice results in a hypoplastic anterior pituitary gland with resultant 10-fold decrease in somatotroph cells and GH production (85). Studies of GHRH receptor (86), and IGF-1 receptor β-subunit (87) in GH-secreting adenomas showed no sequence mutations in the receptors in any of these tumors. In addition, GHRH receptor mRNA levels did not correlate with clinical characteristics of these adenomas (86). However, some GH-producing adenomas expressed a truncated nonfunctioning GHRH receptor through alternative splicing (86), but the pathophysiological relevance of this spliced receptor is yet unclear.

Thyrotropin-releasing hormone (TRH) normally stimulates release of TSH and PRL from pituitary thyrotrophs and lactotrophs, respectively. In addition, TRH can stimulate GH secretion in acromegaly and glycoprotein subunits in nonfunctioning adenomas. Recently, 59 pituitary adenomas, including TSH-, PRL-, and GH-secreting and nonfunctioning tumors were screened for TRH receptor gene mutations (30,88), but all tumors retained the normal wild-type sequence. Dopamine tonically inhibits PRL secretion and lactotroph proliferation via its specific receptor, dopamine type 2 receptor. No mutations in this receptor gene were detected when 79 pituitary tumors (mostly prolactinomas, and several nonfunctioning and TSH-secreting adenomas) were screened (89).

FIBROBLAST GROWTH FACTOR (FGF)

FGF family comprises proteins from at least nine distinct genes (90). These structurally related peptides possess heparin binding sites, and are well-characterized ubiquitous mitogens. The two prototypes of this family are FGF-1 (acidic FGF, a 140 amino acid peptide), and FGF-2 (basic FGF, 146 amino acids) that share a 55% amino acid homology (91). These two peptides do not contain an intact signal peptide, characteristic of secreted proteins, and their secretory pathway is as yet unknown. FGF-4, however, a 206 amino acid protein, encoded by the heparin binding secretory transforming gene (hst), does contain a signal peptide, and is glycosylated and secreted by producing cells. Both FGF-2 and FGF-4 are potent angiogenic factors, which may maintain a rich blood supply to tissues expressing them.

FIBROBLAST GROWTH FACTOR-2 (FGF-2)

Unlike the controversial pituitary expression of FGF-1 (91), FGF-2 is abundantly found in normal pituitary tissue (92), from where it was originally purified (93). Immunohistochemical studies of rat pituitaries localized FGF-2 expression predominantly within folliculostellate cells, using costaining for S-100 protein. Human pituitary adenomas also contain FGF-2 (94,95). This growth factor stimulates PRL secretion from normal rat pituitary cells *(96)* and from cultured human pituitary adenomas *(97)*. However, FGF-2 is not mitogenic for normal or adenomatous anterior pituitary cells in vitro *(96,97)*. Induction of gonadotroph FGF-2 expression by estradiol in Fisher 344 rats *(98)* suggests that the angiogenic activity of FGF-2 may be associated with induced prolactinomas. However, transgenic mice expressing FGF-2 in the anterior pituitary did not develop pituitary tumors *(99)*.

Although MEN 1 syndrome is associated with loss of a tumor suppressor gene on chromosome 11q13, several recent observations have, in addition, identified a disordered pituitary FGF-2 function. Circulating FGF-2, as measured by radioimmunoassay (RIA), is detectable in about 40% of patients with MEN 1 and in most MEN 1 patients with untreated pituitary tumors *(100,101)*. In addition, circulating FGF-2-like autoantibodies have been detected in several MEN 1 prolactinoma patients *(102)*. The pituitary is thus probably the source of plasma FGF-2 immunoreactivity in MEN 1 syndrome, because pituitary tumor resection or medical treatment is followed by lowering of circulating FGF-2 levels *(101)*. These observations suggest that FGF-2 may have a role in stimulating pituitary cell proliferation in association with MEN 1 syndrome, but normal cells are not stimulated to grow, in addition to the hormonal effect *(96,97)*.

FIBROBLAST GROWTH FACTOR-4 (FGF-4) (hst)

The hst gene was first identified as a transforming gene in human stomach cancer *(103)*. hst expression is restricted to embryonic tissue, and in the adult, the growth factor is normally not expressed. Several malignant tumors may express hst, including Kaposi's sarcoma, melanoma, and embryonal carcinoma. Interestingly, hst has been mapped to chromosome 11q13 *(104)*, in proximity to the MEN 1 gene locus.

hst oncogene and FGF-4 peptide induce PRL gene transcription and PRL secretion in rat pituitary cultures *(105)*, and overexpression of hst cDNA in pituicytes also results in enhanced PRL secretion. hst stable transfection of rat pituitary cells induced aggressive and invasive tumors after sc injection to normal rats *(105)*. Moreover, human prolactinomas express transforming sequences of the hst gene *(106)*, and about a third of prolactinomas studied immunostain positively for FGF-4, the protein product of hst *(107)*. Sixty percent of invasive prolactinomas expressed the growth factor, whereas normal pituitary does not express it, and only 5% of other pituitary adenomas positively immunostained for hst. Tumor aggressiveness, as assessed by proliferating cell nuclear antigen (PCNA) staining correlates with prolactinoma hst/FGF-4 expression *(107)*. However, no hst gene rearrangements were demonstrated in 7 PRL-secreting adenomas *(40)*. These observations indicate that in addition to PRL gene transcription induction, FGF-4 may have a mitogenic activity in promoting lactotroph proliferation. Therefore, the unrestrained PRL secretion characterizing prolactinomas may not necessarily reflect merely an increased mass of PRL-secreting cells, but in addition, a direct growth factor-specific induction of hormone transcription.

TRANSFORMING GROWTH FACTOR-α (TGF-α)

Transforming growth factor-α (TGF-α) is a 50 amino acid mitogenic protein that exerts its biological effects through the epidermal growth factor (EGF) receptor. It was detected in several fetal cell types and human malignant tumors *(108)*. In addition, its

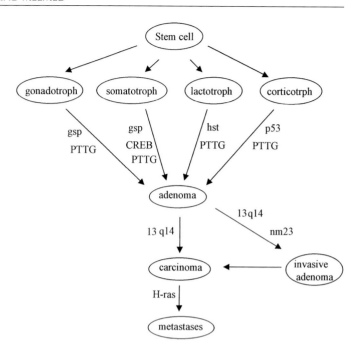

Figure 5-1 Multistep pathogenetic process of pituitary tumorigenesis.

expression has been reported in several normal adult tissues, including brain, gastrointestinal tract, and mammary glands.

TGF-α synthesis was detected in the lactotroph cells of the bovine pituitary by immunohistochemistry *(109)*, and was purified from conditioned medium of bovine pituitary cell cultures *(110,111)*. Moreover, the EGF receptor has also been detected on normal pituitary cells *(111)*. Recently, Finley and Ramsdell *(112)* have demonstrated the essential role of the TGF-α pathway in the pathogenesis of tumors derived from the rat pituitary cell line GH4C1. Others *(113,114)* have studied the expression of TGF-α in normal human pituitary and different types of pituitary adenomas. They detected ubiquitous, but highly variable, expression of the growth factor in normal and adenomatous human pituitary tissues, including ACTH-, GH-, PRL-secreting, and null-cell adenomas. However, TGF-α was not detected in pituitary tumor-conditioned culture media *(114)*. Moreover, the adenomatous expression of this growth factor is insufficient evidence for a causal relationship between pituitary tumorigenesis and TGF-α. To determine the effect of TGF-a overexpression on lactotrophs in vivo, a lactotroph-targeted TGF-α transgenic mouse model was established *(115)*. These mice demonstrated selective pituitary lactotroph hyperplasia and PRL cell adenoma formation, and, thus, may serve as a model for TGF-α-induced prolactinoma pathogenesis. Interestingly, only female mice expressed the transgene and developed adenomas *(115)*.

SUMMARY

Since the observation that pituitary tumors are monoclonal, much evidence has accumulated that multifactorial mechanisms participate in the multistep pathogenetic process of pituitary tumor formation (Figure 1). They include early initiating DNA-altering events (i.e., gsp-activating mutations, 11q13 tumor suppressor chromosomal deletions) (Table 2) that result in mutated pituitary stem cells. These "initiated" cells are subsequently dysregulated and stimulated by multiple endocrine signals, including hypothalamic hormones (GHRH) or their receptors, and paracrine growth factors (FGF-2, FGF-4, TGF-α), leading to clonal expansion of the altered tumor cells. The ultimate tumor biologic behavior in terms of the type of hormone secreted, as well as tumor growth characteristics including invasiveness, may be determined by the initiating oncogenic event or a permissive growth factor effect. Rarely occurring malignant transformation is probably associated with a secondary oncogenic transformation, including H-*ras* mutations and chromosome 13 allelic loss, in a small subset of pituitary adenomas, leading to invasiveness and/or extrapituitary metastatic spread. Thus, the rare pituitary carcinomas may be the result of several genetic alterations.

However, genetic mutations have not yet been detected in most secreting and nonsecreting pituitary adenomas. Therefore, the primary event leading to pituitary clonal growth still requires elucidation in the majority of pituitary tumors.

REFERENCES

1. Sano T, Asa SL, Kovacs K. Growth hormone-releasing hormone-producing tumors: clinical, biochemical, and morphological manifestations. Endocr Rev 1988;9:357–373.
2. Asa SL, Bilbao JM, Kovacs K, Linfoot JA. Hypothalamic neuronal hamartoma associated with pituitary growth hormone cell adenoma and acromegaly. Acta Neuropathol 1980;53:231–234.
3. Billestrup N, Swanson LW, Vale W. Growth hormone-releasing factor stimulates proliferation of somatotrophs in vitro. Proc Natl Acad Sci USA 1986;83:6854–6857.
4. Mayo KE, Hammer RE, Swanson LW, Brinster RL, Rosenfeld MG, Evans RM. Dramatic pituitary hyperplasia in transgenic mice expressing a human growth hormone-releasing factor gene. Mol Endocrinol 1988;2:606–612.
5. Stefaneanu L, Kovacs K, Horvath E, Asa SL, Losinski NE, Billestrup N, et al. Adenohypophysial changes in mice transgenic for human growth hormone-releasing factor: A histological, immunocytochemical, and electron microscopic investigation. Endocrinology 1989;125:2710–2718.
6. Asa SL, Kovacs K, Stefaneanu L, Horvath E, Billestrup N, Gonzales-Manchon C, et al. Pituitary mammosomatotroph adenomas develop in old mice transgenic for growth hormone-releasing hormone. Proc Soc Exp Biol Med 1990;193:232–235.
7. Carey RM, Varma SK, Drake CR Jr, Thorner MO, Kovacs K, Rivier J, et al. Ectopic secretion of corticotropin-releasing factor as a cause of Cushing's syndrome. N Engl J Med 1984;311:13–20.
8. Asa SL, Kovacs K, Tindall GT, Barrow DL, Horvath E, Vecsei P. Cushing's disease associated with an intrasellar gangliocytoma producing corticotropin-releasing factor. Ann Intern Med 1984; 101:789–793.
9. Stenzel-Poore MP, Cameron VA, Vaughan J, Sawchenko PE, Vale W. Development of Cushing's syndrome in corticotropin-releasing factor transgenic mice. Endocrinology 1992;130: 3378–3386.
10. Molith ME. Prolactinoma. In: Melmed S, ed. The Pituitary. Blackwell Science, Cambridge, MA, 1995, pp. 443–477.
11. Ezzat S, Snyder PJ, Young WF, Boyajy LD, Newman C, Klibanski A, et al. Octreotide treatment of acromegaly: a randomized, multicenter study. Ann Intern Med 1992;117:711–718.
12. Herman V, Fagin J, Gonsky R, Kovacs K, Melmed S. Clonal origin of pituitary adenomas. J Clin Endocrinol Metab 1990;71: 1427–1433.
13. Schulte HM, Oldfield EH, Allolio B, Katz DA, Berkman RA, Unnisa Ali I. Clonal composition of pituitary adenomas in patients with Cushing's disease: determination by X-chromosome inactivation analysis. J Clin Endocrinol Metab 1991;73:1302–1308.
14. Biller BMK, Alexander JM, Zervas NT, Hedley-Whyte ET, Arnold A, Klibanski A. Clonal origins of adrenocorticotropin-secreting pituitary tissue in Cushing's disease. J Clin Endocrinol Metab 1992;75:1303–1309.
15. Alexander JM, Biller BMK, Bikkal H, Zervas NT, Arnold A, Klibanski A. Clinically nonfunctioning pituitary tumors are monoclonal in origin. J Clin Invest 1990;86:336–340.
16. Strader CD, Ming Fong T, Tota MR, Underwood D. Structure and function of G protein-coupled receptors. Annu Rev Biochem 1994;63:101–132.
17. Spiegel AM. Genetic basis of endocrine disease. Mutations in G proteins and G protein-coupled receptors in endocrine disease. J Clin Endocrinol Metab 1996;81:2434–2442.
18. Vallar L, Spada A, Giannattasio G. Altered G_s and adenylate cyclase activity in human GH-secreting pituitary adenomas. Nature 1987;330:566–568.
19. Landis CA, Masters SB, Spada A, Pace AM, Bourne HR, Vallar L. GTPase inhibiting mutations activate the α chain of Gs and stimulate adenylyl cyclase in human pituitary tumours. Nature 1989; 340:692–696.
20. Clementi E, Malgaretti N, Meldolesi J, Taramelli R. A new constitutively activating mutation of the Gs protein a subunit-gsp oncogene is found in human pituitary tumours. Oncogene 1990; 5:1059–1061.
21. Spada A, Faglia G. G-protein dysfunction in pituitary tumors. In: Melmed S, ed. Oncogenesis and Molecular Biology of Pituitary Tumors. Front Horm Res, vol. 20. Basel, Krager, pp. 108–121.
22. Landis CA, Harsh G, Lyons J, Davis RL, McCormick F, Bourne HR. Clinical characteristics of acromegalic patients whose pituitary tumors contain mutant Gs protein. J Clin Endocrinol Metab 1990;71:1416–1420.
23. Spada A, Vallar L, Faglia G. G protein oncogenes in pituitary tumors. Trends Endocrinol Metab 1992;3:355–360.
24. Boggild MD, Jenkinson S, Pistorello M, Boscaro M, Scanarini M, McTernan P, et al. Molecular genetic studies of sporadic pituitary tumors. J Clin Endocrinol Metab 1994;78:387–392.
25. Hosoi E, Yokogoshi Y, Hosoi E, Horie H, Sano T, Yamada S, et al. Analysis of the Gs α in growth hormone-secreting pituitary adenomas by the polymerase chain reaction-direct sequencing method using paraffin-embedded tissues. Acta Endocrinol 1993;129:301–306.
26. Weinstein LS, Shenker A, Gejman PV, Merino MJ, Friedman E, Spiegel AM. Activating mutations of the stimulatory G protein in the McCune-Albright syndrome. N Engl J Med 1991;325: 1688–1695.
27. Schwindinger WF, Francomano CA, Levine MA. Identification of a mutation in the gene encoding the alpha subunit of the stimulatory G-protein of adenylyl cyclase in McCune-Albright syndrome. Proc Natl Acad Sci USA 1992;89:5152–5156.
28. Tordjman K, Stern N, Ouaknine G, Yossiphov Y, Razon N, Nordenskjold M, et al. Activating mutations of the G_s α-gene in nonfunctioning pituitary tumors. J Clin Endocrinol Metab 1993; 77:765–769.
29. Williamson EA, Daniels M, Foster S, Kelly WF, Kendall-Taylor P, Harris PE. Gsα and Gi2α mutations in clinically non-functioning pituitary tumours. Clin Endocrinol 1994;41:815–820.
30. Dong Q, Brucker-Davis F, Weintraub BD, Smallridge RC, Carr FE, Battey J, et al. Screening of candidate oncogenes in human thyrotroph tumors: absence of activating mutations of the Gα_q, Gα_{11}, Gα_s, or thyrotropin-releasing hormone receptor genes. J Clin Endocrinol Metab 1996;81:1134–1140.
31. Struthers RS, Vale WW, Arias C, Sawchenko PE, Montminy MR. Somatotroph hypoplasia and dwarfism in transgenic mice expressing a non-phosphorylatable CREB mutant. Nature (Lond) 1991; 350:622–624.
32. Bertherat J, Chanson P, Montminy M. The cyclic adenosine 3', 5'-monophosphate-responsive factor CREB is constitutively activated in human somatotroph adenomas. Mol Endocrinol 1995;9:777–783.
33. Alvaro V, Touraine Ph, Raisman Vozari R, Bai-Grenier F, Birman P, Joubert Bression D. Protein kinase C activity and expression in normal and adenomatous human pituitaries. Int J Cancer 1992; 50:724–730.
34. Alvaro V, Levy L, Dubray C, Roche A, Peillon F, Querat B, et al. Invasive human pituitary tumors express a point-mutated α-protein kinase-C. J Clin Endocrinol Metab 1993;77:1125–1129.

35. Lowy DR, Willumsen BM. Function and regulation of ras. Annu Rev Biochem 1993;62:851–891.

36. Lochrie MA, Hurley JB, Simon MI. Sequence of the alpha subunit of photoreceptor G protein: homologies between transducin, ras, and elongation factors. Science 1985;228:96–99.

37. Bos JL. Ras oncogenes in human cancer: A review. Cancer Res 1989;49:4682–4689.

38. Konkel DA. What do ras oncogenes do? Mol Endocrinol 1988; 2:883–884.

39. Karga HJ, Alexander JM, Hedley-Whyte ET, Klibansky A, Jameson JL. Ras mutations in human pituitary tumors. J Clin Endocrinol Metab 1992;74:914–919.

40. Herman V, Drazin NZ, Gonsky R, Melmed S. Molecular screening of pituitary adenomas for gene mutations and rearrangements. J Clin Endocrinol Metab 1993;77:50–55.

41. Cai WY, Alexander JM, Hedley-Whyte ET, Scheithauer BW, Jameson JL, Zervas NT, et al. Ras mutations in human prolactinomas and pituitary carcinomas. J Clin Endocrinol Metab 1994;78:89–93.

42. Pei L, Melmed S, Scheithauer B, Kovacs K, Prager D. H-ras mutations in human pituitary carcinoma metastasis. J Clin Endocrinol Metab 1994;78:842–846.

43. Pei L, Melmed S. Isolation and characterization of a pituitary tumor-transforming gene (PTTG). Mol Endocrinol 1997;11:433–441.

44. Zhang X, Horwitz GA, Heaney AP, Nakashima M, Prezant TR, Bronstein MD, Melmed S. Pituitary tumor transforming gene (PTTG) expression in pituitary adenomas. J Clin Endocrinol Metab 1999;84:761–767.

45. Heaney AP, Horwitz GA, Wang Z, Singson R, Melmed S. Early involvement of estrogen-induced pituitary tumor transforming gene and fibroblast growth factor expression in prolactinoma pathogenesis. Nat Med 1999;5:1317–1321.

46. Ponder B. Gene losses in human tumours. Nature (Lond) 1988; 335:400–402.

47. Larsson C, Skogseid B, Oberg K, Nakamura Y, Nordenskjold M. Multiple endocrine neoplasia type 1 gene maps to chromosome 11 and is lost in insulinoma. Nature 1988;322:85–87.

48. Fujimori M, Wells SA, Nakamura Y. Fine mapping of the gene responsible for multiple endocrine neoplasia type 1(MEN1). Am J Hum Genet 1992;55:399–403.

49. Friedman E, Sakaguchi K, Bale AE, Falchetti A, Streeten E, Zimering MB, et al. Clonality of parathyroid tumors in familial multiple endocrine neoplasia type 1. N Engl J Med 1989;321:213–218.

50. Thakker RV, Bouloux P, Wooding C, Chotai K, Broad PM, Spurr NK, et al. Association of parathyroid tumors in multiple endocrine neoplasia 1 with loss of alleles on chromosome 11. N Engl J Med 1989;321:218–224.

51. Bystrom C, Larsson C, Blomberg C, Sandelin K, Falkmer U, Skogseid B, et al. Localization of the MEN1 gene to a small region within chromosome 11q13 by deletion mapping in tumors. Proc Natl Acad Sci USA 1990;87:1968–1972.

52. Bale AE, Norton JA, Wong EL, Fryburg JS, Maton PN, Oldfield EH, et al. Allelic loss on chromosome 11 in hereditary and sporadic tumors related to familial multiple endocrine neoplasia type 1. Cancer Res 1991;51:1154–1157.

53. Chandrasekharappa SC, Guru SC, Manickam P, Olufemi S-E, Collins FS, Emmert-Buck MR, Debelenko LV, Zhuang Z, Lubensky IA, Liotta LA, Crabtree JS, et al. Positional cloning of the gene for multiple endocrine neoplasia-type 1. Science 1997;276:404–407.

54. The European Consortium on MEN1. Identification of the multiple endocrine neoplasia type 1 (MEN1) gene. Hum Mol Genet 1997; 6:1177–1183.

55. Agarwal SK, Kester MB, Debelenko LV, Heppner C, Emmert-Buck MR, Skarulis MC, et al. Germline mutations of the MEN1 gene in familial multiple endocrine neoplasia type 1 and related states. Hum Mol Genet 1997;6:1169–1175.

56. Tanaka C, Yoshimoto K, Yamada S, Nishioka H, Moritani M, Yamaoka T, Itakura M. Absence of germ-line mutations of the multiple endocrine neoplasia type 1 (MEN1) gene in familial pituitary adenoma in contrast to MEN1 in Japanese. J Clin Endocrinol Metab 1998;83:960–965.

57. Zhuang Z, Ezzat SZ, Vortmeyer AO, Weil R, Oldfield EH, Park W-S, et al. Mutations of the MEN1 tumor suppressor gene in pituitary adenomas. Cancer Res 1997;57:5446–5451.

58. Prezant TR, Levine J, Melmed S. Molecular characterization of the *Men1* tumor suppressor gene in sporadic pituitary adenomas. J Clin Endocrinol Metab 1998;83:1388–1391.

59. Friend SH, Bernards R, Rogelj S, Weinberg RA, Rapaport JA, Albert DA, et al. A human DNA segment with properties of the gene that predisposes to retinoblastoma and osteosarcoma. Nature (Lond) 1986;323:643–646.

60. Jacks T, Fazeli A, Schmitt EM, Bronson RT, Goodell MA, Weinberg RA. Effects of an RB mutation in the mouse. Nature 1992;359: 295–300.

61. Cryns VL, Alexander JM, Klibanski A, Arnold A. The retinoblastoma gene in human pituitary tumors. J Clin Endocrinol Metab 1993;77:644–646.

62. Zhu J, Leon SP, Beggs AH, Busque L, Gilliliard DG, Black PM. Human pituitary adenomas show no loss of heterozygosity at the retinoblastoma gene locus. J Clin Endocrinol Metab 1994;78: 922–927.

63. Woloschak M, Roberts JL, Post KD. Loss of heterozygosity at the retinoblastoma locus in human pituitary tumors. Cancer 1994; 74:693–696.

64. Pei L, Melmed S, Scheithauer B, Kovacs K, Benedict WF, Prager D. Frequent loss of heterozygosity at the retinoblastoma susceptibility gene (RB) locus in aggressive pituitary tumors: evidence for a chromosome 13 tumor suppressor gene other than RB. Cancer Res 1995;55:1613–1616.

65. Woloschak M, Yu A, Xiao J, Post KD. Abundance and state of phosphorylation of the Rb gene product in human pituitary tumors. Int J Cancer 1996;67:16–19.

66. Levy A, Hall L, Yeudall WA, Lightman SL. p53 gene mutations in pituitary adenomas: rare events. Clin Endocrinol 1994;41:809–814.

67. Sumi T, Stefaneanu L, Kovacs K, Asa SL, Rindi G. Immunohistochemical study of p53 protein in human and animal pituitary tumors. Endocr Pathol 1993;4:95–99.

68. Buckley N, Bates AS, Broome JC, Strange RC, Perrett CW, Burke CW, et al. p53 accumulates in Cushings adenomas and invasive nonfunctional adenomas. J Clin Endocrinol Metab 1994;79:1513–1516.

69. Harvey M, Vogel H, Lee EY-HP, Bradley A, Donehower LA. Mice deficient in both p53 and Rb develop tumors primarily of endocrine origin. Cancer Res 1995;55:1146–1151.

70. Bevilaqua G, Sobel ME, Liotta LA, Steeg PS. Association of low nm23 RNA levels in human primary infiltrating ductal breast carcinomas with lymphnode involvement and other histopathological indicators of high metastatic potential. Cancer Res 1989;49: 5185–5190.

71. Takino H, Herman V, Weiss M, Melmed S. Purine-binding factor (nm23) gene expression in pituitary tumors: marker of adenoma invasiveness. J Clin Endocrinol Metab 1995;80:1733–1738.

72. Weinberg RA. The retinoblastoma protein and cell cycle control. Cell 1995;81:323–330.

73. Woloschak M, Yu A, Xiao J, Post KD. Frequent loss of the p16*ink4a* in human pituitary tumors. Cancer Res 1996;56:2493–2496.

74. Nakayama K, Ishida N, Shirane M, Inomata A, Inoue T, Shishido N, et al. Mice lacking p27[Kip1] display increased body size, multiple organ hyperplasia, retinal dysplasia, and pituitary tumors. Cell 1996;85:707–720.

75. Kiyokawa H, Kineman RD, Manova-Todorova KO, Soares VC, Hoffman ES, Ono M, et al. Enhanced growth of mice lacking the cyclin-dependent kinase inhibitor function of p27*Kip1*. Cell 1996;85:721–732.

76. Fero ML, Rivkin M, Tasch M, Porter P, Carow CE, Firpo E, et al. A syndrome of multiorgan hyperplasia with features of gigantism, tumorigenesis, and female sterility in p27*Kip1*-deficient mice. Cell 1996;85:733–744.

77. Radovick S, Nations M, Du Y, Berg LA, Weintraub BD, Wondisford FE. A mutation in the POU-homeodomain of Pit-1 responsible for combined pituitary hormone deficiency. Science (Wash. DC) 1992;257:1115–1118.

78. Li S, Crenshaw EB, Rawson EJ, Simmons DM, Swanson LW, Rosenfeld MG. Dwarf locus mutants lacking three pituitary cell types result from mutations in the POU-domain gene *pit-1*. Nature (Lond) 1990;347:528–532.

79. Lin C, Lin SC, Chang CP, Rosenfeld MG. Pit-1-dependent expression of the receptor for growth hormone releasing factor mediates pituitary cell growth. Nature (Lond) 1992;360:765–767.

80. Asa SL, Puy LA, Lew AM, Sundmark VC, Elsholtz HP. Cell type-specific expression of the pituitary transcription activator Pit-1 in the human pituitary and pituitary adenomas. J Clin Endocrinol Metab 1993;77:1275–1280.

81. Friend KE, Chiou YK, Laws ER Jr., Lopes MBS, Shupnik MA. Pit-1 messenger ribonucleic acid is differentially expressed in human pituitary adenomas. J Clin Endocrinol Metab 1993;77:1281–1286.

82. Pellegrini I, Barlier A, Gunz G, Figarella-Branger D, Enjalbert A, Grisoli F, et al. Pit-1 gene expression in the human pituitary and pituitary adenomas. J Clin Endocrinol Metab 1994;79:189–196.

83. Delhase M, Vergani P, Malur A, Velkeniers B, Teugels E, Trouillas J, et al. Pit-1/GHF-1 expression in pituitary adenomas: further analogy between human adenomas and rat SMtTW tumours. J Mol Endocrinol 1993;11:129–139.

84. Hoggard N, Callaghan K, Levy A, Davis JRE. Expression of Pit-1 and related proteins in diverse human pituitary adenomas. J Mol Endocrinol 1993;11:283–290.

85. Lin SC, Lin CR, Gukovsky I, Lusis AJ, Sawchenko PE, Rosenfeld MG. Molecular basis of the little mouse phenotype and implications for cell type-specific growth. Nature 1993;364:208–213.

86. Hashimoto K, Koga M, Motomura T, Kasayama S, Kouhara H, Ohnishi T, et al. Identification of alternatively spliced messenger ribonucleic acid encoding truncated growth hormone-releasing hormone receptor in human pituitary adenomas. J Clin Endocrinol Metab 1995;80:2933–2939.

87. Greenman Y, Prager D, Melmed S. The IGF-I receptor sub-membrane domain is intact in GH-secreting pituitary tumours. Clin Endocrinol 1995;42:169–172.

88. Faccenda E, Melmed S, Bevan JS, Eidne KA. Structure of the thyrotrophin-releasing hormone receptor in human pituitary adenomas. Clin Endocrinol 1996;44:341–347.

89. Friedman E, Adams EF, Hoog A, Gejman PV, Carson E, Larsson C, et al. Normal structural dopamine type 2 receptor gene in prolactin-secreting and other pituitary tumors. J Clin Endocrinol Metab 1994;78:568–574.

90. Mason IJ. The ins and outs of fibroblast growth factors. Cell 1994;78:547–552.

91. Gospodarowicz D, Ferrara N, Schweigerer L, Neufeld G. Structural characterization and biological functions of fibroblast growth factor. Endocr Rev 1987;8:95–114.

92. Gospodarowicz D, Neufeld G, Schweigerer L. Fibroblast growth factor. Mol Cell Endocrinol 1986;46:187–204.

93. Bohlen P, Baird A, Esch F, Ling N, Gospodarowicz D. Isolation and partial molecular characterization of pituitary fibroblast growth factor. Proc Natl Acad Sci USA 1984;81:5364–5368.

94. Li Y, Koga M, Kasayama S, Matsumoto K, Arita N, Hayakawa T, et al. Identification and characterization of high molecular weight forms of basic fibroblast growth factor in human pituitary adenomas. J Clin Endocrinol Metab 1992;75:1436–1441.

95. Ezzat S, Smyth HS, Ramyar L, Asa SL. Heterogenous in vivo and in vitro expression of basic fibroblast growth factor by human pituitary adenomas. J Clin Endocrinol Metab 1995;80:878–884.

96. Baird A, Mormede P, Ying SY, Wehrenberg WB, Ueno N, Ling N, et al. A nonmitogenic pituitary function of fibroblast growth factor: regulation of thyrotropin and prolactin secretion. Proc Natl Acad Sci USA 1985;82:5545–5549.

97. Atkin SL, Landolt AM, Jeffreys RV, Diver M, Radcliffe J, White MC. Basic fibroblast growth factor stimulates prolactin secretion from human anterior pituitary adenomas without affecting adenoma cell proliferation. J Clin Endocrinol Metab 1993;77:831–837.

98. Schechter J, Weiner R. Changes in basic fibroblast growth factor coincident with estradiol-induced hyperplasia of the anterior pituitaries of Fischer 344 and Sprague-Dawley rats. Endocrinology 1991;129:2400–2408.

99. Weiner RI, Windle J, Mellon P, Schechter J. Role of FGF in tumorigenesis of the anterior pituitary [Abstract]. J Endocrinol Invest 1991, 14(Suppl. 1):10.

100. Zimering MB, Brandi ML, deGrange DA, Marx SJ, Streeten E, Katsumata N, et al. Circulating fibroblast growth factor-like substance in familial multiple endocrine neoplasia type 1. J Clin Endocrinol Metab 1990;70:149–154.

101. Zimering MB, Katsumata N, Sato Y, Brandi ML, Aurbach GD, Marx SJ, et al. Increased basic fibroblast growth factor in plasma from multiple endocrine neoplasia type 1: relation to pituitary tumor. J Clin Endocrinol Metab 1993;76:1182–1187.

102. Zimering MB, Riley DJ, Thakker-Varia S, Walker AM, Lakshminaryan V, Shah R, et al. Circulating fibroblast growth factor-like autoantibodies in two patients with multiple endocrine neoplasia type 1 and prolactinoma. J Clin Endocrinol Metab 1994;79:1546–1552.

103. Sakamoto H, Mori M, Taira M, Yoshida T, Matsukawa S, Shimizu K, et al. Transforming gene from human stomach cancers and a noncancerous portion of stomach mucosa. Proc Natl Acad Sci USA 1986;83:3997–4001.

104. Yoshida MC, Wada M, Satoh H, Yoshida T, Sakamoto H, Miyagawa K, et al. Human HST1 (HSTF1) gene maps to chromosome band 11q13 and coamplifies with the INT2 gene in human cancer. Proc Natl Acad Sci USA 1988;85:4861–4864.

105. Shimon I, Huttner A, Said J, Spirina O, Melmed S. Heparin-binding secretory transforming gene (hst) facilitates rat lactotrope cell tumorigenesis and induces prolactin gene transcription. J Clin Invest 1996;97:187–195.

106. Gonsky R, Herman V, Melmed S, Fagin J. Transforming DNA sequences present in human prolactin secreting pituitary tumors. Mol Endocrinol 1991;5:1687–1695.

107. Shimon I, Hinton DR, Weiss M, Melmed S. Prolactinomas express human heparin-binding secretory transforming gene (hst) protein product: marker of tumor invasiveness. Clin Endocrinol (Oxf) 1998;48:23–29.

108. Derynck R, Goeddel DV, Ullrich A, Gutterman JU, Williams RD, Bringman TS, et al. Synthesis of messenger RNAs for transforming growth factors α and β and the epidermal growth factor receptor by human tumors. Cancer Res 1987;47:707–712.

109. Korbin MS, Asa SL, Samsoondar J, Kudlow JE. α-Transforming growth factor in the bovine anterior pituitary gland: secretion by dispersed cells and immunohistochemical localization. Endocrinology 1987;121:1412–1416.

110. Samsoondar J, Korbin MS, Kudlow JE. α-Transforming growth factor secreted by untransformed bovine anterior pituitary cells in culture. I. Purification from conditioned media. J Biol Chem 1986;261:14,408–14,413.

111. Mueller SG, Korbin MS, Paterson AJ, Kudlow JE. Transforming growth factor-α expression in the anterior pituitary gland: regulation by epidermal growth factor and phorbol ester in dispersed cells. Mol Endocrinol 1989;3:976–983.

112. Finley EL, Ramsdell JS. A transforming growth factor-α pathway is expressed in GH_4C_1 rat pituitary tumors and appears necessary for tumor formation. Endocrinology 1994;135:416–422.

113. Driman DK, Korbin MS, Kudlow JE, Asa SL. Transforming growth factor-α in normal and neoplastic human endocrine tissues. Hum Pathol 1992;23:1360–1365.

114. Ezzat S, Walpola IA, Ramyar L, Smyth HS, Asa SL. Membrane-anchored expression of transforming growth factor-α in human pituitary adenoma cells. J Clin Endocrinol Metab 1995;80:534–539.

115. McAndrew J, Paterson AJ, Asa SL, McCarthy KJ, Kudlow JE. Targeting of transforming growth factor-α expression to pituitary lactotrophs in transgenic mice results in selective lactotroph proliferation and adenomas. Endocrinology 1995;136:4479–4488.

6 Experimental Models of Pituitary Tumorigenesis

Lucia Stefaneanu, PhD

INTRODUCTION

Pituitary tumors can be induced by chemicals, irradiation, target organ ablation, and genetic manipulations. Despite the availability of these models, pituitary tumorigenesis is still obscure. Depending on the approach, different types of pituitary tumors can be induced, including hormone-secreting or "silent" ones. Conditions similar to those existing in patients with gigantism, amenorrhea, galactorrhea, infertility, Cushing's disease, hypothyroidism, or hypogonadism are created, giving the opportunity not only to obtain a deeper insight into the process of tumorigenesis, but also to test therapeutic modalities. The mouse, especially since the introduction of transgenic technology, is now replacing the rat, which has been the preferred species for inducing different experimental conditions, including pituitary tumors. It is important to emphasize that pituitary tumors arising in rodents are not identical to human ones and that extrapolation of the experimental results to human beings has some limitations. These differences could be attributed not only to the distinct morphologic features of hormone-containing cells of the rodent and human pituitaries but also to differences in the pituitary regulatory mechanisms among species. An important issue is the existence of distinct plurihormonal cells in the normal pituitary, which have been less studied in humans. Bi- or multihormonal tumors are common in rodent and human pituitaries, and they may reflect a normal counterpart or represent a feature achieved by the transformed cells during tumor development and/or progression.

CHEMICALS

ESTROGEN Lactotroph secretion is regulated by hypothalamic-inhibiting and stimulating factors, and peripheral hormones. Among them, dopamine acting via D2 subtype receptor (D2R) plays an inhibitory role, whereas estrogen by binding to estrogen receptor (ER) is the most potent stimulator of prolactin gene transcription, synthesis, and release, as well as multiplication of lactotrophs.

Chronic stimulation with high doses of estrogen represents the first experimental model of pituitary tumor induction, dating back to 1936 *(1–3)*. Since then, natural and synthetic estrogens alone or in association with other chemicals were extensively used in rodents to induce lesions from diffuse lactotroph hyperplasia to nodules and adenomas *(4,5)*. The induction period requires several months to more than a year. Different strains of rats and mice show variable susceptibility to adenoma formation. Gardner and Strong *(6)* reported in 1940 that C57 Black mice are more sensitive to estrogen treatment compared to other strains such as A, C3H, CBA, C12I, and JK. Wiklund et al. *(7)* showed that the Fischer rat is the most sensitive strain to estrogen treatment, but Holtzman rats are relatively resistant. Diethylstilbestrol (DES) is more efficient than 17 β-estradiol (E$_2$) or estrone in inducing pituitary tumors. The efficiency of DES is enhanced when it is administered to weaning rats *(8)*. Extensively studied in the 1950s and 1960s, hormone secretion by pituitary tumors was deduced from the associated changes in target organs, such as mammary glands, adrenals, gonads, and somatic growth. The hormonal potency is more evident in tumor grafting on isologous hosts. Owing to their stimulatory effect on mammary glands, the tumors originally were named mammotrophic. Transplantation studies, followed by bioassays, pioneered by Furth and his colleagues, established that estrogen-induced pituitary tumors possess both mammary gland-stimulating and growth-promoting effects.

In the rat, estrogen-induced adenomas are chromophobic or acidophilic. No compression of nontumorous tissue was reported. The adenoma formation is preceded by massive lactotroph hyperplasia, accompanied by elevated levels of blood prolactin (PRL) *(9)*. After 9 wk of DES, the intensity of hybridization signal for PRL mRNA per cell is increased by 2.3 times, suggesting stimulation of PRL gene transcription *(10)*. In mice, the hyperplasia of lactotrophs is focal or nodular (Figure 1), followed by acidophilic or chromophobic adenomas, with a sinusoid-cystic, rarely solid or trabecular pattern. There are no clear-cut morphologic criteria to distinguish hyperplasia from adenoma. In the rat, pituitary weight >30 mg (normal weight about 10 mg) was arbitrarily used as a criterion to define pituitary adenoma *(11)*. The presence of hemorrhages was reported in association with adenoma. The majority of cells are immunoreactive for PRL, and a minority of cells are positive for growth hormone (GH). Ultrastructurally, the adenoma cells resemble spontaneous lactotroph tumors; however, groups or isolated somatotrophs are present, as well *(12,13)*.

When transplanted, estrogen-induced rat pituitary tumors are growing only in estrogen-conditioned hosts. After one or two passages, autonomous variants arise that grow without estrogen

From: *Diagnosis and Management of Pituitary Tumors* (K. Thapar, K. Kovacs, B. W. Scheithauer, and R. V. Lloyd, eds.), ©Humana Press Inc., Totowa, NJ.

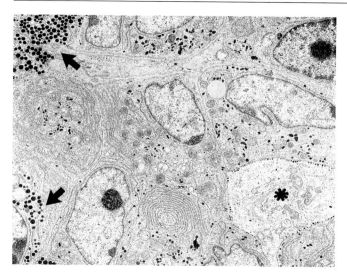

Figure 6-1   Pituitary of a mouse exposed to diethylstilbestrol for 3 mo contains prominent lactotrophs; the lactotrophs are hypertrophied, and contain euchromatic nuclei, enlarged nucleoli, very well-developed rough endoplasmic reticulum, and enlarged Golgi apparatus with numerous forming secretory granules; areas of somatotrophs (arrows) and a corticotroph (asterisk) are also seen. (×5000)

support. Mouse transplanted tumors are becoming autonomous after one passage. After serial passages, tumors can secrete adrenocorticotropin (ACTH) as well *(14)*. The best-studied transplanted tumor-producing GH, PRL, and ACTH is MtT/F4, which originated in a Fischer rat and was successively transplanted for 4 yr. The growth of this tumor is inhibited by estrogen treatment *(15–17)*, whereas PRL and GH gene expression are stimulated *(18,19)*. Two cell lines were established from MtT/F4 tumor, using different culture conditions *(20)*. The growth of one cell line is inhibited by estrogen, but the other is stimulated. These cell lines reveal the heterogeneity of the MtT/F4 tumor.

Although estrogens are widely used to induce lactotroph hyperplasia and pituitary adenoma, the mechanisms responsible for cell proliferation and tumor development are still obscure. Strain differences in pituitary response to estrogen offer the possibility to study the contribution of genetic background to the process of tumorigenesis. The segregation of pituitary tumor formation in Fischer 344xHoltzman hybrids indicated that tumor formation is a polygenetic trait involving two or three as-yet unidentified genetic loci *(21)*. By studying F1 and F2 hybrids between F344 rats in which estrogen or DES induces hemorrhagic adenomas, and Brown Norway rats in which no changes in pituitary weights are seen, Wendell et al. *(22)* concluded that the hemorrhagic phenotype is a recessive, epistatic trait. As in the previous study, it is suggested that two or three genes are involved in the regulation of estrogen effect on lactotroph proliferation and tissue rearrangement, although some additional loci regulating tumor growth are not excluded. In order to identify the underlying mechanism of differential sensitivity between rat strains to estrogen-induced pituitary tumors, Gregg et al. *(23)* investigated pituitary gene expression of carboxypeptidase E (CPE). The role of CPE is to remove basic amino adds from the C-terminus of various pituitary hormones following the cleavage of precursor hormones by endopeptidases, such as proprotein convertases PC2 and PC3. The study revealed that CPE protein is drastically decreased in F344 rats after 10 wk of DES treatment, whereas in Brown Norway rats

CPE shows no change. It appears that CPE is posttranscriptionally regulated in estrogen-sensitive and estrogen-resistant rats. This approach exemplifies the importance of comparative studies of strains with different sensitivities to estrogens. Recently, it was demonstrated that CPE can play the role of a membrane-associated sorting receptor in the Golgi and secretory granules. In *Cpe^{fat}* mutant mouse lacking CPE, pituitary POMC is missorted to the constitutive pathway and secreted in an unregulated manner *(24)*. It remains to be studied whether CPE has such a function in PRL secretion.

Novel data reveal that ER crosstalks with transcription factors, growth factors, and oncogenes *(25)*. The findings in normal and tumorous lactotrophs indicate that regulation of PRL gene transcription and cell proliferation are not coupled. In normal rat pituitary, an early response to E_2 treatment involves increased c-myc and c-fos mRNAs *(26)*. The influence of estrogen on intrinsic pituitary growth factors such as transforming growth factor-beta (TGF-β), basic fibroblast growth factor (bFGF), insulin-like growth factor (IGF-1), and vascular endothelial growth factor (VEGF) are now the focus of emerging studies.

In normal rat pituitary, TGF-β was localized in lactotrophs and melanotrophs *(27)*. Qian et al. *(28)*, applying *in situ* hybridization or *in situ* polymerase chain reaction (PCR) combined with immunocytochemistry for pituitary hormones, revealed TGF-β1 mRNA mainly in lactotrophs, followed by thyrotrophs and gonadotrophs, and less frequently in the other hormone-containing cells of rat pituitary. In general, TGF-β inhibits the growth of epithelial cells *(29)*. In cultured rat pituitary cells, TGF-β1 has a biphasic effect on lactotroph proliferation, with marked inhibition at lower concentration and slight stimulation at a higher one *(28)*. In vitro, TGF-β1 suppresses E_2-induced PRL release and inhibits E_2-induced proliferation of lactotrophs *(27)*. In rats treated chronically with estrogen, the pituitary content of TGF-β1 and TGF-β type II receptor proteins and mRNAs decreases during tumor development *(30)*.

IGF-1 mRNA is present in the pituitary and is diffusely distributed in rat anterior lobe. The role of intrinsic IGF-1 in pituitary secretion and cell proliferation is under investigation. In addition to the inhibition of somatotrophs, IGF-1 plays a role in the stimulation of lactotrophs as demonstrated in mice with inactive IGF-1 *(31)*. Estrogen treatment of ovariectomized rats increases pituitary IGF-1 and IGF binding protein type 2 mRNAs content. The results suggest that IGF-1 may be a modulator of some of the estrogen effects *(32)*.

Estrogen treatment of Fisher rats increases bFGF and VEGF production by pituitary in early phase of PRL cell hyperplasia *(32a,32b)*. Both bFGF and estrogen are inducing a pituitary tumor-derived transforming gene (PTTG) whose role is to inhibit chromatid separation *(32c)*.

Another peptide that can play a role in pituitary adenoma development is galanin. In the rat, galanin is localized in lactotrophs, and its synthesis is markedly stimulated by estrogen treatment *(33)*.

When estrogen administration is associated with a carcinogen or irradiation, the frequency of pituitary tumors is increased. Thus, pituitary tumors can be induced in a relative short time interval, when estrogen is administered with dimethylbenz(a)anthracene (DMBA) assumed to act as initiator of pituitary tumorigenesis *(34)*. Lloyd et al. *(10)* showed that estradiol benzoate- and DMBA-treated F344 rats develop transplantable pituitary tumors within 3 mo. Adenohypophysial tumors with high incidence are evident when estrogen is administered in combination with [90]Sr

(35). The results suggest that ^{90}Sr acts as mutagen on estrogen-stimulated cells.

TRIMETHYLANILINE   2,4,6-Trimethylaniline, a nonsteroidal carcinogen given for 18 mo in the diet of a rat, induced a huge pituitary tumor *(36).* The tumor was transplanted successively and called line 7315. Since all rats with transplants had enlarged mammary glands and lactated, the tumor was named 7315a (active line). During the 7th transfer, some rats did not lactate, and the tumor was named 7315i (inactive line). The tumor TtT-7315a was determined by bioassays to produce PRL, GH, and ACTH, resembling the MtT/F4 transplantable tumor, derived from an estrogen-induced pituitary tumor *(37).* However, the content of GH and ACTH was much lower than in MtT/F4. Ultrastructurally, the 7315a tumor shows large (560–1700 nm) secretory granules resembling those seen in lactotrophs, as well as some very small (160 nm) secretory granules. The 7315i tumor contains only small secretory granules *(38).*

A pituitary tumor cell line, designated MMQ, derived from the 7315a tumor produces only PRL *(39).* The secretory granules of 150–300 nm in diameter are sparse. Since this cell line has functioning dopamine D2 receptor, it can be used to study the regulation of PRL secretion.

CALCITONIN   Administration of high doses of calcitonin to rats for at least 6 mo is associated with high incidence of pituitary tumors *(40,41).* The adenomas express α-subunit mRNA of glycoprotein hormones, and encoded peptide as demonstrated by *in situ* hybridization and immunocytochemistry. Although calcitonin receptor is present in pituitary, it is unknown whether the proliferation of a subset of glycoprotein hormone-producing cells is a direct or indirect effect of calcitonin *(40).*

IONIZING RADIATION

Pituitary tumors can be induced in mice and rats by ionizing radiation *(42–44).* Most of the tumors originated in lactotrophs or corticotrophs.

The incidence of PRL-secreting adenomas increased 17–28 mo after exposure to ionizing radiation from an atomic test detonation or 400–700 r of X-rays in comparison with control LAF1 mice *(45).* The tumors were reddish-brown and hemorrhagic. Histologic examination showed chromophobic adenomas with occasional acidophilic cells disposed in solid nests surrounding spaces filled with blood. Nuclear pleomorphism and giant nuclei were sometime seen. When transplanted, the adenomas were autonomous.

LAF1 mice exposed to ionizing irradiation with ACTH-producing tumors *(46,47)* gained weight and had elevated blood corticosterone levels. The tumors contained ACTH and melanocyte-stimulating hormone (MSH). Transplantable ACTH-producing tumors were derived from these mice *(46,47).* An ACTH-secreting pituitary cell line was established by Sato et al. in 1966 from earlier cultures of one of these transplantable tumors *(48)* and was named AtT-20. AtT-20 pituitary cell line possesses functioning corticotropin-releasing hormone (CRH) receptor and, consequently, can be used to study the regulation of POMC-derived peptides secretion. Cytokines, such as interleukins 1 (IL-1) and 6 (IL-6), macrophage migration-inhibitory factor (MIF), and leukemia-inhibitory factor (LIF) were shown to be produced by AtT-20 cell line and to increase POMC mRNA level and CRH-induced ACTH secretion *(49–51).*

In W/Fu rats exposed to 800 r, pituitary tumors developed in 74% of them within 2 yr. The tumors were hemorrhagic, chromophobic adenomas *(52).* Some of the pituitary tumors were trans-

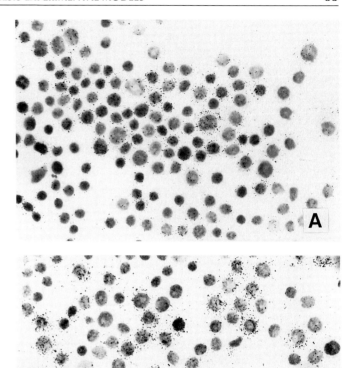

Figure 6-2   Pituitary tumor GH$_3$ cell line grown in complete culture medium, contains signal for both GH **(A)** and PRL **(B)** mRNAs in most cells. Radioactive *in situ* hybridization. (×400)

planted and grew with or without estrogen support. The associated secondary changes in target organs indicated their ability to secrete variable amounts of PRL and GH. One of these tumors was initially called MtT/W5 owing to its ability to secrete prolactin. Three different groups of investigators reported that during serial passages, this tumor ceased to secrete PRL, but maintained that of GH *(53–55).* The tumor became fast-growing and metastasizing. McLeod et al. *(53)* called it St/W5. Hollander and Hollander *(55)* isolated a variant named MtT.W5/OM from an ovarian metastasis. Tashjian et al. *(54)* developed a pituitary tumor cell line, named GH$_3$, which expresses both GH and PRL genes (Figure 2). From the same MtT/W5 tumor, a cell line, GH$_1$, which secretes only GH, was developed *(54).* Further studies of these variants of transplantable tumors showed that all produce high amounts of GH and very little PRL, and by immunocytochemistry GH is present in all tumor cells, but PRL is scarce *(56).* It has been concluded that the tumors originated in a mammosomatotroph, rather than in a lactotroph, which acquired the capacity to produce GH. The interconversion of somatotrophs and lactotrophs with the mammosomatotroph as an intermediate was intensely investigated in the normal pituitary, and the presence of mammosomatotrophs was proven with different techniques *(57).*

Estrogen inhibits the growth of MtT/W15 tumor, and at the same time PRL expression is inhibited as well, but GH gene expression is stimulated *(58).*

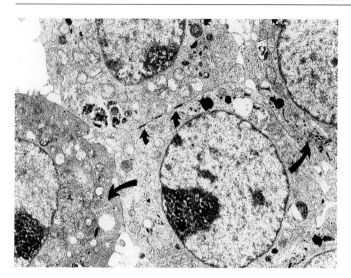

Figure 6-3 Ultrastructurally, GH_3 cells possess euchromatic nuclei with large nucleoli, surrounded by a narrow cytoplasm containing a moderate number of mitochondria, scarce cysternae of rough endoplasmic reticulum, phagolysosomes, and a few, very small secretory granules (large arrows); the cells are attached by tight junctions (small arrows). (×6600)

The pituitary tumor GH_3 cell line is intensely used to characterize the mechanisms of hormone secretion and cell proliferation. Ultrastructurally, GH_3 cells possess very small (50–230 nm) secretory granules, modest Golgi apparatus, bundles of intermediate filaments, phagolysosomes, and tight junctions between cells (Figure 3). GH_3 cells do not transcribe GHRH receptor gene *(58a)*. Extrusion of secretory granules is rarely seen. GH_3 cells contain low-affinity dopamine binding sites *(59)*, despite the presence of D2R mRNA and encoded protein *(60)*. The cell line does not respond to dopamine with increased D2R mRNA as nontumorous lactotrophs, indicating a defective receptor *(61)*. Such an abnormal receptor may offer an explanation for the resistance to bromocriptine treatment of some patients with lactotroph adenomas. When treated with E_2 in culture, the proportion of GH_3 cells secreting both GH and PRL increases, but thyrotropin-releasing hormone (TRH) treatment results in an increased number of cells secreting PRL only, as determined by reverse hemolytique plaque assay *(62)*. PRL secretion is also stimulated by nerve growth factor (NGF), and at the same time, GH secretion is markedly inhibited. NGF treatment of GH_3 cells affects their proliferation as well *(63)*. Basic fibroblastic growth factor (bFGF) stimulates PRL gene expression and proliferation of GH_3 cells, whereas TGF-β stimulates PRL gene expression and inhibits proliferation *(64)*. Estrogen has no effect on bFGF and TGF-β mRNAs *(63)*. The stimulatory effect of bFGF on PRL release by GH_3 cells is enhanced by cotreatment with estrogen *(65)*. Treatment of GH_3 cells with physiological doses of insulin stimulates PRL production and increases PRL mRNA, suggesting a direct effect of insulin on PRL gene transcription or its mRNA stabilization *(66)*. GH_3 cells also produce IGF-1, which is regulated by GH, and T_3 *(67)*. ER can mediate the mitogenic effects of insulin and IGF-1 in the absence of estrogen in culture medium *(68)*.

GH_3C_1 cell line, a subclone of GH_3 cells, also has very small and sparse secretory granules, and responds to estrogen, insulin, and EGF treatment with increased PRL content and decreased GH storage and secretion *(69)*.

TARGET ORGAN ABLATION

THYROIDECTOMY   Thyroid-stimulating hormone (TSH)-producing tumors are induced by chronic thyroid hormone deficiency that can be achieved by radiothyroidectomy, surgical thyroidectomy, antithyroid drugs, or a low-iodine diet. The mouse is the most susceptible mammal in which thyrotroph tumors develop secondary to severe hypothyroidism *(70)*. Gorbman *(71)* was the first to note pituitary tumors after radiothyroidectomy. Complete destruction of thyroid is not essential; pituitary tumors can be found following partial thyroidectomy *(72)* or propylthiouracil administration *(73)*. The pituitaries of LAF_1 mice treated with a low-iodine diet and subsequently with a dose of ^{131}I showed first "thyroidectomy" cells, followed by diffuse thyrotroph hyperplasia, and within 1 yr, multiple nodules *(4,70)*. The hyperplastic and nodular thyrotrophs are immunoreactive for TSH. When transplanted, the nodules are fully hormone-dependent for 3–7 yr growing only in hypothyroid mice; thereafter they become autonomous and proliferate in euthyroid mice. The autonomous tumors secrete low amounts of TSH and variable amounts of gonadotropins. By immunocytochemistry, the transplantable tumors are weakly immunoreactive for TSH and intensely positive for gonadotropins *(74)*. A few transplantable thyrotroph tumors are available, such as TtT 87, TtT 97, MGH 101, and MGH 101A; they are useful models to investigate the regulation of synthesis and release of α- and β-subunits of glycoprotein hormones *(75–79)*. In some of the autonomous tumors, GH immunoreactivity becomes preponderant, whereas TSH immunoreactivity decreases, resembling some human thyrotroph adenomas that coproduced TSH and GH *(80)*.

GONADECTOMY   It was reported that gonadectomy of newborn CE and DBA mice and of F1 hybrids causes pituitary basophilic tumors starting at 14 mo of age *(81,82)*. Pituitary tumors are preceded by adrenal cortical tumors secreting estrogen and also by mammary tumors. Pituitary lesions include opaque or hemorrhagic nodules composed of granular cells with negative image of Golgi complex. These tumors have not been studied by immunocytochemistry. Most probably, they originated in lactotrophs owing to excessive estrogen.

TRANSGENIC MODELS

Transgenic models of pituitary tumors are extremely valuable for the study of the multistep process of tumorigenesis. In order to induce adenohypophysial tumors, different strategies are applied, including insertion of genes encoding releasing hormones, growth factors, or oncogenes fused with appropriate promoters/enhancers, or altering tumor suppressor genes. Usually, the transgene establishes a high predisposition to neoplastic transformation, without directly inducing tumor formation. Spontaneous mutations of genes that interact with the foreign gene are necessary for the tumor development.

ECTOPIC EXPRESSION OF GROWTH HORMONE-RELEASING HORMONE (GHRH)   It is known that GHRH is mitogenic for rat somatotrophs in vitro *(83)* and that in vivo exposure for 1 wk to GHRH is sufficient to induce somatotroph hyperplasia in rat *(84)*. GHRH also induces c-*fos* expression in somatotrophs *(85)*. Mice transgenic for human (h)GHRH fused with the metallothionein promoter express the foreign gene in many tissues, including the adenohypophysis; they have elevated blood levels of GHRH and GH, and develop gigantism *(86)*. Young and adult mice show massive pituitary hyperplasia of acidophils (Figure 4) represented by somatotrophs and some mammo-

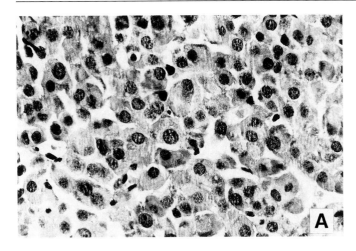

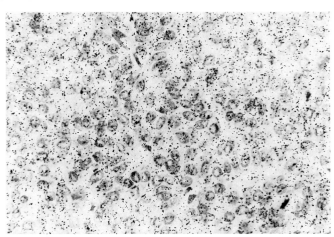

Figure 6-5 Pituitary adenoma found in an old GHRH transgenic mouse contains GH mRNA signal with a diffuse pattern. Radioactive *in situ* hybridization. (×400)

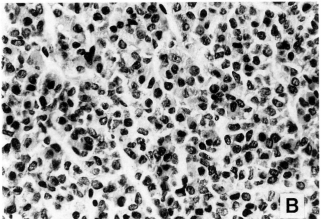

Figure 6-4 The adenohypophysis of a young GHRH transgenic mouse has an increased number of hypertrophied acidophils **(A)**, compared to a control nontransgenic sibling **(B)**. (×400)

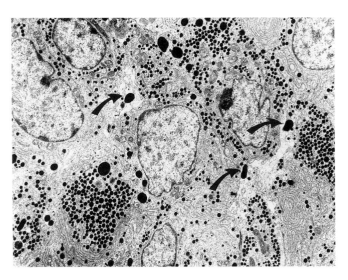

Figure 6-6 By electron microscopy, pituitary adenoma of an old GHRH transgenic mouse is composed of cells resembling the hyperplastic somatotrophs; the cells contain many medium sized secretory granules, and prominent rough endoplasmic reticulum; secretory material extruded into intercellular space is frequently seen (arrows). (×4000)

somatotrophs *(86,87)*. Old mice, 1 yr and over, develop pituitary adenomas composed of cells immunoreactive for GH, and focally for PRL and/or TSH *(88,89)*. *In situ* hybridization reveals a strong, diffuse signal for GH mRNA (Figure 5) and focally for PRL mRNA. Ultrastructurally, two types of adenomas are found *(90)*. The frequent ones contain cells resembling the hyperplastic somatotrophs (Figure 6). The medium-sized cells with slightly eccentric nucleoli are endowed with abundant rough endoplasmic reticulum, and prominent Golgi complexes with forming secretory granules. The secretory granules are abundant and measure 300–500 nm in diameter in many cells. Less frequently, cells with fewer and smaller secretory granules are present. A special feature is the extrusion of secretory granules and of large deposits of secretory material in the intercellular space or toward a capillary. The second adenoma type exhibits cells with sparse, small, secretory granules that have no resemblance to nontumorous somatotroph. Interestingly, in some tumor cells, Golgi apparatus contains secretory granules with bizarre shapes similar to those seen in some human somatotroph adenomas. There are no fibrous bodies—the markers of human sparsely granulated somatotroph adenomas *(80)*. A tumor cell line established from a large tumor of a MT/hGHRH transgenic mouse produces GH and PRL *(90)*. The pathogenesis of adenomas remains to be studied. The presence of high levels of circulating hGHRH suggests that protracted stimulation by GHRH of somatotrophs contributes to the neoplastic process.

It is worth underlining that hGHRH is expressed not only in peripheral organs, but also in the pituitary itself. The heterologous GHRH was localized in different cell types of nontumorous pituitaries *(86,88,90,91)*, and in adenomas *(92)*. The possible involvement of locally produced GHRH to tumorigenesis is not excluded. Recent studies demonstrated that normal human pituitary and many of its tumors express GHRH that may act in an autocrine/paracrine mode to influence the growth and/or hormone secretion of tumor cells *(93–95)*. The contribution of other oncogenes and growth factors remains to be studied.

TARGETED ONCOGENESIS The targeted oncogenesis uses growth factors or viral and cellular oncogenes fused to tissue-specific promoter or enhancer sequence in order to produce experimental models of tumorigenesis. The most frequent viral oncogene used is the large T-antigen of simian virus 40 (SV40), which participates directly in the creation of transformed phe-

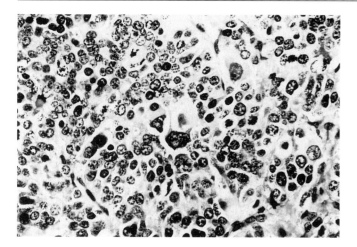

Figure 6-7 Pituitary tumor found in the anterior lobe of a mouse transgenic for AVP/SV40 oncogene is composed of cells with marked nuclear pleomorphism, and frequent mitotic figures. Hematoxylin & eosin. (×400)

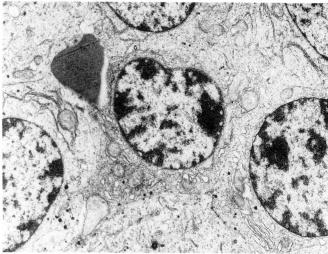

Figure 6-8 Ultrastructurally, the anterior lobe tumors of AVP/SV40 transgenic mice are formed by very undifferentiated cells with rare, tiny secretory granules. (×8400)

notype. Moreover, SV40 large T-antigen, as well as human papillomavirus- (HPV) transforming protein and adenoviral proteins bind p53 and retinoblastoma (Rb) protein. P53 and Rb proteins mediate the arrest of the cell cycle in late G1 phase. The binding to SV40 large T-antigen is believed to inactivate p53 and Rb proteins, allowing progression through the cell cycle. Several lines of evidence indicate that viral or cellular oncogenes interact in multistep events in transformed cell.

Mice Transgenic for Arginine-Vasopressin/SV40 Large T-Antigen   This gene construct was designed to induce hypothalamic tumors. Instead, young mice developed endocrine pancreatic tumors originating in insulin-producing cells and pituitary adenomas *(96)*. Most frequently, the pituitary tumors are localized in anterior lobe, and rarely double adenomas in anterior and intermediate lobes are seen *(97)*. Anterior lobe tumors are very pleomorphic with giant nuclei and multinucleated cells (Figure 7). Mitoses, and hemorrhagic and necrotic areas are frequent. Many tumor cells are immunonegative for adenohypophysial hormones. Some tumors show focal GH and TSH immunostaining. More helpful was the application of *in situ* hybridization, which showed a diffuse signal for GH mRNA in all tumors, indicating their origin in somatotrophs. By electron microscopy, the tumor cells are very undifferentiated (Figure 8), and rare cells have features reminiscent of somatotrophs. Intermediate lobe tumors are immunoreactive for ACTH and contain a strong, diffuse signal for proopiomelanocortin (POMC) mRNA. The tumors are not accompanied by hyperplasia of any cell type. The tumors are immunoreactive for large T-antigen *(95)* and p53 *(98)*, which are not detected in adjacent nontumorous pituitaries.

Mice Transgenic for α-Subunit of Glycoprotein Hormones/SV40 Large T-Antigen   Transgenic mice for α-subunit promoter of glycoprotein hormones fused with SV40 large T antigen develop pituitary tumors transcribing the α-subunit gene *(99)*. The tumors are composed of cells immunoreactive for luteinizing hormone (LH)-β or TSH-β, and α-subunit intermingled with neural tissue, suggesting that a neurotropic factor is secreted by the transformed cells *(100)*. Clonal cell lines derived from these tumors contain α-subunit mRNA and secrete α-subunit, but no β-subunits. Since the cell lines respond to gonadotropin-releasing

hormone (GnRH) stimulation, but not to TRH, the authors concluded that they originated in cells of gonadotroph lineage *(100)*.

Mice Transgenic for Gonadotropin-Releasing Hormone Receptor Gene/SV40 Large T Antigen   The 5'-flanking region (1.2 kb) of the mouse gonadotropin-releasing hormone receptor (mGnRH-R) promoter fused with SV40 large T antigen was used to induce pituitary tumors originating in gonadotrophs *(100a)*. The tumors developed in young and 4–5 months old mice, and showed suprasellar extension and infiltration of brain. The tumors expressed FSHβ, LHβ and α subunit genes, as demonstrated by *in situ* hybridization for their mRNAs. The tumors also expressed GnRH-R mRNA.

Mice Transgenic for Human β-Thyrotropin/SV40T Antigen   Using 1109-bp 5'-flanking sequence of human (h)TSH gene fused to SV40 large T antigen, Maki et al. *(101)* generated a line of transgenic mice transplanting the ovaries of a founder mouse to normal females and crossing them with a normal male. The hemizygous offsprings were dwarfs. Around 7 wk of age, head tumors became visible, and the mice wasted and died within 3 wk. Pituitary tumors are localized in the anterior lobe, and are formed by small, chromophobic cells, and few giant cells with pleomorphic nuclei. A few calcium deposits and mitoses are evident as well. Immunocytochemistry for GH, PRL, TSH, and LH shows immunoreactive cells only in the nontumorous areas and in few tumor-entrapped normal cells. The lack of immunostainings in tumorous cells suggests that they are undifferentiated. The tumor cells exhibit strong nuclear staining for large T-antigen. The authors speculated that the lack of TSH immunoreactivity in the tumor cells could be owing to their origin in a progenitor cell common to somatotrophs, lactotrophs, and thyrotrophs, which share Pit-1 transcription factor. Another possibility could be that they originate in a thyrotroph progenitor cell at the time when transcription factor thyroid embryonic factor (TEF) binds to the 5'-flanking region of TSH-β gene around embryonic day 14. However, the authors did not perform immunostaining for the α-subunit of glycoprotein hormones and/or *in situ* hybridization for α-subunit and TSH-β mRNAs or other hormone mRNAs. The origin of these tumors remains unsolved.

Mice Transgenic for Pit-1/SV40 Large T-Antigen Mice transgenic for SV40 large T-antigen driven by Pit-1 (GHF-1) promoter were produced in order to trigger pituitary tumors originating in the progenitor cells of somatotrophs and lactotrophs (102). GHF-1 (Pit-1) is a transcription factor that is expressed during fetal development before the expression of GH, PRL, and TSH genes. The transgenic mice are dwarfs, and the pituitary tumors express Pit-1, but no GH or PRL. A cell line derived from such a tumor expresses Pit-1 mRNA and encoded protein, and was used to identify an enhancer that activates the Pit-1 gene only during fetal life (102).

Mice Transgenic for Polyoma Early Region/Polyoma Large T-Antigen Symptoms of hypercorticism develop in old mice expressing polyoma large T-antigen. Their pituitaries contain ACTH-immunoreactive adenomas in the anterior lobe (103). Normal mice bearing transplanted tumors have enlarged adrenal cortices, increased body weights, and high levels of blood ACTH. These transgenic mice offer an experimental model of Cushing's disease.

Mice Transgenic for Human β-Actin/HPV Oncogene Type 16 E6/E7 ORFs HPVs types 16, 31, and 35 are found in benign and malignant uterine cervical and anal tumors. In cancers, the viral DNA is integrated into cellular chromosomes causing disruption of the open reading frames (ORFs) of the viral repressors E1 and E2, but leaving E6 and E7 genes intact. E6 and E7 genes encode two oncoproteins with transforming properties. Neuroepithelial tumors appeared in 2.5-mo-old transgenic mice, and by 10 mo of age, in 71% of them. Pituitary tumors developed in 8.7% of mice (104). No attempt to determine the cell of origin of pituitary tumors was carried out. They were called carcinomas, although no metastases were documented.

Mice Transgenic for Prolactin/Transforming Growth Factor-α (TGF-α) Transgenic mice with targeted overexpression of TGF-α to pituitary lactotrophs was created by fusing rat prolactin promoter with the TGF-α structural gene, in order to study the role of this growth factor in adenoma formation (105). The model relies on the observation that lactotroph hyperplasia under estrogen stimulation is associated with increased TGF-α expression in rat pituitary (106). Multiple nodules immunoreactive for PRL and interpreted as adenomas are detected in homozygous female transgenics by 12 mo or an earlier age. The adenomas are preceded by PRL cells hyperplasia. In hyperplastic glands, TGF-α immunoreactivity is stronger than in control ones. The model indicates the contribution of TGF-α to pituitary tumorigenesis. No explanation regarding the absence of pituitary lesions in transgenic males is offered.

INACTIVATION OF TUMOR SUPPRESSOR GENES

Mice with Inactive Retinoblastoma (Rb) Gene Rb gene belongs to the group of tumor suppressor genes which are mutated in a wide range of human tumors. Bilateral retinoblastoma develops in children with mutated Rb allele in germline, and the adults are especially prone to develop osteosarcoma. Despite its ubiquitous expression in adult tissues, Rb mutations were described in a relatively small number of tumor types. A mouse line in which one allele of Rb was disrupted was created in order to understand better the role of this gene in the development of retinoblastoma (107). Unexpectedly, the heterozygous mice are not predisposed to retinoblastoma, but develop large pituitary tumors invading the brain by 8 mo of age. The tumors arise in cells in which the wild-type Rb allele is absent (107). The histologic features together with the

documented diffuse immunoreactivity for ACTH and β-endorphin indicate their origin in the pituitary intermediate lobe (Stefaneanu, et al., unpublished, 1992). The homozygous mice are nonviable owing to neuronal cell death and defective erythropoiesis.

Another well-characterized tumor suppressor gene, p53, seems to play a role in the malignant phenotype of human pituitary tumors (108). However, mice with one or two null alleles of p53 are highly susceptible to malignant lymphomas and sarcomas, and no pituitary tumors were described. Harvey et al. (109) produced hybrid mice by crossing Rb+/− mice with p53+/− or p53−/− mice. Mice heterozygous for mutated Rb and p53 genes (Rb+/−/p53+/−) develop endocrine tumors, including pituitary adenomas, pancreatic islet cell carcinomas, and medullary thyroid carcinomas in addition to lymphomas and sarcomas. The pituitary tumors develop much earlier in Rb+/−/p53−/− compared to Rb+/−/p53+/+ mice, suggesting that Rb and p53 cooperate in pituitary tumorigenesis. This is consistent with the evidence of a direct link between p53 and Rb proteins, both mediating the arrest of the cell cycle in late G1 phase. Thus, p53 activates transcription of p21/WAF1/CIP1, which inhibits cyclin-dependent kinases (cdk) and their complex formation with cyclines. This results in inhibition of Rb phosphorylation. Unphosphorylated Rb binds E2F-1 transcription factor, which is necessary for the entrance into S phase of cell cycle. The dependence of pituitary tumors upon inhibition of E2F-1 was proved by crossing E2F-1−/− mice with Rb+/− mice that resulted in offspring with reduced prevalence of pituitary tumors (110).

Mice with Inactive p27$^{Kip 1}$ Gene Three groups of investigators published at the same time the multiple effects of p27 gene inactivation by targeting in embryonic stem cells. The affected organs include pituitary, thymus, adrenals, and gonads (111–113). The interest in p27 derives from its association with a class of proteins that controls cell-cycle progression by binding to and inactivating cyclin–cdk complexes. When overexpressed, p27 causes cell-cycle arrest in all types of cells tested. In young p27 knockout mice, pituitaries have diffuse hyperplasia of intermediate lobe. At 10–12 wk of age, intermediate lobe tumors of pituitaries are found only in mice lacking p27 protein (111,113), but mice expressing a truncated p27 protein present only nodular hyperplasia of the intermediate lobe (112). The adenomas are composed of basophilic cells with atypical nuclei and occasional hemorrhage. By immunocytochemistry, the adenomas are positive for MSH, β-endorphin, and ACTH (112). These tumors resemble those reported in Rb+/− mice, Rb+/−/p53−/− mice and arginine-vasopressin/SV40 transgenic mice. This similarity may reflect some common process responsible for regulating melanotroph proliferation. Since p27 inhibits D-CDK4 kinase complex, which phosphorylates Rb protein leading to its inactivation, one could speculate that loss of p27 might result in constitutive inactivation of Rb protein owing to hyperphosphorylation (111,113).

Mice with Inactive p18^{Ink4c} Gene P18 protein belongs to the class of Ink4 inhibitors of cyclin-cdk complexes. Mice with inactive p18^{Ink4c} have widespread organomegaly. Pituitary intermediate lobes are hyperplastic in young mice and develop tumors by 10 mo of age. Mice lacking both p18 and p27 die from pituitary adenomas by 3 months of age, indicating that p18 and p27 proteins mediate two separate pathways that suppress pituitary tumorigenesis (114).

CONCLUSIONS

Most experimental human pituitary tumors are benign. Proven malignancy is available only for a transplantable tumor induced by irradiation, which gave distant metastases. The rarity of malignancy among pituitary tumors is intriguing. The current general concept of tumor formation, which is applicable to pituitary, agrees that most tumors originate in a single cell. A somatic mutation in a single cell is probably the initial event in adenoma formation. However, the exact steps leading to initiation and progression are still unknown. Excessive stimulation by a hormone or growth factor is considered to act as promoter of tumor formation.

The available models of pituitary tumorigenesis and the extensive research on pituitary cell lines reveal the complexity of factors involved in this process. The net effect on tumor biology is the result of integration of a variety of extrinsic and intrinsic determinants. A clear picture of tumor formation and progression will be available when this puzzle is solved.

REFERENCES

1. Cramer W, Horning ES. Experimental production by oestrin of pituitary tumors with hypopituitarism. Lancet 1936;1:247–249.

2. McEwen CS, Selye H, Colip JP. Some effects of prolonged administration of oestrin in rats. Lancet 1936;1:775,776.

3. Zondek B. Tumors of the pituitary induced with follicular hormone. Lancet 1936;1:776–8.

4. Furth J, Clifton KH. Experimental pituitary tumors. In: Harris GW, Donovan BT, eds. The Pituitary Gland. University of California Press, Berkeley, 1966, p. 460.

5. Russfield AB. Tumors of endocrine glands and secondary sex organs. US Government Printing Office, Washington DC (Public Health Service Publication No 1332), 1966.

6. Gardner WU, Strong LC. Strain-limited development of tumors of the pituitary gland in mice receiving estrogens. Yale J Biol 1940; 12:543–549.

7. Wiklund JA, Wertz N, Gorski J. A comparison of estrogen effects on uterine and pituitary growth and prolactin synthesis in F344 and Holtzman rats. Endocrinology 1982;109:1700–1707.

8. Lloyd RV. Estrogen-induced hyperplasia and neoplasia in the rat anterior pituitary gland. An immunohistochemical study. Am J Pathol 1983;113:198–206.

9. Lloyd RV, Landefeld TD. Detection of prolactin messenger RNA in rat anterior pituitary by in situ hybridization. Am J Pathol 1986;125:35–44.

10. Lloyd RV, Jin L, Fields K, Kulig E. Regulation of prolactin gene expression in a DMBA-estrogen-induced transplantable rat pituitary tumor. Am J Pathol 1990;137:1525–1537.

11. Clifton KH, Meyer RK. Mechanisms of anterior pituitary tumor induction by estrogen. Anat Rec 1956;125:65–81.

12. Ueda G, Tanizawa O, Hamanaka N, Nishiura H. Changes of growth hormone-containing cells during tumorigenesis and subpassages of estrogen-induced pituitary tumors in rats. Endocrinol Jpn 1970;17:447–452.

13. McComb DJ, Ryan N, Horvath E, et al. Five different adenomas derived from the rat adenohypophysis: immunocytochemical and ultrastructural study. J Natl Cancer Inst 1981;66:1103–1111.

14. Takemoto H, Yokoro K, Furth J, Cohen AI. Adrenotropic activity of mammosomatotropic tumors in rats and mice. I. Biologic aspects. Cancer Res 1962; 22:917–924.

15. Lloyd HM, Meares JD, Jacobi J. Effects of oestrogen and bromocryptine on in vivo secretion and mitosis in prolactin cells. Nature 1975;255:497,498.

16. Morel Y, Albaladejo V, Bouvier J, Andre J. Inhibition by 17 beta-estradiol of the growth of the rat pituitary transplantable tumor MtF4. Cancer Res 1982;42:1492–1497.

17. Lloyd RV, Landefeld TD, Maslar I, Frohman LA. Diethylstilbestrol inhibits tumor growth and prolactin production in rat pituitary tumors. Am J Pathol 1985;118:379–386.

18. Trouillas J, Morel Y, Pharaboz MO, Cordier G, Girod C, Andre J. Morphofunctional modifications associated with the inhibition by estradiol of MtTF4 rat pituitary tumor growth. Cancer Res 1984;44:4046–4052.

19. Jin L, Song JY, Lloyd RV. Estrogen stimulates both prolactin and growth hormone mRNAs expression in the MtT/F4 transplantable pituitary tumor. Proc Soc Exp Biol Med 1989;92:225–229.

20. Joly-Pharaboz MO, Fei ZL, Bouillard B, Andre J. Estradiol stimulation and inhibition of cell growth in new estrogen-sensitive cell lines and tumors established from the MtTF4 tumor. Cancer Res 1990;50:3786–3794.

21. Wiklund J, Rutledge J, Gorski J. A genetic model for the inheritance of pituitary tumor susceptibility in F344 rats. Endocrinology 1981;109:1708–1714.

22. Wendell DL, Herman A, Gorski J. Genetic separation of tumor growth and hemorrhagic phenotypes in an estrogen-induced tumor. Proc Natl Acad Sci USA 1996;93:8112–8116.

23. Gregg D, Goedken E, Gaikin M, Wendell D, Gorski J. Decreased expression of carboxypeptidase E protein is correlated to estrogen-induction of rat pituitary tumors. Mol Cell Endocrinol 1996; 117:219–25.

24. Cool DR, Normant E, Shen F, Chen H-C, Pannell L, Zhang Y, Loh YP. Carboxipeptidase E is a regulated secretory pathway sorting receptor: Genetic obliteration leads to endocrine disorders in CPE^{fat} mice. Cell 1997;88:73–83.

25. Brann DW, Hendry LB, Mahesh VB. Emerging diversities in the mechanism of action of steroid hormones [Review]. J Steroid Biochem Mol Biol 1995;52:113–133.

26. Szijan I, Parma DL, Engel NI. Expression of c-myc and c-fos protooncogenes in the anterior pituitary gland of the rat. Effect of estrogen. Horm Metab Res 1992;24:154–157.

27. Sarkar DK, Kim KH, Minami S. Transforming growth factor-beta 1 messenger RNA and protein expression in the pituitary gland: its action on prolactin secretion and lactotropic growth. Mol Endocrinol 1992;6:1825–1833.

28. Qian X, Jin L, Grande JP, Lloyd RV. Transforming growth factor-beta and p27 expression in pituitary cells. Endocrinology 1996; 137:3051–3060.

29. Roberts AB, Sporn MB. Transforming growth factors [Review]. Cancer Surveys 1985; 4:683–705.

30. Pastorcic M, De A, Boyadjieva N, Vale W, Sarkar DK. Reduction in the expression and action of transforming growth factor beta 1 on lactotropes during estrogen-induced tumorigenesis in the anterior pituitary. Cancer Res 1995; 55:4892–4898.

31. Stefaneanu L, Powell-Braxton L, Won W, Chandrashekar V, Bartke A. Somatotroph and lactotroph changes in the adenohypophyses of mice with disrupted insulin-like growth factor I gene. Endocrinology 1999; 140;3881–3889.

32. Michels KM, Lee W-H, Seltzer A, Saavedra JM, Bondy CA. Up-regulation of pituitary [^{125}I]insulin-like growth factor-I (IGF-I) binding and IGF binding protein-2 and IGF-I gene expression by estrogen. Endocrinology 1993;132:23–29.

32a. Banerjee SK, Sarkar DK, Weston AP, De A, Campbell DR. Overexpression of vascular endothelial growth factor and its receptor during the development of estrogen-induced rat pituitary tumors may mediate estrogen-initiated tumor angiogenesis. Carcinogenesis 1997;6:1155–1161.

32b. Banerjee SK, Zoubine MN, Tran TM, Weston AP, Campbell DR. Overexpression vascular endothelial growth factor and its co-receptor neuropilin-1 in estrogen-induced rat pituitary tumors and GH3 rat pituitary tumor cells. Int J Oncol 2000; 16:253–260.

32c. Heany AP, Horwitz GA, Wang Z, Singson R, Melmed S. Early involvement of estrogen-induced pituitary tumor transforming gene and fibroblast growth factor expression in prolactinoma pathogenesis. Nat Med 1999;11:1317–1321.

33. Vrontakis ME, Yamamoto T, Schroedter IC, Nagy JI, Friesen HG. Estrogen induction of galanin synthesis in the rat anterior pituitary gland demonstrated by in situ hybridization and immunohistochemistry. Neurosci Lett 1989;100:59–64.

34. Kao KJ, Ramirez VD. Induction of pituitary and mammary tumors in male, "fale," and Female rats by either DMBA, estradiol implant or combined treatment. Proc Soc Exp Biol Med 1979;160: 296–301.

35. Nilsson A, Bierke P, Haraldsson I, Broome-Karlsson A. Induction of pituitary tumours by combination of oestrogenic hormones and 90Sr. Acta Radiol—Oncol 1980;19:373–385.

36. Furth J, Ueda G, Clifton KH. The pathophysiology of pituitaries and their tumors: Methodological advances. In: Busch H, ed. Methods in Cancer Research. Academic, New York, 1973, pp. 201–277.

37. Bates RW, Garrison MM, Morris HP. Comparison of two different transplantable mammotropic pituitary tumors. Hormone content and effect on host. Proc Soc Exp Biol Med 1966;123:67–70.

38. Kovi J, Morris HP. Ultrastructure of a mammosomatotrophic and a nonfunctional transplantable pituitary tumor induced in rats by 2,4,6-trimethylaniline. J Nat Cancer Inst 1976;57:197–205.

39. Judd AM, Login IS, Kovacs K, et al. Characterization of the MMQ cell, a prolactin-secreting clonal cell line that is responsive to dopamine. Endocrinology 1988;123:2341–2350.

40. Ishii J, Katayama S, Itabashi A, Takahama M, Kawazu S. Salmon calcitonin induces pituitary tumor in rats. Endocrinol Jpn 1991;38:705–709.

41. Jameson JL, Weiss J, Polak JM, et al. Glycoprotein hormone alpha-subunit-producing pituitary adenomas in rats treated for one year with calcitonin. Am J Pathol 1992;140:75–84.

42. Upton A, Furth J. Spontaneous and radiation-induced pituitary adenomas of mice. J Natl Cancer Inst 1955;15:1005–1021.

43. Durbin PM, Asling CW, Johnston ME, Parrott MW, Jeung N, Williams MH, et al. The induction of tumors in the rat by astatine-211. Radiat Res 1958;9:378–397.

44. VanDyke DC, Simpson ME, Koneff AA, Tobias CA. Long-term effects of deutron irradiation of the rat pituitary. Endocrinology 1959;64:240–257.

45. Furth J, Haran-Ghera N, Curtis HL, Buffett RF. Studies on the pathogenesis of neoplasms by ionizing radiation. I. Pituitary tumors. Cancer Res 1959;19:550–556.

46. Furth J, Godsden EL, Upton AC. ACTH secreting transplantable pituitary tumors. Proc Soc Exp Biol Med 1953;84:253–254.

47. Steelman SL, Kelly TL, Norgello H, Weber GF. Occurrence of melanocyte stimulating hormone (MSH) in a transplantable pituitary tumor. Proc Soc Exp Biol Med 1956;92:392–394.

48. Buonassisi V, Sato G, Cohen AI. Hormone-producing cultures of adrenal and pituitary origin. Proc Natl Acad Sci 1962;48:1184–1190.

49. Spangelo BL, Gorospe WC. Role of the cytokines in the neuroendocrine-immune system axis [Review]. Front Neuroendocrinol 1995;16:1–22.

50. Bernhagen J, Calandra T, Mitchell RA, et al. MIF is a pituitary-derived cytokine that potentiates lethal endotoxaemia. Nature 1993;365:756–759.

51. Ray DW, Ren SG, Melmed S. Leukemia inhibitory factor (LIF) stimulates proopiomelanocortin (POMC) expression in a corticotroph cell line. Role of STAT pathway. J Clin Invest 1996;97:1852–1859.

52. Yokoro K, Furth J, Haran-Ghera N. Induction of mammotropic pituitary tumor by X-rays in rats and mice: the role of mammotropes in development of mammary tumors. Cancer Res 1961;21:178–191.

53. McLeod RM, Smith C, DeWitt GW. Hormonal properties of transplanted pituitary tumors and their relation to the pituitary gland. Endocrinology 1964;75:670–691.

54. Tashjian AH, Yasumura Y, Levine L, Sato GH, Parker ML. Establishment of clonal strains of rat pituitary tumor cells that secrete growth hormone. Endocrinology 1968;82:348–352.

55. Hollander N, Hollander VP. Development of a somatotropic variant of the mammosomatotropic tumor MtT/W5. Proc Soc Exp Biol Med 1971;137:1157–1162.

56. Ito A, Furth J, Moy P. Growth hormone-secreting variants of a mammotropic tumor. Cancer Res 1972;32:48–56.

57. Frawley LS, Boockfor FR. Mammosomatotropes: presence and functions in normal and neoplastic pituitary tissue. Endocr Rev 1991;12:337–355.

58. Song JY, Jin L, Lloyd RV. Effects of estradiol on prolactin and growth hormone messenger RNAs in cultured normal and neoplastic (MtT/W15 and GH3) rat pituitary cells. Cancer Res 1989;49:1247–1253.

58a. Miller TL, Godfrey PA, Dealmeida VI, Mayo KE. The rat growth hormone-releasing hormone receptor gene: structure, regulation, and generation of receptor isoforms with different signaling properties. Endocrinology 1999;140:4152–4165.

59. Cronin MJ, Faure N, Martial JA, Weiner RI. Absence of high affinity dopamine receptor in GH3 cells: a prolactin-secreting clone resistant to the inhibitory action of dopamine. Endocrinology 1980;106:718–723.

60. Johnston JM, Wood DF, Bolaji EA, Johnston DG. The dopamine D2 receptor is expressed in GH3 cells. J Mol Endocrinol 1991;7:131–136.

61. Johnston JM, Wood DF, Read S, Johnston DG. Dopamine regulates D2 receptor gene expression in normal but not in tumorous rat pituitary cells. Mol Cell Endocrinol 1993;92:63–68.

62. Boockfor FR, Schwarz LK. Cultures of GH3 cells contain both single and dual hormone secretors. Endocrinology 1988;122:762–764.

63. Missale C, Boroni F, Sigala S, Zanellato A, Dal Taso R, Balsari A, et al. Nerve growth factor directs differentiation of the bipotential cell line GH3 into the mammotroph phenotype. Endocrinology 1994;135:290–298.

64. Qian X, Jin L, Lloyd RV. Expression and regulation of transforming growth factor b1 in cultured normal and neoplastic rat pituitary cells. Endocr Pathol 1996;7:77–90.

65. Mormede P, Baird A. Estrogens, cyclic adenosine 3',5'-monophosphate, and phorbol esters modulate the prolactin response of GH3 cells to basic fibroblast growth factor. Endocrinology 1988;122:2265–2271.

66. Prager D, Yamashita S, Melmed S. Insulin regulates prolactin secretion and messenger ribonucleic acid levels in pituitary cells. Endocrinology 1988;122:2946–2952.

67. Fagin JA, Pixley S, Slanina S, Ong J, Melmed S. Insulin-like growth factor I gene expression in GH3 rat pituitary cells: messenger ribonucleic acid content, immunocytochemistry, and secretion. Endocrinology 1987;120:2037–2043.

68. Newton CJ, Trapp T, Pagotto U, Renner U, Buric R, Stalla GK. The oestrogen receptor modulates growth of pituitary tumour cells in the absence of exogenous oestrogen. J Mol Endocrinol 1994;12:303–312.

69. Scammell JG, Burrage TG, Dannies PS. Hormonal induction of secretory granules in a pituitary tumor cell line. Endocrinology 1986;119:1543–1548.

70. Furth J, Moy P, Hershman JM, Ueda G. Thyrotropic tumor syndrome. A multiglandular disease induced by sustained deficiency of thyroid hormones. Arch Pathol 1973; 96:217–226.

71. Gorbman A. Tumorous growth in the pituitary and trachea following radiotoxic dosages of I131. Proc Soc Exp Biol Med 1949; 71:237–240.

72. Doniach I, Williams ED. Development of thyroid and pituitary tumors in the rat two years after partial thyroidectomy. Br J Cancer 1962;16:222–231.

73. Moore GE, Backney EL, Bock FG. Production of pituitary tumors in mice by chronic administration of a thiouracil derivative. Proc Soc Exp Biol Med 1953;82:643–645.

74. Furth J, Moy P, Schalch DS, Ueda G. Gonadotropic activities of thyrotropic tumors: demonstration by immunohistochemical staining. Proc Soc Exp Biol Med 1973;142:1180–1184.

75. Gershengorn MC, Marcus-Samuels BE, Geras E. Estrogens increase the number of thyrotropin-releasing hormone receptors on mammotropic cells in culture. Endocrinology 1979;105:171–176.

76. Chin WW, Habner JF, Martorana MA, Keutman HT, Kieffer JD, Maloof F. Thyroid-stimulating hormone: isolation and partial characterization of hormone and subunits from a mouse thyrotrope tumor. Endocrinology 1980;107:1384–1392.

77. Ridgway EC, Kieffer JD, Ross DS, Downing MF, Mover H, Chin WW. Mouse pituitary tumor line secreting only the a-subunit of the glycoprotein hormones: development from a thyrotropic tumor. Endocrinology 1983;113:1597–1601.

78. Ross DS, Kieffer JD, Shupnik MA, Ridgway EC. Pure α-subunit producing tumor derived from a thyrotropic tumor: impaired regulation of α-subunit and its mRNA by thyroid hormone. Mol Cell Endocrinol 1985;39:161–165.

79. Akerblom IE, Ridgway EC, Mellon PL. An α-subunit-secreting cell line derived from a mouse thyrotrope tumor. Mol Endocrinol 1990;4:589–596.

80. Stefaneanu L, Kovacs K, Horvath E, Scheithauer BW. The adenohypophysis. In: Stefaneanu L, Sasano H, Kovacs K, eds. Molecular and Cellular Endocrine Pathology. Arnold, London, 2000, 75–118.

81. Dickie MM, Wooley GW. Spontaneous basophilic tumors of the pituitary glands in gonadectomized mice. Cancer Res 1949; 16:372–384.

82. Dickie MM, Lane PW. Adrenal tumors, pituitary tumors and other pathological changes in F1hybrids of strain DE x DBA. Cancer Res 1956;16:48–52.

83. Billestrup N, Swanson LW, Vale W. Growth hormone-releasing factor stimulates proliferation of somatotrophs in vitro. Proc Nat Acad Sci USA 1986;83:6854–6857.

84. Stefaneanu L, Kovacs K, Horvath E, Clark RG, Cronin MJ. Effect of intravenous infusion of growth hormone-releasing hormone (GRH) on the morphology of rat pituitary somatotrophs. Endocr Pathol 1993;4:131–139.

85. Billestrup N, Mitchell RL, Vale W, Verma IM. Growth hormone-releasing factor induces c-fos expression in cultured primary pituitary cells. Mol Endocrinol 1987;1:300–305.

86. Mayo KE, Hammer RE, Swanson LW, Brinster RL, Rosenfeld MG, Evans RM. Dramatic pituitary hyperplasia in transgenic mice expressing a human growth hormone-releasing factor gene. Mol Endocrinol 1988;2:606–612.

87. Stefaneanu L, Kovacs K, Horvath E, Asa SL, Losinski NE, Billestrup N, et al. Adenohypophysial changes in mice transgenic for human growth hormone-releasing factor: a histological, immunocytochemical, and electron microscopic investigation. Endocrinology 1989;125:2710–2718.

88. Lloyd RV, Jin L, Chang A, Kulig E, Camper SA, Ross BD, et al. Morphologic effects of hGRH gene expression on the pituitary, liver, and pancreas of MT-hGRH transgenic mice. An in situ hybridization analysis. Am J Pathol 1992;141:895–906.

89. Asa SL, Kovacs K, Stefaneanu L, et al. Pituitary adenomas in mice transgenic for growth hormone-releasing hormone. Endocrinology 1992;131:2083–2089.

90. Thiny MT, Antczak C, Fields K, Jin L, Lloyd RV. Effects of estrogen and dexamethasone on a transgenic pituitary cell line. Regulation of hormone and chromogranin/secretogranin expression. Lab Invest 1994;70:899–906.

91. Brar AK, Brinster RL, Frohman LA. Immunohistochemical analysis of human growth hormone-releasing hormone gene expression in transgenic mice. Endocrinology 1989;125:801–809.

92. Osamura R, Oda K, Utsunomiya H, Inada M, Umerura S, Shibuya M, et al. Immunohistochemical expression of Pit-1 protein in pituitary glands of human GRF transgenic mice: Its relationship with hormonal Expressions. Endocr J 1993;40:133–139.

93. Joubert D, Benlot C, Lagoguey A, et al. Normal and growth hormone (GH)-secreting adenomatous human pituitaries release somatostatin and GH-releasing hormone. J Clin Endocrinol Metab 1989;68:572–577.

94. Levy A, Lightman SL. Growth hormone-releasing hormone transcripts in human pituitary adenomas. J Clin Endocrinol Metab 1992;74:1474–1476.

95. Wakabayashi I, Inokuchi K, Hasegawa O, Sugihara H, Minami S. Expression of growth hormone (GH)-releasing factor gene in GH-producing pituitary adenoma. J Clin Endocrinol Metab 1992; 74:357–361.

96. Murphy D, Bishop A, Rindi G, et al. Mice transgenic for a vasopressin-SV40 hybrid oncogene develop tumors of the endocrine pancreas and the anterior pituitary. A possible model for human multiple endocrine neoplasia type 1. Am J Pathol 1987;129: 552–566.

97. Stefaneanu L, Rindi G, Horvath E, Murphy D, Polak JM, Kovacs K. Morphology of adenohypophysial tumors in mice transgenic for vasopressin-SV40 hybrid oncogene. Endocrinology 1992; 130:1789–1795.

98. Sumi T, Stefaneanu L, Kovacs K, Asa SL, Rindi G. Immunohistochemical study of p 53 protein in human and animal pituitary tumors. Endocr Pathol 1993;4:95–99.

99. Windle JJ, Weiner RI, Mellon PL. Cell lines of the pituitary gonadotrope lineage derived by targeted oncogenesis in transgenic mice. Mol Endocrinol 1990;4:597–603.

100. Schechter J, Windle JJ, Stauber C, Mellon PL. Neural tissue within anterior pituitary tumors generated by oncogene expression in transgenic mice. Neuroendocrinology 1992;56:300–311.

100a. Albarracin CT, Frosch MP, Chin WW. The gonadotropin-releasing hormone receptor gene promoter directs pituitary-specific oncogene expression in transgenic mice. Endocrinology 1999; 140:2415–2421.

101. Maki K, Miyoshi I, Kon Y, Yamashita T, Sasaki N, Aoyama S, et al. Targeted pituitary tumorigenesis using the human thyrotropin b-subunit chain promoter in transgenic mice. Mol Cell Endocrinol 1994; 105:147–154.

102. Lew D, Brady H, Klausing K, Yaginuma K, Theill LE, Stauber C, et al. GHF-1-promoter-targeted immortalization of a somatotropic progenitor cell results in dwarfism in transgenic mice. Genes Dev 1993;7:683–693.

103. Helseth A, Haug E, Nesland JM, Siegal GP, Fodstad O, Bautch VL. Endocrine and metabolic characteristics of polyoma large T transgenic mice that develop ACTH-producing pituitary tumors. J Neurosurg 1995;82:879–885.

104. Arbeit JM, Munger K, Howley PM, Hanahan D. Neuroepithelial carcinomas in mice transgenic with human papillomavirus type 16 E6/E7 ORFs. Am J Pathol 1993;142:1187–1197.

105. McAndrew, Paterson A, Asa SL, McCathy KJ, Kudlow JE. Targeting of transforming growth factor-a expression to pituitary lactotrophs in transgenic mice results in selective lactotroph proliferation and adenomas. Endocrinology 1995;136: 4479–4488.

106. Borgundvaag B, Kudlow JE, Mueller SG, George SR. Dopamine receptor activation inhibits estrogen stimulated transforming growth factor-a gene expression and growth in anterior pituitary. Endocrinology 1992;130:3453–3458.

107. Jacks T, Fazeli A, Schmitt EM, Bronson RT, Goodell MA, Weinberg RA. Effects of an Rb mutation in the mouse. Nature 1992;359:295–300.

108. Thapar K, Scheithauer BW, Kovacs K, Pernicone PJ, Laws ER Jr. p53 expression in pituitary adenomas and carcinomas: correlation with invasiveness and tumor growth fractions. Neurosurgery 1996;38:763–870.

109. Harvey M, Vogel H, Lee EY, Bradley A, Donehower LA: Mice deficient in both p53 and Rb develop tumors primarily of endocrine origin. Cancer Res 1995; 55:1146–1151.

110. Yamasaki L, Bronson R, Williams BO, Dyson NJ, Harlow E, Jacks T. Loss of E2F-1 reduces tumorigenesis and extends the lifespan of Rb1(+/–) mice. Nat Genet 1998;4:360–364.

111. Nakayama K, Ishida N, Shirane M, Inomata A, Inoue T, Shishido N, et al. Mice lacking p27(Kip1) display increased body size, multiple organ hyperplasia, retinal dysplasia, and pituitary tumors. Cell 1996;85:707–720.

112. Kiyokawa H, Kineman RD, Manova-Todorova KO, Soares VC, Hoffman ES, Ono M, et al. Enhanced growth of mice lacking the cyclin-dependent kinase inhibitor function of p27(Kip1). Cell 1996; 85:721–732.

113. Fero ML, Rivkin M, Tasch M, Porter P, Carow CE, Firpo E, et al. A syndrome of multiorgan hyperplasia with features of gigantism, tumorigenesis, and female sterility in p27(Kip1)-deficient mice. Cell 1996;85:733–744.

114. Franklin DS, Godfrey VL, Lee H, Kovalev GI, Schoonhoven R, Chen-Kiang S, Su L, Xiong Y. CDK inhibitors p18(IND4c) and p27(Kip1) mediate two separate pathways to collaboratively suppress pituitary tumorigenesis. Genes Dev 1998;18:2899–2911.

7 Pathology of Pituitary Adenomas and Pituitary Hyperplasia

Bernd W. Scheithauer, md, Eva Horvath, PhD,
Ricardo V. Lloyd, md, PhD, and Kalman Kovacs, md, PhD, DSc

INTRODUCTION

Of the diverse neoplasms affecting the sellar region, pituitary adenomas are by far the most common. Their pathologic features are the substance of the present chapter, which is limited to a discussion of benign tumors. The same is true of invasive adenomas and pituitary carcinoma. Discussions of their epidemiology, molecular genetics, endocrine, radiologic, as well as therapeutic aspects are the subjects of separate chapters.

Despite variations in histologic pattern, the basic features of pituitary adenoma are those of a benign endocrine neoplasm. As a result, general pathologists view their assessment as a simple matter of achieving a diagnosis of pituitary adenoma. Given the very high likelihood that a sellar mass is a pituitary adenoma, the diagnosis is often reflexly made on the basis of frozen section or intraoperative smear preparation alone. Providing a more precise, endocrinologically meaningful diagnosis regarding adenoma subtype is at the time of surgery unnecessary. It is no surprise, therefore, that progress in our understanding of the pathobiology of pituitary adenomas is largely owing to the efforts of neuro- and endocrine pathologists who are aware of the diverse clinicopathologic spectrum of such tumors and attuned to differences in their therapy and management based on correlative immunohistochemical and ultrastructural studies. Although to many, simple immunohistochemical confirmation of a major hormonal abnormality is considered adequate, institutions engaged in high-volume pituitary surgery have the standard approach to adenomas, that is, the performance of a wide-spectrum immunobattery for all but Cushing's tumors, and allocation of tissues for possible ultrastructural study. The newly devised World Health Organization Classification of pituitary adenomas (1,2) is based on a multimodality approach incorporating endocrine, radiographic, operative, histo-, and immunochemical data, as well as ultrastructure. It has become clear that with the vagaries and pitfalls of immunohistochemistry, predicting diagnoses entirely on this technology may be misleading, particularly in inexperienced hands. In our opinion, ultrastructural study is mandatory in a significant proportion of cases.

From: *Diagnosis and Management of Pituitary Tumors* (K. Thapar, K. Kovacs, B. W. Scheithauer, and R. V. Lloyd, eds.), ©Humana Press Inc., Totowa, NJ.

Historically, the approach to pituitary adenoma has undergone considerable evolution. High-quality hematoxylin and eosin (H&E) stains, as well as the application of complex histochemical methods, e.g., the Periodic acid-Schiff- (PAS) orange G and Herlant's tetrachrome methods, permitted crude correlation of reactions with endocrine data. The introduction of immunohistochemistry represented a quantum leap. Having undergone a number of modifications to improve sensitivity and specificity, it remains the single most often used method in the workup of pituitary adenomas. The development of all encompassing classifications of pituitary adenomas was, however, the result of correlative immunohistochemical and ultrastructural studies (3). Indeed, these complementary methods are the defining elements of the new 1999 World Health Organization classification (1,2). Assessment of cell proliferation and the demonstration of p53 protein, the product of a tumor suppressor gene, both by immunohistochemical methods, permit the identification of adenomas likely to exhibit aggressive behavior; these too have been incorporated into the diagnostic paradigm (*see* Chapter 22).

A variety of more sophisticated laboratory methods have been applied to pituitary adenomas. These include

1. Immunoelectronmicroscopy for the demonstration of one or more hormones, not only in specific cell types, but also within single secretory granules.
2. *In situ* hybridization permitting the demonstration of hormone messenger RNA.
3. The reverse hemolytic plaque assay for the demonstration of hormone secretion.

Although powerful tools having significantly contributed to our understanding of the pathobiology of pituitary adenomas, they remain in the realm of research rather than diagnostic modalities.

After a preliminary discussion of methods and of the normal pituitary, it is the purpose of this chapter to present a summary of the pathology of pituitary adenomas and of pituitary hyperplasia in a practical, but state-of-the-art manner. It stresses correlation of endocrine, radiologic, and operative data with results of histologic, immunohistochemical, and ultrastructural studies.

TECHNICAL METHODS

HISTOCHEMISTRY Various histochemical techniques, many time-honored, have contributed greatly to the understanding

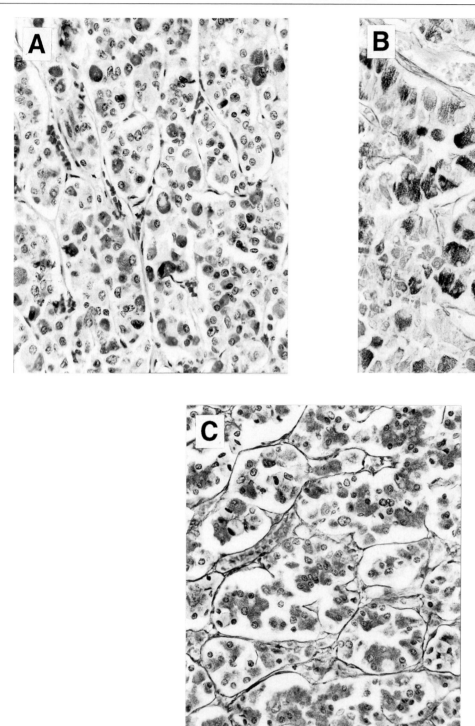

Figure 7-1 On H&E stain, the normal pituitary exhibits acinar architecture, and cellular heterogeneity manifest as variation in cytoplasmic granularity and staining (**A**). Corticotroph and glycoprotein hormone-producing cells are highlighted on PAS stain (**B**). The uniform acinar architecture of the gland is best appreciated on reticulin preparation (**C**). (A, B, C) × 400.

of pituitary diseases. Critically applied, these often provide complementary data. Only the principal stains currently in use are discussed in some detail. Complex histochemical stains, some also termed "trichrome preparations," e.g., PAS-Orange G and Herlant's tetrachrome, representing early attempts at detection

of functionally specific adenohypophysial cell types are no longer in use.

Hematoxylin and Eosin (H&E) This remains the most useful and practical stain for the analysis of normal (Figure 1A) and abnormal pituitary tissues. Eosinophilia is a reflection of granule content, particularly of normal growth hormone (GH) and many prolactin (PRL) cells. Among adenomas, it strongly stains approximately one-half of GH cell adenomas. Mitochondrial accumulation (oncocytic change) produces a coarse "granular" appearance and is also eosinophilic, although less strikingly so. Hematoxylin staining (basophilia) typifies most normal adreno-corticotropin (ACTH) cells and many, but not all cells engaged in glycoprotein hormone (luteinizing hormone [LH], follicle-stimu-lating hormone [FSH], thyroid-stimulating hormone [TSH]) pro-duction. Among adenomas, only ACTH-producing tumors are basophilic. Although chromophobia or lack of staining can be observed to a varying extent in all types of normal adenohypophy-sial cells and adenomas, all are granule-containing.

Periodic Acid-Schiff (PAS)   This method is used to demon-strate primarily carbohydrates, such as glycogen and glycoprotein hormones, e.g., LH, FSH, TSH (Figure 1B). In addition, it reliably stains vascular basal lamina. It is also invaluable for the detection of pro-opiomelanocortin (POMC), the prohormone of ACTH, as well as normal and neoplastic ACTH cells. Among adenomas, those producing glycoprotein hormones stain only when showing sufficient granule content.

Reticulin Stain   The Gomori and the Gordon-Sweet methods are commonly used to assess the integrity of the capillary-rich stromal network surrounding pituitary acini. As such, they aid in the distinction of normal pituitary parenchyma from hyperplastic and adenomatous tissue (Figure 1C). The scant reticulin network of adenoma is also highlighted in cases of "pituitary apoplexy" (*see* Pituitary Apoplexy section).

Trichrome Preparations   The Gomori and Masson trichrome stains, like reticulin preparations, highlight the acinar architecture of the gland and aid in the detection of fibrous connective tissue. Zones of fibrosis in chronic hypophysitis as well as old infarcts are readily detected.

Silver Techniques for Secretory Granules   Endocrine cells containing secretory granules are examined by two principal methods. These are (1) argentaffin methods, which demonstrate primarily enterochromaffin cells of the small intestine, and (2) argyrophil preparations, which stain most neuroendocrine cells. Argentaffin-positive cells take up silver and reduce it to its visible, metallic state without the aid of an extraneous reducing agent. It is of note that alcohol-containing fixatives diminish the argen-taffin reactivity of secretory granules. Argentaffin techniques include the Fontana-Masson, Cherukian-Schenk, and Gomori-Burtner methods (4). The latter method is particularly sensitive in demonstrating neuroendocrine cells, including those of the anterior pituitary (4a). Demonstration of argyrophil granules requires the addition of a reducing agent in order to reduce the impregnated silver to a visible, metallic end product. Examples include the Bodian, Sevier-Munger, and Grimelius techniques (5). As a rule, argyrophil methods are more sensitive, but are less specific than argentaffin stains for the demonstration of endocrine cells. Although reactive cells also include those of the anterior pituitary, both methods have been supplanted by immunohistochemistry.

IMMUNOHISTOCHEMISTRY   Practical Applications
By adding a functional dimension to morphologic studies, immu-nohistochemical techniques have had a major impact on our understanding of the pituitary. We routinely immunostain pitu-itary tissues, tumoral and nonneoplastic, for the full spectrum of pituitary hormones. These include GH, PRL, ACTH, FSH, LH, TSH, and α-subunit, the functionally inactive α-chain of the gly-coprotein hormones. Although general markers of endocrine differentiation, such as chromogranin, synaptophysin, and neu-ron-specific enolase (NSE), are not routinely applied since they provide no more information than immunostains for adenohypo-physial hormones, S-100 protein is a useful marker of stellate cells. Stains for other hormones, as well as peptides, growth fac-tors, oncogenes, tumor suppressor genes, and receptors are of use in only special instances and are mainly of academic interest.

In the assessment of pituitary adenomas, particularly aggres-sive lesions or ones exhibiting more than the occasional mitotic figure (6), we recommend staining for MIB-1, a cell proliferation marker that recognizes the KI-67 antigen in paraffin sections (7). When labeling indices exceed 3%, careful follow-up of the patient is recommended, since such tumors show more aggressive behavior. This includes a faster rate of growth, and a greater tendency to invasion of surrounding tissues (7). Although long-term follow-up is needed, recurrence rates are presumably also increased. Use of proliferating cell nuclear antigen (PCNA) staining (8) is not recommended in that it yields less reliable results. In summary, we have found mitotic activity, MIB-1-labeling indices, and p53 pro-tein immunoreactivity (9,10) to be valuable indicators of tumor behavior and of prognosis. The most useful markers employed in immunohistochemical analysis of pituitary diseases are summa-rized in Table 1.

Overview   Since the early pioneering studies of Coons and coworkers, who localized specific antigens in tissues using anti-bodies labeled with fluorescein isothiocyanate (11), the use of peroxidase and alkaline phosphatase enzymes, as well as of chro-mogens readily visualized on routine light microscopy, has con-tributed greatly to progress in immunocytochemistry (12–16). Various immunohistochemical methods are now in use, including ones applicable to electron microscopy.

Direct Method   Applied by early investigators studying pituitary cells, this was the earliest immunohistochemical method developed (11). It involves attaching the primary antibody directly to an enzyme system or a fluorescent tag and applying it to tissue sections in order to identify specific antigens. Enzyme systems in use include horseradish peroxidase, alkaline phosphatase, glu-cose oxidase, and β-galactosidase. In addition, electron-dense labels, such as ferritin, can be utilized for ultrastructural studies. Although the advantages of this procedure are rapidity and ease of performance, highly purified antibodies are needed to assure specificity.

Indirect or Sandwich Method   More sensitive than the direct method, this approach requires lower concentrations of pri-mary antibody. It involves application of an unlabeled primary antibody followed by a second antibody directed against the first and conjugated to an enzyme system. By increasing the ratio of signal-to-primary antibody, this versatile method permits the iden-tification of antigens present at low levels.

Peroxidase–Antiperoxidase (PAP) Method   This unlabeled method was first developed by Nakane and Pierce for the detection of antitreponemal antibodies (17). The PAP reagent consists of a small, stable immune complex consisting of two molecules of antibody directed against horseradish peroxidase, as well as three molecules of horseradish peroxidase. Although this method is much more sensitive than even the indirect technique, its popular-ity has waned since the development of the avidin–biotin peroxi-dase complex (ABC) technique (18).

Table 1
Broad-Spectrum Immunohistochemical Markers Used in the Study of the Anterior Pituitary and Its Lesions

Antigen	Specific cell type	Reference
Broad-Spectrum Neuroendocrine Markers		
Chromogranin	Most cell types	52,53
Neural cell adhesion molecule (N-CAM)	Most cell types	54
Synaptophysin	Most cell types	55
Neuron-specific enolase	Most cell types	56
Proconvertases	Most cell types	57
Specific pituitary hormone		
PRL	PRL and mammosomatotroph	3
GH	GH and mammosomatotroph	3
ACTH	ACTH	3
LH	LH and FSH	3
FSH	FSH and LH	3
Thyroid-stimulating hormone	TSH	3
Other markers		
S100 protein	Folliculo-stellate cells	58
Galanin	ACTH	59
Keratin	Most cell types	60
Cholecystokinin	ACTH	61
Renin	PRL	62,63
Calcitonin	—	64
Substance P	TSH	65
Vasoactive intestinal polypeptide	PRL cells	66
Thyrotropin-releasing hormone	—	67
GH-releasing hormone	GH, PRL cells	68
Gonadotropin-releasing hormone (GNRH)	Gonadotroph cells	69
Chorionic gonadotropin	Glycoprotein hormone-producing cells	70
Lipocortin	Folliculo-stellate cells	71
MAb lu-5	ACTH	72
Growth factors		
bFGF (Fibroblast growth factor)	Most cell types	73
TGF-α (Transforming growth factor)	PRLa	74
TGF-β	Most cell types	75
Vascular endothelial growth factor (VEGF)	Folliculo-stellate cells	76
Insulin-like growth factor 1 and 2	Most cell types	77,78

ABC Method Developed by Hsu and colleagues, this technique takes advantage of the binding affinity that exists between avidin and biotin in order to detect a primary antibody (18,19). First, avidin is chemically conjugated to horseradish peroxidase. Tight binding then is allowed to take place between avidin and the biotin-associated primary antibody. Finally, peroxidase localization was achieved by its reaction with chromogen. The ABC peroxidase procedure has been shown to be even more sensitive than the PAP method (18,19). Nonspecific staining of tissues containing endogenous biotin can be avoided by such blocking techniques as preincubation with avidin and biotin (13,20). A recent modification of the ABC method employs a streptavidin–biotin–peroxidase complex and affords yet greater sensitivity (20).

Microwave Technology for Morphological Analysis The use of microwave technology has had a significance impact upon histochemical and immunohistochemical analyses. Although microwave fixation was first reported more than two decades ago (21), it is only in recent years that it has been routinely used for tissue fixation and staining (22–25). Systematic analysis of procedural variables has optimized its use in both immunohistochemistry and in situ hybridization (26–30). We recommend caution in the use of this method in that vigorous microwave treatment may result in nonspecific immunoreactivity.

Double Immunostaining Using two different chromogens permits the demonstration of two antigens in not only the same section, but within the same cell. Unfortunately, the method is time-consuming and not uniformly reproducible. As a result, we do not use it routinely and recommend its performance only in special cases of academic interest. The question of whether a tumor is producing two different hormones and if these are present in the same or different cells can usually be resolved by examining consecutive or "mirror" sections.

Controls in Immunocytochemistry It must be emphasized that caution is required in the evaluation of immunocytochemical preparations. Apparent immunopositivity may be owing to nonspecificity of the antibody, crossreaction, poor tissue preservation, or overdiligent antigen retrieval. On the other hand, immunonegativity may be owing to antigen release without storage or to technical problems, such as loss of antigen during fixation, processing, and embedding. Several antigen-retrieval methods are available, including pronase and trypsin digestion, as well as microwave treatment. Although these techniques may unmask antigens, making it easier to demonstrate them by immunocytochemical methods, it is of fundamental importance to perform controls in order to assure staining specificity and reliability. Regardless of whether antigen retrieval is employed, the same need for controls is

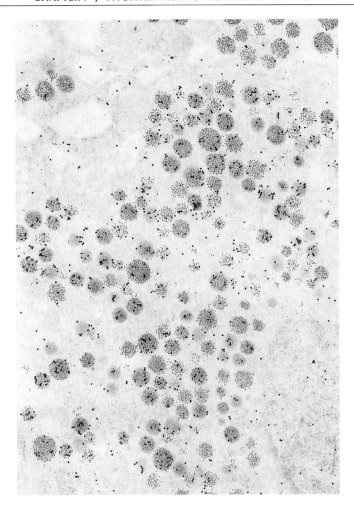

Figure 7-2 Immunoelectron microscopy. Note labeling of granules by silver particles of 10 and 20 mm corresponding to GH and PRL reactivity, respectively (×19,900).

also true of the basic immunostaining method. Negative control methods include elimination of primary antibodies, as well as their replacement with phosphate-buffered saline or antibodies directed against antigens lacking in the specimen. Tissues of known immunoreactivity are typically employed as positive controls. Under optimal circumstances, one should also preabsorb the antibody under conditions of antigen excess in order to abolish immunopositivity. Unfortunately, lack of time and financial resources often preclude the implementation of this very meaningful control procedure.

ELECTRON MICROSCOPY Transmission electron microscopy has been essential to developments in endocrine pathology. Pituitary work in particular has concentrated on correlating morphologic features with specific physiologic functions. Recent applications of immunocytochemical methods at the ultrastructural level has also contributed to rapid progress in the field *(31,32)*. In contrast, scanning electron microscopy has played little or no role.

Ultrastructural studies have had a particular impact on the classification of pituitary tumors. In demonstrating the presence of sometimes distinct varieties of secretory granules, variable organization of cytoplasmic organelles, and a variety of minor, but characteristic features of functional differentiation, this method has been the cornerstone of morphology *(33)*. Correlation of ultra-

structure with secretory activity and therapeutic drug response has also been achieved *(33–36)*.

It should be stressed that electron microscopy cannot determine:

1. Whether any one cell is adenomatous or nonneoplastic.
2. Whether a tumor is benign or malignant, will exhibit a rapid pace of growth, or is invasive.
3. Whether hyperplasia is present.

Despite these shortcomings, ultrastructural investigation is essential to the diagnosis of several adenoma types. Unfortunately, the method is time-consuming, expensive, and requires a level of expertise born of considerable experience. Although the cost-effectiveness of electron microscopy is open to question, we find its use to be indispensable to diagnostic pituitary pathology *(32)*.

Immunoelectron Microscopy This elegant method demonstrates antigens at the ultrastructural level (Figure 2). Using two different size gold particles, it can be used to distinguish the presence of two different antigens, thus answering the question of whether more than one hormone is produced by the same or different cell populations. In some instances, multiple hormones can even be visualized within the same secretory granule. The questions answered by immunoelectron microscopy are more academic

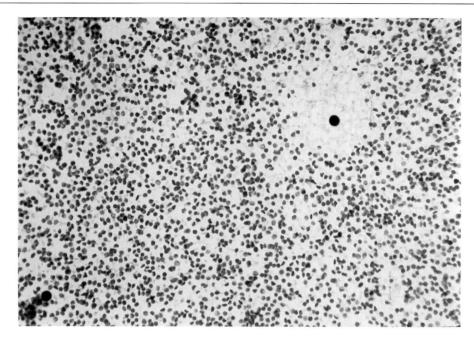

Figure 7-3   RHPA. By way of hemolysis, it demonstrates specific hormone secretion by isolated normal or neoplastic cells.

than practical in nature. Time-consuming and expensive, the technique does not lend itself to routine study of surgical specimens.

REVERSE HEMOLYTIC PLAQUE ASSAY (RHPA)   This method has been applied to the study of pituitary cells and tumors *(37–40)*. In essence, it detects hormone secretion by individual cells (Figure 3) by the classic method used to measure antibody secretion by individual B-lymphocytes. The assay was modified to detect antigen secretion by attaching hormone-specific antibodies to staphylococcal protein A, which binds to the surface of red blood cells. The protein A modification has proven to be effective in detecting hormone secretion by individual cells. Frawley and Neill *(37)* as well as others have shown the method to be very specific and highly sensitive *(37–41)*. Furthermore, it is relatively simple to perform and can be rapidly carried out.

In the identification of specific hormone-secreting cell types, RHPA can confirm the findings of and even substitute for immunocytochemical staining. The following example illustrates the point. Mammosomatotrophs, defined as cells producing both PRL and GH, have been identified in the normal as well as neoplastic rat pituitary. Several investigators have demonstrated their presence by RHPA *(39,40)*. The amount of hormone secreted by individual cells can also be estimated by this method. It has been adapted to correlative ultrastructural studies *(42)*. For example, Vila-Porcile and colleagues found that PRL cells with small (150- to 200-nm) granules are actively secreting and that those with larger (300- to 600-nm) granules are ones stimulated by potassium chloride or thyrotropin-releasing hormone *(42)*.

The cell-blot assay is a variation of the RHPA method in which secretion from individual cells can be measured *(41)*. Cells are incubated on a synthetic material, such as nylon, which takes up the secreted hormones and renders them detectable and measurable using immunoblotting techniques and specific standards. One advantage of cell blots over the traditional RHPA is that lower concentrations of antibodies can be used, thus decreasing the likelihood of crossreactivity *(41)*.

***IN SITU* HYBRIDIZATION TECHNIQUE**   *In situ* hybridization, a recently introduced method in routine use, serves to demonstrate specific messenger RNAs (mRNAs) at the subcellular level. As such, it permits the reliable assessment of gene expression (Figure 4). The procedure involves the application of isotope-labeled probes, a large number of which are commercially available, and visualizing of the end product using autoradiography. This modification of the basic technique, although more complicated, expensive, and time-consuming, is more sensitive than nonisotopic methods, e.g., digoxigenin mRNA localization. *In situ* hybridization can be used to demonstrate the mRNA of receptors, growth factors, oncogenes, and other regulatory peptides. As a result, it has added a whole new dimension to pathology. Used in conjunction with immunocytochemistry, it yields preparations simultaneously demonstrating gene expression and the gene product within the same cell. In such preparations, immunocytochemistry provides information regarding cell hormone content, and *in situ* hybridization confirms the presence of ongoing hormone synthesis. Since various proteins and peptides, especially surface receptors, are easily destroyed during tissue fixation, processing, and embedding, the more sensitive in situ hybridization technique may succeed in demonstrating an mRNA when its gene product has been lost. Under normal circumstances, endocrine cells express the mRNA and its respective hormone. In instances wherein mRNAs are demonstrable, but immunostains for the relatively robust hormones are negative, one may conclude that the hormones were synthesized, but were released rather than stored. Alternatively, in cases wherein hormones are demonstrable, but mRNA cannot be localized by *in situ* hybridization, consideration should be given to the possibility that the hormone was not synthesized, but rather taken up from the extracellular space and stored within the cell.

OTHER METHODS   Various other recently developed research methods are useful in the study of pituitary disease. For example, cyto- and molecular genetic methods demonstrate chro-

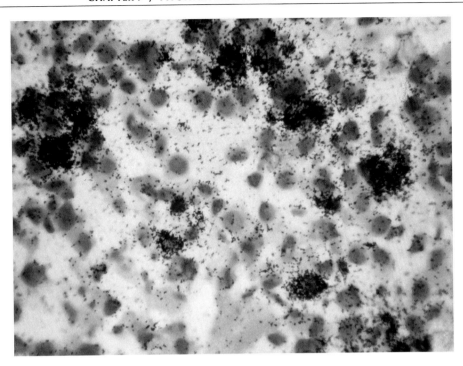

Figure 7-4 *In situ* hybridization. This method is used to demonstrate the presence of either a specific DNA or RNA message in normal or neoplastic cells.

mosomal defects, genetic abnormalities, such as specific mutations, and the presence of oncogenes or of tumor suppressor genes *(43–45)*. Elegant genetic methods in routine use include (1) the fluorescence *in situ* hybridization (FISH) technique, which demonstrates gross genetic abnormalities at the light microscopic level *(46,47)*, and (2) the polymerase chain reaction (PCR), which amplifies genes and permits the analysis of specific intracellular events at the molecular level *(48)*. Molecular biologic methods have also been developed to investigate receptors, signal transduction mechanisms, and intracellular changes that affect hormone synthesis and release. In that pituitary tumors can readily be cultured, various in vitro studies may be undertaken; of these, the RHPA is only one example (*see* Reverse Hemolytic Plaque Assay [RHPA] section). Pituitary tumors can also be transplanted to immunodeficient host animals. For example, the nude mouse model makes it possible to examine tumor growth, endocrine activity, and the effects of drug treatment. Transgenic mice, in which copies of a native or a foreign gene are inserted into the genome, provide experimental models permitting assessment of gene effects in vivo *(49,50)*. In addition, so-called knockout mice represent in vivo experimental models in which specific genes and their effects are eliminated and the resultant pathobiology can be studied by various methods *(51)*. Finally, novel optic methods have come into use, e.g., confocal microscopy and computer image analysis. At present, the various methods serve primarily the basic scientist and do not contribute significantly to diagnosis. As a result, their detailed description is beyond the scope of this chapter.

NORMAL CELL TYPES

The adenohypophysis, or anterior lobe (pars distalis) of the pituitary, consists of cell types that differ not only in distribution (Figure 5) and morphology, but also in terms of their regulation,

hormonal product, physiologic function, and morphology. Their responses to stimulating and inhibitory influences are also variable, thus precluding generalizations regarding adenohypophysial cells. The number of functionally distinctive adenohypophysial cell types is still unsettled. As a corollary, it has yet to be determined what cell(s) gives rise to so-called silent adenomas. In this short account, we refer to the normal adult pituitary as seen in horizontal section (Figure 5). The reader is referred to several lengthy reviews on this subject *(33,79–81)*.

GH Cells These represent the most frequent adenohypophysial cells, accounting for approx 50% of the cell population. Medium-size, ovoid, strongly acidophilic, and GH-immunoreactive, they reside primarily within the lateral wings (Figure 6A), although many also lie scattered throughout the median wedge (Figure 6B). The notion that GH cells are a heterogeneous population is supported by the finding that an indeterminate number of GH-producing cells is also capable of synthesizing prolactin. This observation is supported by immunohistochemistry, *in situ* hybridization, and the RHPA. That a large number of somatotrophs are immunoreactive for α-subunit as well remains unexplained.

Electron microscopy identifies GH cells as ovoid, densely granulated cells (Figure 7). The size range of their secretory granules is broad (200–1000 nm, most frequently 300–500 nm). Although there are also variations in the average size of granules from one cell to another, overlaps preclude the identification of distinct phenotypes. Perhaps the only exception is the cells containing the largest, often irregular granules. These likely represent mammosomatotrophs *(82)*. At the other end of the spectrum, immunoelectron microscopy detects GH-producing cells with small (250-nm and less) secretory granules, ones that could not otherwise be identified as GH-cells.

The morphology of GH cells is not conspicuously altered by stimulation or inhibition. When stimulated by ectopic production

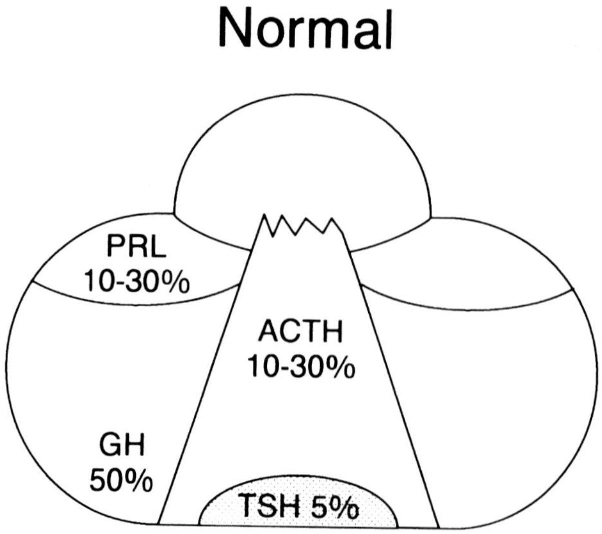

Normal

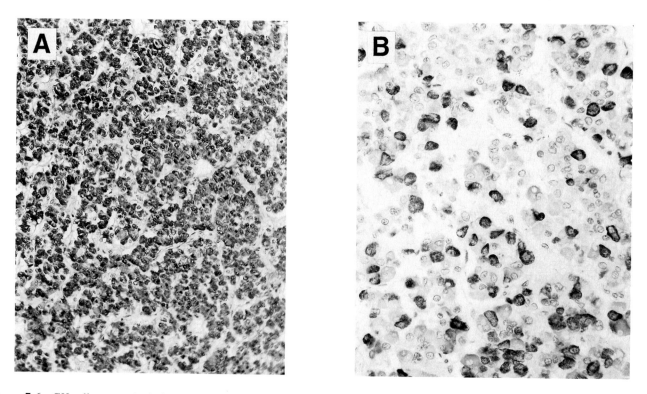

PRL
10-30%

ACTH
10-30%

GH
50%

TSH 5%

Figure 7-5   The distribution of normal adenohypophysial cells, here illustrated in schematic form, is reflected in that of pituitary adenomas, particularly small, endocrinologically functioning examples. Nonfunctioning tumors, on the other hand, are typically macroadenomas that efface pituitary landmarks.

Figure 7-6   GH cells are particularly numerous in the "lateral wings" of the gland (**A**), but also lie dispersed in other portions of the gland (**B**). GH immunostain (A) × 160, (B) × 400.

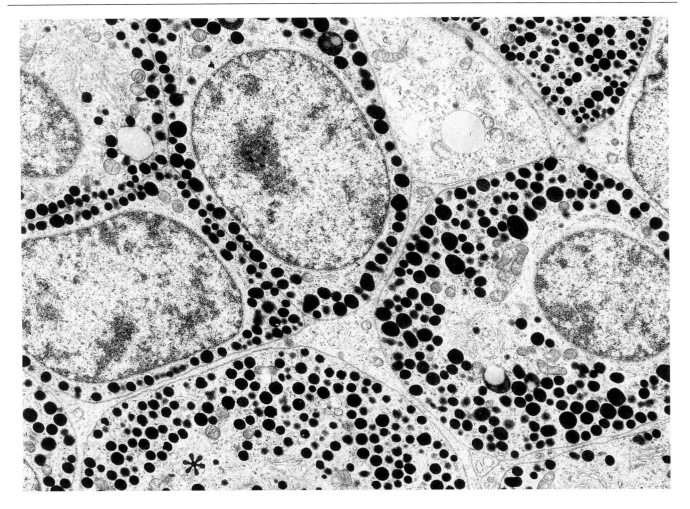

Figure 7-7   Group of normal GH cells. Part of a corticotroph is also shown (asterisk); its secretory granules are of similar size to those of GH cells, but display variation in configuration and in electron density (×8700).

of GHRH, the Golgi apparatus of the somatotrophs does become prominent. On the other hand, on inhibited GH cell adjacent to a GH-producing adenoma may show accumulation of lysosomes, a rather nonspecific response.

The PRL Cell   PLR cell content of the adenohypophysis shows considerable variations (10–30%), being highest in multiparous women. Lactotrophs are scattered throughout the gland, but are heavily represented in the posterolateral rim area of the gland where they are the most frequent cell type. The majority of lactotrophs are small chromophobes with slender processes, displaying strong PRL immunoreactivity over the prominent Golgi region (Figure 8). A small minority of PRL cells are large, densely granulated acidophils showing strong diffuse PRL immunoreactivity throughout the cytoplasm. It is unclear whether this type represents a morphologic variant of PRL cell or a different phenotype. Occasional lactotrophs are in intimate contact with gonadotrophs (Figure 8).

Ultrastructurally, normal sparsely granulated lactotrophs are polyhedral cells with multiple processes. Within the acini, they occur in small groups often removed from the basal lamina, with only their cytoplasmic processes extending to it. The cytoplasm contains moderately to well-developed lamellar rough endoplasmic reticulum (RER) and a sizable Golgi complex containing spherical, pleomorphic secretory granules (Figure 9). Ranging up

to 300 nm in diameter, the sparse cytoplasmic granules may engage in both orthotopic and "misplaced" exocytosis (Figure 9). The ultrastructure of PRL cells reliably reflects their functional activity. Stimulation (pregnancy, estrogen treatment, decline of dopamine transport, increased in thyrotropin-releasing hormone [TRH], β-endorphin secretion) results in a progressive increase in cell size, quantity of RER, and prominence of Golgi complexes. Secretory granules are located primarily within the Golgi region, leaving the rest of cytoplasm nearly devoid of granules. Inhibition (hyperprolactinemia, dopamine agonist treatment) leads to a decrease in cell size and in the quantity of membranous organelles.

ACTH Cells or Corticotrophs   These are regarded as the major component of the proopiomelanocortin- (POMC) producing cell population. Although they occur chiefly in groups or clusters in the anterior two-thirds of the median wedge (Figure 10), corticotrophs also lie scattered throughout the remainder of the gland. Deeply basophilic and PAS-positive, these ovoid cells often contain an unstained vacuole and are thus quite distinctive. Strong immunoreactivity is noted for various POMC peptides, such as ACTH, β-endorphin, β-lipotropin, CLIP, and so forth (Figure 4). Corticotrophs are easily recognized at the ultrastructural level as well (Figure 11). Although the size of the secretory granules of densely granulated ACTH cells lies within the same range as those of GH cells, it is the distinctive morphology of POMC granules

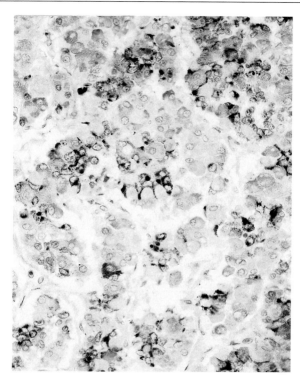

Figure 7-8 Normal lactotrophs occur in densely and sparsely granulated form and show a tendency to surround or "hug" gonadotrophs. PRL immunostain × 640.

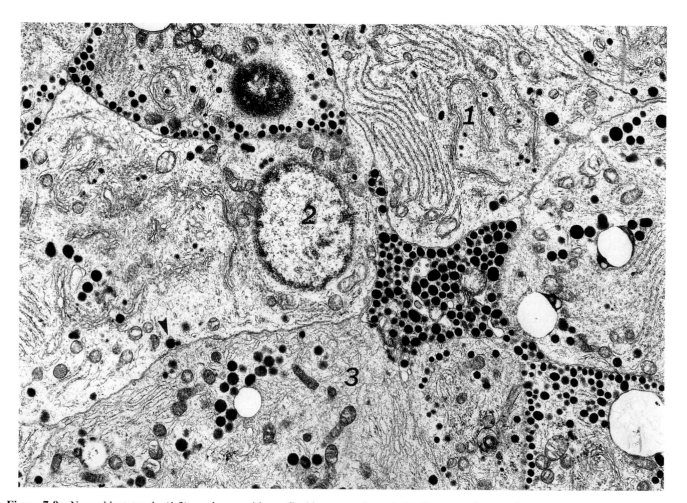

Figure 7-9 Normal lactotrophs (1,2) are shown, with one flanking a gonadotroph (3). Note granule extrusion (arrowhead), a typical feature of PRL cells (×8700).

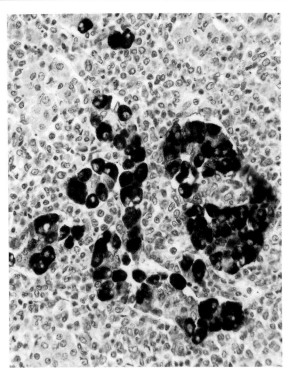

Figure 7-10 Corticotrophs often lie in aggregates and should not be mistaken for pathologic hyperplasia or microadenoma formation. Immunostain for ACTH ×400.

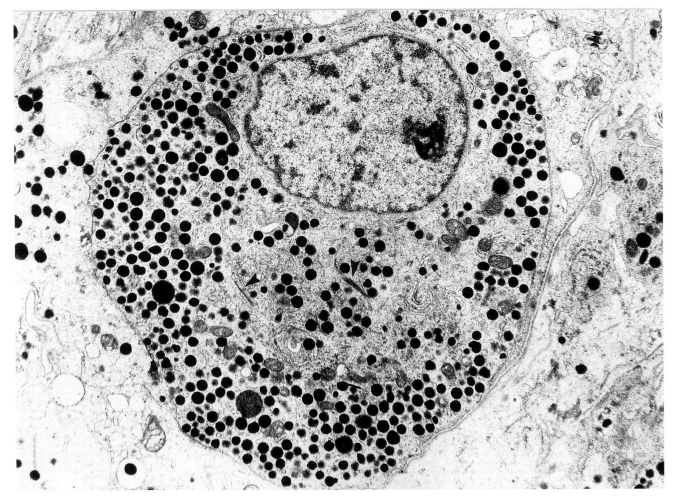

Figure 7-11 Normal corticotroph cell showing the characteristic indented or heart-shaped morphology of its secretory granules. Note bundles of cytokeratin filaments (arrowheads) (×6800).

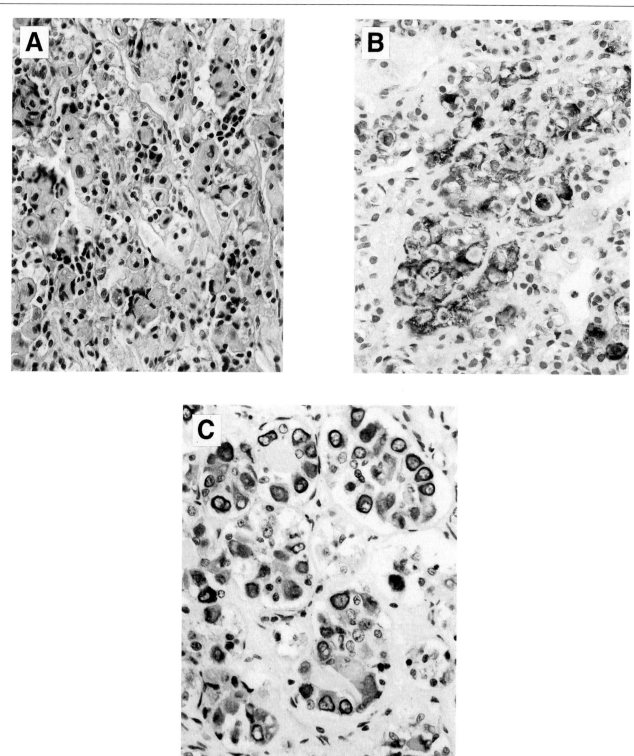

Figure 7-12   Crooke's hyaline change occurs in normal corticotrophs in the setting of cortisol excess. Note pale perinuclear rings of the filamentous material on H&E stain **(A)**. The hyaline rings lack ACTH reactivity **(B)**, but show strong cytokeratin staining **(C)**. (A) H&E × 640; (B, C) immunostain × 640.

that aids in their identification. The 250- to 450-nm (mostly 300- to 350-nm) secretory granules are often dented, irregular or heart-shaped, and may show variable electron density. The other reliable marker is the presence of cytokeratin filament bundles in the peri-nuclear region. The electron lucent vacuole evident at the light microscopic level is a large lysosomal body. Whereas no qualitative changes in cytoplasmic organization result from functional stimu-lation, functional suppression owing to negative feedback effects of elevated glucocorticoid levels (Cushing's disease/syndrome, iatro-genic hypercorticism) induces Crooke's hyalinization (Figure 12).

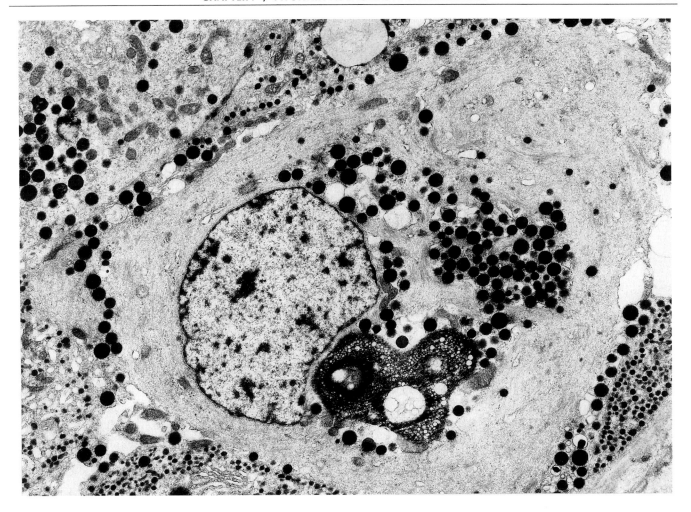

Figure 7-13 Corticotrophs exhibiting Crooke's hyalinization, i.e., excessive accumulation of cytokeratin filaments. Note central displacement of secretory granules and the presence of a large lysosome, the "enigmatic body" (×6720).

The alteration represents abundant cytokeratin production (Figure 12). At the ultrastructural level, it consists of perinuclear ring-like accumulation of intermediate filaments (Figure 13).

As previously alluded to, POMC-producing cells of the human adenohypophysis are heterogeneous. Instead of forming an anatomically distinct zone, the cells of the intermediate zone (pars intermedia) are intermingled with other cell types of the pars distalis and often extend into the neural lobe ("basophil invasion") (Figure 14). Owing to their morphologic similarity (Figure 15) and shared immunoreactivities, ACTH cells and pars intermedia-derived cells cannot be distinguished under normal conditions. The physiologic role of POMC-derived cells of the human pars intermedia and neural lobe as well as the normal hormone content is unknown. Such cells do not undergo Crooke's hyaline change. Their nonneoplastic proliferation is rare under 40 yr of age, but common in elderly subjects. Pathologists should be aware of this change, since it holds the answer to the puzzle of nodular basophilic and ACTH-immunoreactive POMC cell hyperplasia (often incorrectly diagnosed as corticotroph hyperplasia) in the absence of Cushing's disease.

TSH Cells or Thyrotrophs These account for an estimated 5% of adenohypophysial cells. Located chiefly within the anterior one-third of the median wedge, they show moderate basophilia

and PAS positivity. Immunostaining for TSH confirms the nature of these medium-size or large, distinctly angular cells with their long cytoplasmic processes (Figure 16). Ultrastructurally, they exhibit an interface with the acinar basal lamina. Thyrotrophs possess a spherical nucleus, a spherical Golgi apparatus associated with numerous Golgi vesicles, and slightly dilated RER as well as variably dense 100- to 250-nm secretory granules (Figure 17). Similar cells, but with irregular, drop-shaped secretory granules may also be seen. It is not known whether these two cell forms are mere morphologic variants or have functional implications.

Sustained stimulation (thyroidectomy, hypothyroidism) evokes highly distinctive changes. By light microscopy, the "thyroid deficiency" or "thyroidectomy" cells are large, pale, polyhedral cells often containing coarse, PAS-positive globules (lysosomes) and exhibiting variable TSH immunoreactivity. Electron microscopy shows that enlargement of these cells is mainly owing to proliferation and dilation of RER filled with a proteinaceous, low-density substance. In addition, the Golgi complex is prominent. With progression of changes, the number of secretory granules tends to decrease, thus explaining the variable, often weak TSH immunoreactivity. Suppressed thyrotrophs encountered in the nontumorous gland adjacent to thyrotroph adenoma are small cells with heterochromatic nuclei, poorly

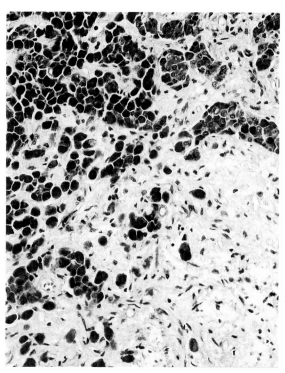

Figure 7-14   Basophil invasion. The presence of numerous POMC-producing cells in the posterior lobe of the pituitary is a common finding of no pathologic significance. ACTH immunostain ×250.

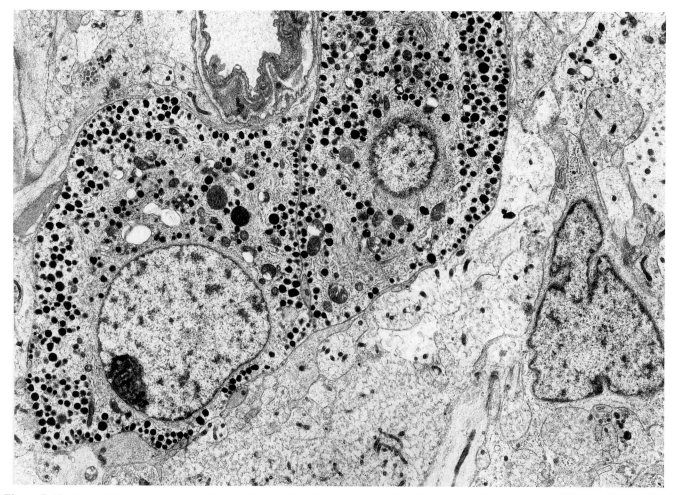

Figure 7-15   Basophil invasion showing the granulated cells to lie among posterior lobe neurites. Their general features resemble those of anterior lobe corticotrophs (×5750).

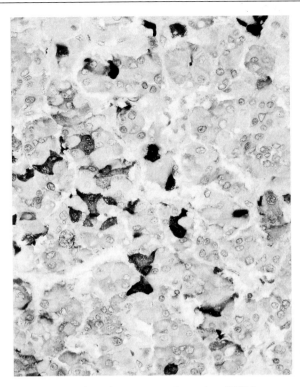

Figure 7-16   Thyrotrophs vary in configuration and often show process formation. TSH immunostain ×400.

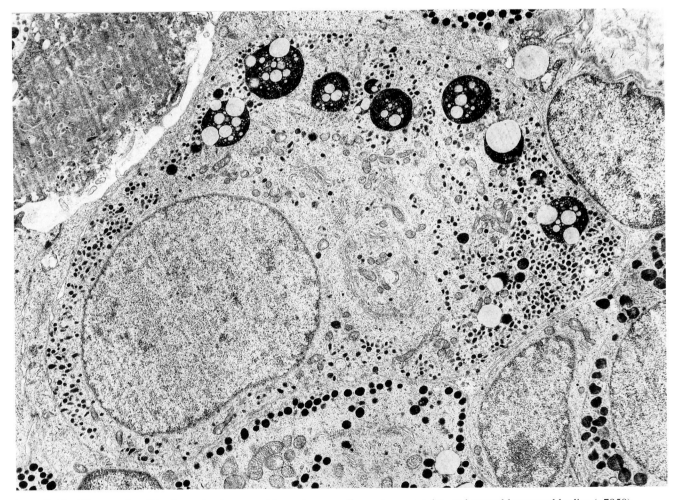

Figure 7-17   Thyrotroph cell is shown having eccentric nucleus, small secretory granules, and several lysosomal bodies (×7950).

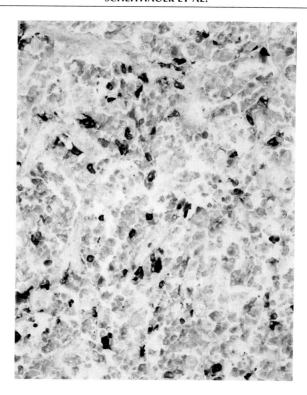

Figure 7-18   Normal gonadotroph cells occur singly and lie uniformly distributed in the pituitary gland. LH immunostain × 400.

developed membranous organelles, several lysosomes, and small secretory granules.

Gonadotroph Cells   These represent an estimated 15–20% of adenohypophysial cells. The middle-sized or large, ovoid, PAS-positive and FSH-LH immunoreactive cells are quite evenly scattered throughout the pars distalis (Figure 18). They exhibit a large interface with the basal lamina. Their ultrastructure is characterized by a spherical, euchromatic nucleus, cytoplasm of low electron density containing slightly dilated RER, a large ring-shaped Golgi complex, and 200- to 500-nm secretory granules variable in shape, texture, and electron density (Figure 19).

Prolonged stimulation owing to primary hypogonadism or surgical ablation of the gonads results in the development of "castration" or "gonadectomy" cells. The alteration is characterized by a gradual increase in cell size, progressive proliferation and dilation of RER, and prominence of the Golgi complex (Figure 20). With advancement of changes, secretory granule numbers tend to decrease and dilation of RER increases, the result being formation of so-called signet ring cells.

Physiologic suppression of gonadotrophs is observed during advanced stages of pregnancy (83). As estrogen levels surge around term, immunoreactivity for FSH and LH may no longer be detectable in gonadotrophs. The ultrastructural aspects of suppression are only poorly documented in rare cases of hypogonadotrophic hypogonadism (Kallmann's syndrome) and in the nontumorous adenohypophysis around gonadotroph adenomas. Suppressed cells are small and feature a heterochromatic nucleus, numerous cytoplasmic lysosomal bodies, and few small secretory granules.

Null Cells   Cells with ultrastructural features resembling those of null adenoma (*see below*) occur in the normal pituitary (Figure 21). Their origin, nature, and relation to other cell types, as well as to null cell adenomas for that matter, is unclear.

Stellate Cells   In addition to the functionally distinctive cell types noted above, cells termed "stellate" or "folliculostellate" also occur within the normal pituitary. Immunoreactive for S-100 protein (Figure 22) and glial fibrillary acidic protein (GFAP), stellate cells lack secretory granules as well as hormone secretion and are characterized by processes that either surround pituitary acini or insinuate themselves between adenohypophysial cells (Figure 23). The physiologic role of stellate cells is uncertain. They are thought to be supporting or sustentacular in nature and have been found to contain growth factors and cytokines. Furthermore, they are thought to be implicated in paracrine regulation (81,84,85). To date, no convincing evidence of neoplastic transformation of stellate cells has been reported.

A common feature of the normal anterior pituitary is follicles composed of adenohypophysial cells (Figure 24). These structures are often filled with an eosinophilic, proteinaceous substance. ACTH cells frequently contribute to follicle formation. On immunohistochemistry, the cell apices of the follicles are epithelial membrane antigen- (EMA) immunoreactive (Figure 24). At the ultrastructural level, the cell apices are linked by junctional complexes (Figure 25).

Rathke's Cleft Remnants (Figure 26)   At the interface of the anterior and posterior pituitary lobes, remnants of Rathke's cleft may be encountered as glands or cleft-like spaces composed of cuboidal, columnar, mucin-producing, or ciliated epithelium. Occasional pituitary hormone-producing cells may also be encountered. Accumulation of secretions within the cyst gives rise to small cysts, a frequent incidental autopsy findings (86). Symptomatic cysts are far less common.

Miscellaneous Cells   Squamous metaplasia of adenohypophysial cells is a common occurrence in the pars tuberalis (87) (Figure 27), in the surrounding of healed pituitary infarcts, and so forth.

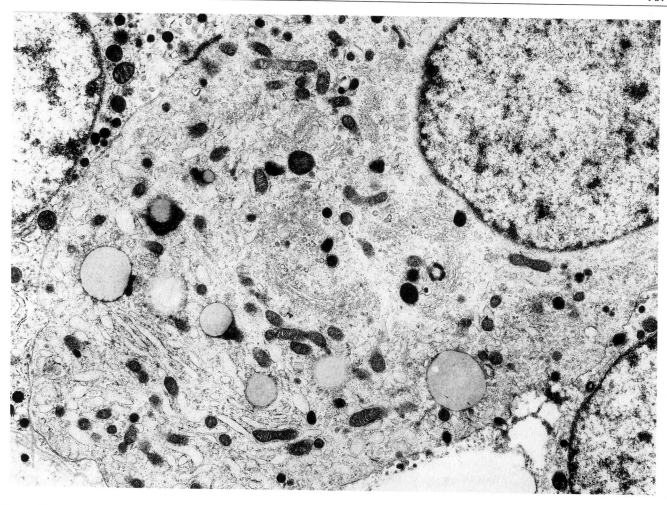

Figure 7-19 Gonadotroph cell showing signs of active secretion: well-developed, slightly dilated RER and prominent Golgi complex (×11,440).

Vasculature The adenohypophysis is a well-vascularized organ in which low-pressure capillaries or sinusoids predominate. Arterial blood flow is minor. Like the endothelial cells of most endocrine organs, those of the pituitary form fenestrations consisting of apposed cell membranes without interposed cytoplasm.

Salivary Gland Remnants In view of the origin of the adenohypophysis from stomatodeum, the finding of foci of ectopic salivary gland tissue in association with the gland is not a surprise *(88)*. The remnants typically occur on the posterosuperior aspect of the pituitary and microscopically resemble serous acini (Figure 28). Such rests presumably give rise to rare salivary gland tumors in the sellar region.

PITUITARY ADENOMAS

During the last two decades, unprecedented progress has been made to obtain deeper insight into the morphologic features of pituitary tumors, to understand their cytogenesis and etiology better, and to correlate their ultrastructural findings with growth rate, therapeutic responsiveness, as well as biologic behavior. Recently applied molecular methods have provided new data on clonality *(89–92)*, mutation *(93,94)*, and chromosomal abnormalities *(95–97)*. A minority are MEN-I-associated *(98)*. It has become evident that pituitary adenoma cells not only contain the well-known pituitary hormones, but also produce hypothalamic hormones, various growth factors, cytokines, and oncogenes. It is thought that the local production of these peptides and proteins may, by a paracrine or autocrine mechanism, influence their endocrine activity, proliferating potential, and aggressiveness. The significance of angiogenesis to the pathobiology of pituitary adenomas is unsettled *(99,100)*. Benign adenomas arising in all types of adenohypophysial cells are frequently occurring lesions. Small functional tumors can be localized to those parts of the pituitary wherein their respective cell types are normally most concentrated (Figure 29). Although most adenomas are solitary, multiple examples do occur in the clinical setting *(101,102)*. Small, incidental adenomas can be found in 10–20% of adult autopsy pituitaries *(3,103,104)*; multiplicity is common *(105)* (Figure 30). Their radiographic detection has also been reported *(106)*.

In the clinical setting, pituitary adenomas occur over a wide age range, including children *(107–110)*. Although the vast majority arise in the sella, occasional examples originate from the pituitary stalk or are truly ectopic *(111–114)*. One rare example arose in a teratoma *(115)*.

Pituitary adenomas can also be classified according to size, an approach commonly used by imaging specialists and neurosurgeons. Tumors <10 mm in diameter are termed "micro-

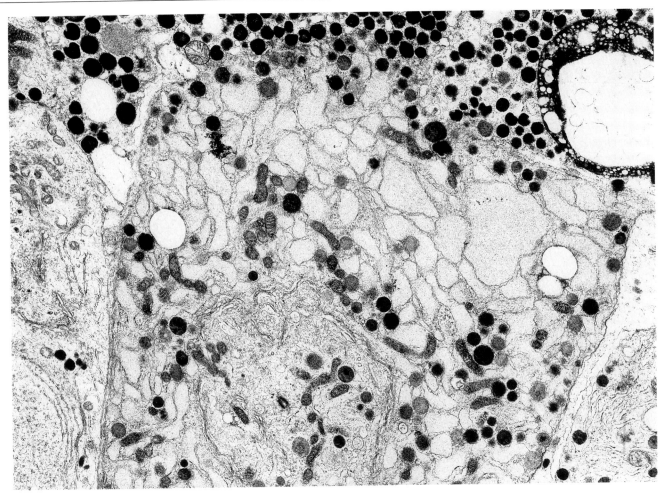

Figure 7-20   Castration cell. Note prominent Golgi complex as well as abundance and dilatation of RER (×9000).

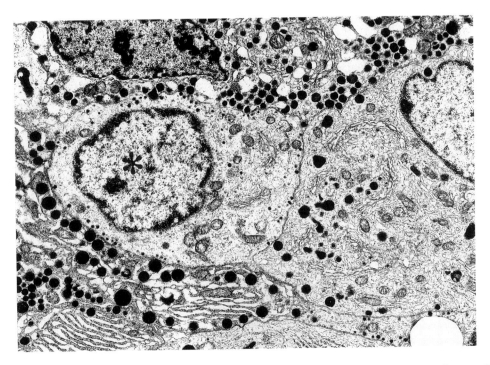

Figure 7-21   Null cell (asterisk). In the normal pituitary, such cells are few and feature poorly developed organelles as well as scant secretory granules (×7200).

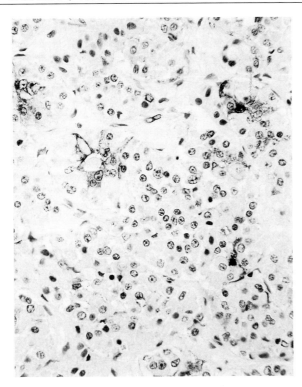

Figure 7-22 Stellate cells are best seen on S-100 protein immunostain wherein they feature processes that either follow the contours of other cells or of the periphery of acini (×250).

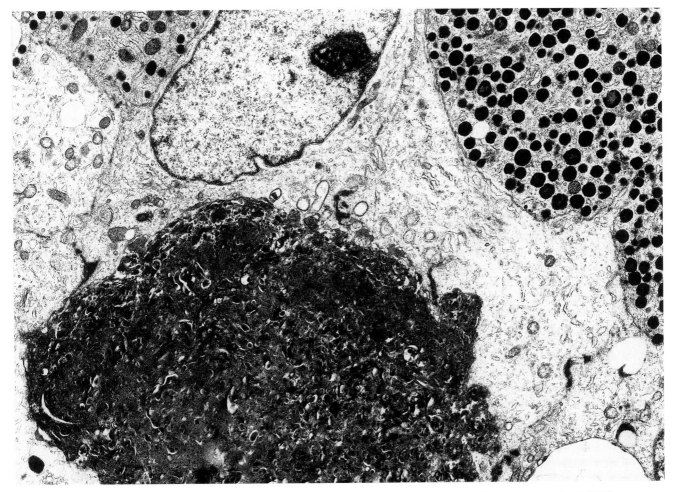

Figure 7-23 Stellate cells surrounding electron-dense, "colloid" in the acinar lumen. Note lack of secretory granules (×8400).

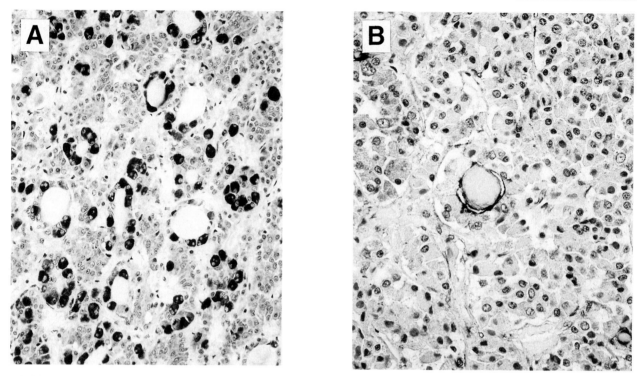

Figure 7-24 Unrelated to age or disease, follicle formation is a common feature of the normal pituitary. Secretory cells of various types contribute to their formation (**A**). Luminal aspects of follicles are EMA-positive (**B**). (A) ACTH immunostain × 400; (B) EMA immunostain × 400.

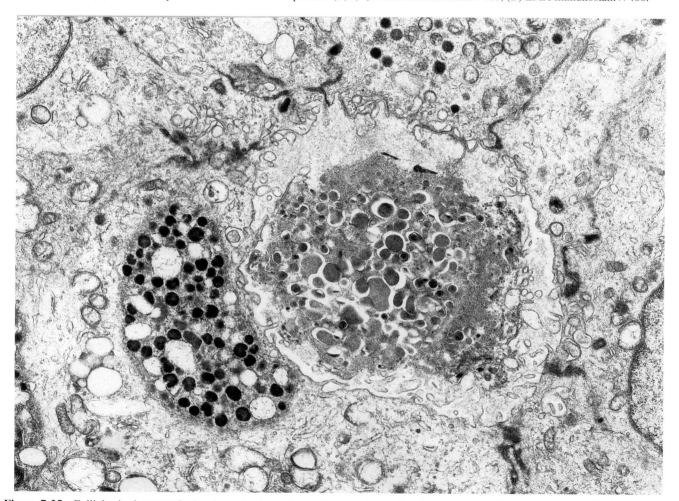

Figure 7-25 Follicles in the normal adenohypophysis are formed by secretory cells of various types. Note the presence of apical terminal bars (×12,600).

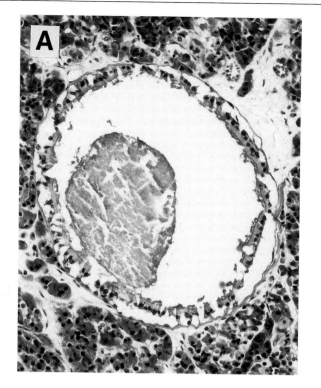

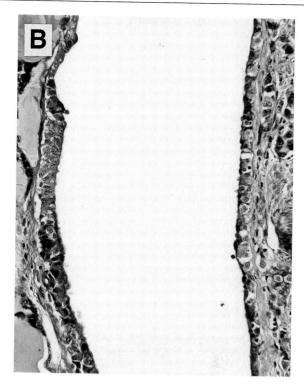

Figure 7-26 Rathke's cleft remnants take the form of microcysts **(A)** or clefts **(B)** at the interface of the anterior and posterior lobes. Although the epithelium is often ciliated (A), it may include mucin-producing as well as adenohypophysial cells (B). (A,B) H&E × 250.

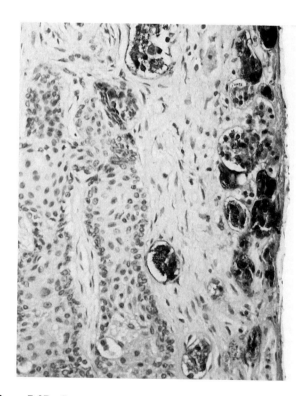

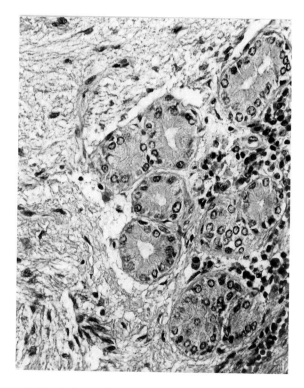

Figure 7-27 Squamous metaplasia in the pars tuberalis affects various cell types, particularly gonadotrophs (H&E × 250).

Figure 7-28 Salivary gland rests are uncommonly seen on the superior surface of the pituitary gland, usually posterior to the pituitary stalk. These rarely give rise to salivary gland tumors of the sellar region. H&E × 100.

ADENOMAS

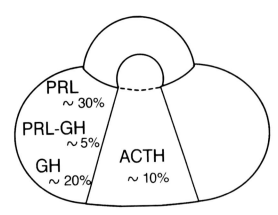

Figure 7-29   The localization and frequency of functioning microadenomas reflects the maximal concentration of their corresponding normal pituitary cells (*see* Figure 5).

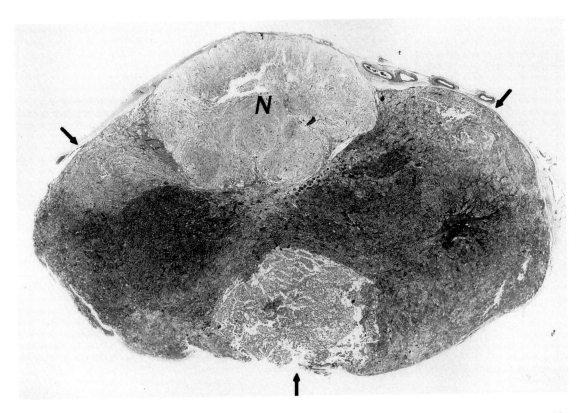

Figure 7-30   Multiple incidental pituitary adenomas (arrows). Such tumors, particularly those in the gland, often are lactotrophic tumors. The remainder are mainly null-cell adenomas (N, neurohypophysis).

adenomas," whereas those larger than 10 mn in diameter are designated "macroadenomas." Based on the results of neuroimaging, four grades of pituitary adenomas can be distinguished *(116)* (*see also* Chapter 12). According to Hardy's scheme, grade I adenomas are intrapituitary tumors, <10 mm in diameter; grade II adenomas are larger than 10 mm, but are still contained within the intact sella; grade III lesions are larger, so-called diffuse adenomas associated with focal sellar erosions and extension beyond the boundaries of the sella; and grade IV adenomas infiltrate such parasellar structures as the sphenoid and cavernous sinuses, compress the pitu-

itary stalk, optic chiasm and/or cranial nerves, and in some instances, even invade adjacent brain *(116)*.

For both practical and theoretical purposes, several pathologic classifications of pituitary adenomas have been developed. Early classifications divided pituitary adenomas into acidophilic, basophilic, and chromophobic types. This separation of pituitary adenomas based on tinctorial characteristics has been found to be of little value *(3)*. For example, cytoplasmic acidophilia may denote production of GH, PRL, or merely oncocytic change. Although basophilia is a typical feature of ACTH-producing

Table 2
Immunohistochemical Classification
of Adenohypophysial Tumors 1999 WHO Classification (1,2)

Principal immunoreactivity	Secondary immunoreactivity[a]
GH	PRL, α-SU(f)[c], TSH, FSH, LH(i)[d]
PRL	α-SU(i)
GH and PRL	α-SU(f), TSH(i)
ACTH	LH, α-SU(i)
TSH	α-SU(f), GH, PRL(i)
FSH/LH/α-SU	PRL, GH, ACTH(i)
Plurihormonal[b]	
Hormone immunonegative	

[a]Secondary hormone immunoreactivities are commonly observed. Although most are not clinically expressed, the hormones may be biochemically detected in blood.

[b]The most common combinations of immunoreactivities are GH/PRL/TSH and/or α-subunit (SU). Other combinations are rare, e.g., ACTH-LH, GH-ACTH, PRL-TSH, and so forth.

[c]f: frequent.

[d]i: infrequent.

adenomas, basophilic tumors can be functionally "silent," and some ACTH-producing adenomas are chromophobic. More than 60% of surgically removed adenomas are chromophobic. Such tumors may be clinically non-functioning or may secrete GH, PRL, ACTH, or glycoprotein hormones *(3)*.

The most frequently used classification is based upon the immunohistochemical demonstration of hormone content supported by correlative ultrastructural data (Table 2). This combination, the backbone of the new World Health Organization classification *(1,2)*, distinguishes GH, PRL, ACTH, TSH, FSH/LH, and α-subunit-producing tumors as well as other, less common, but distinctive adenoma types. Of these, some are endocrinologically functional, and others are not (inactive adenomas). Tumors are frequently bi- or plurihormonal, producing two or more hormones. It should be noted that every adenohypophysial cell type appears capable of neoplastic transformation and that all known adenohypophysial hormones can be produced and secreted in excess. The immunophenotype of pituitary adenomas in terms of conventional, nonhormonal markers has also been studied in detail *(96,117)*. Finally, a number of substances of unknown pituitary–hypothalamic function have been demonstrated in the normal pituitary as well as adenomas (Table 1).

Another useful classification attempts to separate adenomas based on their aggressiveness. Thus, particularly with respect to dura and parasellar structures, pituitary adenomas can be divided into expansively growing or invasive tumors *(118)*. Tumors with expansive growth are demarcated and grossly noninfiltrative. Pituitary adenomas lack a true capsule. This is readily apparent at the microscopic level where the border between tumor and normal adenohypophysis is at most a well-defined zone of condensed reticulin fibers derived from surrounding acini ("pseudocapsule") (*see* Figure 34). Invasive adenomas are not grossly demarcated; to a varying extent, they infiltrate and destroy surrounding tissues. Although invasive adenomas are likely to be large, even microadenomas may radiographically or grossly invade *(118)*. It must be stressed that the presence of invasion in the context of our discussion refers not to microscopic dural invasion, an all too common occurrence *(119)*, but to radiographic or grossly (operatively) apparent invasion *(118)*. We believe that invasion is most

reliably assessed by the imaging specialist or by the neurosurgeon. Whereas gross invasion cannot be missed by a combination of imaging, microscopic invasion is easily overlooked and may not be sampled.

Pituitary adenomas can also be separated on the basis of their growth potential. Mitotic index or immunocytochemical cell proliferation markers can be applied. Currently, MIB-1 is the most extensively used antibody, which detects the KI-67 antigen on formalin-fixed and paraffin-embedded sections. In our practice, tumors with MIB-1 index lower than 3% are usually slowly growing tumors, whereas in those with MIB-1-index more than 3%, one usually notes rapidly growing aggressive tumors *(7)*. Although overlaps and exceptions exist, the investigation of MIB-1 index is a valuable method that helps to assess prognosis. Mitotic counts are also useful. Mitoses are usually rarely encountered in pituitary adenomas, but mitotic counts are higher in rapidly growing adenomas and carcinomas *(6)*. Although not currently popular and largely displaced by other methods, DNA ploidy and S-phase determinations on flow cytometry have been studied *(120)*. Adenomas with excessive proliferative activity demonstrate p53 protein immunoreactivity *(10)*, despite infrequency of mutations in this gene *(121)*.

The new 1999 WHO classification of pituitary adenomas *(2)* is based not only on the morphologic features of the tumor, e.g., histology, immunohistochemical profile, and ultrastructural appearance, but also includes endocrine as well as radiographic/operative data regarding tumor size and invasiveness. The classification includes histologic, immunocytochemical (Table 2), ultrastructural (Table 3), endocrine, and neurologic/operative data *(1,2)*.

APPROACH TO THE SPECIMEN

The scope of this section is limited to morphologic methods useful in the assessment of pituitary lesions. Nevertheless, detailed clinical and endocrinologic data, such as blood hormone levels, before and after stimulation and suppression tests, are essential to arriving at a correct diagnosis. It is also self-evident that neuroimaging techniques, primarily magnetic resonance imaging (MRI), provide essential data regarding tumor localization, size, and extent. On the basis of MRI, even microadenomas as small as 3 mm can be confidently identified.

INTRAOPERATIVE METHODS Of morphologic techniques routinely applied to tumor diagnosis, few can be usefully employed by pathologists at the time of pituitary surgery. Gross inspection, although crucial to the examination of tumors in other organs, only occasionally provides diagnostic information. Pituitary tumors are often small and are removed as minute fragments intermingled with blood, fibrin, and crushed nontumoral tissue. Indeed, in some instances, it is not all apparent whether the specimen contains tumor or only nontumoral pituitary gland. Despite these shortcomings, pituitary or sellar specimens should be examined macroscopically by both the neurosurgeon and pathologist. Gross inspection may still be rewarding, especially in instances wherein the lesion is other than an adenoma, e.g., craniopharyngioma (calcification, cholesterol-rich "machine oil"-like fluid), Rathke's cleft cysts (mucus), abscess (fibrinopurulent exudate), and so on.

Frozen Section A debated and controversial issue is whether intraoperative frozen section examination should be performed on freshly removed tissue. Its practical value is limited in that endocrine and imaging data usually make the diagnosis obvious, as do operative findings. Furthermore, histologic variation (Figure 31)

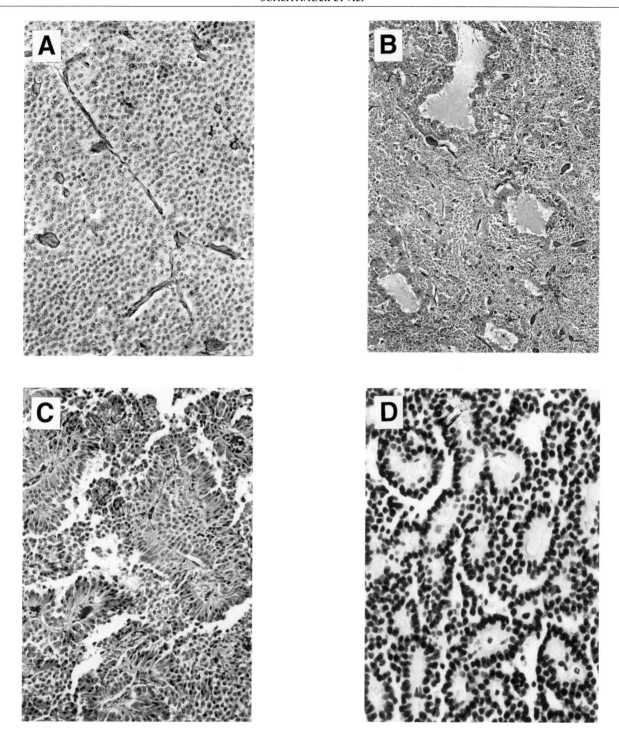

Figure 7-31 *(continued on next page)* Pattern variation in pituitary adenomas is considerable and invites misdiagnosis at frozen section and on routine histochemical stains. **(A–E)** Cellular pleomorphism and atypia **(F)** in the absence of mitoses is of no clinical significance. (A–E) H&E × 160–320; (F) H&E × 400.

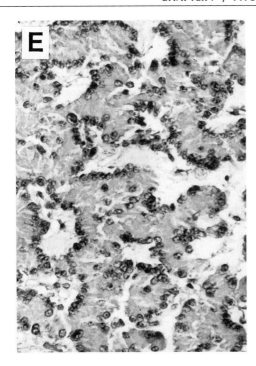

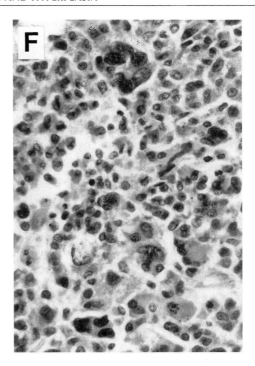

Table 3
Ultrastructural Classification of Adenohypophosial Tumors
1999 WHO Classification *(1,2)*

Tumor type	Variant
GH cell adenoma	Densely granulated
	Sparsely granulated
PRL cell adenoma	Sparsely granulated
	Densely granulated
Adenomas with GH	Mixed GH-PRL cell adenoma
and PRL cell	Mammosomatotroph cell adenoma
differentiation	Acidophil stem-cell adenoma
ACTH cell adenoma	Densely granulated
	Sparsely granulated
	Crooke cell variant
TSH cell adenoma	
FSH-LH cell adenoma	Male type
	Female type
Null-cell adenoma	Nononcocytic
	Oncocytic
Other adenomas	Silent "corticotroph" subtype 1
	Silent "corticotroph" subtype 2
	Silent adenoma subtype 3
	Plurimorphous adenomas, e.g.,
	GH-PRL-TSH, PRL-ACTH,
	and so forth
	Unclassified

may actually cause diagnostic confusion, particularly in technically suboptimal preparations. This approach is favored by neurosurgeons, but by few discerning pathologists who find that in fresh frozen section preparations, morphologic details are often suboptimal. Not only are cytologic details obscured, but in some instances, it is difficult to distinguish conclusively adenoma from nontumoral adenohypophysis (Figure 32). Furthermore, the effects of freezing seriously compromise subsequent histochemical and immunocytologic studies. By definition, ultrastructural evaluation cannot be performed on tissues previously frozen. Thus, we strongly recommend that frozen section examination be considered only when tissue is abundant and permits sacrifice of a small portion of the specimen. Instead, we promote the use of tissue imprints or smears stained by H&E. Although various other staining methods are suitable (hemalum-phloxine, modified Papanicolau), some are not. Specifically, stains involving air-drying of preparations (Romanovsky stains, such as May-Grünwald Giemsa or Diff-quick) are to be avoided. We prefer H&E stains in that cytoplasmic granularity and tinctorial characteristics of adenoma preparations correlate well with those seen in routine H&E-stained sections.

Smear Preparations The smear or touch techniques are simple, fast, and provide a whole other dimension in the assessment of tissue specimens. In typical cases, they readily distinguish adenoma from nontumoral adenohypophysial cells (Figure 33). Immunocytochemical methods can also be applied to smear preparations. The same is true of FISH analysis.

Permanent Sections For optimal assessment of pituitary adenomas, we recommend not only an H&E, PAS, and reticulin stain, the latter for demonstration of loss of acinar architecture (Figure 34), but also 10 unstained sections for performance of a complete pituitary hormone immunobattery.

THE ADENOMAS

GH-PRODUCING PITUITARY ADENOMAS The pathogenesis of growth hormone excess is varied *(122–124)*. Approximately 15% of all pituitary adenomas produce GH in excess *(3,31,33)*. Clinically, the vast majority of patients are adults presenting with acromegaly. If GH overproduction becomes manifest before puberty, the result is gigantism. These tumors arise in the "acidophilic cell line" and include five distinct, well-defined entities *(3,31,33,80,123)*. Under this heading, the two most common tumor types are the densely and sparsely granulated

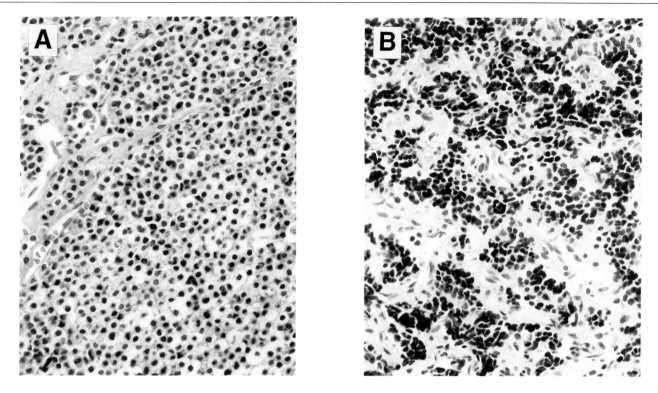

Figure 7-32   Frozen section artifacts obscure cytologic detail and negatively affect immunoreactivity **(A)**. Mechanical artifacts, such as compression, may produce hyperchromasia and a small-cell carcinoma-like appearance, respectively **(B)**. (A and B) H&E × 400.

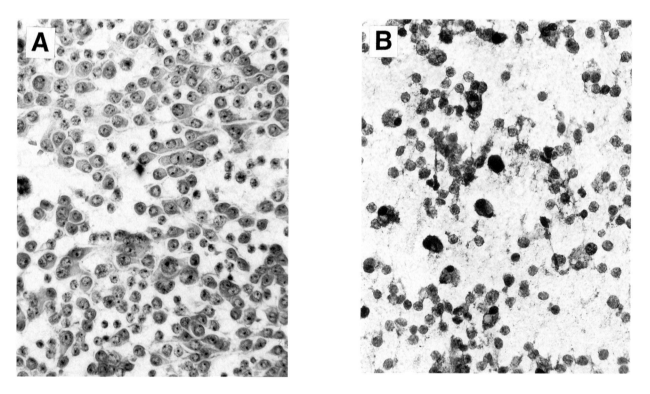

Figure 7-33   In smear preparations **(A)**, pituitary adenomas are characterized by uniform cytoplasmic staining and often by the emergence of distinct nucleoli. On occasion, a mitotic figure is also apparent. By comparison, normal gland yields low cellularity, cellular heterogeneity, and lack of nuclear abnormalities **(B)**. (A, B) H&E × 640.

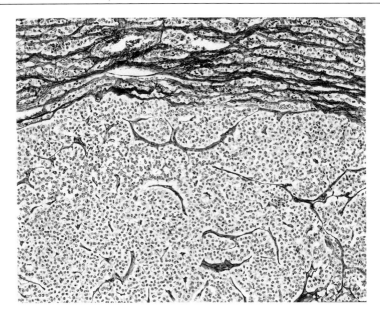

Figure 7-34 On reticulin stain, adenomas are characterized by loss of acinar architecture. Note compression of surrounding tissue, the basis of "pseudoencapsulation" (above) (×400).

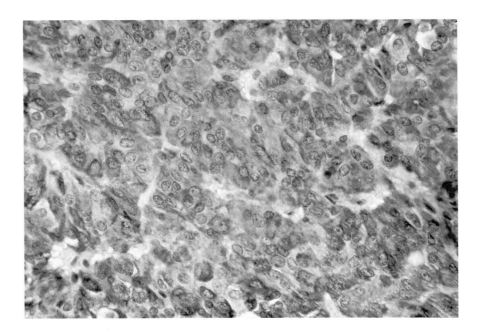

Figure 7-35 Of the two forms of somatotroph adenomas, the acidophilic, densely granulated adenoma is strongly immunoreactive for GH (×400).

somatotroph adenomas. Each consists of a single cell population. The three remaining tumor types, variably associated with acromegaly and bihormonal in also expressing PRL, will be discussed under a separate heading.

Densely Granulated Somatotroph Adenomas These are acidophilic, PAS-negative tumors that often exhibit a diffuse or trabecular growth pattern *(3,31,33,80)*. Mitotic figures are very rare, and the MIB-1-labeling index, a useful measure of cell proliferation, is very low *(6,7)*. Slowly growing and usually well-demarcated tumors, their rate of invasion is relatively low. Immunocytochemistry shows diffuse, strong positivity for GH throughout the cytoplasm (Figure 35). Although ultrastructurally

monomorphous (Figure 36), such adenomas are very often plurihormonal *(125,126)*. Aside from GH, the most frequently seen immunoreactivities are for PRL and/or α-subunit, less frequently for β TSH, and only occasionally for FSH/LH. These less common immunoreactivities are usually not reflected in terms of blood hormone levels or clinical symptoms. In only a few cases do goiter and hyperthyroidism develop in the course of acromegaly. It is of note that TSH production by a bihormonal GH- and TSH-producing adenoma apparently occurs only in the densely granulated variant.

Electron microscopy shows that the adenoma cells are similar to normal nonadenomatous somatotrophs *(3,33,79,127,128)*

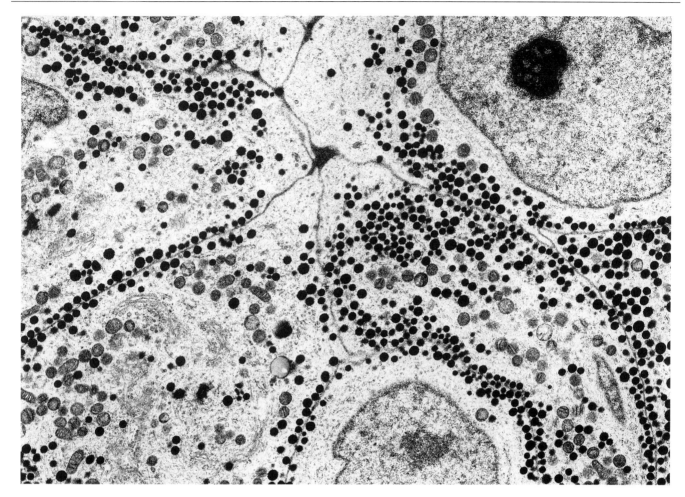

Figure 7-36   Densely granulated somatotroph adenoma. Note abundance of large, dense secretory granules with tight-filling membranes (×8100).

(Figure 36). They are spherical or polyhedral in configuration and possess a fairly uniform, centrally located nucleus with a prominent nucleolus, abundant cytoplasm with peripherally disposed and slender RER cisternae, a spherical Golgi apparatus containing immature secretory granules, and round or ovoid mitochondria (Figure 36). Secretory granules are numerous, randomly distributed, evenly electron-dense, and measure 150–1000 nm (mostly 300–450 nm). Exocytosis is not seen. Endocrine amyloid deposition, crystallization of the secretory material, and tubuloreticular aggregates within endothelial cells may also be seen.

Sparsely Granulated Somatotroph Adenomas   These are chromophobic, PAS-negative tumors exhibiting a diffuse growth pattern. Varying degrees of cellular and nuclear pleomorphism may be apparent. In some tumors, characteristic pale, eosinophilic "fibrous bodies" can readily be identified (Figure 37). Paranuclear in location, these structures are spherical and often appear to indent the nucleus. Fibrous bodies are strongly immunopositive for cytokeratin *(129)*, but lack staining for adenohypophysial hormones. Immunocytochemistry for GH is always positive, but the reaction varies from weak, focal immunopositivity reflecting the location of the Golgi complex to diffuse strong cytoplasmic staining (Figure 37). A few scattered cells may be positive for PRL but unlike the densely granulated variant, other immunoreactivities are usually not detected. Mitotic figures are rarely encountered, and the MIB-1 index is generally low (<3%). Although some

tumors are indolent and expansive, others are more rapidly growing and exhibit local invasion. Sparsely granulated somatotroph adenomas are often operated on at an earlier age, and both grow more rapidly as well as recur more often than densely granulated somatotroph adenoma *(130)*.

Ultrastructurally, sparsely granulated somatotroph adenomas consist of a single cell type not normally seen in the adult pituitary *(3,33,79,127,128)* (Figure 38). Spherical or irregular in configuration, they possess either an eccentric, flattened, or crescentic nucleus or peripherally situated lobulated or multiple nuclei. Cytoplasm is abundant and usually contains randomly scattered short profiles of RER; longer parallel cisternae or concentric whorls are far less common. The Golgi region is often occupied by the spherical fibrous body, a diagnostic marker composed of aggregates of cytokeratin immunoreactive filaments and smooth endoplasmic reticulum (Figure 38). The Golgi complex is either enmeshed within this filamentous mass, which also contains mitochondria, secretory granules, and lysosomes, or is displaced by it. Mitochondria are ovoid, spherical, or slightly irregular. Paired or multiple centrioles may be seen in the Golgi area. Secretory granules are randomly distributed, sparse, and measure 100–250 nm. The vascular endothelium may contain tubuloreticular aggregates. Endocrine amyloid deposition also rarely occurs. An additional feature in a few tumors is the presence of nerve cells and neuropil. They are regarded as a sign of neuronal metaplasia of adenomatous somatotrophs *(131)*.

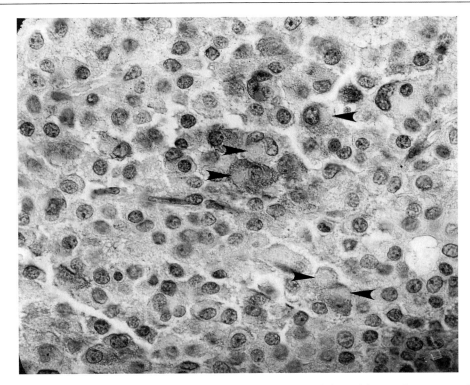

Figure 7-37 Sparsely granulated somatotroph adenomas are weakly GH-immunoreactivity and feature the presence of paranuclear intermediate filament (cytokeratin) whorls termed "fibrous bodies." Immunostain for GH × 640.

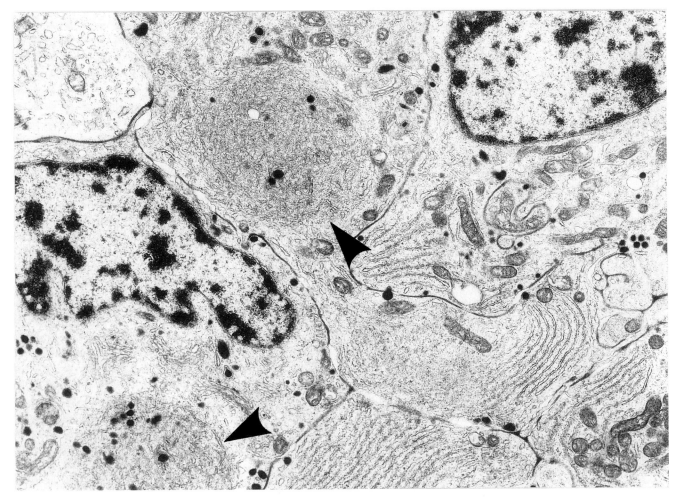

Figure 7-38 Sparsely granulated somatotroph adenoma with characteristic fibrous bodies (arrowheads) (×13,200).

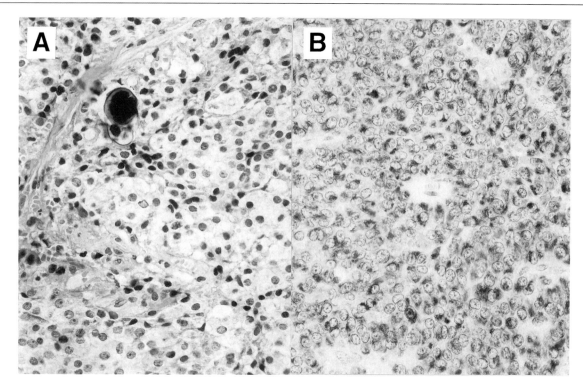

Figure 7-39   Lactotroph cell adenomas are typically chromophobic and often feature calcospherite (psammoma body) formation **(A)**. Strong paranuclear (Golgi zone) reactivity for PRL **(B)** is a characteristic feature. H&E × 400; (B) × 400.

ADENOMAS PRODUCING PRL   Lactotroph adenomas represent the most frequent pituitary tumor (3,33,79,80,132,133). In the recent past, their incidence was noted to be increasing (134). Although occurring in every age group, in the surgical material, they are most common in young females. In autopsy material, however, this gender-related difference in frequency is not obvious. Clinically, females present with amenorrhea, galactorrhea, and infertility. In males, symptoms, such as decreased libido and impotence, are less apparent. PRL cell adenomas are often well-demarcated microadenomas. Nonetheless, some are more aggressive, have a rapid growth rate, and even in microadenoma form are grossly seen to invade dura or adjacent structures (118). Macroadenomas are the rule in both postreproductive females and males in whom local symptoms may be conspicuous. These include headache owing to increased intracranial pressure as well as visual defects and cranial nerve palsies related to compressive effects or invasion. Such tumors have higher proliferation indices than the microadenomas of young females (135).

Morphologically, lactotroph adenomas can be divided into chromophobic, slightly acidophilic, and strongly acidophilic tumors. The latter are rare, densely granulated lactotroph tumors that present and behave like other, more ordinary lactotrophic adenomas

The sparsely granulated lactotroph adenoma is the most frequent tumor type in the human pituitary (3). Such tumors are chromophobic (Figure 39), slightly acidophilic, and PAS-negative. Surgically removed examples usually show a diffuse growth pattern (Figure 18). In contrast, the rare papillary pattern occurs in autopsy material wherein lactotrophic tumors are the most frequent of "incidentalomas" (Figure 30). Cellular and nuclear pleomorphism is variable, and it does not correlate with biologic

behavior. Particularly in reproductive-age females, mitotic figures are rare, and the MIB-1 index is low (6,7,135). Although calcification is very rare in other adenoma types, it is encountered in approximately 15% of lactotroph adenomas (136). In some tumors, only a few small calcospherites are seen (Figure 39), whereas in other instances, large psammoma bodies are numerous and accompanied by a fibrous reaction. It is unclear why calcification is frequent in lactotroph adenomas. Rarely does bone formation occur in lactotroph adenomas. These adenomas, called pituitary stones (137), are extremely hard and accompanied by calcifications, fibrosis, and an inflammatory response.

The pattern of immunoreactivity for PRL is stereotypic in being paranuclear ("Golgi pattern immunopositivity") (Figure 39). Diffuse cytoplasmic staining is not seen since secretory granules are sparse. With the rare exception of variable α-subunit reactivity in some macroadenomas, stains for other hormones are negative. Thus, the tumors are primarily monohormonal and are composed of but a single cell type.

The ultrastructural features of sparsely granulated lactotroph adenomas are characteristic and diagnostic (127,128,132). The adenoma cells are spherical, oval, or irregular. Their predominantly euchromatic nucleus may be spherical or irregular and contains a large, dense nucleolus. Cytoplasm is abundant and contains long parallel cisternae and concentric whorls of RER ("Nebenkerns"). Prominence of RER membranes is more conspicuous in lactotroph adenomas than in other adenoma types. Golgi complexes are extensive and harbor numerous spherical or pleomorphic maturing secretory granules. Overall, secretory granules are sparse and small (100–300 nm). The most characteristic ultrastructural marker of lactotroph adenoma cells is exocytosis of secretory granules. Extrusion of secretory granules may be ortho-

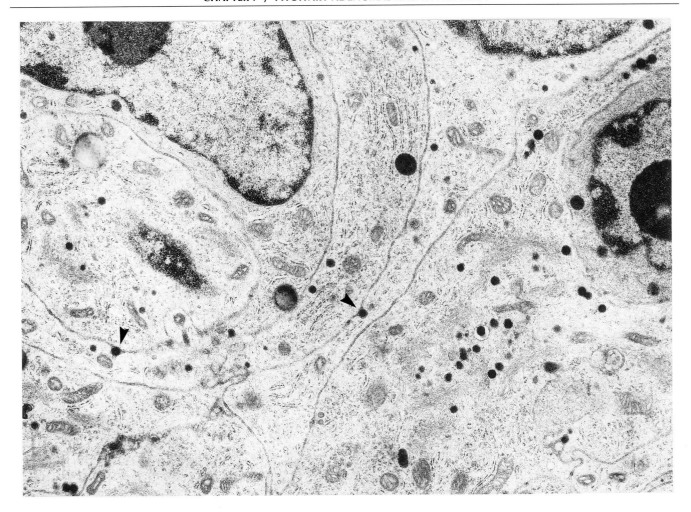

Figure 7-40 Sparsely granulated lactotroph adenoma with well-developed RER and Golgi complex. Note misplaced exocytoses (arrowheads) (×12,750).

topic (at the capillary interface of the cell) or misplaced, i.e., occurring on the lateral cell membrane distant from capillaries and basal lamina (Figure 40). A relatively frequent occurrence in lactotroph adenomas is the production of endocrine amyloid *(127,138,139)*. Its deposition may be mild and evident only on electron microscopy. In these instances, amyloid fibrils appear as intracytoplasmic membrane-bound aggregates within dilated cisternae of RER. If extensive, amyloid deposition may also be seen in the extracellular space. In rare cases, the amyloid forms large, slightly acidophilic, PAS-positive spheres obvious in histologic section or even grossly (Figs. 41,42). Neuronal metaplasia is a rare event in lactotroph adenomas *(140)*.

In contrast to sparsely granulated tumors, the rare, densely granulated lactotroph adenoma ultrastructurally features smaller cells and abundance of secretory granules of larger size (400–450 nm; occasionally 700 nm) and more varied shape (Figure 43). Granule extrusion is seen. Some granules may feature uneven electron density.

ADENOMAS PRODUCING GH AND PRL   Mixed Somatotroph-Lactotroph Adenomas These are bimorphous, bihormonal tumors consisting of both somatotrophs and lactotrophs *(3,123,141)*. Clinically, they are accompanied by acromegaly or gigantism as well as varying degrees of hyperprolactinemia and its

sequela. Although benign, some mixed adenomas show accelerated growth and local invasion. Total surgical removal may be difficult, and recurrences are common.

Histologically, most tumors are composed of an admixture of acidophilic and chromophobic cells. Immunocytochemistry shows the acidophilic cells to be immunoreactive for GH and the chromophobic cells for PRL (Figure 44). The two cell types may be seen intermingled as individual cells or forming small monomorphous cell nests.

Electron microscopy shows mixed GH cell–PRL cell adenomas to be bimorphous and to consist of two different cell types, most often densely granulated somatotrophs and sparsely granulated lactotrophs *(127,128)* (Figure 45). Immunoelectron microscopy and *in situ* hybridization provide additional evidence that the tumor is formed of two different cell types. In a number of tumors, however, cells with transitional features are identified, suggesting that these unusual tumors arise either from a common precursor cell or that their cells can transform one to the other *(142)*.

Mammosomatotroph Adenomas These are monomorphous tumors composed of a single GH- and PRL-producing cell type known to occur in the normal pituitary *(82,143)*. Clinically, these tumors are associated with acromegaly or gigantism and varying degrees of hyperprolactinemia and its sequela. They are

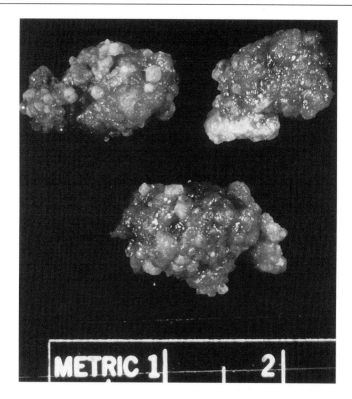

Figure 7-41   Coarse, "caviar-like" amyloid bodies are an occasional feature of lactotroph adenomas (*see also* Figure 42).

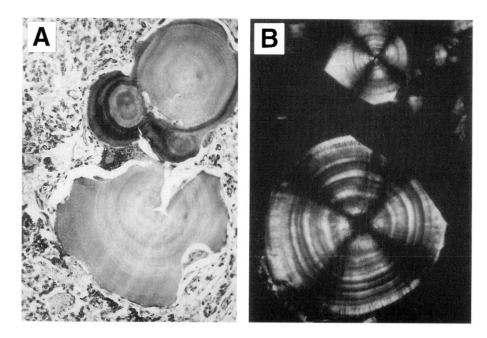

Figure 7-42   Lactotroph cell adenoma with massive, spherical amyloid bodies showing a tendency to radial cracking. These are Congo red-positive **(A)** and show birefringence under polarized light **(B)** (*see also* Figure 41). (A, B) ×200.

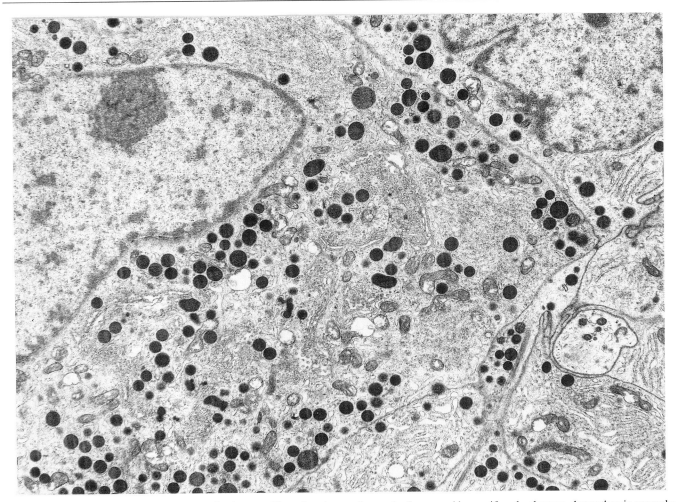

Figure 7-43 Densely granulated lactotroph adenoma. Note abundance of granules larger and less uniformly electron-dense than in sparsely granulated tumors (*see also* Figure 40). Golgi and RER are conspicuous (×7900).

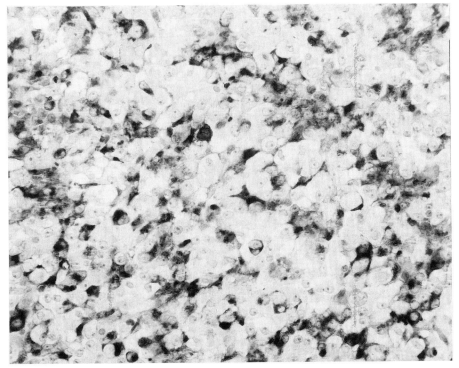

Figure 7-44 Mixed GH cell-PRL cell adenoma. Note variable, paranuclear to diffuse cytoplasmic staining of lactotrophs, but absence of reactivity in somatotrophs. PRL immunostain × 400.

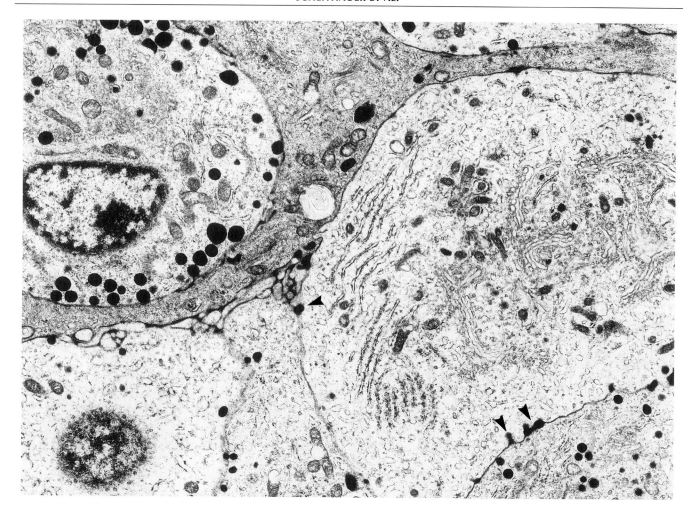

Figure 7-45   Mixed GH cell-PRL cell adenoma consisting of densely granulated somatotrophs (upper left) and sparsely granulated lactotrophs. Note several granule extrusions in a PRL cell (arrowheads) (×9300).

slowly growing tumors with very occasional mitotic figures and very low MIB-1-labeling indices. Being immunoreactive for GH, α-subunit, PRL, and sometimes TSH, its biological behavior as well as immunohistochemical profile is very similar to that of densely granulated somatotroph adenomas. Thus, it is questionable whether the distinction between these two tumor types is of any clinical significance.

Ultrastructurally, mammosomatotroph adenomas resemble densely granulated somatotroph adenomas. In some tumors, the large size (1000–1500 nm) of its ovoid to irregular secretory granules may be conspicuous. Extrusion of secretory granules with uneven mottled texture is also a distinguishing feature of mammosomatotroph cell adenomas (Figure 46). Cells producing both GH and PRL are readily demonstrated by the RHPA assay *(82)*. Furthermore, immunoelectron microscopy demonstrates both hormones within the same secretory granules *(127)*.

Acidophil Stem-Cell Adenomas   These are potentially bihormonal tumors, but are most often associated with elevation of PRL alone, hormone levels being disproportionally low for the size of the lesion *(144)*. Physical stigmata of GH overproduction, elevated GH levels, and especially full-blown acromegaly are rare. Acidophil stem-cell adenomas are monomorphous tumors exhibiting a diffuse growth pattern. Their cells are chromophobic PAS-

negative. A characteristic finding is the presence of clear cytoplasmic vacuoles, the light microscopic equivalents of giant mitochondria (Figure 47). Despite the fact that these tumors may exhibit a rapid growth and invasiveness, mitotic figures are infrequent, and MIB-1 indices are not high. Immunocytochemistry demonstrates varying degrees of PRL immunoreactivity, whereas GH stain is usually weak, focal, or entirely absent (Figure 48).

Electron microscopy reveals a monomorphous tumor displaying lactotrophic and somatotrophic features, specifically the presence of fibrous bodies and misplaced exocytoses *(127,128)*. In the majority of tumors, lactotrophic features predominate. RER may be poorly or well developed, but Golgi bodies are not conspicuous. Secretory granules are sparse, randomly distributed, or peripherally situated and rarely exceed 200 nm. Generalized oncocytic change is a frequent finding and is always associated with formation of giant mitochondria and lack or loss of lamellae (Figure 49). Thus, the ultrastructural appearance of this adenoma is unique and easily distinguished from that of other tumor types. We consider electron microscopy essential to achieving the diagnosis.

PITUITARY ADENOMAS PRODUCING ACTH   Corticotroph Adenomas   These pose challenges to clinical endocrinologists, imaging specialists, neurosurgeons, and pathologists alike. Clinically, they are associated with pituitary-dependent Cushing's

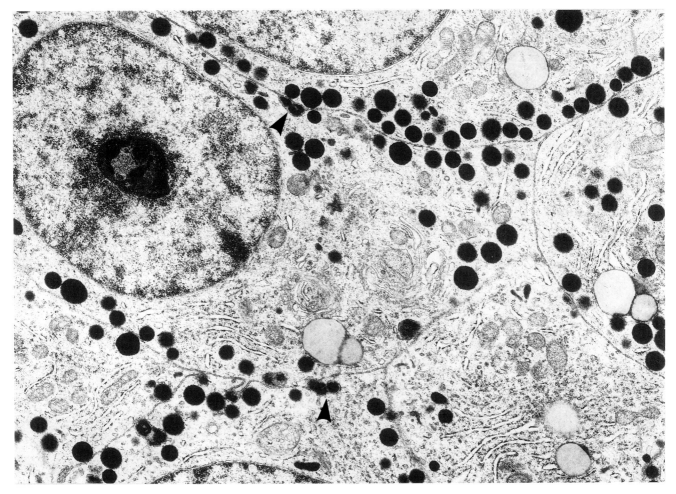

Figure 7-46 Mammosomatotroph adenoma. Its appearance is similar to that of densely granulated GH cell adenoma with added features of mottled secretory granules and granule extrusions (arrowheads) (×12,750).

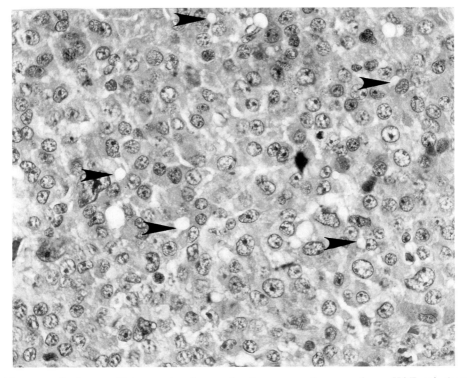

Figure 7-47 Acidophil stem-cell adenoma. Only occasional examples show paranuclear vacuoles on H&E stain (arrows), the light microscopic correlate to giant mitochondria (*see* Figure 49) (×400).

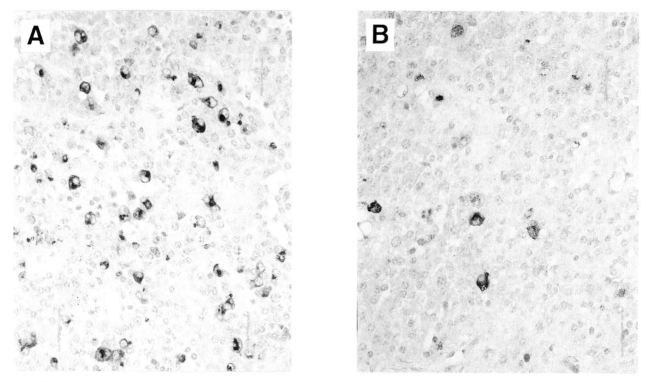

Figure 7-48   Acidophil stem-cell adenoma typically shows more abundant PRL reactivity **(A)** than GH staining **(B)**. (A and B) Immunostain × 400.

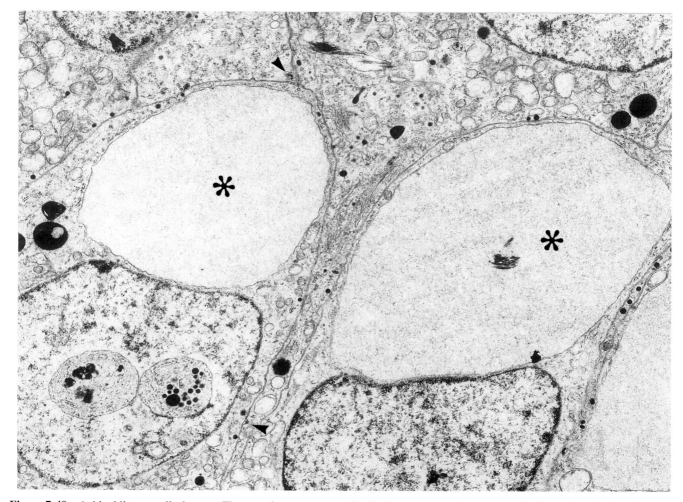

Figure 7-49   Acidophil stem-cell adenoma. The rare adenoma type usually displays oncocytic change as well as formation of giant mitochondria (asterisks). Note granule extrusions (arrowheads) (×9300).

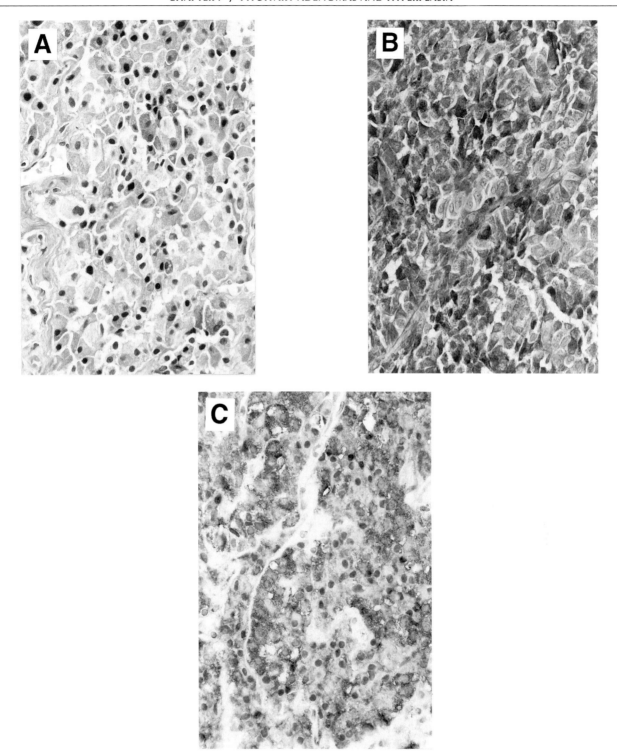

Figure 7-50 Corticotroph cell adenomas feature polygonal cells with amphophilic cytoplasm **(A)**, PAS positivity **(B)**, and variable ACTH staining **(C)**. (A, B, C) × 400.

disease, the now rare Nelson's syndrome in patients who underwent previous bilateral adrenalectomy for hypercorticism. The nonfunctioning ("silent") adenomas *(3,145)* are discussed separately. Corticotroph adenomas occur more frequently in women; the female-to-male ratio is approximately 5:1. The majority are small microadenomas with high hormonal activity. Even very small tumors, ones undetectable by the most advanced of imaging

techniques, may cause severe clinical symptoms. If untreated, corticotroph adenomas can lead to serious disease and to patient demise. Thus, a correct diagnosis and appropriate treatment, primarily surgery, are essential.

By histology, most corticotroph adenomas are basophilic and exhibit strong, diffuse cytoplasmic PAS positivity *(145)* (Figure 50). Generally well-demarcated, they show very little or no cellular

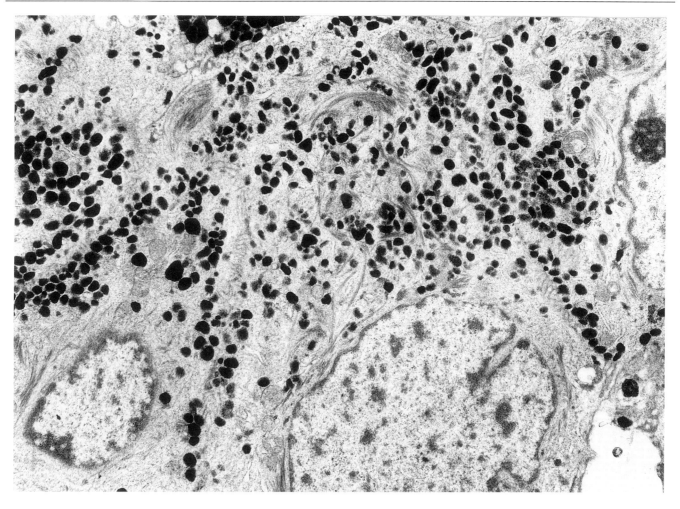

Figure 7-51   Corticotroph cell adenoma possessing numerous irregular and heart-shaped secretory granules as well as bundles of cytokeratin filaments (×7950).

and nuclear pleomorphism. Mitotic figures are rare, and the MIB-1 index is low. Occasionally, no tumor is found in frozen or permanent sections of the fragmented surgical specimen. The minute adenoma might not have been removed, may have been lost during the surgical procedure or tissue processing, or may remain unsampled in paraffin blocks. Alternatively, the hypercorticism might have been caused by corticotroph hyperplasia or ectopic ACTH syndrome instead of an adenoma *(146,147)*. In such instances, it is essential to collect and process all available tissues, including that in suction bottles as well as unstained sections for PAS, reticulin, and ACTH stains. Few corticotroph adenomas are large. Such tumors are generally chromophobic and show little or no PAS positivity. They may be aggressive, have a rapid growth rate, and invade surrounding structures. Although they also secrete ACTH, their endocrine activity is less pronounced than that of the small, basophilic microadenomas. Adenomas associated with Nelson's syndrome are usually large, aggressive, and difficult to treat owing to a propensity for invasion and recurrence *(3,33,118)*.

To varying extents, all corticotroph adenomas are immunoreactive for ACTH (Figure 50) and other peptides derived from proopiomelanocortin, the prehormone of ACTH. These include β-endorphin, β-LPH, CLIP, and so forth. Immunostains are usu-

ally negative for other pituitary hormones. In some cases, especially in macroadenomas, focal immunoreactivity may be seen for α-subunit *(148)* LH, or galanin, a neuropeptide produced mainly in gut and hypothalamus *(33)*. Corticotrophic adenomas are also cytokeratin-reactive, the degree of staining being a reflection of their intermediate filament content *(see below)*.

By electron microscopy, the basophilic variant of corticotroph adenoma is composed of polyhedral, often elongated, spindle-shaped cells with a spherical or ovoid nucleus, prominent nucleolus, and abundant and somewhat electron-dense cytoplasm *(127,128)* (Figure 51). RER is moderately developed and may show focal, uneven dilation. The Golgi complex is spherical or elongated and contains several maturing secretory granules. Corticotroph granules are numerous, vary in shape and electron density, and measuring 200–450 nm. Although most are randomly distributed throughout the cytoplasm, some form a single or double row beneath the cell membrane. In addition to spherical forms, others are indented, irregular, drop-shaped, or heart-shaped (Figure 51). Another marker of corticotroph cells is the presence of cytokeratin filaments forming small bundles in the perinuclear region *(149)*. Adenomas associated with Nelson's syndrome have similar ultrastructure features but lack or exhibit only rare microfilaments *(3,33,79,127,128)*.

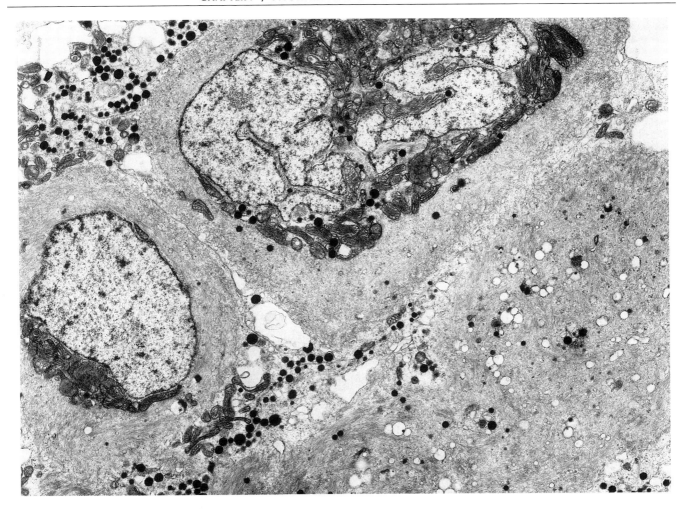

Figure 7-52 Crooke's cell adenoma is a morphologic variant of corticotroph adenoma displaying excessive accumulation of cytokeratin filaments (×6600).

On the other hand, the chromophobic variant of corticotroph adenoma shows a lesser degree of differentiation, possessing less cytoplasm, only poorly developed membranous organelles, sparse and smaller secretory granules measuring 200–300 nm, a few large lysosomes, and only occasional cytokeratin filaments *(33,79,127,128)*.

Crooke's hyalinization *(150)* or the excessive deposition of cytokeratin filaments is generally considered an attribute of the nonneoplastic corticotrophs exposed to elevated levels of circulating glucocorticoids *(81,149)*. For unclear reasons, a minority of corticotroph adenomas display focal or generalized Crooke's hyaline change ("Crooke's cell adenoma") *(151–153)* (Figure 52). The adenomas thereby affected differ in tumor as well as in cell size and in markers of hormonal activity. The clinical severity of Cushing's disease associated with Crooke's cell adenomas also shows some variations; occasional patients lack Cushingoid features and present only with mass effects or psychiatric symptoms. Crooke's hyalinization in corticotroph adenomas is of no particular clinical relevance. Amyloid deposition is infrequently observed in corticotroph adenomas *(154)*.

ADENOMAS SECRETING TSH   Thyrotroph Adenomas
These are the least frequent of adenohypophysial tumors, representing about 1% of cases *(3,33,79,155,157)*. They occur with

equal frequency among the sexes and occur at any age. Clinically, thyrotroph adenomas may occur in the setting of hyperthyroidism, long-standing primary hypothyroidism, or euthyroidism *(155–161)*. The most important association is with increased endocrine activity, i.e., characteristic clinical symptoms of hyperthyroidism *(161)*. Tumors associated with long-standing primary hypothyroidism are probably preceded by thyrotroph cell hyperplasia. Tumors associated with euthyroidism belong to the group of "functionally silent" tumors that synthesize the hormones, but do not secrete them in quantities necessary to induce increased activity of the target gland.

At surgery, most thyrotroph adenomas are macroadenomas showing evidence of invasion *(118,162)*. Histologically, most are chromophobic and show a sinusoidal pattern or the formation of perivascular pseudorosette, a nonspecific histologic finding, often by elongated cells (Figure 53). Only rare thyrotroph adenomas contain an abundance of secretory granules and are basophilic as well as PAS-positive. Sizable PAS-positive cytoplasmic globules are often seen and represent lysosomes. Perivascular and interstitial fibrosis is an occasional, but unexplained finding. Immunocytochemistry demonstrates conclusive immunoreactivity for TSH and less often for α-subunit (Figure 53). In some instances, occasional adenoma cells may contain GH or PRL. As a rule,

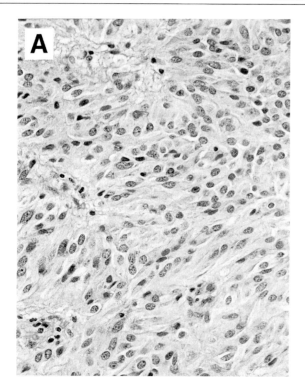
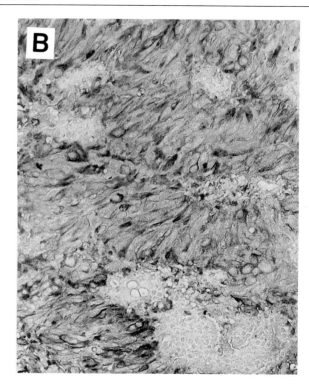

Figure 7-53 Thyrotroph cell adenomas are often composed of elongated cells **(A)** showing variable, often patchy TSH immunoreactivity **(B)**. Note vague perivascular pseudorosetting. (A) H&E × 400; (B) TSH immunostain × 400.

immunostains for other adenohypophysial hormones are negative. Despite occasional cellular and/or nuclear pleomorphism, mitotic figures are infrequently encountered, and the MIB-1 index is usually low *(6,7)*.

By electron microscopy, the adenoma cells are often elongated or fusiform, their polar configuration resembling that of nontumorous thyrotrophs *(127,157)*. Nuclei are spherical, oval, or irregular and are mainly euchromatic. RER may be prominent, featuring short ribosome-studded stacks, and slightly dilated cisternae. Golgi complexes are prominent, globoid, and contain several maturing secretory granules. As a rule, secretory granules are sparse, small, and tend to form a single layer beneath the cell membrane (Figure 54). Variably electron-dense, they are spherical, rod-shaped, or irregular and measure 150–250 nm. In some cells, secretory granules accumulate within the cell processes. There appears to be no correlation between ultrastructural features and endocrine activity, i.e., findings are often the same in tumors associated with hyper-, hypo-, or euthyroidism. A minority of thyrotroph adenomas appear less differentiated with poorly developed membranous organelles. Such tumors may closely resemble null-cell adenomas. Given the often uneven expression of differentiation in glycoprotein hormone-producing adenomas, as reflected in both immunoreactivities and at the ultrastructural level, this may be owing to vagaries of sampling. It is of note that the presence of "thyroidectomy" or "thyroid deficiency cells" is very rare in tumors.

PLURIHORMONAL ADENOMAS Tumors producing multiple hormones diverse in chemical composition and biologic action are termed plurihormonal adenomas *(125,126)*. The one-cell, one-hormone theory, dominant in endocrine pathology for decades, has of necessity been revised given data derived largely

from immunocytochemical studies. It became evident that many endocrine cells, nontumorous and neoplastic, are capable of producing more than a single hormone.

Plurihormonal adenomas can be divided into monomorphous and plurimorphous forms, the latter consisting of more than one cell type (Figure 55). The cytogenesis of plurihormonal adenomas is entirely unclear. It may be that they originate in uncommitted precursor cells, which owing to obscure factors undergo multidirectional differentiation. Another explanation is that plurihormonal clones existing in the nontumorous pituitary give rise to such tumors.

The most frequent combination of plurihormonality is exemplified by densely granulated somatotroph adenomas, which feature concomitant production of GH and PRL as well as of glycoproteins, such as α-subunit or less often β TSH. It recently became apparent that Pit-1, a common transcription factor, plays an important role in differentiation and maturation of somatotrophs, lactotrophs, and thyrotrophs *(96,163–165)*. Whether Pit-1 plays a role in the adenoma plurihormonality remains to be determined.

In addition to their principal hormones (TSH, FSH/LH), glycoprotein adenomas often show minor immunoreactivities for the other hormones, such as GH, PRL, or even ACTH. Although the association of gonadotropins with ACTH is uncommon, occasional gonadotroph adenomas, particularly in women, exhibit minor staining for ACTH and β-endorphin *(33)*. It is of note that a small proportion of corticotroph adenomas, usually macroadenomas, exhibit immunopositivity for LH and/or α-subunit *(148,166)*. Rare combinations, such as GH and ACTH, or of PRL and gonadotrophic hormones, do occasionally occur *(125,126)*. In most instances, plurihormonality is expressed only as multiple immunoreactivities, rarely exerting a clinical influence.

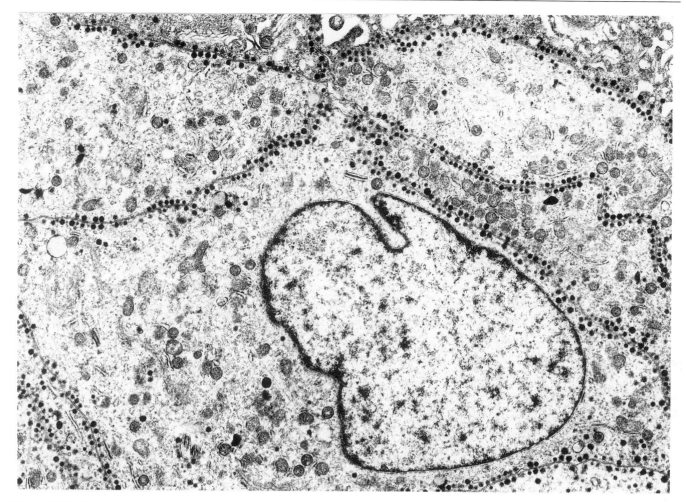

Figure 7-54 Thyrotroph adenoma showing peripheral accumulation of small secretory granules outlining cell borders (×8700).

The extent to which plurihormonality exists and its prognostic significance are unknown. Inasmuch as a number of growth factors, oncogenes, and other proteins/peptides have recently been demonstrated in pituitary cells, it may be that all pituitary adenomas are plurihormonal. Studies based on limited patient numbers seem to suggest that plurihormonal tumors grow more rapidly, are more aggressive and invasive, and recur more frequently than do monohormonal variants. In our experience, no close correlation seems to exist between plurihormonality and biologic behavior.

CLINICALLY NONFUNCTIONING PITUITARY ADENOMAS Adenomas that appear clinically to be nonfunctioning include several distinct morphologic entities. These patients have no obvious symptoms or laboratory alterations related to hormone excess. The mild hyperprolactinemia so often seen may be owing to increased PRL release from the nontumorous pituitary. Termed "stalk section effect," it is thought to result from compression of the pituitary stalk and resultant interference with hypothalamic dopamine transport. Alternatively, secretory products of the growing adenoma may induce release of PRL from the nontumorous gland. With the possible exception of PRL, the blood levels of other pituitary hormones are either within the normal range or abnormally low. Owing to lack of endocrine symptoms, functionally silent pituitary tumors become large and compress or destroy the remaining pituitary, thereby resulting in various degrees of selective or general hypopituitarism.

Several morphologically distinct entities can be distinguished among clinically nonfunctioning adenoma. Among these are gonadotroph adenomas, null-cell adenomas of ordinary or oncocytic type, and three subtypes of silent adenomas. It should be kept in mind that various lesions, tumorous and nontumorous, e.g., meningioma, metastatic carcinoma, craniopharyngioma, lymphoma, plasmacytoma, chordoma, pituitary hyperplasia, hypophysitis, and granulomatous disease, may clinically and by neuroimaging mimic nonfunctioning pituitary adenomas.

Gonadotroph Adenomas These occur more frequently than was previously thought (167–169). In large surgical series, they account for approx 10% of all adenomas. Most occur in the elderly; gonadotroph adenomas rarely occur in patients under 40 yr of age. It is difficult to set precise diagnostic criteria for this tumor type. Since most are associated with FSH/LH levels normal for patient age, gonadotroph adenomas appear to be clinically rare. Because of lack of endocrine symptoms, the patients usually present with visual disturbances, headache, hypopituitarism, or cranial nerve palsy owing to a large sellar mass. At the light microscopic and even the immunohistochemical level, the diagnosis may also be tentative, since minor FSH/LH immunoreactivity may be seen in null-cell adenomas. Thus, some authors consider these two tumor types to be but ends of a continuous spectrum. From the practical point of view, the merging of the two tumor types may be justified, since their clinical presentation, laboratory findings, and

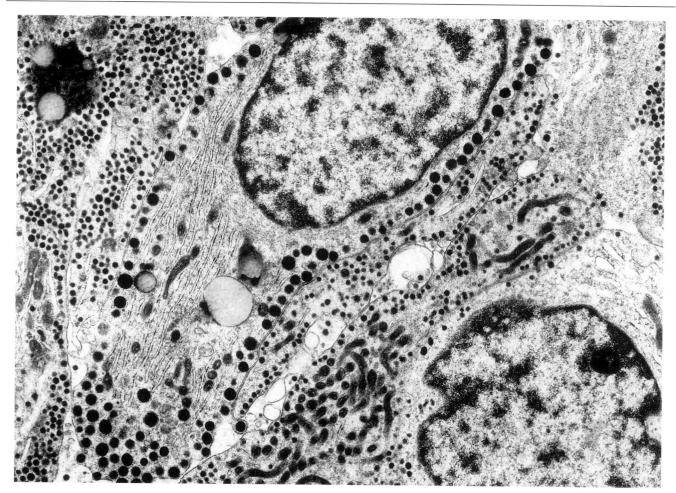

Figure 7-55   Bimorphous plurihormonal clinically functioning adenoma consisting of densely granulated GH cells (central cell) and of thyrotroph cells (×11,900).

treatment are the same *(169)*. From the theoretical point of view, however, the distinction seems to be justified.

Histologically, gonadotroph adenomas are chromophobic. A minority show varying degrees of acidophilia. The tumor cells are usually PAS-negative, although at high magnification, one often sees a tracery of sparse, PAS-positive granules along the cell membrane. The histologic pattern is often diffuse or features pseudorosette formation around vessels (Figure 56). Papilla formation is rarely seen. The cells show no significant cellular and/or nuclear pleomorphism. Despite the large size of most gonadotroph adenomas, mitotic figures are only occasional *(6)*, and the MIB-1-labeling index is low *(7)*. Immunoreactivity for FSH and LH is highly variable and often patchy (Figure 56), a frequent finding in all types of glycoprotein hormone-producing adenomas. There appears to be no consistent correlation between FSH/LH immunoreactivity and blood hormone values *(169)*. It is puzzling that several highly differentiated gonadotroph adenomas, especially the so-called female types *(see below)*, show scant or no FSH/LH or α-subunit immunoreactivity. Furthermore, these same lesions occasionally display minor ACTH immunoreactivity, thus rendering their correct diagnosis at the light microscopic level unfeasible. α-Subunit, the enhanced secretion of which is a good clinical indicator of a glycoprotein hormone-producing adenoma, is also a poor marker, since null-cell adenomas of conventional or

oncocytic type may exhibit more extensive α-subunit immunoreactivity than gonadotroph tumors fully expressed with ultrastructural features and high secretory activity. A plausible explanation of this finding is that gonadotroph adenomas are characterized by increased production of α-subunit as well as high rates of secretion, whereas the more inactive null-cell adenomas store more of the synthesized hormones.

As previously alluded to, gonadotroph adenomas show sex-related differences in their ultrastructure *(167)*. Typical gonadotroph adenomas occurring in males consist of elongated polar or irregular cells with well-developed RER and prominent Golgi complexes. Secretory granules are small (<200 nm), unevenly distributed, and tend to accumulate in cell processes (Figure 57). Oncocytic change is common, occurring in approx 50% of male gonadotroph adenomas.

In females, the majority of gonadotroph adenomas are composed of highly differentiated polar cells with long attenuated processes. Their ultrastructural marker is vacuolar, "honeycomb transformation" of the prominent Golgi complex *(167,170)*. It consists of clusters of uniform spheres filled with low-density proteinaceous material containing occasionally maturing secretory granules (Figure 58). The overwhelming majority of the secretory granules are small, measuring 100–150 nm. They accumulate in cell processes and are almost completely absent in the peri-

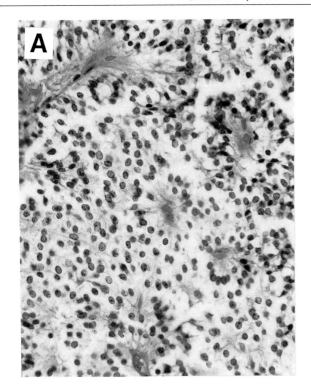
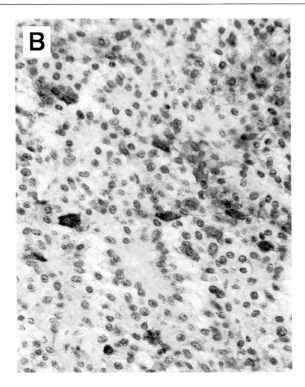

Figure 7-56 Gonadotroph cell adenomas are chromophobic and commonly show rosette formation (**A**). Staining for gonadotropic hormones (LH/FSH) may be weak or patchy (**B**). (A) H&E × 400; (B) LH immunostain × 400.

nuclear regions. The almost total absence of immature secretory granules suggests defective packaging of secretory material, possibly accounting for poor immunostaining or lack of immunoreactivity in some cases. Oncocytic change is less common than in gonadotroph adenomas of males. In a few cases, highly differentiated gonadotroph cells alternate with null-cell-like cells. In these tumors, honeycomb transformation is less conspicuous or absent. The cause of the vacuolar transformation of the Golgi complex is unknown.

A small contingent of gonadotroph tumors occurring in both sexes consists partly or entirely of polyhedral, usually strongly FSH/LH-immunoreactive cells. They possess a variable number of randomly distributed medium-size (up to 400–450 nm) secretory granules of spherical or irregular shape and variable electron density. Such cells are remarkably similar to nontumorous gonadotrophs.

Two additional morphologic markers may be present in gonadotroph adenomas *(127,167)*. One is follicle formation, a feature readily detectable at the light microscopic level owing to the strong PAS positivity of the follicular content (Figure 59). The other is the inconsistent presence of the so-called light bodies. These spherical or ovoid structures, although usually similar in size to mitochondria, are bound by a slightly ruffled, single membrane surrounding their ill-defined, granular-tubular content. The origin and function of light bodies are not known, but their presence is very indicative of gonadotroph differentiation.

Null-Cell Adenomas Like gonadotroph adenomas, these are usually large at the time of diagnosis and unassociated with hormone excess, short of mild hyperprolactinemia in some cases. The name null-cell adenoma was borrowed from immunology (B-, T-, and null-lymphocytes), indicating that the cell type and its

origin could not be clearly defined *(171,172)*. Null-cell adenomas occur in nononcocytic and oncocytic form ("pituitary oncocytoma").

Histologically, nononcocytic null-cell adenomas are composed of chromophobic (Figure 60), PAS-negative cells that often exhibit a diffuse growth pattern. Pseudorosette formation around capillaries may also be seen. As a rule, immunocytochemistry shows either complete absence of immunoreactivity for all known adenohypophysial hormones or minor, focal staining for FSH, LH, or α-subunit. In a minority of cases, scant staining for other hormones, such as GH, PRL, ACTH, and/or TSH and PRL, is noted *(172–174)*. Not surprisingly, in vitro studies have demonstrated the capacity for hormone secretion by null-cell adenomas *(175,176)*. Chromogranin immunoreactivity is a reliable feature of this as well as of glycoprotein adenomas *(52)*.

By electron microscopy, nononcocytic null-cell adenomas are composed of small, polyhedral, or nonuniform cells possessing an irregularly outlined nucleus, and poorly developed RER and Golgi *(3,33,81,127,128)* (Figure 61). The secretory granules are sparse, spherical, or rod-shaped, measure 100–250 nm, and are randomly distributed within the cytoplasm. In some cells, accumulation of mitochondria (oncocytic change) is a common finding. Based on ultrastructural findings, the "cell of origin" of null-cell adenoma cannot be defined.

The oncocytic variant of null-cell adenoma, often termed simply "pituitary oncocytoma," also occurs mainly in men and women over 40 yr of age. They show a slight male preponderance, but this is not evident in all studies.

By light microscopy, oncocytic null-cell adenomas are chromophobic or variably acidophilic owing to accumulation of mitochondria (Figure 62). Their cells are spherical, oval, or irregular in configuration and are usually larger than null cells. No major cel-

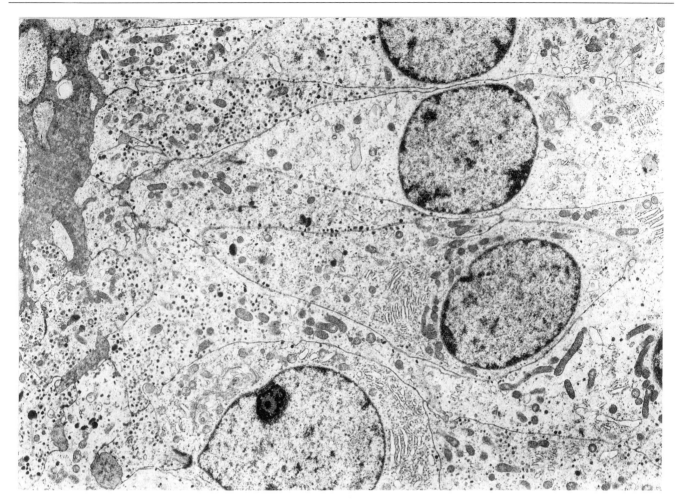

Figure 7-57   Gonadotroph adenoma in a male patient. The polarity of cells and accumulation of small secretory granules within cell processes are characteristic features (×6300).

lular and nuclear pleomorphism is evident. Mitotic figures are only occasionally seen, and the MIB-1-labeling index is very low. Like conventional null-cell adenomas, they are usually large and grow at a slow rate. Their histologic pattern is nearly always diffuse. Similar to conventional, nononcocytic null-cell adenomas, immunostainings may be entirely negative for all adenohypophysial hormones. In other cases, focal immunopositivity may be seen for FSH, LH, and α-subunit. As in nononcocytic examples, scant reactivity for GH, TSH, PRL, or ACTH suggests heterogeneity of immunophenotype or of the cellular differentiation of null-cell tumors *(174,177–179)*.

By electron microscopy, the cardinal feature of oncocytomas is their abundance of mitochondria (Figure 63). Mitochondrial accumulation may be focal or diffuse and may vary in extent. We classify a tumor as oncocytoma if at least 50% of adenoma cells show a high mitochondrial content. In contrast to nononcocytic null cells, in which the mitochondria occupy 8–10% of the cytoplasmic volume, mitochondria in the oncocytic variant occupy 15–50% of the cytoplasm *(180)*.

It should be mentioned that mitochondrial accumulation occurs not only in oncocytic null-cell adenomas. Mitochondrial abundance is also seen in most acidophil stem cell, numerous gonadotroph, and in infrequent adenomas of other types. These tumors, however, also bear the morphologic markers appropriate to their cellular derivation.

"SILENT ADENOMAS"   In addition to null-cell adenomas, which account for 25% of surgically removed pituitary tumors, other types of adenomas may also be clinically nonfunctioning. As has been alluded to, a high proportion of gonadotroph and some of thyrotroph adenomas are unaccompanied by signs of hormone hypersecretion. A small number, approx 2–3%, of sparsely granulated GH cell adenomas are also clinically silent. None of these tumors should be confused with the three subtypes of silent adenomas *(181,182)*, neoplasms morphologically well defined and having characteristic ultrastructural features as well as patterns of immunoreactivity. They are not only functionless, but cytogenetically appear unassociated with any of the five known anterior pituitary cell types. Owing to the lack of specific endocrine symptoms, these tumors are likely to be macroadenomas at presentation. Two of the three subtypes consist of POMC-producing cells and probably arise in the cells of the pars intermedia region (*see* Normal Cell Types, *above*). The cellular derivation of the third subtype of silent adenoma is open to conjecture, although the salient ultrastructural features of this resemble those of glycoprotein hormone-producing adenomas *(182)*.

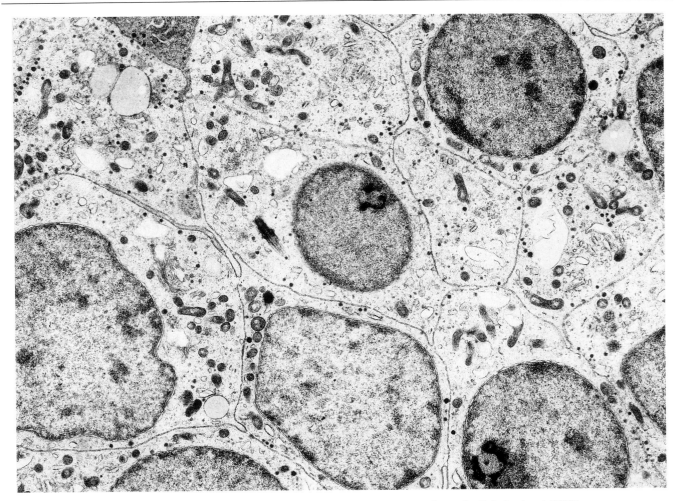

Figure 7-61   Null-cell adenoma showing signs of endocrine differentiation, but no markers of cell derivation (×8700).

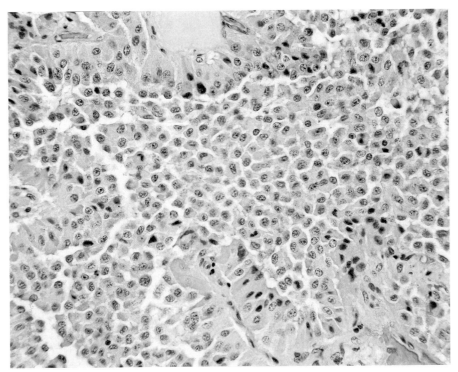

Figure 7-62   Null-cell adenoma, oncocytic-type. Their acidophilic cytoplasm is coarse-textured owing to accumulation of mitochondria rather than secretory granules. H&E × 400.

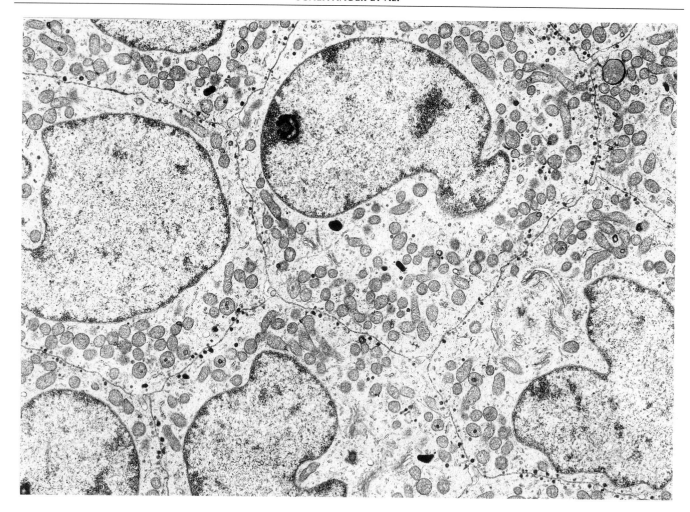

Figure 7-63 Pituitary oncocytoma, the oncocytic form of null-cell adenoma (×8400).

most women are operated on between 20 and 35 yr of age, whereas a young age predilection is lacking in males. In female patients, the tumors are accompanied by mild or moderate hyperprolactinemia and often present at the microadenoma stage. In men, on the other hand, they are almost always macroadenomas, causing local mass effects rather than endocrine symptoms. The basis for hyperprolactinemia in female patients is likely oversecretion of PRL by nontumorous lactotrophs, but is not readily explained on the basis of stalk section effect. It is not surprising that a clinical diagnosis of prolactinoma is often made and results in patients being treated with dopamine agonists. Although these agents normalize blood PRL levels, tumor cell proliferation is not suppressed, and the lesion continues to grow relentlessly.

Histologically, subtype 3 silent adenomas consist of chromophobic, slightly acidophilic cells, often large, irregular, and containing sparse, small, PAS-positive cytoplasmic granules. The overall pattern of growth is typically diffuse. Cellular and nuclear pleomorphism may be considerable, but the MIB-1-labeling index is low. Attention to immunocytochemistry alone may lead to misleading conclusions. Some tumors show few or no cells immunopositive for known adenohypophysial hormones, whereas in others, the presence of several hormones can be demonstrated. In contrast to rather weak, focal, or negative immunostaining, ultrastructural investigation reveals a highly differentiated and functionally active-appearing adenoma (Figure 65 and 66). Its cells resemble mainly active glycoprotein hormone-producing cells, which are large, elongated, or irregular in configuration and possessing a large, somewhat pleomorphic nucleus often containing conspicuous, multiple spheridia (Figure 65). Cytoplasm is abundant and filled with well-developed RER, varying quantities of smooth endoplasmic reticulum (Figure 66), an elaborate, prominent, and often tortuous Golgi complex, and fair numbers of mitochondria forming clusters and often displaced by proliferating endoplasmic reticulum. Secretory granules are sparse, predominantly spherical, and measure 150–250 nm. In some examples, a conspicuous finding is the interdigitation of adjacent cell membranes. Adenomas with less conspicuous differentiation consist of cells containing less in the way of membranous organelles and resembling those of thyrotroph adenomas. The cytogenesis of subtype 3 silent adenoma is unknown. More studies are required to clarify their cellular derivation, endocrine function, as well as the discrepancy between their clinical presentation and immunocytochemical/ultrastructural features.

NEURONAL METAPLASIA IN PITUITARY ADENOMAS

Ganglion cell-containing lesions of the sellar region include a pathogenetic spectrum varying from presumably developmental or dysplastic processes to glioneuronal neoplasms. Their characterization is not always possible, since (1) architectural variation

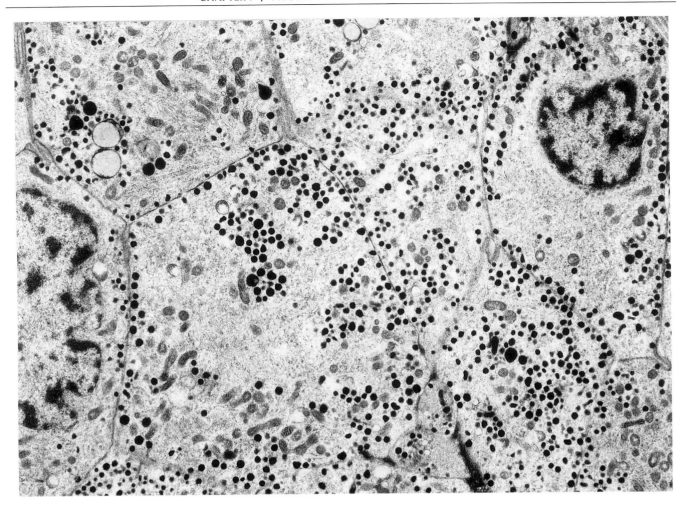

Figure 7-64   Silent "corticotroph" adenoma subtype 2. The morphology of secretory granules resembles that of corticotroph granules, but are much smaller (×8700).

is broad and confounds a clear distinction of malformation and neoplasm, and (2) no sharp line divides tumors composed entirely of ganglion cells (gangliocytoma) from similar lesions with a glial element (ganglioglioma). Herein we focus on ganglion cells occurring in pituitary adenomas, usually but not exclusively *(140,186,187)* those that are GH-producing *(131,188,189–191)*. Recent evidence, however, suggests that they are not developmental lesions, i.e., neuronal choristomas that by production of hypothalamic-releasing hormones induce adenoma formation *(188,189)*, but rather the result of metaplasia of adenoma cells *(131)*. Supporting this interpretation are morphologic studies demonstrating cells with transitional immunocytologic evidence of pituitary hormone production by ganglion cells and lack of an accompanying precursor lesion (pituitary hyperplasia) features *(131,140)*. The recent demonstration of hypothalamic hormones in pituitary adenomas *(192,193)* also promotes this concept.

Morphologically, ganglion cells may be few or numerous, and are accompanied by variable amounts of neuropil (Figure 67). In most instances, adenoma cells lie clustered among neurons. Transitional cells feature relative abundance of cytoplasm and vesicular nuclei with an often sizable central macronucleolus. As in other ganglion cell lesions, binucleation may be observed. Fully developed neurons exhibit variable quantities of Nissl substance and

processes. In addition to the immunophenotype of the adenoma cells, neurons feature not only class III β tubulin and occasionally neurofilament protein, but also epithelial markers, such as cytokeratin *(140)*. Nerve growth factor receptor has also been demonstrated in both components *(140)*. Ultrastructural studies have clearly documented the morphologic transition of adenoma to ganglion cells. With rare exception, such as one pituitary carcinoma in which the primary tumor was neuron-containing *(140)*, adenohypophysial tumors with neuronal metaplasia are benign and behave like ordinary adenomas. This also held true in one rare case wherein the neuronal element appeared to be immature *(190)*.

PITUITARY APOPLEXY   Hemorrhagic infarction of pituitary adenomas is relatively uncommon. When massive, it represents a surgical emergency. Apoplexy most often affects large, nonfunctional adenomas, but small, endocrinologically active tumors are not spared *(194–198)*. On occasion, the process destroys an entire adenoma and results in resolution of endocrine symptoms. In rare instances, apoplexy is precipitated by stimulatory endocrine testing *(199–201)*. Although large series have found clinically apparent apoplexy to occur in only about 1–2% of all adenomas *(195,197)*, organized hemorrhage, necrosis, or cystic change indicative of prior tissue injury is microscopically apparent in up

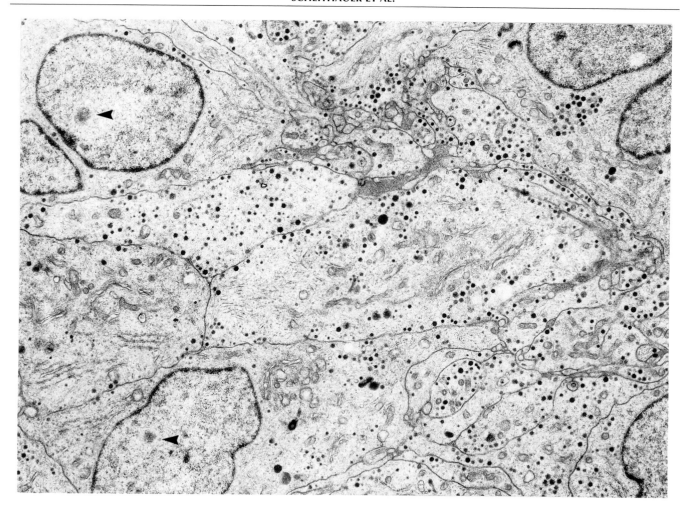

Figure 7-65 Silent adenoma subtype 3. The cellular polarity and uneven distribution of secretory granules are similar to those seen in glycoprotein hormone-producing adenomas. Note prominent nuclear spheridia (arrowheads) (× 6950).

to 10% *(195)*. These effects of apoplexy are typically widespread within adenoma tissue and may affect an entire specimen. In acute apoplexy, the basic architecture of the infarcted adenoma and its stroma is best demonstrated on reticulin stain (Figure 68). Laminar thrombus with polymorphonuclear leukocytes is also a common feature. Only in a minority of cases is viable adenoma or adjacent normal pituitary tissue sampled. These may show capillary reaction or even granulation tissue formation, depending on the stage at which the process is sampled.

AGGRESSIVE ADENOHYPOPHYSIAL TUMORS For a detailed discussion of invasive adenomas *(118)* and metastasizing adenohypophysial tumors ("pituitary carcinoma"), the reader is referred to Chapter 22, as well as to select recent references on the subject *(162,202)*.

TREATMENT EFFECTS ON ADENOMAS

Pituitary adenomas are common lesions causing a wide range of endocrine and local symptoms. Although most are slow-growing, some reach considerable size and affect quality of life. Clinical effects may be owing to endocrine hyper- or hypofunction or to mass effects on or invasion of sellar region structures. Any one of these, if not treated, may result in demise of the patient.

Although considerable effort has been invested in the development of treatment modalities, the relative benefits of medical therapies vs surgery remain controversial. Treatment has three basic objectives:

1. Normalization of hormone levels associated with functional tumors.
2. Elimination or diminution of mass effects.
3. Hormone replacement in patients having developed hypopituitarism.

Herein, we deal only with the first two objectives; restoration of endocrine equilibrium is not in the domain of pathology. Three forms of treatment are available, including surgery, radiation therapy, and medical treatment. The way in which these modalities relate to pathology is the subject of our discussion.

SURGERY Resection of tumor is the first option in patients with Cushing's disease as well as with endocrinologically nonfunctioning tumors, such as null-cell and gonadotroph adenomas. Somatotroph, lactotroph, and thyrotroph adenomas are also frequently treated by surgery *(203)*, especially in instances wherein medical therapy fails. The aim of surgery is selective adenomectomy, most often by the transsphenoidal approach. The objective is gross total tumor removal while leaving sufficient

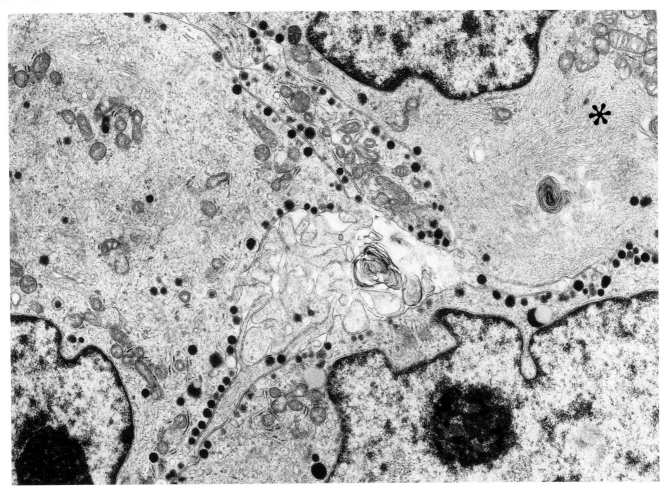

Figure 7-66 Silent adenoma subtype 3. In addition to nuclear irregularity and nucleolar prominence, note abundance of smooth endoplasmic reticulum (asterisk) (×12,600).

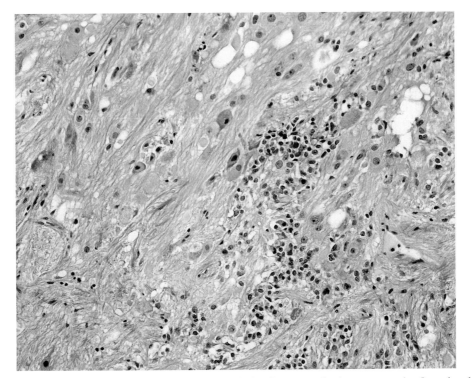

Figure 7-67 Pituitary adenoma with neuronal metaplasia. The small, dark cells are neoplastic somatotrophs. Occasional neurons showed GH immunoreactivity. The patient was acromegalic. H&E × 400 (courtesy Nancy Karpinski, San Diego, CA).

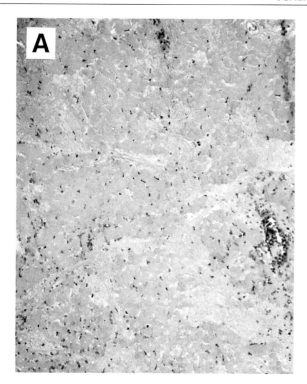
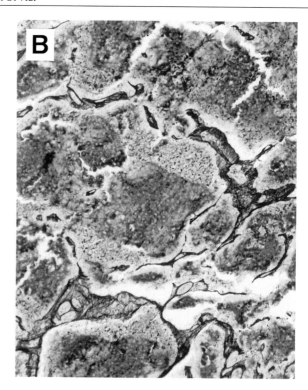

Figure 7-68   Pituitary apoplexy. Note lack of diagnostic features on H&E **(A)**, but the presence of an adenoma-like pattern on reticulin stain **(B)**. (A and B) × 160.

adenohypophysial tissue to avoid hypopituitarism. Postoperative macrophage influx with removal of blood is followed by formation of granulation tissue and finally of a fibrous scar. When tumor persists, its further growth is often intimately associated with this fibrous tissue. Clinically evident recurrence often necessitates repeat surgery. Resected adenomas are morphologically analyzed for the purpose of functional subclassification and prognostication.

RADIATION THERAPY   Irradiation is only occasionally the first form of treatment. If surgery is contraindicated, medical therapy fails, or the tumor is large or invasive, radiotherapy should be considered. Although in most cases sellar irradiation is unnecessary, it is often indicated when an invasive adenoma is subtotally removed, when endocrine and/or local symptoms persist, or in instances of tumor recurrence. It is of note that adenoma cells are not particularly radiosensitive. Relatively large doses must be administered to relieve endocrine and/or local symptoms or to achieve tumor shrinkage or destruction. Therapeutic side effects include:

1. Radiation injury of surrounding tissues *(204–206)*.
2. Partial or total hypopituitarism, which may be mild, moderate, or severe in degree and permanent.
3. Typically after an interval of years, the development of postirradiation neoplasms, usually fibro- or osteosarcomas.

The incidence of gliomas is also increased after radiotherapy of the sellar region *(207)*.

With regard to the pituitary, pathologic alterations following irradiation are not dramatic. A varying degree of fibrosis is the most conspicuous finding, as is vascular injury and degeneration of pituitary cells. Regardless of which of the radiation modalities

is employed, their morphologic effects are similar. Those of a new therapeutic method, Gamma Knife "surgery," remain to be fully documented *(208–210)*.

MEDICAL THERAPY   The most controversial of medical therapies to come into use was developed only a few decades ago. Two main types of drugs are the basis of this discussion, dopamine agonists and somatostatin analogs. Attempts to introduce several other agents have been far less encouraging and are not dealt with herein.

Dopamine Agonists   It is of note that dopamine (D_2) receptors mediate the effects of dopamine agonists and are present not only on the surface of PRL cells, but also on various other adenoma cells. Thus, although it was logical to attempt dopamine agonist medication in the treatment of other adenomas, results were not encouraging *(211)*. Currently, few centers use dopamine agonists in the treatment of patients with other than lactotrophic adenomas. The various agents under consideration have been found to be effective in the treatment of approx 90% of PRL cell adenomas *(212)*.

A large number of dopamine agonists and related compounds are commercially available. In that all have similar clinical, endocrinologic, and morphologic effects, they will be jointly discussed herein. These agents significantly reduce tumor size, restore menstrual function and fertility, stem galactorrhea, increase libido, and eliminate impotence *(213)*. Unfortunately, the effects of dopamine agonists are reversible; on discontinuance of treatment, tumors regrow and clinical as well as endocrine symptoms reappear. Although "complete cure" has been reported, it is very rare and may have its basis in pituitary apoplexy, which has been observed in patients undergoing dopamine agonist therapy. Finally, occasional tumors are or become bromocryptine-resistant *(214)*.

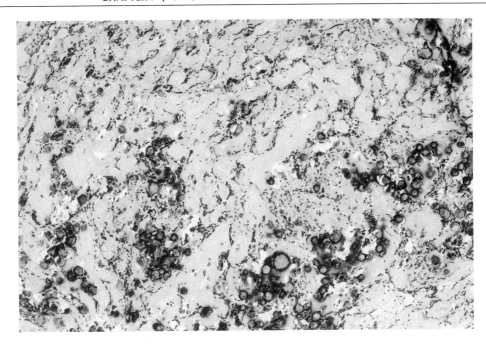

Figure 7-69   Dopamine agonist effect on a lactotroph adenoma. Note the "small-cell" appearance of the tumor as well as stromal fibrosis. H&E × 160.

Morphologic alterations related to dopamine agonist treatment are consistently seen and can be spectacular *(34,35,215)*. Compared to lactotroph adenomas of untreated patients, they include marked tumor cell shrinkage. Morphometry has documented the change, which is owing chiefly to loss of cytoplasmic volume. In that cytoplasm shrinks more markedly than does the nucleus, the nuclear:cytoplasmic ratio is increased and may produce an appearance of a "small-cell tumor" (Figure 69). Reduction in volume densities of RER and Golgi complexes is dramatic. Mitochondrial and lysosomal volume densities are unaltered. Although secretory granule diameters remain unchanged, granule volume densities are slightly increased. In patients undergoing longer-term treatment, tumors often show extensive perivascular and interstitial fibrosis. Individual cell necrosis may be seen, but apoptosis as assessed by light and electron microscopy is not a conspicuous feature. In view of this "cellular shutdown," it is intriguing that granule exocytoses are still evident (Figure 70). Immunocytochemistry generally demonstrates cytoplasmic PRL reactivity, but in some cases, especially in cases wherein diminution of blood PRL levels is dramatic, massive tumor involution may be seen, immunoreactivity being decreased or focally lacking. *In situ* hybridization shows a marked decrease in estrogen receptor mRNA and an increase in D_2 receptor mRNA *(216)*. In some cases, microhemorrhage or even sizable foci of hemorrhage are noted.

We have investigated the light microscopic, immunocytochemical, and ultrastructural features of other adenoma types, such as somatotroph and null-cell adenomas subject to dopamine agonist therapy. These showed no recognizable differences when compared to untreated tumors of similar type. Although, as previously noted, pituitary adenomas other than lactotroph tumors also possess D_2 receptors, they appear to show no therapeutic response. This is in accordance with clinical and neuroimaging studies that have shown no reduction in tumor size in patients with treated somatotroph adenomas *(211)*.

The effect of dopamine agonists on lactotroph adenomas is reversible. Although in some instances tumor shrinkage is permanent and the adenoma does not regrow, discontinuance of treatment is typically followed by a rise in blood PRL levels, tumor regrowth, and the reappearance of clinical and endocrine symptoms. The morphology of once, but no longer, treated adenoma cells is indistinguishable from that of tumors never exposed to dopamine agonists. Conclusively, immunopositive for PRL, the adenoma cells are large and contain:

1. Conspicuous RER as well as Golgi complexes.
2. Many free ribosomes and polysomes.
3. Few randomly distributed spherical, oval, or irregular-shaped secretory granules, some undergoing granule extrusions.

Furthermore, *in situ* hybridization also reveals PRL mRNA, estrogen receptor mRNA, and D_2 receptor mRNA at levels comparable to those of adenoma cells never exposed to dopamine agonists. In tumors that were treated long-term, the fibrotic response remains an obvious indicator of previous therapy.

Some lactotroph adenomas appear to display a variable response to dopamine agonist treatment. Histologically, this is expressed by alternating small-cell and large-cell areas also differing in PRL immunoreactivity receptor status *(35)*. An alternate explanation for this finding may be that groups of suppressed cells in treated lactotroph adenomas do not revert to their original state following cessation of dopamine agonist administration, thus resulting in a patchwork of large- and small-cell areas *(217)*.

Somatostatin Analogs   Another drug effectively used in the treatment of certain pituitary adenomas is octreotide, a long-acting somatostatin analog. Somatostatin, a hypothalamic hormone known to inhibit GH secretion, appears to be an obvious choice for the treatment of somatotroph adenomas. However, its short half-life in the circulation excluded its therapeutic use. On the other

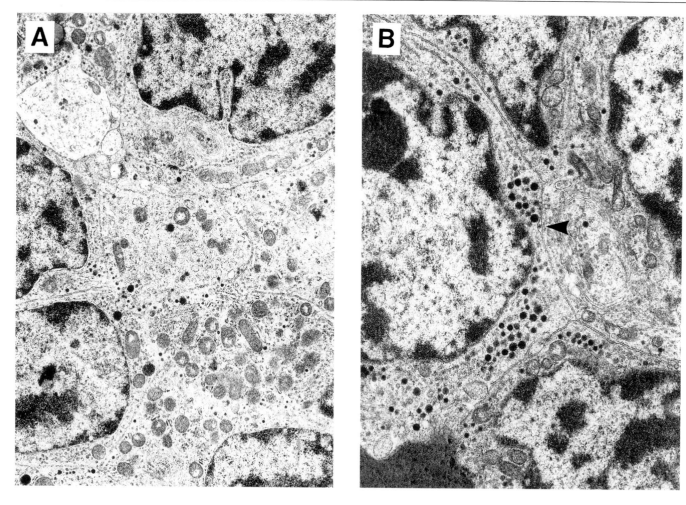

Figure 7-70   Sparsely granulated PRL cell adenoma showing effects of dopamine agonist (bromocriptine) treatment, including heterochromatic nucleus, and marked involution of RER as well as Golgi membranes resulting in shrinkage of adenoma cells **(A)**. Note storage of granules and their occasional exocytosis **(B)**. (A) × 9000; (B) × 13,650.

hand, the somatostatin analog octreotide has a half-life of approx 12 h, thus permitting its use in the treatment of patients with acromegaly or gigantism. Somatostatin receptors are not limited to somatotrophs or even adenohypophysial cells. Indeed, they are present on the cell surfaces of many endocrine and nonendocrine tumors. Octreotide is, therefore, widely used in the treatment of endocrine neoplasms. Among pituitary adenomas, GH- and TSH-producing tumors respond favorably to treatment *(218–220)*. Somatostatin analogs are of no efficacy in other adenoma types, despite the presence of receptors.

In acromegalic patients, octreotide therapy ameliorates signs and symptoms of disease, causing almost immediate cessation of headache, a decrease in blood GH and TSH levels, and slows or reverses the physical signs of acromegaly *(221,222)*. Interestingly, despite intensive octreotide treatment, no significant tumor shrinkage is seen in most cases. Slight to moderate tumor involution occurs in only a minority *(223)*.

The clinical and morphologic effects of octreotide have been well studied *(224–226)*. Many adenomas of octreotide-treated patients are morphologically indistinguishable from those of untreated patients. Where alterations are evident, the cells typically contain more numerous and larger secretory granules. In some instances, many large lysosomes containing secretory granules are apparent, a process termed "crinophagy" (Figure 71). No vascular changes are evident, such as platelet accumulation, endothelial damage, thrombosis, or capillary occlusion. Neither tumor cell necrosis nor apoptosis is seen. Amyloid deposition may be noted, but can be seen in untreated tumors as well. Only occasionally do tumor cells appear smaller, but this change is inconspicuous. The most consistent, although rarely prominent finding is mild to moderate perivascular and interstitial fibrosis. Cell shrinkage and fibrosis are certainly much less conspicuous than in dopamine agonist-treated lactotroph adenomas. GH and TSH immunoreactivity remains unchanged despite intensive treatment. GH gene expression also remains unaltered. At present, no data are available regarding the reversibility of these morphologic changes. In any event, since treatment effects are not striking and do not occur in every case, the issue of their reversibility would be difficult to address.

Medical treatment of pituitary adenomas obviously has great future potential. The above-noted systematic studies of the effects of dopamine agonists and somatostatin analogs have provided valuable experience and have set the stage for the evaluation of new agents that will no doubt be discovered.

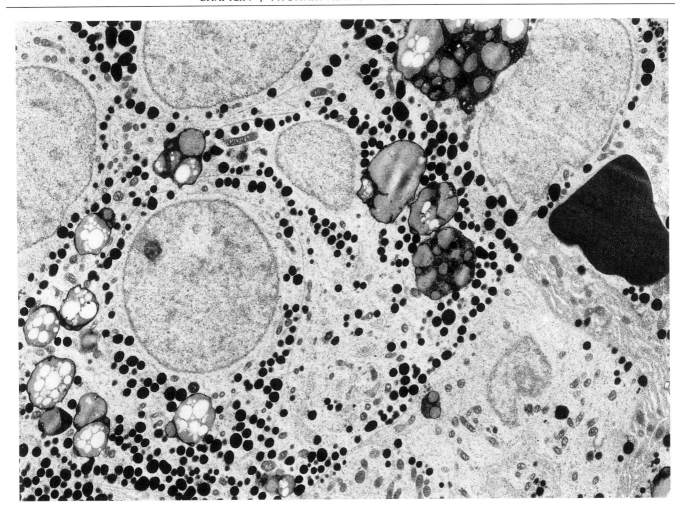

Figure 7-71 Somatostatin analog effect on a lactotroph adenoma. Note relatively scant organelles and the presence of prominent lysosomes suggesting ongoing crinophagy (×6500).

PITUITARY HYPERPLASIA

All known adenohypophysial cell types may undergo hyperplasia. Depending on circumstances, pituitary hyperplasia may be physiologic as in pregnancy, compensatory as in hypothyroidism, or pathologic. The latter is rare, but may result in clinically manifest disease *(128,227,228)*. From the diagnostic viewpoint, pituitary hyperplasia represents a major problem, since it is unsuspected on clinical or radiographic grounds and may be difficult, if not impossible to diagnose or to distinguish from adenoma (*see* Figure 74) in fragmented surgical specimens *(128,227,228)*. Histologically, it can be nodular or diffuse. Of the two patterns, nodular hyperplasia is most readily evident in microsections. Confirmation of diffuse hyperplasia requires laborious cell counting, preferably in large tissue fragments or in the intact pituitary. It is of note that the distinction of hyperplasia from adenoma is made on histochemical and immunostains (*see* Figure 74), not at the ultrastructural level (Figure 72).

SOMATOTROPH HYPERPLASIA This is rare and occurs primarily in pituitaries of patients with growth hormone-releasing hormone (GHRH)-secreting extracranial tumors, such as endocrine neoplasms of the pancreas, pheochromocytomas, and various carcinoid tumors *(124,229,230)*. It has also been reported in patients with the McCune-Albright syndrome *(231)* and in occasional cases of gigantism with onset in childhood *(232,233)*. Somatotroph hyperplasia is most often diffuse, but may rarely be nodular, expansion of the acinar pattern being evident on reticulin stains. The hyperplastic cells are principally acidophils immunoreactive for GH. Ultrastructure demonstrates stimulated, actively secreting somatotrophs (Figure 72). Adenoma formation may rarely supervene on the hyperplasia accompanying ectopic GHRH production *(234)*.

LACTOTROPH HYPERPLASIA This is a normal, well-characterized feature of pregnancy and lactation *(83)*, and is obviously much more common than somatotroph hyperplasia. The pituitaries of pregnant women are often enlarged two-fold and contain a vastly increased number of chromophobic lactotrophs exhibiting PRL immunostaining and ultrastructural evidence of high endocrine activity. Such "pregnancy cells" are formed partly by multiplication of pre-existing lactotrophs and partly by recruitment of somatotrophs, which have the capacity to transform to lactotrophs *(83,235)*. Lactotroph hyperplasia is rarely seen in the nontumorous adenohypophysis of patients harboring a PRL-producing pituitary adenoma. Although not a consistent finding, it is more commonly seen in association with long-standing primary hypothyroidism and in Cushing's disease *(33,128,236,237)*. Lactotroph hyperplasia is also a common finding in patients treated with estrogens for a protracted period of time *(238)* (Figure 73). Proliferation of lactotrophs

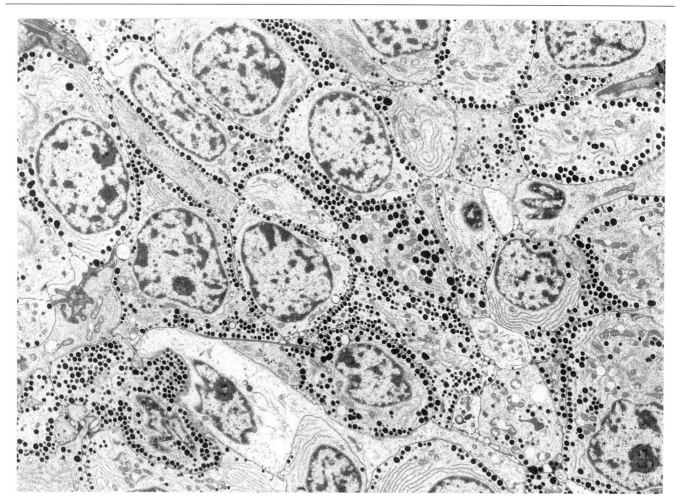

Figure 7-72   Somatotroph hyperplasia, as in this example in association with gigantism, cannot be distinguished from adenoma at the ultrastructural level. An occasional cell in this GH- and PRL-producing lesion contains large granules typical of mammosomatotroph cells (×4500).

may also occur when the synthesis or release of hypothalamic dopamine, the main PRL-inhibiting factor (PIF), is defective or when its downward flow to the adenohypophysis is disrupted. The latter mechanism is thought to underlie "stalk section effect."

Gestational lactotroph hyperplasia is diffuse and massive. The process is reversible, regressing after delivery, but persisting if lactation is elected. Postpartum or postlactational regression is often incomplete. As a result, pituitary weights are usually higher in multiparous women than in nulliparas. In contrast to gestational lactotroph hyperplasia, that caused by various pathologic processes in the sella region is often multifocal or nodular. Idiopathic lactotroph hyperplasia is extremely rare *(239)*.

The occurrence of neoplastic transformation of hyperplastic lactotrophs has not been proven. Of interest, however, is the case of a male-to-female transsexual who after prolonged and excessive estrogen treatment developed hyperprolactinemia and was found to have a PRL-secreting pituitary adenoma *(240)*. It is uncertain whether the adenoma was causally related to estrogen treatment or a coincidental lesion. Finally, one retrospective study of estrogen effect on the human pituitary documented hyperplasia, but found no statistically significant increase in PRL cell adenomas *(238)*.

CORTICOTROPH HYPERPLASIA   This is known to occur in patients with corticotropin-releasing hormone (CRH) secreting

extracranial tumors *(241,242)*, in long-standing untreated Addison's disease *(243)*, as well as in some patients with pituitary-dependent Cushing's disease *(146,244,245)*. In the latter condition, hyperplasia may occur alone or in association with a corticotroph adenoma. It is of note that in an estimated 10–15% of patients with pituitary-dependent Cushing's disease, no adenoma is detected despite a careful search. In some of these, striking corticotroph hyperplasia may be seen and is likely responsible for the Cushing's disease. Corticotroph hyperplasia may be focal, nodular, or diffuse. In some cases, the hyperplastic corticotrophs show the presence of Crooke's hyaline change, whereas in others, none is evident. No doubt, transition of nodular hyperplasia to adenoma may occur *(246)*, but the morphologic distinction between nodular hyperplasia and microadenoma is not possible in all instances.

THYROTROPH HYPERPLASIA   This is known to develop in patients with long-standing, untreated primary hypothyroidism *(128,236,247)*. Such patients often have hyperprolactinemia and galactorrhea, their pituitaries being enlarged and simulating lactotroph adenoma. Thus, thyrotroph hyperplasia may not be recognized. Instead, an erroneous diagnosis of prolactinoma is often made. The clinical recognition of thyrotroph hyperplasia is of practical importance, since failure to make the diagnosis may result in unnecessary surgery. Thyrotroph hyperplasia is a poten-

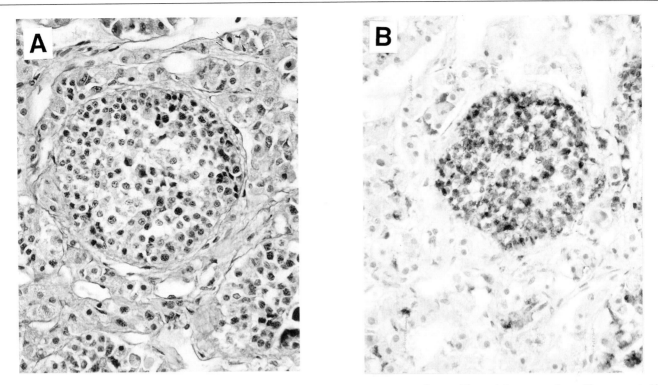

Figure 7-73 Lactotroph hyperplasia in chronic estrogen administration for prostate carcinoma. The nodular pattern is readily apparent. **(A)** H&E × 400; **(B)** PRL immunostain × 400.

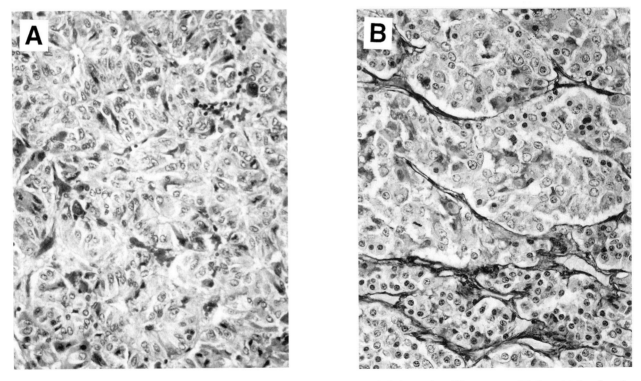

Figure 7-74 Pituitary hyperplasia, such as this example of thyrotroph hyperplasia in hyperthyroidism, can readily be mistaken for adenoma **(A)**. Its nodular architecture is best seen on reticulin stain, which unlike that of normal gland (*see* Figure 1), shows acinar expansion **(B)**. (A) H&E × 400; (B) reticulin × 400.

tially reversible process that often regresses on replacement doses of thyroid hormone. It is clearly owing to excessive TRH secretion resulting from absence of negative feedback effects of thyroid hormones. Although the process is readily mistaken for adenoma on H&E stain, its nodular, and thus nonneoplastic nature is readily evident in reticulin preparations (Figure 74). Proliferating thyrotrophs are large and feature an eccentric nucleus as well as abundant, vacuolated cytoplasm containing several large, PAS-positive globules (lysosomes). Such so-called thyroidectomy or thyroid deficiency cells are readily recognized, and their presence facilitates the diagnosis (81,128). Ultrastructurally, these cells feature abundant cytoplasm, prominence of dilated profiles of RER, conspicuous Golgi complexes, several large lysosomes, and sparse, small secretory granules. Occasionally, thyrotroph adenomas occurring in patients with long-standing hypothyroidism are associated with thyrotroph hyperplasia.

GONADOTROPH HYPERPLASIA This is said to occur in patients with long-standing primary hypogonadism, particularly when loss of gonadal steroid production begins at a young age. For example, gonadotroph hyperplasia may be seen at autopsy in cases of life-long hypogonadism, such as Klinefelter's syndrome. An intriguing, but unresolved question is why gonadotroph hyperplasia is not apparent in old age, a time when the negative feedback effect of gonadal hormones is lacking. Thus, although the regular occurrence of gonadotroph adenomas in the elderly and their development in rare patients with long-standing hypogonadism suggest a tumorigenic role of target organ deficiency, a causal relationship has not conclusively been proven.

There are several reasons why it is often difficult to make the diagnosis of hyperplasia. In the normal pituitary, the various adenohypophysial cell types are unevenly distributed, and if the surgical specimen consists only of small fragments, whose precise location within the pituitary is unknown, the diagnosis of hyperplasia remains uncertain. Furthermore, hyperplasia can be focal and may not have been included in the specimen. Finally, surgically removed tissue is subject to technical artifacts, such as mechanical compression, cautery, and frozen section effects, all of which interfere with critical histologic assessment. The infrequency with which pituitary hyperplasia comes to surgical attention, as well as lack of experience on the part of all but a few pathologists, further complicates the problem of diagnosis.

REFERENCES

1. Kovacs K, Scheithauer BW, Horvath E, Lloyd RV. The World Health Organization classification of adenohypophysial neoplasms. A proposed five-tier scheme. Cancer 1996;78:502–510.
2. Kovacs K, Scheithauer BW, Horvath E, Lloyd RV. The adenohypophysis. In: Solcia E, Klöppel G, Sobin LH, eds. The World Health Organization Classification of Endocrine Tumours, 2nd ed. Springer-Verlag, Berlin, 1999, pp. 15–28, 75–90.
3. Kovacs K, Horvath E. Tumors of the pituitary gland. Atlas of tumor pathology, 2nd Ser. Fasc. 21. Armed Forces Institute of Pathology, Washington, DC, 1986, pp. 1–264.
4. Sheenhan DC, Hropchak BB. Theory and Practice of Histochemistry. CV Mosby, St. Louis, 1980, pp. 276–279.
4a. Smith DM Jr, Haggitt RC. A comparative study of generic stains for carcinoid secretory granules. Am J Surg Pathol 1983;7:61–68.
5. Pearse AGE. The APUD concept and its implications in pathology. Pathol Annu 1974;9:27–41.
6. Thapar K, Yamada Y, Scheithauer B, Kovacs K, Yamada S, Stefaneanu L. Assessment of mitotic activity in pituitary adenomas and carcinomas. Endocr Pathol 1996;7:215–221.
7. Thapar K, Kovacs K, Scheithauer BW, Stefaneanu L, Horvath E, Pernicone PJ, et al. Proliferative activity and invasiveness among pituitary adenomas and carcinomas: an analysis using the MIB-1 antibody. Neurosurgery 1996;38:99–106.
8. Hsu DW, Hakim F, Biller BMK, de la Monte S, Zervas NT, Klibanski A, et al. Significance of proliferating cell nuclear antigen index in predicting pituitary adenoma recurrence. J Neurosurg 1993;78:753–761.
9. Buckley N, Bates AS, Broome JC, Strange RC, Perrett CW, Burke CW, et al. p53 protein accumulates in Cushing's adenomas and invasive non-functional adenomas. J Clin Endocrinol Metab 1994;79:1513–1516.
10. Thapar K, Scheithauer BW, Kovacs K, Pernicone PJ, Laws ER Jr. p53 expression in pituitary adenomas and carcinomas: correlation with invasiveness and tumor growth fractions. Neurosurgery 1996;38:763–771.
11. Coons AH, Creech HJ, Jones RN. Immunological properties of an antibody containing a fluorescent group. Proc Soc Exp Biol Med 1941;47:200–202.
12. Sternberger LA, Hardy PH Jr., Cuculis JJ, Meyer HG. The unlabeled antibody enzyme method to immunohistochemistry: preparation and properties of soluble antigen-antibody complex (horseradish peroxidase-antihorseradish peroxidase) and its use in identification of spirochetes. J Histochem Cytochem 1970;18:315–333.
13. Taylor CR. Immunoperoxidase techniques. Practical and theoretical aspects. Arch Pathol Lab Med 1978;102:113–121.
14. Childs GV, Unabia G. Application of avidin-biotin-peroxidase complex (ABC) method to the light microscopic localization of pituitary hormones. J Histochem Cytochem 1982;30:713–716.
15. Gosselin EJ, Cate CC, Pettengill OS, Sorenson GD. Immunocytochemistry: its evolution and criteria for its application in the study of epon-embedded cells and tissues. Am J Anat 1986;175:135–160.
16. Sternberger L. Immunocytochemistry, 3rd ed. John Wiley, New York, 1986.
17. Nakane PK, Pierce GB Jr. Enzyme-labelled antibodies: preparation and application for localization of antigen. J Histochem Cytochem 1966;14:929–931.
18. Hsu SM, Raine L, Fanger H. A comparative study of the peroxidase-antiperoxidase method and avidin-biotin complex method for studying polypeptide hormones with radioimmunoassay antibodies. Am J Clin Pathol 1981;75:734–738.
19. Hsu SM, Raine L, Fanger H. Use of avidin-biotin-peroxidase complex (ABC) in immunoperoxidase techniques: a comparison between ABC and unlabeled antibody (PAP) procedures. J Histochem Cytochem 1981;29:577–580.
20. Taylor CR. Immunomicroscopy: A Diagnostic Tool for the Surgical Pathologist. WB Saunders, Philadelphia, 1986.
21. Mayers CP. Histological fixation by microwave heating. J Clin Pathol 1970;23:273–275.
22. Leong ASY, Dayman ME, Milos J. Microwave irradiation as a form of fixation for light and electron microscopy. J Pathol 1985;146:313–321.
23. Boon ME, Kok LP. Microwave Cookbook of Pathology. The Art of Microscopic Visualization, 2nd ed. Coubomb, Leyder, 1988.
24. Shi SR, Key ME, Kalra KL. Antigen retrieval in formalin-fixed paraffin-embedded tissues: an enhancement method for immunohistochemical staining based on microwave oven heating of tissue sections. J Histochem Cytochem 1991;39:741–748.
25. Leong ASY. Microwave technology for morphological analysis. Cell Vision 1994;1:278–288.
26. Bourinbaiar AS. Microwave irradiation-stimulated in situ hybridization procedure with biotinylated DNA probe. Eur J Morphol 1991;29:213–128.
27. Volkers HH, van den Brink WJ, Rook R, van den Berg FM. Microwave label detection technique for DNA in situ hybridization. Eur J Morphol 1991;29:59–62.
28. Allan GM, Smyth JA, Todd D, McNulty MS. In situ hybridization for the detection of chicken anemia virus in formalin-fixed paraffin-embedded section. Avian Dis 1993;37:177–182.
29. Evers P, Vylings HBM. Microwave-stimulated antigen retrieval is pH and temperature dependent. J Histochem Cytochem 1994;42:1555–1563.
30. Sperry A, Jin L, Lloyd RV. Microwave treatment enhances detection of RNA and DNA by in situ hybridization. Diagn Mol Pathol 1996;5:291–296.

31. Kovacs K, Horvath E. Pathology of growth-hormone-producing tumors of the human pituitary. Semin Diagn Pathol 1986;3:18–33.

32. Horvath E. Ultrastructural markers in the pathologic diagnosis of pituitary adenomas. Ultrastruct Pathol 1994;18:171–179.

33. Horvath E, Scheithauer BW, Kovacs K, Lloyd RV. Regional neuropathology: hypothalamus and pituitary. In: Graham DI, Lantos PL, eds. Greenfield's Neuropathology, 6th ed., Arnold, London, 1997, pp. 1007–1094.

34. Tindall GT, Kovacs K, Horvath E, Thorner MO. Human prolactin-producing adenomas and bromocriptine: a histological, immunocytochemical, ultrastructural and morphometric study. J Clin Endocrinol Metab 1982;55:1178–1183.

35. Kovacs K, Stefaneanu L, Horvath E, Lloyd RV, Lancranjan I, Buchfelder M, et al. Effect of dopamine agonist medication on prolactin producing pituitary adenomas. A morphologic study including immunocytochemistry, electron microscopy and in situ hybridization. Virchows Arch Pathol Anat 1991;418:439–446.

36. Tougard C, Picart R. Use of pre-embedding ultrastructural immunocytochemistry in the localization of a secretory product and membrane proteins in cultured prolactin cells. Am J Anat 1986; 175:161–177.

37. Frawley LS, Neill JD. A reverse hemolytic plaque assay for microscopic visualization of growth hormone release from individual cells: evidence for somatotrope heterogeneity. Neuroendocrinology 1984;39:484–487.

38. Childs GV, Burke JA. Use of the reverse hemolytic plaque assay to study the regulation of anterior lobe adrenocorticotropin (ACTH) secretion by ACTH-releasing factor, arginine vasopressin, angiotensin II and glucocorticoids. Endocrinology 1987;120:439–444.

39. Lloyd RV, Coleman K, Fields K, Nath V. Analysis of prolactin and growth hormone production in hyperplastic and neoplastic rat pituitary tissue by the hemolytic plaque assay. Cancer Res 1987;47:1087–1092.

40. Lloyd RV, Anagnostou D, Cano M, Barkan AL, Chandler WF. Analysis of mammosomatotropic cells in normal and neoplastic human pituitary tissue by the reverse hemolytic plaque assay and immunocytochemistry. J Clin Endocrinol Metab 1988;66: 1103–1110.

41. Kendall ME, Hymer WC. Measurement of hormone secretion from individual cells by cell blot assay. Methods Enzymol 1989; 168:327–338.

42. Vila-Porcile E, Picart R, Tougard C. Adaptation of the reverse hemolytic plaque assay to electron microscopy: a study of one individual secretory activity in prolactin cell subpopulations. J Histochem Cytochem 1994;42:11–22.

43. Alvaro V, Levy L, Dubray C, Roche A, Peillon F, Querat B, et al. Invasive human pituitary tumors express a point-mutated alpha-protein kinase-C. J Clin Endocrinol Metab 1993;77:1125–1129.

44. Thakkar RV, Pook MA, Wooding C, Boscaro M, Scanarini M, Clayton RN. Association of somatotrophinomas with loss of alleles on chromosome 11 and with gsp mutations. J Clin Invest 1993;91:2815–2821.

45. Lloyd RV, Jin L, Chandler WF, Horvath E, Stefaneanu L, Kovacs K. Pituitary specific transcription factor messenger ribonucleic acid expression in adenomatous and nontumorous human pituitary tissues. Lab Invest 1994;69:570–575.

46. Cowan JM. Fishing for chromosomes. The art and its applications. Diagn Mol Pathol 1996;3:224–226.

47. Kontogeorgos G, Kapranos N. Interphase analysis of chromosome 11 in human pituitary somatotroph adenomas by direct fluorescence in situ hybridization. Endocr Pathol 1996;7:203–206.

48. Templeton NS. The polymerase chain reaction. History, methods, and applications. Diagn Mol Pathol 1992;1:58–72.

49. Asa SL, Kovacs K, Stefaneanu L, Horvath E, Billestrup N, Gonzalez-Manchon C, et al. Pituitary adenomas in mice transgenic for growth hormone-releasing hormone. Endocrinology 1992; 131:2083–2089.

50. Stefaneanu L, Kovacs K. Transgenic models of pituitary disease. Microsc Res Tech 1997;39:194–204.

51. Harvey M, Vogel H, Eva YH, Lee P, Bradley A, Donehower LA. Mice deficient in both p53 and Rb develop tumors primarily of endocrine origin. Cancer Res 1995;55:1146–1151.

52. Lloyd RV, Wilson BS, Kovacs K, Ryan N. Immunohistochemical localization of chromogranin in human hypophyses and pituitary adenomas. Arch Pathol Lab Med 1985;109:515–517.

53. Lloyd RV, Cano M, Rosa P, Hille A, Huttner WB. Distribution of chromogranin A and secretogranin I (chromogranin B) in neuroendocrine cells and tumors. Am J Pathol 1988;130:296–304.

54. Jin L, Hemperly JJ, Lloyd RV. Expression of neural cell adhesion molecule (N-CAM) in normal and neoplastic human neuroendocrine tissues. Am J Pathol 1991;138:961–969.

55. Stefaneanu L, Ryan N, Kovacs K. Immunocytochemical localization of synaptophysin in human hypophyses and pituitary adenomas. Arch Pathol Lab Med 1988;112:801–804.

56. Asa SL, Ryan N, Kovacs K, Singer W, Marangos PJ. Immunohistochemical localization of neuron-specific enolase in the human hypophysis and pituitary adenomas. Arch Pathol Lab Med 1984;108:40–43.

57. Lloyd RV, Jin L, Qian X, Scheithauer BW, Young WF Sr., Daus DH. Analysis of the chromogranin. A post-translational cleavage product pancreastatin and the prohormone convertase PC2 and PC3 in hormonal and neoplastic human pituitaries. Am J Pathol 1995;146:1188–1199.

58. Marin F, Kovacs K, Stefaneanu L, Horvath E, Cheng Z. S-100 protein immunopositivity in human nontumorous hypophyses and pituitary adenomas. Endocr Pathol 1992;3:28–38.

59. Vrontakis ME, Sano T, Kovacs K, Friesen HG. Presence of galanin-like immunoreactivity in non-tumorous corticotrophs and corticotroph adenomas of the human pituitary. J Clin Endocrinol Metab 1987;66:804–810.

60. Ironside JW, Royds JA, Jefferson AA, Timperley WR. Immunolocalization of cytokeratins in the normal and neoplastic human pituitary gland. J Neurol Neurosurg Psychiatry 1987;50:57–65.

61. Rehfeld JF, Lindholm J, Andersen BN, Bardram L, Canter P, Fenger M, et al. Pituitary tumors containing cholecystokinin. N Engl J Med 1987;316:1244–1247.

62. Mizuno K, Ojima M, Hashimoto S, Watari H, Tani M, Satoh M, et al. Multiple forms of immunoreactive renin in human pituitary tissue. Life Sci 1985;37:2297–2304.

63. Saint-Andre JP, Rohmer V, Alhenc-Gelas F, Menard J, Bigorgne J-C, Corvol P. Presence of renin, angiotensinogen and converting enzyme in human pituitary lactotroph cells and prolactin adenomas. J Clin Endocrinol Metab 1986;63:231–237.

64. Deftos LJ. Pituitary cells secrete calcitonin in the reverse hemolytic plaque assay. Biochem Biophys Res Commun 1987;146: 1350–1356.

65. Roth KA, Krause JE. Substance-P is present in a subset of thyrotrophs in the human pituitary. J Clin Endocrinol Metab 1990;71:1089–1095.

66. Hsu DW, Riskind PN, Hedley-Whyte TE. Vasoactive intestinal peptide in the human pituitary gland and adenomas. An immunocytochemical study. Am J Pathol 1989;135:329–338.

67. Le Dafniet M, Grouselle D, Li JY, Kujas M, Bression D, Barret A, et al. Evidence of thyrotropin-releasing hormone (TRH) and TRH-binding sites in human nonsecreting pituitary adenomas. J Clin Endocrinol Metab 1987;65:1014–1019.

68. Rauch C, Li JY, Croissandeau G, Berthet M, Peillon F, Pages P. Characterization and localization of an immunoreactive growth hormone-releasing hormone precursor form in normal and tumoral human anterior pituitaries. Endocrinology 1995;136:2594–2601.

69. Miller GM, Alexander JM, Klibanoki A. Gonadotropin-releasing hormone messenger RNA expression in gonadotroph tumors and normal human pituitary. J Clin Endocrinol Metab 1996;81:80–83.

70. Odell WD, Griffin J, Bashey HM, Snyder PJ. Secretion of chorionic gonadotropin by cultured human pituitary cells. J Clin Endocrinol Metab 1990;71:1318–1321.

71. Johnson MD, Gray ME, Pepinsky RB, Stahlman MT. Lipocortin-1 immunoreactivity in the human pituitary gland. J Histochem Cytochem 1990;38:1841–1845.

72. Kovacs K, Ryan N, Stefaneanu L. Identification of corticotrophs in the human pituitary with mAB lu-5, a novel immunocytochemical marker. Pathol Res Pract 1987;182:775–779.

73. Silverlight JJ, Prysor-Jones RA, Jenkins JS. Basic fibroblast growth factor in human pituitary tumours. Clin Endocrinol 1990;32:669–676.

74. Kobrin MS, Asa SL, Samsoondar J, Kudlow JE. α-transforming growth factor in the bovine anterior pituitary gland: secretion by dispersed cells and immunohistochemical localization. Endocrinology 1987;121:1412–1416.

75. Jin L, Qian X, Kulig E, Sanno N, Scheithauer BW, Kovacs K, et al. Transforming growth factor-β, transforming growth factor beta receptor II and p27^{Kip1} expression in nontumorous and neoplastic human pituitaries. Am J Pathol 1997;151:509–519.

76. Ferrara N, Henzel WJ. Pituitary follicular cells secrete a novel heparin-binding growth factor specific for vascular endothelial cells. Biochem Biophys Res Commun 1989;161:851–858.

77. Alberti VN, Takita LC, de Mesquita MI, Percario S, Maciel RM. Immunohistochemical demonstration of insulin-like growth factor I (IGF-I) in normal and pathological human pituitary gland. Pathol Res Pract 1991;187:541–542.

78. Budd GC, Pansky B, Budd NJ. Insulin or insulin-like peptides in the human pituitary. Ann Clin Lab Sci 1987;17:111–115.

79. Scheithauer BW, Kovacs K, Horvath E. The adenohypophysis. In: Lechago J, Gould VE, eds. Bloodworth's Endocrine Pathology, 3rd ed. 1997, Williams and Wilkins, Baltimore, MD, pp. 85–152.

80. Horvath E, Kovacs K. The adenohypophysis. In: Kovacs K, Asa SL, eds. Functional Endocrine Pathology, 2nd Edition, Blackwell, Boston, 1998, pp. 247–281.

81. Horvath E, Kovacs K. Fine structural cytology of the adenohypophysis in rat and man. J Electron Microsc Tech 1988;8:401–432.

82. Lloyd RV. Analysis of mammosomatotropic cells in normal and neoplastic human pituitaries. Pathol Res Pract 1988;183:577–579.

83. Scheithauer BW, Sano T, Kovacs K, Young WR Jr, Ryan N, Randall RV. The pituitary gland in pregnancy, a clinicopathologic and immunohistochemical study of 69 cases. Mayo Clin Proc 1990;65:461–474.

84. Allaerts W, Carmeliet T, Denef C. New perspectives in the function of pituitary folliculo-stellate cells. Mol Cell Endo 1990;71:73–81.

85. Marin F, Stefaneanu L, Kovacs K. Folliculo-stellate cells in the pituitary. Endocr Pathol 1991;2:180–192.

86. McGrath P. Cysts of sellar and pharyngeal hypophyses. Pathology 1971;3:123–131.

87. Asa SL, Kovacs K, Bilbao JM. The pars tuberalis of the human pituitary. A histologic, immunohistochemical, ultrastructural and immunoelectron microscopic analysis. Virchow Arch A, Pathol Anat Histopathol 1983;399:49–59.

88. Schochet SS Jr, McCormick WF, Helmi NS. Salivary gland rests in the human pituitary. Light and electron microscopic study. Arch Pathol 1974;98:193–200.

89. Herman V, Fagin J, Gonsky R, Kovacs K, Melmed S. Clonal origin of pituitary adenomas. J Clin Endocrinol Metab 1990;71:1427–1433.

90. Jacoby LB, Hedley-Whyte ET, Pulaski K, Seizinger BR, Martuza RL. Clonal origin of pituitary adenomas. J Neurosurg 1990;73:731–735.

91. Schulte HM, Oldfield EH, Allolio B, Katz DA, Berkman RA, Ali IU. Clonal composition of pituitary adenomas in patients with Cushing's disease: determination by X-chromosome inactivation analysis. J Clin Endocrinol Metab 1991;73:1302–1308.

92. Biller BM, Alexander JM, Zervas NT, Hedley-Whyte ET, Arnold A, Klibanski A. Clonal origins of adrenocorticotropin-secreting pituitary tissue in Cushing's disease. J Clin Endocrinol Metab 1992;75:1303–1309.

93. Karga HJ, Alexander JM, Hedley-Whyte ET, Klibanski A, Jameson JL. Ras mutations in human pituitary tumors. J Clin Endocrinol Metab 1992;74:914–919.

94. Cyrns VL, Alexander JM, Klibanski A, Arnold A. The retinoblastoma gene in human pituitary tumors. J Clin Endocrinol Metab 1993;77:644–646.

95. Herman V, Drazin NZ, Gonsky R, Melmed S. Molecular screening of pituitary adenomas for gene mutations and rearrangements. J Clin Endocrinol Metab 1993;77:50–55.

96. Lloyd RV. Molecular biological analysis of pituitary disorders. In: Lloyd RV, ed. Surgical Pathology of the Pituitary Gland. WB Saunders, Philadelphia, 1993, pp. 85–93.

97. Boggild MD, Jenkinson S, Pistorello M, Boscaro M, Scanarini M, McTernan P, et al. Molecular genetic studies of sporadic pituitary tumors. J Clin Endocrinol Metab 1994;78:387–392.

98. Scheithauer BW, Laws ER Jr, Kovacs K, Horvath E, Randall RV, Carney JA. Pituitary adenomas of the multiple endocrine neoplasia type I syndrome. Semin Diagn Pathol 1987;4:205–211.

99. Jugenburg M, Kovacs K, Stefaneanu L, Scheithauer BW. Vasculature in nontumorous hypophyses, pituitary adenomas, and carcinomas: A quantitative morphologic study. Endocr Pathol 1995;6(2):115–124.

100. Jugenburg M, Kovacs K, Jungenburg I, Scheithauer BW. Angiogenesis in endocrine neoplasms. Endocr Pathol 1997;8(4):259–272.

101. Kontogeorgos G, Scheithauer BW, Horvath E, Kovacs K, Lloyd RV, Smyth HS, et al. Double adenomas of the pituitary: a clinicopathologic study of 11 tumors. Neurosurgery 1992;31:840–849.

102. Wynne AG, Scheithauer BW, Young W, Kovacs K, Ebersold M. Coexisting prolactinoma and corticotropinoma: a case report with reference to the relationship of corticotropin and prolactin excess. Neurosurgery 1992;30:919–923.

103. Costello RT. Subclinical adenoma of pituitary gland. Am J Pathol 1936;12:205–216.

104. McComb DJ, Ryan N, Horvath E, Kovacs K. Subclinical adenomas of the human pituitary: new light on old problems. Arch Pathol Lab Med 1983;107:488–491.

105. Kontogeorgos G, Kovacs K, Horvath E, Scheithauer BW. Multiple adenoma of the pituitary gland. A retrospective autopsy study with clinical implications. J Neurosurg 1991;74:243–247.

106. Burrow GN, Wortzman G, Rewcastle NB, Holgate RC, Kovacs K. Microadenomas of the pituitary and abnormal sellar tomograms in an unselected autopsy series. N Engl J Med 1981;304:156–158.

107. Kane LA, Leinung MG, Scheithauer BW, Bergstralh EJ, Laws ER Jr, Groover RV, et al. Pituitary adenomas in childhood and adolescence. J Clin Endocrinol Metab 1994;79(4):1135–1140.

108. Partington MD, Davis DH, Laws ER Jr, Scheithauer BW. Pituitary adenomas in childhood and adolescence: results of transsphenoidal surgery. J Neurosurg 1994;80:209–216.

109. Leinung MC, Kane LA, Scheithauer BW, Carpenter PC, Laws ER Jr, Zimmerman D. Long-term treatment of Cushing's disease in childhood. J Clin Endocr Metab 1995;80:2475–2479.

110. Mindermann T, Wilson CB. Pediatric pituitary adenomas. Neurosurgery 1995;36:259–269.

111. Lloyd RV, Chandler WF, Kovacs K, Ryan N. Ectopic pituitary adenomas with normal anterior pituitary glands. Am J Surg Pathol 1986;10;546–552.

112. Kleinschmidt-DeMasters BK, Winston KR, Rubinstein D, Samuels MA. Ectopic pituitary adenoma of the third ventricle. Case report. J Neurosurg 1990;72:139–142.

113. Kikuchi K, Kowada M, Sasaki J, Sageshima M. Large pituitary adenoma of the sphenoid sinus and the nasopharynx: report of a case with ultrastructural evaluations. Surg Neurol 1994;42:330–334.

114. Takahata T, Katayama Y, Tsubokawa T, Oshima H, Yoshino A. Ectopic pituitary adenoma occurring in the interpeduncular cistern. J Neurosurg 1995;83:1092–1094.

115. Palmer PE, Bogojavlensky S, Bhan AK, Scully RE. Prolactinoma in wall of ovarian dermoid cyst with hyperprolactinemia. Obstet Gynecol 1990;75:540–543.

116. Hardy J. Transsphenoidal microsurgery of the normal and pathological pituitary. Clin Neurosurg 1969;16:185–217.

117. Lloyd RV, Scheithauer BW, Kovacs K, Roche PC. The immunophenotype of pituitary adenomas. Endocr Pathol 1996;7:145–150.

118. Scheithauer BW, Kovacs KT, Laws ER Jr, Randall RV. Pathology of invasive pituitary tumors with special reference to functional classification. J Neurosurg 1986;65:733–744.

119. Selman WR, Laws ER Jr, Scheithauer BW, Carpenter SM. The occurrence of dural invasion in pituitary adenomas. J Neurosurg 1986;4:402–407.

120. Anniko M, Tribukait B, Wersall J. DNA ploidy and cell phase in human pituitary tumors. Cancer 1984;53:1708–1713.

121. Levy A, Hall L, Yeudall WA, Lightman SL. p53 gene mutations in pituitary adenomas: rare events. Clin Endocrinol 1994;41: 809–814.

122. Laws ER Jr, Scheithauer BW, Carpenter S, Randall RV, Abboud CF. The pathogenesis of acromegaly. Clinical and immunocytochemical analysis in 75 patients. J Neurosurg 1984;63:35–38.

123. Scheithauer BW, Kovacs K, Randall RV, Horvath E, Laws ER Jr. Pathology of excessive production of growth hormone. J Clin Endocrinol Metab 1986;15:655–681.

124. Sano T, Asa SL, Kovacs K. Growth hormone-releasing hormone-producing tumors: clinical, biochemical, and morphological manifestations. Endocr Rev 1988;9:357–373.

125. Horvath E, Scheithauer BW, Kovacs K, Randall RV, Laws ER Jr, Thorner MO, et al. Pituitary adenomas producing growth hormone, prolactin, and one or more glycoprotein hormones: a histologic, immunohistochemical, and ultrastructural study of four surgically removed tumors. Ultrastruct Pathol 1983;5:171–183.

126. Scheithauer BW, Horvath E, Kovacs K, Laws ER Jr, Randall RV, Ryan N. Plurihormonal pituitary adenomas. Semin Diagn Pathol 1986;3:69–82.

127. Horvath E, Kovacs K. Ultrastructural diagnosis of human pituitary adenomas. Microsc Res Tech 1992;20:107–135.

128. Horvath E, Kovacs K. Ultrastructural diagnosis of pituitary adenomas and hyperplasias. In: Lloyd RV, ed. Surgical pathology of the Pituitary Gland. WB Saunders, Philadelphia, 1993, pp. 52–84.

129. Neuman PE, Goldman JE, Horoupian DS, Hess MA. Fibrous bodies in growth hormone-secreting adenomas contain cytokeratin filaments. Arch Pathol Lab Med 1985;109:505–508.

130. Robert F. Electron microscopy of human pituitary tumors. In: Tindall GT, Collins WF, eds. Clinical Management of Pituitary Disorders. Raven, New York, 1979, pp. 113-131.

131. Horvath E, Kovacs K, Scheithauer BW, Lloyd RV, Smyth HS. Pituitary adenoma with neuronal choristoma (PANCH): composite lesion or lineage infidelity? Ultrastruct Pathol 1994;18:565–574.

132. Horvath E, Kovacs K. Pathology of prolactin cell adenomas of the human pituitary. Semin Diagn Pathol 1986;3:4–17.

133. Randall RV, Scheithauer BW, Laws ER Jr, Abboud CF, Ebersold MJ, Kao PC. Pituitary adenomas associated with hyperprolactinemia: a clinical and immunohistochemical study of 97 patients operated on transsphenoidally. Mayo Clin Proc 1985; 60:753–762.

134. Annegers JF, Coulam CB, Abboud CF, Laws ER Jr, Kurland LT. Pituitary adenoma in Olmstead County, Minnesota, 1935–1977. A report of an increasing incidence of diagnosis in women of childbearing age. Mayo Clin Proc 1978;53:641–643.

135. Calle-Rodrigue R, Giannini C, Scheithauer BW, Lloyd RV, Kovacs K, Stefaneanu L, et al. Prolactinomas in male and female patients: a comparative clinicopathologic study. Mayo Clin Proc 1998; 73:1046–1052.

136. Rilliet B, Mohr G, Robert F, Hardy J. Calcification in pituitary adenomas. Surg Neurol 1981;15:249–255.

137. Webster J, Peters JR, John R, Smith J, Chan V, Hall R, et al. Pituitary stone: two cases of densely calcified thyrotrophin-secreting pituitary adenoma. Clin Endocrinol (Oxford) 1984;40: 137–143.

138. Hinton DR, Polk RK, Linse KD, Weiss MH, Kovacs K, Garner JA. Characterization of spherical amyloid protein from a prolactin-producing pituitary adenoma. Acta Neuropathol 1997;93:43–49.

139. Landolt AM, Kleihues P, Heitz PU. Amyloid deposits in pituitary adenomas. Differentiation of two types. Arch Pathol Lab Med 1987;111:453–458.

140. Scheithauer BW, Horvath E, Kovacs K, Lloyd RV, Stefaneanu L, Buchfelder M, et al. Prolactin-producing pituitary adenoma and carcinoma with neuronal components—a metaplastic lesion. Pituitary 1999;1:197–206.

141. Corenblum B, Sirek AM, Horvath E, Kovacs K, Ezrin C. Human mixed somatotrophic and lactotrophic pituitary adenomas. J Clin Endocrinal Metab 1976;42:857–863.

142. Li J, Stefaneanu L, Kovacs K, Horvath E, Smyth HS. Growth hormone (GH) and prolactin (PRL) gene expression and immunoreactivity in GH- and PRL-producing human pituitary adenomas. Virchows Arch Pathol Anat 1993;422:193–201.

143. Horvath E, Kovacs K, Singer W, Smyth HS, Killinger DW, Ezrin C. Mammosomatotroph cell adenoma of the human pituitary: a morphologic entity. Virchows Arch Pathol Anat 1983;398:277–289.

144. Horvath E, Kovacs K, Singer W, Smyth HS, Killinger DW, Ezrin C, et al. Acidophil stem cell adenoma of the human pituitary: clinicopathological analysis of 15 cases. Cancer 1981;47:761–771.

145. Robert F, Hardy J. Human corticotroph cell adenomas. Semin Diagn Pathol 1986;3:34–41.

146. McNicol AM. Patterns of corticotropic cells in the adult human pituitary in Cushing's disease. Diagn Histopathol 1981;4:335–341.

147. Lloyd RV, Chandler WF, McKeever PE, Schteingart DE. The spectrum of ACTH-producing pituitary lesions. Am J Surg Pathol 1986;10:618–626.

148. Berg KK, Scheithauer BW, Felix I, Kovacs K, Horvath E, Klee GG, et al. Pituitary adenomas that produce adrenocorticotropic hormone and α-subunit; clinicopathological, immuno-histochemical, ultrastructural, and immunoelectron microscopic studies in nine cases. Neurosurgery 1990;26:357–403.

149. Neuman PE, Horoupian DS, Goldman JE, Hess MA. Cytoplasmic filaments of Crooke's hyaline change belong to the cytokeratin class. An immunocytochemical and ultrastructural study. Am J Pathol 1984;116:214–222.

150. Crooke A. A change in the basophil cells of the pituitary gland common to conditions which exhibit the syndrome attributed to basophil adenoma. J Pathol Bacteriol 1935;41:339–349.

151. Felix IA, Horvath E, Kovacs K. Massive Crooke's hyalinization in corticotroph cell adenoma of the human pituitary. A histological, immunocytochemical, and electron microscopic study of three cases. Acta Neurochirurg (Wien) 1982;58:235–243.

152. Horvath E, Kovacs K, Josse R. Pituitary corticotroph cell adenoma with marked abundance of microfilaments. Ultrastruct Pathol 1983;5:249–255.

153. Jaap AJ, Scheithauer BW, Kovacs K, Horvath E, Lloyd RV, Meyer FB, et al. A clinicopathologic study of silent corticotroph adenoma. Endocr Pathol 1998;9:393–394.

154. Bilbao J, Kovacs K, Horvath E, Higgins HP, Horsey WJ. Pituitary melanocorticotrophinoma with amyloid deposition. Can J Neurol Sci 1975;2:199–202.

155. Gharib H, Carpenter PC, Scheithauer BW, Service FJ. The spectrum of inappropriate pituitary thyrotropin secretion associated with hyperthyroidism. Mayo Clin Proc 1982;57:556–563.

156. Fatourechi V, Gharib H, Scheithauer BW, et al. Pituitary thyrotropic adenoma associated with congenital hypothyroidism. Am J Med 1984;76:725–728.

157. Girod C, Trouillas J, Claustrat B. The human thyrotropic adenoma: pathologic diagnosis in five cases and critical review of the literature. Semin Diagn Pathol 1986;3:58–68.

158. Wajchenberg BL, Tsanaclis AMC, Marino R Jr. TSH-containing pituitary adenoma associated with primary hypothyroidism manifested by amenorrhea and galactorrhea. Acta Endocrinol (Kbh) 1984;106:61–66.

159. Gesundheit N, Petrick PA, Nissim M, Dahlberg PA, Doppman JL, Emerson CH, et al. Thyrotropin-secreting pituitary adenomas: Clinical and biochemical heterogeneity. Case reports and follow-up of nine patients. Ann Intern Med 1989;111:827–835.

160. Kuzuya N, Inoue K, Ishibashi M, et al. Endocrine and immunohistochemical studies on thyrotropin (TSH)-secreting pituitary adenomas: responses of TSH, α-subunit, and growth hormone to hypothalamic releasing hormones and their distribution in adenoma cells. J Clin Endocrinol Metab 1990;71:1103–1111.

161. Wynne AG, Gharib H, Scheithauer BW, et al. Hyperthyroidism due to inappropriate secretion of thyrotropin in 10 patients. Am J Med 1992;92:15–24.

162. Pernicone PJ, Scheithauer BW. Invasive pituitary adenomas and pituitary carcinomas. In: Lloyd RV, ed. Surgical Pathology of the Pituitary Gland. Saunders, Philadelphia, Major Probl Pathol 1993, pp. 121–136.

163. Friend KE, Chiou YK, Laws ER Jr, Lopes MB, Shupnik MA. Pit-1 messenger ribonucleic acid is differentially expressed in human pituitary adenomas. J Clin Endocrinol Metab 1993;77;1281–1286.

164. Sanno N, Teramoto A, Matsuno A, Osamura Y. Expression of human Pit-1 product in the human pituitary and pituitary adenomas. Arch Pathol Lab Med 1996;120:73–77.

165. Yamada S, Takahashi M, Hara M, Hattori A, Sano T, Ozawa Y, et al. Pit-1 gene expression in human pituitary adenomas using the reverse transcription polymerase chain reaction method. Clin Endocrinol 1996;45:263–272.

166. Sano T, Kovacs K, Asa SL, Smyth HS. Immunoreactive luteinizing hormone in functioning corticotroph adenomas of the pituitary. Immunohistochemical and tissue culture studies of two cases. Virchows Arch Pathol Anat 1990;417:351–367.

167. Horvath E, Kovacs K. Gonadotroph adenomas of the human pituitary: sex-related fine structural dichotomy. A histologic, immunohistochemical and electron microscopic study of 30 tumors. Am J Pathol 1984;117:429–440.

168. Trouillas J, Girod C, Sassolas G, Claustrat B. The human gonadotropic adenoma: pathologic diagnosis and hormonal correlations in 26 tumors. Semin Diagn Pathol 1986;3:42–57.

169. Young WF Jr, Scheithauer BW, Kovacs KT, Horvath E, Davis DH, Randall RV. Gonadotroph adenoma of the pituitary gland: a clinicopathologic analysis of 100 cases. Mayo Clin Proc 1996;71:649–656.

170. Kontogeorgos G, Horvath E, Kovacs K. Sex-linked ultrastructural dichotomy of gonadotroph adenomas of the human pituitary: an electron microscopic analysis of 145 tumors. Ultrastruct Pathol 1990;14:475–482.

171. Kovacs K, Horvath E, Ryan N, Ezrin C. Null cell adenoma of the human pituitary. Virchows Arch Pathol Anat 1980;387:165–174.

172. Kovacs K, Asa SL, Horvath E, Ryan N, Singer W, Killinger DW, et al. Null cell adenomas of the pituitary: attempts to resolve their cytogenesis. In: Lechago J, Kameya T, eds. Endocrine Pathology Update, Field and Wood, Philadelphia, 1990, pp. 17–31.

173. Saeger W, Gunzl H, Meyer M, Schulze C, Ludecke DK. Immunohistological studies on clinically silent pituitary adenomas. Endocr Pathol 1990;1:37–44.

174. Kontogeorgos G, Kovacs K, Horvath E, Scheithauer BW. Null cell adenomas, oncocytomas, and gonadotroph adenomas of the human pituitary: an immunocytochemical and ultrastructural analysis of 300 cases. Endocrinol Pathol 1993;4:20–27.

175. Asa SL, Gerrie B, Singer W, Horvath E, Kovacs K, Smyth HS. Gonadotropin secretion in vitro by human pituitary null cell adenomas and oncocytomas. J Clin Endocrinol Metab 1986;62:1011–1019.

176. Asa SL, Cheng Z, Ramyar L, Singer W, Kovacs K, Smyth HS, et al. Human pituitary null cell adenomas and oncocytomas in vitro: effects of adenohypophysiotropic hormones and gonadal steroids on hormone secretion and tumor cell morphology. J Clin Endocrinol Metab 1992;74:1128–1134.

177. Jamieson JL, Klibanski A, Black McL, et al. Glycoprotein hormone genes are expressed in clinically non-functioning pituitary adenomas. J Clin Invest 1987;80:1472–1478.

178. Sakurai T, Seoh H, Yamamoto N, et al. Detection of mRNA of prolactin and ACTH in clinically non-functioning adenomas. J Neurosurg 1988;69:653–659.

179. Matsuno A, Teramoto A, Takekoshi S, et al. HGH, PRL and ACTH gene expression in clinically non-functioning adenomas detected with nonisotopic in situ hybridization method. Endocr Pathol 1995;6:13–20.

180. Yamada S, Asa SL Kovacs K. Oncocytomas and null cell adenomas of the human pituitary: morphometric and in vitro functional comparison. Virchows Arch Pathol Anat 1988;413:333–339.

181. Horvath E, Kovacs K, Killinger DW, Smyth HS, Platts ME, Singer W. Silent corticotropic adenomas of the human pituitary gland; a histologic, immunocytologic and ultrastructural study. Am J Pathol 98:617–638, 1980.

182. Horvath E, Kovacs K, Smyth HS, Killinger DW, Scheithauer BW, Randall R, et al. A novel type of pituitary adenoma: morphological features and clinical correlations. J Clin Endocrinol Metab 1988;66:1111–1118.

183. Lloyd RV, Fields K, Jin L, Horvath E, Kovacs K. Analysis of endocrine active and clinically silent, corticotropic adenomas by in situ hybridization. Am J Pathol 1990;137:479–488.

184. Nagaya T, Seo H, Kuwayama A, et al. Proopiomelanocortin gene expression in silent corticotroph cell adenoma and Cushing's disease. J Neurosurg 1990;72:262–267.

185. Stefaneanu L, Kovacs K, Horvath E, Lloyd RV. In situ hybridization study of pro-opiomelanocortin (POMC) gene expression in human pituitary corticotrophs and their adenomas. Virchows Arch Pathol Anat 1991;419:107–113.

186. Asa SL, Kovacs K, Tindall GT, Barrow DL, Horvath E, Vecsei P. Cushing's disease associated with an intrasellar gangliocytoma producing corticotrophin-releasing factor. Ann Intern Med 1984;101:789–793.

187. Saeger W, Puchner MJ, Ludecke DK. Combined sellar gangliocytoma and pituitary adenoma in acromegaly or Cushing's disease. Virchows Arch Pathol Anat 1994;425:93–99.

188. Asa SL, Scheithauer BW, Bilbao JM, Horvath E, Ryan N, Kovacs K, et al. A case for hypothalamic acromegaly: a clinicopathologic study of six patients with hypothalamic gangliocytomas producing growth hormone-releasing factor. J Clin Endocrinol Metab 1984;58:796–803.

189. Scheithauer BW, Kovacs K, Randall RV, Horvath E, Okazaki H, Laws ER Jr. Hypothalamic neuronal hamartoma and adenohypophyseal neuronal choristoma: their association with growth hormone adenoma of the pituitary gland. J Neuropathol Exp Neurol 1983;42:648–663.

190. Lach B, Rippstein P, Benoit BG, Staines W. Differentiating neuroblastoma of pituitary gland: neuroblastic transformation of epithelial adenoma cells. Case report. J Neurosurg 1996;85:953–960.

191. Towfighi J, Salam MM, McLendon RE, Powers S, Page RB. Ganglion cell containing tumors of the pituitary gland. Arch Pathol Lab Med 1996;120:369–377.

192. Levy A, Lightman SL. Growth hormone-releasing hormone transcripts in human pituitary adenomas. J Clin Endocrinol Metab 1992;74:1474–1476.

193. Thapar K, Kovacs K, Stefaneanu L, Scheithauer BW, Killinger DW, Lloyd RV, et al. Overexpression of the growth hormone-releasing hormone gene in acromegaly associated pituitary tumors: an event associated with neoplastic progression and aggressive behavior. Am J Pathol 1997;151:769–784.

194. Wakai S, Fukushima T, Teramoto A, Sano K. Pituitary apoplexy: its incidence and clinical significance. J Neurosurg 1981;55: 187–193.

195. Mohr G, Hardy J. Hemorrhage, necrosis, and apoplexy in pituitary adenomas. Surg Neurol 1982;18:181–189.

196. Ebersold MJ, Laws ER Jr., Scheithauer, BW, Randall RV. Pituitary apoplexy treated by transsphenoidal surgery: a clinicopathology and immunocytochemical study. J Neurosurg 1983; 58:315–320.

197. Bills DC, Meyer FB, Laws ER Jr, Davis DH, Ebersold MJ, Scheithauer BW, et al. A retrospective analysis of pituitary apoplexy. Neurosurgery 1993;33:602–609.

198. Bonicki W, Kasperlik-Azluska A, Koszewski W, Zgliczynski W, Wislawski J. Pituitary apoplexy: endocrine, surgical and oncological emergency. Incidence, clinical course and treatment with reference to 799 cases of pituitary adenomas. Acta Neurochirurgica 1993;120:118–122.

199. Shirataki K, Chihara K, Shibata Y, Tamaki N, Matsumoto S, Fujita T. Pituitary apoplexy manifested during a bromocriptine test in a patient with a growth hormone- and prolactin-producing pituitary adenoma. Neurosurg 1988;23:395–398.

200. Masago A, Eueda Y, Kanai H, Magal H, Umemura S. Pituitary apoplexy after pituitary function test: a report of two cases and review of the literature [review]. Surg Neurol 1995; 43:158–164.

201. Reznik Y, Chapon F, Lahlou N, Deboucher N, Mahoudeau J. Pituitary apoplexy of a gonadotroph adenoma following gonadotrophin-releasing hormone agonist therapy for prostatic therapy. J Endocr Invest 1997;20:566–568.

202. Pernicone PJ, Scheithauer BW, Sebo TJ, Kovacs KT, Horvath E, Young WF, et al. Pituitary carcinoma. A clinicopathologic study of 15 cases. Cancer 1997;79:804–812.

203. Davis DH, Laws ER Jr., Ilstrup DM, Speed JK, Caruso M, Shaw EG, et al. Results of surgical treatment for growth hormone-secreting pituitary adenomas. J Neurosurg 1993;79:70–75.

204. Fisher BJ, Gaspar Le, Noone B. Radiation therapy of pituitary adenoma: delayed sequelae. Radiology 1993;187:843–846.

205. Bliss P, Kerr GR, Gregor A. Incidence of second brain tumours after pituitary irradiation in Edinburgh 1962-1990. Clin Oncol 1994;6:361–363.

206. Rauhut F, Stolhe D. Combined surgery and radiotherapy of invasive pituitary adenomas—problems of radiogenic encephalopathy. Acta Neurochir, Suppl 1996;65:37–40.

207. Simmons NE, Laws ER Jr. Glioma occurrence after sellar irradiation: case report and review. Neurosurgery 1998;42:172–178.

208. Marks LB. Conventional fractionated radiation vs. radiosurgery for selected benign intracranial lesions (arteriovenous malformations, pituitary adenomas, and acoustic neuromas). Review. J Neuro-Oncol 1993;17:223–230.

209. Pollock BE, Kondziolka D, Lunsford LD, Flickinger JC. Stereotactic radiosurgery for pituitary adenomas: imaging, visual and endocrine results. Acta Neurochir Suppl 1994;62:33–38.

210. Motti ED, Losa M, Pieralli S, Zecchinelli A, Longobardi B, Giugni E, et al. Stereotactic radiosurgery of pituitary adenomas. Review. Metabolism: Clin Exp 1996;45(8 Suppl 1):111–114.

211. Schaardenburg D van, Roelfsema F, Srters AP van, Vielvoye GJ. Bromocriptine therapy for non-functioning pituitary adenoma. Clin Endocrinol 1989;30:475–484.

212. Ciccarelli E, Camanni F. Diagnosis and drug therapy of prolactinoma. Review Drugs 1996;51:954–965.

213. Fahlbusch R, Buchfelder M, Schrell U. Short-term preoperative treatment of acroprolactinomas by dopamine agonists. J Neurosurg 1987;67:807–815.

214. Pellegrini I, Rasolonjanahary R, Gunz G, Bertrand P, Delivet S, Jedynak CP, Kordon C, Peillon F, Jaquet P, Enjalbert A. Resistance to bromocriptine in prolactinomas. J Clin Endocrinol Metab 1989;69:500–509.

215. Saeger W, Mohr K, Caselitz J, Ludecke DK. Light and electron microscopical morphometry of pituitary adenomas in hyperprolactinemia. Path Res Pract 1986;181:544–550.

216. Bevan JS, Webster J, Burke CW, Scanlon MF. Dopamine agonists and pituitary tumors shrinkage. Endocr Rev 1992;13:220–240.

217. Horvath E, Kovacs K, Killinger DW, Gonzalez J, Smyth HS. Diverse ultrastructural response to dopamine agonist medication in human pituitary prolactin cell adenomas. In: Hoshino K, ed. Prolactin Gene Family and Its Receptors. Elsevier, Amsterdam, 1988, pp. 307–311.

218. Barkan AL, Lloyd RV, Chandler WF, Hatfield MK, Gebarski SS, Kelch RP, et al. Preoperative treatment of acromegaly with long-acting somatostatin analog SM S 201-995: shrinkage of invasive pituitary macroadenomas and improved surgical remission rate. J Clin Endocrinol Metab 1988;67:1040–1048.

219. Bertherat J, Brue T, Enjalbert A, Gunz G, Rasolonjanahary R, Warnet A, et al. Somatostatin receptors on thyrotropin-secreting pituitary adenomas: comparison with the inhibitory effects of octreotide upon in vivo and in vitro hormonal secretions. J Clin Endocrinol Metab 1992;75:540–546.

220. Chanson P, Weintraub BD, Harris AG. Octreotide therapy for thyroid-stimulating hormone-secreting pituitary adenomas. Ann Intern Med 1993;119;236–240.

221. Newman CB, Melmed S, Snyder PJ, et al. Safety and efficacy of long term octreotide therapy of acromegaly: results of a multicenter trial in 103 patients—a clinical research center study. J Clin Endocrinol Metab 1995;80:2768–2775.

222. Lamberts SWJ, van der Lely AJ, de Herder WW, Hofland LJ. Octreotide. N Engl J Med 1996;334:246–254.

223. Thapar K, Kovacs KT, Stefaneanu L, Scheithauer BW, Horvath E, Lloyd RV, et al. Antiproliferative effect of the somatostatin analogue octreotide on growth hormone-producing pituitary tumors: results of a multicenter randomized trial. Mayo Clin Proc 1997;72:893–900.

224. Vance ML, Harris AG. Long-term treatment of 189 acromegalic patients with the somatostatin analog octreotide. Results of the International Multicenter Acromegaly Study Group. Arch Intern Med 1991;151:1573–1578.

225. Ezzat S, Snyder PJ, Young WF, Boyajy LD, Newman C, Klibanski A, et al. Octreotide treatment of acromegaly: a randomized, multicenter study. Ann Intern Med 1992;117:711–718.

226. Ezzat S, Horvath E, Harris AG, Kovacs K. Morphologic effects of octreotide on growth hormone-producing pituitary adenomas. J Clin Endocrinol Metab 1994;79:113–118.

227. Saeger W, Ludecke DK. Pituitary hyperplasia. Definition, light and electron microscopic structures and significance in surgical specimens. Virchows Arch Pathol Anat 1983;399:277–287.

228. Horvath E, Kovacs K, Scheithauer BW. Pituitary hyperplasia. Pituitary 1999;1:169–180.

229. Thorner MO, Perryman RL, Cronin MJ, Rogol AD, Draznin M, Johanson A, et al. Somatotroph hyperplasia. J Clin Invest 1982;70:965–977.

230. Ezzat S, Asa SL, Stefaneanu L, Whittom R, Smyth HS, Horvath E, et al. Somatotroph hyperplasia without pituitary adenoma associated with a long-standing growth hormone-releasing hormone-producing bronchial carcinoid. J Clin Endocrinol Metab 1994;78:555–560.

231. Kovacs K, Horvath E, Thorner MO, Rogol AD. Mammosomatotroph hyperplasia associated with acromegaly and hyperprolactinemia in a patient with the McCune-Albright syndrome: a histologic, immunocytologic and ultrastructural study of the surgically removed adenohypophysis. Virchows Arch Pathol Anat 1984;403:77–86.

232. Moran A, Asa SL, Kovacs K, et al. Gigantism due to pituitary mammosomatotroph hyperplasia. N Engl J Med 1990;323:322–326.

233. Zimmerman D, Young WF Jr, Ebersold MJ, et al. Congenital gigantism due to growth hormone-releasing hormone excess and pituitary hyperplasia with adenomatous transformation. J Clin Endocrinol Metab 1993;46:216–222.

234. Scheithauer BW, Carpenter PC, Block B. Ectopic secretion of a growth hormone releasing factor: report of a case of acromegaly with bronchial carcinoid tumor. Am J Med 1984;76:605–616.

235. Stefaneanu L, Kovacs K, Lloyd R, Scheithauer BW, Sano T, Young W. Pituitary lactotrophs and somatotrophs in pregnancy: a correlative in situ hybridization and immunocytochemical study. J Clin Endocrinol Metab 1992;62:291–296.

236. Pioro EP, Scheithauer BW, Laws ER Jr, Randall RV, Kovacs K, Horvath E. Combined thyrotroph and lactotroph cell hyperplasia simulating prolactin-secreting pituitary adenoma in long-standing primarily hypothyroidism. Surg Neurol 1988;29:218–226.

237. Scheithauer BW, Kovacs KT, Young WF Jr, Randall RV. The pituitary gland in hypothyroidism. Mayo Clin Proc 1992;67:22–26.

238. Scheithauer BW, Kovacs KT, Randall RV, Ryan N. Effects of estrogen upon the human pituitary: a clinicopathologic study. Mayo Clin Proc 1989;64:1077–1084.

239. Jay V, Kovacs K, Horvath E, Lloyd RV, Smyth HS. Idiopathic prolactin cell hyperplasia of the pituitary mimicking prolactin cell adenoma: a morphological study including immunocytochemistry, electron microscopy and in situ hybridization. Acta Neuropathol 1991;82:147–151.

240. Kovacs K, Stefaneanu L, Ezzat S, Smyth HS. Prolactin-producing pituitary adenoma in a male-to-female transsexual patient with protracted estrogen administration. A morphologic study. Arch Pathol Lab Med 1994;118:562–565.

241. Carey RM, Varma SK, Drake CR Jr, Thorner MO, Kovacs K, Rivier J, et al. Ectopic secretion of corticotropin releasing factor as a cause of Cushing's syndrome: a clinical, morphologic, and biochemical study. N Engl J Med 1984;311:13–20.

242. Schteingart DE, Lloyd RV, Akil H, et al. Cushing's syndrome secondary to ectopic corticotropin-releasing hormone-adrenocorticotropin secretion. J Clin Endocrinol Metab 1986;63:770–775.

243. Scheithauer BW, Kovacs K, Randall RV. The pituitary gland in untreated Addison's disease. A histologic and immunocytologic study of 18 adenohypophyses. Arch Pathol Lab Med 1983;107:484–487.

244. Saeger W, Geisler F, Lüdecke DK. Pituitary pathology in Cushing's disease. Pathol Res Pract 1988;183:592–595.

245. Young WF Jr, Scheithauer BW, Gharib H, Laws ER Jr, Carpenter PC. Cushing's syndrome due to primary multinodular corticotrope hyperplasia. Mayo Clin Proc 1988;63:256–262.

246. Kovacs K, Stefaneanu L, Horvath E, Buchfelder M, Fahlbusch R, Althoff PH, et al. Pituitary corticotroph adenoma in a woman with long-standing Addison's disease: a histologic, immunocytochemical, electron microscopic and in situ hybridization study. Endocr Pathol 1996;7:91–97.

247. Khalil A, Kovacs K, Sima AAF, Burrow GN, Horvath E. Pituitary thyrotroph hyperplasia mimicking prolactin-secreting adenoma. J Endocrinol Invest 1984;7:399–404.

8 Molecular Pathology of Pituitary Tumors

Ricardo V. Lloyd, MD, PhD

INTRODUCTION

Molecular biological methods have been used to study pituitary disorders in recent years. Techniques, such as Southern and Northern hybridization, *in situ* hybridization (ISH), polymerase chain reaction (PCR), single-strand confirmation polymorphism (SSCP) analysis, and clonal analysis, have been used to examine normal and neoplastic pituitary tissues. These methods have contributed greatly to advances in the understanding of pituitary disorders. This chapter will review some basic molecular biological techniques and illustrate their applications to the study of pituitary disorders.

HYBRIDIZATION METHODS

Hybridization involves pairing of complementary strands of nucleic acids, such as DNA–DNA, DNA–RNA, or RNA–RNA hybrids. The various forms of hybridizations include:

1. Solution hybridization in which the annealing of nucleic acids occurs in a liquid state.
2. Northern and Southern blots in which the DNA and RNA are immobilized to an inert support, such as nylon membranes or nitrocellulose filters, and are analyzed on these solid matrices.
3. ISH in which hybridization occurs in cytologic or histologic preparations.

In situ hybridization is the ideal method of analysis for morphologists who study pituitary gene expression, because the probe hybridizes to the messenger RNA or DNA fixed *in situ* within cells (Figure 1). Thus, the relationship of cells expressing specific gene products to other cells in the sections can be readily appreciated. A combination of ISH analysis and immunohistochemistry can be used to localize gene transcripts and the translated protein products within the same cell or in adjacent cells.

TISSUE PREPARATION AND PROCESSING FOR ISH

The preservation of nucleic acid is one of the important first steps in any ISH study *(1,2)*. Previous studies have shown that messenger RNA is much better preserved in frozen tissue sections than in paraffin-embedded tissues. Fixatives, such as paraformaldehyde and neutral buffered formalin, are excellent for messenger RNA preservation, whereas ethanol-acetic acid fixation results in

From: *Diagnosis and Management of Pituitary Tumors* (K. Thapar, K. Kovacs, B. W. Scheithauer, and R. V. Lloyd, eds.), ©Humana Press Inc., Totowa, NJ.

less than optimal preservation of nucleic acid for ISH. After fixation, tissues can be sectioned and stored at –70°C for a few weeks to months without loss of mRNA in the tissues.

Formalin fixation provides satisfactory results for ISH analysis to localize DNA and RNA. The messenger RNA signal detected in paraffin sections is usually less than that seen in frozen sections of the same tissues used for ISH. Archival materials have been used successfully to localize messenger RNA after many years of storage at room temperature in paraffin-embedded blocks *(3)*.

A variety of probes can be used for ISH including cDNA, cRNA (riboprobes), and synthetic oligonucleotide probes. These latter probes, which are readily generated by automated synthesizers, offer several advantages, including ease of penetration into cells in paraffin sections and availability in large amounts of long-term usage. Complementary RNA probes or riboprobes are frequently used for ISH studies *(2,4)*. These cRNA or antisense probes form stable hybrids with cellular RNA, and the background signal or nonspecific binding can be reduced after hybridization with the use of the enzyme ribonuclease A, since ribonuclease A digests single-stranded, but not double-stranded RNA hybrids.

SIGNAL DETECTION

Use of reporters to detect the hybrid of probe and nucleic acid of interest within cells can be done with radioactive or nonradioactive methods. Radioactive reporters include ^{32}P-, ^{33}P-, ^{35}S-, ^{125}I-, and ^{3}H-labeled nucleotides. The suboptimal resolution with signal detectors, such as ^{32}P, is compensated by its greater sensitivity and the feasibility of readily quantifying the results. The obvious hazards of working with radioactive isotopes is a major drawback to their use, and many nonisotopic methods have been developed in the past few years for ISH. These have included digoxigenin, biotin, and fluorescein-labeled probes. The excellent resolution in tissues and cytologic preparations of the nonisotopic probe makes up for their relative insensitivity compared to the radioactive probe. In recent years, the sensitivity of nonisotopic detection methods has been improved with techniques, such as utilizing probe cocktails, using multiple biotin tails with oligonucleotide probes and by a combination of *in situ* polymerase chain reaction (PCR) *(5–8)*.

CONTROLS NEEDED FOR ISH STUDIES

A variety of controls can be utilized in performing ISH analyses. These should include:

1. Northern and Southern hybridization analysis to characterize the molecular sizes of the nucleic acids of interest.

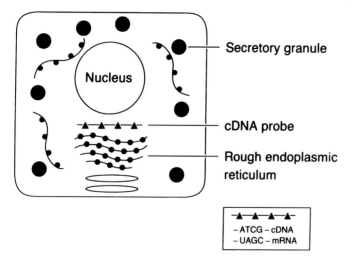

Secretory granule

cDNA probe

Rough endoplasmic
reticulum

$-$ ATCG $-$ cDNA
$-$ UAGC $-$ mRNA

Figure 8-1 Schematic diagram showing the detection of specific messenger RNA (mRNA) in a pituitary cell by ISH. The reporter or signal detector of the probe can be isotopic, such as ^{35}S, or nonisotopic, such as digoxigenin. The cDNA probe hybridizes to the complementary mRNA. The mRNA is detected in the cell cytoplasm.

2. Treatment of cells with ribonuclease or deoxyribonuclease for hybridization to decrease the hybridization signal.
3. Localization of protein products within the cell in which the messenger RNA is localized.
4. Use of sense probes with oligonucleotide and riboprobes.
5. Performing ISH in tissues known not to express the messenger RNA or DNA under investigation.
6. Competition experiments with unlabeled probe before performing the hybridization reaction.

PROBLEMS IN THE INTERPRETATION OF ISH ANALYSES

ISH is very technically demanding and requires numerous controls, especially when localizing nucleic acids that are present in low copy numbers within cells. In analyzing tissues with low to moderate copy numbers of specific genes or gene products, false-negative results can be readily obtained. Ribonuclease can be a major contaminant, which can diminish or abolish the hybridization signal when RNA probes are used or when RNA within tissues or cells is analyzed. The use of RNase-free conditions when performing the assay can decrease this problem significantly. Contamination of enzymes, such as proteolytic enzymes and nucleases, which are commonly used during prehybridization treatment, can lead to false-negative results. The specificity of the probe used in the analysis, especially oligonucleotide probes, must be carefully analyzed. Crosshybridization can be readily reduced using high-stringency conditions, such as elevated temperatures or very low-salt concentrations, during hybridization and in the posthybridization washes.

The presence of endogenous biotin and endogenous alkaline phosphatase can lead to false-positive reactions. Pretreatment with levamisole may help to reduce endogenous alkaline phosphatase. The use of radioactive probes presents other problems in interpretation. Chemography, the creation of reduced crystals in the emulsion, which alter the role of latent images by chemicals present in the specimen during autoradiography, may lead to false interpretation of the results. Appropriate controls, including slides without radioactive probes, should be utilized to avoid this problem.

HYBRIDIZATION ANALYSES OF THE PITUITARY

There have been many studies of ISH localization of gene products in growth hormone- and prolactin-secreting tumors and normal growth hormone and prolactin cells (Figures 2A,B,C and Color Plates). This may be related to the relative abundance of these tumor types in surgically excised pituitary neoplasms. In one of the early studies of human pituitary tumors by ISH Pixley et al. *(9)* analyzed dissociated cells from growth hormone-producing pituitary tumors using a cDNA probe. They noted a decrease in the percentage of cells expressing growth hormone messenger RNA in the cells that were cultured for 2–3 d. Various investigators have used formalin-fixed, paraffin-embedded tissue sections to examine gene expression in the pituitary. Lloyd et al. *(10,11)* observed that most growth hormone- (GH) secreting pituitary tumors expressed both GH and prolactin mRNA. Prolactin-producing cells and tumors commonly express only prolactin, but not growth hormone message, supporting the concept that prolactin-producing cells and tumors are terminally differentiated. Levy and Lightman *(12,13)* examined the effects of GH-releasing hormone (GHRH) and somatostatin on GH gene expression in human pituitary tumors by quantitative ISH. When two GH adenomas were studied in culture, GHRH and hydrocortisone did not change GH messenger RNA level expression, although the GH messenger RNA transcript could be readily detected in the tumors. Kovacs et al. *(14)* and Trouillas et al. *(15)* examined GH tumors that expressed immunoreactive growth hormone in which the patients do not have clinical evidence of acromegaly using ISH immunohistochemistry and electron microscopy. They showed that the GH gene and protein products were expressed in the tumor cells, although the patients did not have acromegaly. The functional state of the GH message and proteins in patients with silent GH tumors is currently unknown. Saeger et al. *(16)* studied 40 pituitary adenomas from patients with acromegaly and compared immunohistochemistry and ISH. They found 100% correlation for GH and 60% for prolactin of the hybridization signal and the hormone content. Their findings that 87% of the growth hormone tumors express prolactin messenger RNA is in agreement with earlier studies by Lloyd et al. *(11)*.

Stefaneanu et al. *(17)* studied pituitaries from pregnant and lactating women. They found that GH cells expressed prolactin messenger RNA during pregnancy, and these findings were more marked during the latter part of pregnancy. These important observations suggested that there was a transformation of cell types with the development of mammosomatotroph cells expressing both prolactin and GH in this altered physiological state. In a study of the effects of bromocriptine treatment on prolactin-secreting pituitary adenomas by ISH, Kovacs et al. observed that prolactin messenger RNA was decreased by bromocriptine in a population of small cells, indicating that these cells responded to the drug with decreased cytoplasmic volume. However, a subpopulation of larger prolactin cells expressed significant amounts of prolactin messenger RNA, in spite of bromocriptine therapy, indicating a resistance to this dopamine agonist *(18)*.

ISH analyses of adrenocorticotropic hormone (ACTH)-secreting tumors have been reported by several investigators (Figure 2D). Lloyd et al. *(19)* analyzed a series of ACTH-immunoreactive pituitary tumors for pro-opiomelanocortin (POMC) messenger RNA expression and found that most of the functional tumors that were classified as type 1 silent adenomas, which were morphologically similar to functional pituitary tumors in patients with Cushing's disease, expressed POMC mRNA. Only a few of the

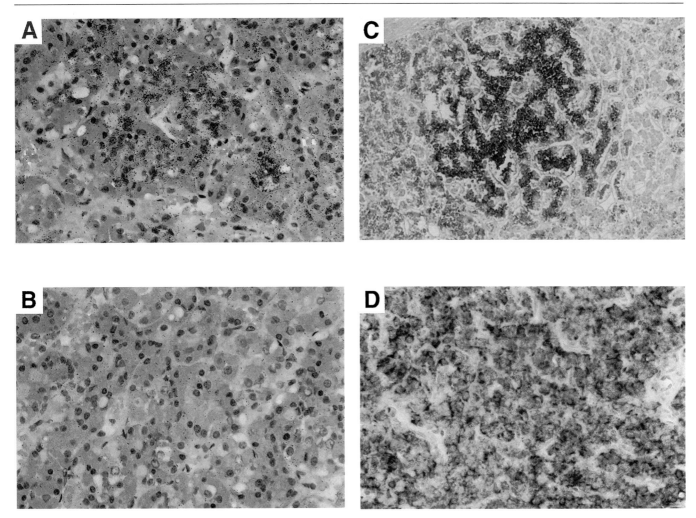

Figure 8-2 ISH applications in the pituitary. (**A**) Detection of PRL mRNA in normal pituitary with a ^{35}S-labeled oligonucleotide probe (×250); (**B**) the sense control probe is negative (×250); (**C**) incidental PRL adenoma detected by ISH with a digoxigenin-labeled oligonucleotide probe in an autopsy pituitary (×200); (**D**) an ACTH adenoma expressing pro-opiomelanocortin detected with a digoxigenin-labeled oligonucleotide probe (×300). (*See* Color Plates, following p. 176.)

type 2 and type 3 tumors, which are subtypes of ACTH silent tumors subclassified by electron microscopy, had detectable levels of POMC messenger RNA. Stefaneanu et al. *(20)* reported similar findings in an analysis of 22 functional and silent ACTH-secreting tumors. These studies strongly suggested that the morphological features of corticotroph tumors may be related to POMC production in functional and in subtype 1 silent adenomas. Nagaya et al. *(21)* reported that the size of the POMC transcript in a case of a silent ACTH tumor was similar to that in functional ACTH adenomas when analyzed by Northern hybridization. This observation suggests that in silent tumors, the messenger RNA may not be an abnormal molecule, unlike the longer POMC mRNA transcript present in some neuroendocrine tumors *(22)*. Other investigators have used digoxigenin-labeled oligonucleotide probes to show that the messenger RNA for POMC as well as for prolactin and GH could be readily detected with this nonisotopic technique in human pituitary tumors *(23)*. In a recent follow-up study by Fehn et al. *(24)*, pituitaries from 16 patients with Cushing's disease and 10 patients with Nelson's syndrome were analyzed by ISH with digoxigenin-labeled probes. They showed that the signal was significantly greater in Nelson's syndrome than in Cushing's disease, suggesting differences in POMC transcript expression in these two conditions.

Studies of nonneoplastic pituitaries for POMC gene expression by Mengod et al. *(25)* showed that POMC messenger RNA could be detected in postmortem pituitaries up to 66 h after death. Lopez et al. in a recent study *(26)* used quantitative ISH to show that there was an increase in POMC messenger RNA in suicide victims compared to patients who had cardiac death.

A few studies of ISH analyses of gonadotrophic, null-cell, and oncocytic adenomas have been reported. These tumors share some immunophenotypic and ultrastructural features. Lloyd et al. *(27)* examined follicle-stimulating hormone (FSH)-β and luteinizing hormone (LH)-β and α-subunit of glycoprotein hormone messenger RNA in gonadotroph, null-cell, and oncocytic tumors. α-Subunits of glycoprotein hormones, FSH-β and/or LH-β messenger RNA were seen in most gonadotroph and null-cell tumors, but in very few oncocytomas. The findings led these investigators to postulate that gonadotroph and null-cell tumors are probably closely related and the oncocytomas may represent a dedifferentiated tumor related to null-cell adenomas. In a study of 40 clinical and nonfunctional pituitary tumors, Bäz et al. *(28)* found that about one-third of the tumors expressed beta subunit of human chorionic gonadotropin (βHCG)/βLH. A small number of the tumors express prolactin or GH messenger RNA. Other workers *(29)* also detected

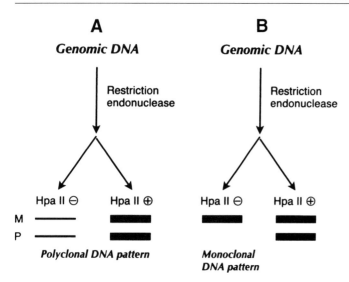

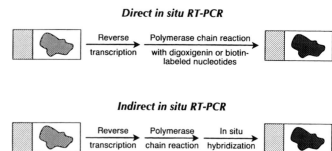

Figure 8-4 Schematic diagram of *in situ* RT-PCR in tissue sections to detect mRNA with low copy numbers. The direct method is more specific, but less sensitive in detecting the amplified cDNA. The RT reaction converts the mRNA to cDNA. The indirect method uses a separate ISH step to detect the amplified product and is more specific than the direct method. Controls used for *in situ* RT-PCR include omitting *Taq* polymerase, RT, and/or primers that should result in low level or absent staining in the indirect procedure.

Figure 8-3 Schematic diagram of DNA restriction analysis by enzyme digestion and Southern hybridization for clonality of pituitary tumors. Normal tissues, such as white blood cells or nonneoplastic pituitary (**A**), or a pituitary adenoma (**B**) DNA is digested with the RFLP enzyme and an additional enzyme to detect the distal end of the alletic restriction fragment. A portion of genomic DNA is cut with *Hpa*II to determine X-inactivation of the maternal (M) or paternal (P) X-linked gene. Polyclonal tissues are partially resistant to *Hpa*II, so the intensity of the band on Southern blot is reduced by 50%. The monoclonal pituitary adenoma in β has a single pattern of X-inactivation, which makes it completely resistent to *Hpa*II digestion in one X chromosome, whereas the second X chromosome is cut completely, resulting in a single band on Southern blotting.

prolactin and POMC messenger RNA in a group of nonfunctional adenomas, indicating the heterogeneous nature of these neoplasms.

A wide variety of other messenger RNA transcripts have been analyzed in pituitary tissues by ISH. These have ranged from the transcripts for secretory granule protein messenger RNAs, such as the chromogranin/secretogranin family *(30–33)*, to hypothalamic hormones *(34–36)*, to hormone receptors, and transcription factors, such as Pit-1 *(37,38)*. These studies have demonstrated the utility of ISH in localizing gene transcripts in individual cells and in separating expression of specific genes in neoplastic or normal pituitary tissues. The increasing numbers of messenger RNA transcripts analyzed by ISH in the pituitary reflects the rapid proliferation of available probes and the broad interest of many investigators in analyzing normal and neoplastic pituitary tissues.

CLONAL ANALYSIS

The monoclonal nature of most pituitary adenomas can be demonstrated by clonal analysis *(39–41)*. In these studies, restriction fragment-length polymorphism (RFLP) analysis is performed on genomic DNA after enzyme digestion (Figure 3). Commonly used markers include the specific X chromosome genes, such as hypoxanthine phosphoribosyltransferase (HPRT), and phosphoglycerate kinase (PGK). With RFLP analysis, nucleotide sequences between two or more individuals can be detected by differences in the restriction sites after digestion using specific restriction enzymes. Southern analysis is subsequently used to examine the banding pattern of the digested products. The use of methylation-sensitive enzymes, such as *Hpa*II and *Hha*I, is advantageous, since these enzymes do not cut methylated sequences and do not digest

inactivated X chromosomes. According to the Lyon hypothesis of X chromosome inactivation, the inactive X chromosome is usually hypermethylated *(42)*. Since one X chromosome is randomly inactive in each cell of a female during early embryonic development, the RFLP fragment remains intact in an informative subject, whereas the other X chromosome fragment is degraded. By performing clonal analysis after enzyme digestion in normal tissues, one detects polyclonal populations of both alleles, but in neoplastic proliferations in which one allele is inactive, a monoclonal population or one band is detected by RFLP (Figure 4). Normal peripheral lymphocyte DNA is often used as a control tissue to compare to the neoplasm that is being studied in these analyses, since it is polyclonal.

More recent approaches to clonal analyses have used methods based on polymorphism of the X chromosome-linked androgen receptor and on random inactivation of these gene by methylation *(43,44)*.

Many studies of clonal analysis in pituitary adenomas have been reported *(45–48)*. Herman et al. *(45)* analyzed various pituitary adenomas and found that somatotroph adenomas, lactotroph adenomas, and corticotroph adenomas, and gonadotroph adenoma were all monoclonal, whereas normal pituitary tissue was polyclonal. These data suggested that somatic cell mutations occurred before clonal expansion of the neoplasm. Jacoby et al. *(46)* reported similar findings in a study of 12 adenomas from selected female patients. In this analysis, three pituitary adenomas were informative for the clonal analysis and these included one mixed prolactin–GH adenoma, one gonadotroph adenoma, and a nonfunctional adenoma. Alexander et al. *(47)* found monoclonal inactivation in six clinically nonfunctional pituitary tumors. Not all clonal analysis of pituitary tumors have found monoclonal populations. For example, in the study by Schulte et al., *(48)* six tumors from patients with Cushing's disease, including four with macroadenomas and two microadenomas, showed monoclonal population. There were three additional pituitary adenomas, including one microadenoma and two macroadenomas, which showed a polyclonal pattern of X chromosome inactivation. The latter findings and occasional reports of polyclonal tumors in other studies suggest that some corticotroph adenomas may arise from a single cell or possibly from more than one cell.

PCR ANALYSIS OF ONCOGENES, SUPPRESSOR GENES AND OTHER GENE PRODUCTS IN PITUITARY ADENOMAS

DNA amplification by the PCR has greatly influenced the study of pituitary disorders. In a typical PCR reaction, small amounts of DNA can be amplified up to 1 million fold and the final product analyzed by various techniques, including polyacrylamide gel electrophoresis with ethidium bromide staining of the bands and Southern hybridization (49). Messenger RNA expression in cells can also be analyzed by PCR by a combination of reverse transcriptase to generate cDNA with subsequent amplification of the cDNA. This approach has been used in the study of pituitary disorders by many investigators (50–53). The primers are oligonucleotides of 18–30 bases, with sense and antisense orientations relative to the DNA sequence, which are added to the target DNA samples along with *Taq* DNA polymerase. The primers hybridize to the target to provide a starting point for the polymerase to begin synthesizing the second strand of DNA. The DNA is heated to denature the two strands after synthesis is completed and then cooled to allow reannealing of the primers. Repeating of the cycles from 10 to 40 times results in specific target sequences that are greatly amplified and can be readily detected by polyacrylamide gel analysis. Approximately 10^5 or 10^6 amplifications of the target DNA can be performed in a few hours after 20–40 cycles. Advantages of the PCR technique include:

1. The ability to use very small samples to produce amplified DNA.
2. The great flexibility of this technique in its application to many problems in molecular biology.
3. The ease of automating this technology.

PCR analyses have been used extensively in the study of pituitary disorders (48,50–71). Analysis of GH-secreting adenomas showed mutations of the α gene of the guanine nucleotide binding protein G_s, which stabilizes the protein active conformation by inhibiting the intrinsic guanosine triphosphatase activity. GH tumors with this mutation had increased secretory activity; ultrastructural studies showed densely granulated cells with prominent rough endoplasmic reticulum and Golgi regions. The mutated GH tumors were smaller than other GH tumors without the G_s mutation and were more sensitive to inhibitory agents, such as somatostatin and dopamine. PCR techniques characterized the G mutant proteins at two critical sites, namely arginine 201 and glycine 227. This G_s mutation was present in approx 40% of patients with GH-secreting tumors. Although patients with prolactin, TSH, ACTH, and nonfunctional tumors did not have this mutation, more recent studies have found G_s mutations in ACTH and nonfunctional adenomas (67,68). These findings have suggested that G_s mutations in pituitary GH tumors may arise from a yet-to-be characterized specific oncogene. Yoshimoto et al. (53) found G_s α-mutations in 4 of 53 pituitary tumors, in a small percentage of thyroid neoplasm as well as adrenocortical adenomas. In contrast, many other endocrine tumors including parathyroid, pancreatic endocrine and pheochromocytomas did not have G_s mutation, indicating that specific subsets of endocrine tumors have G_s mutations.

In an in vitro analysis of GH tumors with and without gsp mutations by Adams et al. (71), GHRH stimulated gsp-negative tumors strongly, and the basal phosphatidylinusitol turnover rate was elevated in some gsp-negative tumors, suggesting that defects in this second messenger system were present in a subset of gsp-negative GH tumors (52).

PCR techniques have been used to analyze other types of mutations in pituitary tumors. Alvaro et al. (51) recently found that there was a point mutation in position 294 of the protein in the B3 region of protein kinase C-α isoform that resulted in overexpression of the PKC α-isoform in human pituitary tumors. This mutation was seen more commonly in invasive tumor compared to noninvasive tumors.

The presence of hypothalamic releasing hormones have been detected in the pituitary gland by PCR in recent years. Pagesy et al. (35) detected gonadotropic hormone releasing hormone (GnRH) messenger RNA in the anterior pituitary of the rat. Other studies have detected GHRH messenger RNA in human pituitary tumors using PCR techniques (53). As discussed earlier GHRH messenger RNA was localized by Levy and Lightman, by ISH in human pituitary tumors (34). PCR techniques have also been helpful in analyzing molecular heterogeneity in pituitary hormone genes. Kamijo and Phillips (54) studied isolated GH deficiency type Ia, which is caused by deletion in GH-1 genes. These investigators confirmed the heterogeneity of GH-1 gene deletions by showing differences for each of the three deletion sizes studied. They reported that the location and the sizes of all deletions agreed with previous size estimates based on Southern blot analysis, and that the clinical differences observed in the development of anti-GH antibodies and poor growth responses after GH treatment were unexplained since they observe discordant outcomes in patients who had deletions of the same size and approximate locations of the GH-1 gene. Another GH deficiency by PCR (55) detected GH type IA deficiency in subjects with severe growth retardation. In a cohort of seven Chinese subjects with severe growth retardation, they identified two subjects with isolated GH deficiency type IA, suggesting that this approach could be used to detect this type of GH deficiency in children with severe GH deficiency of early onset.

The combination of ISH and PCR should be ideal for the morphologist to visualize low abundant messages in cells. Ongoing studies in various laboratories are using this approach to examine gene expression in pituitary cells and tumors (8). *In situ* reverse transcriptase-(RT)PCR works best with cytospin preparation and frozen tissue sections compared to paraffin sections. Localization of the amplified product by the indirect technique utilizing a separate ISH step is more specific than direct incorporation of deoxynucleotides during PCR amplification (5,8) (Figs. 4 and 5 and Color Plates).

SSCP ANALYSIS

The SSCP technique is a powerful and rapid way to detect gene mutations in DNA (56). It can be performed with fresh tissues or with paraffin blocks. This technique permits detection of sequence changes in single-stranded DNA fragments. The DNA fragment migrate on a nondenaturing polyacrylamide gel in a manner that is dependent on its conformation, which is related to ionic strength and temperature. Fragments between 50 and 400 bp are usually analyzed. After electrophoresis, mutations in the DNA appear as shifts in the single-strand DNA bands when compared with the wild-type control sequence. In the typical analysis, samples are run at several temperatures with and without glycerol and then analyzed by autoradiography or by nonisotopic methods. SSCP has been used to screen pituitary tumors for G-protein mutations (57), mutations of *ras* oncogene, p53, and retinoblastoma suppressor genes (58,59). These recent studies have shown that although typical adenomas do not express these mutations commonly, occasional aggressive adenomas and pituitary carcinomas may have mutations in p53. Retinoblastoma suppressor genes muta-

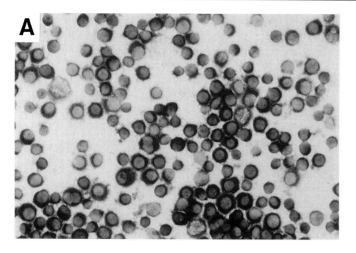

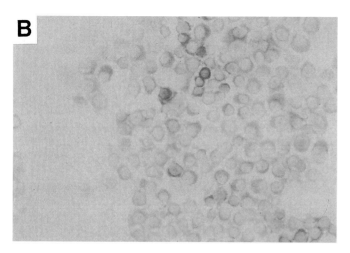

Figure 8-5   Comparison of *in situ* RT-PCR and ISH to detect PRL mRNA in GH₃ cells grown in serum-free media with low PRL mRNA levels. **(A)** *In situ* RT-PCR detects a strong signal for PRL by the indirect method in all of the tumor cells (×250). **(B)** There is a weak and focal hybridization signal for PRL mRNA detected by ISH in the same population of GH₃ cells (×250). (*See* Color Plates, following p. 176.)

tions have been reported to be uncommon in human pituitary tumors *(60,61)*. However, loss of heterozygosity of 13q markers in pituitary carcinomas has been reported to suggest another tumor suppressor gene on 13q *(70)*.

Analysis of oncogene mutation in pituitary tumors, especially H-*ras* has shown rare point mutations of *ras* in aggressive adenomas *(59,62)*, but in few pituitary carcinomas *(66)*.

MOLECULAR ANALYSIS OF GROWTH FACTORS IN THE PITUITARY

The role of growth factors in pituitary tumor proliferation and differentiation is currently under intense investigation. A variety of growth factors have been examined in human pituitary cells in vitro *(48,72,73)*. These polypeptide molecules can stimulate or inhibit cell proliferation and modulate cell differentiation. Growth factors that have been identified in the pituitary include: epidermal growth factor (EGF), transforming growth factor (TGF) α and β, insulin-like growth factors (IGF-1 and IGF-2), nerve growth factor (NGF), and

fibroblast growth factor (FGF) among others *(74,75)*. Receptors for many of these growth factors have also been identified in the pituitary.

EGF receptors have been found in normal human pituitary cells *(76)* using biochemical assays. Although EGF binding was readily detected in normal human pituitary tissues obtained from postmortem specimens, it was not detected in any of the 22 pituitary adenomas studied. One possible explanation was the possibility of an altered c-*erb*-B proto-oncogene, which normally encodes the wild-type EGF receptor. Basic fibroblast growth factor (bFGF), and angiogenic and mitogenic factor in many cells have been found in the bovine and human pituitary gland tissues. Silverlight et al. *(73)* observed that bFGF was more abundant in normal human pituitaries than in pituitary adenoma as evaluated by immunohistochemistry, which suggests that reduction in the levels of this growth factor in many pituitary tumors may favor the stimulation of pituitary growth.

Other growth factors, including IGF, have been analyzed in human pituitaries using molecular and cell biological techniques. The IGFs are homologous to proinsulin and share metabolic properties with insulin, growth stimulation, and metabolic effects. IGF-1 and somatostatin-C have been found in normal and neoplastic rat pituitary tissues. IGF may be under the control of GH, and probably participates in the endocrine and paracrine pathways in the regulation of GH synthesis and secretion *(77)*. In vitro studies have shown that various growth factors can stimulate differentiation in cultured pituitary cells *(78,79)*. Atkin et al. *(78)* showed that IGF-1 in cultured gonadotroph pituitary adenomas stimulated FSH secretion as well as the number of glycoprotein-secreting cells entering the S-phase of proliferation cycle. This is one of the few examples in which growth factors stimulated cell proliferation in human pituitary tumors.

OTHER MOLECULAR BIOLOGICAL STUDIES

Cytogenetic analyses of pituitary tumors have contributed to our knowledge about these neoplasms. Rock et al. *(63)* recently examined the karyotypes of 18 resected pituitary tumors, and found abnormalities associated with chromosomes 1, 4, 7, and 19 in some tumors. Thakker et al. *(64)* observed lesions involving 11q13 in 4 of 12 sporadic GH-producing pituitary tumors. The 11q13 region of chromosome 11 is associated with tumor development with multiple endocrine neoplasia type I, including tumors of the pituitary, parathyroid, and pancreas. In a subsequent study, Boggild et al. *(65)* analyzed pituitary tumors from 88 patients and found activating dominant mutations of G$_s$α by PCR in 36% of the tumors. They found deletions of chromosome 11 in 16 tumors (18%). These deletions were found in all four major subtypes of pituitary tumors, including GH, prolactin, ACTH, and nonfunctional tumors. Deletions on other autosomal chromosomes were found in <6% of the tumors. In addition, they found multiple autosomal losses in two aggressive adenomas and suggested that there may be a multistep progression in the development of these more aggressive neoplasms. Interestingly, they did not find amplification or rearrangement of various cellular oncogenes examined, including N-*ras*, *myc*, H-*ras*, and *fos* in the adenomas.

More recent studies have used new techniques such as comparative genomic hybridization (CGH) to detect new genetic abnormalities in pituitary adenomas *(65a)*.

Dysregulation of pituitary cell cycle proteins such as p27 and p16 have been reported in pituitary adenomas *(65b,65c)*.

Table 1
Transcription Factors in the Pituitary Gland[a]

Class	Examples	Examples in pituitary
Helix-turn-helix	Homeobox or homeodomain	Pit-1/GHF-1
Zinc finger	Steroid hormone receptors	Estrogen receptor, Ad4 BP/SF1
	Thyroid hormone receptor	
	Retinic acid receptor	
Leucine zipper	c *Jun*, c *fos*	c-*Jun*, c-*fos*
	CREB	CREB
Helix-loop-helix	Muscle transcription factors (MyoD)	TEF
	c-*myc* gene	c-*myc*

[a]CREB—cyclic AMP response element binding protein.
TEF—thyrotroph embryonic factor.

TRANSCRIPTION FACTORS AND PITUITARY DISEASES

Transcription factors are proteins that bind to regulatory elements in the promoter and enhancer regions of DNA. They have critical roles in gene regulation during development, in cellular growth, and in differentiation. After interacting with DNA, transcription factors can stimulate (or inhibit) gene expression, RNA, and protein production. The study of transcription factors is a rapidly developing area of molecular biology *(80–83)*. Analysis of these factors have contributed to our understanding of various molecular diseases in a relatively short period.

Various transcription factors have been described in the pituitary gland (Table 1). The pit-1, helix-turn-helix transcription factor has been one of the most studied DNA regulatory proteins in recent years *(84–92)*. Pit-1 is widely distributed in normal and neoplastic cells in the anterior pituitary, but the highest levels are in GH, prolactin, and thyroid-stimulating hormone cells and tumors. Deficiencies of pit-1 in humans, which are usually caused by mutations in codons 271, 185, 172, and 24, are associated with dwarfism and/or cretinism *(84–92)*. The role of pit-1 in pituitary tumor development is uncertain. Although pit-1 may be important for pituitary cell proliferation in experimental system *(84)*, there is no increased expression of this transcription factor in pituitary tumors. The role of the other transcription factors listed in Table 1 in diseases involving the pituitary gland is uncertain at this time. The cyclic adenosine monophosphate response element binding protein (CREB), a member of the leucine zipper group, is widely distributed in many tissues, including the pituitary gland. Mutations in CREB have resulted in dwarfism and somatotroph hypoplasia in transgenic mice *(93)*.

Recent studies of the *MEN1* tumor suppressor gene in sporadic pituitary tumors have suggested that mutation or imprinting does not play a prominent role in sporadic pituitary adenoma pathogenesis *(94)*, although they may be important in a subgroup of these tumors *(95)*.

The occasional observation of genetic instability, including autosomal deletions in pituitary tumors, suggests a multistep model of neoplasia in these tumors. However, unlike many tumors, such as colonic carcinoma in which multistep progression is common with subsequent metastatic tumor development, this progression is extremely uncommon in human pituitary tumors and the mechanisms inhibiting tumor progression in pituitary and other endocrine tumors are currently unknown *(96)*.

This overview of molecular analysis of pituitary disorders highlights the rapid progress that has been made during the past few years in understanding the molecular basis of pituitary diseases. We can anticipate an ever-increasing amount of information about the molecular basis of pituitary diseases during the coming years.

REFERENCES

1. Lloyd RV, Iacangelo A, Eiden LE, Cano M, Jin L, Grimes M. Chromogranin A and B messenger ribonucleic acids in pituitary and other normal and neoplastic human endocrine tissues. Lab Invest 1989;60:548–556.
2. Singer RH, Lawrence JB, Villnave C. Optimization of *in situ* hybridization using isotopic and non-isotopic detection methods. Biotechniques 1986;4:230–259.
3. Gee CE, Roberts JL. *In situ* hybridization histochemistry; a technique for the study of gene expression in single cells. DNA 1983;2:157–163.
4. Hankin RC, Lloyd RV. Detection of messenger RNA in routinely processed tissue sections with biotinylated oligonucleotide probes. Am J Clin Pathol 1989;92:166–171.
5. Bagasra O, Seshamma T, Pomerantz RJ. Polymerase chain reaction *in situ*: intracellular amplification and detection of HIV-1 proviral DNA and other specific genes. J Immunol Methods 1993;158:131–145.
6. Chen RH, Fuggle SV. In situ cDNA polymerase chain reaction. A novel technique for detecting mRNA expression. Am J Pathol 1993;143:1527–1534.
7. Nuovo GJ, MacConnell P, Forde A, Delvonne P. Detection of human papilloma virus DNA in formalin-fixed tissues by *in situ* hybridization after amplification by polymerase chain reaction. Am J Pathol 1991;139:845–854.
8. Jin L, Qian X, Lloyd RV. Comparison of mRNA expression detected by in situ PCR and in situ hybridization in endocrine cells. Cell Vision 1995;2:314–321.
9. Pixley S, Weiss M, Melmed S. Identification of human growth hormone messenger ribonucleic acid in pituitary adenoma cells by *in situ* hybridization. J Clin Endocrinol Metab 1987;65:575–580.
10. Lloyd RV, Cano M, Chandler WF, Barkan AL, Horvath E, Kovacs K. Human growth hormone and prolactin secreting pituitary adenomas analyzed by *in situ* hybridization. Am J Pathol 1989;134:605–613.
11. Lloyd RV. Analysis of human pituitary tumors by *in situ* hybridization. Pathol Res Pract 1988;183:558–560.
12. Levy A, Lightman SL. Quantitative *in situ* hybridization histochemistry studies on growth hormone (GH) gene expression in acromegalic somatotrophs: effects of somatostatin, GH-releasing factor and cortisol. J Mol Endocrinol 1988;1:19–26.
13. Levy A, Lightman SL. Relationship between somatostatin and growth hormone messenger ribonucleic acid in human pituitary adenomas: an *in situ* hybridization histochemistry study. Clin Endocrinol 1990;32:661–668.
14. Kovacs K, Lloyd RV, Horvath E, Asa SL, Stefaneanu L, Killinger DW, et al. Silent somatotroph adenomas of the human pituitary. A morphologic study of three cases including immunocytochemistry, electron microscopy, *in vitro* examination and *in situ* hybridization. Am J Pathol 1989;134:345–353.

15. Trouillas J, Sassolas G, Loras B, Velkeniers B, Raccurt M, Chotard L, et al. Somatotropic adenomas without acromegaly. Pathol Res Pract 1991;187:943–949.

16. Saeger W, Uhlig H, Bäz E, Fehr S, Ludecke DK. *In situ* hybridization for different mRNA in GH-secreting and in inactive pituitary adenomas. Pathol Res Pract 1991;187:559–563.

17. Stefaneanu L, Kovacs K, Lloyd RV, Scheithauer BW, Young WF Jr, Sano T, et al. Pituitary lactotrophs and somatotrophs in pregnancy: a correlative in situ hybridization and immunocytochemical study. Virchows Arch [B] 1992;62:291–296.

18. Kovacs K, Stefaneanu L, Horvath E, Lloyd RV, Lancranjan I, Buchfelder M, et al. Effect of dopamine agonist medication and prolactin-producing pituitary adenomas: A morphological study including immunocytochemistry, electron microscopy and *in situ* hybridization. Virchows Arch [A] Pathol Anat Histopathol 1991; 418:439–446.

19. Lloyd RV, Fields K, Jin L, Horvath E, Kovacs K. Analysis of endocrine active and clinically silent corticotropic adenomas by *in situ* hybridization. Am J Pathol 1990;137:479–488.

20. Stefaneanu L, Kovacs K, Horvath E, Lloyd RV. *In situ* hybridization study of pro-opiomelanocortin (POMC) gene expression in human pituitary corticotrophs and their adenomas. Virchows Arch [A] 1991;419:107–113.

21. Nagaya T, Seo H, Kuwayama A, Sakurai T, Tsukamoto N, Nakane T, et al. Proopiomelanocortin gene expression in silent corticotroph cell adenoma and Cushing's disease. J Neurosurg 1990;72:262–267.

22. de Keyzer Y, Bertagna X, Luton JP, Kahn A. Variable modes of proopiomelanocortin gene transcription in human tumors. Mol Endocrinol 1989;3:215–223.

23. McNicol AM, Farquharson MA, Walker E. Non-isotopic *in situ* hybridization with digoxigenin and alkaline-phosphatase-labeled oligodeoxynucleotide probes. Applications in pituitary gland. Pathol Res Pract 1991;187:556–558.

24. Fehn M, Farquharson MA, Sautner P, Saeger W, Lüdecke DK, McNicol AM. Demonstration of pro-opiomelanocortin mRNA in pituitary adenomas and para-adenomatous gland in Cushing's disease and Nelson's Syndrome. J Pathol 1993;169:335–339.

25. Mengod G, Vivanco MM, Christnacher A, Probst A, Palacios JM. Study of pro-opiomelanocortin mRNA expression in human postmortem pituitaries. Mol Brain Res 1991;10:129–137.

26. Lopez JF, Palkovits M, Arato M, Mansour A, Akil H, Watson SJ. Localization and quantification of pro-opiomelanocortin mRNA and glucocorticoid receptor mRNA in pituitaries of suicide victims. Neuroendocrinology 1992;56:491–501.

27. Lloyd RV, Jin L, Fields K, Chandler WF, Horvath E, Stefaneanu L, et al. Analysis of pituitary hormones and chromogranin A mRNAs in null cell adenomas, oncocytomas and gonadotroph adenomas by *in situ* hybridization. Am J Pathol 1991;139:553–564.

28. Bäz E, Saeger W, Uhlig H, Fehr S, Lüdecke DK. HGH, PRL and βHCG/βLH gene expression in clinically inactive pituitary adenomas detected by *in situ* hybridization. Virchows Arch [A] 1991;418:405–410.

29. Sakurai T, Seo H, Yamamoto N, Nagaya T, Nakane T, Kuwayama A, et al. Detection of mRNA of prolactin and ACTH in clinically nonfunctioning pituitary adenomas. J Neurosurg 1988;69:653–659.

30. Lloyd RV, Jin L. Analysis of chromogranin/secretogranin messenger RNAs in human pituitary adenomas. Diagn Mol Pathol 1994; 3:38–45.

31. Song JY, Jin L, Chandler WF, England BG, Smart JB, Landefeld TD, et al. Gonadotropin-releasing hormone regulates gonadotropin beta-subunit and chromogranin B mRNA in cultured chromogranin A positive pituitary adenomas. J Clin Endocrinol Metab 1990; 71:622–630.

32. Kilar F, Muhr C, Funa K. *In situ* hybridization histochemistry of mRNAs for hormones and chromogranins in normal pituitary tissue and pituitary adenoma. Acta Endocrinol 1991;125:628–636.

33. Jin L, Chandler WF, Smart JB, England BG, Lloyd RV. Differentiation of human pituitary adenomas determines the pattern of chromogranin/secretogranin messenger ribonucleic acid expression. J Clin Endocrinol Metab 1993;76:728–735.

34. Levy A, Lightman SL. Growth hormone releasing hormone transcripts in human pituitary adenomas. J Clin Endocrinol Metab 1992;74:1474–1476.

35. Pagesy P, Li JY, Berthet M, Peillon F. Evidence of gonadotropin-releasing hormone mRNA in the rat anterior pituitary. Mol Endocrinol 1992;6:523–528.

36. Li JY, Pagesy P, Berthet M, Racadot O, Kujas M, Racadot J, et al. Somatostatin cells in human somatotropic adenoma. Virchows Arch [A] 1992;420:95–101.

37. Lloyd RV, Jin L, Chandler WF, Horvath E, Stefaneanu L, Kovacs K. Pituitary specific transcription factor messenger ribonucleic acid expression in adenomatous and non-tumorous human pituitary tissues. Lab Invest 1993;69:570–575.

38. Asa SL, Puy LA, Lew AM, Sundmark VC, Elsholtz HP. Cell type-specific expression of the pituitary transcription activator pit-1 in the human pituitary and pituitary adenomas. J Clin Endocrinol Metab 1993;77:1275–1280.

39. Vogelstein B, Fearon ER, Hamilton SR, Feinberg AP. Use of restriction fragment length polymorphisms to determine the clonal origin of human tumors. Science 1985;227:642–645.

40. Hicks DG, LiVolsi VA, Neidich JA, Puck JM, Kant JA. Clonal analysis of solitary follicular nodules in the thyroid. Am J Pathol 1990;137:553–562.

41. Keshet I, Lieman-Hurwitz J, Cedar H. DNA methylation affects the formation of active chromatin. Cell 1986;44:535–543.

42. Lyon MF. X-chromosome inactivation and developmental patterns in mammals. Biol Rev Cambridge Philosophic Soc 1972;47:1–35.

43. Noguchi S, Motomura K, Inaji H, Imaoka S, Koyama H. Clonal analysis of human breast cancer by means of polymerase chain reaction. Cancer Res 1992;52:6594–6597.

44. Allen RC, Zoghbi HY, Moseley AB, Rosenblatt HM, Belmont JW. Methylation of Hpa II and HhaI sites near the polymorphic CAG repeat in the human androgen-receptor gene correlates with X chromosome inactivation. Am J Hum Genet 1992;51:1229–1239.

45. Herman V, Fagin J, Gonsky R, Kovacs K, Melmed S. Clonal origin of pituitary adenomas. J Clin Endocrinol Metab 1990;71: 1427–1433.

46. Jacoby LB, Hedley-Whyte T, Pulaski K, Seizinger BR, Martuza RL. Clonal origin of pituitary adenomas. J Neurosurg 1990;73:731–735.

47. Alexander JM, Biller BM, Bikkal H, Zervas NT, Arnold A, Klibanski A. Clinically nonfunctioning pituitary tumors are monoclonal in origin. J Clin Invest 1990;86:336–340.

48. Asa SL, Ezzat S. The cytogenesis and pathogenesis of pituitary adenomas. Endocr Rev 1998;19:798–827.

49. Mullis KB, Faloona FA. Specific synthesis of DNA in vitro via a polymerase-catalyzed chain reaction. Methods Enzymol 1987;155: 335–350.

50. Landis CA, Masters SB, Spada A, Pace AM, Bourne HR, Vallar L. GTPase inhibiting mutations activate the α chain of G_s and stimulate adenylyl cyclase in human pituitary tumors. Nature 1989;340: 692–696.

51. Alvaro V, Levy L, Dubray C, Roche A, Peillon F, Querat B, et al. Invasive human pituitary tumors express a point-mutated α-protein kinase-C. J Clin Endocrinol Metab 1993;77:1125–1129.

52. Spada A, Arosio M, Bochicchio D, Bazzoni N, Vallar L, Bassetti M, et al. Clinical, biochemical and morphological correlates in patients bearing growth hormone-secreting pituitary tumors with or without constitutively active adenylyl cyclase. J Clin Endocrinol Metab 1990;71:1421–1426.

53. Wakabayashi I, Inokuchi K, Hasegawa O, Sugihara H, Minami S. Expression of growth hormone (GH)-releasing factor gene in GH-producing pituitary adenoma. J Clin Endocrinol Metab 1992; 74:357–361.

53. Yoshimoto K, Iwahana H, Fukuda A, Sano T, Itakura M. Rare mutations of the G_s alpha subunit gene in human endocrine tumors. Mutation detection by polymerase chain reaction-primer-introduced restriction analysis. Cancer 1993;72:1386–1393.

54. Kamijo T, Phillips JA III. Detection of molecular heterogeneity in GH-1 gene deletions by analysis of polymerase chain reaction amplification products. J Clin Endocrinol Metab 1992;74:786–789.

163

55. Vnencak-Jones CL, Phillips JA, DeFen W. Use of polymerase chain reaction in detection of growth hormone gene deletions. J Clin Endocrinol Metab 1990;70:1550–1553.

56. Orita M, Iwahana H, Kanazawa H, Hayashi K, Sekiya T. Detection of polymorphisms of human DNA by gel electrophoresis as single-strand conformation polymorphisms. Proc Natl Acad Sci USA 1989;86:2766–2770.

57. Drews RT, Gravel RA, Collu R. Identification of G protein a subunit mutations in human growth hormone (GH)- and GH/prolactin-secreting pituitary tumors by single-strand conformation polymorphism (SSCP) analysis. Mol Cell Endocrinol 1992;87:125–129.

57. Herman V, Drazin NZ, Gonsky R, Melmed S. Molecular screening of pituitary adenomas for gene mutations and rearrangements. J Clin Endocrinol Metab 1993;77:50–55.

59. Pei L, Melmed S, Scheithauer BW, Kovacs K, Prager D. H-ras mutations in human pituitary carcinoma metastases. J Clin Endocrinol Metab 1994;78:842–846.

60. Cryns VL, Alexander JM, Klibanski A, Arnold A. The retinoblastoma gene in human pituitary tumors. J Clin Endocrinol Metab 1993;77:644–646.

61. Zhu J, Leon SP, Beggs AH, Busque L, Gilliland DG, Black PM. Human pituitary adenomas show no loss of heterozygosity at the retinoblastoma gene locus. J Clin Endocrinol Metab 1994;78:922–927.

62. Karga HJ, Alexander JM, Hedley-Whyte ET, Klibansky A, Jameson JL. Ras mutation in human pituitary tumors. J Clin Endocrinol Metab 1992;74:914–919.

63. Rock JP, Babu VR, Drumheller T, Chason J. Cytogenetic findings in pituitary adenoma: Results of a pilot study. Surg Neurol 1993;40:224–229.

64. Thakker RV, Pook MA, Wooding C, Boscaro M, Scanarini M, Clayton RN. Association of somatotrophinomas with loss of alleles on chromosome II and with gsp mutations. J Clin Invest 1993;91:2815–2821.

65. Boggild MD, Jenkinson S, Pistorello M, Boscaro M, Scanarini M, McTernan P, et al. Molecular genetic studies of sporadic pituitary tumors. J Clin Endocrinol Metab 1994;78:387–392.

65a. Daniel M, Aviram A, Adams EF, Buchfelder M, Barkai G, Fahlbusch R, et al. Comparative genomic hybridization analysis of nonfunctioning pituitary tumors. J Clin Endocrinol Metab 1998;83:1801–1805.

65b. Lloyd RV, Jin L, Qian X, Kulig E. Aberrant p27^{Kip1} expression in endocrine and other tumors. Am J Pathol 1997;150:401–407.

65c. Woloschak M, Yu A, Post KD. Frequent inactivation of the p16 gene in human pituitary tumors by gene methylation. Mol Carcinogenesis 1997;19:221–224.

66. Cai WY, Alexander JM, Hedley-Whyte ET, et al. Ras mutations in human prolactinomas and pituitary carcinomas. J Clin Endocrinol Metab 1994;78:89–93.

67. Williamson EA, Daniels M, Foster S, et al. Giα alpha and gi2 alpha mutations in clinically non-functioning pituitary tumours. Clin Endocrinol 1994;41:815–820.

68. Williamson EA, Ince PG, Harrison D, et al. G-protein mutations in human pituitary adrenocorticotrophic hormone-secreting adenomas. Eur J Clin Invest 1995;25:128–131.

70. Pei L, Melmed S, Scheithauer B, Kovacs K, Benedict WF, Prager D. Frequent loss of heterozygosity at the retinoblastoma susceptibility gene (RB) locus in aggressive pituitary tumors: evidence for a chromosome 13 tumor suppressor gene other than RB. Cancer Res 1995;55:1613–1616.

71. Adams EF, Lei T, Buchfelder M, Petersen B, Fahlbusch R. Biochemical characteristics of human pituitary somatotrophinomas with and without gsp mutations: in vitro cell culture studies. J Clin Endocrinol Metab 1995;80:2077–2081.

72. Ezzat S, Melmed S. The role of growth factors in the pituitary. J Endocrinol Invest 1990;13:691–698.

73. Silverlight JJ, Prysor-Jones RA, Jenkins JS. Basic fibroblast growth factor in human pituitary tumors. Clin Endocrinol 1990;32:669–676.

74. Halper J, Parnell PG, Carter BJ, Reu P, Scheithauer BW. Presence of growth factors in human pituitary. Lab Invest 1992;66:639–645.

75. Jin L, Song J, Chandler WF, England BG, Smart JB, Barkan A, et al. Hybridization studies of cultured human pituitary PRL- and GH-producing adenoma cells: Effects of thyrotropin-releasing hormone, somatostatin and phorbol ester. Endocr Pathol 1990;1:25–36.

76. Birman P, Michard M, Li JY, Peillon F, Bression D. Epidermal growth factor-binding sites, present in normal human and rat pituitaries, are absent in human pituitary adenomas. J Clin Endocrinol Metab 1987;65:275–281.

77. Fagin JA, Pixley S, Slanina S, Ong J, Melmed S. Insulin-like growth factor I gene expression in GH3 rat pituitary cells: Messenger ribonucleic acid content, immunocytochemistry and secretion. Endocrinology 1987;120:2037–2043.

78. Atkin SL, Landolt AM, Jeffreys RV, Hipkin L, Radcliffe J, Squire CR, et al. Differential effects of insulin-like growth factor 1 on the hormonal product and proliferation of glycoprotein-secreting human pituitary adenomas. J Clin Endocrinol Metab 1993;77:1059–1066.

79. Chaidarun SS, Eggo MC, Stewart PM, Barber PC, Sheppard MC. Role of growth factors and estrogen as modulators of growth, differentiation and expression of gonadotropin subunit genes in primary cultured sheep pituitary cells. Endocrinology 1994;134:935–944.

80. Pabo CO, Sauer RT. Transcription factors: structural families and principles of DNA recognition. Ann Rev Biochem 1992;61:1053–1095.

81. Papavassilious AG. Molecular medicine. Transcription factors. N Engl J Med 1995;332:45–47.

82. Vellanoweth RL, Suprakar PC, Roy AK. Transcription factors in development growth and aging. Lab Invest 1994;70:784–799.

83. Nakamura S, Ohtsaru A, Takamura N, Kitange G, Tokunaga Y, et al. Prop-1 gene expression in human pituitary tumors. J Clin Endocrinol Metab 1999;84:2581–2584.

84. Castrillo JL, Theill LE, Karin M. Function of the homeodomain protein GHF-1 in pituitary cell proliferation. Science 1991;253:199.

85. Hoggard N, Callaghan K, Levy A, Davis JR. Expression of Pit-1 and related proteins in diverse human pituitary adenomas. J Mol Endocrinol 1993;11:283–290.

86. Voss JW, Rosenfeld MG. Anterior pituitary development: short tales from dwarf mice. Cell 1992;70:527–530.

87. Lloyd RV, Jin L, Chandler WF, Horvath E, Stefaneanu L, Kovacs K. Pituitary specific transcription factor messenger ribonucleic acid expression in adenomatous and nontumorous human pituitary tissues. Lab Invest 1993;69:570–575.

88. Sanno N, Inada K, Utsunomiya H, Umemura S, Itoh Y, Matsuno A, et al. Expression for pit-1 product in human pituitaries: histochemical studies using an antibody against synthetic human pit-1 protein. Med Sci Res 1994;22:685–687.

89. Ohta K, Nobukani Y, Mitsubuchi H, Fujimoto S, Matsuo N, Inagaki H, et al. Mutations in the pit-1 gene in children with combined pituitary hormone deficiency. Biochem Biophys Res Commun 1992;189:851–855.

90. Pfaffle RW, DiMattia GE, Parks JS, Brown MR, Wit JM, Jansen M, et al. Mutation of the POU-specific domain of Pit-1 and hypopituitarism without pituitary hypoplasia. Science (Washington) 1992;257:1118–1121.

91. Radovick S, Nations M, Du Y, Berg LA, Weintraub BD, Wondisford FE. A mutation in the POU-homeodomain of Pit-1 responsible for combined pituitary hormone deficiency. Science (Washington) 1992;257:1115–1118.

92. Tatsumi K, Miyai K, Natomi T, Kaibe K, Amino N, Mizuno Y, et al. Cretinism with combined hormone deficiency caused by a mutation in the Pit-1 gene. Nature Genet 1992;1:56–58.

93. Struthers RS, Vale WW, Arias C, Sawchenko PE, Montminy MR. Somatotroph hypoplasia and dwarfism in transgenic mice expressing a nonphosphorylatable CREB mutant. Nature 1991;350:622–624.

94. Prezant TR, Levine J, Melmed S. Molecular characterization of the MenI tumor suppressor gene in sporadic pituitary tumors. J Clin Endocrinol Metab 1998;83:1388–1391.

95. Zhuang Z, Ezzat SZ, Vortmeyer AO, West R, Oldfield EH, Park W-S, et al. Mutations of the MEN I tumor suppressor gene in pituitary tumors. Cancer Res 1997;57:5446–5451.

96. Farrell WE, Clayton RN. Molecular biology of human pituitary adenomas. Ann Med 1998;30:192–198.

9 Diagnosis, Management, and Prognosis of Pituitary Tumors

General Considerations

MARY LEE VANCE, MD

INTRODUCTION

The identification and management of a pituitary tumor is straightforward once the potential diagnosis is entertained. The greatest difficulty in clinical medicine is the delay in diagnosis because of a nonspecific clinical feature, such as headache, which is attributed to "stress" or a migraine syndrome. Similarly, nonspecific complaints of decreased energy, libido, and weight gain may be attributed to depression or aging. Thus, the greatest challenge to the physician is to entertain the possibility that a patient's symptoms may be related to a pituitary tumor and/or pituitary dysfunction. Because of excellent imaging technology, magnetic resonance imaging (MRI), many patients are now found to have a pituitary lesion incidentally—the study was obtained to "rule out" intracranial pathology because of trauma or headaches. Once a pituitary tumor is considered or found, it is then necessary to determine the type of tumor (secretory, nonsecretory), pituitary function (hypo- and hyperfunction), the need for hormone replacement, and the status of the visual system before recommending appropriate therapy.

PREVALENCE

Pituitary adenomas and other pituitary masses are common. A review of 13 autopsy studies of 9737 pituitary glands from patients without suspected pituitary disease demonstrated that a microadenoma (<10 mm) was present in 1072 glands (11%). The tumor detection rate varied among studies ranging from 1.5 to 27% *(1)*. In studies in which immunostaining for prolactin was performed, 42% of tumors were positive for prolactin. A macroadenoma (>10 mm) was present in three (0.03%) specimens *(2)*.

In several studies of subjects with normal endocrine function who underwent an imaging study, a focal hypodensity of >3 mm on computed tomography (CT) scan was found in 4–20%; MRI studies revealed a focal hypodensity 3–6 mm in 10% and 2–5 mm in 38% of normal subjects *(3,4)*. Such a lesion in the setting of normal endocrine function is termed an "incidentaloma." The natural history of such lesions was characterized in 31 patients

From: *Diagnosis and Management of Pituitary Tumors* (K. Thapar, K. Kovacs, B. W. Scheithauer, and R. V. Lloyd, eds.), ©Humana Press Inc., Totowa, NJ.

followed for an average of 6.4 yr with serial CT scans. In 15 patients with a microadenoma, no change in size was noted during follow-up, but in 16 patients with a macroadenoma, 4 (25%) tumors enlarged and required surgical removal *(5)*. The most common types of pituitary adenomas are either nonfunctioning or prolactin-producing. A nonfunctioning tumor does not secrete a detectable hormone into the circulation, but tumor immunostaining is often positive for gonadotropins (luteinizing hormone [LH], follicle-stimulating hormone [FSH]) and/or the α-subunit. In Table 1 the types of lesions found in the sellar and parasellar areas is shown.

DIAGNOSIS

The biochemical diagnosis of pituitary hypersecretion and pituitary deficiency can usually be accomplished in the outpatient setting with blood and urine samples. Table 2 shows the necessary screening studies that should be performed at the initial visit to determine if there is excessive hormone production and to identify hormone deficiencies. Tables 3 and 4 show the dynamic studies that may be necessary as indicated clinically. The diagnosis of a pituitary tumor is both biochemical (endocrine studies) and anatomic (imaging studies)—both types of studies are necessary to provide maximal information and to direct appropriate therapy.

A patient with a pituitary tumor may experience the effects of a mass lesion, endocrine effects, or both. The most common manifestation of a mass lesion is headache, which may or may not be relieved with analgesic medication. The type of headache is nonspecific. Pain may occur in the orbital, frontal, temporal, or occipital region—there is no precise feature of a headache caused by a pituitary lesion. This lack of specificity may result in a clinical misdiagnosis of migraine or tension headache. Although headache is commonly ascribed to the lesion in a patient with a macroadenoma (>10 mm), a less-recognized phenomenon is that patients with a microadenoma (<10 mm) may also experience headache. The headache caused by a pituitary mass is thought to originate from tumor expansion within a small space with transmission of pressure to the surrounding dura, which contains nerve fibers.

The other prominent feature of the mass effect of a pituitary lesion is development of visual abnormalities. The classical abnormality occurs with superior extension of a tumor and compression of the optic chiasm resulting in a bitemporal loss of vision. In this setting, the first abnormality is a superior temporal quadrant

Table 1
Lesions of the Sella and Parasellar Regions

Pituitary adenoma
   Prolactin
   GH
   ACTH
   LH, FSH
   α-Subunit
   Nonsecretory
   Null cell
   Silent ACTH
   Silent GH
Cell rest tumors
   Craniopharyngioma
   Rathke's cleft cyst
   Epidermoid
   Chordoma
   Lipoma
Germ-cell tumors
   Germinoma
   Dermoid
   Teratoma
   Atypical teratoma (dysgerminoma)
Gliomas
   Chiasmatic-optic nerve glioma
   Oligodendroglioma
   Ependymoma
   Astrocytoma
   Microglioma
Metastatic tumor
Internal carotid artery aneurysm
Granuloma, infection, inflammatory lesions
   Sarcoid
   Giant-cell granuloma
   Histiocytosis X
   Lymphocytic hypophysitis
   Abscess
   Echinococcal cyst
   Mucocoele
Meningioma
Gangliocytoma
Hypothalamic hamartoma
Colloid cyst
Arachnoid cyst

Table 2
Screening Studies for Evaluation of a Pituitary Lesion

Hormone excess	Serum prolactin
	Serum IGF-1
	Serum LH, FSH
	Serum α-subunit
	Serum TSH
	24-h urine-free cortisol
Hormone deficiency	Serum cortisol (AM)
	Serum thyroxine (T4) or free T4
	Serum testosterone (men)
	Serum estradiol (premenopausal women)

Table 3
Dynamic Tests to Identify Pituitary Hormone Hypersecretion

Acromegaly (GH)	Oral glucose tolerance test
Cushing's syndrome/	Low-dose dexamethasone test
Cushing's disease	Low dose dexamethasone + CRH[a] test
	High-dose dexamethasone test
	Inferior petrosal sinus sampling + CRH[a]

[a]CRH: corticotropin-releasing hormone.

Table 4
Dynamic Tests to Identify Pituitary Deficiency

ACTH deficiency	Insulin tolerance test
	Metyrapone test
GH deficiency	Insulin tolerance test
	L-DOPA test
	Arginine test
	GHRH[a] test
	GHRP[b] test
Antidiuretic hormone (ADH) deficiency	Water deprivation test
Gonadotropin (LH, FSH) deficiency	GnRH[c] test

[a]GHRH: growth hormone-releasing hormone.
[b]GHRP: growth hormone-releasing peptide.
[c]GnRH: gonadotropin-releasing hormone.

defect, which may not be appreciated by the patient. If the tumor extends superiorly, anteriorly, and laterally, the patient may develop loss of vision in one eye, both nasal and temporal fields. Visual acuity may be affected adversely in both situations. Tumor extension laterally may impair oculomotor function, resulting most commonly in a third nerve palsy with ptosis and opthalmoplegia. A less frequent occurrence is a fourth nerve palsy with the inability to move the eye laterally. An area of misdiagnosis is attributing loss of visual acuity in older patients to macular degeneration or a cataract. The ophthalmologic evaluation in a patient with visual loss should include fundoscopy, assessment of acuity, and the visual field determination using automated perimetry (Goldmann, Humphries, Octopus).

Endocrine effects of a pituitary mass are classified according to hormone deficiency and hormone hypersecretory syndromes. In general, the larger the mass, the greater the probability of compromise of normal pituitary function. The exception to this observa-

tion is the adverse effect of hyperprolactinemia, even a mild elevation, on gonadal function. The most serious effect of a pituitary tumor on normal pituitary function is the loss of adrenocorticotropic hormone (ACTH) or thyroid-stimulating hormone (TSH) production resulting in secondary adrenal insufficiency and secondary hypothyroidism, respectively. These conditions are potentially life-threatening and require prompt diagnosis and treatment. Hypogonadism from loss of normal pulsatile LH and FSH secretion is a common pituitary deficiency associated with a pituitary tumor, although growth hormone (GH) deficiency is also common. Loss of cyclic menses or infertility in premenopausal women usually results in an early diagnosis, since these patients have an obvious marker of gonadal function and tend to seek medical consultation early in the course. Men develop loss of libido and erectile dysfunction, but may not seek medical advice early if these symptoms are attributed to "aging" or "stress." Thus, although there are hormonal manifestations of pituitary dysfunction in men, the diagnosis of a pituitary tumor may occur because of visual loss or evaluation for headache. Since postmenopausal women no longer have menses to indicate pituitary dysfunction, they are most frequently diagnosed because of the mass effect (visual loss, headache). Development of diabetes insipidus (DI), polyuria, and polydipsia are not common clinical features of a pituitary adenoma, but they may occur. Diabetes insipidus is characterized by frequent urination (often hourly), especially at night; hypernatremia occurs if the patient does not ingest enough fluid to compensate for the urinary loss. The most common lesions causing DI include metastatic tumors, granuloma, and a craniopharyngioma, which impair hypothalamic production of antidiuretic hormone (ADH). Another infrequent disturbance of posterior pituitary function is the syndrome of inappropriate antidiuretic hormone secretion (SIADH), causing hyponatremia with symptoms of fatigue, nausea, vomiting, and headache.

A pituitary adenoma producing an excessive amount of a hormone or hormones causes a distinct clinical syndrome. A feature common to any type of lesion is interference with gonadotropin secretion, resulting in hypogonadism. The precise determinant of how an adenoma interferes with gonadotropin secretion is not known, but may occur as a result of compression of normal gonadotropes. The exception is excessive production of prolactin, which has a direct inhibitory effect on pulsatile LH secretion causing disordered LH release and inadequate gonadal stimulation; reduction in prolactin with a dopamine agonist drug restores the pattern of pulsatile LH secretion to normal with resultant return of gonadal function.

Excessive prolactin secretion in premenopausal women causes amenorrhea, oligomenorrhea, or regular menses with infertility; galactorrhea, spontaneous or expressible, also occurs. Postmenopausal women may also develop galactorrhea if they are taking estrogen replacement, but it is uncommon in long-standing estrogen deficiency (estrogen is necessary to produce breast milk). Men may develop gynecomastia as well as galactorrhea. The gynecomastia may be unilateral or bilateral and always requires evaluation. Hypogonadism is the hallmark of hyperprolactinemia, and loss of libido occurs both in men and women. In men, diminished erectile function may occur without development of complete impotence. The causes of hyperprolactinemia are numerous and must be excluded before concluding that a patient has a prolactin-secreting tumor. A common cause of an elevated serum prolactin is ingestion of drugs that interfere with normal dopaminergic inhibition of prolactin. In Table 5 causes of hyperprolactinemia are listed. Obtaining a thorough history of medication use is necessary before embarking on a time-consuming and expensive evaluation; discontinuation of the causative medication should result in reduction in prolactin to normal. The precise and accurate serum prolactin concentration in conjunction with the MRI findings must be correlated in order to make the correct diagnosis. In a patient with a macroadenoma, the serum prolactin is usually >200 ng/mL if the tumor is a prolactinoma. A mild to moderate elevation of prolactin (<200 ng/mL) often occurs in the presence of a large tumor: this is secondary hyperprolactinemia. Secondary hyperprolactinemia is thought to occur because of interference with dopamine transport to lactotrope cells, resulting in loss of inhibition of prolactin secretion. The correct diagnosis is critical since the treatment is different for a prolactinoma (medical therapy) and a nonsecretory tumor with secondary hyperprolactinemia (surgery).

Excessive GH production causes acromegaly in adults and gigantism if it occurs before epiphyseal closure. Acromegaly is usually identified because of acral and facial enlargement, but it is actually a systemic disease causing considerable morbidity and

**Table 5
Causes of Hyperprolactinemia**

Medications
  Psychotropic (e.g., haloperidol, resperidol)
  Antidepressants (e.g., amoxapin)
  Estrogen
  Opiates
  Calcium channel blocker (verapamil)
  Antihypertensives (α methyldopa, reserpine)
  Dopamine antagonists (domperidome, metoclopramide)
Pituitary adenoma
  Prolactin-secreting adenoma
  GH-secreting adenoma
  Secondary hyperprolactinemia, usually a macroadenoma
Other pituitary lesion, e.g., metastatic, sarcoid, aneurysm
Hypothalamic lesion
Head trauma
Pregnancy
Spinal cord lesions
Chest wall trauma
Nipple stimulation

premature mortality, most frequently from cardiovascular disease. Disorders caused by acromegaly include hypertension, diabetes mellitus or glucose intolerance, sleep apnea, increased risk of colon polyps and colorectal cancer, renal stones, carpal tunnel syndrome, osteoarthritis, goiter and thyroid nodules, dental malocclusion, hyperhidrosis, and enlargement of the hands, feet, tongue, nose, lips, and facial bones. The problem with acromegaly is the delay in diagnosis despite treatment of the associated conditions; the estimated time from the onset of symptoms to diagnosis ranges from 7 to 10 yr. It is usual for the patient to have undergone surgery for carpal tunnel syndrome, and treatment for arthritis, hypertension, and diabetes before the diagnosis of acromegaly is considered. This is understandable since the physical changes in the face, hands, and feet are gradual, and it may be years before the "classical" features are evident. Patients and family members often attribute the facial changes and medical conditions to normal "aging." Another clinical feature that may lead to an incorrect diagnosis is the finding of hyperprolactinemia with the conclusion that the patient has a prolactinoma. Patients with early acromegaly may not have the classical physical features, the diagnosis is not entertained, and the patient is treated medically for a prolactinoma. Although medical therapy may lower prolactin to normal, the tumor does not shrink as expected with a prolactinoma that responds to a dopamine agonist drug. Since GH-producing tumors may also secrete excessive amounts of prolactin (bihormonal tumor), it is necessary to exclude acromegaly before concluding that the tumor is solely prolactin-secreting. The diagnosis of acromegaly is made by obtaining a serum insulin-like growth factor 1 (IGF-1) concentration. IGF-1 is produced by the liver and other tissues in response to GH and serves as an indicator of overall GH secretion. The definitive test for acromegaly is an oral glucose tolerance test. In normal subjects, GH decreases to <1 ng/mL. In patients with acromegaly there may be a decline in GH (not to <1 ng/mL), no change, or a paradoxical increase in GH. Measurement of a single GH level is not an appropriate test—a patient with acromegaly may have a normal random GH level and still have the disease. Figure 1 shows 24-h serum GH concentrations measured every 5 min in a normal woman and in a woman with acromegaly. In

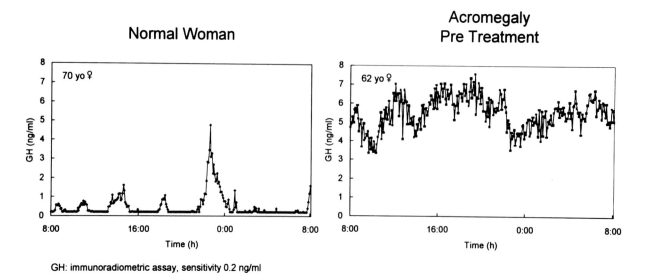

GH: immunoradiometric assay, sensitivity 0.2 ng/ml

Figure 9-1 Twenty-four-hour serum GH profiles in a normal woman and a woman with acromegaly. Note that in acromegaly, GH is detectable throughout the 24-h period.

normal subjects, there are periods of relative secretory quiescence with intermittent GH pulses, but in patients with acromegaly, GH is secreted continuously without periods of very low or undetectable GH levels. The continuous exposure to GH instead of intermittent concentrations is likely the basis for the features of this disease. Successful treatment results in decreasing the mortality rate to that of the normal population, but treatment of this and other types of pituitary tumors may require several types of therapies. Even if a patient achieves a cure of the disease, the effects of long-standing excessive GH secretion often require continued treatment. The most obvious example is the need for joint replacement, usually large joints, hips, and knees because of long-standing osteoarthritis and the need to monitor the patient for colon polyps and colorectal cancer.

Pituitary hypersecretion of ACTH results in excessive stimulation of the adrenal glands, resulting in hypercortisolism and Cushing's syndrome. Cushing's syndrome is the term applied to the clinical features of excess glucocorticoid exposure and does not connote etiology. The most common cause of Cushing's syndrome is iatrogenic—the administration of glucocorticoid drugs as treatment for various disorders. Endogenous hypercortisolism occurs as a result of excessive cortisol production from an adrenal lesion (adenoma or carcinoma) or from excessive stimulation by ACTH from the pituitary or an ectopic source, such as a bronchial or thymic carcinoid, a pancreatic tumor (adenoma, carcinoma), or a small-cell carcinoma. The etiology is classified as ACTH-dependent (pituitary, ectopic) or ACTH-independent (adrenal) Cushing's.

Cushing's syndrome is a multisystem disorder that is associated with significant morbidity and premature mortality. Symptoms and signs of Cushing's include weight gain (central, abdominal obesity, supraclavicular, posterior cervical), difficulty losing weight despite strict dieting, mood changes (most commonly depression), hirsutism, frontal and temporal hair loss, acne, oligomenorrhea or amenorrhea, muscle weakness (usually proximal), hypertension, diabetes, osteopenia, osteoporosis, bone fractures, skin infections (tinea versicolor, furuncles), vaginal candidiasis, facial plethora, and thin skin with ecchymoses. Hypokalemia may occur with elevated serum ACTH concentra-

tions. The difficulty in diagnosing Cushing's occurs because obesity and depression are common and Cushing's is relatively uncommon. Cushing's occurs more often in women, and the high prevalence of obesity and depression in this group may be mistakenly attributed to simple depression.

The first step in evaluating a patient with possible Cushing's is to determine if cortisol production is increased. Measurement of serum cortisol values may be misleading—serum cortisol concentrations vary according to the time of day and night and are affected by stress, which may abolish the normal diurnal cortisol rhythm. The most accurate way to assess cortisol production is measurement of a 24-h urine-free cortisol (UFC) concentration, which is an integrated measure of adrenal cortisol secretion, and the most precise method of measuring UFC is by high-performance liquid chromatography (HPLC). In earlier studies, measurement metabolites of cortisol and adrenal androgens, 17 hydroxysteroids and 17 ketosteroids, respectively, were used to diagnose Cushing's; these tests are less precise because of crossreactivity with other substances and have been replaced by measurement of UFC. It is prudent to measure two 24-h samples for UFC (and creatinine to assess the adequacy of the collections) before embarking on dynamic tests to establish the diagnosis and etiology of excessive cortisol production. If the UFC concentrations are elevated, a serum ACTH should then be measured to determine if Cushing's is ACTH-dependent (pituitary or ectopic ACTH etiology) or ACTH-independent (adrenal etiology). The ACTH sample must be collected in a specific manner (chilled heparin-containing tube, placed on ice, cold centrifuged immediately) in order to obtain a valid result. If serum ACTH is detectable or elevated, localization of a pituitary or ectopic source is then in order. The dynamic studies for Cushing's syndrome/Cushing's disease are listed in Table 3. After the dynamic studies are performed and if the results suggest a pituitary etiology, then an MRI study should be performed. A caveat regarding imaging studies in patients with pituitary-dependent Cushing's is that 40–50% have a normal imaging study. The use of inferior petrosal venous sinus sampling with corticotropin-releasing hormone (CRH) administration and the simultaneous measurement of bilateral inferior petrosal and peripheral serum ACTH concentrations increases the accuracy of the diagnosis *(6)*.

Petrosal sinus sampling does not distinguish among normal subjects, patients with pseudo-Cushing's syndrome, and patients with Cushing's disease; thus, it is only helpful to confirm that the pituitary is the source of abnormal ACTH production (7). It is less successful in localizing the side of the lesion and is only 40–50% accurate. The diagnosis of pituitary-dependent Cushing's is one of the most problematic endeavors in clinical endocrinology. None of the tests have a diagnostic accuracy of 100%. Thus, some patients must undergo several studies before the etiology is established with reasonable accuracy.

A gonadotropin-secreting adenoma causes the clinical syndrome of hypogonadism as described previously. The syndrome is identifiable more readily in men and premenopausal women who note changes in sexual function and menstrual cycles, respectively. However, the most common clinical presentation in a patient with a gonadotrope-producing tumor is that of the mass effect—headache or visual loss or a clinically unsuspected finding on an imaging study. The diagnosis of a gonadotropin or α-subunit-producing tumor is made by measuring serum LH, FSH, and α-subunit concentrations. These measurements, if elevated, are important as a tumor marker to assess the effects of treatment.

The clinically nonfunctioning pituitary adenoma, which does not secrete an excessive amount of hormone, is usually diagnosed because of the mass effect (headache, visual loss) or because of hypogonadism in men and premenopausal women. These patients, particularly men and postmenopausal women, usually have a macroadenoma at the time of diagnosis and have a greater risk of having pituitary hormone deficiency. The diagnosis in these patients is established by an imaging study and by measuring pituitary and target gland hormones to determine if there is pituitary hypersecretion and/or pituitary deficiency. The precise diagnosis is made by pathologic examination of the surgical specimen and by immunostaining of the tissue. Many of these tumors are positive by immunostaining for gonadotropins (LH, FSH) or the α-subunit even though there is no excessive hormone in the circulation.

A TSH-secreting tumor is the rarest type of adenoma and causes hyperthyroidism with symptoms of tachycardia, tremor, weight loss, difficulty sleeping, heat intolerance, and hyperdefecation. The correct diagnosis is achieved by measuring serum TSH and serum T4 or free T4. A detectable or elevated TSH in a hyperthyroid patient is diagnostic since TSH should be suppressed with primary hyperthyroidism.

Other sellar lesions, nonpituitary adenomas, are also associated with the clinical effects of a pituitary adenoma, i.e., mass effect and hypopituitarism. As with nonsecretory tumors, the precise diagnosis is made by pathologic examination of the surgical specimen.

The anatomic diagnosis of a pituitary lesion requires an optimal imaging study. The most precise method of imaging the sellar, suprasellar, and parasellar areas is by MRI. Although a properly performed CT scan of the pituitary is equally sensitive in detecting a pituitary lesion, the limitation of a CT scan is the inability to image precisely the optic chiasm, the cavernous sinus, and the relationship to the pituitary lesion. If an MRI cannot be performed (ferrous metal in the body, marked obesity, claustrophobia), then a CT must be ordered and performed to image the sella optimally. Optimal imaging is achieved by obtaining thin sections (1.5 mm) through the pituitary in the coronal plane, before and after intravenous contrast. If the patient is unable to extend his or her neck

adequately for coronal sections, then the scan should be reformatted in the coronal plane. If this is not possible, images reformatted in the sagittal plane may provide useful information. The "standard" method of cranial CT imaging is axial sections obtained every 5 mm—this method will fail to detect a small and sometimes a large pituitary lesion, emphasizing the necessity for requesting specifically that thin sections through the pituitary gland be obtained. Since subjects with normal pituitary function may have incidental small lesions, the clinical significance of a small lesion must be interpreted in light of symptoms and endocrine function. The finding of an incidental small lesion does not require treatment if there are no clinical symptoms or endocrine dysfunction. Such a patient should be followed clinically, with hormone studies and by obtaining a yearly MRI study for 3–5 yr. If there are no changes, a study can then be obtained every 2 yr.

MANAGEMENT OF PITUITARY ADENOMAS

The goals of treatment of a pituitary lesion are straightforward and include: reduction or elimination of the lesion, restoration of vision if abnormal, reduction in hormone hypersecretion to normal, and preservation of normal pituitary gland function, thus avoiding the need for hormone replacement. Realistically, this may not always occur with single therapy; many patients, particularly those with a large adenoma, require several therapies, including surgery, medical therapy, and radiation therapy. The patient must be informed that a single therapy may not be adequate to treat the adenoma before embarking on any treatment. Even if single therapy is effective in achieving the goals of treatment, a patient must receive regular, lifelong follow-up because of the risk of tumor recurrence, the need to monitor hormone replacement, and the need to monitor the response to medical therapy for the tumor. There is always a risk of tumor recurrence even if the tumor has been resected successfully. The reported symptomatic recurrence rate, requiring additional treatment, in patients with a nonsecretory tumor is on the order of 16% within 8 yr of the initial surgery and approx 25% within 10 yr in patients undergoing successful surgery for a prolactinoma (8). Recurrence of a secretory tumor is diagnosed by following the originally elevated hormone (IGF-1, 24-h UFC, prolactin, LH, FSH, α-subunit, TSH). If hypersecretion reoccurs, then an MRI study is indicated. Since there is no serum marker for nonsecretory tumors, a yearly MRI study is necessary for early detection of recurrence.

The initial treatment of a pituitary tumor is either surgical resection or medical therapy to effect prompt reduction in tumor mass and decompression of the optic chiasm or cavernous sinus. Transsphenoidal surgery is the preferred approach for all tumors, except prolactin-secreting adenomas with medical treatment being the first choice. The transsphenoidal approach is associated with less risk, less morbidity, and with more rapid recovery than is a craniotomy. The surgical approach is determined by the area of suprasellar tumor extension, i.e., superior and lateral extension may require craniotomy. The most important aspect of pituitary surgery is the choice of the neurosurgeon. In a general neurosurgery practice, pituitary surgery is only a minor portion of total surgeries, usually <10 operations/yr. In contrast, neurosurgeons who have a particular interest and expertise in pituitary surgery usually perform more than 100 pituitary operations/yr. It is also important to note that the published reports of surgical results originate from neurosurgeons with extensive experience and expertise with pituitary surgery. Thus, it is inappropriate to conclude that every neurosurgeon has similar expertise and outcomes. The referring physician has the responsibility to inform the patient of the necessity to seek neurosurgical consultation with an experienced pituitary neurosurgeon.

Prolactin-secreting tumors were treated surgically until the development of dopamine agonist drugs in the 1970s and 1980s. Hypothalamic dopamine inhibits prolactin secretion; administration of a dopamine agonist drug, such as bromocriptine, pergolide, quinagolide, or cabergoline, reduces serum prolactin and effects tumor shrinkage in the majority of patients with a prolactinoma (9–13). Medical therapy is now considered the preferred initial treatment since complete resection of a large tumor is rarely possible and requires postoperative medical therapy. All of the available drugs are effective, but some are better tolerated than others. The most common side effects are nausea, vomiting, and orthostatic symptoms, all of which can be minimized by beginning treatment with a small dose and increasing it gradually to the recommended dose. These medications should always be taken with food to reduce the risk of side effects. Patients should be followed closely to assure that serum prolactin and tumor size are decreasing. If the patient has visual abnormalities, frequent ophthalmologic follow-up is necessary. Although approx 90% of patients have a reduction in prolactin and tumor size, in patients with large tumors and markedly elevated prolactin, e.g., 2000 ng/mL, months to years of medical therapy may be necessary to lower prolactin to normal (<20 ng/mL). Persistently elevated prolactin *per se* is not harmful, but the patient usually remains hypogonadal and may require gonadal steroid replacement. Surgery is recommended for the patient who does not respond to medical therapy, who cannot tolerate medical therapy, and as a personal preference. In this situation, the patient must be informed of a possible need for medical therapy if surgery is not curative. Similarly, dopamine agonist treatment is not curative in the strict sense of the term—reduction in prolactin, tumor shrinkage, and restoration of normal pituitary function occur, but only if the medication is taken continuously. The dopamine agonist drugs do not destroy the tumor, and discontinuation of medical therapy usually results in return of hyperprolactinemia and tumor expansion.

The management of a patient with a TSH-secreting adenoma must first be directed toward reducing thyroid hormone levels to normal before subjecting the patient to surgery because of the risk of arrhythmia with anesthesia. A TSH-secreting tumor may be treated with medical therapy, octreotide, or by surgical removal. Medical therapy with octreotide lowers serum TSH to normal, resulting in normal thyroid hormone levels, and in reduction in tumor size. Surgical resection is an option, but patients with a large tumor have a high probability of having persistent disease and will require chronic medical therapy (octreotide) after surgery.

The endocrine management of a patient undergoing surgery involves providing an adequate glucocorticoid milieu to avoid adrenal insufficiency during the stress of anesthesia, surgery, and the perioperative period. Even if the patient has a normal serum cortisol before surgery, the amount of ACTH reserve may not provide adequate protection during this stress. All patients, with the exception of patients with Cushing's disease, should be given adequate glucocorticoid doses during and at least 24 h after surgery to avoid adrenal insufficiency. Patients with Cushing's disease do not require glucocorticoid treatment (unless being treated with a drug to lower adrenal cortisol production). In non-Cushing's patients, a reasonable steroid regimen is hydrocortisone, 100 mg

intravenously on call to the operating room and every 6 h for 24 h, followed by 50 mg very 6 h for 24 h. Serum cortisol should be measured 8 h after the last hydrocortisone and every morning until discharge for hospital. If the morning serum cortisol is >10 µg/dL, the patient may be discharged without hydrocortisone replacement, but should be given a supply of tablets to take if symptoms of adrenal insufficiency occur. If the morning serum cortisol is <10 µg/dL, replacement should be given and formal assessment of need for chronic replacement carried out after recovery from surgery, usually 4–6 wk later. The glucocorticoid replacement dose has decreased with demonstration that the prior doses caused excessive bone loss. Suggested replacement regimens include hydrocortisone, 15 mg on awakening and 5 mg at 6 PM, or prednisone, 5 mg on awakening. Although this is a fairly standard regimen, the variability in steroid metabolism requires that some patients receive a higher dose or more frequent dosing. The dose and frequency of glucocorticoid replacement are determined by clinical symptoms and empiric adjustment. There is no reliable blood or urine test to assess the adequacy of replacement. Mineralocorticoid replacement is unnecessary in patients with pituitary disease since aldosterone secretion is regulated primarily by volume status and serum potassium. If a patient is given glucocorticoid replacement after surgery, it may be necessary to perform a stimulation test to determine the need for lifelong therapy. The easiest test is administration of synthetic ACTH with measurement of serum cortisol. This test provides inferential information, i.e., a normal cortisol response implies normal ACTH production. However, ACTH administration does not stimulate the entire hypothalamic–pituitary–adrenal axis and may result in misleading conclusions. The metyrapone or insulin hypoglycemia tests are the best tests of pituitary reserve. The insulin hypoglycemia test must be performed with physician supervision and should not be conducted in a patient with coronary artery disease, seizure disorder, or generalized debility. The normal cortisol response to stimulation tests is a serum cortisol of 18 µg/dL or greater.

In the immediate postoperative period, the patient must be monitored closely for development of DI, which occurs in approx 12% of patients (transient DI) and which is permanent in approx 3%. DI is characterized by polyuria and hyposthenuria. A very low urine specific gravity level in the setting of excessive urine output (after accounting for the volume of intravenous fluids administered during and after surgery) suggests DI. This is treated by allowing unlimited oral fluid intake and by administering the synthetic vasopressin analog, desmopressin acetate (dDAVP). dDAVP can be administered intravenously or orally in the perioperative period. Intranasal administration is not possible in patients who have had a transsphenoidal operation since the nares will be packed with gauze for 2–3 d after surgery. dDAVP should only be administered as needed according to the urine output since DI may be transient. One caveat about polyuria after pituitary surgery is the patient with acromegaly. A brisk diuresis can be expected with reduction in circulating GH levels and should not be interpreted as DI, emphasizing the importance of regular measurement of urine specific gravity in conjunction with the hourly urine output and oral and intravenous intake. If a patient requires dDAVP replacement, dose and frequency of administration are determined by the clinical response, i.e., control of urinary frequency. If the thirst mechanism is intact, the patient can recognize the need for the next dose. Measurement of serum sodium or serum osmolality is usually not helpful since both will be normal if the patient is ingesting an adequate amount of fluid. Chronic replacement with dDAVP can be intranasal (rhinal tube or spray), oral, or subcutaneous.

In approx 9% of patients, transient symptomatic hyponatremia develops 8–10 d after surgery. Symptoms include nausea, weakness, headache, and generalized fatigue. These symptoms are also consistent with adrenal insufficiency. Since the patient is usually at home when this occurs, he or she should immediately have serum sodium and cortisol (if not receiving replacement) measured. If hyponatremia occurs, fluid restriction of 800 cc/24 h for 2–3 d is indicated.

The need for thyroid hormone replacement is determined by measuring the serum thyroxine (T4) or free thyroxine concentration. Measurement of serum TSH is not an accurate test to determine the need for thyroid hormone replacement in a patient with pituitary disease—the TSH concentration may be normal in the setting of a very low thyroxine level. If the serum T4 or free T4 level is below normal prior to surgery, thyroid hormone replacement is indicated. In the patient with a normal preoperative serum T4, the hormone should be measured at the postoperative evaluation, usually 4–6 wk after surgery. As with glucocorticoid replacement, the thyroid hormone replacement dose is adjusted according to clinical criteria. Measuring the T4 or free T4 level can serve as a guideline, but the normal range for this hormone is fairly broad, and dose adjustment requires assessment of symptoms and body weight.

Gonadal steroid replacement in men is determined by clinical features in conjunction with the serum testosterone concentration, measured in the morning. A low serum testosterone indicates the need for testosterone replacement, which is administered either by intramuscular injection or with a transdermal patch. Oral testosterone is to be avoided because of potential liver toxicity. If the patient is receiving intramuscular testosterone, adjustment of dose and frequency is based on clinical symptoms and measuring the nadir serum testosterone level—the day before the next dose. The transdermal preparations provide more consistent physiologic testosterone concentrations without the supra and subphysiologic levels observed with intramuscular administration. It is prudent to measure a serum prostate-specific antigen (PSA) level before beginning testosterone therapy and to follow prostate size and serum PSA levels once a year. Even if a man is not interested in sexual function, testosterone replacement is necessary to prevent osteoporosis and for its beneficial effects on muscle mass and bone marrow function.

Estrogen and progesterone replacement in hypogonadal women is also necessary to prevent osteoporosis, to reduce the risk of premature cardiovascular disease, and to treat hot flashes, decreased libido, and vaginal dryness. If the patient is premenopausal, it is reasonable to wait 2–3 mo after surgery for gonadal function to resume. If menses does not return, gonadal steroid replacement should be given. Postmenopausal women should receive replacement for the reasons noted above. The exception is the patient with a history of breast cancer or a strong family history of breast cancer. In this situation, a drug, such as alendronate, should be considered as protection against accelerated bone loss. If the woman has had a hysterectomy, administration of progesterone is not necessary. Whichever regimen is selected, adequate calcium supplementation, 1200–1500 mg of elemental calcium/d, is indicated. A pelvic examination and pap smear and mammogram should be performed and repeated yearly.

Over the past 15 years, the subject of GH deficiency in adults has received a great deal of attention from the medical and non-medical communities. GH deficiency in adults results in a distinct syndrome which includes an increase in body fat, particularly intra-abdominal visceral fat, decreased muscle mass, diminished exercise tolerance and strength, and psychosocial disturbances including decreased energy, social isolation, disturbances of sleep, and a diminished sense of well-being. Three epidemiologic studies indicate that GH deficiency in adults is associated with premature mortality from cardiovascular disease. Administration of GH to adults causes an increase in muscle mass, a decrease in fat mass, particularly intra-abdominal visceral fat, a decrease in bone density, and improvement in muscle strength and endurance. Several of the psychological disturbances also improve significantly with GH therapy. There are no outcome studies on the benefits and risks of long-term GH replacement in adults, because it has only been used therapeutically for <15 years. The diagnosis of GH deficiency requires a stimulation test, such as insulin-induced hypoglycemia, L-DOPA, arginine, growth hormone-releasing hormone (GHRH) or growth-hormone-releasing peptide (GHRP). If GH replacement is recommended, the patient should be followed regularly with clinical assessments, and measurement of serum IGF-1 concentrations (to avoid overreplacement) and serum lipid concentrations (GH replacement decreases LDL and increases HDL cholesterol).

In patients with persistent hormone hypersecretion after surgery, medical therapy is indicated for hyperprolactinemia and for persistent GH excess. As mentioned, dopamine agonist drugs are effective therapy for a prolactinoma, and they may be beneficial for excessive GH secretion. However, the most effective current medical treatment for persistent acromegaly is a somatostatin analog. Somatostatin is the hypothalamic hormone that inhibits GH production, and somatostatin analogs, octreotide and lanreotide, improve clinical symptoms and lower GH and IGF-1 concentrations in approx 90% of patients. Reduction in serum IGF-1 to normal, however, occurs in 40–50% of patients and is most likely related to the number and binding affinity of tumor somatostatin receptors. Reduction in tumor size to <50% occurs in 30–40% of patients *(14–18)*. Some patients have a better response to a combination of a dopamine agonist and somatostatin analog, and this should be given if there is only a partial response to a somatostatin analog. Medical therapy for persistent Cushing's is directed at reducing adrenal cortisol production with drugs, such as ketoconazole or metyrapone. Unfortunately, there is no effective medication to treat the primary problem—excessive ACTH production. If surgery is not curative, the preferred method to treat the pituitary tumor is by pituitary radiation, which may require months to years to be effective. While awaiting the beneficial effect of pituitary radiation, it is important to control excessive cortisol production to prevent the morbidity and premature mortality associated with Cushing's. Bilateral adrenalectomy has been used to eliminate excessive cortisol production, which also produces adrenal insufficiency, requiring lifelong glucocorticoid and mineralocorticoid replacement. Resection of the adrenal glands may also result in Nelson's syndrome in which there is expansion of the previously unidentified pituitary adenoma. Unfortunately, this is an exchange of one problem for another since patients who develop Nelson's syndrome often have large tumors, which are not amenable to complete resection as well as very elevated serum ACTH levels, resulting in marked hyperpigmentation.

Pituitary radiation is used as adjunctive therapy if surgical resection is not successful or if the tumor exhibits aggressive behavior, e.g., recurrence, refractory to medical therapy (acromegaly, prolactinoma). Pituitary radiation may be delivered via three ports (bitemporal, frontal) in multiple fractions, usually 20–30 over 4–5 wk, or by stereotactic single-dose methods, such as proton beam, Lineac, or the Gamma-knife. Pituitary radiation of any type is not suitable as primary therapy because of the delay in reducing tumor size and reducing excessive hormone levels to normal. For example, conventional fractionated radiation for acromegaly may require 10–20 yr to reduce GH levels to normal, and the average time to biochemical cure for Cushing's disease is 3 yr. It is not yet known if the recently developed focused approaches, the Lineac or the Gamma-knife, reduce excessive hormone levels to normal more rapidly, but the advantage is minimizing exposure of brain tissue to radiation. A limitation of the focused techniques is their application for only small or residual tumors—the radiation dose and radiation scatter have a risk of damaging vision if there is not adequate distance between the tumor and optic chiasm. If a patient receives conventional fractionated radiation, there is a high risk of developing pituitary insufficiency, which occurs from damage to the hypothalamic regulatory neurons. It is not yet known if a similar incidence of pituitary deficiency occurs with the stereotactic methods. Any patient who receives pituitary radiation of any type must receive regular follow-up to assess the effects of the treatment and to diagnose and treat pituitary deficiency.

PROGNOSIS

The prognosis for recovery and cure of a pituitary tumor depends on the type and size of the tumor. As noted, surgical resection of large tumors is successful in debulking the mass, but less effective in eliminating the tumor completely or in reducing pituitary hypersecretion to normal. Thus, many patients require multimodality therapy: surgery, medical treatment, and pituitary radiation, to achieve a cure. In patients with acromegaly or Cushing's disease, it is imperative to reduce the excessive hormone to normal to reduce the risk of premature mortality and ongoing resulting morbidity. Reduction in excessive GH or ACTH production should, and probably does, reduce the risk of premature mortality, although information on outcomes in patients with Cushing's disease is lacking. Once a patient has had a pituitary tumor, irrespective of type or treatments, lifelong medical follow-up is necessary to detect early recurrence, to monitor hormone replacement, and to treat any complications related to the adenoma.

SUMMARY

The optimal diagnosis and treatment of a patient with pituitary disease require a cooperative team of medical specialists from the fields of endocrinology, neurosurgery, neuroradiology, neuroophthalmology, neuropathology, and radiation therapy. With careful diagnostic and therapeutic regimens, a patient should be able to lead a normal, productive life with regular medical follow-up and treatment of tumor recurrence or pituitary deficiency. The presence of a pituitary tumor should not result in premature mortality if attention is given to all aspects of the disease

REFERENCES

1. Moltich ME, Russell EJ. The pituitary "incidentaloma." Ann Intern Med 1990;112:925–931.
2. Burrow GN, Wortzman G, Rewcastle NB, Holgate RC, Kovacs K. Microadenomas of the pituitary and abnormal sellar tomograms in an unselected autopsy series. N Engl J Med 1981;304:156–158.
3. Chong BW, Kucharczyk W, Singer W, George S. Pituitary gland MR: A comparative study of healthy volunteers and patients with microadenomas. AJNR Am J Neuroradiol 1994;15:675–679.
4. Elster AD. Modern imaging of the pituitary. Radiology 1993; 187:1–14.
5. Donovan LE, Corenblum B. The natural history of the pituitary incidentaloma. Arch Intern Med 1995;155:181–183.
6. Oldfield EH, Doppman JL, Nieman LK, Chrousos GP, Miller DL, Katz DA, et al. Petrosal sinus sampling with and without corticotropin-releasing hormone for the differential diagnosis of Cushing's Syndrome. N Engl J Med 1991;325:897–905.
7. Yanovski JA, Cutler GB, Doppman JL, Miller DL, Chrousos GP, Oldfield EH, et al. J Clin Endocrinol Metab 1993;77:503–509.
8. Ebersold MJ, Quast LM, Laws ER, Scheithauer B, Randall RV. Long-term results in transsphenoidal removal of nonfunctioning pituitary adenomas. J Neurosurg 1986;64:713–719.
9. Kleinberg DL, Boyd AE, Wardlaw S, et al. Pergolide for the treatment of pituitary tumors secreting prolactin or growth hormone. N Engl J Med 1983; 309:704–709.
10. Vance ML, Lipper M, Klibanski A, et al. Treatment of prolactin-secreting pituitary macroadenomas with the long-acting non-ergot dopamine agonist CV 205-502. Ann Intern Med 1990;112:668–673.
11. Ciccarelli E, Giusti M, Miola C, et al. Effectiveness and tolerability of long term treatment with cabergoline, a new long-lasting ergoline derivative, in hyperprolactinemic patients. J Clin Endocrinol Metab 1989; 69:725–728.
12. Webster J, Piscitelli G, Polli A, et al. A comparison of cabergoline and bromocriptine in the treatment of hyperprolactinemic amenorrhea. Cabergoline Comparative Study Group [see comments]. N Engl J Med 1994; 331:904–909.
13. Biller BMK, Molitch ME, Vance ML, et al. Treatment of prolactin-secreting macroadenomas with the once-weekly dopamine agonist cabergoline. J Clin Endocrinol Metab 1996; 81:2338–2343.
14. Sassolas G, Fossati P, Chanson P, et al. Experience of a six-month treatment with sandostatin at increasing doses in acromegaly. Horm Res 1989; 31:51–54.
15. Vance ML, Harris AG. Long-term treatment of 189 acromegalic patients with the somatostatin analog octreotide. Results of the International Multicenter Acromegaly Study Group. Arch Int Med 1991; 151:1573–1578.
16. Newman CB, Melmed S, Snyder PJ, et al. Safety and efficacy of long term octreotide therapy of acromegaly-results of a multicenter trial in 103 patients. J Clin Endocrinol Metab 1995; 80:2768–2775.
17. Reubi JC, Landolt AM. The growth hormone responses to octreotide in acromegaly correlate with adenoma somatostatin receptor status. J Clin Endocrinol Metab 1989;68:844–850.
18. Ezzat S, Snyder PJ, Young WF, et al. Octreotide treatment of acromegaly: a randomized, multicenter study. Ann Intern Med 1992; 117:711–718.

10 Neuro-Ophthalmologic Evaluation of Pituitary Tumors

SHIRLEY I. STIVER, MD, PhD AND JAMES A. SHARPE, MD

INTRODUCTION

The intricate anatomy of the fiber pathways within the optic chiasm, nerves, and tracts manifests itself in a myriad of visual symptoms. Sir Isaac Newton (cited by Rucker) *(1)* first speculated about the crossing of the fiber tracts within the chiasm in 1704. Since then, through the landmark writings of Harvey Cushing *(2)* and Traquair *(3)*, and to the present time, the effects of pituitary and related tumors on the visual pathway have intrigued neurosurgeons, ophthalmologists, and neurologists. Several excellent reviews of the neuro-ophthalmologic features of the optic chiasm and pituitary tumors have been published *(4–12)*. This chapter reviews new developments in the embryology of the optic chiasm, the nature and pathogenesis of visual symptoms in relation to relevant anatomy of the chiasm and optic nerves, visual syndromes caused by pituitary and related tumors, and the recovery of visual dysfunction following various management strategies.

EMBRYOLOGY OF THE OPTIC CHIASM

In the 22-d human embryo optic vesicles begin to form as outpouchings of the forebrain. The optic vesicles subsequently invaginate to form the optic cups, connected to the brain by optic stalks. Before 3 wk of gestation, the anlage of the optic chiasm is present as a thickening on the floor of the forebrain *(13)*. By the 4th wk, retinal ganglion cell axons start to grow from the optic cup toward the brain, transforming the optic stalk into an optic nerve. As the retinal axons pass along the optic nerve they disperse so that all or most of their retinotopic order is lost *(14,15)*.

The first retinal axons from the two eyes exit the optic nerves and meet at the ventral diencephalon to form a primordial X-shaped optic chiasm at approximately 8 wk of gestation *(13,16)*. Zones of regulatory genes expressed in the chiasmatic region provide guidance information for retinally projected axons *(17)*. Prior to the arrival of retinal axons, early-differentiated neurons migrate to the region of the developing hypothalamus where the optic chiasm will form. They pattern themselves into an inverted V-shaped array, which marks the posterior boundary of the X-shaped chiasm *(18,19)*. Retinal axons encountering these neurons do not grow through this cell population; rather, they are deflected along the

anterior boundary of these neurons into the optic tracts, thereby patterning the X-shape of the chiasm. Antibodies to the surface molecule, CD44, on these embryonal neurons ablates chiasm formation *(16)*. At this early stage, the majority of axons within the chiasm are crossed. It is not until the 11th wk that uncrossed fibers appear in the chiasm *(20,21)*, and retinal axons arriving at the chiasm from the temporal and nasal retinal fields grow into the ipsilateral or contralateral aspect of the chiasm, respectively. The decussation pattern seen in adults is present at approximately the 13th wk *(20,21)*.

Axon routing in the chiasm during embryogenesis derives from interactions between receptors on the retinal axon growth cones and inhibitory and promoting signals from within the optic chiasm *(15,16,18,22–24)*. Crossed and uncrossed axons respond differently to these signals. Monoclonal antibody markers for radial glia in embryonic mouse have demonstrated a palisade of radial glial fibers about the midline of the chiasm and a morphologically distinct thin raphe of cells at the midline *(22)*. These localized chiasm structures are inhibitory to uncrossed, but not to crossed axons, and serve to establish the decussation of the chiasm. Video microscopy of dye-labeled axons as they grow through the chiasm demonstrates that both nasal and temporal retinal fibers show long pauses in growth at the midline *(24)*. Although nasal fibers eventually cross the midline, temporal fibers develop highly branched growth cones, and ultimately growth is directed towards the ipsilateral optic tract by transformation of a backward-directed filopodium into a new growth cone *(24,25)*.

In animal models, enucleation of one eye just before or during the time when the first axons reach the chiasm severely impairs development of the uncrossed fibers from the other eye *(26–28)*. This suggests that normal development of the uncrossed pathway is dependent upon interaction between axons of the two eyes at the optic chiasm. Once they pass the midline, crossed fibers affiliate with uncrossed retinal axons from the opposite eye. The crossed fibers play a role in guiding the uncrossed axons from the chiasm into the optic tract *(15,28)*. GAP-43, a membrane protein found in growth cones, is important for mediating axonal growth into the optic tract. In GAP-43–deficient mice, axon trajectories within the chiasm are circuitous, optic tract formation is delayed, and retinal axons exit the chiasm randomly to enter the optic tract *(29)*.

The optic tracts passing posteriorly from the chiasm are seen by the 12th gestational week *(13)*. During the second month, the fetal eyes move to assume a more frontal position. This is accompanied

From: *Diagnosis and Management of Pituitary Tumors* (K. Thapar, K. Kovacs, B. W. Scheithauer, and R. V. Lloyd, eds.), ©Humana Press Inc., Totowa, NJ.

173

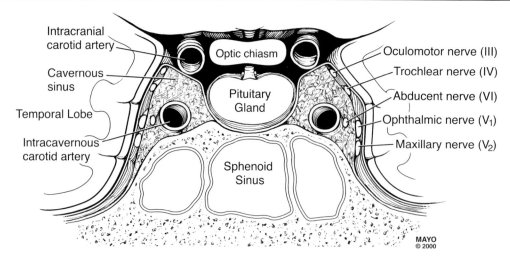

Figure 10-1   Coronal section of the cavernous sinus showing the relationship of the oculomotor (III), trochlear (IV), trigeminal ophthalmic and maxillary divisions (V_1 and V_2), and abducent (VI) cranial nerves to the pituitary gland.

by narrowing of the anterior chiasmal angle, which has been invoked as the source of the looping of fibers in the formation of Wilbrand's knee *(vide infra) (5)*. Myelination of the fibers of the visual pathway begins at approximately the 6th or 7th mo and continues on until sometime after birth.

ANATOMY

ANATOMY OF THE SELLAR REGION   At birth, the pituitary gland is approximately 1/5 the size and weight of the adult gland *(30)*. It grows to fill 3/4 of the sella in adulthood, measuring 10 mm in the anterior-posterior, 15 mm in the sagittal, and 5 mm in the superior-inferior dimensions *(31)*. The gland is generally 20% larger in females than in males, and increases in size with each pregnancy since there is incomplete involution of the gland following delivery *(8,31)*.

The diaphragma is thinnest centrally around the infundibulum and increases peripherally usually to the thickness of at least one layer of dura *(7)*. The thickness and the degree of incompetence of the diaphragma sella may determine the ease and rapidity of suprasellar growth of pituitary tumors *(32)*.

The oculomotor (III) and trochlear (IV) nerves run between the two leaves of dura that constitute the lateral wall of the cavernous sinus, whereas the abducent (VI) nerve is suspended by fibrous trabeculae within the more medial aspect of the sinus itself (Figure 1). These nerves may be affected by lateral expansion of pituitary tumors. Pituitary tumors extending into and around the clivus may damage the abducent nerve (VI) as it traverses the posterior aspect of the clivus to enter Dorello's canal.

ANATOMY OF THE CHIASM   The intracranial optic nerves and chiasm rise from the optic canals at a 45° angle relative to the diaphragma (Figure 2) *(7)*. The chiasm is separated from the underlying diaphragma and dorsum sella by the subarachnoid space of the chiasmatic cistern, the height of which measures between 0 and 10 mm *(7)*. Thus, suprasellar tumor extension generally greater than 10 mm above the diaphragma is present before the chiasm is affected. Consequently, visual dysfunction in the setting of a small tumor is related to unilateral optic nerve rather than chiasmal compression *(7,33)*.

In approximately 80% of cases the optic chiasm lies directly over the central diaphragma and pituitary gland, but it may be

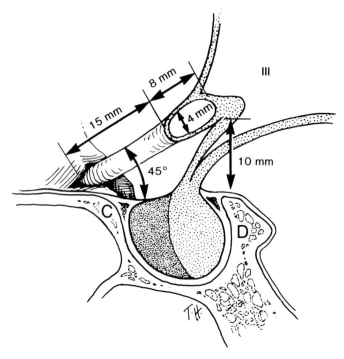

Figure 10-2   Sagittal view of the optic nerve and chiasm demonstrating their angled relation to the sella. III = third ventricle; C = anterior clinoid; D = dorsum sellae. (From Slamovits TL. Anatomy and Physiology of the Optic Chiasm. In: Miller NR, Newman NJ, eds. Walsh and Hoyt's Clinical Neuro-Ophthalmology. vol. 1, 5th ed. Williams & Wilkins, Baltimore, 1998, pp. 85–100.

"prefixed," lying over the tuberculum sella in ~9%, or "postfixed," situated over the dorsum sella in ~11% of patients (Figure 3) *(34)*. This variability of positioning of the optic chiasm plays a role in the myriad of visual syndromes seen in association with pituitary and sellar tumors. Classic bitemporal hemianopia may not be observed in the setting of a pre- or postfixed chiasm. The rostral position of a prefixed chiasm causes compression to occur on the optic tract leading to an incongruous homonymous hemianopia, and an anterior chiasmal syndrome or a monocular field defect

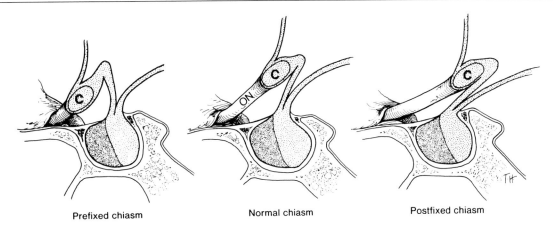

Prefixed chiasm   Normal chiasm   Postfixed chiasm

Figure 10-3   Sagittal view of the optic chiasm illustrating prefixed, normal and postfixed positions. ON = optic nerve; C = chiasm. (From Slamovits TL. Anatomy and Physiology of the Optic Chasm. In: Miller NR, Newman NJ, eds. Walsh and Hoyt's Clinical Neuroophthalmology. Vol. 1, 5th Ed. Wilkins, Baltimore, 1998, pp. 85–100. With permission from Harcourt Publishers Ltd.)

can arise from compression of a postfixed chiasm. Ikeda and Yoshimoto *(35)* have argued that visual symptomatology is unrelated to the position of the chiasm, but is determined by the degree of suprasellar extension of the tumor.

ANATOMY OF AXONAL PATHWAYS WITHIN THE OPTIC NERVES, CHIASM, AND TRACTS

As axons from the retinal ganglion cells enter the optic nerve they lose their retinotopic order *(14,15)*. Just before they enter the chiasm, fibers of the optic nerve disperse into nasal and temporal aggregates *(36,37)*. Bilateral connections underlying binocular vision arise from the segregation of the approx 2.2×10^6 axons traversing the optic chiasm *(38)* in an organized fashion such that the fibers from the nasal half of each retina decussate in the chiasm to the contralateral optic tract, while fibers from the temporal retina destined for the ipsilateral optic tract do not cross (Figure 4). The vertical meridian, dividing the nasal and temporal retina, passes through the fovea. The ratio of crossed to uncrossed fibers is 53:47 *(38)*. Superior retinal quadrant fibers remain superiorly within the chiasm, inferior quadrant fibers inferiorly, going on to assume medial and lateral dispositions in the optic tracts, respectively (Figure 4) *(39–43)*.

The chiasm is largely a macular structure with approximately 90% of the axons in the chiasm originating in the retina near the fovea (Figure 5) *(41,44)*. Macula fibers within the chiasm are both crossed and uncrossed. While concentrated towards the posterior aspect of the chiasm, only the anterior inferior and posterior inferior chiasms are devoid of macular fibers *(5)*. Textbook renditions of the chiasm represent rationalizations for the clinically manifest visual fields, and despite extensive studies, the precise fiber tract anatomy of the chiasm has not been elucidated *(7,37,45)*.

It has been accepted that fibers of the inferior nasal retinal field cross in the anterior aspect of the chiasm and loop forward for a distance of 3–4 mm into the contralateral optic nerve as Wilbrand's knee, before passing back to the contralateral optic tract (Figure 6) *(5,7,46)*. Fibers from the superior nasal retina decussate posteriorly in the chiasm and do not form a similar loop, possibly because of the obtuse angle of the optic tracts at the posterior chiasm *(5)*. Wilbrand's knee fibers are more prominent in the human than in monkeys, an animal whose retinal projections are thought to be similar to those in humans. The difference has been attributed to the narrower angle between the converging optic nerves in humans

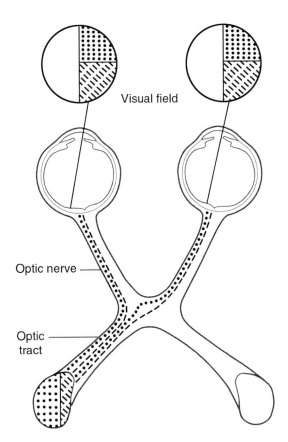

Visual field

Optic nerve

Optic tract

Figure 10-4   Retinotopic organization of the visual system demonstrating (1) crossing of the nasal retinal fibers and uncrossed temporal retinal fibers in the chiasm and (2) segregation of the superior retinal fibers (corresponding to the inferior visual field) medially and inferior retinal fibers (representing the superior visual field) laterally in the optic tract. ©The Mayo Clinic 2000.

(5). Wilbrand's knee has become synonymous with the clinical phenomenon of anterior chiasmal syndrome *(vide infra)*.

The finding of aberrant looping of crossed nasal fibers into the contralateral optic nerve, known as Wilbrand's knee, was based on post mortem studies of patients with a history of remote monocular enucleation *(47)*. Horton *(47)* has suggested that the anterior loop-

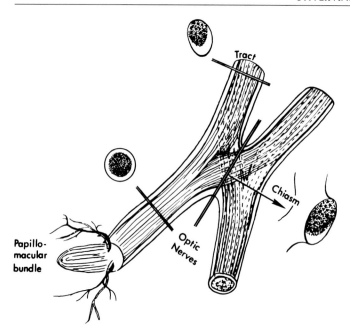

Figure 10-5 Cross-sectional representations of the optic nerves, chiasm, and tracts illustrating that the papillomacular bundle subserving central vision forms an extensive component of the fiber tracts within each system. (From Glaser JS. Neuro-ophthalmology, 2nd ed. J.B. Lippincott, Philadelphia, 1990, p. 71. With permission from Harcourt Publishers Ltd.)

ing fibers of Wilbrand's knee are not present in normal optic pathways; rather, they represent an artifact of long-term enucleation. A study of eight rhesus monkeys, examined following injection of tritiated proline to label the axons of the retinal ganglion cells from the eye to the lateral geniculate, failed to show any evidence of Wilbrand's knee fibers. Enucleation of one eye in each of two monkeys was carried out with similar examination at 6 mo and 4 yr following enucleation. Myelin staining of the visual pathway was done also in three patients who had undergone enucleation 5 mo, 27 mo, and 28 yr before death. Wilbrand's knee fibers were not seen 5–6 mo following enucleation but were present in the specimens examined 2 or more yr following enucleation. Horton (47) concluded that after 6 mo, atrophy develops in the nerve of the enucleated eye, distorting the chiasm slightly and causing the fibers of the normal optic nerve to spill into the entry zone of the atropic nerve.

Axonal fibers within the optic tracts are segregated such that the medial optic tract carries fibers from the superior quadrants of both the uncrossed temporal retinal field and crossed nasal retinal field, whereas the lateral tract comprises inferior quadrant retinal fields of the uncrossed temporal and crossed nasal fields.

VASCULAR SUPPLY OF THE CHIASM AND INTRACRANIAL OPTIC NERVE

The optic chiasm traverses obliquely through the Circle of Willis with the anterior cerebral and communicating arteries residing superiorly, the internal carotid arteries situated laterally, and the posterior cerebral, posterior communicating, and basilar arteries lying below the chiasm (Figure 7) (48). This oblique course gives a framework for the main elements of the arterial supply to the chiasm (48–52). The dorsal aspect of the chiasm is supplied primarily by the A1 segments of the anterior cerebral artery. Branches of the anterior communicating and internal carotid arteries contribute variably, and dorsal supply to the

central chiasm is relatively sparse. Arteriolar branches of the internal carotid arteries and anterior cerebral arteries supply the lateral aspects of the chiasm. Supply to the ventral chiasm is predominantly through branches of the internal carotid artery augmented by the posterior cerebral, posterior communicating, and basilar arteries that supply the infundibulum and extend small branches to the chiasm (48,52). Bergland and Ray (48) have reported that the blood supply to the central chiasm comes solely from the ventral aspect of the chiasm via these vessels. Selective ventral supply to the central chiasm renders it vulnerable to ischemia from below due to pituitary tumor growth.

Supply to the intracranial optic nerves is from the internal carotid, anterior cerebral, and anterior communicating arteries (50). The capillary network is less dense and potentially more susceptible to compression or injury on the temporal aspect of the optic nerve (53).

Venous drainage from the dorsal aspect of the chiasm is via the anterior cerebral veins, whereas the ventral chiasm drains through a "preinfundibular venous arch," which subsequently passes laterally into the basal veins of Rosenthal at the sides of the interpeduncular fossa (49).

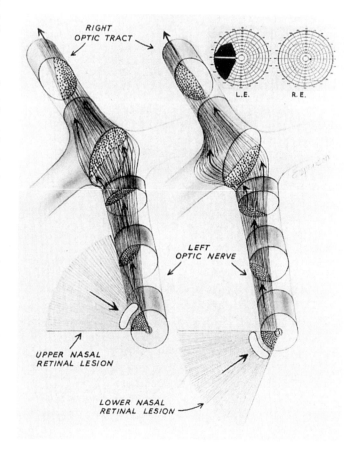

Figure 10-6 Schematic demonstrating the course of the crossed inferior nasal fibers through the inferior aspect of the chiasm and looping forward into the contralateral optic nerve as Wilbrand's knee. The superior nasal fibers cross in the superior aspect of the chiasm and do not loop forward. (From Slamovits TL. Anatomy and Physiology of the Optic Chiasm. In: Miller NR, Newman NJ, eds. Walsh and Hoyt's Clinical Neuro-Ophthalmology. vol. 1, 5th ed. Williams & Wilkins, Baltimore, 1998, pp. 85–100.

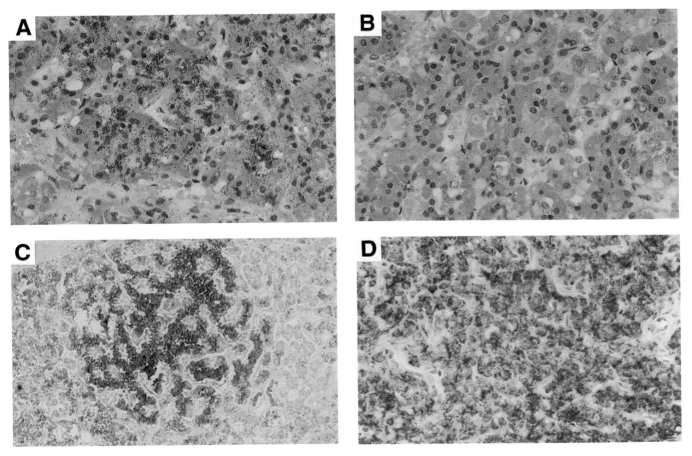

Figure 8-2. (See discussion on p. 156.) ISH applications in the pituitary. **(A)** Detection of PRL mRNA in normal pituitary with a ^{35}S-labeled oligonucleotide probe (×250); **(B)** the sense control probe is negative (×250); **(C)** incidental PRL adenoma detected by ISH with a digoxigenin-labeled oligonucleotide probe in an autopsy pituitary (×200); **(D)** an ACTH adenoma expressing pro-opiomelanocortin detected with a digoxigenin-labeled oligonucleotide probe (×300).

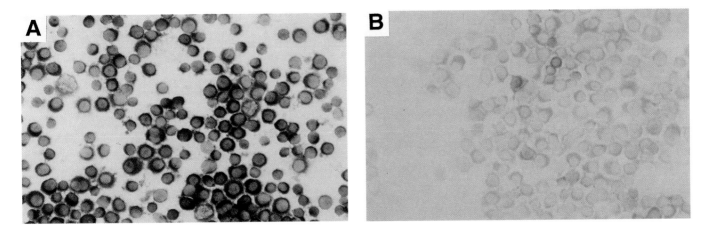

Figure 8-5. (See complete caption and disussion on pp. 159, 160.) Comparison of *in situ* RT-PCR and ISH to detect PRL mRNA in GH$_3$ cells grown in serum-free media with low PRL mRNA levels. **(A)** *In situ* RT-PCR detects a strong signal for PRL by the indirect method in all of the tumor cells (×250). **(B)** There is a weak and focal hybridization signal for PRL mRNA detected by ISH in the same population of GH$_3$ cells (×250).

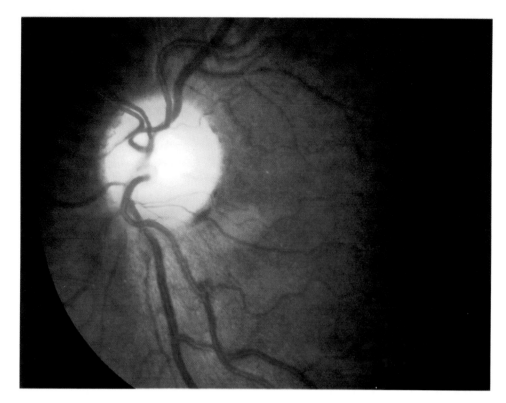

Figure 10-13. (See discussion on pp. 181, 184.) Fundoscopic image demonstration band or bowtie atrophy in a patient with temporal hemanopia and acuity 20/20 in the ipsilateral eye and no light perception in the contralateral eye.

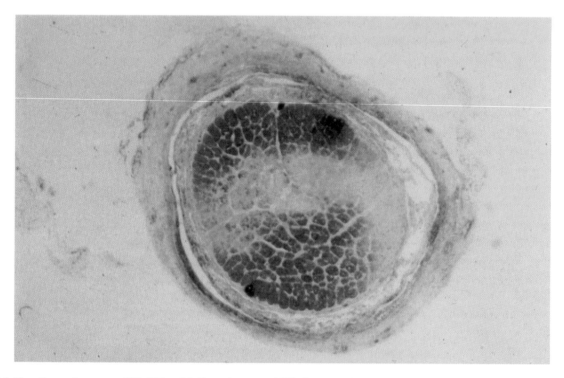

Figure 10-14. (See discussion on pp. 184, 185 and full caption on p. 185.) Cross-section mount of optic nerve stained for myelin, illustrating band atrophy of nerve fibers from the nasal retina.

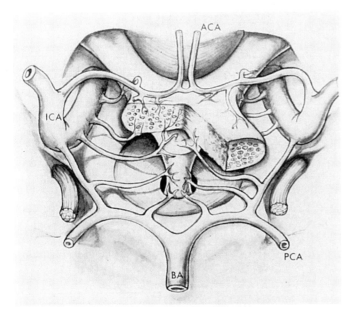

Figure 10-7 Arterial supply to the chiasm illustrating supply to the dorsal chiasm from the anterior cerebral arteries, supply to the lateral chiasm from branches of the internal carotid artery, and supply to the ventral chiasm via the internal carotid, posterior cerebral, posterior communicating, and basilar arteries. ACA = anterior cerebral artery; ICA = internal carotid artery; PCA = posterior cerebral artery; BA = basilar artery. (From ref. *48* with permission.)

PATHOPHYSIOLOGY OF OPTIC NERVE AND CHIASM DYSFUNCTION

Arguments favoring both mechanical and vascular mechanisms of optic nerve and chiasmal dysfunction from tumor compression have been debated in the literature for years. It is difficult to explain bitemporal hemianopia, with involvement of the crossing nasal fibers and complete sparing of the uncrossed temporal fibers, strictly by a mechanical mechanism. Preferential stretching of the central chiasm has been invoked *(54)* and supported by balloon compression models in cadavers *(55)*. These studies demonstrated involvement of the inferior crossing followed by superior crossing fibers with relative sparing of the lateral fibers. Others have proposed that the central part of the chiasm is selectively vulnerable to mechanical compression because of the concentration of small macular fibers within it *(56)*. The absence of fibrous tissue and the presence of interweaving fibers within the chiasm may contribute also to the relative susceptibility of the central chiasm to mechanical compression *(54)*.

The rich collateral vascular supply to the chiasm has been presumed to protect it from arterial ischemic damage. Based on their finding of central chiasmal supply solely from a ventral group of vessels (*vide supra*), Bergland and Ray *(48)* have suggested that bitemporal field deficits arise from pituitary tumor growth through compromise of this supply, rather than by direct neural compression. Hoyt *(5)* has argued that pressure from a tumor is insufficient to impede arterial flow, proposing instead that tumor compression obstructs capillary and venous flow, leading to stagnant, anoxic blood and consequent physiologic blockade of axonal conduction. Relative sparing of capillary and venous compression at the lateral aspects of the chiasm was thought to account for preservation of the uncrossed temporal fibers in bitemporal field deficits. Lao and

co-workers' report *(57)* of a sparse capillary supply to the central chiasm further supports vulnerability of the crossing fibers on a vascular basis. They hypothesize that vascular steal (diversion of blood flow) from the chiasmal capillary network to supply the pituitary tumor may unmask this susceptibility.

Ischemic mechanisms have been criticized because they do not account for the rapid recovery of visual function that typically follows surgical decompression *(58)*. Recovery from neural compression has been modeled in histological studies of cat optic nerve undergoing balloon compression. Demyelination is evident early, and continued compression leads to further progressive demyelination accompanied by axonal degeneration. Beginning at 5 wk, evidence of remyelination can be seen despite ongoing balloon compression *(56,59)*. Visual impairment secondary to tumor compression is suggested to result from a combination of Wallerian nerve fiber loss, demyelination with conduction block, and "physiologic block" in normal and remyelinated fibers, which would be able to conduct if they were not compressed *(56,59)*. Recovery following decompression occurs in two phases. An initial rapid return of function occurs due to restoration of conduction by relief of the "physiologic block" in normal and remyelinated fibers, and a slower phase taking weeks to months follows as fibers of the remaining intact pathway undergo remyelination and functional reorganization possibly by way of collateral spouting *(56,59,60)*.

Pituitary tumor compression is said to cause selective impairment of the magnocellular (M) visual system, important for the perception of fast motion stimuli, as compared to the parvocellular (P) pathway, which mediates perception of stimuli that are stationary or in slow motion *(61)*. M and P fibers have been shown to segregate at the level of the optic chiasm in primates and likely in humans as well *(37,62)*. M axons predominantly occupy a ventral subpial position in the optic chiasm and thus are the first axons to experience compression. In addition, the larger M axons are thought to be more susceptible than the smaller P axons to compression injury.

Contrast sensitivity testing has been reported to be a very sensitive indicator of visual dysfunction and, by using appropriate paradigms, the parvocellular and magnocellular visual pathways can be individually assessed. Porciati et al. *(63)* have documented contrast sensitivity losses in the presence of normal visual acuity and normal fields in a series of 28 patients with pituitary adenoma. Contrast sensitivity losses were found to be independent of adenoma size, extent of adenoma impingement on the optic chiasm, or degree of pituitary stalk deviation, suggesting that mechanisms beyond chiasmal compression and vascular involvement are important in visual dysfunction caused by pituitary tumors *(63,64)*. In their study, parvocellular loss was more frequent than magnocellular pathway impairment *(63)*.

CLINICAL SYNDROMES

OVERVIEW Pituitary and parasellar tumors present with a wide variety of visual signs and symptoms, ranging from the classical bitemporal hemianopias to the rare and fascinating phenomena of visual hallucinations and see-saw nystagmus. Over the years, increased clinical awareness and modern neuroimaging have significantly decreased the number of patients exhibiting severe field or acuity loss at the time of diagnosis *(65,66)*. At the other end of the spectrum, pituitary adenomas with significant suprasellar extension can exist without visual symptoms and with normal visual fields (Figure 8) *(67)*. Visual evoked potentials in

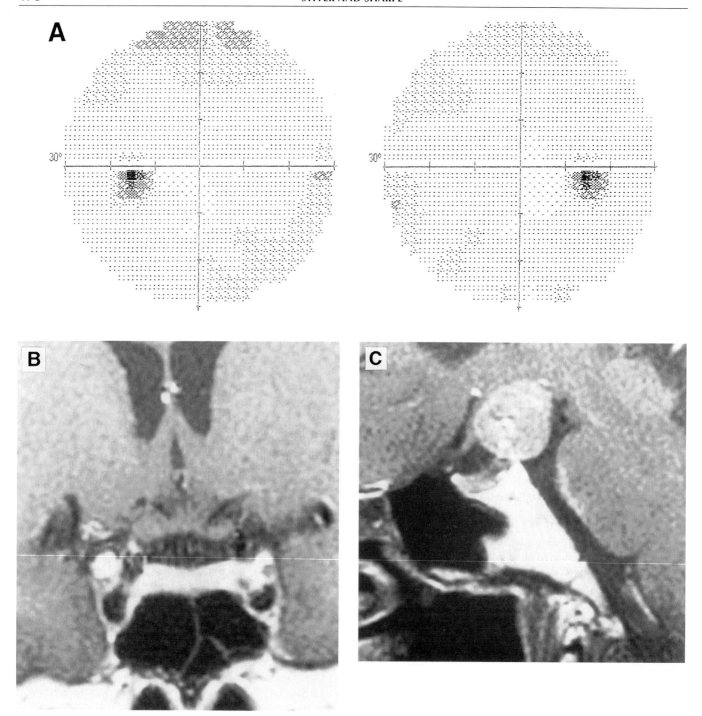

Figure 10-8 Fifty-six-year-old female with a several-year history of headaches, visual acuity 20/20 bilaterally, and normal disks to fundoscopy. **(A)** Her visual fields were normal and remained stable over 9 yr of follow-up without treatment. **(B)** Coronal and **(C)** sagittal MRI demonstrates a posteriorly situated tumor. The chiasm is splayed over the tumor.

these cases may be abnormal *(68,69)*, and latency abnormalities have been described as sensitive indicators of visual pathway impingement *(68)*. More recently, contrast sensitivity testing has been found to be sensitive to visual dysfunction from pituitary tumors even in the setting of normal visual acuity and fields *(63,64)*. It has been proposed as a method for early detection and monitoring of visual compromise in patients with pituitary adenoma. The subtleties of the neuro-ophthalmologic examination and field testing methods have been well described *(6,9,70,71)* and reviewed by Arnold *(4)*.

Small pituitary tumors can give rise to visual dysfunction long before they cause chiasmal compression, if they extend anteriorly to involve the optic nerve *(72,73)*. Isolated cases of visual loss from pituitary tumors that are entirely intrasellar have been reported *(74,75)*. In general, though, a tumor that causes chiasmal compression is usually of considerable size, having grown to traverse the approx 10 mm of subarachnoid space between the diaphragma and the chiasm *(vide supra)* (Figure 9) *(3,7)*. In a series of 50 patients, Ikeda and Yoshimoto *(35)* have shown that

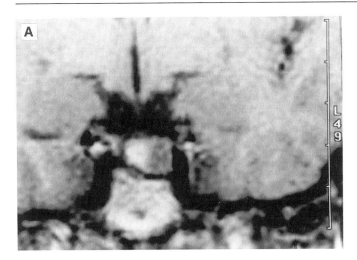

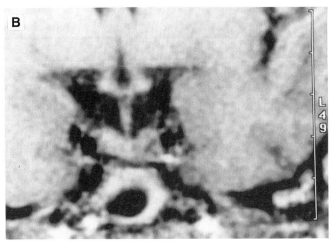

Figure 10-9   A thirty-three-year-old female had amenorrhea for 7 yr, a prolactin level of 170 ng/mL, and no visual symptoms or signs. **(A)** and **(B)** T1-weighted coronal MRI images demonstrating a left-sided adenoma that histologically proved to be a null-cell tumor. In (B) the subarachnoid space outlines the pituitary stalk. The intervening subarachnoid space between the sella and chiasm measures approx 10 mm.

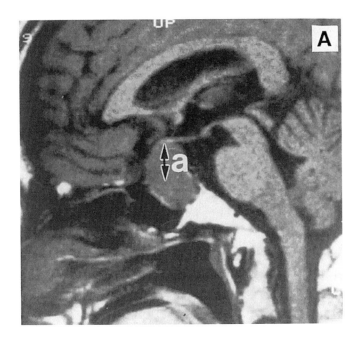

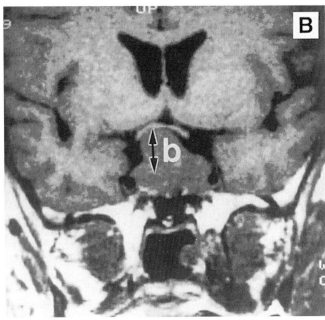

Figure 10-10   MRI demonstrating measurement guidelines to predict visual impairment if the chiasm is displaced **(A)** more than 8 mm above a reference line between the frontal base and posterior clinoid on the sagittal view or **(B)** more than 13 mm above a reference line between the upper surfaces of the cavernous internal carotid arteries on the coronal view. (From Ikeda H, Yoshimoto T. Visual disturbances in patients with pituitary adenoma. Acta Neurol Scand 1995;92:157–160. With permission from Munksgaard International Publishers Ltd.)

the degree of tumor extension present on high resolution MRI correlates with visual disturbance as evaluated by Goldmann perimetry. Visual impairment occurs only if displacement of the chiasm exceeds 8 mm above a reference line drawn between the frontal base and posterior clinoid on the sagittal view and 13 mm above a reference line between the upper surfaces of the cavernous internal carotid arteries on the coronal view (Figure 10) *(35)*. This method is reported to be sufficiently reliable to predict when tumor growth will affect visual function.

Endocrinologically active pituitary tumors manifest themselves before they grow to such a size. Thus, it is generally the non-secreting adenomas, less frequently prolactinomas, and

rarely growth hormone tumors, that first present with visual symptoms *(58,76,77)*.

The course of visual deterioration is usually slow and insidious. It may affect one or both eyes initially. Tumor hemorrhage or infarction can precipitate an acute and sometimes catastrophic decline in vision. Hormonal influences during pregnancy can accelerate the temporal profile of visual impairment.

VISUAL FIELD SYNDROMES   The incidence of visual field deficits, either as the presenting complaint or as an associated finding at the time of diagnosis, is summarized from review of the literature in Table 1 *(58,67,74–82)*. Many of these studies are influenced by referral bias. The more recent larger studies of

Table 1
Incidence of Visual Field Deficits in Patients with Pituitary Tumors *(58,67,74–82)*

Author	Study years	No. patients	Study group	No. (%) visual field defect	No. (%) symptomatic
Comtois et al. (1991) *(78)*	1962–87	126	Nonsecretory pituitary adenomas	93 (74%)	—
Mohr et al. (1990) *(67)*	1962–87	77	Giant macroadenomas	74 (96%)	—
Cohen et al. (1985) *(75)*	1974–84	100	Pituitary adenomas and visual dysfunction	—	88 (88%)
Trobe et al. (1984) *(79)*	1976–82	49	Pituitary adenoma and visual dysfunction	—	37 (76%)
Trautmann and Laws (1983) *(74)*	1971–82	714	Pituitary adenomas	230 (32%)	—
Halle (1983) *(58)*	1974–81	50	Pituitary adenomas	34 (68%)	20/34 (59%)
Anderson et al. (1983) *(76)*	1976–81	200	Pituitary adenomas	18 (9%)	13/18 (72%)
Symon (1979) *(80)*	1968–78	101	Consecutive pituitary adenomas; giants excluded	100 (99%)	94/101 (93%)
Wilson and Dempsey (1978) *(77)*	1970–76	250	Pituitary adenomas	60 (24%)	28/60 (47%)
Wray (1976) *(81)*	1974–76	100	Pituitary adenomas	31 (31%)	—
Hollenhorst and Younge (1973) *(82)*	1940–62	1000	Pituitary adenomas	(70%)	(84%)

Trautmann and Laws *(74)*, Anderson et al. *(76)*, and Wilson and Dempsey *(77)* would suggest that somewhere between 10 and 30% of patients with pituitary tumors present to practicing neuro-ophthalmologists and neurosurgeons today with a visual field deficit. Approx 75% of patients with a visual field defect are symptomatic (Table 1).

The spectrum of visual field defects produced by pituitary tumors is summarized in Table 2 *(58,67,75,78,79,82–84)*. Bitemporal hemianopia, generally present in 55–75% of cases, is the most common type of field loss. Patterns of field loss may not always be easy to interpret. As the tumor grows and exerts increasing mass effect from below, both compression by the anterior cerebral arteries and compression of the optic nerves against the bony optic foramen can lead to complex fields *(85)*. Decreased visual acuity correlates with the extent of extrafoveal visual field loss *(86,87)*.

Bitemporal Hemianopia This classic field pattern, which has become synonymous with visual loss in pituitary tumors, begins first with field depression in the superior temporal quadrants and expands in a clockwise direction in the right eye and in counterclockwise fashion in the left eye *(3,8)*. The superonasal quadrant is last affected. Visual fields losses with sloping margins usually indicate a slowly progressive lesion, while those with steep margins and uniform density suggest a more static lesion *(85)*. Asymmetrical field loss between the two eyes is usual *(2,3,6,85)*.

Bitemporal field defects may be scotomatous or nonscotomatous. The large representation of macular fibers within the chiasm leads to involvement of the central 30° of the visual field in over 95% of cases *(4)*. Scotomatous defects may split or spare the macula, usually the former *(85)*. The characteristic cut-off at the vertical meridian is key to differentiating scotomatous defects due to chiasmal interference from other causes of scotoma. Of note, Younge *(88)* has described bitemporal field defects with 2½–3°, and in some cases up to 10°, of midline tilting from the vertical meridian. The presence of scotoma suggests active tumor growth, whereas a scotoma tends to be absent when the tumor is slow growing or stable *(3,89)*. Nonscotomatous bitemporal hemianopia involves field changes largely in the peripheral isopters, and no scotomata are present *(85)*.

As noted by Cushing *(2)*, visual acuity can remain normal even in the face of a severe bitemporal field deficit. If the fibers from the temporal fovea are spared, the patient can be totally unaware of even a dense temporal deficit.

Anterior Chiasmal Syndrome The anterior chiasmal syndrome results from compression of one optic nerve near its junction with the optic chiasm, leading to a field deficit on the side of the lesion and a superotemporal field cut, attributable to involvement of the inferior nasal fibers of Wilbrand's knee, in the fellow eye *(vide supra)* (Figure 11). The ipsilateral field defect can be variable ranging from a paracentral scotoma to an extensive field defect and even blindness of the homolateral eye. The danger with these presentations is to miss the superior field defect in the eye opposite the patient's complaints and thereby misdiagnose the problem as an isolated optic neuropathy. In this regard, visual evoked potentials using selective nasal and temporal half-field stimulation may be useful *(69)*, but they are superfluous to detailed perimetry.

The precise localizing value of anterior chiasmal syndromes often leads falsely to the assumption that the lesion causing the defect is small. The tumor can be quite large and yet cause this exquisitely defined field loss. The superior temporal field loss in the anterior chiasmal syndrome has been classically attributed to involvement of the crossed inferior nasal fibers of Wilbrand's knee *(90,91)*. The possibility that Wilbrand's knee may not exist in the normal human optic pathway has led Horton *(47)* to suggest that the anterior chiasmal syndrome arises from superimposition of a temporal hemianopia in one eye from prechiasmal optic nerve

Table 2
Types of Visual Field Defects in Patients with Pituitary Tumors (58,67,75,78,79,82–84)

Field defect	Elkington (1968) (83) %	Hollenhorst and Younge (1973) (82)	Halle et al. (1983) (58)	Trobe et al. (1984) (79)	Cohen et al. (1985) (75)	Mohr et al. (1990) (67)	Sullivan et al. (1991) (84)	Comtois et al. (1991) (78)
Bitemporal hemianopia	71	57	18	45	54	53	67	54
Bitemporal quadrantopsia	—	—	35	—	17	10	13	15
Junctional syndrome	—	20	—	39	7	10	2	—
Monocular temporal loss	9	5	9	4	—	8	—	—
Homonymous hemianopia	5	6	3	4	1	1	2	—
Other	15	—	—	8	21	18	16	—

compression and an early superior bitemporal quadrantopsia from chiasmal involvement.

Of note, Traquair first used the term "junctional scotoma" to describe a unilateral temporal field defect due to compression of the ipsilateral optic nerve at the anterior angle of the chiasm, at a site where the crossed and uncrossed fibers have segregated (3). The "junctional scotoma of Traquair," with a normal field in the fellow eye, should be distinguished from an anterior chiasmal syndrome (92).

Monocular Hemianopia Monocular temporal visual loss represents approx 4–9% of visual field defects caused by pituitary tumors (Table 2). Involvement of solely the paracentral temporal visual field is unusual and comprises 1–2% of visual field defects due to pituitary adenomas (93). Hershenfeld and Sharpe (92) reported a series of 24 patients with monocular temporal hemianopia, in which 15 (64%) were caused by pituitary adenomas, 4 (16%) were related to other tumors of the sellar region, and the remainder were attributable to optic disk dysversion 2 (8%), functional disorder 2 (8%), and optic neuritis 1 (4%). Segregation of the fibers of the nasal and temporal fields within the optic nerve begins before the fibers enter the chiasm (36,37). Thus monocular temporal hemianopia has been attributed to compression of the medial aspect of the optic nerve close enough to the chiasm that the nasal and temporal fibers have started to part but far enough along the nerve so as to miss the crossing nasal fibers of Wilbrand's knee from the contralateral eye (Figure 12) (46,92).

In most cases, a relative afferent pupillary defect (RAPD) accompanies the monocular temporal field loss (92). The presence of normal pupillary reactions in association with a monocular field complaint has been interpreted variably. Hershenfeld and Sharpe (92) argue that the two are incompatible, and the presence of a monocular temporal field loss with normal pupillary reaction provides evidence of a functional disorder. A linear relationship between the magnitude of the RAPD and degree of field loss by Goldmann perimetry has been demonstrated, and discordance between the two should be carefully checked (94). Kosmorsky et al. (46) have suggested that the presence of temporal hemianopia in the absence of an RAPD implies that the visual fibers are functionally and perhaps anatomically distinct from the pupillary pathways, and caution not to disregard these patients as functional.

Homonymous Hemianopia Homonymous hemianopias signify involvement of the optic tract. An incongruous homonymous hemianopia in association with decreased visual acuity suggests posterior chiasmal involvement (3). Frequently the homonymous hemianopia may be masked by superimposition of a chiasmal bitemporal defect and manifests itself solely by the presence of a less dense nasal field loss ipsilateral to the lesion (6).

Binasal Hemianopia Binasal hemianopia is a rare visual field defect which has been attributed to chiasmal involvement in primary empty sella (95). As the chiasm descends into the pituitary fossa, traction may compromise blood flow from small feeding branches of the carotid arteries that supply the lateral aspect of the chiasm and thereby cause this unusual deficit (95).

VISUAL ACUITY AND OPTIC ATROPHY Detailed clinical examination and modern neuroimaging have decreased the frequency of visual acuity loss and optic atrophy at the time of diagnosis by providing early detection of pituitary tumors. Loss of visual acuity in 70% and findings of optic atrophy in 34% of patients in Hollenhorst and Younge's series from 1940 to 1962 (82) contrasts with Anderson et al.'s 1976–1981 series (76) in which decreased visual acuity was seen in 4% and optic atrophy was present in 2% of patients. Abnormalities in pseudoisochromatic plate testing may be evident before there is any detectable visual acuity loss, but normal color vision does not exclude significant extrafoveal visual field loss (9). It is well accepted that the degree of optic atrophy may not correlate with visual acuity (58). In very slowly compressive lesions, there may be no optic atrophy despite severely impaired acuity. Optic disk pallor signifies loss of axons, but visual loss can persist for months, perhaps years, without visible loss of axons. The width of the chiasm evaluated 3 mm anterior to the pituitary stalk on a coronal MRI and measuring less than 13.5 mm has been correlated with fundoscopic evidence of optic atrophy (96).

Retrograde axonal degeneration from chiasmal compression may lead to attrition of the retinal nerve fibers in advance of optic disk color changes. Rake defects, most easily identified as dull, dark red streaks in the supero- and infero- temporal arcuate nerve fiber layer, correlate with nerve fiber loss and are the earliest manifestation of optic atrophy (97,98). Pituitary and related tumors with chiasmal compression affecting only the crossing fibers in the chiasm cause a characteristic horizontal band or bowtie pattern

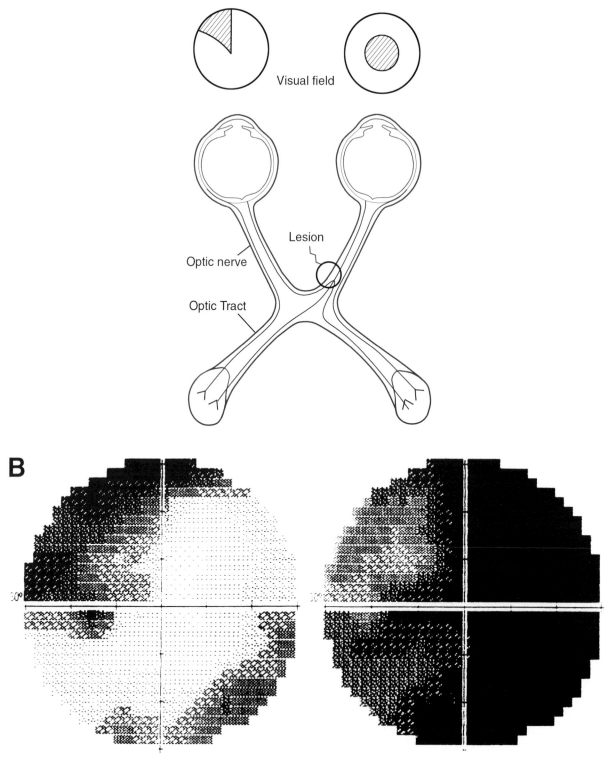

Figure 10-11   (**A**) Schematic of the anterior chiasmal syndrome, classically attributed to compression of one optic nerve adjacent to the chiasm leading to an ipsilateral field loss and compression of the crossed inferior nasal fibers from the opposite eye giving rise to a contralateral superotemporal field loss. (**B**) Example of visual fields in a patient with anterior chiasmal syndrome demonstrating extensive ipsilateral loss and a superotemporal field cut in the fellow eye. A ©The Mayo Clinic 2000.

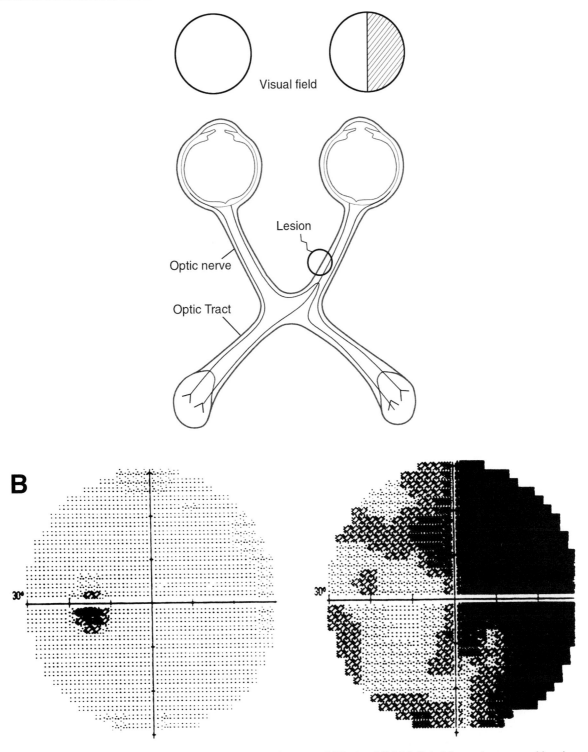

Figure 10-12 Monocular temporal hemianopia. **(A)** anatomic pathways and **(B)** visual field deficit. Monocular temporal hemianopia arises from compression of the medial optic nerve far enough along the nerve such that the nasal and temporal fibers have begun to segregate, but sparing the chiasm so that the crossing inferior nasal fibers from the opposite eye are not involved. A, ©The Mayo Clinic 2000. B, From Hershenfeld SA, Sharpe JA. Br J Ophthalmol 1993; 77:424–427. With permission from BMJ Publishing Group.

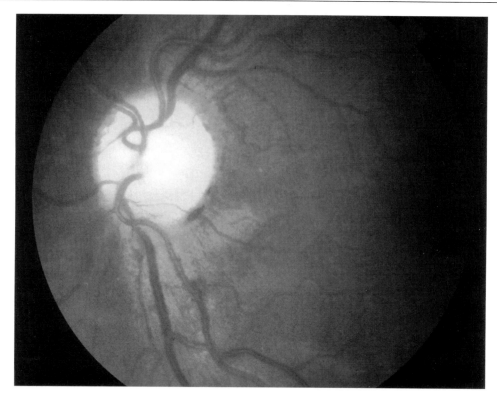

Figure 10-13 Fundoscopic image demonstrating band or bowtie atrophy in a patient with temporal hemanopia and acuity 20/20 in the ipsilateral eye and no light perception in the contralateral eye. (*See* Color Plates, following p. 176.)

of optic atrophy (Figures 13 and 14 and Color Plates; *36,99*). Selective loss of nasal nerve fibers causes optic disk pallor in a band sparing the upper and lower poles of the optic disk. Unilateral band atrophy correlates with from contralateral compression of the optic tract and is usually accompanied by diffuse temporal disk atrophy in the eye ipsilateral to the tumor. The unilateral band atrophy is in the eye opposite to the side of optic tract damage. Bilateral band atrophy specifies chiasmal tumor compression *(4)*.

Papilledema in the setting of a pituitary tumor large enough to cause hydrocephalus and deterioration of visual acuity now rarely seen *(8)*.

INCIPIENT OPTIC NERVE COMPRESSION   Pituitary adenomas and parasellar tumors extending into the prechiasmal space can precipitate a distinct syndrome of incipient optic nerve compression *(73)*. The patient complains specifically of dimming of vision in one eye, yet demonstrates near normal Snellen acuity and a normal optic disk. Dyschromatopsia as detected with pseudoisochromatic color test plates is dramatically abnormal, a relative afferent pupillary defect can be demonstrated, and subtle monocular field defects are found. Imaging confirms tumor compression at the prechiasmal portion of the optic nerve on the symptomatic side and surgical decompression restores vision promptly.

DIPLOPIA   Nonparetic Diplopia (Hemifield Slide Phenomena)   Patients with bitemporal hemianopia may complain of blurring or loss of vision with intermittent diplopia. The duplicated images may be horizontally or vertically disposed. This phenomena in the setting of normal ocular muscle function is referred to as hemifield slide (Figure 15) *(83,100–102)*. This nonparetic type of diplopia in association with pituitary tumors is actually more common than that from cranial nerve compression arising

from tumor expansion into the cavernous sinus *(58)*. In Elkington's series *(83)* of 184 patients with bitemporal hemianopia, 84 complained of diplopia without evidence of extraocular muscle palsy.

The mechanism of hemifield slide has been shown to be loss of binocular fusion stability and overlap of the preserved visual fields (Figure 16) *(101)*. With the bitemporal field deficit, there is insufficient visual stimuli to correlate corresponding and overlapping points. Loss of the linkage maintaining binocularity between the nasal field of one eye and the temporal field of the opposite eye occurs. Any tendency for the eyes to drift is not compensated, and overlap of the remaining fields leads to diplopia (Figure 16). Intermittent blurring or loss of vision at a depth of 2 to 3 feet may accompany hemifield slide. Patients have difficulty with depth perception, particularly with precision tasks that require anterior-posterior alignment, such as threading a needle. This arises from overlap of each nonseeing temporal hemifield to form a wedge of visual loss that has its apex at the fixation point (Figure 17) *(103)*. The limited field from each eye causes the fixation point to shift easily. As fixation moves closer, letters in reading may be skipped and as the fixation point shifts further away when the eyes diverge, letters or objects may appear twice in the middle field of vision due to hemifield slide *(104)*.

Paretic Diplopia   Diplopia arising from compression of one or more of the third, fourth, or sixth cranial nerves is seen generally with cavernous sinus invasion in association with advanced tumor growth. Consequently, it is a relatively uncommon complaint (Table 3) *(74,76–78,81–83,105)*. It is usually accompanied by other signs or symptoms of visual impairment, but cases of sellar lesions presenting with isolated oculomotor nerve paresis have been reported *(106)*. The third cranial nerve is involved first and most frequently *(74)*; the pupil may be dilated and poorly reactive,

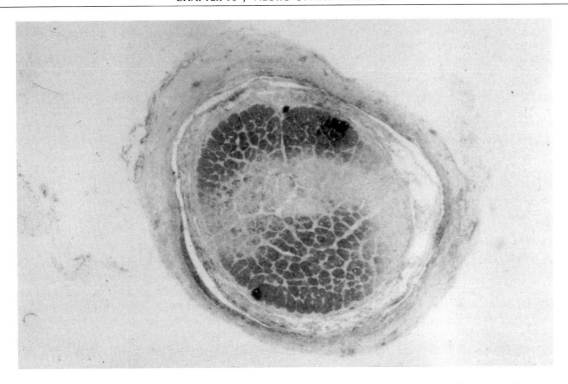

Figure 10-14 Cross-section mount of optic nerve stained for myelin, illustrating band atrophy of nerve fibers from the nasal retina. (From Sharpe JA. Visual dysfunction with basal skull tumours. Can J Neurol Sci 1985;12:332–335. With permission. *See* Color Plates.)

or it may be normal. If the oculosympathetic system is concomitantly affected, the pupil may be smaller than that of the fellow eye and constrict poorly to light and dilate weakly in darkness *(9)*.

SEE-SAW NYSTAGMUS See-saw nystagmus, a binocular synchronous alternating depression and extorsion of one eye with elevation and intorsion of the fellow eye, is an uncommon manifestation of pituitary tumors. The "see-saw" descriptor of the nystagmus denotes dysconjugate movement in the vertical plane while simultaneous torsional movements are conjugate. In Drachman's 1966 review *(107)* of see-saw nystagmus, 9 of 15 cases involved tumors in the region of the optic chiasm and diencephalon. Visual impairment due to bitemporal hemianopia and severe compromise of visual acuity was present in 11 of the 15 cases. In 2 cases the fields and acuity were normal, and the nystagmus was only transitory. See-saw nystagmus arises from visual deprivation and optic chiasm dysfunction, as well as from diencephalon and brainstem dysfunction. Drachman *(107)* suggested that a combination of these, rather than a single lesion, precipitates the clinical syndrome of see-saw nystagmus. More recently, however, see-saw nystagmus has been identified as a manifestation of isolated structural defects of the optic chiasm in patients with achiasma *(108–110)*. Furthermore, loss of vision alone has been shown to result in see-saw nystagmus *(111)*.

VISUAL HALLUCINATIONS Spontaneous visual phenomena are associated with pituitary tumors *(112,113)*. Both simple, unformed patterns of shapes and flashes of light, as well as complex, formed hallucinations of objects and people can occur. The pathophysiology of visual hallucinations has been summarized by Ram et al. *(112)* into stimulation and release phenomena. Release phenomena result from visual cortical sensory deprivation, develop and subside slowly, and can be aborted by eye movement. Homonymous hemianopias and acute visual deterioration are more

likely to precipitate release phenomena, as compared to a slowly progressive bitemporal hemianopia, which is accompanied by only partial cortical deprivation. Blindness arising at a level from the cornea to striate cortex can cause visual hallucinations attributed to sensory deprivation *(114)*. Stimulation phenomena are related to seizure activity and give rise to paroxysmal, stereotyped hallucinations that are unaffected by eye movement. In the context of pituitary tumors, they result from tumor extension and compression of the frontal and temporal lobes *(113)*.

FOSTER KENNEDY SYNDROME A single case of an extensive pituitary adenoma causing a Foster Kennedy syndrome with primary optic atrophy in one eye and papilledema in the fellow eye has been reported *(115)*.

VISUAL PRESENTATIONS WITH TUMORS OTHER THAN PITUITARY ADENOMAS **Craniopharyngiomas** The hypophyseal duct runs between the arms of the optic tracts and thus craniopharyngiomas cause early compression of the posterior chiasm *(85)*. Field changes frequently begin in the lower temporal quadrants *(85)*. In addition, a dilated third ventricle from hydrocephalus can exert pressure on the chiasm from above with the earliest field defect being a small bilateral inferior temporal quadrant scotoma close to fixation *(85)*.

The afferent visual system is affected at presentation in most cases of craniopharyngioma *(116,117)*. In Baskin and Wilson's series *(118)* of 74 childhood and adult patients with craniopharyngiomas, 53 (72%) had visual field deficits and 5 (7%) had third or sixth cranial nerve palsies. The distribution of field deficits showed bitemporal hemianopias to be the most common type of field loss (49%), but relative to studies of pituitary adenomas, there was a higher incidence of homonymous hemianopias (19%) and unilateral or bilateral blindness (11%) *(118)*. A review of papillary craniopharyngiomas reported an 84% incidence of visual loss *(119)*.

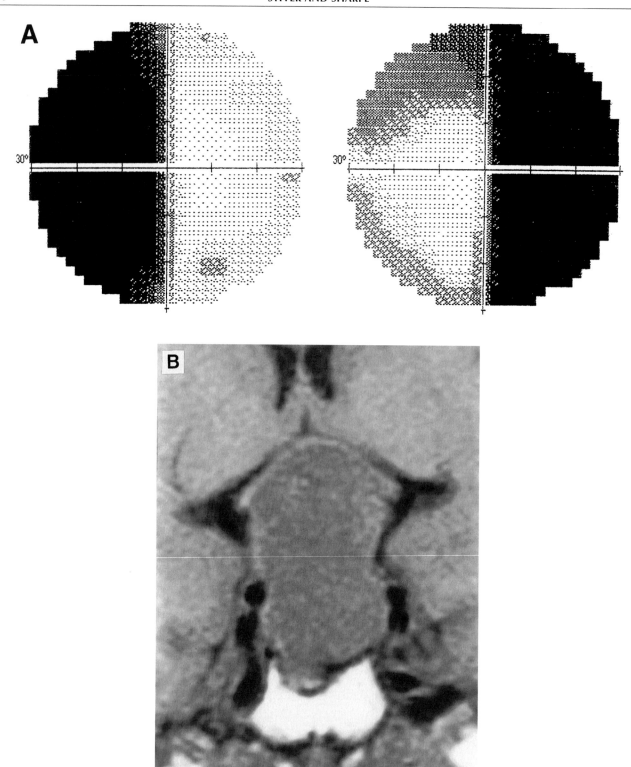

Figure 10-15   Fifty-year-old female presenting with hemifield slide phenomena. She had a 1½-yr history of difficulty reading and complained that letters would be doubled, jumbled, and/or missing. (**A**) Visual fields demonstrating bitemporal hemianopia. (**B**) Coronal MRI showing a large intrasellar mass with suprasellar extension and compression and thinning of the chiasm. Pathologically, the tumor was a pituitary adenoma with immunoreactivity for prolactin and adrenal corticotropin hormone (ACTH).

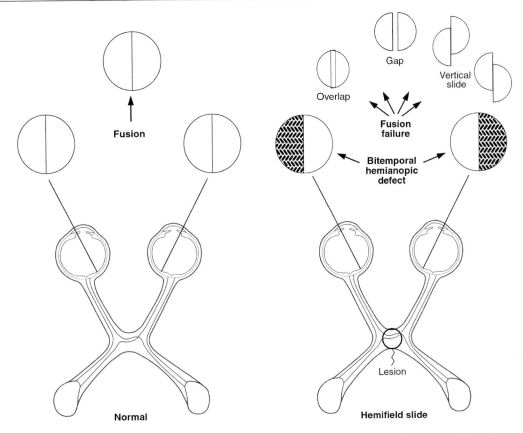

Figure 10-16 Hemifield slide phenomena arising in the setting of bitemporal hemianopia from fusion instability. The nasal and temporal fields lose their linkage, and overlap of the preserved visual fields occurs. ©The Mayo Clinic 2000.

Comparison of childhood and adult populations traditionally has reported more extensive visual loss in children related to delayed recognition of the problem (Table 4) *(116)*. Others, however, have noted a higher incidence of visual signs and symptoms in adults (Table 4) *(117,120)*.

Tuberculum and Diaphragma Sella Meningiomas Tuberculum sella meningiomas are situated in close proximity to the anterior aspect of the chiasm and therefore produce chiasmal dysfunction, typically bitemporal inferior quadrantopsia, even when they are quite small *(85)*. In a series of 88 tuberculum sella meningiomas, all but 9 were associated with visual symptoms *(121)*.

A small series of 12 diaphragma sella meningiomas, a more uncommon lesion, evidenced visual acuity deficits in 9 and field defects in 7 patients, including 5 bitemporal hemianopias and 2 monocular temporal hemianopias *(122)*.

VISUAL SYNDROMES IN SELLAR NON-TUMOROUS LESIONS Rathke's Cleft Cysts Rathke's cleft cysts are being more frequently detected by MRI and have been reported as incidental findings in up to 33% of autopsy cases *(123)*. Although usually asymptomatic, visual disturbance is a common presentation in those cysts that do become symptomatic *(124–126)*. In a series of 16 Rathke's cleft cysts treated surgically, 6 patients (38%) had visual disturbance, most commonly intermittent visual blurring *(125)*. A review of 147 cases of symptomatic Rathke's cleft cysts indicated that visual disturbance, present in 56%, was second only to pituitary dysfunction as a presenting feature *(126)*. El-Mahdy and Powell *(127)* found that only 4 patients (14%) in a series of 28 symptomatic Rathke's cleft cysts presented with visual complaints. However, examination found visual acuity impairment in 36% and field defects in 46% of patients.

Intrasellar Arachnoid Cysts Intrasellar arachnoid cysts are uncommon lesions, distinct from Rathke's cysts and empty sella. They arise by growth of a diverticulum between the layers of arachnoid in the subdiaphragmatic space or as an arachnoid diverticulum that has herniated through the diaphragma *(128)*. Unlike empty sella, free communication with the subarachnoid space does not exist, and these cysts can cause symptoms by way of local mass effect. In a surgical series of 13 biopsy-proven intrasellar arachnoid cysts, 7 (54%) patients presented with visual loss, most frequently a bitemporal hemianopia (6 of 7) *(129)*. A study of cystic pituitary lesions supports the higher incidence of visual complaints as a presenting feature in arachnoid cysts (60% of 5 patients) as compared to Rathke cleft cysts (38% of 26 patients) *(130)*.

Pregnancy During pregnancy the pituitary gland enlarges in size 70% *(131)*. Increased parity and pituitary hyperplasia, with partial but incomplete resolution following pregnancy, does not seem to be a risk factor for the development of pituitary tumors *(132)*. The issue of whether women with normal pituitary glands can develop visual field defects from enlargement of the gland during pregnancy has been debated *(8)*. The number of women with occult undiagnosed pituitary tumors who go through pregnancy without symptoms related to their tumor is unknown. For women with a known pituitary adenoma, >96% complete the pregnancy without any permanent visual sequelae *(133)*. In a series of 91 pregnancies in 73 women with untreated pituitary tumors, 25% developed symptoms or signs of visual disturbance during their

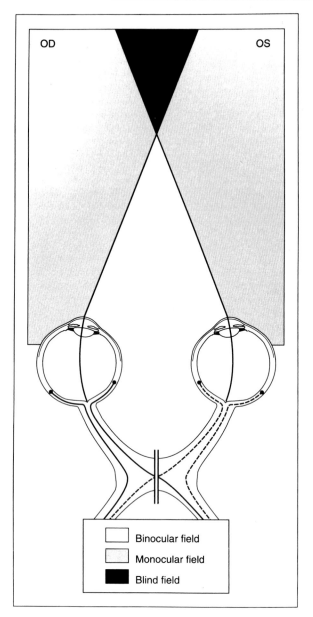

Figure 10-17 With complete bitemporal hemianopia, overlap of the nonseeing temporal fields forms a wedge of visual loss beyond the point of fixation. (From Slamovits TL, Burde R, Neuro-ophthalmology, Mosby, St. Louis, 1994, p. 4.3. With permission from Harcourt Publishers Ltd.)

radiotherapy. The risk, therefore, of visual dysfunction from enlargement of a pituitary adenoma during pregnancy depends on whether the tumor is a microadenoma or a macroadenoma. In a series of 54 prolactin microadenomas in which suprasellar extension was excluded based on perimetry, pneumoencephalography, or computed tomography, 4 patients (7.4%) developed visual symptoms during pregnancy, 2 with bitemporal hemianopsia at 37–38 wk gestation and 2 with symptoms but no field defects on examination *(136)*. This is consistent with the incidence of visual symptoms during pregnancy for microadenomas in the reports of Gemzell and Wang (5.5%) *(137)*, Molitch (1.6%) *(138)*, and Melmed et al. (6.7%) *(139)*, which suggest a relatively low risk of visual problems from microadenomas in pregnancy. Kupersmith et al. *(131)* found not a single case of visual loss in 57 cases of microadenomas. When visual symptoms and signs manifest from enlargement of a microadenoma, they typically present late in pregnancy and can be managed by waiting for resolution of the visual deficit with postpartum shrinkage of the adenoma. An isolated example of a small adenoma giving rise to a significant field impairment beginning at 24 wk gestation has been reported *(140)*. By comparison, reports of the risk of visual dysfunction from macroadenomas during pregnancy vary from 15.5% (Molitch, ref. *138*) and 16.7% (Melmed et al., ref. *139*) to 75% (Kupersmith et al., ref. *131*).

Following delivery, there is incomplete involution of the gland and each subsequent pregnancy leads to further enlargement *(8)*. Kupersmith and associates *(131)* noted that even with multiple pregnancies, no patient with a microadenoma became symptomatic. Based on reports of patients who experienced visual disturbance, not with the first but with subsequent pregnancies, others have cautioned that the risk of visual problems may increase with each pregnancy *(8)*.

Pituitary Apoplexy Pituitary apoplexy, a clinical syndrome of headache, visual loss, ophthalmoplegia, and altered mental state arises from hemorrhage or infarction of the pituitary gland usually in the setting of a pre-existing pituitary adenoma (Figure 18). It occurs in approx 2–10% of patients with pituitary tumors, more commonly macroadenomas *(141)*. Wakai et al. *(142)* have reported a 6.8% incidence of major attacks and a 2.3% incidence of minor attacks of pituitary apoplexy, as well as a 7.5% incidence of asymptomatic hemorrhage in pituitary adenoma patients. Histologic retrospective review of 783 surgically resected pituitary adenomas showed focal abnormalities of hemorrhage, ischemic infarction, or necrosis in 113 (14.4%) *(143)*. Clinically 19 (2.5%) manifested themselves as an acute syndrome that could be readily recognized as pituitary apoplexy *(143)*.

Visual symptomatology arising from pituitary apoplexy ranges from subtle and subacute complaints, slowly progressive over days of weeks, to an acute, dramatic presentation with rapid visual failure within hours. On occasion, reduction or resolution of the underlying tumor can accompany the hemorrhage and necrosis of the apoplectic event, leading to spontaneous improvement in visual symptoms caused by pre-existing tumor compression *(8,144,145)*. Pituitary apoplexy has been proposed as a marker of tumor invasiveness *(143)*.

Review of a number of case series of pituitary apoplexy by Rolih et al. *(141)* reveals an incidence of visual disturbance in 62% of patients, second only to headache as a presenting complaint. Ophthalmoplegia was present in 40–70% with third nerve palsy being most common *(141,146–149)*. Ophthalmoplegia resulting from

pregnancy. The time course for the development of visual symptoms was distributed almost evenly between the three trimesters: 36% in the first, 27% in the second, and 36% in the third trimester *(133)*. Signs and symptoms of visual dysfunction may progress more rapidly in the pregnant state. Visual problems are usually preceded by complaints of headache. The median time for the development of antecedent headache is approx at 10 wk gestation and for the onset of visual symptoms it is 14 wk gestation *(133,134)*.

Following review of data from numerous series, Molitch *(135)* has estimated the risk of symptomatic adenoma growth during pregnancy (after discontinuation of bromocriptine) to be 1% for microadenomas, 23% for macroadenomas, and 2.8% for residual tumors that have undergone prepregnancy tumor debulking or

Table 3
Incidence of Extra-ocular Muscle (EOM) Palsy in Pituitary Tumors *(74,76–78,81–83,105)*

Study	Incidence of EOM palsy	Cranial nerve(s) involved
Elkington (1968) *(83)*	14/260 (5.4%)	—
Comtois et al. (1991) *(78)*	15/126 (11.9%)	60% cranial nerve III
		20% cranial nerves IV or VI
Anderson et al. (1983) *(76)*	2/200 (1%)	—
Wilson and Dempsey (1978) *(77)*	12/250 (4.8%)	—
Trautmann and Laws (1983) *(74)*	12/851 (1.4%)	11/12 (92%) cranial nerve III
		1/12 (8%) cranial nerve VI
Wray (1976) *(81)*	1.4%	—
Hollenhorst and Younge (1973) *(82)*	46/1000 (4.6%)	—
Randall et al. (1983) *(105)*	3/100 (3%)	—

Table 4
Comparison of Visual Signs in Adult and Childhood Craniopharyngiomas *(116,120)*

	Study			
	Repka et al. (116)		*Cherninkova et al.* (120)	
Visual sign	*Children*	*Adults*	*Children*	*Adults*
Decreased visual acuity	50%	36%	70%	82%
Dyschromatopsia	82%	59%	—	—
Optic atrophy	50%	30%	52%	62%
Visual field defects	57%	91%	68%	82%

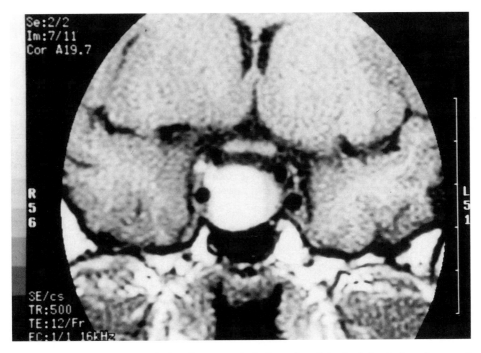

Figure 10-18 Coronal T1 MRI (without contrast) showing normal pituitary (gray) in the left pituitary fossa and a large bright signal corresponding to hemorrhage in a patient with pituitary apoplexy.

pituitary apoplexy can occur without any tumor extension into the cavernous sinus *(150)*. Thompson et al. *(151)* have described a form of pituitary apoplexy presenting primarily with extraocular muscle palsies, in which visual acuity and fields are normal and headache is only a minor complaint. All 3 cases of what they termed "non-apoplectic" pituitary apoplexy were histologically confirmed to show infarction or necrosis in addition to hemorrhage. Pituitary apoplexy has been diagnosed in a patient presenting with blurred vision due to a bitemporal hemianopic field deficit in the absence of any headache *(152)*, and a case of pituitary apoplexy presenting as an isolated third nerve palsy has also been reported *(153)*.

Lymphocytic Hypophysitis Lymphocytic hypophysitis is an uncommon disorder, typically of women in the latter stages of pregnancy or postpartum, characterized by chronic inflammation and progressive destruction of the anterior pituitary *(154,155)*. Patients present with anterior pituitary hypofunction or less commonly diabetes insipidus *(156)*. Isolated examples of visual dysfunction and field loss associated with lymphocytic hypophysitis have been reported *(157–161)*.

Pituitary Abscess Pituitary abscess may be primary, arising within a previously healthy gland, or secondary, in association with an existing pituitary lesion. Contiguous spread from meningitis, sphenoid sinusitis, or cavernous sinus thrombophlebitis has been reported, but most often a source of infection cannot be identified. Presentation with visual disturbance is common. In a series of 6 pituitary abscesses, all presented with visual symptoms *(162)*, and Domingue and Wilson *(163)* reported 7 cases of pituitary abscess in which 4 patients had complaints and evidence of visual disturbance. In many cases, the presence of an associated pituitary lesion confounds assessment of whether the abscess or the underlying sellar mass lesion was responsible for the visual loss. Given the proximity of the sphenoid sinus and the possible occurrence of CSF leak during surgical intervention, it is somewhat surprising that intrasellar abscess is not a more common complication of transsphenoidal surgery *(164)*.

Empty Sella Empty sella syndrome has traditionally been classified as primary or idiopathic, and secondary as a consequence of surgical intervention or radiation therapy of a pituitary adenoma. Visual defects are characteristically manifested more commonly in secondary empty sella and are reported to be uncommon in primary empty sella *(95,165)*. Gallardo et al. *(166)*, however, have reported an unusually high incidence of visual defects in 76 patients of whom 73 were diagnosed with primary empty sella and 3 as secondary empty sella. Visual field defects were observed in 19.7%, optic atrophy in 10.5%, papilledema in 5.3%, and extraocular muscle palsies in 4% of patients in his series *(166)*. Bjerre *(167,168)* notes that the most common field defect associated with primary empty sella is bitemporal hemianopia seen in 3 patients in his series of 20 patients with empty sella. Two cases of binasal hemianopia have been reported in primary empty sella *(vide supra)* *(95)*. Empty sella can also arise as a complication of pseudotumor cerebri and can be associated with optic atrophy from chronic papilledema *(167)*.

Classically, visual field abnormalities in empty sella syndrome have been attributed to herniation of the chiasm into the empty sella *(169)*. Ischemia has been implicated as an alternative mechanism to chiasmal herniation, but it has not been overwhelmingly adopted *(170)*. A number of studies have noted an association between coexisting pituitary adenomas and empty sella syndrome

and it has been postulated that primary empty sella syndrome arises from infarction of a preexisting pituitary adenoma *(166,168, 171,172)*. Radiologic demonstration of the evolution of a pituitary adenoma into an empty sella has been reported *(171)*. Bjerre *(167)* has argued that field defects in primary empty sella arise as a result of compression of the optic apparatus from the preexisting tumor, prior to its apoplectic transformation, or via compression brought about by the apoplexy.

MANAGEMENT OUTCOMES **Conservative Therapy** In general, pituitary tumors grow slowly over time. The 9–27% incidence of previously undiagnosed pituitary tumors found at autopsy *(173,174)* implies that not all pituitary tumors need to be treated. Indeed, large (> 2.5 cm), asymptomatic pituitary adenomas causing gross distortion of the optic nerves and chiasm have been reported as incidental autopsy findings *(175)*. Conservative management with clinical and radiological follow-up for evidence of growth and impingement on the optic pathway is appropriate for endocrinologically and visually silent tumors. Attempts to correlate the risk of visual impairment with neuroradiological imaging remain to be validated *(35,96)*. When a macroadenoma is managed conservatively, one must always be cognizant of the 2–10% incidence of pituitary apoplexy with risk of abrupt visual loss. In addition, growth of a microadenoma to a macroadenoma during 10 mo of estrogen therapy has been reported *(176)*.

Medical Management and Outcome Bromocriptine, a dopamine receptor agonist, has proved efficacious in the treatment of prolactin-secreting pituitary tumors. A multicenter study by Molitch et al. *(177)* of 27 patients with prolactin macroadenomas showed tumor size reduction in 19 patients at 6 wk and in another 8 patients at 6 mo. Prolactin levels fell to less than 11% of basal values in all but 1 patient, and normalized in 18 of the 27. The extent of tumor size reduction was equal to or greater than 50% in 18 patients (64%) but did not correlate with reduction in serum prolactin. In their study, 9 of 10 patients with abnormal visual fields had significant improvement following bromocriptine therapy *(177)*. In Moster et al.'s series *(178)* of 10 patients with prolactin macroadenomas and visual dysfunction, 6 had return of their visual acuity and fields to normal, 3 patients had persisting minor deficits after an average 15 mo follow-up on bromocriptine, and 1 patient had no response after 9 mo of therapy. In this study, 4 patients whose visual acuity was limited to finger counting or hand motion recovered useful visual function. Improvement in vision with bromocriptine treatment was noted also by Lesser et al. *(179)* in all 8 patients, 6 with blurred vision and all 8 with a field cut. In this study, improvements in visual acuity were dramatic in 2 patients with improvement of their visual acuity from finger counting to 20/25 and 20/20. In all of these studies, subjective or objective improvement in vision was noted within days of initiating therapy *(177–179)*. Radiologically, a significant reduction in tumor size has been demonstrated at 1 wk and often continues for years *(180)*. Reduction in tumor size may however be delayed, and in the absence of progressive visual field deficits, it is recommended that a trial of therapy be continued for 6 mo before a lack of response is deemed a failure *(177)*.

Long-acting injectable forms of bromocriptine have been tested against oral bromocriptine in a double blind randomized fashion *(181)*. Despite higher serum bromocriptine levels, the injectable form was well tolerated and led to a more rapid decline in prolactin levels. Use of monthly injectable bromocriptine in the treatment of 13 patients with macroprolactinomas, 5 of whom had visual field

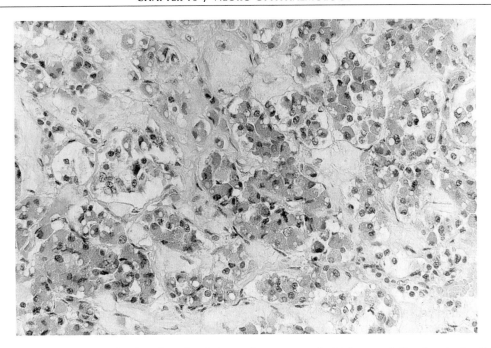

Figure 10-19   Hematoxylin and eosin stained section of a pituitary adenoma treated with bromocriptine showing hyaline fibrosis.

defects, led to improvement of visual fields in 3 and return to normal vision in 2 *(182)*. Cabergoline, a new oral dopamine agonist with duration of action up to 14 d, led to normalization of pretreatment visual field defects in 70% of patients *(183)*.

Isolated cases of visual loss during bromocriptine therapy have been ascribed to the development of postural hypotension with a decrease in perfusion pressure to a compromised visual system *(184)*. Chiasmal herniation into the sella during bromocriptine-induced macroadenoma involution can be clinically silent or may present with worsening of visual function *(180,185)*. Bromocriptine therapy of a prolactinoma induces a fibrotic reaction within the tumor (Figure 19) *(186)*. Surgeons have debated whether this fibrotic change makes surgical resection of a prolactinoma, previously treated with bromocriptine, more or less difficult *(179,187)*. Bromocriptine therapy needs to be continued indefinitely, and rapid regrowth associated with severe visual loss after discontinuation of therapy has been reported *(188,189)*. Anecdotal accounts of pituitary apoplexy during bromocriptine treatment have been reported, but a causal relationship remains speculative *(142)*. Furthermore, up to 36% of tumors will decrease in size minimally or only modestly with bromocriptine treatment *(177)*, and therefore it is important that ongoing visual assessment be carried out during therapy.

Assessment by CT and MRI suggests that approximately 20–30% of growth hormone tumors shrink with bromocriptine therapy and that this is accompanied by decreased growth hormone levels *(190)*. Rarely do growth hormone levels return to normal. However, concomitant hypersecretion of prolactin in approx 20–25% of acromegalic patients confounds a clear definition of which cells are responsive to the bromocriptine *(190,191)*. Data for the response of visual symptoms to bromocriptine treatment in acromegalic patients is sparse. In a large series of 73 acromegalic patients treated with bromocriptine, two patients with upper quadrant defects for red vision showed improvement over 3 mo of therapy, although the treatment regimen in one case was confounded by the addition of radiation therapy *(192)*. By con-

Table 5
Visual Outcome after Surgical Resection of Pituitary Macroadenomas in Relation to Preoperative Optic Disk Appearance *(84)*

Optic Disk	Visual acuity improvement	Visual field improvement
Bilateral pallor	65%	63%
Unilateral pallor	63%	55%
No atrophy	85%	72%

trast, 70–92% of acromegalic patients treated with bromocriptine experience subjective improvement of their systemic symptoms of headache, perspiration, soft tissue swelling, and articular pain, and show evidence of decreased urinary hydroxyproline excretion and improved glucose tolerance *(190,191,193,194)*.

The somatostatin analogue, octreotide, induces 10–33% tumor shrinkage in acromegalics *(195,196)*. A patient with visual loss from a growth hormone secreting macroadenoma has been documented to respond to treatment with octreotide with subjective improvement in vision beginning at 72 h, recovery of a bitemporal hemianopsia following four months of treatment, and a 20–25% reduction in tumor size by CT scan *(197)*. Octreotide has been reported also to improve visual function in nonfunctioning and gonadotropin-secreting pituitary adenomas *(198)*.

Surgical Treatment Results   Visual outcome results following surgical resection of macroadenomas in patients with preoperative visual dysfunction are summarized in Table 5 *(84)*. In general, improvement or restoration of extrafoveal visual fields can be expected in 66–97% of patients, and a smaller percentage, 42–79%, experience an improvement or return to normal of their visual acuity. Improvement of visual function is usually apparent within the first few days of decompression and continues for months afterward *(77,80,199)*. A significant improvement in visual acuity does not occur without a concomitant improvement in extrafoveal visual fields *(87)*. By contrast, the extrafoveal visual fields may improve significantly with no change in visual acuity *(87)*.

Although recovery of visual function is usually evident in the immediate postoperative period *(200)*, it is important to be aware of the possibility of delayed visual recovery when considering reoperation or radiation therapy for patients who have not responded quickly to surgical intervention *(80,201)*. Abrupt improvement in visual fields at 10 wk following subtotal tumor resection has been correlated with CT imaging demonstrating delayed collapse of the tumor capsule *(201)*. The possibility of gradual resolution of postoperative hematoma and/or residual tumor edema could not be strictly excluded. Postoperative imaging shows that it may take several months for the chiasm to return to normal position following complete tumor removal *(202)*.

The response of extraocular muscle paresis to therapy has been less extensively reported. In Wilson and Dempsey's series *(77)* of 250 adenomas, 12 patients (4.8%) had preoperative ocular muscle palsies of which 5 (41.6%) recovered fully following trans-sphenoidal surgery. These results contrast with those of Comtois et al. *(78)*, who noted complete resolution of ophthalmoplegia in 14 of 15 cases (93%) following transsphenoidal surgery. Similarly, in a series of 84 nonsecreting pituitary adenomas, 8 of 9 patients (89%) with diplopia improved following transsphenoidal resection *(203)*.

Comparative reports between visual outcome results of transsphenoidal and transcranial resection are sparse. Sullivan et al. *(84)* retrospectively reviewed 45 cases of macroadenomas with preoperative visual deficits. A transfrontal approach was used in 23 and transsphenoidal in 22, the former being done from 1968 to 1983 and the later between 1983 and 1987. Visual fields improved in 81% of transsphenoidal decompressions as compared to 56% of transcranial surgeries, whereas visual acuity results improved following transfrontal surgery in 76% as compared to 71% of transsphenoidal surgeries. Nakane et al. *(204)* reported improved visual acuity in 91% and improved visual fields in 84% after transsphenoidal procedures versus improved visual acuity in 60% and improved visual fields in 45% of patients after transfrontal craniotomy. In none of these series were patients randomized. Paracentral scotomata are considered by some surgeons to implicate a pre-fixed chiasm or retrochiasm extension of the tumor, and to thereby favor transsphenoidal as compared to transcranial decompression *(77)*.

Prognostic Factors for Visual Outcome in Surgically Treated Pituitary Adenomas   Predictors of visual recovery following surgical therapy for pituitary adenomas include severity of preoperative deficit, duration of symptoms, age of the patient, and the presence of optic atrophy. Tumor size does not appear to correlate with degree of recovery.

Preoperative Visual Loss   Preoperative visual function has been found to correlate with postoperative recovery *(75,80,86)*, and the severity of the preoperative visual loss is considered by many to be the most important predictive factor of visual outcome *(87)*. Mild preoperative dysfunction predicts complete recovery, while the degree of recovery of patients with severe loss is unpredictable *(87)*.

The nonlinearity of both visual acuity and extrafoveal field function and the uncertainty of their relative predictive importance have thwarted attempts to simplify prediction of visual outcome *(75,87)*. Efforts have been directed towards developing a unified

score to record visual field and acuity function *(80,86,87)*. Using a unified scoring system, full recovery of vision correlated with good preoperative vision, whereas significant preoperative deficit was associated with poor recovery. Outcome in cases with intermediate preoperative function was dependent on other factors such as age, duration of symptoms, and size of tumor *(86)*.

VISUAL ACUITY   Preoperative visual acuity is predictive of outcome. Significant recovery can be expected in 77–89% of eyes with preoperative acuity of 20/100 or better, but below this there is only a 62–69% chance of meaningful recovery *(75,84)*. A preoperative visual field deficit without loss of acuity indicates more limited compression and therefore a better prognosis *(75)*.

VISUAL FIELDS   In contrast to the predictive value of preoperative visual acuity, the degree of preoperative extrafoveal visual field deficit does not correlate as rigorously with visual outcome *(75)*. Blaauw et al. *(86)* have developed a scoring system for visual fields, weighted towards the central fields, which correlates preoperative deficit with the degree of postoperative recovery. Despite this, it has been observed that patients with severe field loss can experience dramatic improvements in vision *(75)*. Scotomatous types of field defects are thought to indicate rapid tumor growth and have been typified as a good prognostic sign, with 62–72% of patients experiencing full recovery of their visual fields following decompression *(205,206)*.

OPTIC ATROPHY   In general, the prognostic importance of the color of the optic disk has been debated, except that most agree that visual outcome will not improve in the setting of a preoperative frankly atrophic disk *(75,205)*. In El-Azouzi et al.'s series of 41 patients, 6 of 7 with evidence of optic atrophy showed no change in vision after surgery *(207)*. In contrast to studies noted above, Sullivan et al. *(84)* found no association between visual recovery and preoperative visual acuity and extrafoveal fields in their study of 45 symptomatic macroadenomas. They reported, however, an association between preoperative optic atrophy and poor recovery of acuity and fields, but it did not reach statistical significance due to limitations of sample size (Table 5).

Patients with poor visual function without changes in the optic disk may still experience good recovery, if the preoperative optic disk is normal or shows only temporal pallor (Table 6) *(205)*. Hajda and Pásztor *(205)* have argued that the appearance of the optic disk is a better indicator of visual outcome than preoperative acuity or field function. They suggested that the prognostic importance of field or acuity status is confounded by (1) the association of peripheral field defects and good visual acuity with normal optic disks and (2) the relationship between central field defects and poor visual acuity with optic disk pallor.

Duration of Symptoms   An inverse correlation between the duration of both field and acuity loss with postoperative visual prognosis has been noted by a number of authors *(75,80,87)*. In Symon and Jakubowski's series *(80)* of 94 patients with visual dysfunction from a pituitary adenoma, 50 had a history of symptoms less than 1 year, 22 a history between 1–2 yr, and 22 a history of 2–10 yr. The group with full recovery of vision had a mean symptomatic period less than 1 year, and as the duration of symptoms increased, the recovery declined. Duration may, however, not be an independent risk factor, but rather may simply reflect the severity of preoperative visual loss *(75)*.

Age   Studies have reported an inverse correlation of age and outcome *(75,80,87)*. In the setting of a large tumor, Symon and Jakubowski *(80)* noted a proportional decrease in visual recovery

Table 6
Visual Outcome Following Transsphenoidal Resection
of 117 Pituitary Adenomas in Relation
to Preoperative Optic Disk Appearance *(205)*

Visual outcome	Normal	Improved	Unchanged	Worsened
Optic disk normal	59%	25%	13.6%	2.3%
Temporal pallor	28.6%	62.8%	8.6%	—
Optic atrophy	0	47.5%	42.5%	10%

Table 7
Visual Outcome Following Transsphenoidal Resection
of Suprasellar Nonsecretory
and Prolactin Secreting Pituitary Tumors *(74)*

	Improvement in visual function	
	Nonsecretory	Secretory
Visual acuity	35/82 (43%)	15/21 (71%)
Visual fields	106/149 (71%)	49/56 (87%)

with each consecutive decade and a sharper decline in outcome after 60 years. Neither age nor tumor size alone had prognostic significance in their study. Others have not found a correlation between age and visual outcome *(84)*.

Tumor Size Most studies have failed to find a correlation between tumor size or degree of suprasellar extension and postoperative visual recovery *(80,87,200)*. Hudson et al. *(33)* prospectively studied preoperative and postoperative visual fields in relation to tumor volume calculated from thin cuts on CT imaging. Preoperative visual field loss in the superonasal, but not inferonasal, superotemporal or inferotemporal quadrants correlated with tumor volume. Intuitively this is reasonable since the superonasal field is involved late in the course of chiasmal compression. Tumor volume could not be correlated with postoperative visual field recovery with the exception that it predicted inferonasal field recovery in small tumors whose volume was 5 cm^3 or less *(33)*.

Tumor Type In a comparison of suprasellar prolactinomas and nonsecretory tumors, Trautmann and Laws *(74)* noted that patients with nonsecretory tumors had a poorer visual outcome attributed to the larger size of these tumors at the time of diagnosis (Table 7).

Reoperation Symptomatic patients undergoing surgery for the first time have been reported to experience an overall improvement in their visual acuity in 87% of cases, while repeat surgery yields a 68% chance of visual acuity improvement *(75)*. Visual fields also responded with a similar trend. Comparison of preoperative vision between the two groups was not detailed.

Postoperative Visual Deterioration **Immediate** The incidence of visual worsening after surgical decompression in the hands of experienced pituitary surgeons varies from 0–4% *(75,200,208)*. Extrafoveal visual fields almost never deteriorate postoperatively without accompanying significant loss of visual acuity *(75)*.

In Trautman and Laws' large series of 1003 patients *(74)*, in which 851 had a diagnosis of pituitary adenoma, 18 patients' vision worsened with surgery. Thirteen experienced visual loss, two visual loss and extraocular palsy, and three extraocular palsy without visual loss *(74)*. In Wilson and Dempsey's *(77)* series of 250 transsphenoidal operations, permanent postoperative visual impairment occurred in a single case, from an intrasellar hematoma. Temporary monocular loss of vision occurred in an additional 5 cases and was attributed to edema in 3 and to intracapsular hematoma in 2. Evacuation of the two hematomas led to subsequent improvement in vision. Three patients in this series acquired new extraocular palsies, 2 of which recovered fully. Transient oculomotor or abducens nerve palsies have been noted in 1–4% of transsphenoidal approaches *(77,209)*.

Visual complications after transsphenoidal resection of pituitary adenomas in patients with normal fields, acuity, and ocular motility preoperatively are unusual *(77,84)*. In Trautmann and Laws' series *(74)*, 5 of 581 patients undergoing transphenoidal pituitary resection had normal vision preoperatively but not postoperatively.

Visual deterioration following surgery is most commonly a result of a postoperative hematoma *(208)*. In the setting of significant residual tumor following resection, postoperative swelling can also worsen vision and can be a precipitating factor in the formation of a postoperative hematoma. In 100 transsphenoidal surgeries, Cohen et al. *(75)* reported a 3% incidence of early postoperative visual deterioration, of which 1 was caused by an intrasellar hematoma and 2 were related to residual tumor. Early reexploration improved vision in 2 patients, but reexploration at 2 wk in a third patient failed to bring about any change in vision.

Visual evoked potentials monitored during chiasmal decompression show that deterioration in cortical response with manipulation of the chiasm does not predict a postoperative visual deficit *(210,211)*. In contrast, the absence of any deterioration of evoked potentials intraoperatively is a reliable prognostic sign of a good outcome *(210,211)*. In transcranial approaches, the vulnerability of a compressed chiasm to frontal lobe retraction may be a factor in postoperative visual deterioration *(54)*. The vascular supply to the chiasm is at greater risk during transcranial surgery *(80)*, whereas the transsphenoidal approach does not breech the arachnoid and spares the blood supply to the chiasm *(75)*.

Slavin et al. *(212)* have reported two cases of visual deterioration attributed to inadvertent packing of fat into the suprasellar cistern during closure of the transsphenoidal approach. Wilson and Dempsey *(77)* comment on a single case of a third nerve palsy secondary to excessive packing of the sella. Although reports of this complication are rare, Slavin et al. *(212)* suggest that it may be a more common occurrence, and argue that failure of chiasmal decompression to improve vision quickly or a new postoperative visual deficit should lead one to consider that excessive fat has been placed in the sella.

Delayed Delayed visual dysfunction following surgical resection is a sign of tumor recurrence, radionecrosis, chiasmal arachnoiditis, or empty sella syndrome. Recurrent tumor is the most common cause of delayed visual deterioration following pituitary tumor resection *(4)*. Recurrence rates vary widely from 1–21% *(74,78,200)* usually becoming clinically evident at an average of 4–8 yr after treatment *(200)*. Radiation, near the time of initial surgery, delays the time to recurrence *(200)*.

The development of empty sella syndrome is frequently quoted as a cause of delayed visual deterioration following pituitary treatment. Visual change has been attributed to descent of the chiasm into the empty sella. Adams *(213)* has cogently argued that secondary empty sella is not a cause of postoperative visual deterioration. He suggests that progressive visual loss in the setting of an empty sella is more often attributable to delayed radiation induced vascular changes *(213)*. However, a few cases of empty sella with visual dysfunction following surgical tumor resection and without radiation treatment argue against this theory *(214)*.

Outcome Results for Tumors and Conditions Other Than Pituitary Adenomas *Craniopharyngiomas* Visual outcome after surgical treatment of craniopharyngiomas is not as favorable as for pituitary adenomas. This has been attributed to the adherent character of these tumors and their relative posterior location making removal more difficult *(116)*. In a series of 40 craniopharyngiomas treated by transsphenoidal surgery in whom 34 had abnormal vision preoperatively, normalization of vision occurred in only 7, improvement in 2, no change in 23, and worsening in 2 *(74)*. Baskin and Wilson *(118)* report a series of 74 patients operated on through transcranial (61%) or transsphenoidal (39%) routes with complete resection achievable in only 7 patients. They were able, however, to accomplish stabilization or improvement of ophthalmologic status in 91% of patients with subtotal resection and radiation. Using a transcranial approach in adult patients, Repka et al. *(116)* reported that visual acuity loss present in 42% of eyes preoperatively decreased to 23% of eyes postoperatively, and that fields improved from 9% with normal fields preoperatively to 48% with normal fields postoperatively. Visual acuity but not extrafoveal field recovery was the same between adults and children. A recent long-term outcome analysis of surgically resected craniopharyngiomas demonstrated that preoperative visual deterioration was significantly associated with poor outcome *(215)*. In this study 62% of patients had preoperative visual field deficits and approx 45% had pallor of at least one optic disk. After surgical intervention by transcranial and transsphenoidal routes, vision improved in approx 25%, was unchanged in 50%, and worsened in 25% *(215)*.

In a pediatric series, Abrams and Repka *(216)* also reported that preoperative visual symptoms were associated with a poor visual outcome following surgical treatment. Children presenting at less than 6 yr of age did significantly worse than older children, due to the higher incidence of unrecognized visual loss in the younger group. Comparative studies of visual outcome in children versus adults have documented more severe visual loss at presentation and poorer recovery following treatment in visually symptomatic childhood craniopharyngiomas *(120)*.

Konig et al. *(217)* compared the results of transnasal and transcranial approaches to craniopharyngioma resection. Following transnasal resection, full recovery or improvement of vision occurred in 94% of patients with preoperative visual dysfunction. After transcranial surgery, only 65% of patients had improvement of their visual status, and there was an associated 26% incidence of visual deterioration with the transcranial approach *(217)*. Fahlbusch et al. *(117)* also report a more favorable visual outcome following transsphenoidal as compared to transcranial resection. Transcranial resection in 75 patients with visual symptoms led to vision normalization in 36%, improvement in 35%, no change in 15%, and worsened function in 15%. Furthermore, 7% of preoperatively asymptomatic patients incurred a new deficit. Transsphenoidal resection was not associated with any worsened visual function or new deficits; 47% of symptomatic patients normalized, 40% improved, and 13% had no change in their visual

status *(117)*. For patients with severely impaired vision, cyst aspiration followed by a waiting period to allow vision to stabilize prior to definitive surgery has been reported to improve visual outcome *(218)*.

Rathke's Cleft and Intrasellar Cysts Visual symptoms from Rathke's cleft and intrasellar cysts respond well to surgical intervention. Meyer et al. *(129)* reported improved visual outcome in all 7 patients with visual field loss secondary to an intrasellar arachnoid cyst following transsphenoidal exploration and marsupialization of the cyst wall.

Review of 137 Rathke's cleft cysts treated by a comparable mix of transsphenoidal and transcranial procedures, showed that of 76 patients with preoperative visual field defects, 8 resolved, 31 improved, 6 remained unchanged, and none worsened following surgical intervention *(126)*. Similarly, of 40 patients with impaired visual acuity, 6 experienced resolution, 15 improved, 5 remained unchanged, and none worsened with surgical treatment *(126)*. (In this study, not all patients had both pre- and postoperative testing.) Transfrontal (9) or transsphenoidal (1) decompression with partial cyst resection (and one radical cyst excision) led to normalization of vision in 4, improvement in 2, and residual deficit in 3, with 2 patients being lost to follow-up in Repka et al.'s *(116)* study of 11 visually symptomatic Rathke's cleft cysts.

Complete evacuation of the cyst contents and extensive opening of the cyst wall has been recommended, as simple cyst aspiration frequently led to recurrence *(126)*. Unless the cyst is entirely suprasellar, the transsphenoidal approach is preferred since the recurrence rate is approximately one-half that of a transcranial procedure and the risk of aseptic meningitis from spillage of the cyst contents into the subarachnoid space is lower *(126)*. All five patients of Ross et al. *(123)* with Rathke's cleft cysts achieved full recovery of their vision following cyst decompression and fenestration via a transsphenoidal route. In El-Madhy's and Powell series *(127)* operated through a transsphenoidal approach with partial cyst wall excision and cyst drainage, 67% of preoperative visual acuity deficits and 68% of field defects improved or normalized with surgery. Postoperative improvement correlated inversely with the degree of preoperative field or acuity loss.

Tuberculum Sella and Diaphragma Meningiomas Craniotomy and resection of 88 tuberculum sella meningiomas, in which all but 9 were associated with visual symptoms, led to improvement in vision in 54%, no change in 27%, and worsening of vision in 19% *(121)*. In the Kinjo et al. *(122)* series of 12 diaphragma meningiomas all were reported to have a good outcome following surgical resection.

Pregnancy Management of pituitary adenomas with visual dysfunction during pregnancy depends on the nature of the tumor, the stage of pregnancy at presentation of visual symptoms, and the severity and temporal profile of the visual impairment. Symptoms presenting in the first two trimesters from tumors other than prolactinomas are usually managed surgically unless the visual deficit is minimal and stable *(133)*. Patients presenting with visual symptoms in the third trimester can usually be followed without surgery. Treatment is delivery as soon as the fetus is viable.

If the tumor is a prolactinoma a trial of bromocriptine can be undertaken with careful monitoring of visual status. Mashima and Oguchi *(219)* have used visual evoked potentials (VEP) to monitor the reversibility of visual dysfunction in pregnancy. Normal latencies correlated with full recovery of field defects and visual acuity loss, but delayed latencies were associated with permanent visual impairment. A women who presented with bitemporal hemianopia and blurred vision at 22 wk was carried to 38 wk before induction of delivery based on normal VEP latencies; as predicted her seriously impaired visual function returned to normal after childbirth. Prolactin levels are not useful for following prolactinomas with visual symptoms *(136)*. A lack of response to bromocriptine (with anything but a mild visual deficit) or visual deterioration is an indication for surgical intervention. During pregnancy, concerns raised about the safety of bromocriptine need to be considered *(8,135,136,220)*.

Surgical intervention during pregnancy does not carry a higher complication rate *(133)*. In Magyar and Marshalls' review *(133)* of 91 pregnancies in 73 women with untreated pituitary tumors, 23 (25%) became symptomatic with visual dysfunction, 22 of whom underwent surgical or radiation treatment, and only 1 experienced a persistent visual deficit.

Pituitary Apoplexy The strongest indication for emergent surgical intervention of pituitary apoplexy is acute severe visual deterioration. Early but not emergent surgery is favored for most other indications *(221)*. In a series of 12 cases, surgery performed up to 3 wk after the apoplectic event was associated with progression of visual symptoms in only 1 case *(221)*. In Bills et al.'s *(148)* series of 38 patients, all but one of whom was treated by transsphenoidal decompression, improvement in visual acuity occurred in 88%, in visual fields in 95%, and in ocular paresis in 100% of patients, with only 1 patient experiencing a worsening of visual acuity. Bills et al. *(148)* have suggested that delay in decompression beyond 1 wk may retard visual recovery.

In a study of 35 patients with an acute apoplectic episode symptomatic with headache or visual disturbance, Randeva et al. *(149)* demonstrated the clear benefit to transsphenoidal surgery within 8 d of the event. Overall, visual acuity deficits improved in 86%, field deficits in 76%, and ocular paresis in 91%. Visual acuity normalized in 100% of patients treated within 8 d, whereas normal acuity was restored in only 46% and partially improved in 31% of those treated beyond 8 d. Visual fields normalized in 75% of those undergoing early surgery and in only 23% of those decompressed after 8 d. Ocular paretic deficits responded better as well, with normalization after early surgery in 73% as compared to only 42% decompressed by late surgery *(149)*.

It has been argued that patients solely with ophthalmoplegia or those who present in a delayed fashion relative to the apoplectic event do not necessarily require surgery *(146,222)*. Opthalmoplegia is well documented to recover without intervention, although the recovery may be incomplete. A trial of conservative therapy with decadron for 7 d, with surgical intervention at that time if recovery was incomplete or earlier if there was progression of symptoms, showed resolution of ophthalmoplegia in 6 of 7 patients *(223)*. Transsphenoidal surgery was performed in 5 patients, with normalization of vision in 1, partial recovery in 1, and minimal change in 2 (1 patient not accounted for). The poor outcome from surgery was attributed to the severity of visual loss at presentation, not to the delay in surgical intervention *(223)*. Onesti et al. *(147)* reported improved visual function following surgery in 13 of 16 patients, 56% with preoperative visual acuity loss, 69% with field loss, and 44% with ophthalmoplegia. Of note, 3 patients with monocular or binocular blindness decompressed at 2–5 d after the apoplectic event, showed no recovery of vision. This may support the concept that severity of visual loss is a prognostic determinant of outcome in pituitary apoplexy.

Empty Sella Progressive visual field loss is an indication for surgical intervention in empty sella syndrome. Outcome results are equivocal with a significant number of patients experiencing no improvement in their vision. Gallardo et al. *(166)* reported that only 46% of patients had improvement of their visual disturbance after transsphenoidal packing of 56 cases of empty sella. Surgical exploration of eight empty sella syndromes demonstrated two patients with descent of the chiasm who improved postoperatively without any packing of muscle or fat into the sella *(169)*. Six of the 8 patients were found to have arachnoid adhesions and had no significant improvement in their vision *(169)*. Others have suggested that the finding of dense scar tissue at surgery correlates with visual improvement following detethering *(214)*. In a single case report, detethering and packing of the empty fossa led to improvement in visual function even when carried out 18 mo after the onset of visual dysfunction *(224)*.

Radiation Therapy Recent monographs have reviewed radiation and radiosurgical treatment of pituitary tumors *(225,226)*. Single dose tolerance of the optic chiasm is 8–10 Gy with a required clearance of 3–5 mm *(227)*. The optic pathway is spared with total radiation doses of 45 Gy given in fractions of 1.8 Gy over 35 d in 25 sessions *(213)*, and injury is more frequently associated with total doses exceeding 50 Gy with fractions of 2.5 Gy *(4)*. Patients vary in their sensitivity to radiation-induced damage. The development of visual symptoms during the course of the radiation treatments is unusual *(6)*.

Visual loss associated with radiation optic neuropathy is usually profound and of acute onset. Field defects may accompany the acuity loss. Visual deficits typically present within 3 yr, with a peak incidence at 8–18 mo, following treatment *(228)*. Risk factors for visual loss following stereotactic Gamma Knife radiotherapy include a dose to the optic apparatus exceeding 8 Gy and pretreatment visual dysfunction *(228)*. MRI studies at the time of visual deterioration show enlargement and gadolinium contrast enhancement of the optic chiasm *(228,229)*. Follow-up studies demonstrate atrophy of the optic chiasm and contrast enhancement has been shown to persist even 1 yr later *(229)*. Fundoscopy may be normal or show swelling of the optic nerve head in the acute setting, with atrophy not becoming evident until 4–8 wk later *(4)*.

CONCLUSION

Recent fascinating developments have been achieved in the study of the embryological development of the optic chiasm. The complex nature of fiber pathways laid down *in utero* come to light with many interesting clinical signs and symptoms when the optic complex is compressed by pituitary lesions. Over the years significant advances have been made in both the medical and surgical management of pituitary lesions. In more recent years, emphasis has turned to critical appraisal of outcome results and determination of prognostic factors.

REFERENCES

1. Rucker CW. The concept of a semidecussation of the optic nerves. Arch Ophthalmol 1958;59:159–171.
2. Cushing H. The chiasmal syndrome of primary optic atrophy and bitemporal field defects in adults with a normal sella turcica. Arch Ophthalmol 1930;3:704–735.
3. Scott GI. Traquair's Clinical Perimetry, 7th ed. Henry Kimpton, London, England, 1957, pp. 218–252.
4. Arnold AC. Neuroophthalmologic evaluation of pituitary disorders. In: Melmed S, ed. The Pituitary. Blackwell Scientific, Cambridge, MA, 1995, pp. 687–707.

5. Hoyt WF. Correlative functional anatomy of the optic chiasm. Clin Neurosurg 1970;17:189–208.

6. Melen O. Neuro-ophthalmologic features of pituitary tumors. Endocrinol Metab Clin 1987;16:585–608.

7. Slamovits TL. Anatomy and Physiology of the Optic Chiasm. In: Miller NR, Newman NJ, eds. Walsh and Hoyt's Clinical Neuro-Ophthalmology. vol. 1, 5th ed. Williams & Wilkins, Baltimore, 1998, pp. 85–100.

8. Gittinger JW, Jr. Tumors of the Pituitary Gland. In: Miller NR, Newman NJ, eds. Walsh and Hoyt's Clinical Neuro-Ophthalmology. vol. 2, 5th ed. Williams & Wilkins, Baltimore, 1998, pp. 2141–2221.

9. Wormington CM. Pituitary adenoma: diagnosis and management. J Am Optom Assoc 1989;60:929–935.

10. Lesser RL. Neuro-ophthalmic aspects of pituitary disease. In: Goodrich I, Lee KJ, eds. The Pituitary. Clinical Aspects of Normal and Abnormal Function. Elsevier Science, Amsterdam, The Netherlands, 1987, pp. 67–85.

11. Alleyne Jr CH, Newman N. Neuro-Ophthalmology of Pituitary Tumors. In: Krisht AF, Tindall GT, eds. Pituitary Disorders. Lippincott Williams & Wilkins, Baltimore, 1999, pp. 165–185.

12. Chung SM. Neuro-ophthalmic manifestations of pituitary tumors. Neurosurg Clin N Am 1999;10:717–729.

13. Barber AN, Ronstrom GN, Muelling Jr RJ. Development of the visual pathway: optic chiasm. Arch Ophthalmol 1954;52:447–453.

14. Horton JC, Greenwood MM, Hubel DH. Non-retinotopic arrangement of fibres in the cat optic nerve. Nature 1979;282:720–722.

15. Guillery RW, Mason CA, Taylor JSH. Developmental determinants at the mammalian optic chiasm. J Neurosci 1995;15:4727–4737.

16. Sretavan DW, Puré E, Siegel MW, Reichardt LF. Disruption of retinal axon ingrowth by ablation of embryonic mouse optic chiasm neurons. Science 1995;269:98–101.

17. Marcus RC, Shimamura K, Sretavan D, Lai E, Rubenstein JLR, Mason CA. Domains of regulatory gene expression and the developing optic chiasm: correspondence with retinal axon paths and candidate signaling cells. J Comp Neurol 1999;403:346–358.

18. Mason CA, Sretavan DW. Glia, neurons, and axon pathfinding during optic chiasm development. Curr Opin Neurobiol 1997;7:647–653.

19. Sretavan DW, Feng L, Puré E, Reichardt LF. Embryonic neurons of the developing optic chiasm express L1 and CD44, cell surface molecules with opposing effects on retinal axon growth. Neuron 1994;12:957–975.

20. Sakamoto H. Development of the trigeminus, with particular reference to the ophthalmic nerve. Acta Soc Ophthal Jap 1952;56:1355–1357.

21. Sakamoto H. Embryology of the third, fourth, and sixth cranial nerves. Acta Soc Ophthal Jap 1953;57:146–148.

22. Marcus RC, Blazeski R, Godement P, Mason Ca. Retinal axon divergence in the optic chiasm: Uncrossed axons diverge from crossed axons within a midline glial specialization. J Neurosci 1995;15:3716–3729.

23. Sretavan DW, Reichardt LF. Time-lapse video analysis of retinal ganglion cell axon pathfinding at the mammalian optic chiasm: Growth cone guidance using intrinsic chiasm cues. Neuron 1993;10:761–777.

24. Godement P, Mason CA. Retinal axon divergence in the optic chiasm: Dynamics of growth cone behavior at the midline. J Neurosci 1994;14:7024–7039.

25. Chan SO, Wong KF, Chung KY, Yung WH. Changes in morphology and behavior of retinal growth cones before and after crossing the midline of the mouse chiasm—a confocal microscopy study. Eur J Neurosci 1998;10:2511–2522.

26. Godement P, Vanselow J, Thanos S, Bonhoeffer F. A study of the developing visual systems with a new method of staining neurons and their processes in fixed tissue. Development 1987;101:697–713.

27. Taylor JSH, Guillery RW. The effect of a very early monocular enucleation upon the development of the uncrossed retinofugal pathway in ferrets. J Comp Neurol 1995;357:331–340.

28. Chan SO, Chung KY, Taylor JSH. The effects of early prenatal monocular enucleation on the routing of uncrossed retinofugal axons and the cellular environment at the chiasm of mouse embryos. Eur J Neurosci 1999;11:3225–3235.

29. Stretavan DW, Kruger K. Randomized retinal ganglion cell axon routing at the optic chiasm of GAP-43-deficient mice: association with midline recrossing and lack of normal ipsilateral axon turning. J Neurosci 1998;18:10502–10513.

30. Kaplan SL, Grumbach MM, Aubert ML. The orthogenesis of pituitary hormones and hypothalamic factors in the human fetus: Maturation of central nervous system regulation of anterior pituitary functions. Recent Prog Horm Res 1976;32:161–243.

31. Sabshin JK. The pituitary gland—anatomy and embryology. In: Goodrich I, Lee KJ, eds. The Pituitary. Clinical Aspects of Normal and Abnormal Function. Elsevier Science, Amsterdam, The Netherlands, 1987, pp. 19–27.

32. Robinson F, Goodrich I. Neurological manifestations of extrasellar expanding pituitary adenomas. In: Goodrich I, Lee KJ, eds. The Pituitary. Clinical Aspects of Normal and Abnormal Function. Elsevier Science, Amsterdam, The Netherlands, 1987, pp. 55–65.

33. Hudson H, Rissell C, Gauderman WJ, Feldon SE. Pituitary tumor volume as a predictor of postoperative visual field recovery. J Clin Neuroophthalmol 1991;11:280–283.

34. Bergland RM, Ray BS, Torack RM. Anatomical variations in the pituitary gland and adjacent structures in 255 human autopsy cases. J Neurosurg 1968;28:93–99.

35. Ikeda H, Yoshimoto T. Visual disturbances in patients with pituitary adenoma. Acta Neurol Scand 1995;92:157–160.

36. Unsöld R, Hoyt WF. Band atrophy of the optic nerve: the histology of temporal hemianopsia. Arch Ophthalmol 1980;98:1637–1638.

37. Naito J. Retrogeniculate projection fibers in the monkey optic chiasm: a demonstration of the fiber arrangement by means of wheat germ agglutinin conjugated to horseradish peroxidase. J Comp Neurol 1994;346:559–571.

38. Kupfer C, Chumbley L, Downer JC. Quantitative histology of optic nerve, optic tract and lateral geniculate nucleus of man. J Anat 1967;101:393–401.

39. Brouwer B, Zeeman WPC. Experimental anatomical investigations concerning the projection of the retina of the primary optic centers in apes. J Neurol Psychopathol 1925;6:1–10.

40. Brouwer B, Zeeman WPC. The projection of the retina in the primary optic neuron in monkeys. Brain 1926;49:1–35.

41. Hoyt WF, Lois O. The primate chiasm: Details of visual fiber organization studied by silver impregnation techniques. Arch Ophthalmol 1963;70:69–85.

42. Hoyt WF, Tudor RC. The course of the parapapillary temporal retinal axons through the anterior optic nerve: A Nauta degeneration study in the primate. Arch Ophthalmol 1963;69:503–507.

43. Hoyt WF, Lois O. Visual fiber anatomy in the infrageniculate pathway of the primate. uncrossed and crossed retinal fiber projection studied by Nauta silver stain. Arch Ophthalmol 1962;68:94–106.

44. Glaser JS. Neuro-ophthalmology, 2nd ed. J.B. Lippincott, Philadelphia, 1990, p. 71.

45. Reese BE. Clinical implications of the fibre order in the optic pathway of primates. Neurol Res 1993;15:83–86.

46. Kosmorsky GS, Tomsak RL, Diskin DK. Absence of the relative afferent pupillary defect with monocular temporal visual field loss. J Clin Neuroophthalmol 1992;12:181–191.

47. Horton JC. Wilbrand's knee of the primate optic chiasm is an artefact of monocular enucleation. Trans Am Ophthalmol Soc 1997;95:579–609.

48. Bergland R, Ray BR. The arterial supply of the human optic chiasm. J Neurosurg 1969;31:327–334.

49. Dawson BH. The blood vessels of the human optic chiasma and their relation to those of the hypophysis and hypothalamus. Brain 1958;81:207–217.

50. Miller NR. Vascular supply of the visual pathways. In: Miller NR, ed. Walsh and Hoyt's Clinical Neuro-ophthalmology. vol. 1, 4th ed. 1982, pp. 104–107.

51. Perlmutter D, Rhoton AL. Microsurgical anatomy of the anterior cerebral-anterior communicating recurrent artery complex. J Neurosurg 1976;45:259–272.

52. Wollschlaeger P, Wollschlaeger G, Ide C, Hart W. Arterial blood supply of the human optic chiasm and surrounding structures. Ann Ophthalmol 1971;3:862–869.

53. Francois J, Neetens A, Collette JM. Vascularization of the primary optic pathways. Br J Ophthalmol 1958;42:65–80.

54. O'Connell JEA. The anatomy of the optic chiasma and heteronymous hemianopia. J Neurol Neurosurg Psychiatry 1973;36:710–723.

55. Hedges TR. The preservation of the upper nasal field in the chiasmal syndrome: An anatomic explanation. Trans Am Ophthalmol Soc 1969;67:131–141.

56. McDonald WI. The symptomatology of tumours of the anterior visual pathways. Can J Neurol Sci 1982;9:381–390.

57. Lao Y, Gao H, Zhong Y. Vascular architecture of the human optic chiasma and bitemporal hemianopia. Chin Med Sci J 1994;9:38–44.

58. Halle AA, Drewry RD, Robertson JT. Ocular manifestations of pituitary adenomas. South Med J 1983;76:732–735.

59. Clifford-Jones RE, McDonald WI, Landon DN. Chronic optic nerve compression: An experimental study. Brain 1985;108:241–262.

60. Jacobson SG, Eames RA, McDonald WI. Optic nerve fibre lesions in adult cats: Pattern of recovery of spatial vision. Exp Brain Res 1979;36:491–508.

61. Tassinari G, Marzi CA, Lee BB, Di Lollo V, Campara D. A possible selective impairment of magnocellular function in compression of the anterior visual pathways. Exp Brain Res 1999;127:391–401.

62. Tassinari G, Campara D, Balercia G, Chilosi M, Martignoni G, Marzi CA. Magno- and parvocellular pathways are segregated in the human optic tract. Neuroreport 1994;5:1425–1428.

63. Porciatti V, Ciavarella P, Ghiggi MR, D'Angelo V, Padovano S, Grifa M, Moretti G. Losses of hemifield contrast sensitivity in patients with pituitary adenoma and normal visual acuity and visual field. Clin Neurophysiol 1999;110:876–886.

64. Gutowski NJ, Heron JH, Scase MO. Early impairment of foveal magno- and parvocellular pathways in juxta chiasmal tumours. Vision Res 1997;37:1401–1408.

65. Garfield J, Neil-Dwyer G. Delay in diagnosis of optic nerve and chiasmal compression presenting with unilateral failing vision. Br Med J 1975;1:22–25.

66. Segal AJ, Fishman RS. Delayed diagnosis of pituitary tumors. Am J Ophthalmol 1975;79:77–81.

67. Mohr G, Hardy J, Comtois R, Beauregard H. Surgical management of giant pituitary adenomas. Can J Neurol Sci 1990;17:62–66.

68. Gott PS, Weiss MH, Apuzzo M, Van Der Meulen JP. Checkerboard visual evoked response in evaluation and management of pituitary tumors. Neurosurgery 1979;5:553–558.

69. Brecelj J. A VEP study of the visual pathway function in compressive lesions of the optic chiasm. Full-field versus half-field stimulation. Electroencephalogr Clin Neurophysiol 1992;84:209–218.

70. Harrington DO. The Visual Fields. A Textbook and Atlas of Clinical Perimetry, 3rd ed. C.V. Mosby Co., Saint Louis, 1971, pp.14–47.

71. Harrington DO. The Visual Fields. A Textbook and Atlas of Clinical Perimetry, 3rd ed. C.V. Mosby, Saint Louis, 1971, pp. 48–69.

72. Sharpe JA. Visual dysfunction with basal skull tumours. Can J Neurol Sci 1985;12:332–335.

73. Knight CL, Hoyt WF, Wilson CB. Syndrome of incipient prechiasmal optic nerve compression. Arch Ophthalmol 1972;87:1–11.

74. Trautmann JC, Laws E, Jr. Visual status after transsphenoidal surgery at the Mayo Clinic, 1971–1982. Am J Ophthalmol 1983;96:200–208.

75. Cohen AR, Cooper PR, Kupersmith MJ, Flamm ES, Ransohoff J. Visual recovery after transsphenoidal removal of pituitary adenomas. Neurosurgery 1985;17:446–452.

76. Anderson D, Faber P, Marcovitz S, Hardy J, Lorenzetti D. Pituitary tumors and the ophthalmologist. Ophthalmology 1983;90:1265–1270.

77. Wilson CB, Dempsey LC. Transsphenoidal microsurgical removal of 250 pituitary adenomas. J Neurosurgery 1978;48:13–22.

78. Comtois R, Beauregard H, Somma M, Serri O, Aris-Jilwan N, Hardy J. The clinical and endocrine outcome to trans-sphenoidal micro-

surgery of nonsecreting pituitary adenomas. Cancer 1991;68:860–866.

79. Trobe JD, Tao AH, Schuster JJ. Perichiasmal tumors: Diagnostic and prognostic features. Neurosurgery 1984;15:391–399.

80. Symon L, Jakubowski J. Transcranial management of pituitary tumours with suprasellar extension. J Neurol Neurosurg Psychiatry 1979;42:123–133.

81. Wray SH. Neuro-ophthalmologic manifestations of pituitary and parasellar lesions. Clin Neurosurg 1976;24:86–117.

82. Hollenhorst RW, Younge BR. Ocular manifestations produced by adenomas of the pituitary gland: analysis of 1000 cases. In: Kohler PO, Ross GT, eds. Diagnosis and Treatment of Pituitary Tumours. Excerpta Medica, Amsterdam, 1973, pp. 53–64.

83. Elkington SG. Pituitary adenoma: pre-operative symptomatology in a series of 260 patients. Br J Ophthalmol 1968;52:322–328.

84. Sullivan LJ, O'Day J, McNeill P. Visual outcomes of pituitary adenoma surgery. St. Vincent's Hospital 1968–1987. J Clin Neuroophthalmol 1991;11:262–267.

85. Harrington DO. The Visual Fields. A Textbook and Atlas of Clinical Perimetry, 3rd ed. C.V. Mosby Co, Saint Louis, 1971, pp. 251–298.

86. Blaauw G, Braakman R, Çuhadar M, Hoeve LJ, Lamberts SWJ, Poublon RML, Singh R, Wijngaarde R. Influence of transsphenoidal hypophysectomy on visual deficit due to a pituitary tumour. Acta Neurochir (Wien) 1986;83:79–82.

87. Findlay G, McFadzean RM, Teasdale G. Recovery of vision following treatment of pituitary tumours: Application of a new system of visual assessment. Trans Ophthalmol Soc UK 1983;103 (pt 2):212–216.

88. Younge BR. Midline tilting between seeing and nonseeing areas in hemianopia. Mayo Clin Proc 1976;51:562–568.

89. Sugita K, Sato O, Hirota T, Tsugane R, Kageyama N. Scotomatous defects in the central visual field in pituitary adenomas. Neurochirurgia 1975;18:155–162.

90. Bird A. Field loss due to lesions at the anterior angle of the chiasm. Proc Royal Soc Med 1972;65:519–520.

91. Karanjia N, Jacobson DM. Compression of the prechiasmatic optic nerve produces a junctional scotoma. Am J Ophthalmol 1999;128:256–258.

92. Hershenfeld SA, Sharpe JA. Monocular temporal hemianopia. Br J Ophthalmol 1993;77:424–427.

93. Mojon DS, Odel JG, Rios RJ, Hirano M. Pituitary adenoma revealed by paracentral junctional scotoma of Traquair. Ophthalmologica 1997;211:104–108.

94. Thompson HS, Montague P, Cox TA, Corbett JJ. The relationship between visual acuity, pupillary defect, and visual field loss. Am J Ophthalmol 1982;93:681–688.

95. Charteris DG, Cullen JF. Binasal field defects in primary empty sella syndrome. J Neuroophthalmol 1996;16:110–114.

96. Parravano JG, Toledo A, Kucharczyk W. Dimensions of the optic nerves, chiasm, and tracts: MR Quantitative comparison between patients with optic atrophy and normals. J Comput Assist Tomogr 1993;17:688–690.

97. Newman NM. Ophthalmoscopic observation of the retinal nerve fiber layer. Trans Am Acad Ophthalmol Otolaryngol 1977;83:786–796.

98. Newman NM, Tornambe PE, Corbett JJ. Ophthalmoscopy of the retinal nerve fiber layer. Use in detection of neurologic disease. Arch Neurol 1982;39:226–233.

99. Lundstrom M, Frisen L. Atrophy of optic nerve fibers in compression of the chiasm-degree and distribution of ophthalmoscopic changes. Acta Ophthalmol 1976;54:623–640.

100. Kubie LS, Beckmann JW. Diplopia without extra-ocular palsies, caused by heteronymous defects in the visual fields associated with defective macular vision. Brain 1929;52:317–333.

101. Borchert MS, Lessell S, Hoyt WF. Hemifield slide diplopia from altitudinal visual field defects. J Neuroophthalmol 1996;16:107–109.

102. Chamlin M, Davidoff LM, Feiring EH. Ophthalmologic changes produced by pituitary tumors. Am J Ophthalmol 1955;40:353–368.

103. Slamovits TL, Burde R. Neuro-ophthalmology, Mosby, St. Louis, 1994, p. 4.3.

104. Wertenbaker C, Gutman I. Unusual visual symptoms. Surv Ophthalmol 1985;29:297–299.

105. Randall RV, Laws E, Jr, Abboud CF, Ebersold MJ, Kao PC, Scheithauer BW. Transsphenoidal microsurgical treatment of prolactin-producing pituitary adenomas. Results in 100 patients. Mayo Clin Proc 1983;58:108–121.

106. Neetens A, Selosse P. Oculomotor anomalies in sellar and parasellar pathology. Ophthalmologica 1977;175:80–104.

107. Drachman DA. See-saw nystagmus. J Neurol Neurosurg Psychiatry 1966;29:356–361.

108. Dell'Osso LF, Daroff RB. Two additional scenarios for see-saw nystagmus: achiasma and hemichiasma. J Neuroophthalmol 1998;18:112–113.

109. Apkarian P. Chiasmal crossing defects in disorders of binocular vision. Eye 1996;10:222–232.

110. Leitch RJ, Thompson D, Harris CM, Chong K, Russell-Eggitt I, Kriss A. Achiasma in a case of midline craniofacial cleft with see-saw nystagmus. Br J Ophthalmol 1996;80:1023–1027.

111. May EF, Truxal AR. Loss of vision alone may result in seesaw nystagmus. J Neuroophthalmol 1997;17:84–85.

112. Ram Z, Findler G, Gutman I, Tadmor R, Sahar A. Visual hallucinations associated with pituitary adenoma. Neurosurgery 1987;20:292–296.

113. Dawson DJ, Enoch BA, Shepherd DI. Formed visual hallucinations with pituitary adenomas. Br Med J 1984;289:414.

114. Cogan DG. Visual hallucinations as release phenomena. Albrecht Von Graefes Arch Klin Exp Ophthalmol 1973;188:139–150.

115. Ruben S, Elston J, Hayward R. Pituitary adenoma presenting as the Foster-Kennedy syndrome. Br J Ophthalmol 1992;76:117–119.

116. Repka MX, Miller NR, Miller M. Visual outcome after surgical removal of craniopharyngiomas. Ophthalmology 1989;96:195–199.

117. Fahlbusch R, Honegger J, Paulus W, Huk W, Buchfelder M. Surgical treatment of craniopharyngiomas: experience with 168 patients. J Neurosurg 1999;90:237–250.

118. Baskin DS, Wilson CB. Surgical management of craniopharyngiomas: A review of 74 cases. J Neurosurg 1986;65:22–27.

119. Crotty TB, Scheithauer BW, Young WF, Davis DH, Shaw EG, Miller GM, Burger PC. Papillary craniopharyngioma: a clinicopathological study of 48 cases. J Neurosurg 1995;83:206–214.

120. Cherninkova S, Tzekov H, Karakostov V. Comparative ophthalmologic studies on children and adults with craniopharyngiomas. Ophthalmologica 1990;201:201–205.

121. Gokalp HZ, Arasil E, Kanpolat Y, Ralim T. Meningiomas of the tuberculum sella. Neurosurg Rev 1993;16:111–114.

122. Kinjo T, Al-Mefty O, Ciric I. Diaphragma sellae meningiomas. Neurosurgery 1995;36:1082–1092.

123. Ross DA, Norman D, Wilson CB. Radiologic characteristics and results of surgical management of Rathke's cysts in 43 patients. Neurosurgery 1992;30:173–178.

124. Rao GP, Blyth CPJ, Jeffreys RV. Ophthalmic manifestations of Rathke's cleft cysts. Am J Ophthalmol 1995;119:86–91.

125. Kleinschmidt-DeMasters BK, Lillehei KO, Stears JC. The pathologic, surgical, and MR spectrum of Rathke cleft cysts. Surg Neurol 1995;44:19–27.

126. Voelker JL, Campbell RL, Muller J. Clinical, radiographic, and pathological features of symptomatic Rathke's cleft cysts. J Neurosurg 1991;74:535–544.

127. El-Mahdy W, Powell M. Transsphenoidal management of 28 symptomatic Rathke's cleft cysts, with special reference to visual and hormonal recovery. Neurosurgery 1998;42:7–17.

128. Hornig GW, Zervas NT. Slit defect of the diaphragma sellae with valve effect: observation of a "slit valve". Neurosurgery 1992;30:265–267.

129. Meyer FB, Carpenter SM, Laws ER, Jr. Intrasellar arachnoid cysts. Surg Neurol 1987;28:105–110.

130. Shin JL, Asa SL, Woodhouse LJ, Smyth HS, Ezzat S. Cystic lesions of the pituitary: clinicopathological features distinguishing craniopharyngioma, Rathke's cleft cysts, and ararachnoid cyst. J Clin Endocrinol Metab 1999;84:3972–3982.

131. Kupersmith MJ, Rosenberg C, Kleinberg D. Visual loss in pregnant women with pituitary adenomas. Ann Int Med 1994;121:473–477.

132. Coogan PF, Baron JA, Lambe M. Parity and pituitary adenoma risk. J Natl Cancer Inst 1995;87:1410–1411.

133. Magyar DM, Marshall JR. Pituitary tumors and pregnancy. Am J Obstet Gynecol 1978;132:739–751.

134. Nelson PB, Robinson AG, Archer DF, Maroon JC. Symptomatic pituitary tumor enlargement after induced pregnancy. J Neurosurg 1978;49:283–287.

135. Molitch ME. Management of prolactinomas during pregnancy. J Reprod Med 1999;12(suppl):1121–1126.

136. Divers W, Jr, Yen SSC. Prolactin-producing microadenomas in pregnancy. Obstet Gynecol 1983;62:425–429.

137. Gemzell C, Wang CF. Outcome of pregnancy in women with pituitary adenoma. Fertil Steril 1979;31:363–372.

138. Molitch ME. Pregnancy and the hyperprolactinemic woman. N Engl J Med 1985;312:1364–1370.

139. Melmed S, Braunstein GD, Chang RJ, Becker DP. Pituitary tumors secreting growth hormone and prolactin. Ann Intern Med 1986;105:238–253.

140. Van Dalen JTW, Greve EL. Rapid deterioration of visual fields during bromocriptine-induced pregnancy in a patient with a pituitary adenoma. Br J Ophthalmol 1977;61:729–733.

141. Rolih CA, Ober KP. Pituitary apoplexy. Endocrinol Metab Clin North Am 1993;22:291–302.

142. Wakai S, Fukushima T, Teramoto A, Sano K. Pituitary apoplexy: its incidence and clinical significance. J Neurosurg 1981;55:187–193.

143. Bonicki W, Kasperlik-Zaluska A, Koszewski W, Zgliczyński W, Wislawski J. Pituitary apoplexy: endocrine, surgical and oncological emergency. Incidence, clinical course and treatment with reference to 799 cases of pituitary adenomas. Acta Neurochir (Wien) 1993;120:118–122.

144. Wright RL, Ojemann R, Drew JH. Haemorrhage into pituitary adenomata; report of 2 cases with spontaneous recovery. Arch Neurol 1965;12:326–330.

145. Schatz NJ, Job OM, Glaser JS. Spontaneous resolution of pituitary adenoma after apoplexy. J Neuroophthalmol 2000;20:42–44.

146. Reid RL, Quigley ME, S.S.C.Yen. Pituitary apoplexy: A review. Arch Neurol 1985;42:712–719.

147. Onesti ST, Wisniewski T, Post KD. Clinical versus subclinical pituitary apoplexy: presentation, surgical management, and outcome in 21 patients. Neurosurgery 1990;26:980–986.

148. Bills DC, Meyer RB, Laws ER, Jr, Davis DH, Ebersold MJ, Scheithauer BW, Ilstrup DM, Abboud CF. A retrospective analysis of pituitary apoplexy. Neurosurgery 1993;33:602–609.

149. Randeva HS, Schoebel J, Byrne J, Esiri M, Adams CBT, Wass JAH. Classical pituitary apoplexy: clinical features, management and outcome. Clin Endocrinol 1999;51:181–188.

150. Markowitz S, Sherman L, Kolodny HD, Baruh S. Acute pituitary vascular accident (pituitary apoplexy). Med Clin North Am 1981;65:105–116.

151. Thompson D, Powell M, Foster O. Atypical presentation of vascular events in pituitary tumours: "non-apoplectic" pituitary apoplexy. J Neurol Neurosurg Psychiatry 1994;57:1441–1442.

152. Lohmann CP, Köhler M, Ullrich OW. Incomplete bitemporal hemianopia without headache: an unusual case of pituitary apoplexy. Eye 2000;14:116–117.

153. Rossitch E, Carrazana EJ, Black PM. Isolated oculomotor nerve palsy following apoplexy of a pituitary adenoma. J Neurosurg Sci 1992;36:103–105.

154. McDermott MW, Griesdale DE, Berry K, Wilkins E. Lymphocytic adenohypophysitis. Can J Neurol Sci 1988;15:38–43.

155. Cosman F, Post KD, Holub DA, Wardlaw SL. Lymphocytic hypophysitis. Report of 3 new cases and review of the literature. Medicine 1989;68:240–256.

156. Thodou E, Kontogeorgos G, Kovacs K, Horvath E, Ezzat S. Clinical case seminar: lymphocytic hypophysitis: clinicopathological findings. J Clin Endocrinol Metab 1995;80:2302–2311.

157. Stelmach M, O'Day J. Rapid change in visual fields associated with suprasellar lymphocytic hypophysitis. J Clin Neuroophthalmol 1991;11:19–24.

158. Levine SN, Benzel EC, Fowler MR, Shroyer JV, Mirfakhraee M. Lymphocytic adenohypophysitis: clinical, radiological, and magnetic resonance imaging characterization. Neurosurgery 1988;22: 937–941.

159. Kerrison JB, Lee AG, Weinstein JM. Acute loss of vision during pregnancy due to a suprasellar mass. Surv Ophthalmol 1997;41: 402–408.

160. Katano H, Umemura A, Kamiya K, Kanai H, Yamada K. Visual disturbance by lymphocytic hypophysitis in a non-pregnant woman with systemic lupus erythematosus. Lupus 1998;7:554–556.

161. Farah JO, Rossi M, Foy PM, MacFarlane IA. Cystic lymphocytic hypophysitis, visual field defects and hypopituitarism. Int J Clin Pract 1999;53:643–644.

162. Jain KC, Varma A, Mahapatra AK. Pituitary abscess: a series of six cases. Br J Neurosurg 1997;11:139–143.

163. Domingue JN, Wilson CB. Pituitary abscesses. Report of seven cases and review of the literature. J Neurosurg 1977;46:601–608.

164. Henegar MM, Koby MB, Silbergeld DL, Rich KM, Moran CJ. Intrasellar abscess following transsphenoidal surgery. Surg Neurol 1996;45:183–188.

165. Buckman MT, Husain M, Carlow TJ, Peake GT. Primary empty sella syndrome with visual field defects. Am J Med 1976;61: 124–128.

166. Gallardo E, Schächter D, Caceres E, Becker P, Colin E, Martinez C, Henriques C. The empty sella: results of treatment in 76 successive cases and high frequency of endocrine and neurological disturbances. Clin Endocrinol 1992;37:529–533.

167. Bjerre P. The empty sella: a reappraisal of etiology and pathogenesis. Acta Neurol Scand Suppl 1990;130:1–25.

168. Bjerre P, Gyldensted C, Riishede J, Lindholm J. The empty sella and pituitary adenomas. A theory on the causal relationship. Acta Neurol Scand 1982;66:82–92.

169. Mortara R, Norrell H. Consequences of a deficient sellar diaphragm. J Neurosurg 1970;32:565–573.

170. Kirkali P, Kansu T, Erzen C, Cial A. A radiological insight into primary empty sella syndrome with visual dysfunction. Neuro-ophthalmology 1989;9:259–265.

171. Robinson DB, Michaels RD. Empty sella resulting from the spontaneous resolution of a pituitary macroadenoma. Arch Int Med 1992;152:1920–1923.

172. Domingue JN, Wing SD, Wilson CB. Coexisting pituitary adenomas and partially empty sellas. J Neurosurg 1978;48:23–28.

173. Burrow GN, Wortzman G, Rewcastle NB. Microadenomas of the pituitary and abnormal sellar tomograms in an unselected autopsy series. N Engl J Med 1981;304:156–158.

174. McCormick WF, Halmi NS. Absence of chromophobe adenomas from a large series of pituitary tumors. Arch Pathol 1971;92: 231–238.

175. Auer RN, Alakija P, Sutherland GR. Asymptomatic large pituitary adenomas discovered at autopsy. Surg Neurol 1996;46:28–31.

176. Garcia MM, Kapcala LP. Growth of a microprolactinoma to a macroprolactinoma during estrogen therapy. J Endocrinol Invest 1995;18:450–455.

177. Molitch ME, Elton RL, Blackwell RE, Caldwell R, Chang RJ, Jaffe R, Joplin G, Robbins RJ, Tyson J, Thorner MO. Bromocriptine as primary therapy for prolactin-secreting macroadenomas: results of a prospective multicenter study. J Clin Endocrinol Metab 1985; 60:698–705.

178. Moster ML, Savino PJ, Schatz NJ, Snyder PJ, Sergott RC, Bosley TM. Visual function in prolactinoma patients treated with bromocriptine. Ophthalmology 1985;92:1332–1341.

179. Lesser RL, Zheutlin JD, Boghen D, Odel JG, Robbins RJ. Visual function improvement in patients with macroprolactinomas treated with bromocriptine. Am J Ophthalmol 1990;109:535–543.

180. Lundin P, Bergstrom K, Nyman R, Lundberg PO, Muhr C. Macroprolactinomas: serial MR imaging in long-term bromocriptine therapy. Am J Neuroradiol 1992;13:1279–1291.

181. Ciccarelli E, Grottoli S, Miola C, Avataneo T, Lancranjan I, Camanni F. Double blind randomized study using oral or injectable bromocriptine in patients with hyperprolactinaemia. Clin Endocrinol 1994;40:193–198.

182. Ciccarelli E, Miola C, Grottoli S, Avataneo T, Lancranjan I, Camanni F. Long term therapy of patients with macroprolactinoma using repeatable injectable bromocriptine. J Clin Endocrinol Metab 1993;76:484–488.

183. Verhelst J, Abs R, Maiter D, van den bruel A, Vandeweghe M, Velkeniers B, Mockel J, Lambrigts G, Petrossians P, Coremans P, Mahler C, Stevenaert A, Verlooy J, Raftopoulos C, Beckers A. Cabergoline in the treatment of hyperprolactinemia: a study in 455 patients. J Clin Endocrinol Metab 1999;84:2518–2522.

184. Couldwell WT, Weiss MH. Visual loss associated with bromocriptine. Lancet 1992;340:1410–1411.

185. Taxel P, Waitzman DM, Harrington JF, Fagan RH, Rothfield NF, Chen HH, Malchoff CD. Chiasmal herniation as a complication of bromocriptine therapy. J Neuroophthalmol 1996;16:252–257.

186. Mori H, Maeda T, Saitoh Y, Onishi T. Changes in prolactinomas and somatotropinomas in humans treated with bromocriptine. Pathol Res Pract 1988;183:580–583.

187. Perrin G, Treluyer C, Trouillas J, Sassolas G, Goutelle A. Surgical outcome and pathological effects of bromocriptine preoperative treatment in prolactinomas. Pathol Res Pract 1991;187:587–592.

188. Clark J, Wheatley T, Edwards OM. Rapid enlargement of non-functioning pituitary tumor following withdrawal of bromocriptine. J Neurol Neurosurg Psychiatry 1985;48:287.

189. Thorner MO, Perryman RL, Rogol AD, Conway BP, Macleod RM, Login IS. Rapid changes of prolactinoma volume after withdrawal and reinstitution of bromocriptine. J Clin Endocrinol Metab 1981;53:480–483.

190. Jaffe CA, Barkan AL. Treatment of acromegaly with dopamine agonists. Endocrinol Metab Clin North Am 1992;21:13–35.

191. Vance ML, Evans WS, Thorner MO. Bromocriptine. Ann Int Medicine 1984;100:78–91.

192. Wass JAH, Thorner MO, Morris DV, Rees ZH, Mason AS, Jones AE, Besser GM. Long-term treatment of acromegaly with bromocriptine. Br Med J 1977;1:875–878.

193. Melmed S. Acromegaly. In: Melmed S, ed. The Pituitary. Blackwell Science, Inc., Cambridge, MA, 1995, pp. 413–442.

194. Thorner MO, Besser GM. Successful treatment of acromegaly with bromocriptine. Postgrad Med J 1976;52 suppl 1:71–74.

195. Barnard LB, Grantham WG, Lamberton P, O'Dorisio TM, Jackson IMD. Treatment of resistant acromegaly with a long-acting somatostatin analogue (SMS 201-995). Ann Int Med 1986;105:856–61.

196. Jackson IMD, Barnard LB, Lamerton P. Role of long-acting somatostatin analogue (SMS 201-995) in the treatment of acromegaly. Am J Med 1986;81(suppl 6B):94–101.

197. Cobb W, Jackson IMD. Short-term recovery of visual field loss in acromegaly during treatment with a long-acting somatostatin analogue. Am J Med 1989;86:496–497.

198. Warnet A, Harris AG, Renard E, Martin D, James-Deidier A, Chaumet-Riffaud P. A prospective multicenter trial of octreotide in 24 patients with visual defects caused by nonfunctioning and gonadotropin-secreting pituitary adenomas. Neurosurgery 1997;41: 786–795.

199. Kayan A, Earl CJ. Compressive lesions of the optic nerves and chiasm. Brain 1975;98:13–28.

200. Ciric I, Mikhael M, Stafford T, Lawson L, Garces R. Transsphenoidal microsurgery of pituitary macroadenomas with long-term follow-up results. J Neurosurg 1983;59:395–401.

201. Goldman JA, Hedges III T, Shucart W, Molitch ME. Delayed chiasmal decompression after transsphenoidal operation for a pituitary adenoma. Neurosurgery 1985;17:962–964.

202. Teng MM, Huang CI, Chang T. The pituitary mass after transsphenoidal hypophysectomy. Am J Neuroradiol 1988; 9:23–26.

203. Colao A, Cerbone G, Cappabianca P, Ferone D, Alfieri A, Di Salle F, Faggiano A, Merola B, de Divitiis E, Lombardi G. Effect of surgery and radiotherapy on visual and endocrine function in nonfunctioning pituitary adenomas. J Endocrinol Invest 1998;21: 284–290.

204. Nakane T, Kuwayama A, Watanabe M, Kageyama N. Transsphenoidal approach to pituitary adenomas with suprasellar extension. Surg Neurol 1981;16:225–229.

205. Hajda M, Pásztor E. Significance of the appearance of the optic disc for predicting visual function following removal of pituitary adenomas. Neurolog Med Chir (Tokyo) 1983;23:561–565.

206. Wilson P, Falconer MA. Patterns of visual failure with pituitary tumours. Br J Ophthalmol 1968;52:94–110.

207. El-Azouzi M, Black PM, Candia G, Zervas NT, Panagopoulos KP. Transsphenoidal surgery for visual loss in patients with pituitary adenomas. Neurol Res 1990;12:23–25.

208. Black PM, Zervas NT, Candia GL. Incidence and management of complications of transsphenoidal operation for pituitary adenomas. Neurosurgery 1987;20:920–924.

209. Laws E, Jr, Kern EB. Complications of transphenoidal surgery. Clin Neurosurg 1976;23:401–416.

210. Lorenz M, Renella RR. Intraoperative monitoring: visual evoked potentials in surgery of the sellar region. Zentralbl Neurochir 1989;50:12–15.

211. Wilson WB, Kirsch WM, Neville H, Stears J, Feinsod M, Lehman RAW. Monitoring of visual function during parasellar surgery. Surg Neurol 1976;5:323–329.

212. Slavin ML, Lam BL, Decker RE, Schatz NJ, Glaser JS, Reynolds MG. Chiasmal compression from fat packing after transsphenoidal resection of intrasellar tumor in two patients. Am J Ophthalmol 1993;115:368–371.

213. Adams CBT. The management of pituitary tumours and post-operative visual deterioration. Acta Neurochir (Wien) 1988;94:103–116.

214. Czech T, Wolfsberger S, Reitner A, Görzer H. Delayed visual deterioration after surgery for pituitary adenoma. Acta Neurochir (Wien) 1999;141:45–51.

215. Duff JM, Meyer FB, Ilstrup DM, Laws E, Jr, Schleck CD, Scheithauer BW. Long-term outcomes for surgically resected craniopharyngiomas. Neurosurgery 2000;46:291–305.

216. Abrams LS, Repka MX. Visual outcome of craniopharyngioma in children. J Pediatr Ophthalmol Strabismus 1997;34:223–228.

217. Konig A, Ludecke DK, Herrman HD. Transnasal surgery in the treatment of craniopharyngiomas. Acta Neurochir (Wien) 1986;83:1–7.

218. Pierre-Kahn A, Sainte-Rose C, Renier D. Surgical approach to children with craniopharyngiomas and severely impaired vision: special considerations. Pediatr Neurosurg 1994;21 Suppl 1:50–56.

219. Mashima Y, Oguchi Y. Visual evoked potential in the management of pituitary tumor during pregnancy. Doc Ophthalmol 1987;65:57–64.

220. Griffith RW, Trukalj I, Braun P. Outcome of pregnancy in mothers given bromocriptine. Br. J. Clin. Pharmacol 1978;5:227.

221. Vidal E, Cevallos R, Vidal J, Ravon R, Moreau JJ, Rogues AM, Loustaud V, Liozon F. Twelve cases of pituitary apoplexy. Arch Intern Med 1992;152:1893–1899.

222. Lloyd MH, Belchetz PE. The clinical features and management of pituitary apoplexy. Postgrad Med J 1977;53:82–85.

223. Maccagnan P, Macedo CLD, Kayath MJ, Nogueira RG, Abucham J. Conservative management of pituitary apoplexy: a prospective study. J Clin Endocrinol Metab 1995;80:2190–2197.

224. Hamlyn PJ, Baer R, Afshar F. Transsphenoidal chiasmopexy for long standing visual failure in the secondary empty sella syndrome. Br J Neurosurg 1988;2:277–279.

225. Laws ER, Jr, Vance M. Radiosurgery for pituitary tumors and craniopharyngiomas. Neurosurg Clin N Am 1999;10:327–336.

226. Kondziolka DS, Flickinger JC, Lunsford LD. Radiation Therapy and Radiosurgery of Pituitary Tumors. In: Krisht AF, Tindall GT, eds. Pituitary Disorders. Lippincott Williams & Wilkins, Baltimore, 1999, pp. 407–415.

227. Hall WA. Stereotactic Radiosurgery in Perspective. In: Cohen AR, Haines SJ, eds. Concepts in Neurosurgery. 7, Williams & Wilkins, Baltimore, 1995, p. 114.

228. Girkin CA, Comey CH, Lunsford LD, Goodman ML, Kline LB. Radiation optic neuropathy after stereotactic radiosurgery. Ophthalmology 1997;104:1634–1643.

229. Piquemal R, Cottier JP, Arsene S, Lioret E, Rospars C, Herbreteau D, Jan M, Renard JP. Radiation-induced optic neuropathy 4 years after radiation: report of a case followed up with MRI. Neuroradiology 1998;40:439–441.

11 Imaging of Pituitary Tumors

DEREK EMERY, MD AND WALTER KUCHARCZYK, MD

INTRODUCTION

Magnetic resonance imaging (MRI) and computed tomography (CT) have largely replaced all other imaging modalities in the diagnostic evaluation of the pituitary gland and surrounding structures. Plain film radiography has proven to be both insensitive and nonspecific in the evaluation of pituitary lesions, and is rarely utilized in the investigation of pituitary disease. At best, an abnormality of the sella turcica seen on a skull radiograph will lead to further imaging with CT or MRI. Polytomography, previously used extensively, is sensitive to minor abnormalities in the contour of the bony sella. However, these abnormalities correlate poorly with lesions of the pituitary gland (1,2), and therefore, the use of polytomography has also been abandoned.

CT is a much better method of evaluating the pituitary than either plain skull radiographs or polytomography, and remains the imaging modality of choice in centers where access to MRI is limited or where there is a contraindication to MRI. The major advantage of CT is that it provides detailed images of bone and calcifications. However, there are several disadvantages to CT: patient positioning for coronal scans is uncomfortable; the injection of intravenous contrast agents is usually required; images of the pituitary gland may be degraded by beam-hardening artifacts; and most importantly, there is less soft tissue image contrast than with MRI. Thus, the gland and the adjacent soft tissues, such as blood vessels and optic chiasm, are not optimally visualized.

MRI is now the imaging method of choice for patients suspected of having pituitary pathology. MRI is superior to CT in the delineation of lesions within the pituitary gland as well as in determining the relationship of tumors with parasellar soft tissue structures (3–6). The greater soft tissue image contrast and clarity of the MRI images results in better interobserver agreement on the imaging findings (6). MRI also has the advantage of better multiplanar imaging capabilities. On the other hand, MRI is relatively insensitive to bony erosion and calcification, which are occasionally important markers of disease.

Angiography is no longer used in the routine evaluation of pituitary lesions. In special circumstances, angiography is used for venous sampling from the petrosal sinuses in evaluation of occult tumors, particularly adrenocorticotropic hormone (ACTH)-secreting microadenomas.

From: *Diagnosis and Management of Pituitary Tumors* (K. Thapar, K. Kovacs, B. W. Scheithauer, and R. V. Lloyd, eds.), ©Humana Press Inc., Totowa, NJ.

THE NORMAL PITUITARY GLAND

The pituitary gland is best evaluated on high-resolution coronal images, whether these be CT or MRI (Figure 1). High spatial resolution requires slices 3 mm or less in thickness (1.5 mm for CT), and pixels no larger than 1 mm on the side. Coronal images minimize partial volume averaging artifacts from parasellar vessels and cerebral spinal fluid in the basal cisterns, and allow for comparisons of midline symmetry. For CT, coronal imaging requires that the patient's neck be extended and the gantry tilted; for MRI, no special positioning is required. On MRI, coronal images are supplemented with sagittal views; sagittal views are not possible with CT. A variety of MRI sequences can be used, the most frequent now being T1-weighted spin-echo, and T2-weighted fast spin echo images.

The size, shape, and internal characteristics of the pituitary gland are features that are used in the diagnosis of pituitary disease. There is a normal variation of these features with the age and sex of the patient. On MRI, the normal adult anterior pituitary gland is of relatively homogeneous signal intensity and is isointense to white matter on both T1- and T2-weighted images (7). On CT, the attenuation of the gland is also similar to white matter.

In the normal adult, the height of the gland ranges from 3 to 9 mm. The superior surface of the gland may be concave, flat, or convex. It should be bilaterally symmetrical about the midline. After contrast administration, the anterior lobe and pituitary stalk enhance intensely. If dynamic scanning is performed, a typical temporal pattern of enhancement is seen to occur. First, the stalk and the area around where the stalk attaches to the gland (the "pituitary tuft") enhance. Then the enhancement spreads peripherally, reaching the lateral margin of the gland about 1 min later (8).

The posterior pituitary gland does not have a distinctive appearance on CT, but on MRI, it is distinguished by hyperintense signal intensity on T1-weighted images (Figure 1). The exact cause of the hyperintense signal within the posterior pituitary gland remains undetermined. It is almost certainly linked to stored neurosecretory material, and its presence is an important sign of an functionally intact neurohypophysis.

The infundibulum of the gland is usually midline, but even in normals may be asymmetrically positioned (9). This may be secondary to lateral eccentricity of the gland with respect to the brain, or less often owing to eccentric insertion of the stalk into the gland. Thus, lateral placement of the stalk on coronal images, as an isolated finding, is a poor indicator of pituitary pathology.

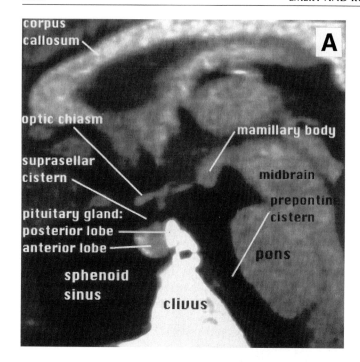

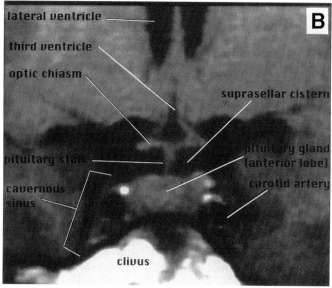

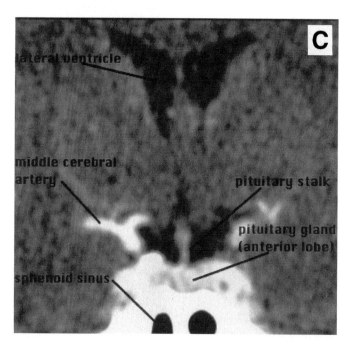

Figure 11-1 Normal pituitary gland, sella turcica, and parasellar region. **(A)** Sagittal T1W MRI. **(B)** Coronal T1W MRI. **(C)** Coronal enhanced CT.

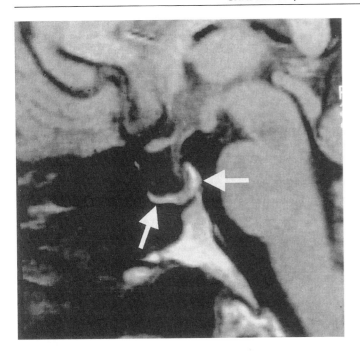

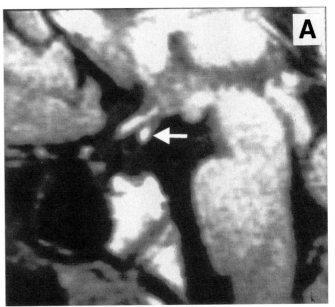

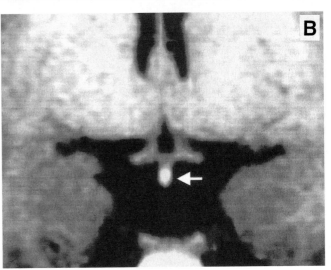

Figure 11-2 Empty sella turcica. Sagittal T1W MRI. The sella turcica is enlarged and filled with CSF. The pituitary gland (arrows) is flattened inferiorly.

The size, shape, and signal of the pituitary gland vary with age *(10)*. The superior surface of the gland is typically convex in neonates and young infants, and then flattens out in older infants. The signal intensity of the anterior lobe is increased in neonates. This starts to decrease at about 2 mo of age and should equal that of the adult gland by 6 mo of age. Until puberty, there is no significant size difference in the pituitary gland of males and females, all being less than or equal to 6 mm in height. With puberty, the gland enlarges, the female gland up to 10 mm in height and the male up to 7 mm in height *(11)*. Following puberty the gland decreases slightly in size, and then continues a gradual decline in size throughout adulthood. The female gland remains larger than that of the male until after 70 yr of age *(12)*.

Pregnancy causes a significant increase in the size of the pituitary gland. There is a progressive increase in gland height and superior convexity throughout gestation with a maximum size reached in the immediate postpartum period. At this time, the gland may reach a height of 12 mm *(13)*. The signal intensity is also slightly increased in pregnant subjects *(14)*.

Frequently an "empty sella" is detected incidentally on CT or MRI. This consists of an enlarged sella turcica with a flattened pituitary gland along its floor and a normal pituitary stalk (Figure 2). This is owing to a patulous diaphragma sella that allows cerebrospinal fluid to enter and enlarge the superior aspect of the sella turcica. In almost all instances, it should be considered a normal variant, although in rare instances, it may be associated with a cerebrospinal fluid leak, endocrinopathy, or entrapment of the optic chiasm. Rarely, herniation of the subarachnoid space into the sella is caused by an elevation of intracranial pressure.

CONGENITAL ANOMALIES

Congenital anomalies of the pituitary gland are uncommon. When present, they may be associated with other midline anoma-

Figure 11-3 Pituitary dwarfism. **(A)** Sagittal T1W MRI. **(B)** Coronal T1W MRI. The pituitary gland itself is small. There is no evidence of the high signal of the posterior pituitary within the sella turcica. The pituitary stalk is not continuous with the gland. There is a nodule of hyperintense signal at the inferior tip of the truncated pituitary stalk (arrow).

lies of both the face and intracranial structures. Hypoplasia of the gland may be seen on CT and MRI as a small, but otherwise normal gland within a small shallow sella turcica. Duplication of the pituitary has also been reported in association with varying degrees of median cleft face syndrome *(15)*.

Growth hormone-deficient dwarfism has now been recognized as a specific imaging entity. Until the late 1980s, the diagnosis of growth hormone-deficient dwarfism was achieved purely on clinical and biochemical criteria. Imaging of the pituitary gland played no part in the diagnosis. In 1988, a series of papers were published that described a unique group of findings concerning this disorder on T1-weighted MRI. These consisted of an abnormally small anterior lobe, absence of high signal from the posterior lobe, truncation of the infundibulum in the suprasellar cistern, and a nodule of high signal at the tip of the truncated stalk (Figure 3) *(16,17)*.

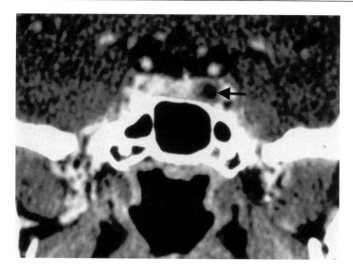

Figure 11-4 Pituitary microadenoma. Contrast-enhanced coronal CT scan. There is a small area of hypoattenuation within the gland (arrow), confirmed at surgery to be an adenoma. This case illustrates the typical CT finding in microadenomas. (Courtesy of Dr. Perry Cooper.)

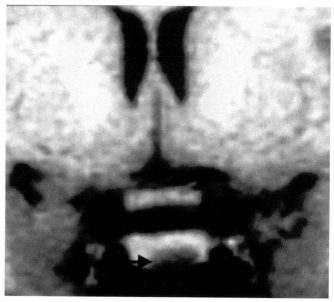

Figure 11-5 Pituitary microadenoma. Coronal T1W MRI. The adenoma is apparent as a focus of decreased signal in the pituitary gland (arrow).

Since the initial reports, hundreds of similar cases have been recognized worldwide, and now MRI plays a important function in demonstrating the morphologic abnormalities of the hypothalamic–pituitary axis in this disorder. Many of these patients have deficiencies of other adenohyophyseal hormones, and a small percentage have other intracranial midline anomalies.

PITUITARY ADENOMAS

Pituitary adenomas are the most common tumor of the sella turcica and are by far the most common indication for pituitary imaging. On CT, adenomas usually appear as an area of hypoattenuation within the gland on both nonenhanced and enhanced studies (Figure 4) *(18)*. Additional CT findings that may be supportive of the diagnosis include focal erosion of the sellar floor or a focal convexity of the superior surface. MRI is better than CT in predicting the presence, position, and size of an adenoma in the pituitary fossa *(19)*. On MRI, most microadenomas will be hypointense to the normal gland on unenhanced and enhanced T1-weighted images (Figures 5 and 6). One third to one half will be hyperintense on T2 weighted images. The visibility of a lesion on MRI is influenced by both the size and the composition of the lesion *(20)*. Cystic degeneration or necrosis will facilitate the detection of a lesion on both T1 and T2. MRI is superior to CT in delineating cystic degeneration or hemorrhage within tumors. Any evidence of mass effect from microadenomas is usually quite subtle. The most common change will be an asymmetric convexity of the superior surface of the gland. This should be considered significant only if the convexity is off the midline and different from the contralateral side of the gland *(7)*.

No one MRI method is consistently best for detecting microadenomas. Thus, combinations of sequences are frequently employed, with the most extensive protocols reserved for patients who are surgical candidates. Intravenous contrast enhancement provides some increase in sensitivity in the detection of microadenomas *(21–23)*. However, unless the patient is a surgical candidate, the localization and size of a microadenoma are of little importance. Our own imaging strategy depends on the treatment plan for the patient. If surgery is being contemplated, such as in a case of Cushing's disease, then more extensive imaging is performed, including contrast-enhanced scans. If medical treatment alone is planned, less extensive imaging is done. In the case of macroadenomas or other large tumors, imaging in multiple scan planes is performed to determine the relationship of the tumor to the surrounding structures for surgical planning.

A useful supplement to conventional contrast-enhanced MRI is the performance of dynamic studies (Figure 6) *(24,25)*. The strategy for dynamic MRI is based on differential enhancement rates between the normal pituitary gland and adenomas. The normal pituitary gland reaches peak enhancement sooner than most adenomas. Thus, early images will show the greatest difference in signal intensity between the tumor and the normal gland. Later, contrast in the normal gland will wash away faster than from the adenoma, and the signal difference will no longer be apparent. Thus dynamic contrast-enhanced studies may be used to emphasize the differences in the rate of enhancement between the normal gland and adenomas (Figure 6).

There is no difference in the imaging features of secretory and nonsecretory adenomas, nor is there a difference between the various secretory types *(7)*. On average, functioning adenomas present as smaller lesions than nonfunctioning tumors. The latter typically grow to a relatively large size prior to presenting with signs of compression of the pituitary gland, the optic pathway, or the hypothalamus.

Pars intermedia cysts and certain technical artifacts may simulate the appearance of a microadenoma, both on MRI and CT *(26)*. Magnetic susceptibility artifact caused by the air/soft tissue interface between the sphenoid sinus and floor of the sella turcica may simulate a microadenoma, particularly at the junction of the midline sphenoid sinus septum with the sella floor. Thus very small lesions lying immediately over the septum should be interpreted with caution *(27)*.

Macroadenomas (over 10 mm) are easily detected on both CT and MRI (Figures 7 and 8). CT is superior in determining the

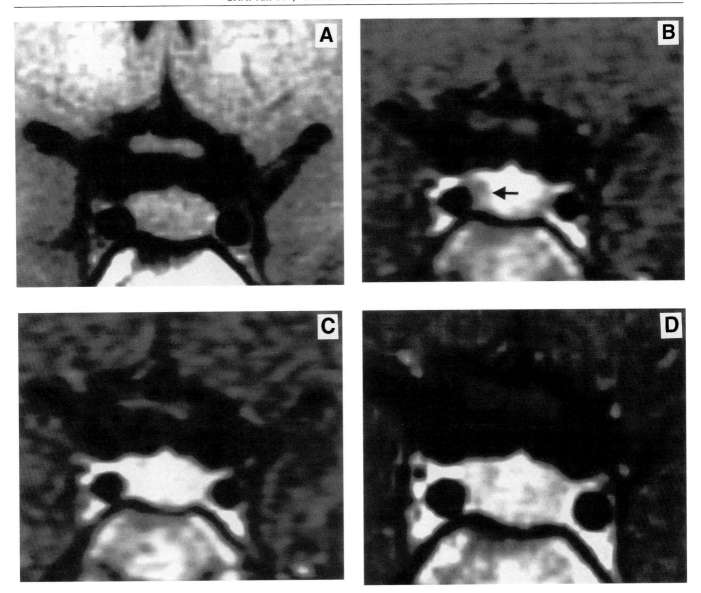

Figure 11-6   Cushing's disease. Dynamic MRI. **(A)** Nonenhanced coronal T1W MRI. **(B)** Early phase dynamic enhanced MRI. **(C)** Late phase of dynamic enhanced MRI. **(D)** Delayed image dynamic enhanced MRI. The pituitary adenoma (arrow) is seen only on the early phase of the dynamic study. The gland is homogeneous in signal intensity on both the nonenhanced image (A) and the later images (C and D).

presence of bony erosion and calcification, whereas MRI is more useful in determining the relationship of the gland to the surrounding structures, including the cavernous sinuses, the optic pathway, and the floor of the third ventricle. Sagittal and axial planes in addition to the routine coronal plane are useful for surgical planning. Dynamic enhancement may be useful in differentiating the residual normal pituitary tissue from the surrounding tumor *(28)*. The internal features of a macroadenoma may be useful in surgical planning. It has been suggested that those tumors that are soft and easily aspirated at surgery are hyperintense on T2W, whereas firm tumors tend to be isointense *(29)*.

The determination of cavernous sinus involvement is problematic. Because the medial wall of the cavernous sinus is thin and not clearly seen with either CT or MRI, it is difficult to determine when tumors cross this barrier. One author has suggested that the most reliable sign is obliteration of the vein of the carotid sulcus on dynamic contrast-enhanced MRI *(30)*. Another sign of cavern-

ous sinus invasion is that pituitary adenomas tend to enhance less than the adjacent cavernous sinus *(31)*. The most sensitive sign of cavernous sinus invasion is an asymmetry in the signal intensity between the two sides. This, however, is not specific *(32)*. Encasement of the intracavernous carotid artery is a specific, but not a sensitive sign of cavernous sinus invasion (Figure 9). Our own opinion is that subtle degrees of sinus invasion cannot yet be reliably predicted. The only accurate sign to indicate that the cavernous sinus is not involved is the presence of normal pituitary gland between the tumor and the cavernous sinus.

Acute hemorrhage or infarction of a pituitary adenoma may result in significant swelling of the gland, and the clinical syndrome of pituitary apoplexy with severe headache, hypotension, and sudden visual loss. More commonly, hemorrhage into an adenoma will be asymptomatic. Over 20% of all pituitary adenomas show evidence of hemorrhage on MRI. This is most common in patients treated with bromocriptine for a prolactinoma (Figure 10)

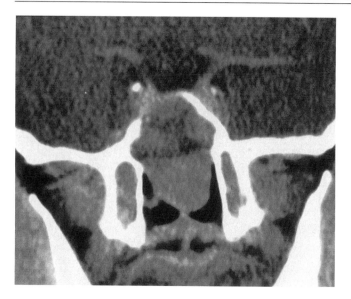

Figure 11-7 Macroadenoma. Coronal contrast-enhanced CT scan. There is a large mass within the sella turcica, which has eroded through the bony sellar floor and fills the sphenoid sinus.

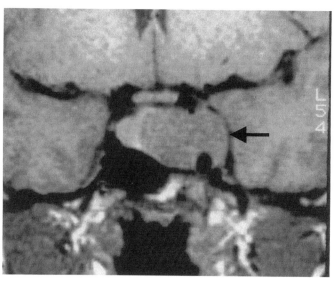

Figure 11-9 Cavernous sinus invasion. Coronal T1W MRI showing encasement of the left intracavernous internal carotid by a pituitary adenoma (arrow). Although cavernous sinus invasion is readily apparent in this patient, more subtle degrees of invasion are difficult to detect.

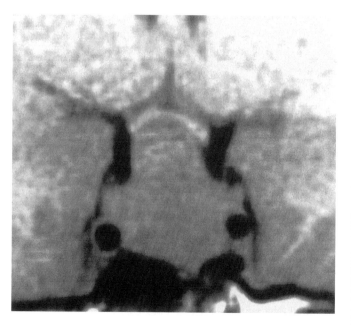

Figure 11-8 Macroadenoma. Coronal T1W MRI. There is a homogeneous sellar and suprasellar mass that elevates and compresses the optic chiasm.

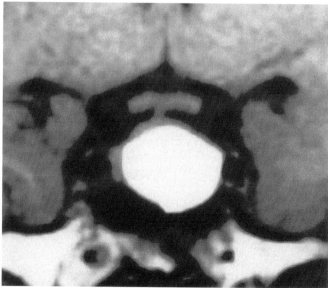

Figure 11-10 Hemorrhage into an adenoma. Coronal T1W MRI. This 22-yr-old female was being treated with bromocriptine for a prolactinoma. The large area of increased signal within the sellar mass represents subacute hemorrhage.

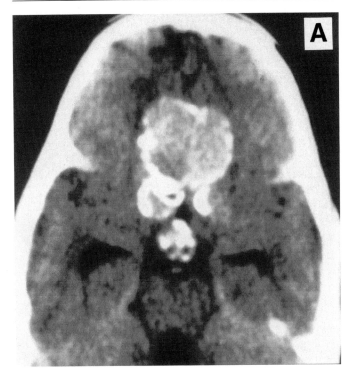
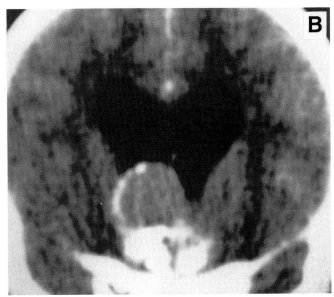

Figure 11-11   Craniopharyngioma. **(A)** Axial nonenhanced CT. **(B)** Coronal enhanced CT. There is a heterogeneous sellar and suprasellar mass with large areas of calcification within the sella as well as partial calcification of the rim.

(33–35). Hemorrhage within an adenoma results in a marked change of the imaging characteristics. On CT, acute hemorrhage (first 3 d) into a pituitary adenoma is seen as an area of increased attenuation within the gland on noncontrast images. Subacute or chronic hemorrhage may have the same appearance as areas of necrosis or fluid *(36)* and cannot be definitively identified on a single CT study. On MRI, very acute hematomas appear hypointense on T2-weighted images owing to the presence of deoxyhemoglobin. The signal intensity will then change owing to the progressive breakdown of red cells and the formation of methemoglobin, becoming noticeably bright on both T1- and T2-weighted images in the subacute phase. This appearance persists for well over a year. Postpartum ischemic necrosis of the pituitary gland (Sheehan's syndrome) will have a similar appearance to pituitary apoplexy, except there will be no evidence of an adenoma.

Rarely, pituitary adenomas can occur in an ectopic location. These are most commonly found in the sphenoid sinus *(37–39).* Other possible locations include the suprasellar cistern, superior orbital fissure, parasellar regions, the nasal cavity, and the skull base. These appear as a soft tissue mass isointense to brain on T1 weighted images.

The postsurgical appearance of the pituitary gland depends on the surgical approach, the size of the lesion removed, and the presence and type of implanted material *(40,41).* Early postoperative imaging may show an increase in the height of the gland compared to the preoperative studies. MRI scans done within 4 mo of surgery will often reveal the presence of gelatin foam implanted during the procedure. This will appear as a sellar mass, which is isointense to gray matter and somewhat heterogeneous on T1-weighted images. Gadolinium-enhanced studies reveal marked peripheral enhancement of the gelatin foam. This is likely secondary to the presence

of granulation tissue. In later postoperative studies (4–15 mo), the gelatin foam may decrease in size or disappear. Muscle and fat implanted within the sella have a heterogeneous appearance. Following trans-sphenoidal surgery, the sphenoid sinus is usually partially or completely opacified, and there is marked peripheral enhancement, secondary to the swollen mucosa. The sinus will gradually clear. However, signs of mucosal swelling may persist up to 12 mo after surgery.

CRANIOPHARYNGIOMAS

Craniopharyngiomas account for approx 3% of primary intracranial brain tumors. They are most common in children between 5 and 10 yr of age with a second peak in incidence in the sixth decade *(42).* They present with headaches, visual symptoms, or hypothalamic/pituitary dysfunction.

Craniopharyngiomas most commonly have both sellar and suprasellar components (75%), or are entirely suprasellar (20%). Uncommonly they are entirely intrasellar (5%) *(43).* Rarely, they are entirely within the third ventricle *(44).*

Pediatric craniopharyngiomas are most often composed of a solid nodule and a cystic component (Figures 11 and 12). The vast majority of pediatric craniopharyngiomas have some degree of calcification *(45).* Calcification and cyst formation are less prevalent in adult craniopharyngiomas.

The calcifications may be nodular and extensive, or may be fine and rim-like. These are best seen on CT and may be missed entirely on MRI. Solid areas of dense calcification are usually dark on MRI, resulting in a heterogeneous appearance to the solid component of the tumor on both the T1- and T2-weighted MRI images. The solid component will enhance with contrast administration.

Cystic components of craniopharyngiomas may be very large, and are often well defined and internally uniform. Uncommonly,

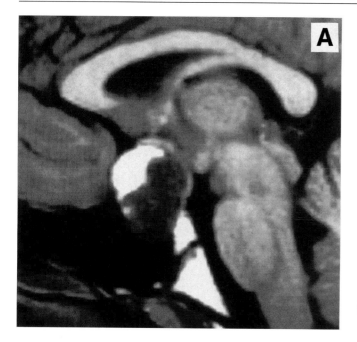

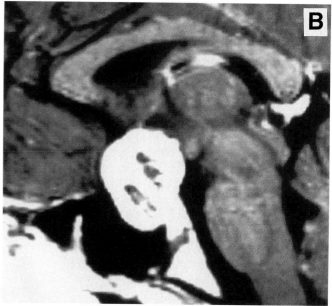

Figure 11-12 Craniopharyngioma. **(A)** Sagittal T1W MRI. **(B)** Sagittal enhanced MRI. There is a heterogeneously enhancing sellar and suprasellar mass. The cystic component is of homogeneous high signal. The rim of the cystic component is somewhat irregular and enhances on the postcontrast images.

there will be septations or fluid–fluid levels within the cysts. The cystic component may be superior to the solid nodule, or it may wrap around the sides. The cystic components are of decreased attenuation on CT. The cystic components of these tumors contain differing amounts of blood products, proteinaceous debris, or cholesterol, resulting in a variable appearance on T1-weighted images *(46,47)*. In most cases, the cystic component will be of high or intermediate signal on T1-weighted images. In some cases, the cystic component will be isointense or hypointense on T1-weighted images *(46,48)*. On T2-weighted images, the cystic component is hyperintense.

GERM-CELL TUMORS   Intracranial germ-cell tumors most commonly occur in the pineal region (48%). The suprasellar cistern is the second most common site (37%); in some cases, both sites will be involved simultaneously (6%) (Figure 13) *(49)*. Germinomas are the most common intracranial germ-cell tumors. However, nongerminomatous germ-cell tumors, including teratomas, embryonal carcinomas, endodermal sinus tumors, and choriocarcinomas, may also involve the sellar region *(49,50)*. Germinomas involving the sellar region may present with diabetes insipidus, visual disturbance, or endocrinopathy. Germ-cell tumors tend to disseminate within the neuraxis, or less commonly systemically.

Germinomas are usually solid, but may contain cystic regions *(51)*. On nonenhanced CT scans, germinomas are usually of increased attenuation relative to brain matter and may contain obvious calcifications. There is intense enhancement on postcontrast images *(50,52)*. The tumor is usually iso- or slightly hypointense to white matter on T1-weighted MRI images and increased signal on T2-weighted MRI *(51)*.

MENINGIOMAS   Five to 10% of meningiomas occur in a parasellar location (Figures 14 and 15). They may originate from the tuberculum sellae, the dorsum sella, or the cavernous sinus dura. Parasellar meningiomas may grow into the sella

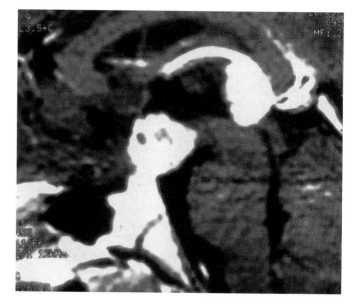

Figure 11-13 Germinoma. Sagittal enhanced T1W MRI. There are well-circumscribed enhancing lesions in the pineal region as well as in the suprasellar cistern. Synchronous pineal and suprasellar masses are highly typical of germinoma.

making it difficult to differentiate these lesions form a pituitary macroadenoma.

Meningiomas tend to be well circumscribed and isointense to gray matter on T1-weighted images. Signal on T2-weighted images is variable with about 50% being isointense and most of the remainder being hyperintense. Those tumors that are isointense on both T1- and T2-weighted images may be difficult to identify on noncontrast studies. Evidence of mass effect with displacement of adjacent structures or thickening of adjacent dura may be recog-

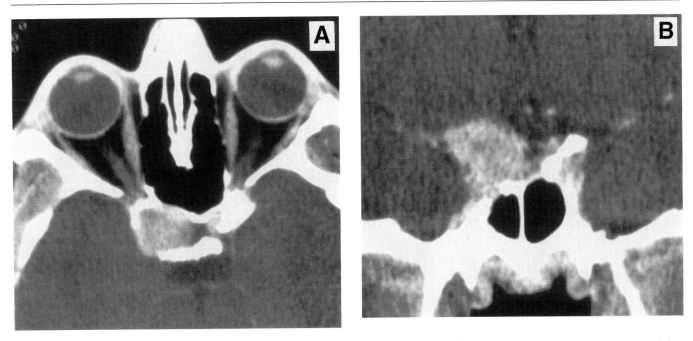

Figure 11-14 Meningioma. **(A)** Axial enhanced CT scan. **(B)** Coronal enhanced CT scan. There is a homogeneous enhancing mass arising from the tuberculum sellae and extending into the sella turcica.

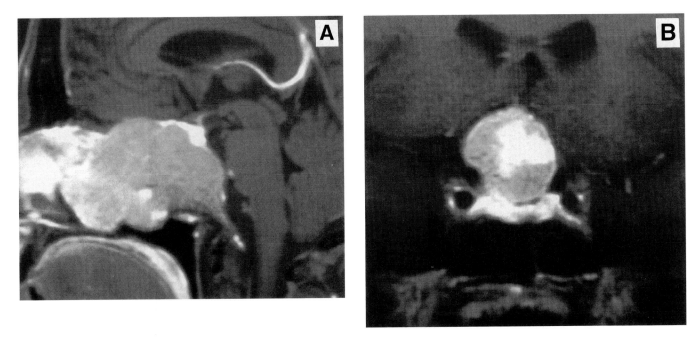

Figure 11-15 Meningioma. **(A)** Sagittal enhanced T1W MRI. **(B)** Coronal enhanced T1W MRI. A large brightly enhancing mass fills the sella turcica, the suprasellar cistern, and extends into the anterior cranial fossa.

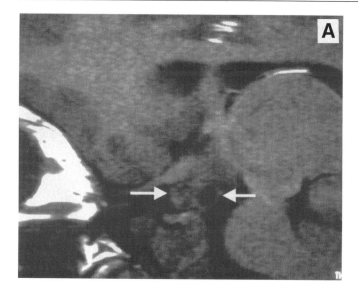

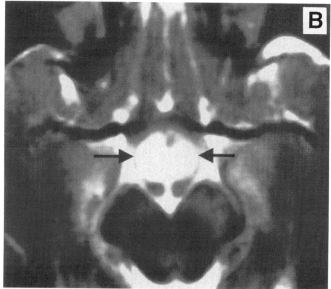

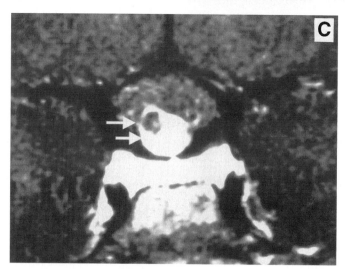

Figure 11-16 Chiasmatic glioma in a patient with neurofibromatosis type 1. (**A**) Sagittal T1W MRI. (**B**) Axial T2W MRI. (**C**) Enhanced coronal MRI. There is a mass centered on the optic chiasm. The mass contains solid and cystic components. The solid component is isointense on T1-weighted images and hyperintense on T2-weighted images. A portion of the mass enhances.

nized. There may be white matter edema within adjacent brain tissue. There is intense and homogeneous enhancement of meningiomas on postcontrast images. This is one of the most useful features to differentiate these tumors from macroadenomas, which tend to enhance more heterogeneously and to a lesser extent than meningiomas *(53)*. Other features of meningiomas are a wide dural base of attachment and enhancement of the perilesional dura (the "dural tail sign"). If the diaphragma sellae can be identified, it should be depressed in the case of a suprasellar meningioma and elevated in the case of an intrasellar macroadenoma. Bony hyperostosis and calcification (best seen on CT scan) are further clues that a suprasellar lesion is a meningioma.

CHIASMATIC AND HYPOTHALAMIC GLIOMAS Gliomas may originate from the hypothalamus or the optic chiasm. These tumors are often large at the time of presentation, and it may be impossible to determine whether the origin is from the hypothalamus or optic chiasm. Large tumors may completely fill the suprasellar cistern. Chiasmatic and hypothalamic gliomas are more

common in children where they make up 10–15% of supratentorial tumors *(54)*. There is an association between these tumors and neurofibromatosis type I.

Chiasmatic and hypothalamic gliomas may be identified on CT scans as a mass or an abnormal area of enhancement. Enlargement of the optic nerves may result in widening of the optic canals, which can be clearly identified on CT images. These tumors are isointense to brain on T1-weighted images and hyperintense on T2-weighted images (Figure 16). Larger tumors may contain cysts and areas of necrosis, resulting in a heterogeneous appearance. Enhancement on postcontrast images is variable. There is a tendency to invade brain along the optic pathways, which will be seen as areas on increased signal on the T2-weighted images.

GRANULAR CELL MYOBLASTOMA Primary tumors of the posterior pituitary gland are rare. Both gliomas (pilocytic astrocytomas) and granular cell myoblastoma's (choristoma) have been reported. Because of the rarity of these lesions, reports of imaging findings are based on just a few cases. Noncontrast CT of a granular cell myoblastoma has shown a hyperattenuating mass that enhances on postcontrast images *(55)*. MRI has been reported to show a mass isointense to brain tissue on T1- and T2-weighted images (Figure 17) *(55)*. We have a single case in which the tumor is homogeneously hyperintense on T1-weighted images and heterogeneous on T2-weighted images.

METASTASIS TO THE PITUITARY Metastasis to the pituitary gland is commonly found at autopsy *(56)*. They are rarely symptomatic and, hence, rarely subject to antemortem imaging investigation. The most common sources of pituitary metastases are breast and lung carcinomas. Metastatic deposits to the pituitary result in a sellar mass that is difficult to differentiate from a large, but otherwise normal pituitary gland. It is unusual for hematogenous metastases to the pituitary to cause sellar enlargement or bony erosion *(56)*. Suprasellar extension may be accompanied by a distinct indentation at the site of the diaphragma sella. The metastasis is usually isointense to brain on T1 and moderately hyperintense on T2. Enhancement on postgadolinium images is variable.

PRIMARY SELLAR MELANOMA Primary melanoma is another rare lesion found in this area *(57)*. On CT, these appear as homogeneous hyperattenuating lesions entirely in the sella or with suprasellar extension. The characteristic MRI appearance is one of high signal on T1-weighted images and low signal on T2-weighted images. This pattern differentiates these lesions from a subacute hemorrhage, which is usually hyperintense on both T1- and T2-weighted images.

CYSTIC LESIONS

Benign cystic lesions located in the sella are most commonly Rathke's cleft cysts or pars intermedia cysts. Less commonly, epidermoid, dermoid (Figure 18), and arachnoid cysts (Figure 19), as well as cystircercosis may involve the sella. All of these nonneoplastic cysts, with the possible exception of the epidermoid cyst, tend to be well defined on CT and MRI, but they vary in size, shape, and location. They may be entirely intrasellar, intra- and suprasellar, or less commonly entirely suprasellar *(58)*.

Most Rathke's cleft cysts are of intermediate attenuation on CT, hyperintense on T1- and T2-weighted MRI, and do not enhance, although it may be difficult to differentiate enhancing adjacent normal pituitary tissue from the cyst wall (Figure 20). Dynamic enhanced studies may be useful in this differentiation, because pituitary tissue enhances earlier that of the cyst wall. Craniopharyngiomas and cystic pituitary adenomas show enhancement of the cyst walls and tend to be larger, more irregular, and more heterogeneous in signal intensity. A smaller number of Rathke's cleft cysts contain serous-type, low-protein fluid. These tend to be low attenuation on CT, hypointense on T1-weighted MRI, and strongly resemble the appearance of CSF. Rarely, complex Rathke's cleft cysts contain a high proportion of inspissated secretions or desquamated cells. These have a heterogeneous internal appearance with regions of wall thickening and contrast enhancement, and very low signal on T2-weighted images. These can be mistaken for solid tumors *(59)*.

TUMOR-LIKE LESIONS

PITUITARY HYPERPLASIA Reactive hyperplasia of the pituitary gland may occur in cases of endocrine failure, such as primary hypothyroidism and hypogonadism *(60–62)*. Hyperplasia is identified on CT and MRI as diffuse, uniform, and bilaterally symmetric enlargement of the gland, which may extend superiorly

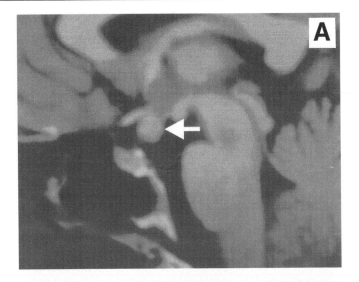

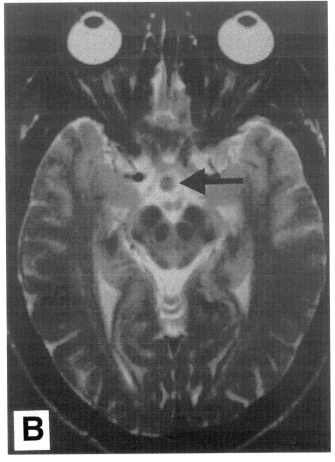

Figure 11-17 Granular cell myoblastoma (choristoma). **(A)** Sagittal T1W MRI. **(B)** Axial T2W MRI. There is a suprasellar mass (arrow) that is isointense to white matter on both T1W and T2W images. (Courtesy of Dr. Blake McClarty.)

into the suprasellar cistern. The resultant pituitary mass homogeneously enhances on contrast-enhanced images. Treatment with appropriate exogenous hormone replacement results in a return of the pituitary to a normal size and configuration.

HAMARTOMA OF THE TUBER CINEREUM Hypothalamic hamartomas are masses that usually originate from the poste-

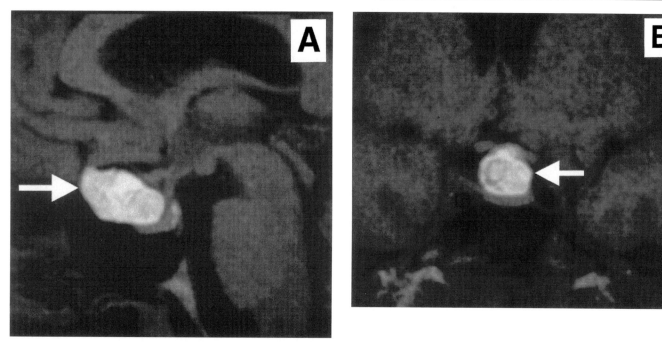

Figure 11-18   Dermoid. **(A)** Sagittal T1W MRI. **(B)** Coronal T1W MRI. There is a heterogeneously hyperintense sellar and suprasellar mass. The increased signal intensity on nonenhanced images is typical of a fat-containing mass.

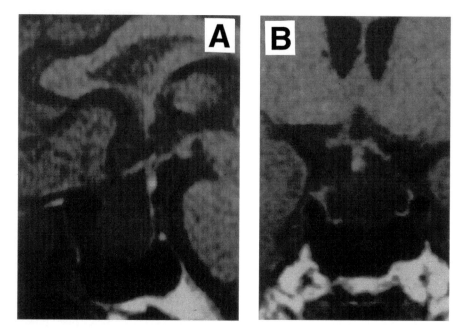

Figure 11-19   Arachnoid cyst. **(A)** Sagittal T1W MRI. **(B)** Coronal T1W MRI. There is a sellar and suprasellar mass, which is isointense to CSF.

rior aspect of the hypothalamus, most typically from the floor of the third ventricle between the pituitary stalk and the mamillary bodies (Figure 21). On CT scans, these lesions have attenuation characteristics similar to that of normal gray matter. Small lesions may be missed on CT, but identified on MRI. On MRI, hamartomas are isointense to gray matter on T1-weighted images and are usually of increased signal intensity on T2-weighted images *(63)*. Rarely, these hamartomas enhance with contrast or show evidence of calcification, fat, or cyst formation *(64)*. Het-

erogeneous signal may occur in lesions containing fat, calcium, or areas of necrosis.

LANGERHANS CELL HISTIOCYTOSIS   Langerhans cell histiocytosis (eosinophilic granulomatosis) involves the structures around the suprasellar cistern more frequently than any other part of the neuraxis (Figure 22). The most common manifestation is infiltration of the pituitary stalk, which is identified as thickening and increased enhancement. Frequently, the normal high signal of the posterior pituitary gland will be also absent, and the patients

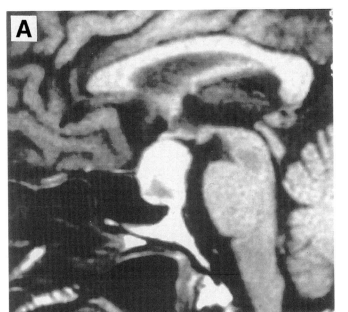

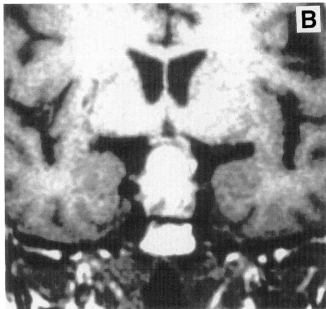

Figure 11-20 Rathke's cleft cyst. **(A)** Sagittal T1W MRI. **(B)** Coronal T1W MRI. This intra- and suprasellar cyst is well defined and is of increased signal intensity on these nonenhanced images.

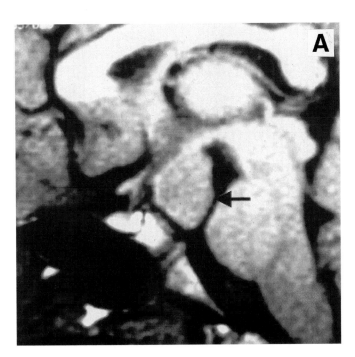

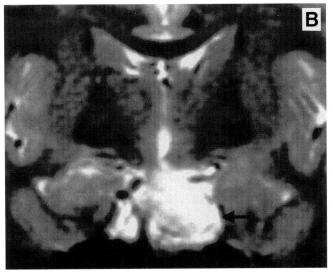

Figure 11-21 Hypothalamic hamartoma. **(A)** Sagittal T1W MRI. **(B)** Coronal T2W MRI. The homogeneous mass extending from the floor of the third ventricle causes anterior displacement of the pituitary stalk. The mass is isointense to gray matter on T1W images and of increased signal intensity on T2W images.

will clinically have diabetes insipidus. Other causes of a thickened stalk include germinoma, sarcoidosis, tuberculosis, metastasis, and infiltration from adjacent neoplasms (65).

INFLAMMATORY LESIONS

LYMPHOCYTIC ADENOHYPOPHYSITIS Lymphocytic adenohypophysitis is a rare inflammatory disorder that presents with hypopituitarism. This disorder is most common in gravid and

postpartum females. There are reports of this rare disorder occurring in males and nongravid females.

Imaging reveals a homogeneous intrasellar mass with or without suprasellar extension. On MRI, it is isointense or slightly hyperintense to gray matter on T1-weighted images (66). The pituitary stalk is thickened (65). The mass enhances markedly on postgadolinium images. In most cases, abnormal enhancement will extend to the infundibulum (67) and to the surrounding dura. Histologic specimens

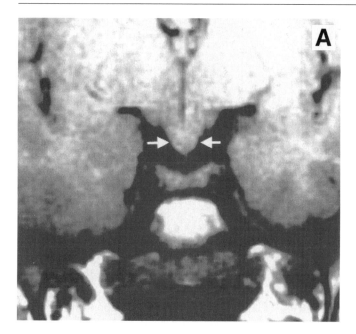

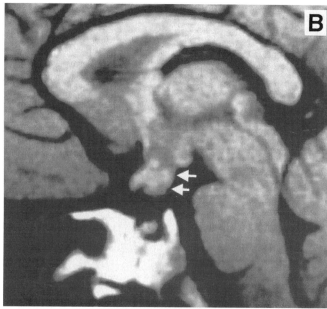

Figure 11-22 Langerhan's cell histiocytosis. (**A**) Coronal T1W MRI. (**B**) Sagittal T1W MRI. The pituitary stalk is thickened (arrows). The normal high signal from the posterior pituitary gland is absent.

have shown that the enhancing dura is infiltrated with inflammatory cells *(66)*. Although the pituitary mass may be mistaken for a pituitary adenoma, the dural enhancement can be used to differentiate this inflammatory disorder from an adenoma or hyperplasia. Neither a pituitary adenoma nor hyperplasia of the pituitary normally results in enhancement of adjacent soft tissues. An exception to this rule may occur in cases of an adenoma complicated by necrosis or infarction. Other inflammatory processes, such as sarcoidosis, and fungal or tuberculous infection *(68)*, may also result in an MRI appearance similar to that of lymphocytic adenohypophysitis.

ABSCESS   Pituitary abscesses are uncommon lesions that result from secondary infection of pre-existing lesions, following surgery, or rarely *de novo* in a previously healthy gland. Bacterial, fungal *(69)*, and tuberculous abscesses have been reported. Most pituitary abscesses are spread from an adjacent septic focus, such as sphenoid sinusitis, meningitis, osteomyelitis, or cavernous sinus thrombophlebitis. Occasionally the septic focus will be remote from the pituitary and spread hematogenously. An abscess appears as a sellar mass (Figure 23) similar to an adenoma on noncontrast MRI and CT. One distinctive feature is that the rim of the mass enhances on enhanced studies, MRI, and CT, but the central portion remains hypointense.

METABOLIC DISORDERS

DIABETES INSIPIDUS   Central diabetes insipidus may be caused by damage to the hypothalamus, by neoplastic or infiltrative lesions, by surgery, by trauma, or it may be idiopathic *(70)*. Central diabetes insipidus is rarely inherited *(71)*. The diagnosis of diabetes insipidus is usually made clinically. Imaging by means of MRI or CT is useful in determining the etiology of this disorder; most importantly, imaging is needed to rule out a neoplastic or infiltrative lesion of the neurohypophyseal structures. MRI may also be used to help distinguish between central diabetes insipidus and psychogenic polydipsia, since the presence of the high signal within the posterior pituitary on T1-weighted MRI is evidence of a functionally intact neurohypophyseal system *(72)*. If vasopressin

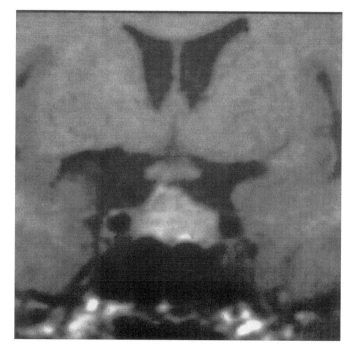

Figure 11-23 Abscess. Coronal T1W MRI. There is a sellar and suprasellar mass that cannot be differentiated from normal pituitary gland.

stores are depleted, as in central diabetes insipidus, the normal high signal of the posterior pituitary disappears *(73,74)*. The normal high signal of the posterior pituitary will remain in patients with psychogenic or nephrogenic diabetes insipidus.

VASCULAR AND ISCHEMIC LESIONS

Berry aneurysms from the cavernous or supraclinoid portions of the internal carotid arteries may protrude into the sella. Tortuous carotid arteries may meet in the midline ("kissing carotids").

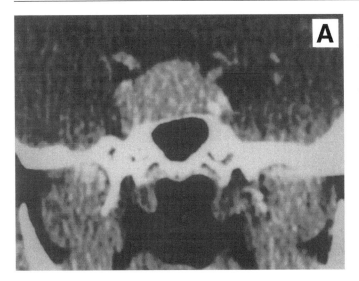

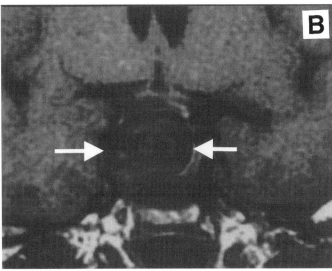

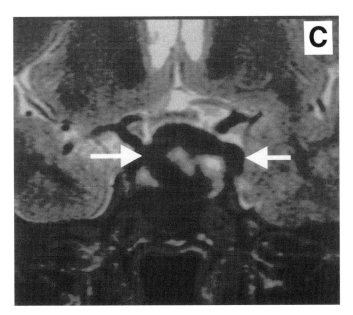

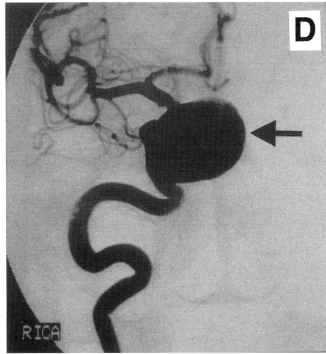

Figure 11-24   Aneurysm. **(A)** Coronal enhanced CT. **(B)** Coronal T1W MRI. **(C)** Coronal T2W MRI. **(D)** Right internal carotid angiogram. The aneurysm cannot be differentiated from a nonvascular sellar mass on CT (A). On MRI there is a large, well-circumscribed mass (arrows) of predominantly decreased signal on both T1W and T2W images (B and C). The angiogram shows the aneurysm arising from the intracavernous portion of the internal carotid artery.

Anterior communicating, posterior communicating, and basilar tip aneurysms may project into the suprasellar cistern. Large or calcified aneurysms may be recognized on nonenhanced CT as an area of increased density or curvilinear calcification. Nonthrombosed portions of the aneurysm will enhance densely and homogeneously. Small, noncalcified, or thrombosed aneurysms may be missed on CT images. Aneurysms involving the sella turcica and suprasellar cistern are easily identified on MRI (Figure 24). T1-weighted images will reveal a well-defined lesion that lacks internal signal (signal void) *(75)*. There may also be significant

artifacts from the flowing blood, resulting in multiple ghosts in the phase-encoding direction. Thrombus within the aneurysm will appear on T1-weighted images as a multilamellated high signal that completely or partially fills the lumen.

REFERENCES

1. Burrow GN, Wortzman G, Rewcastle NB, Holgate RC, Kovacs K. Microadenomas of the pituitary and abnormal sellar tomograms in an unselected autopsy series. N Engl J Med 1981;304:156–158.
2. Wortzman G, Rewcastle NB. Tomographic abnormalities simulating pituitary microadenomas. Am J Neuroradiol 1982;3:305–512.

3. Kulkarni MV, Lee KF, McArdle CB, Yeakley JW, Haar FL. 1.5T MR imaging of pituitary microadenomas: technical considerations and CT correlation. Am J Neuroradiol 1988;9:5–11.

4. Webb SM, Ruscalleda J, Schwarzstein D, et al. Computerized tomography versus magnetic resonance imaging: a comparative study in hypothalamic-pituitary and parasellar pathology. Clin Endocrinol 1992;1992:459–465.

5. Lundin P, Bergstom K, Thuomas KA, Lundberg PO, Muhr C. Comparison of MR imaging and CT in pituitary macroadenomas. Acta Radiolol 1991;32:189–196.

6. Johnson MR, Hoare RD, Cox T, et al. The evaluation of patients with a suspected pituitary microadenoma: computer tomography compared to magnetic resonance imaging. Clin Endocrinol 1992;36:335–338.

7. Kucharczyk W, Davis DO, Kelly WM, Sze G, Norman D, Newton TH. Pituitary adenomas: high-resolution MR imaging at 1.5 T. Radiology 1986;161:761–765.

8. Sakamoto Y, Takahashi M, Korogi Y, Bussaka H, Ushio Y. Normal and abnormal pituitary glands: gadopentetate dimeglumine-enhanced MR imaging. Radiology 1991;178:441–445.

9. Ahmadi H, Larsson EM, Jinkins JR. Normal pituitary gland: coronal MR imaging of infundibular tilt. Radiology 1990;1990:389–392.

10. Cox TD, Elster AD. Normal pituitary gland: changes in shape, size, and signal intensity during the 1st year of life at MR imaging. Radiology 1991;179:721–724.

11. Elster AD, Chen MYM, Williams DW, Key LL. Pituitary gland: MR imaging of physiologic hypertrophy in adolescence. Radiology 1990;174:681–685.

12. Suzuki M, Takashima T, Kadoya M, et al. Height of normal pituitary gland on MR imaging: age and sex differentiation. J Computer Assisted Tomogr 1990;14:36–39.

13. Elster AD, Sanders TG, Vines FS, Chen MYM. Size and shape of the pituitary gland during pregnancy and post partum: measurement with MR imaging. Radiology 1991;181:531–535.

14. Miki Y, Asato R, Okumura R, et al. Anterior pituitary gland in pregnancy: hyperintensity at MR. Radiology 1993;187:229–231.

15. Ryals BD, Brown DC, Levin SW. Duplication of the pituitary gland as shown by MR. Am J Roentgenology 1993;14:137–139.

16. Kelly WM, Kucharczyk W, Kucharczyk J, et al. Posterior pituitary ectopia: an MR feature of pituitary dwarfism. Am J Neuroradiol 1988;9:453–460.

17. Kikuchi K, Fujisawa I, Momoi T, et al. Hypothalamic–pituitary function in growth hormone-deficient patients with pituitary stalk transection. J Clin Endocrinol Metab 1988;67(4):817–823.

18. Wolpert SM. The radiology of pituitary adenomas. Semin Roentgenology 1984;14:53–69.

19. Mikhael MA, Ciric IS. MR imaging of pituitary tumors before and after surgical and/or medical treatment. J Computer Assisted Tomog 1988;12:441–445.

20. Dwyer AJ, Frank JA, Doppman JL, et al. Pituitary adenomas in patients with Cushing disease: initial experience with Gd-DTPA-enhanced MR imaging. Radiology 1987;163:421–426.

21. Newton DR, Dillon WP, Norman D, Newton TH, Wilson CB. Gd-DTPA-enhanced MR imaging of pituitary adenomas. Am J Neuroradiol 1989;10:949–954.

22. Davis PC, Gokhale KA, Joseph GJ, et al. Pituitary adenoma: correlation of half-dose gadolinium-enhanced MR imaging with surgical findings in 26 patients. Radiology 1991;180:779–784.

23. Macpherson P, Hadley DM, Teasdale E, Teasdale G. Pituitary microadenomas. Neuroradiology 1989;34:293–298.

24. Miki Y, Matsuo M, Nishizawa S, et al. Pituitary adenomas and normal pituitary tissue: enhancement patterns on gadopentetate-enhanced MR imaging. Radiology 1990;177:35–38.

25. Kucharczyk W, Bishop JE, Plewes DB, Keller MA, George S. Detection of pituitary microadenomas: comparison of dynamic keyhole fast spin-echo, unenhanced, and conventional contrast-enhanced MR imaging. Am J Roentgenology 1994;163:671–679.

26. Peck WW, Dillon WP, Norman D, Newton TH, Wilson CB. High-Resolution MR imaging of pituitary microadenomas at 1.5 T: experience with Cushing disease. Am J Roentgenology 1989;152:145–151.

27. Elster AD. Sellar susceptibility artifacts: theory and implications. Am J Neuroradiol 1993;14:120–136.

28. Lundin P, Bergstrom K. Gd-DTPA-enhanced MR imaging of pituitary macroadenomas. Acta Radiol 1992;33:323–332.

29. Snow RB, Johnson CE, Morgello S, Lavyne MH, Patterson RH. Is magnetic resonance imaging useful in guiding the operative approach to large pituitary tumors. Neurosurgery 1990;26:801–803.

30. Lee B, Cho J, Kim DI. Dynamic MR imaging of the cavernous sinus. Radiol Soc North Am: Radiol 1995;197 (Suppl):135.

31. Nakamura T, Schorner W, Bittner RC, Felix R. The value of paramagnetic contrast agent gadolinium-DTPA in the diagnosis of pituitary adenomas. Neuroradiology 1988;30:481–486.

32. Scotti G, Yu C-Y, Dillon WP, et al. MR imaging of cavernous sinus involvement by pituitary adenomas. Am J Roentgenology 1988;151:799–806.

33. Yousem DM, Arrington JA, Zinreich SJ, Kumar AJ, Bryan RN. Pituitary adenomas: possible role of bromocriptine in intratumoral hemorrhage. Radiology 1989;170:239–243.

34. Kyle CA, Laster RA, Burton EM, Stanford RA. Subacute pituitary apoplexy: MR and CT appearance. J Computer Assisted Tomogr 1990;14:40–44.

35. Lazaro CM, Guo WY, Sami M, et al. Haemorrhagic pituitary tumours. Neuroradiology 1994;36:111–114.

36. Ostrov SG, Quencer RM, Hoffman JC, Davis PC, Hasso AN, David NJ. Hemorrhage within pituitary adenomas: how often associated with pituitary apoplexy syndrome. Am J Neuroradiol 1989;10:503–510.

37. Matsumura A, Meguro K, Doi M, Tsurushima H, Tomono Y. Suprasellar ectopic pituitary adenoma: case report and review of the literature. Neurosurgery 1990;26:681–685.

38. Slonim SM, Haykal HA, Cushing GW, Freidberg SR, Lee AK. MRI appearances of an ectopic pituitary adenoma: case report and review of the literature. Neuroradiology 1993;35:546–548.

39. Hattori N, Ishihara T, Saiwai S, et al. Ectopic prolactinoma on MRI. J Computer Assisted Tomogr 1994;18:936–938.

40. Dina TS, Feaster SH, Laws ER, Davis DO. MR of the pituitary gland postsurgery: serial MR studies following transspenoidal resection. Am J Neuroradiol 1993;14:763–769.

41. Steiner E, Knosp E, Herold CJ, et al. Pituitary adenomas: findings of postoperative MR imaging. Radiology 1992;185:521–527.

42. Carmel PW, Antunes JL, Chang CH. Craniopharyngiomas in children. Neurosurgery 1982;11:382–389.

43. Harwood-Nash DC. Neuroimaging of childhood craniopharyngioma. Pediatr Neurosurg 1994;21 (Suppl):2–10.

44. Matthews FD. Intraventricular craniopharyngioma. Am J Neuroradiol 1983;4:984–985.

45. Hoffman HJ, De Silva M, Humphreys RP, Drake JM, Smith ML, Blaser SI. Aggressive surgical management of craniopharyngiomas in children. J Neurosurg 1992;76:47–52.

46. Pusey E, Kortman KE, Flannigan BD, Tsuruda J, Bradley WG. MR of craniopharyngiomas: tumor delineation and characterization. Am J Neuroradiol 1987;8:439–444.

47. Ahmadi J, Destian S, Apuzzo MLJ, Segall HD, Zee C-S. Cystic fluid in craniopharyngiomas: MR imaging and quantitative analysis. Radiology 1992;182:783–785.

48. Freeman MP, Kessler RM, Allen JH, Price AC. Craniopharyngioma: CT and MR imaging in nine cases. J Computer Assisted Tomogr 1987;11:810–814.

49. Jennings MT, Gelman R, Hochberg F. Intracranial germ-cell tumors: natural history and pathogenesis. J Neurosurg 1985;63:155–167.

50. Hoffman HJ, Otsubo H, Hendrick B, et al. Intracranial germ-cell tumors in children. J Neurosurg 1991;74:545–551.

51. Sumida M, Uozumi T, Kiya K, et al. MRI of intracranial germ cell tumours. Neuroradiology 1995;37:32–37.

52. Takeuchi J, Handa H, Nagata I. Suprasellar germinoma. J Neurosurg 1978;49:41–48.

53. Michael AS, Paige ML. MR imaging of intrasellar meningiomas simulating pituitary adenomas. J Computer Assisted Tomogr 1988;12:944–946.

54. Barkovich AJ. Pediatric Neuroimaging, 2nd ed. Raven, New York, 1995.

55. Cone L, Srinivasan M, Romanul FCS. Granular cell tumor (choristoma) of the neurohypophysis: two cases and a review of the literature. Am J Neuroradiol 1990;11:403–406.

56. Schubiger O, Haller D. Metastases to the pituitary–hypothalamic axis An MR study of 7 symptomatic patients. Neuroradiology 1992;34:131–134.

57. Chappell PM, Kelly WM, Ercius M. Primary sellar melanoma simulating hemorrhagic pituitary adenoma: MR and pathologic findings. American Journal of Neuroradiol 1990;11:1054–1056.

58. Hua F, Asato R, Miki Y, et al. Differentiation of suprasellar nonneoplastic cysts from cystic neoplasms by Gd-DTPA MRI. J Computer Assisted Tomogr 1992;16:744–749.

59. Kucharczyk W, Peck WW, Kelly WM, Norman D, Newton T. Rathke cleft cysts: CT, MR imaging and pathologic features. Radiology 1987;165:491–495.

60. Kuroiwa T, Okabe Y, Hasuo K, Yasumori K, Mizushima A, Masuda K. MR imaging of pituitary hypertrophy due to juvenile primary hypothyroidism: a case report. Clin Imaging 1991;15:202–205.

61. Hutchins WW, Crues JV, Miya P, Pojunas KW. MR Demonstration of pituitary hyperplasia and regression after therapy for hypothyroidism. Am J Neuroradiol 1990;11:410.

62. Dadachanji MC, Bharucha NE, Jhankaria BG. Pituitary hyperplasia mimicking pituitary tumor. Surg Neurol 1994;42:397–399.

63. Hahn FJ, Leibrock LG, Huseman CA, Makos MM. The MR appearance of hypothalamic hamartoma. Neuroradiology 1988;30:65–68.

64. Burton EM, Ball WS, Crone K, Dolan LM. Hamartoma of the tuber cinereum: a comparison of MR and CT findings in four cases. Am J Neuroradiol 1989;10:497–501.

65. Tien RD, Newton TH, McDermott MW, Dillon WP, Kucharczyk J. Thickened pituitary stalk on MR images in patients with diabetes insipidus and Langerhans cell histiocytosis. American Journal of Neuroradiology 1990;11:703–708.

66. Ahmadi J, Meyers GS, Segall HD, Sharma OP, Hinton DR. Lymphocytic adenohypophysitis: contrast-enhanced MR imaging in five cases. Radiology 1995;195:30–34.

67. Abe T, Matsumoto K, Sanno N, Osamura Y. Lymphocytic hypophysitis: case report. Neurosurgery 1995;36:1016–1019.

68. Pereira J, Vaz R, Carvalho D, Cruz C. Thickening of the pituitary stalk: a finding suggestive of intrasellar tuberculoma? Case report. Neurosurgery 1995;36:1013–1016.

69. Heary RF, Maniker AH, Wolansky LJ. Candidal pituitary abscess: case report. Neurosurgery 1995;36:1009–1013.

70. Moses AM, Streeten DHP. Disorders of the Neurohypophysis. In: Wilson JD, Braunwald E, Isselbacher KJ, eds. Harrison's Principles of Internal Medicine, 12th ed. McGraw-Hill, New York: 1991, pp. 1682–1691.

71. Martin MR. Familial diabetes insipidus. Q J Med 1959;28:573–582.

72. Moses AM, Clayton B, Hochhauser L. Use of T1-weighted MR imaging to differentiate between primary polydipsia and central diabetes insipidus. Am J Neuroradiol 1992;13:1273–1277.

73. Fujisawa I, Nishimura K, Asato R, et al. Posterior lobe of the pituitary in diabetes insipidus: MR findings. J Computer Assisted Tomogr 1987;11:221–225.

74. Maghnie M, Villa A, Arico M, et al. Correlation between magnetic resonance imaging of posterior pituitary and neurohypophyseal function in children with diabetes insipidus. J Clin Endocrinol Metab 1992;74:795–800.

75. Atlas SW, Mark AS, Fram EK, Grossman RI. Vascular intracranial lesions: applications of gradient-echo MR imaging. Radiology 1988;169:455–461.

12 Positron Emission Tomography in Sellar Tumors

In Vivo Metabolic, Receptor, and Enzyme Characterization

CARIN MUHR, MD, PHD

INTRODUCTION

Positron emission tomography (PET) is now a well-recognized technique for research as well as clinical practice. The PET technique has been in use for more than 20 years in a wide range of scientific areas and now has also proven to be of great value in clinical practice. We have used the PET technique for 16 years to investigate intracranial tumors and especially sellar tumors of which pituitary adenomas are the most common tumor type. PET has been used to characterize in vivo these tumors with respect to metabolism, receptor properties, and enzyme content like. The characterization has been used for diagnosing and outlining the tumors, in differential diagnostic perspective, and in the follow-up of treatment (1,2).

METABOLIC STUDIES

For metabolic studies, ^{11}C-L-methionine and ^{18}F-fluorodeoxyglucose have been used. ^{11}C-L-methionine will relate to the amino acid metabolism in the tumor and only accumulate in viable tumor tissue. The uptake in the tumor is usually higher than in the surrounding brain, which will make a delineation of the active tumor tissue possible. ^{18}F-fluorodeoxyglucose will give the actual glucose metabolism in the tumor. Just as for ^{11}C-L-methionine, ^{18}F-fluorodeoxyglucose will accumulate in viable tumor tissue and reflect the degrees of metabolic activity within this tissue. However, the glucose metabolism in the brain is also high—usually about the same level as in the pituitary tumor—which means that delineation of the tumor can be difficult (Figure 1).

DOPAMINE RECEPTOR STUDIES

Dopamine receptor studies were performed with the specific dopamine D_2 antagonist ^{11}C-raclopride. The two stereoisomers, the r-form and the s-form of raclopride, were used. The s-form will show the total binding, and the r-form the nonspecific binding. By subtracting the nonspecific binding from the total binding, the specific D_2 binding was determined. The striatum, the region in the brain that contains the highest amounts of D_2 receptor binding,

was always included in the area examined as a reference. The cerebellum was also used as a reference tissue since the cerebellum contains almost no D_2 binding.

MAO-B ENZYME CHARACTERIZATION

PET with ^{11}C-L-deprenyl was used for measuring the MAO-B enzyme content in the tumor tissue. Deprenyl is an irreversible MAO-B inhibitor, and the binding of ^{11}C-L-deprenyl will be dependent on the amount of the MAO-B enzyme content in the tumors.

PATIENT MATERIAL

One hundred twenty patients with a pituitary expansive process were examined with PET to characterize the lesions. All the patients except one were adults. Around 30% of the patients had a prolactinoma, 50% a clinically nonsecreting pituitary adenoma, 10% growth hormone- (GH), adrenocorticopic hormone (ACTH)-, follicle-stimulating hormone (FSH)-, or thyroid-stimulating hormone (TSH)-secreting adenomas and the remaining 10% meningiomas, chordomas, craniopharyngiomas, cystic malformations or abscesses. Out of the adenomas the majority of the patients, had a macroadenoma, and only five patients a microadenoma.

PET METHODS

The PET studies were performed in two types of PET brain scanners, the earlier studies in a Scanditronix PC 384-3B and the later in a GEMS 2048B. The PC-384-3B camera simultaneously produced three slices with a slice thickness of about 11 mm and spacing of 14 mm. The spatial resolution was 8 mm full-width, half-maximum (FWHM). The GEMS 2048B camera was of a later generation and technically more advanced, and produced 15 slices with a slice thickness of 6.5 mm and spacing of about 6.5 mm. The spatial resolution was 5 mm (FWHM).

The radiolabeled substance, synthesized for each examination, was given in a dose from 100 to 250 MBq, as an iv bolus injection. Each batch was tested for sterility and radiochemical purity. The PET study was started at the time of the bolus injection and undertaken as dynamic examination sequences with 10–17 scans obtained during 30–50 min.

A region of interest (ROI) was marked with a cursor to represent the tumor, and the activity of the labeled substance within this ROI was measured, and the ratio to the activity in normal brain

From: *Diagnosis and Management of Pituitary Tumors* (K. Thapar, K. Kovacs, B. W. Scheithauer, and R. V. Lloyd, eds.), ©Humana Press Inc., Totowa, NJ.

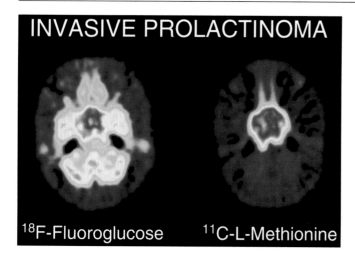

Figure 12-1 PET of a patient with a pituitary adenoma. Uptake in the adenoma is high with both ^{11}C-L-methionine and ^{18}F-fluorodeoxyglucose (FDG), but the uptake of FDG is also high in the brain. The outlining of the adenoma is better with methionine becasue the uptake of methionine is lower in the brain.

tissue was calculated. For the dopamine receptor studies, the reference area was the cerebellum, which is in practice void of D_2 binding. For detailed information, see our article (1,3).

The PET technique enables in vivo evaluation of the tumor metabolism, and repeat examinations can be performed within a relatively short time. The amount of radiation is dependent on the radionuclide used. ^{11}C has a half-life of 20 min. A ^{11}C-labeled substance will cause an amount of radiation that is comparable to a regular CT scan. For patients with a tumor, also benign, the radiation from the PET examination thus is a minor problem. The amount of radioactive substance can also be adjusted, and for clinical examinations, there is often the possibility to simplify the procedures. The costs involved with PET studies are still high, and special facilities with high technology and highly specialized personal are required, but when applied, PET yields very valuable data.

PET EXAMINATIONS

All patients were examined with PET with ^{11}C-L-methionine, most of the prolactinoma patients were also examined with ^{11}C-raclopride for D_2 receptor determination, some patients were also examined with ^{18}F-fluorodeoxyglucose for glucose metabolism estimation, and some with ^{11}C-L-deprenyl for determination of the MAO-B enzyme content. All patients evaluated during treatment were examined with PET before and at regular intervals during treatment. Each patient was in this respect his or her own control.

CLINICAL AND HORMONAL EVALUATION

All the patients were clinically examined, receiving a neurological examination, including neuroophthalmology, evaluation of hypothalamo-pituitary, thyroid, adrenal, and gonadal functions, evaluation of GH (usually including a 24-h profile, and insulin-like growth factor 1 [IGF-1] and α-subunit determination).

COMPUTED TOMOGRAPH (CT) AND MAGNETIC RESONANCE IMAGING (MRI)

All patients were examined with CT and, with few exceptions, also with MRI including contrast enhancement.

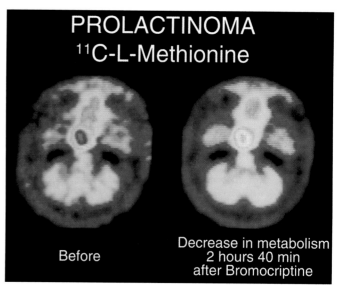

Figure 12-2 PET image of a patient with a prolactinoma demonstrating the rapid decrease in metabolism in the prolactinoma already 2 h and 40 min after im bromocriptine injection.

PET IN PROLACTINOMAS

METABOLIC STUDIES WITH ^{11}C-L-METHIONINE AND ^{18}F-FLUORODEOXYGLUCOSE IN PROLACTINOMAS The prolactinomas are metabolically very active and usually have such a high metabolic index using ^{11}C-L-methionine that they can be distinguished from the other pituitary adenomas. Using ^{18}F-fluorodeoxyglucose will also show a high metabolism in the prolactinomas, but as discussed above, the contrast to the surrounding brain is usually higher with ^{11}C-L-methionine than with ^{18}F-fluorodeoxyglucose (Figure 1), which is essential when outlining the tumor extension. The metabolic activity as measured with PET correlates well to the amount of prolactin secretion. The metabolic activity will decrease considerably when the adenoma responds to medical treatment as discussed below, and metabolic PET studies are in this respect very valuable in the follow-up of treatment. This decrease in the ^{11}C-L-methionine uptake in the prolactinoma after initiation of bromocriptine treatment is observed early and is marked (Figure 2). This is also true for nonsecreting adenomas and of special value since there are no hormonal markers in serum that might help.

DOPAMINE RECEPTOR BINDING STUDIES WITH ^{11}C-RACLOPRIDE IN PROLACTINOMAS Using ^{11}C-raclopride for determination of D_2 binding demonstrated high amounts of D_2 binding in all the prolactinomas that were examined before the start of treatment. The amounts measured with PET corresponded well to what has been described from in vitro studies. The D_2 binding within the group of prolactinomas varies, and high D_2 binding seems to be a prerequisite for response to dopamine agonist therapy (3–5). In some prolactinomas, the dopamine binding has shown to exceed the amounts found in the striatum in the brain (Figure 3).

The prolactinomas that were investigated with PET for dopamine receptor binding were investigated before treatment with dopamine agonist therapy. These prolactinomas investigated with ^{11}C-raclopride all demonstrated high D_2 binding. All these patients responded well to treatment with a considerable

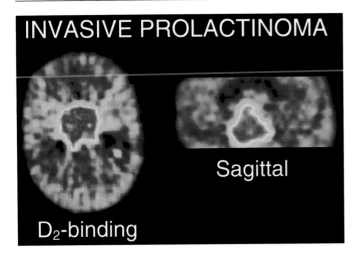

Figure 12-3 PET images with the specific dopamine antagonist ^{11}C-L-raclopride of a patient with a prolactinoma. High dopamine-D_2-binding is demonstrated in the prolactinoma.

decrease or normalization of serum prolactin and later tumor volume decrease.

D_2 BINDING DURING DOPAMINE AGONIST TREATMENT IN PROLACTINOMAS The PET technique allows repeat studies to follow, for example, receptor occupancy after administration of a medication. The D_2 binding was studied after initiation of dopamine agonist treatment. The patient was examined with ^{11}C-raclopride before start of treatment and re-examined after given a 50-mg im injection of bromocriptine retard. Three and a half hours after the injection, the number of free receptors had decreased by 20–30%, and by 13 h, a decrease of 50% in the number of free D_2 receptors was seen. This demonstrates that it is only necessary to interfere with about 20–50% of the D_2 receptors to achieve a dramatic effect of the bromocriptine with decreased metabolism as measured with PET and decreased serum prolactin levels *(1)*.

MICROPROLACTINOMAS The visualization of small volumes like a microprolactinoma with PET is dependent on the ratio between the uptake of the labeled substance within the microadenoma and the uptake in the surrounding structures. For ^{11}C-L-methionine, this ratio in prolactinomas is favorable, and even small adenomas are possible to diagnose (Figure 4). It is also possible to determine the D_2 binding in the microadenomas. After initiation of treatment with a dopamine agonist, if the prolactinoma responds, a repeat PET examination with ^{11}C-methionine will demonstrate a considerable decrease in the amino acid metabolism (Figure 3).

DOPAMINE AGONIST THERAPIES IN PROLACTINOMAS

BROMOCRIPTINE Bromocriptine is the dopamine agonist medication most commonly used for prolactinomas. Bromocriptine has been used since the early 1970s and is therefore also the medication with which we have the most experience *(6,7)*. Bromocriptine has been used in a large number of pregnant women from the moment of conception to full-term pregnancy. No teratogenic or hormonal disturbances have been seen when these children have been examined *(8)*. This gives us great confidence in the safety of bromocriptine. Positive effect from bromocriptine treatment is readily demonstrated by a considerable decrease in the

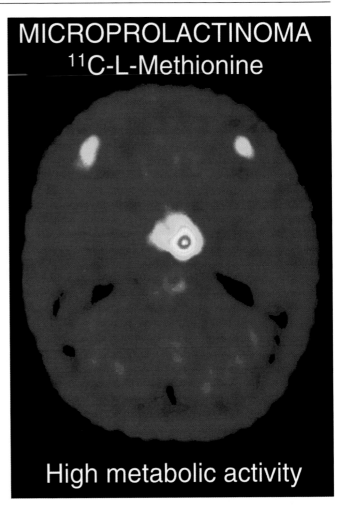

Figure 12-4 PET image with ^{11}C-L-methionine showing a female patient with a microprolactinoma with high metabolism.

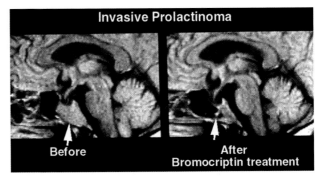

Figure 12-5 MRI images in sagittal projection from a patient with an invasive prolactinoma before *(left)* and after 6 mo bromocriptine treatment *(right)*.

amino acid metabolism studied with PET (Figure 3). We have also demonstrated the very rapid effect of bromocriptine retard given as an im injection *(9,9a)*. Dramatic effects can be observed a few hours after the injection with a considerable decrease in amino acid metabolism combined with a considerable decrease in the serum prolactin levels. This is later followed by tumor volume decrease (Figure 5) *(7)*.

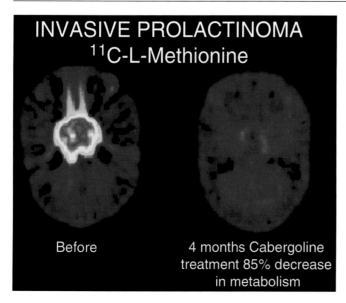

Figure 12-6   PET-images with ^{11}C-L-methionine demonstrating a middle-aged female patient with an invasive prolactinoma with high metabolism before *(left)* and the considerably decreased metabolism (85%) after 4 mo treatment with a dopaminagonist, cabergoline *(right)*.

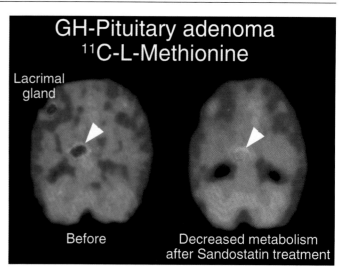

Figure 12-7   Pet images with ^{11}C-L-methionine demonstrating a patient with a GH-pituitary adenoma before *(left)* and after *(right)* Sandostatin treatment showing the decrease in metabolism within the adenoma and (also the lacrimal gland).

NEWER DOPAMINE AGONIST THERAPIES   We have also examined prolactinomas treated with Quinagolide (Norprolac) and Pergolide and observed a considerable decrease in the amino acid metabolism evaluated by PET. Cabergoline with a somewhat different profile and a longer half-life for an oral preparation has also been studied with PET and shown a considerable decrease in the amino acid metabolism in the prolactinomas (Figure 6). It is also well known that there can be a difference in response between these dopamine agonist medications for the same patient with a prolactinoma. The tolerability of the different medications may also vary.

PROLACTINOMAS RESISTANT TO DOPAMINE AGONIST THERAPY

In total, we have had three prolactinoma patients who were resistant to dopamine agonist therapy. All three were examined with PET for dopamine binding, but only after a resistance had been diagnosed. Two of these patients, one female and one male, demonstrated low amounts of D_2 binding. However, the third patient had moderately high D_2 binding. This demonstrates that there is also a possible disturbance of the receptor system that might not severely interfere with the D_2 binding as such.

Each of these three patients had prolactin values that proved the tumors to be prolactinomas. Two of the patients had also been operated on, and the tumor tissue demonstrated positive immunoreactivity for prolactin. These patients had tried several dopamine agonist therapies and shown resistant patterns. It was also the experience that during the development of resistance, a change in the dopamine agonist medication may give a response, but only sometimes for a limited time. One patient showed after developing resistance to bromocriptine a positive response to Quinagolide (Norprolac) for a year and then became resistant to this dopaminagnist also. Bromocriptine is by far the most commonly used dopamine agonist. The injectable retard im preparation was shown to have very rapid effect, and already within a few hours, a dramatic decrease in the metabolic activity within the

tumor was seen by PET as well as a decrease in serum prolactin levels *(9a,9b)*.

SOMATOSTATIN ANALOGUE TREATMENT OF GH ADENOMAS AND TSH ADENOMAS   In the prolactinomas, we have demonstrated that the metabolic activity as measured with ^{11}C-methionine correlates well to the endocrine activity of the tumor. This was also true for GH-secreting adenomas (Figure 7) and the two TSH adenomas we have examined. Sandostatin, which inhibits the GH secretion, will thus give a rapid decrease in the metabolic activity within the adenoma when a positive response is seen. With a short-lasting preparation, even the duration of each injection can be demonstrated *(1)*.

MEDIUM-LARGE ADENOMAS WITH HYPERPROLACTINEMIA

Many endocrine tumors still have some of the regulatory systems intact that control normal glands. Many pituitary tumors will therefore respond with stimulation or inhibition to these regulatory factors. Prolactin secretion is regulated by dopamine from the hypothalamus. Prolactin is the only pituitary hormone that is primarily regulated via an inhibition. This means that when dopamine somehow is interfered with, an increase in serum prolactin levels will occur since the inhibition on prolactin secretion via the dopamine receptors of the prolactinoma cells cannot take place. Any type of tumor or other lesion that interfere with dopamine from the hypothalamus might thus cause a hyperprolactinemia.

When inhibition of dopamine is interfered with, the normal pituitary will cause a moderate hyperprolactinemia with values up to 200 µg/L. However, a small prolactinoma might also cause a moderate hyperprolactinemia in this same range, and there is therefore a differential diagnostic problem. Using PET with ^{11}C-L-methionine and ^{11}C-raclopride will solve these problems.

In the prolactinomas, ^{11}C-L-methionine will demonstrate a high metabolic index, and the dopamine receptor study will show high dopamine D_2 binding in the prolactinoma. If dopamine agonist therapy is given, a positive response will be observed as a dramatic

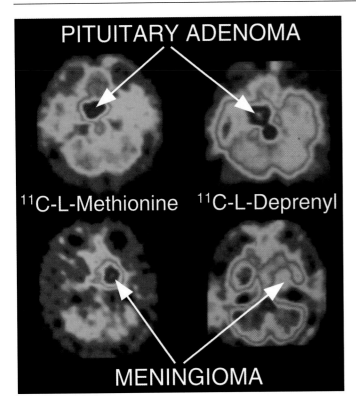

Figure 12-8 PET images of two patients, one with a pituitary adenoma *(above)* and one with a suprasellar meningioma *(below)*. Both tumors have high uptake of ^{11}C-L-methionine *(left)* but only the pituitary adenoma demonstrates high uptake *(upper right)* of ^{11}C-L-deprenyl and can thus be differentiated from the meningioma *(lower right)*.

and rapid decrease in the amino acid metabolism, which provides support for the prolactinoma diagnosis *(10)* (Figure 3).

DIFFERENTIAL DIAGNOSIS NONSECRETING PITUITARY ADENOMAS—SUPRASELLAR MENINGIOMAS

The nonsecreting pituitary adenomas might be difficult to differentiate from suprasellar meningiomas with extension into the sella turcica. For this differential diagnostic procedure, we have found that the MAO-B content in the nonsecreting adenomas differs distinctly from that in the meningiomas. The nonsecreting adenomas will have high levels of MAO in contrast to the very low amounts found in the meningiomas. PET with ^{11}C-L-deprenyl will reveal the amount of MAO-B in the tumor and thus make the differential diagnosis possible *(11)* (Figure 8).

METABOLIC INDEX WITH PET

By combining ^{11}C-L-methionine and ^{18}F-fluorodeoxyglucose, the differential diagnosis between a nonsecreting pituitary adenoma and a chordoma can be achieved. In all the pituitary adenomas, the ratio between the uptake of ^{11}C-L-methionine and ^{18}F-fluorodeoxyglucose is always higher than 1 and is usually above 1.5 in comparison to chordomas, in which the ratio is always below 1 *(1,2,10)*. We have also used PET with ^{11}C-L-methionine to help in the differential diagnose between scull base neuromas and meningiomas as the meningiomas will always have a higher tumor/normal brain ratio than the neuromas *(12)*. PET with ^{18}F-fluorodeoxyglucose has also been used for malignancy grad-

ing and differentiation of intracranial tumors by other groups (for example, *13,14,14a*).

MAO-B CONTENT

Within the group of nonsecreting pituitary adenomas, the MAO-B content will vary with higher levels in some patients than in others. It is not known what these very high levels represent, but it may well be owing to some characteristic properties that would be of interest in developing an understanding of the tumor's behavior.

D_2 BINDING IN A CLINICALLY HORMONALLY INACTIVE PITUITARY ADENOMA

In the clinically hormonally inactive adenomas as a group, PET with ^{11}C-L-raclopride for D_2 receptor binding revealed sparse to no D_2 binding. It is well known that a few of the clinically hormonally inactive adenomas respond partially to dopamine agonist treatment. Our findings with sparse D_2 binding might well fit with this partial response in the patients with the hormonally inactive adenoma. The patients that respond to dopamine agonist therapy were the ones who showed measurable amounts of D_2 binding in their tumors. One of these patients has a macroadenoma. She has rejected both surgical intervention and radiotherapy and has been given dopamine agonist treatment. She feels very well and has therefore twice stopped her medication herself. On these occasions, within 3 mo off the medication, her bitemporal visual field defects have reappeared. When she again started medication, the visual fields normalized.

DIAGNOSIS OF RECURRENT TUMOR TISSUE

As mentioned, PET with ^{11}C-L-methionine will visualize all viable tumor tissue and will also diagnose tumor recurrence at an early stage. PET with ^{11}C-L-methionine is also sensitive in visualizing small volumes of metabolically active tumor masses. A recurrent tumor, especially growing invasive pituitary adenomas extending into the cavernous sinus and into the bony structures like the clivus, may be difficult to visualize with MRI. In these situations, PET with ^{11}C-L-methionine will outline the metabolically active tumor portions.

DISCUSSION

PET enables in vivo characterization of pituitary tumors. Almost any substance can be labeled with a positron-emitting radionuclide by skilled radiochemists, and the field and possibilities for PET studies are vast. Examples of metabolic studies for characterization of the pituitary adenomas and differential diagnosis have been presented. We find PET especially useful in visualizing metabolically active tumor masses and for further differential diagnostic aids. The diagnosis of a pituitary mass with MRI is usually performed with high precision, but the value of PET in determining the precise nature of the mass has been demonstrated. D_2 receptor bindings are also of interest in this differentiation and to predict the outcome of dopamine agonist therapy. However, it is not known if there are differences between the prolactinoma patients that are of importance in the clinical handling, for example, with regard to the more recent dopamine agonist therapies. This might be of interest for further study using PET. Using a combination of metabolic studies with ^{11}C-L-methionine and ^{18}F-fluorodeoxyglucose showed differences that might represent important characteristic features of these tumors. This is also of interest for further study.

There is an increased number of patients, including older patients, who are examined using a CT or MRI of the brain for various reasons and in whom an asymptomatic pituitary tumor is diagnosed, but does not necessarily require treatment. These patients are also important to study in vivo for evaluation of the metabolic activity and proliferation markers that have just begun to be used. If possible, markers for apoptosis, the normal cell death mechanism, would also add to the evaluation of these tumors. Of course, the same is true for initiation of new treatment in all adenomas, such as the very fascinating angiostatic treatment of tumors that is now beginning. It might even be possible to find a marker for angiogenic activity in the tumors.

The PET technique demands highly specialized facilities and experienced staff and is thus expensive, but is also very valuable when used correctly both for clinical practice and for advanced research. PET is certainly one of the most fascinating techniques available today.

ACKNOWLEDGMENTS

The PET examinations have been performed in the PET Center, at the University Hospital, Uppsala, Sweden, in collaboration with Bengt Långström and his team and their great contribution is hereby acknowledged. This work was supported by grants from the Swedish Medical Research Council, the Swedish Cancer Society, and Söderbergs Foundation.

REFERENCES

1. Muhr C, Bergström M. Positron emission tomography applied in the study of pituitary adenomas. J Endocrinol Invest 1991;14:509–528.
2. Muhr C. Positron emission tomography (PET) in pituitary adenomas. In: Landolt AM, Reilly PL, Vance ML, eds. Pituitary Adenomas. Churchill Livingstone, Medical Division of Longman Group UK Ltd, 1996, pp. 229–238.
3. Muhr C, Bergström M, Lundberg P-O, Bergström K, Hartvig P, Lundqvist H, et al. Dopamine receptors in pituitary adenomas: PET visualization with C-11-N-methylspiperone. J Comput Assist Tomogr 1986;10:175–180.
4. Muhr C, Bergström M, Lundberg PO, Bergström K, Långström B. In vivo measurement of dopamine receptors in pituitary adenomas using positron emission tomography. Acta Radiol. Proceedings: Symposium Neuroradiologicum 1986.
5. Muhr C, Bergström M, Lundberg P O, Hartman M, Bergström K, Pelletieri L, et al. Malignant prolactinoma with multiple intracranial metastases studied with positron emission tomography. Neurosurgery 1988;22:374–379.
6. Benker G, Gieshoff B, Freundlieb O, Windeck R, Schulte H M, Lancranjan I, et al. Parenteral bromocriptine in the treatment of hormonally active pituitary tumors. Clin Endocrinol 1986;24:505–513.
7. Lundin P, Bergström K, Nyman R, Lundberg PO, Muhr C. Macroprolactinomas: Serial MR imaging in long-term bromocriptine therapy. AJNR 1992;13:1279–1291.
8. Raymond JP, Goldstein E, Konopka P, Leleu MF, Merceron RE, Loria Y. Follow up of children born of bromocriptine-treated mothers. Hormone Res 1985;22:239–246.
9. Bergström M, Muhr C, Lundberg PO, Bergström K, Lundqvist H Antoni G, et al. In vivo study of amino acid distribution and metabolism in pituitary adenomas using positron emission tomography with ^{11}C-D-methionine and ^{11}C-L-methionine. J Comput Assist Tomogr 1987;11:384–389.
9a. Bergström M, Muhr C, Lundberg P O, Bergström K, Gee A D, Fasth K-G, et al. Rapid decrease in amino acid metabolism in prolactin-secreting pituitary adenomas after bromocriptine treatment—a PET study. J Comput Assist Tomogr 1987;11:815–819.
10. Muhr C. PET in endocrinology. In: Higgins CB, Auffermann W, eds. Endocrine Imaging. Thieme Medical Publishers, New York, 1994, pp. 344–352.
11. Bergström M, Muhr C, Lundberg PO, Jossan S, Gati I, Lilja A, et al. Differentiation of pituitary adenoma an meningioma: visualization with positron emission tomography and 11C-deprenyl. Neurosurgery 1992;30:855–861.
12. Nyberg G, Bergström M, Enblad P, Lilja A, Muhr C, Långström B. PET-Methionine of Skull Base Neuromas and Meningiomas. Acta Otolaryngol 1997;117:482–489.
13. Di Chiro G, Oldfield E, Wright DC, de Michele D, Katz DA, Patronas NJ, et al. Cerebral necrosis after radiotherapy and/or intraarterial chemotherapy for brain tumors: PET and neuropathologic studies. Am J Roentgenol 1988;150:189–197.
14. Delbecke D, Meyerowitz C, Lapidus RL, Maciunas RJ, Jennings MT, Moots PL, et al. Optimal cutoff levels of F-18 fluorodeoxyglucose uptake in the differentiation of low-grade from high-grade brain tumours with PET. Radiology 1995;195:47–52.
14a. Di Chiro G, Hatazawa J, Katz DA, Rizzoli HV, de Michele D. Glucose utilization by intracranial meningiomas as an index of tumor aggressivity and probability of recurrence: a PET study. Radiology 1987;164:521–526.

13   Pituitary Surgery

Kamal Thapar, md, phd, and Edward R. Laws, Jr.

INTRODUCTION

Despite ongoing advances in the pharmacologic management of pituitary tumors, surgery remains the therapy of choice for a large majority of pituitary tumors. Even though surgical efficacy is now being judged by more rigorous technical standards and by more stringent endocrine criteria than ever before, such scrutiny has only served to reinforce the fundamental role of surgery in the management of pituitary adenomas and other lesions of the sellar region. In this chapter, the surgical management of pituitary tumors is reviewed. Emphasis is placed on indications for surgery, the selection of operative approach, details of operative technique, avoidance and management of surgical complications, and the results of surgery for pituitary adenomas.

PITUITARY SURGERY: HISTORICAL CONSIDERATIONS

Most accounts of the history of pituitary surgery begin with an operation performed more than a century ago (1892), when a general surgeon, F. T. Paul (1851–1941), undertook the surgical management of an acromegalic patient *(1)*. The patient, a 34-yr-old woman, suffered from headache, facial pain, and visual loss. At the suggestion of Sir Victor Horsely, Paul performed a subtemporal decompression, however, the tumor itself proved inaccessible. The patient's symptoms, presumably those of elevated intracranial pressure, were alleviated. The patient died about 3 mo later, and the autopsy revealed a tangerine-sized pituitary tumor. The histologic diagnosis was that of a "round cell sarcoma," the prevailing nosology (Virchow's) for pituitary adenomas at the time. Horsely subsequently used both the temporal and subfrontal approaches to treat 10 patients with pituitary tumors, reporting his series in 1906 *(2)*.

The next major advance, both technical and conceptual, arose from Vienna, where a number of surgeons devised and successfully applied extracranial approaches to the sella. Schloffer (1868–1937) was the first, employing an extensive lateral rhinotomy-type incision with resection of the septum and turbinates en route to the sella *(3)*. A variation of this approach was advocated by von Eisenberg (1860–1939) *(4)*, only to be further modified by von Hochenegg (1859–1940) who accessed the sella through the frontal sinus *(5)*. Shortly thereafter (1909), Cushing (1869–1939) used a variation of Schloffer's method in an acromegalic patient, later refining the technique and adopting the sublabial incision that was soon to be described by Halstead (1869–1926) and Kanavel (1874–

1938) *(6–8)*. Contemporaneously, major contributions to the evolution of the transsphenoidal approach were provided by Oscar Hirsch, who described the endonasal approach in 1910 and, later, the submucosal, transseptal transsphenoidal approach *(9)*.

As cranial neurosurgery continued to evolve, so too did transcranial approaches to pituitary tumors. Indeed, the second decade of this century brought with it an escalating enthusiasm for transcranial approaches, so much so that transsphenoidal approaches were all but abandoned, particularly in North America. Technical contributions by Heuer (1882–1950), Frazier (1870–1936), Krause (1857–1937), Cushing, and others led to adoption of transcranial approaches to the pituitary as routine, eclipsing, almost to the point of extinction, the transsphenoidal approach. Fortunately, transsphenoidal methods were sustained by a few. Most notable among these was Norman Dott (1897–1973) of Edinburgh, who continued to practice, refine, and teach transsphenoidal techniques. One of his students, Gerard Guiot (1912–1996), popularized the procedure in France, becoming one of its major advocates *(10)*. In turn, Guiot passed on transsphenoidal methodologies to Jules Hardy of Montreal, who reintroduced this approach to the neurosurgical mainstream in North America *(11)*. In doing so, Hardy merged the procedure with the operating microscope, illuminating, for the first time, microsurgical aspects of the technique, the concept of microadenomas, and the feasibility of selective tumor removal, while preserving normal pituitary tissue and function. Together, Guiot and Hardy popularized their work in the 1960s, establishing those technical and conceptual aspects of the procedure that form the basis of transsphenoidal microsurgery as it is practiced today. Transsphenoidal microsurgery now represents the preferred approach for more that 95% of pituitary tumors, and for a large proportion of other sellar pathologies as well.

PITUITARY TUMORS: GENERAL CONSIDERATIONS

CLINICAL PRESENTATION   The clinical presentation of pituitary adenomas usually centers on one or more of three clinical scenarios *(12,13)*. The first involves pituitary hyperfunction in the form of several characteristic hypersecretory states. Hypersecretion of prolactin (PRL), growth hormone (GH), adrenocorticotropic hormone (ACTH), and rarely thyroid-stimulating hormone (TSH), will produce their corresponding clinical phenotypes: amenorrhea-galactorrhea syndrome, acromegaly or gigantism, Cushing's disease, and secondary hyperthyroidism, respectively. Because as many as 70% of pituitary adenomas are endocrinologically active, the presence of a hypersecretory endocrine state is the most common mode of presentation.

From: *Diagnosis and Management of Pituitary Tumors* (K. Thapar, K. Kovacs, B. W. Scheithauer, and R. V. Lloyd, eds.), ©Humana Press Inc., Totowa, NJ.

The second mode of presentation involves pituitary insufficiency, and is typically associated with larger tumors, which compress either the nontumorous pituitary gland or its stalk, or, as in the case of giant pituitary adenomas, compress hypophysiotrophic areas of the hypothalamus (HT). In general, the pituitary gland displays remarkable functional resilience to even extreme degrees of chronic compression and distortion. Eventually, however, anterior pituitary failure will supervene. In the face of such compression, the various secretory elements differ in their functional reserve. Gonadotrophs, being the most vulnerable, are affected first. Thereafter, thyrotroph, somatotroph, and eventually corticotroph function is sequentially compromised. Curiously, regardless of how large the tumor is or how extreme the glandular or stalk compression may be, posterior pituitary failure (i.e., diabetes insipidus [DI]) is very rarely a presenting feature of pituitary adenomas; its preoperative presence virtually excludes a diagnosis of pituitary adenoma. As described, hypopituitarism that accompanies pituitary adenomas is usually a chronic process, however, in the setting of pituitary apoplexy, it can be an acute, unexpected, and immediately life-threatening event.

A third pattern of presentation is based on mass effects, with or without co-existing endocrinopathy. Given its location at the skull base and its proximity to various anatomic structures, a growing adenoma will produce a predictable array of neurologic signs and symptoms. Headache is commonly an early symptom, one that has been attributed to stretching of the overlying diaphragma sellae; its presence or severity of headache does not necessarily correlate with tumor size. The most common objective feature of these tumors is visual loss, a consequence of suprasellar growth and compression of the anterior visual pathways. An asymmetric bitemporal hemianopsia is the classically observed deficit, although other patterns of visual dysfunction can and commonly do occur. With continued suprasellar growth, pituitary tumors can encroach on the HT, causing alterations of sleep, alertness, eating, behavior, and emotion. Transgression of the lamina terminalis can bring these tumors into the region of the third ventricle, wherein foraminal obstruction may produce hydrocephalus. Lateral growth, with penetration of the cavernous sinus, is not uncommon among pituitary adenomas. As the interstices of the sinus are progressively invaded, the carotid artery and cranial nerves transiting therein may become ensheathed by tumor tissue. Onset of ptosis, facial pain, or diplopia indicate such cranial nerve involvement. With lateral intracranial growth, compression and/or irritation of the mesial temporal lobe can result in seizures of a partial complex type. Finally, some pituitary tumors can assume truly gigantic proportions, so that involvement of the anterior, middle, and posterior cranial fossae produces the full spectrum of neurologic signs and symptoms.

An additional, but diagnostically important, mass-related feature, common to any pituitary or non-pituitary sellar mass, is moderate hyperprolactinemia (<150 ng/mL). This phenomenon, frequently referred to as the stalk section effect, is the result of compressive or destructive lesions involving the pituitary stalk or HT. In health, PRL secretion is under tonic HT inhibitory control, as mediated by various prolactin inhibitory factors. Dopamine, the most important of these inhibitory factors, is released by the HT, and descends via the portal circulation to the anterior pituitary where it suppresses PRL release by pituitary lactotrophs. Processes that impair dopamine's HT release (compressive or destructive lesions involving the HT), or with its adenohypophyseal transfer (compressive or destructive lesions of the stalk), place pituitary lactotrophs in a disinhibited state. The result is moderate elevation in the serum PRL level. The importance of the phenomenon lies primarily in its recognition. Because virtually any structural, infiltrative, neoplastic, or inflammatory process involving the sella can produce this effect, the mere presence of a moderately elevated PRL level, in association with a sellar mass, should not immediately prompt a diagnosis of prolactinoma. Generally, PRL levels in excess of 150 ng/mL are the result of PRL-producing tumor. Below this level, the lesion may still be a small prolactinoma, however, any of a variety of other sellar pathologies could also be culpable.

Finally, pituitary tumors may occasionally be discovered incidentally, typically in a patient suffering from headache or other nonspecific symptoms, in whom routine brain imaging reveals a abnormality in the size, shape, or contents of the sella. The situation is especially common today, because of the superior resolution of magnetic resonance imaging (MRI). When carefully sought, subtle signal changes in the pituitary gland can be identified in approx 10–12% or more of routine MRI scans; thus, the mere presence of an incidental abnormality on MRI does not necessary imply the presence of an adenoma nor an immediate need for intervention (14,15). Instead, careful clinical and endocrinologic correlation are required for such "incidentalomas."

RADIOLOGIC CLASSIFICATION OF PITUITARY TUMORS   From a surgical standpoint, pituitary tumors can be classified on the basis of their size and growth characteristics, as determined by imaging studies. The most enduring classification was that devised by Hardy about 25 yr ago (11). This five-tiered radiologic classification first distinguishes tumors as microadenomas or macroadenomas (Figure 1). The former are less than 1 cm in diameter and the latter are greater than 1 cm in diameter. Microadenomas are designated as grade 0 or grade I tumors, depending on whether the sellar appearance is normal or whether minor sellar changes are present, respectively. Macroadenomas, causing diffuse enlargement, focal destruction, and extensive destruction of sella, are referred to as grade II, grade III, and grade IV tumors, respectively. Macroadenomas are further subclassified on the degree and direction of extrasellar extension (Figure 1).

DIAGNOSIS AND THERAPY OF PITUITARY ADENOMAS: GENERAL PRINCIPLES

It is important to recognize that pituitary tumors represent a clinical problem that stands at the interface of several medical and surgical disciplines. Calling upon the expertise of individuals from the fields of endocrinology, neurosurgery, neuroradiology, otolaryngology, ophthalmology, pathology, and radiation therapy, the optimal and comprehensive management of pituitary tumors often relies on a truly interdisciplinary effort.

In patients in whom a pituitary adenoma is suspected, a coordinated two-step diagnostic approach is required. The first step involves establishing an endocrine diagnosis and the second relates to securing an anatomic diagnosis.

STEP 1: ESTABLISH ENDOCRINE DIAGNOSIS   Ordinarily, the history and physical examination will provide some indication as to the endocrine status of the patient. Suspicions of hormone excess and/or deficiency must then be validated by careful endocrine testing. An endocrine diagnosis is reached by measuring pituitary and target gland hormones in both basal and dynamic states. These measurements are very sensitive indicators of dis-

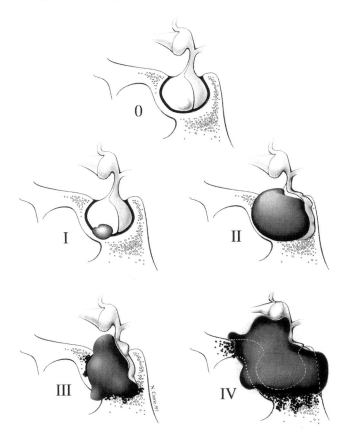

Figure 13-1 Hardy classification of pituitary tumors. Grade 0: Intra-pituitary microadenoma; normal sellar appearance. Grade I: Intra-pituitary microadenoma; focal bulging of sellar wall. Grade II: Intrasellar macroadenoma; diffusely enlarged sella; no invasion. Grade III: Macroadenoma; localized sellar invasion and/or destruction. Grade IV: Macroadenoma; extensive sellar invasion and/or destruction.

turbed pathophysiologic activity, and will generally indicate whether or not a pituitary tumor is present, and, if so, its secretory type. As an initial endocrine screen, basal measurements of PRL, GH, ACTH, luteinizing hormone, follicle-stimulating hormone, thyroid-stimulating hormone, α-subunit, thyroxine, cortisol, insulin-like growth factor-I (IGF-I), testosterone, and estrogen should be obtained. By identifying states of relative excess or deficiency, this survey will provide a preliminary estimate of the integrity of various pituitary–target gland axes. Thereafter, additional provocative, dynamic, and special hormonal assays are performed to define precisely a specific endocrinopathy.

STEP 2: ESTABLISH ANATOMIC DIAGNOSIS Once an endocrine diagnosis has been established, an anatomic diagnosis must be obtained. Formerly based on skull radiographs, and later by computed tomography scanning, the anatomic diagnosis is now provided by high-resolution, gadolinium-enhanced MRI. This technique will allow the identification of up to 70% of microadenomas, including those as small as 3 mm. For macroadenomas, high diagnostic sensitivity is less of an issue, and the merits of MRI lie in its capacity to identify important relationships between the tumor and surrounding neurovascular structures. The position of the carotid arteries, the status of the optic chiasm, and the extent of supra- and parasellar extension are of particular operative concern, and each is fully delineated by MRI.

In certain circumstances, such as those involving Cushing's disease and acromegaly, extracranial imaging may also be required, to secure the correct anatomic diagnosis. In such situations, exclusion of an ectopic hormone-secreting tumor in the chest, abdomen, or retroperitoneum may be necessary to confirm a pituitary-dependent source of hormonal excess.

TREATMENT Once a diagnosis of pituitary adenoma has been established on the basis of clinical examination, endocrinologic testing, and imaging studies, optimal therapy begins with a clear assessment of the treatment objectives. In general, therapy for pituitary tumors should be directed at the following goals:

1. Reversal of endocrinopathy and restoration of normal pituitary function.
2. Elimination of mass effect and restoration of normal neurologic function.
3. Eliminate or minimize the possibility of tumor recurrence.
4. Obtain a definitive histological diagnosis.

Given the current era of pituitary tumor management, absolute realization of these goals has become increasingly feasible for a growing proportion of pituitary tumor patients. For some of the more difficult tumors, such as certain large and locally invasive endocrine-active tumors, only partial realization of these goals will be possible. In such cases, disease control will supersede cure as the most reasonable therapeutic expectation.

Therapeutic options for pituitary tumors include surgical resection, receptor-mediated pharmacotherapy, and radiation therapy (conventional and stereotactic). Although each is effective to various degrees in various situations, the merits and limitations of these modalities must be carefully considered, thoughtfully individualized, and a comprehensive plan of management provided to each patient. Surgical considerations are discussed here; the use of other therapies, in the context of individual tumor types, is discussed in this chapter.

SURGERY FOR PITUITARY ADENOMAS

INDICATIONS FOR SURGERY

1. Perhaps the most urgent indication for surgical intervention relates to instances of pituitary apoplexy *(16–18)*. Patients may present with either hemorrhage into an existing pituitary tumor or with acute necrosis of the tumor with subsequent swelling (Figure 2). In either case, the presentation includes sudden headache, precipitous visual loss, altered level of consciousness, and collapse from acute adrenal insufficiency. An often dramatic event, pituitary apoplexy may lead to serious neurological deficits and even death, without timely intervention. In such situations, urgent glucocorticoid replacement and surgical decompression constitute the most reliable and effective form of therapy.

2. A second clear surgical indication is progressive mass effect (usually visual loss) from a large macroadenoma. These patients should always have a serum PRL determination, because prompt and dramatic shrinkage of prolactinomas can occur with appropriate pharmacologic management. More often, the PRL level is only modestly elevated, and the patient has a clinically nonfunctioning pituitary tumor or other sellar mass. Such patients will be in need of surgical decompression.

3. Among the hyperfunctioning pituitary adenomas, surgery is the treatment of choice for Cushing's disease, acrome-

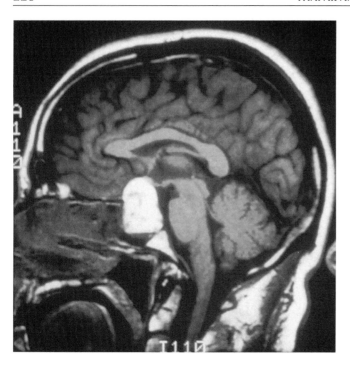

Figure 13-2 Pituitary apoplexy. Sagittal MRI shown intratumoral hemorrhage and mass effect.

galy, and secondary hyperthyroidism. In the case of Cushing's disease, medical management is invariably suboptimal, and surgery provides the best means of obtaining prompt and lasting remission. In the case of somatotroph and thyrotroph adenomas, some latitude exists for the use of somatostatin analogs as the initial intervention, however, surgery remains the preferred, primary, and definitive treatment for these condition. For most prolactinomas, medical therapy will be the preferred option. There are, however, several important surgical indications for prolactinomas; these are discussed in the subheading Results of Surgery.

4. Failure of prior therapy often represents an indication for surgical intervention and usually occurs in one of several situations. Some patients treated with radiotherapy (RT) have a favorable initial response, followed by recurrence of symptoms, either in the form of mass effect or recurrent hormonal hypersecretion. Others will have been treated with pharmacologic therapy, however, the response may have been suboptimal. For example, in some patients with a presumed prolactinoma, medical therapy can normalize PRL levels, but progressive tumor growth continues. At surgery, these patients usually have lesions other than prolactinoma. In other patients with genuine prolactinomas and very high PRL levels, a suboptimal response to medical therapy may take the form of persistently elevated PRL levels. Surgery may reduce tumor burden and lead to a more effective pharmacologic response. The same also applies to acromegalic patients treated with somatostatin analogs.

5. A final and somewhat generic surgical indication relates to need for a tissue diagnosis. Although seldom required in the case of functioning pituitary adenomas, this indication

may be exercised when confronted with a nonfunctioning sellar mass whose pathologic identity cannot be confirmed without histologic examination *(19)*.

SURGICAL CONTRAINDICATIONS Contraindications for surgery are few. The most important relate to the general medical condition of the patient, which, in the face of florid Cushing's disease, acromegaly, or secondary hyperthyroidism, can pose a significant anesthetic risk. In most cases, however, the medical condition of the patient can be stabilized without undue delay. Similarly, profound hypopituitarism can also be a temporary contraindication to surgery, although it will be fully responsive to steroid and thyroid replacement. Active sinus infection may also contraindicate the transsphenoidal approach, although this is generally responsive to appropriate antibiotic therapy. Very rarely, the MRI may reveal ectatic and tortuous carotid arteries that protrude from the region of the cavernous sinus and obstruct transsphenoidal access. If significant, such a situation can also contraindicate this approach.

PREOPERATIVE EVALUATION Once an anatomic diagnosis and an endocrine diagnosis have established the patient as a surgical candidate, a comprehensive preoperative evaluation is undertaken. Attention is first turned to optimizing the medical condition of the patient. The general medical examination should address issues such as hypertension, cardiac disease, diabetes, thyroid status, and pituitary endocrine function, because such perturbations commonly occur in pituitary tumor patients, and most are, to a significant degree, responsive to pharmacologic management. In all patients with an adenoma, some consideration should be given to the possibility of multiple endocrine neoplasia type 1. Soliciting the family history and measuring serum calcium levels is important in this regard.

Because visual dysfunction frequently complicates the course of many pituitary tumors, a complete ophthalmologic evaluation is mandatory in all patients with visual complaints, and for those whose tumors exhibit suprasellar extension. In addition to the asymmetrical bitemporal hemianopic defect classically associated with pituitary tumors, other forms of visual dysfunction also occur. Depending on the anatomic status of the chiasm (prefixed, normal, or postfixed), the size of the tumor, its precise direction of tumor growth, and the chronicity of the process, junctional scotomas, various monocular field defects, impaired acuity, afferent pupillary defects, papilledema, and optic atrophy may all be observed. Assessment of visual fields and acuity on a serial basis are often necessary to document disease progression and response to therapeutic intervention.

In some instances of microadenoma, particularly those involving Cushing's disease, MRI of the sella may fail to reveal a definite adenoma. Still, a confirmatory endocrine diagnosis of Cushing's disease ensures a high level of confidence that a corticotroph adenoma is indeed present, and that it can be identified and selectively removed via the transsphenoidal approach. When sellar exploration is undertaken under such circumstances, it is important for the surgeon to have some appreciation of pituitary gland cytoarchitecture and the topological organization of the anterior pituitary gland. As shown in Figure 3, each of the various secretory types of pituitary adenomas have a preferential site of origin, reflecting the density and distribution of normal hormone-secreting cells of the pituitary. A general awareness of this arrangement can be helpful when one is dissecting through a seemingly normal gland in search for a presumed microadenoma.

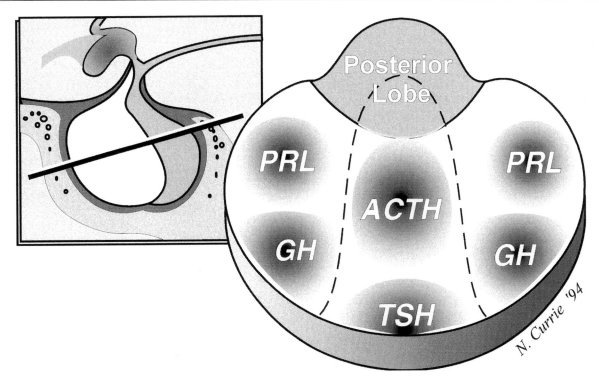

Figure 13-3 Topological organization of the anterior pituitary gland. The distribution of the various secretory cells in the pituitary is not random: Different hormone-secreting cells preferentially accumulate at different intraglandular sites. When viewed in horizontal cross-section, the gland is comprised of a central mucoid wedge and two lateral wings. Occupying the anterior and posterior portions of the central wedge are thyrotrophs and corticotrophs, respectively. Within the lateral wings, somatotrophs are situated anteriorly; lactotrophs have a more posterior location. These locations also correspond to the intraglandular sites of origin for the respective types of pituitary adenomas. Gonadotrophs are diffusely distributed throughout the gland, thus gonadotroph adenomas have no preferential site of origin.

Table 1
Surgical Approaches for Pituitary Tumors

Standard Transsphenoidal Approaches
    Endonasal, submucosal, transseptal transsphenoidal approach
    Endonasal, submucosal, septal pushover approach
    Sublabial transseptal transsphenoidal approach
    Endoscopic transsphenoidal approach

Standard Transcranial Approaches
    Pterional craniotomy
    Subfrontal craniotomy
    Subtemporal craniotomy

Alternative Skull Base Approaches
    Cranio-orbito-zygomatic osteotomy approach
    Transbasal approach of Derome
    Extended transsphenoidal approach
    Lateral rhinotomy/paranasal approaches
    Sublabial transseptal approach with nasomaxillary osteotomy
    Transethmoidal and extended transethmoidal approaches
    Sublabial transantral approach

CHOICE OF SURGICAL APPROACH Surgical approaches to the sellar region can be broadly categorized into three basic groups: transsphenoidal approaches, conventional craniotomy, and alternative skull base approaches (Table 1). For historical completeness, one might also include stereotactic approaches as a fourth category; however, this is now so seldom, if ever, indicated that it is not discussed further. Within each of the three groups, there is one or more standard procedure, as well as a menu of technical variations and options that allow the operation to be precisely tailored to the situation at hand. Currently, some 96% of all pituitary adenomas can be approached through a transsphenoidal approach. The remainder will require transcranial approaches, consisting of either standard pterional or subfrontal craniotomy or various skull base approaches, which may be transcranial, extracranial, or a combination of the two.

The choice of surgical approach will depend on a number of factors. The most important of these include the size of the sella, its degree of mineralization, the size and pneumatization of the sphenoid sinus, the position and tortuosity of the carotid arteries, the presence and direction of any intracranial tumor extensions, whether or not any uncertainty exists as to the pathology of the lesion; and whether or not any prior therapy has been administered (surgery, pharmacologic, or radiotherapeutic). As a rule, a transsphenoidal approach is preferred in all but the following circumstances: a tumor with significant anterior extension into the anterior cranial fossa or lateral and/or posterior extension into the middle or posterior cranial fossae; a tumor with suprasellar extension and an hour-glass configuration that is constrained by a small diaphragmatic aperture; when there is reason to believe that the consistency of a tumor having suprasellar extension is sufficiently fibrous, so as to prevent its collapse and descent into the sella when resected from below; and if there is some doubt as to the actual nature of the pathology (i.e., meningioma). If any of these features are present, a transcranial procedure would be required.

There will be the occasional circumstance when the configuration of the tumor will be such that a single approach, either transsphenoidal or transcranial, will be insufficient to effect com-

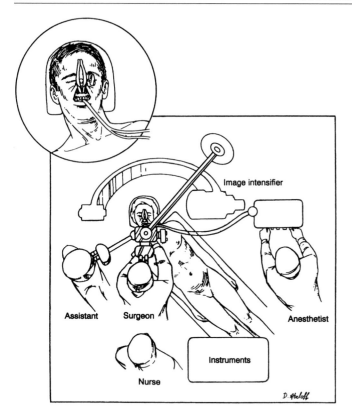

Figure 13-4 Operating room setup for transsphenoidal surgery.

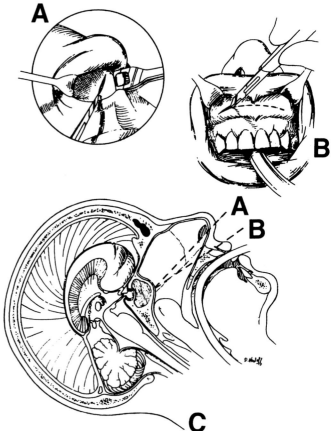

Figure 13-5 Endonasal (**A**) and sublabial (**B**) incisions, and the direction of approach (**C**) afforded by each.

plete tumor removal. The situation is uncommon, and is typically associated with dumbbell-shaped tumors having a significant intrasellar component that has grown up through, and has been narrowed by, the diaphragmatic aperture. The suprasellar component in such cases may be inaccessible from below; the infrasellar component may not be safely and readily accessible from above. Similarly, such bicompartimentalization occurs when an intrasellar component is associated with anterior, lateral, and retrosellar intracranial extensions into the anterior, middle, and posterior cranial fossae. In such situations, a combined transsphenoidal–transcranial approach can be used. Barrow et al. *(20)* describe the simultaneous performance of both approaches by two surgical teams. Alternatively, the two may be performed in a staged fashion. In considering such combined approaches, it is important to be certain that the risks of aggressive surgery are justified by the benefits of radical tumor removal. In some instances, particularly those involving elderly patients with large, slow-growing, nonfunctioning tumors, a less radical and safer subtotal decompression may be preferable. Still, in carefully selected patients, the combined approach can represent an effective alternative.

TRANSSPHENOIDAL APPROACHES

For the overwhelming majority of pituitary tumors, one or another variation of the transsphenoidal approach will represent the most appropriate route *(21,22)*. Ordinarily, this will imply a standard microsurgical, submucosal, transseptal transsphenoidal procedure. The virtues of the transsphenoidal approach are many, but most important, it represents the most physiologic and minimally traumatic corridor of surgical access to the sella, providing direct and superior visualization of the pituitary gland and adjacent pathology.

POSITIONING The patient is placed in a semirecumbent position, the head being supported with a horseshoe headrest (Figure 4). Because the head is not fixed, gentle lateral movements of the head can be used to optimize intraoperative visualization, especially of the cavernous sinus area. The patient is positioned so that the left ear points toward the left shoulder, allowing the surgeon a more comfortable midline approach to the nose and head. If significant suprasellar extension is present, a malleable needle or catheter may be placed into the lumbar subarachnoid space, into which an infusion of air may be used to facilitate descent of the tumor's superior extent into the sella. Once the endotracheal tube is in place, the oropharynx is carefully packed with cotton gauze, to prevent the accumulation of blood into the throat and eventually into the stomach. Details of anesthetic management have been described *(23)*.

At this point, some consideration should be given to the eventual issue of sellar reconstruction and the potential need for fat, fascia lata, and rarely, bone grafts. Depending on the anticipated need, these tissue grafts will either be obtained at this point, or the donor sites will be included in the sterile field, should the need arise. The videofluoroscopic apparatus is then brought into position.

Because pituitary reserve for the pituitary–adrenal axis may be impaired, it remains customary to administer a regimen of stress-dose exogenous corticosteroids, both during surgery and in the immediate postoperative (p/o) period. Antibiotic prophylaxis is usually employed.

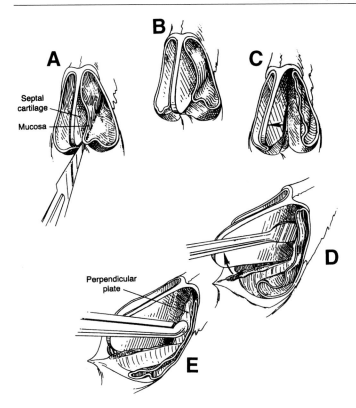

Septal cartilage

Mucosa

Perpendicular plate

Figure 13-6 The nasal tunnels are connected (**A**) and elevated (**B**). Displacement of the nasal septum to the right (**C**) and disarticulation from the maxillary ridge (**D**). Removal of the perpendicular plate of the ethmoid (**E**).

SPHENOID SINUS ACCESS AND EXPOSURE The next major consideration in the transsphenoidal procedure will be the precise route of entry into the sphenoid sinus. The two basic options are the endonasal approach or the sublabial approach (Figure 5). Selection of one over the other depends on the size of the nostril, the size of the lesion, and the preference of the surgeon. The authors favor the basic endonasal approach in most instances, reserving the sublabial incision for larger and more difficult lesions, when a broader corridor of surgical access is required. Endoscopic methods of access are also being more often employed.

Endonasal Approaches After the skin of the face is prepared with an aqueous antiseptic solution, the nostrils are packed with pledgets of cotton gauze soaked in 5% cocaine, and inserted with a nasal speculum and bayonet forceps. The pledgets are allowed to remain in contact with the nasal mucosa for 5–10 min, while draping of the patient is completed. A solution of 0.5% xylocaine in 1:200,000 epinephrine is injected submucosally. Using a 25-gage needle, 10–20 mL of the solution is infiltrated, first along the upper gingiva, then along the inferior portion of the nasal septum, and finally along the lateral aspects of the nasal septum. A conscious effort is made to dissect the nasal mucosa away from the cartilaginous septum with the injection solution. This step is performed under direct vision with the aid of a nasal speculum, headlight, and loupes.

The authors have adopted the initial approach of the rhinologist, i.e., a right-sided hemitransfixion in the nostril, because this method greatly simplifies the dissection of the left anterior nasal mucosal tunnel away from the septum (Figures 5A and 6). The incision is made along the inferior border of the nasal septum. The columella is retracted laterally to the patient's left. The inferior

border of the cartilaginous septum is exposed with sharp dissection, and the left side of the septum is exposed submucosally with a combination of sharp and blunt dissection, thereby creating the left anterior tunnel. The premaxillary region is then undermined by blunt dissection with small scissors. The dissection continues posteriorly, elevating the nasal mucosa away from the cartilaginous septum, back to the junction of the cartilaginous and bony septi. A vertical incision is then made at this junction point, and bilateral posterior submucosal tunnels are created on either side of the perpendicular plate of the ethmoid. The articulation of the cartilaginous septum with the maxilla is then dissected free, and an attempt is made to raise the inferior mucosal tunnel on the opposite side, so that the cartilaginous septum can be displaced laterally without creating inferior mucosal tears. A self-retaining nasal speculum can then be introduced to straddle the perpendicular plate of the ethmoid, exposing the face of the sphenoid sinus. Sometimes, the nostril may be too small to accommodate a standard speculum. In such instances, an inferior extension of the hemitransfixion incision within the alar ring is often adequate for exposure. If the nose is small or if more generous exposure is needed, an alar incision, along the right inferior ala, is usually sufficient to accommodate a standard speculum. At closure, the alarotomy must be closed with the usual plastic technique.

In some patients, particularly children and those who have had previous nasal, septal, or transsphenoidal surgery, the authors have used an alternative endonasal approach called the endonasal septal pushover technique *(24)*. Instead of a submucosal incision for creation of an anterior nasal tunnel, the nostril is entered, and an incision is made through the lateral mucous membrane of the nasal septum at the base of the septal insertion onto the maxillary ridge. The incision is carried back to the junction of the cartilaginous and bony septi, or back to the face of the sphenoid, if this bone has previously been removed. The nasal septum is carefully disarticulated, an opposite-sided inferior tunnel is developed, and the septum, together with the two layers of attached mucous membrane, is reflected laterally, to expose the perpendicular plate of the ethmoid and the sphenoid face. This rapid method may lack the elegance of the standard submucosal approach, but can be very effective when the conventional approach proves difficult. If necessary, it may also be converted to a sublabial approach.

Endoscopic Approach Although the transsphenoidal approach has always been considered minimally invasive, particularly when compared to conventional transcranial approaches, the concept has been redefined in the context of endoscopic approaches to the sella *(25)*. These approaches utilize straight and angled endoscopes as either the sole visualization tool or as a supplement to the operating microscope (hybrid approach). The approach is usually performed through an entirely endonasal route in a fashion identical to that described above. Proponents of the technique emphasize its superior and panoramic intrasellar visualization, its less-traumatic nature, the avoidance of p/o nasal packs, and the need for shorter hospital stays. Although preliminary results are encouraging, additional experience and follow-up will be required to determine if the efficacy of this approach is comparable to standard microsurgical transsphenoidal approaches.

Sublabial Approach Under loupe magnification, the upper lip is retracted, and an incision is made in the buccogingival junction from one canine tooth to the other (Figure 7). Subperiosteal dissection is used to carefully elevate the mucosa from the maxillary ridge and the anterior nasal spine, until the inferior border of

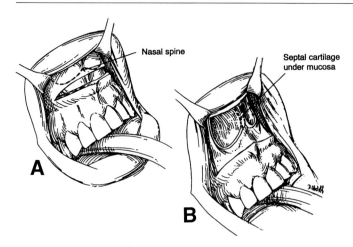

Figure 13-7 The sublabial approach. Relationships of the initial incision (**A**) and exposure of the pyriform aperture and the cartilaginous septum (**B**).

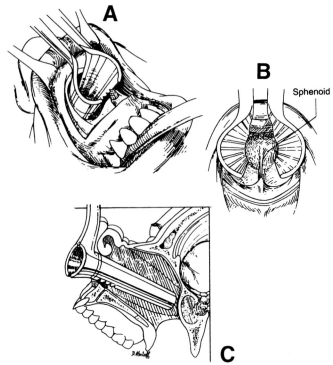

Figure 13-8 Insertion of the transsphenoidal speculum (**A**); surgeon's view of the sphenoid (**B**); and operative approach (**C**).

the pyriform aperture is exposed (Figure 7B). Using curved dissectors and working from the lateral border medially, the two inferior nasal tunnels are created by dissecting the mucosa away from the superior surface of the hard palate. With sharp dissection, the left anterior tunnel and the left inferior tunnels are connected, and the entire left side of the nasal septum is exposed, back to the perpendicular plate of the ethmoid. Using firm, blunt dissection along the left side of the base of the nasal septum, the cartilaginous portion of the nasal septum is dislocated and reflected to the right, and a right posterior mucosal tunnel is developed along the right side of the bony septum (Figure 6). At this point, it should be possible to insert the transsphenoidal retractor (Figure 8). It should be spread gently, and care should be taken to place all mucosal tears in the nasal mucosa lateral to the retractor blades. As the retractor is opened, the turbinates will fracture; it is unwise to apply a great deal of force in opening the retractor. Once the retractor is in place, the vomer, with its distinctive keel shape, should be visualized.

SPHENOIDOTOMY AND SELLAR ENTRY Having reached the anterior face of the sphenoid sinus by one of the above routes, videofluoroscopy or neuronavigational image guidance is used to make any necessary adjustments to the final position and trajectory of the retractor blades. Midline orientation is crucial at this stage; computed tomography images of the sphenoidal region are helpful in delineating the bony anatomy and in planning sphenoidal entry. Portions of the bony nasal septum present in the operative field should be resected with a Lillie-Koeffler tool or a Ferris-Smith punch. Any cartilage and bone that has been resected should be preserved, so that it can be used during closure. For experienced surgeons, the nasal spine anteriorly does not represent a major obstacle, and, from a cosmetic standpoint, it is preferable to preserve this structure, rather than chisel it away. With the sphenoid retractors in position, the keel of the vomer and the face of the sphenoid are seen (Figure 8B). On either side of the central ridge, the ostia of the sphenoid sinuses can be identified.

The operating microscope having been introduced, the anterior wall of the sphenoid is now opened. Fracturing into the sphenoid sinus is usually possible by grasping the vomer with a Lillie-Koeffler forceps, Ferris-Smith punch, or chisel, if necessary. Once within the sphenoid sinus, the exposure is widened with a right-angled punch. The mucosa within the sinus is resected with a cup

forceps. Resection of the mucosa aides in reducing bleeding, and decreases the risk of p/o mucocele formation. With all internal bony landmarks now clearly visible, the surgeon now reorients him/herself with respect to the position of the carotid arteries, the sellar floor, the anterior fossa floor and the clivus, correlating the operative anatomy with the real-time fluoroscopic images, and ensuring that the appropriate midline trajectory is maintained.

The sellar floor should be clearly visible. With some tumors, the sellar floor will be eroded or will be extraordinarily thin, so that it can be fractured with a blunt hook (Figure 9A). Occasionally, a midline septum within the sphenoid sinus can be used to gain entry into the sella, simply by grasping its base and gently twisting as the bone is removed. If the floor of the sella is thick, a small chisel can be used to remove a square of bone. In cases of an even thicker sellar floor and when the sphenoid sinus is poorly pneumatized, a high-speed drill can be used to provide exposure. In the setting of recurrence, the appearance of the sellar floor can vary considerably. In the more difficult instances, it may consist entirely of scar tissue, seemingly in continuity with the scarring encountered in the sphenoid sinus. In other cases, the sellar floor may have been fully reconstituted, appearing as though no prior procedure had been performed. The surgeon should, once again, use careful videofluoroscopic control or image guidance to continually monitor sellar entry, exposure, and trajectory. Once the sellar floor has been penetrated, the opening is widened with a Kerrison-type punch. An adequate bony exposure is crucial to the success of the transsphenoidal approach, particularly when dealing with large tumors. For recurrent tumors, in particular, a wide bony opening will allow virgin dura to be uncovered. Identification of the latter will be a real comfort, and will assist in establishing a plane between scar tissue. In general, the authors favor a wide removal in virtually every case, and this should extend from one cavernous

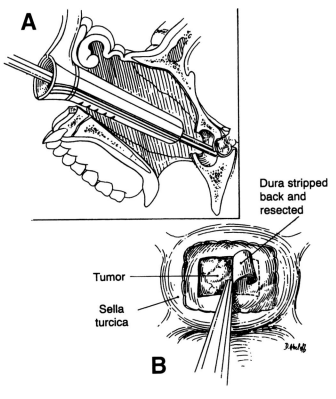

Dura stripped back and resected

Tumor

Sella turcica

Figure 13-9 Removal of the floor of the sella (**A**), and opening of the dural window (**B**).

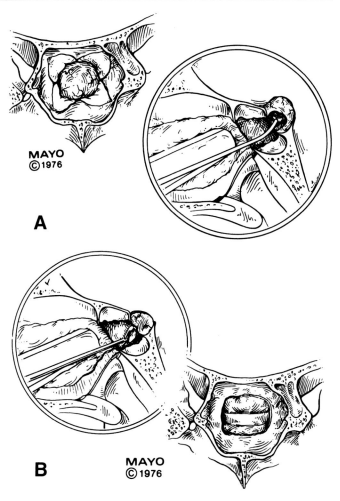

MAYO
©1976

A

MAYO
©1976

B

Figure 13-10 Removal of the adenoma with a ring curette (**A**). At closure, the sella is packed with fat or Gelfoam, and the floor is reconstructed with a stent of nasal cartilage (**B**).

sinus to the other. A small bony margin of the sellar floor should be left, however, because this facilitates sellar reconstruction at the end of the procedure.

Exposure within the sella proper is carried out with the use of the operating microscope, with a 350–400 mm objective distance and oculars with a magnification of ×12.5. The magnification should be adjusted so that the sella fills the entire field of vision once the intrasellar portion of the operation has begun. An invasive tumor may erode through the anterior dura of the sella, but, in most cases, the dura will be intact. It is exposed as widely as is feasible, and careful attention is paid to its appearance. Transverse, blue intracavernous sinuses traversing the sella at the top and bottom of the anterior dura are common, particularly in microadenomas. The anterior dura may appear totally blue and very thin, indicating the possible presence of an empty sella. Once the dura is exposed completely, it should be opened with great care. A partial empty sella is sometimes present, and a cerebrospinal fluid (CSF) leak early in the operation can be a major deterrent to success. Before the dural incision is made, it is prudent to review the imaging studies once again, to note the position of the carotid arteries, so that they are not injured upon durotomy. In dealing with some cystic pituitary adenomas, a helpful maneuver is to use a long needle to evacuate and evaluate cyst contents prior to dural opening. These issues having been considered, the site of dural opening is selected, cauterized, and incised in either a cruciate fashion or with the excision of a dural window (Figure 9B). Next, an attempt is made to establish a definite subdural cleavage plane between the pituitary gland or tumor and the underlying dura. A plane of dissection between the two leaves of the dura should be carefully avoided, because this allows entrance into the cavernous sinus, and heavy venous bleeding will result. The dural perimeter

is widened by shrinking the dural margins with cautery, providing an unobstructed view into the sella.

TUMOR REMOVAL For the typical macroadenoma, the tumor is entered with a ring curette, tissue is loosened, and then removed with a relatively blunt curette (Figure 10A). One should attempt tumor removal in an orderly fashion. The authors' practice has been to first remove tumor in the inferior aspect, then to proceed laterally, from inferior to superior on both sides, removing tumor along the medial side of the cavernous sinus. One must resist coring out the central and most accessible portion of the tumor first, because this may cause premature descent of the diaphragma and entrapment of more laterally situated tumor. It is also important to delay the superior dissection until the lesion is relatively free elsewhere, because this minimizes trauma to the pituitary stalk and secondarily transmitted trauma to the HT. It is recognized that the surgeon may, on occasion, be required to follow tumor into one cavernous sinus or the other, or to deal with tumor directly involving the diaphragma. In either instance, any maneuver more forceful than gentle curetting may be a dangerous move; pulling of adherent fragments must be avoided. Decompression of the intrasellar portion of the tumor frequently permits a suprasellar extension to prolapse into view within the sella. Once this has been resected, the diaphragma subsequently prolapses and generally signifies that the resection is complete. When spontaneous prolapse of tumor capsule and/or diaphragma do not occur, instillation of 15–20 mL of air or lactated Ringer's solution into a lumbar subarachnoid catheter may facilitate descent. Alternatively, bilateral jugular vein compression can also help in delivering suprasellar tumor. If the tumor still fails to descend, a ring curette can be used cautiously in the intracranial space, but only under direct fluoroscopic control. Verification that no residual tumor remains is provided by direct inspection, or with the help of dental mirror, a nasopharyngoscope, or a small fiberoptic endoscope. Bleeding from the tumor bed can usually be controlled by precise tamponade with cotton patties or Gelfoam.

In all cases, a concerted effort is made to preserve normal pituitary tissue. In a large diffuse adenoma, normal glandular tissue usually appears as a thin membrane, situated superolaterally against the sellar wall. The orange-yellow color of the gland, together with its firm consistency, distinguishes it from the greyish color and finely granular texture typical of the tumor. A biopsy of the suspected glandular remnant may be taken for confirmation, but the appearance is often so typical that this tissue can be left behind with confidence.

Microadenomas necessitate a different operative strategy, since it is well recognized that many will not be immediately visualized upon opening of the dura. Instead, a systematic search through a seemingly normal-appearing gland is often required. The authors begin with a transverse glandular incision, followed by subdural dissection and mobilization of the lateral wings. If the incision in the gland is deep enough, lateral pressure with a Hardy dissector usually causes the microadenoma to herniate into the operative field. Its location can, therefore, be delineated, its cavity entered, and its removal completed by use of a small ring curette and cup forceps. All suspicious tissue is removed, and a biopsy specimen is occasionally obtained from the residual, and presumably normal, pituitary gland.

Treatment of the tumor bed with absolute alcohol or Zenker's solution may be used, although there is not evidence to indicate that it improves the immediate result or the risk of recurrence. Understandably, this step is contraindicated when an intraoperative CSF leak has been encountered.

RECONSTRUCTION AND CLOSURE   After the tumor has been removed and hemostasis has been achieved, the sella must be carefully evaluated regarding reconstruction and closure. The authors prefer not to leave dead space in the sella. If no CSF leak has occurred, the sella is loosely packed with Gelfoam (Figure 10B). If, however, a CSF leak has been encountered, then some form of tissue graft becomes mandatory. Reconstruction of the sellar roof can be attempted with a piece of homologous dural graft material or fascia lata; however, this step probably adds little to the security of the seal. Current practice favors simple packing of the sella with fat taken from the right lower quadrant of the abdomen. The fat is soaked in chloramphenicol solution, may be rolled in Avitene, is trimmed to appropriate size, and is snugly placed within the sella. In either case, the sellar floor is then carefully reconstructed using a suitably trimmed piece of cartilage or bone. In cases in which previous surgery has been performed and no bone is available, alternative materials for closure include banked bone allograft, or, rarely, iliac crest autograft or methylmethacrylate. Some surgeons utilize fibrin glue as part of the closure in patients who have had CSF leaks, but this has not been found to be especially useful in the authors' experience. An impressive mound of fibrin glue is a poor

substitute for an inadequate structural repair, because it is the integrity of the latter, and not the adhesive properties of the former that is the essential deterrent of p/o CSF leaks. Likewise, the authors do not use lumbar drainage in patients who have had p/o CSF leaks; instead, a policy has been adopted of immediate reexploration, repacking of the sella, and reconstruction of the floor.

In closing the nasal portion of the procedure, careful attention is paid to achieving anatomic and physiologic restoration. If an intraoperative CSF leak has occurred, the sphenoid sinus is packed with fat, but, in the absence of a leak, it is left free of foreign material. The posterior septal space may be reimplanted with crushed nasal bone and cartilage. The septal flaps are reapproximated, the nasal septum is returned to its midline insertion and any accessible mucosal tears are repaired with fine catgut sutures. Bilateral endonasal packs, consisting of gauze packing within the fingers of a rubber glove that has been lubricated with petroleum jelly or antibiotic ointment, are placed in the nostrils. The nasal and/or gingival incisions are closed with interrupted 4-0 catgut sutures, and a gauze moustache dressing is applied. Prophylactic antibiotics are continued until the nasal packing is removed, usually on the second p/o day.

POSTOPERATIVE CARE   Because most patients awaken promptly and are fully alert, the authors have not found it necessary to utilize a urinary catheter or intensive care monitoring following most routine transsphenoidal procedures. In all patients, however, vigilant p/o monitoring of water and electrolyte balance is mandatory. Diuresis of varying degrees regularly occurs in the p/o period, but does not necessarily imply a diagnosis of diabetes insipidus nor a need for vasopressin. However, this state must, be distinguished from true DI, which is accompanied by a brisk diuresis, defined by characteristic alterations in the serum sodium and serum/urine osmolalities, and for which prompt fluid replacement and vasopressin are crucial. When it does occur, DI is usually temporary. Exogenous stress level steroids are rapidly tapered, beginning on the first p/o day. If there is any doubt about the functionality of the pituitary-adrenal axis, steroid replacement in physiologic doses (hydrocortisone 20 mg/d) should be administered until formal endocrine testing is undertaken.

Prophylactic antibiotics are continued until the nasal packing is removed, usually on the second p/o day. In uncomplicated cases, the patient can be discharged from hospital by the fourth day. The first follow-up visit occurs about 6 wk after surgery, at which time endocrine testing is performed and endocrine replacement therapy administered for any deficiencies identified. Follow-up gadolinium enhanced MRI of the sella is usually performed at approx 3 mo postoperatively, and then on an annual basis, as necessary. Formal visual field examinations are also performed at the 3-mo visit for patients who presented with any preoperative visual deficits.

COMPLICATIONS OF TRANSSPHENOIDAL APPROACH Of the many virtues of the transsphenoidal approach, its safety and low complication rate are among the most important. With its lack of visible scars, lower mortality and morbidity, compared to conventional transcranial approaches, and its greater patient tolerance, transsphenoidal surgery is appealing to both patient and physician. As determined by several retrospective cumulative series, operative mortality and major morbidity rates are 0.5 and 2.2%, respectively (26). Operative deaths are usually the result of intracranial hemorrhage, HT damage, or meningitis related to CSF

Table 2
Complications of Transsphenoidal Surgery

Operative mortality (30 d)		
Hypothalamic injury/hemorrhage	5	
Meningitis	2	
Vascular injury/occlusion	4	
CSF leak/pneumocephalus, SAH/spasm, MI	1	
Postoperative MI, postoperative seizure	2	
Total	14	(1.0%)
Major morbidity		
Vascular occlusion/stroke/SAH/spasm	5	
Visual loss (new)	11	
Vascular injury (repaired)	8	
Meningitis (nonfatal)	8	
Sellar abscess	1	
Sellar pneumatocele	1	
Sixth cranial nerve palsy	2	
Third cranial nerve palsy	1	
CSF rhinorrhea	49	
Total	86	(3.4%)
Lesser morbidity		
Hemorrhage (intraoperative or postoperative)	9	
Postoperative psychosis	5	
Nasal septal perforation	16	
Sinusitis, wound infection	5	
Transient cranial nerve palsy (III or IV)	5	
Diabetes insipidus (usually transient)	35	
Cribiform plate fracture	2	
Maxillary fracture	2	
Hepatitis	1	
Symptomatic SIADH	37	
Total	117	(4.6%)

Authors' series of 2562 pituitary adenomas. MI, myocardial infarction; SAH, subarachnoid hemorrhage; SIADH, syndrome of inappropriate secretion of antidiuretic hormone.

fistulae. Although infrequent, a wide variety of other complications can also occur with this approach (Table 2); *(27)*. The classic technical complications associated with the transsphenoidal approach are discussed below. To these, one could also regard failure to achieve endocrine control of a hypersecretory state as a complication of the procedure; this issue is discussed in the subheading Results of Surgery, below.

Hypothalamic Injury Damage to the HT may result from direct surgical injury, and also from hemorrhage or ischemia provoked by the procedure. Clinical manifestations of HT damage include death, coma, DI, memory loss, and disturbances of vegetative functions (morbid obesity, uncontrollable hunger or thirst, and disturbances in temperature regulation). Such complications are more frequent in patients with prior craniotomy or radiation *(28)*. Gentle surgical technique, and avoidance of traction on the tumor capsule and pituitary stalk, will minimize the occurrence of such injuries.

Visual Damage Damage to the optic nerves and chiasm can also occur from direct surgical trauma, hemorrhage, or ischemia. Fractures of bony structures at the base of the skull can damage optic nerves, and can occur from misdirected placement and aggressive opening of transsphenoidal retractors. Many patients have preoperative compromise of visual function, making them more vulnerable to further damage. Such complications are more

likely to occur in patients with adhesions from prior cranial surgery or radiation *(28)*. Assessment of the bony anatomy, careful and gentle technique, confirmation of surgical landmarks, and effective use of flouroscopic guidance to direct the approach are the major methods of avoiding these complications. Finally, at the time of sellar reconstruction, overpacking the sella can cause chiasmal compression; underpacking can lead to a secondary empty sella, with the late onset of visual loss caused by chiasmatic prolapse.

Arterial Damage Although rare, arterial injury is a well-known complication of transsphenoidal surgery, and is one of the chief sources of operative mortality accompanying the procedure. Virtually every larger transsphenoidal series includes at least one example of arterial injury, most of which have proven fatal. The intracavernous portion of the carotid tends to be the most vulnerable, followed by other components of the circle of Willis. Because the tumor may be quite adherent to arterial structures, arteries may be lacerated, perforated, avulsed, or damaged, so that they develop spasm or intraluminal thrombosis. Intracranial hemorrhage, thrombotic stroke and embolic stroke, and the development of false aneurysms or carotid-cavernous fistulae are the usual sequelae of such injuries. When vascular injury is suspected, tamponade should be used to control hemorrhage and an immediate postoperative angiogram should be obtained. Again, gentle technique devoid of aggressive traction on the tumor capsule, not deviating from the midline, and repeated assessment of bony landmarks are the most effective means of avoiding these frequently devastating complications.

CSF Rhinorrhea CSF rhinorrhea and meningitis are among the more common serious complications associated with transsphenoidal surgery. They are the result of disruption of the sellar diaphragm, which is usually thinned, adherent to tumor, and susceptible to direct or traction injury. Among microadenomas, small arachnoid diverticula may be the site of leakage. In most instances, this can be avoided, with gentle microtechnique. In other instances, however, the diaphragm may have been invaded by tumor, and its disruption may be a necessary and unavoidable consequence of complete tumor removal. That being the case, careful closure of the sella becomes a crucial part of the procedure; the authors' method of doing so has been outlined above. In the p/o period, ready acknowledgment of a CSF leak is essential, as is early recognition and therapy of meningitis, if and when such leaks occur. Postoperative CSF leaks usually manifest at the time nasal packing is removed. These are best managed by prompt transsphenoidal re-exploration, identification of the leak, and resealing. CSF fistulae may occasionally manifest beyond the immediate p/o period. The authors have found the transethmoidal approach particularly useful in the management of these late CSF leaks.

Cavernous Sinus Injury Pituitary tumors involve the cavernous sinus with some regularity. In some cases, the tumor may be adherent to the medial wall of the sinus only; in other more invasive tumors, frank invasion of the sinus interstices occurs. In the process of stripping the tumor from the medial dura, in the course of following the tumor into the sinus, or with overzealous packing of sinus bleeding, injury to the cavernous sinus and its contents can occur. The carotid artery and the sixth cranial nerve are most vulnerable to such maneuvers; the third and fourth cranial nerves are damaged less frequently. Again, gentle technique, good visualization of anatomic structures, and accurate hemostasis with Gelfoam and tamponade, help to avoid such complications.

Iatrogenic Hypopituitarism In most instances, existing pituitary function can usually be preserved. Among microadenomas, the authors' recent experience indicates that loss of one or more anterior pituitary functional axes occurs in approx 3% of cases *(29)*; for macroadenomas, anterior pituitary function can be preserved in more than 95% of cases, provided that pituitary function was normal preoperatively. In contrast, patients with established preoperative endocrine deficits, partial or complete restoration of endocrine deficits is achieved in only 16–30%. DI occurs temporarily in as many as one-third of all patients, but posterior pituitary failure is permanent in no more than 3% of patients. As a rule, p/o endocrine deficits tend to be more frequent and more severe in patients who have undergone reoperation, or in those treated by craniotomy.

Brainstem Injury Damage to the brainstem may occur with a misdirected approach that violates the clivus, or, more commonly, when a larger tumor erodes the clivus, exposing the underlying dura.

Nasal Complications Although generally less immediate and rarely fatal, complications relating to the nasofacial aspect of the procedure can be annoying and persist for some time after surgery. Imprudent use of the retractor may result in diastasis or fracture of the hard palate, optic canals, or the cribiform plate, the latter also being a source of CSF rhinorrhea. In the p/o period, the mucosa of the sphenoid sinus may become infected, giving rise to a febrile sinusitis and the eventual development of a mucocele. Inadequate hemostasis in the nasal portion of the procedure may lead to superficial wound hemorrhage and swelling. Technical errors in handling the nasal mucosa, the nasal septum, and the nasal spine may result in an external nasal deformity that may be distressing, both cosmetically and functionally. Loss of smell can also occur, presumably because of damage to nerve endings in the nasal mucosa. Finally, overaggressive enlargement of the basal pyriform aperture can damage distal branches of the alveolar nerves and/or vessels, which may devitalize or desensitize the teeth and gums of the maxilla. Virtually all of these local complications can be avoided with careful nondestructive surgical technique during the exposure and meticulous reconstruction at the time of closure.

Complications Associated with Reoperation It is generally true in neurosurgery, and certainly true for pituitary tumors, that reoperations carry higher complication rates and outcomes less favorable than initial operations *(30)*. This issue was carefully studied in a series of 158 patients, most of whom had pituitary tumors, and all of whom required secondary transsphenoidal surgery for recurrence, persistent disease, or treatment of complications relating to unsuccessful prior therapy of one form or another *(28)*. Although the scope of that study extended beyond the single issue of repeat surgery for recurrent pituitary tumors, many of the conclusions are still applicable in the current context. Of the 158 patients treated with repeat transsphenoidal surgery, operative mortality was 2.5%, and the new complication rate was 29%; this contrasts with the 0.5% mortality and 2.2% morbidity rates that are frequently quoted for initial transsphenoidal operations *(28)*.

Operative complications are notably more frequent and more serious in those patients in whom the initial procedure was a transcranial one. In such situations, the diaphragma may be partially or totally absent, leading to scarring and dense arachnoidal adhesions between the tumor and the optic apparatus, HT, and basal vasculature, all of which add to the hazards of a transsphenoidal procedure *(28)*. For patients in whom the original approach was transsphenoidal, scarring, adhesions, and distorted anatomy also predispose to complications, although to a lesser degree. Prior RT or pharmacologic therapy may be expected to induce fibrotic changes in the tumor, although the authors have not found this to be a consistently adverse effect nor an overly important predisposing factor for surgical complications. Most instances of operative mortality have generally been the result of intracranial hemorrhage, HT damage, or meningitis related to CSF fistulae.

CONVENTIONAL TRANSCRANIAL APPROACHES FOR PITUITARY TUMORS

Given the effectiveness and safety of the transsphenoidal approach, together with its suitability for more than 95% of pituitary adenomas, current indications for transcranial approaches have become few and infrequent. Still, several important situations can arise for which transcranial surgery will be the most advisable. The most common of these relates to tumors that have extended up from the sella, and have spilled into the anterior, middle, or posterior cranial fossae. For such extensions, the transcranial approach affords superior access. A second situation is that of the dumbbell-shaped tumor, whose suprasellar portion is disproportionately larger than is its intrasellar component. Particularly if the intrasellar component and sella are small, a transcranial approach is ordinarily the most effective means of dealing with the suprasellar component. A transcranial procedure may also be indicated if residual tumor remains after a transsphenoidal procedure and complete resection is still the desired goal. This would also include those tumors whose fibrous nature prevented tumor descent during a transsphenoidal procedure. Finally, a transcranial approach will be the procedure of choice when doubt exists as to the diagnosis of pituitary adenoma and the possibility of meningioma, craniopharyngioma, chordoma, or other pathology is suspected. The major advantage of the craniotomy approach is that it affords the surgeon a complete view of the effect of the pituitary tumor on intracranial structures. Specifically, the optic nerves and chiasm, unusual intracranial extensions into the anterior and middle cranial fossae, as well as retrosellar clival extensions, can all be visualized and accessed. Similarly, when sufficiently large, some suprasellar extensions will involve third ventricular structures; craniotomy allows such extensions to be dealt with directly. The major limitation of the transcranial approach, however, is that the intrasellar portion of the tumor can be more difficult to remove, particularly when a prefixed chiasm also exists. As discussed below, strategies are available to deal with this situation.

There are three basic transcranial microsurgical approaches to pituitary tumors: pterional, subfrontal, and subtemporal. Selection of one approach over the others depends on the precise geometry and growth trajectory of the tumor, as well as the preference and experience of the surgeon. Probably the most versatile approach, and the one that the authors prefer, is the pterional approach.

THE PTERIONAL APPROACH For most tumors, except those with significant left-sided extensions, the authors use a right-sided pterional approach. The placement of a lumbar drain is optional, but can help with brain relaxation during the intradural portion of the procedure. The head is placed in a three-point pinion headrest and turned 20 degrees to the left side, so that the lateral aspect of the malar eminence is brought to an uppermost position. The position of the neck relative the body is such that venous drainage of the head is uncompromised.

The scalp incision is placed behind the hairline, using a coronal or curved Dandy incision. A small lateral frontal or frontotemporal bone flap is usually sufficient, although it is frequently desirable to extend the frontal portion inferiorly to the supraorbital ridge. The sphenoid ridge is generously drilled from lateral to medial. The dura is opened in a C-shaped fashion and reflected anteriorly.

Attention is then turned to achieving adequate brain relaxation. This requires either osmotic diuresis and/or withdrawal of CSF, either through a lumbar drain, or directly from the basal cisterns, or from the lateral ventricle if hydrocephalus coexists. Ordinarily, the authors begin by gently elevating the frontal lobe, identifying the optic nerve and carotid artery, and sharply incising their respective arachnoid cisterns. This step is performed with patience, gradually withdrawing sufficient CSF to optimize brain relaxation and minimize retraction pressures. Microdissection and opening of the Sylvian fissure is almost always worthwhile, because it releases the frontal lobe and allows it to fall more freely backward with gravity. Self-retaining retractors are placed as necessary.

In most instances, obvious tumor will be encountered behind the tuberculum and between the optic nerves. The pituitary stalk, with its portal vessels producing a characteristic vertically striated appearance, can usually be identified behind the tumor in the triangle between the lateral border of the right optic nerve and the carotid triangle. Every effort is made not to disturb this structure. The tumor capsule is then carefully dissected away from surrounding structures. Great care should be exercised in dealing with portions of the tumor attached to the optic apparatus, the dissection of which may damage these structures or their microvasculature. The tumor can be entered through several operative corridors. Usually, the capsule is incised between the optic nerves. The tumor is entered and its contents removed by curettes, suction, or, for unusually fibrous tumor, with sharp dissection. Manipulation of the capsule and additional internal decompression can be performed through the opticocarotid triangle as well. A translamina terminalis approach can also be performed, should a third ventricular component fail to descend. If the intrasellar portion of the tumor is difficult to remove because of its consistency, a prefixed chiasm, or other factors, a transtuberculum transsphenoidal corridor can be used (31). This requires drilling just behind the jugum sphenoidale to expose the sphenoid sinus, followed by opening the anterior wall of the sella. When such a maneuver is anticipated, a subfrontal approach is preferred, rather than a pterional one.

Once the tumor has been removed, and hemostasis assured, particularly from within the sella, the dura is closed in a watertight fashion. If the frontal sinus has been transgressed, it should be exenterated and isolated with a pericranial flap. The bone flap is replaced, the temporalis muscle reapproximated, and the scalp closed in the usual two-layered fashion.

Postoperatively, the patient is observed overnight in the intensive care unit. The p/o care of these patients, like those undergoing transsphenoidal surgery, centers on careful monitoring of fluid and electrolytes, recognition and management of DI, should it develop, and replacement therapy for pituitary insufficiency. In addition, these patients, like all patients undergoing craniotomy for any reason, must also be monitored for brain swelling, p/o

hemorrhage, seizures, CSF leak, and infection. Mortality and major morbidity with transcranial procedures are generally less than 3%, and the overall complication rate is usually less than 10%.

ALTERNATIVE SKULL BASE APPROACHES TO PITUITARY TUMORS

Few situations will arise when pituitary tumors cannot be removed by either the transsphenoidal or transcranial techniques just described. When such situations do occur, most will involve giant invasive pituitary tumors with intracranial projections that are unusual in extent or direction. In these circumstances, several skull base approaches can be tailored to the specific need at hand. Because such approaches are not specific to pituitary adenomas, they are only mentioned briefly: The interested reader is referred to accompanying references. An essential caveat that must always be kept in mind, particularly when contemplating such radical resective procedures for pituitary adenomas, is that the goal of surgery should be clear and justifiable. Just because a radical resection is technically possible, that does not necessarily imply that it will be biologically or prognositically meaningful. Because most pituitary adenomas are histologically benign and slow-growing, and since subtotal resection followed by radiation often affords satisfactory disease control and progression-free survival, the benefits of pursuing a more radical surgical course must be carefully weighed with the alternatives of management.

EXTRACRANIAL APPROACHES When the standard transsphenoidal corridor proves too restrictive for tumors that extend widely beyond the confines of the sella, several extracranial approaches can be used. For pituitary tumors that involve the upper and mid-clivus, an extended transsphenoidal approach can be used (32). The authors have found this approach very effective for chordomas of the clivus, and have adapted its use for similarly situated pituitary adenomas (33). This approach involves a wider sphenoid sinus and sellar opening than does the standard transsphenoidal approach, especially inferiorly. In doing so, bony removal can extend as far inferiorly as the epipharynx, which generally approximates the roof of the hard palate. Because the corridor of access for this sublabial approach is the pyriform aperture, it is the walls of this structure that represent the lateral limits of this approach, with the hard palate representing the inferior limits. The addition of a maxillotomy will allow wider opening of the pyriform aperture and more lateral maneuverability. Fundamentally, however, it remains essentially a midline approach that is appropriate for midline lesions only. More extensive extracranial approaches, such as the lateral rhinotomy approach (34,35), transethomoidomaxillary approach (35), transmaxillary approach (36), or various craniofacial midface degloving procedures, can also be used when lateral extracranial extensions exist, depending on the precise anatomic extent of the tumor.

TRANSCRANIAL APPROACHES Of intracranial extensions that may be difficult to access through conventional craniotomy, particularly when tumor resection from within the cavernous sinus is desired, or when large parasellar extensions exist, a combined cranio-orbito-zygomatic osteotomy can provide the necessary basal exposure (37). For more anteriorly situated tumors involving the anterior fossa floor and extending posteriorly along the clivus, the subfrontal transbasal approach, popularized by Derome, can provide an effective route (38,39).

Table 3
Summary of P/O Remission and Recurrence After Transsphenoidal Surgery for Pituitary Adenomas

Clinical entity	Number[a]	Remission rate[b] %		Recurrence[c] %	
Acromegaly	468	Microadenoma	72	8	
		Macroadenoma	50		
Prolactinoma	871	Microadenoma	87	13	
		Macroadenoma	50		
Cushing's disease	381	Microadenoma	91	12	(adults)
		Macroadenoma	56	42	(children)
Nelson-Salassa syndrome	62	Microadenoma	70		
		Macroadenoma	40	40	
Clinically nonfunctioning and miscellaneous PIT adenomas	883	—[d]		16	(radiographic)
				6	(symptomatic)

Authors' series, 1972–1997, (n = 2665).

[a]Includes total number of cases in each category (micro- and macroadenomas).

[b]Remission criteria as follows: Acromegaly: basal GH <2.5 ng/mL; GH <1.0 ng/mL on oral glucose tolerance test; and normalization of serum IGF-I level. Prolactinoma: serum PRL level <20 ng/mL. Cushing's disease: normalization of 24-h urinary free cortisol. Nelson-Salassa syndrome: normalization of serum ACTH level.

[c]Recurrence rates based on a cohort of 100 patients in each category, each of whom were followed for a period of 10 yr or more.

[d]Among clinically nonfunctioning tumors, recovery of vision was used as one end point of therapeutic success. Objective changes in visual status were as follows: improved 81%; unchanged 15%; deterioration 4%.

RESULTS OF SURGERY

Just as pituitary tumors are, pathologically, endocrinologically, and biologically, a heterogeneous group of lesions, so too are the results of surgery for pituitary tumors, which vary among the different pituitary tumor subtypes. The results of the authors' series of over 2600 pituitary adenomas are summarized in Table 3 *(29)*. Results of surgery and special considerations for each major type of pituitary tumor are described below.

PROLACTIN-PRODUCING PITUITARY ADENOMAS   Once the primary mode of therapy for prolactinomas, operative treatment has been justifiably usurped by dopaminergic therapy as the initial treatment of choice for most prolactinomas. Despite its secondary and more selective role in prolactinoma management, surgery remains an essential component of the therapeutic armamentarium against these tumors, because there are a number of situations in which surgery will be the most appropriate first-line option, and, in some instances, the only effective option *(40)*.

Indications for surgical management of prolactinomas are several (Table 4). One of the clearest indications for operative intervention is pituitary apoplexy. When the MRI indicates that the bulk of the tumor is composed of hemorrhagic and/or necrotic material, dopamine agonists are unlikely to provide a satisfactory reduction in tumor volume. Cystic prolactinomas, sharing a similarly poor volumetric response to dopamine agonists, are best treated surgically. A small percentage of patients will be intolerant to the side effects of bromocriptine. In these situations, surgery is indicated, and can be highly successful. Another indication is patients resistant to dopaminergic therapy. Resistance usually manifests in one of two ways. The first is when the PRL levels fail to normalize; in such a situation, there is still a risk that the patient may suffer the adverse effects of hyperprolactinemia, and there is the threat that the tumor may continue to enlarge, despite continued pharmacologic management. The second type of hyporesponder is the patient who has a good response to medical management in terms of normalization of hyperprolactinemia, but in whom, there is little or no volumetric response, and mass effects remain.

Table 4
Surgical Indications for Prolactinomas

Microprolactinomas
   Resistance or suboptimal response to dopamine agonist therapy
   Intolerance to dopamine agonist therapy
   Patient preference against long-term dopamine agonist therapy

Macroprolactinomas
   Pituitary apoplexy
   Cystic prolactinoma
   Resistance or suboptimal response to dopamine agonist therapy
   Reduction of tumor burden as an adjuvant to enhancing the effectiveness of dopamine agonist therapy, RT, or radiosurgery
   Prolactinoma with extensive erosion into the sphenoid sinus, in which the risk of a CSF leak is high, with dopamine agonist-induced tumor shrinkage
   In the female patient desiring pregnancy, surgery is undertaken with the objective of reducing the eventual risk of pregnancy-induced tumor enlargement
   Mass effects presenting during pregnancy
   When the diagnosis of prolactinoma is uncertain and a tissue diagnosis is required

Included in such situations are the pseudoprolactinomas, which are sellar masses other than genuine prolactinomas that produce hyperprolactinemia on the basis of stalk compression. Both types of hyporesponders represent legitimate indications for surgical management. Surgery may also be indicated in the patient with a large invasive prolactinoma, in whom a successful response to dopaminergic therapy can be anticipated, but in whom extensive erosion of the skull base may be the source of a CSF leak with pharmacologic tumor shrinkage. As discussed below, surgical issues and indications also arise in the context of infertility and planned or established pregnancy; these are discussed in the section, Surgical Issues Relating to Fertility and Pregnancy.

The strongest argument in favor of surgical resection for prolactinomas has been, and continues to be, that surgery is a definitive mode of therapy, which, in contradistinction to medical therapy, provides the only opportunity for potential cure. In fact, however, curative resections are achieved in only a minority of patients with macroprolactinomas, and, among all prolactinomas of all sizes, curative resections are associated with a progressive recurrence rate over time.

Microprolactinomas The rate of curative resections, as defined by p/o normalization of PRL levels, are highest among microadenomas, particularly those accompanied by PRL levels less than 100 ng/mL. In the Mayo Clinic series involving 100 patients with prolactinomas, 32 of which met these criteria, normalization of PRL levels was achieved in 88% (41). Larger tumors, and/or those accompanied by higher PRL elevations, suffered a dramatic reduction in surgical cure rate. Among microadenomas having preoperative PRL levels in excess of 100 ng/mL, a curative result was observed in only 50%. Similar results have been reported by others (42). In his summary of 31 published series involving 1224 patients with microprolactinomas, Molitch (43) calculated an overall endocrinologic cure rate of 71.2%, independent of preoperative PRL levels. Similarly, in a multicenter international survey involving 1518 patients with microprolactinomas, Zervas (26) reported an overall surgical cure rate of 74%.

Macroprolactinomas The surgical outcome for patients with PRL-secreting macroadenomas has proved far less encouraging. In a second report of the Mayo Clinic experience (44), only 53% of surgically treated patients with macroadenomas experienced normalization of PRL levels. Among locally invasive macroadenomas, the surgical cure rate was further reduced to 28% (44). Comparable results have also been shown in other surgical series. In the aforementioned literature review of 31 published series, Molitch calculated an overall curative resection rate of 31.8% among 1256 macroadenomas (43). Similarly, in the aforementioned international survey, which analyzed outcomes of 1022 operated macroadenomas, Zervas (26) reported an overall surgical cure rate of 30%. Of patients who have failed medical therapy, relief of mass effects can be expected in the overwhelming majority, even though biochemical remission is not easily achieved.

Because the degree of hyperprolactinemia reflects both the size and invasiveness of the tumor, the preoperative serum PRL level has proven an especially reliable predictor of surgical outcome. As a general rule, curative resection rates drop precipitously when preoperative PRL levels exceed 200 ng/mL. This has been validated by several series in which surgical cure rates varied between 74 and 88% when PRL levels were below this threshold, but dropped to 18–47% when PRL levels exceeded 200 ng/mL (43). When the preoperative PRL level exceeds 1000 ng/mL, seldom does surgery alone result in cure.

Although preoperative PRL levels are predictive of potential surgical curability, PRL determinations obtained in the immediate p/o period are useful indicators of whether or not surgical cure actually has been achieved. Subnormal p/o PRL levels, particularly those less than 10 ng/mL, virtually guarantee a durable and longlasting curative result. Although p/o values between 11 and 20 ng/mL also qualify as curative, these patients appear at some risk for future tumor recurrence (45).

As a strategy to improve surgical outcomes in prolactinomas, some have suggested that preoperative treatment with bromocriptine may improve operative results. In one retrospective report (46) examining the surgical outcomes of 20 patients with bromocriptine pretreatment and 20 patients treated with surgery alone, bromocriptine treatment was associated with more favorable out-

comes among both microprolactinomas (87 vs 50%) and macroadenomas (33 vs 17%). The report of Weiss et al. (46a) suggests a similar trend. In 10/19 macroadenomas pretreated with bromocriptine, tumor shrinkage of >30% was noted, and subsequent surgery resulted in normalization of PRL levels in 70%. Of the remaining nine patients in whom bromocriptine failed to induce shrinkage of this degree, only 22% had normalization of PRL levels with surgery. In other reports, no beneficial effect of bromocriptine pretreatment has been observed (47,48). This concept of medical pretreatment has theoretical appeal, but the authors' experience suggests that improvements in surgical results with this strategy, if they occur at all, are modest at best.

Postoperative Recurrence In evaluating the overall effectiveness of surgical therapy, some consideration must be given to the issue of tumor recurrence (49). Ordinarily, tumor recurrence manifests endocrinologically with return of hyperprolactinemia; radiologically evident tumor regrowth is neither necessarily, nor is it commonly present. The reported frequency of biochemical recurrence has varied greatly. Serri et al. (45), reported recurrence rates of 50% for microadenomas and 80% for macroadenomas, following mean remission periods of 4 yr and 2.5 yr, respectively. Although that is one of the most frequently quoted studies to date, these recurrence rates are among the highest in the literature. In his review, Molitch (43) observed more favorable results; recurrent hyperprolactinemia was observed in 17.4% (82/471) of microadenomas and in 18.6% (48/235) of macroadenomas. Similarly, Post and Habas (50) reported 17 and 20% recurrence rates for microadenomas and macroadenomas, respectively, for patients followed longer than 5 yr. These data more accurately approximate the authors' experience: In a surgical series, that currently includes 771 patients with prolactinomas, there has been a 24% recurrence rate in patients followed for 10 yr or more (51).

Worthy of reiteration is the fact that, in the majority of recurrences, particularly in the setting of microprolactinomas, the relapse tends to biochemical, rather than radiologic. For example, in a 10-yr follow-up study of 58 women with microprolactinomas, all of whom were successfully treated with transsphenoidal surgery, 43% experienced a relapse of moderate hyperprolactinemia; only two patients showed radiologic evidence of tumor recurrence (52). This peculiar phenomenon of delayed hyperprolactinemia is poorly understood, and is believed to be a variant of the stalk section effect. In most instances, the hyperprolactinemia is only of a modest degree, is not always symptomatic, may spontaneously resolve, is only rarely associated with radiologically evident recurrence, and does not necessarily warrant therapy.

Surgical Issues Relating to Fertility and Pregnancy Prolactinomas pose three basic problems regarding planned or established pregnancy: infertility, risk of tumor growth during pregnancy, and effects of therapy on fetal development. Infertility is the result of functional anovulation caused by hyperprolactinemia, and, in the case of larger pituitary tumors associated with glandular compression and hypopituitarism, it may also be complicated by hypogonadotrophism caused by irreversible loss of pituitary gonadotrophs. It is important to recognize that by the time the latter has supervened, normalization of PRL hypersecretion by either medical or surgical means will not restore anovulation. In such patients, ovulation can only be induced by exogenous gonadotrophin therapy.

Because hyperplasia of normal pituitary lactotrophs is a normal physiological response during pregnancy, and one associated with a doubling in size of the normal pituitary, it follows that a corresponding response may also occur in neoplastic lactotrophs, producing an increase in tumor size. For microadenomas, the risk of tumor enlargement is small: Symptomatic enlargement occurs in 1.6% of cases, and radiologically evident enlargement occurs in 4.5% (53). In contrast, macroadenomas have a significantly greater propensity for pregnancy-induced growth, because symptomatic and nonsymptomatic enlargement occurs in 15.5 and 8.5% of cases, respectively (53). Among macroadenomas that have previously undergone surgical or RT ablation prior to pregnancy, the risk of regrowth during pregnancy is significantly less (4.3%).

A final issue that must be considered in caring for patients harboring prolactinomas, in whom pregnancy is either planned or established, concerns the effects of therapy on the fetus. Experience has clearly shown that bromocriptine therapy, when used as primary therapy to normalize PRL levels and restore fertility in patients who eventually conceived and discontinued bromocriptine during early pregnancy (3–4 wk), is not associated with any increased risk of spontaneous abortions or congenital abnormalities (43). Even when used throughout pregnancy, bromocriptine appears unassociated with teratogenic effects. In a review of approx 100 patients in whom bromocriptine therapy was carried out throughout pregnancy, the only abnormalities were an undescended testicle in one infant and a talipes deformity in another (43). As a general principle, fetal exposure to bromocriptine should be as short as possible; however, the available data do suggest that exposure throughout pregnancy is probably safe. Similar reassuring data are not available concerning the safety of other dopamine agonists. Regarding surgery during pregnancy, it is known that surgery of any type carries some risk of fetal loss. When performed during the first trimester, a 1.5-fold increase in fetal loss can be expected, which increased to fivefold increase during the latter part of pregnancy (54). Based on the available data, it can be argued that surgery places the fetus at greater risk than does continuous bromocriptine therapy during pregnancy.

Management In the patient with a microprolactinoma who desires pregnancy, both bromocriptine and surgery have comparable rates (80–85%) of restoring fertility. In patients treated with bromocriptine, therapy should be stopped at the first sign of pregnancy. Such patients should have careful clinical examinations throughout pregnancy to identify the exceptional microadenoma that might enlarge. Because PRL levels normally rise during the first trimester, these are uninformative regarding to the status of the tumor.

In the patient with a macroprolactinoma who desires pregnancy, several management options exist, each of which is directed at avoiding the 15–35% risk of tumor enlargement that occurs during pregnancy. The more conservative approach, one preferable to the authors, begins with primary resection of the macroprolactinoma, with the objective of a curative resection. Should hyperprolactinemia and ovulatory failure persist postoperatively, bromocriptine is used to restore fertility. Pregnancy in this setting will be associated with a greatly reduced risk (4.5%) of tumor expansion. A second approach involves treating the patient initially with bromocriptine to restore fertility, withdrawing therapy at the first sign of pregnancy, and carefully monitoring the patient throughout the pregnancy with serial clinical and neuro-ophthalmologic evaluations. Should symptomatic tumor enlargement occur, the options include urgent surgical resection or reinstitution of bromocriptine for the duration of the pregnancy. Although it is

true that bromocriptine has been safely taken throughout pregnancy, not all patients or their physicians will be comfortable with this option. For such patients, transsphenoidal surgery, even with the aforementioned risks of fetal loss, will be a preferable alternative.

Clearly, the management of prolactinomas in preparation of or during pregnancy is a complicated issue for which there is no right answer that will be applicable in all situations. The approach must be highly individualized and will ultimately rest on the preferences of a well-informed patient with whom the alternatives of management have been clearly discussed.

GH-SECRETING PITUITARY ADENOMAS

In the overwhelming majority of acromegalic patients, including all those in whom biochemical remission has been achieved, as well as those in whom GH levels have been significantly reduced but not normalized, prompt regression of several symptoms can be expected postoperatively. Headache frequently improves immediately, which, over the next few days, is followed by improvements in hyperhydrosis, paresthesias, and regression of soft tissue swelling. Such responses tend to be the rule, being observed to some degree in 97% of surgically treated patients (55). Diabetes also responds to surgery in a predictably favorable fashion: For patients in whom GH levels are normalized, resolution of diabetes and/or glucose intolerance have been reported in up to 80–100% of cases (56,57). Significant improvements in glucose tolerance can also be expected in patients in whom surgery reduces, but fails to normalize, GH levels. Hypertension tends to be considerably less responsive to surgery than are the other acromegalic features (56,57). Although some improvement in blood pressure has been noted postoperatively, hypertension often persists, sometimes even after successful surgery.

Hyperprolactinemia, accompanying approx 40–50% of somatotroph adenomas, is frequently the result of a bihormonal tumor capable of both GH and PRL hypersecretion. Of acromegalic women of child-bearing age, approx one-half will have amenorrhea (58). The authors previously reported on a series of six such amenorrheic females, of whom four experienced p/o resumption of menses; two of these eventually conceived (59). A comparable response has been reported by others (60).

Symptomatic mass effects can be expected to respond to surgery in the majority of instances. Improvements in visual fields have been reported in 90–100% of patients (59,61,62).

Defining Endocrinologic Remission Although it has been recognized for some time that the completeness of surgical resection must ultimately be judged on the basis of measurable endocrinologic parameters, there has been a distinct lack of uniformity in the specific endocrinologic criteria that investigators have used to define remission or cure. It is now clear that the criteria employed to define remission in earlier series, such as reduction of basal GH levels to less than 10 ng/mL, may have been too liberal; patients thought to have been cured on this basis were in fact not cured, and continued to have active acromegaly (63–65). As a result, and particularly during the past decade, the concept of cure in acromegaly has evolved considerably, and some consensus now exists about the minimum biochemical criteria that must underlie its definition. First, it is preferable to speak in terms of remission rather than cure, because the long-term outcome of surgically treated somatotroph adenomas is still not definitively known, and no endocrinologic criteria, however stringent, can absolutely guarantee that the patient will remain free of disease in the future.

Table 5
Results of Primary Transsphenoidal Surgery for GH-secreting Pituitary Adenomas

Series	Number	Remission rates				Remission criteria
		Total series	Microadenomas	Macroadenoma		
Teasdale et al., 1982 *(75)*	28	19/28 (68%)	N/A	N/A		GH <5.0 ng/mL
Serri et al., 1985 *(76)*	25	21/25 (84%)	8/8 (100%)	13/17 (77%)		GH <5 ng/mL; and GH <2.5 ng/mL on OGTT
Roelfsema et al., 1985 *(77)*	60	37/60 (62%)	6/9 (67%)	31/51 (61%)		GH ≤2.5 ng/mL
Grisoli et al., 1985 *(62)*	100	60/100 (60%)	N/A	N/A		GH <5 ng/mL
van't Verlaat et al., 1988 *(78)*	25	14/25 (56%)	N/A	N/A		GH <5 ng/mL and GH ≤2 ng/mL on OGTT
Ross and Wilson, 1988 *(73)*	153[a]	86/153 (56%)	N/A	N/A		GH <5 ng/mL
Losa et al., 1989 *(79)*	29	16/29 (55%)	N/A	N/A		GH <1 ng/mL on OGTT and normal IGF-I level
Valdemarsson et al., 1991 *(72)*	38	28/38 (74%)	11/13 (85%)	17/25 (68%)		GH <5 ng/mL and/or GH <3.0 ng/mL on OGTT
Fahlbusch et al., 1992 *(69)*	222	126/222 (57%)	53/74 (72%)	73/150 (49%)		GH <2 ng/mL during OGTT
		158/222 (71%)	60/74 (81%)	98/150 (65%)		GH <5 ng/mL
Tindall et al., 1993 *(80)*	91[b]	75/91 (82%)	N/A	N/A		GH <5 ng/mL and/or normal IGF-I level
Davis et al., 1993[c] *(81)*	174	(52%)	N/A	N/A		GH ≤2 ng/mL (basal or during OGTT)
Sheaves et al., 1996 *(66)*	100	42/100 (42%)[d]	(61%)	(23%)		GH ≤2.5 ng/mL
Authors' series (1988–97)	117	64/117 (55%)	16/22 (73%)	48/95 (50.5%)		GH ≤2.5 ng/mL; and GH ≤1 ng/mL during OGTT; and normal IGF-I level

[a]Results from 153 patients who did not have prior therapy, from a total series of 214 patients, are included here.
[b]Results from 91 patients who did not have prior therapy, from a total series of 103 patients, are included here.
[c]2.25% of patients in this series had p/o radiation therapy.
[d]Six patients achieving surgical remission were also given p/o radiation therapy.

Currently, and in addition to a favorable clinical response, the operational definition of endocrinologic remission in acromegaly requires suppression of GH levels to less than 1 ng/mL during an oral glucose tolerance test and normalization of the age-adjusted plasma IGF-I levels *(64–69)*. In virtually all instances, patients fulfilling these criteria will also have basal GH levels of less than 5 ng/mL, but, because the converse is often, but not necessarily, true, there has been a move away from using this, or, for that matter, any specific basal or random GH level as the sole remission criterion. Moreover, it can be argued that the value of a GH level <5 ng/mL, despite its widespread use in reporting surgical results historically, is still an arbitrary therapeutic end point. If remission is to be based on any critical GH level, the only prognostically justifiable criterion is a mean GH level <2.5 ng/mL. Reductions of mean GH levels below this threshold have been identified as the most important factor associated with reducing mortality in acromegaly *(70)*. Accordingly, if lowering of GH levels is to be used as a measure of surgical success, reduction below this value would, in this context, represent a reasonable therapeutic end point. Other endocrinologic outcome criteria have been proposed, such as p/o normalization of a previously paradoxical response to thyrotropin-releasing hormone (TRH) or the somewhat laborious verification that the 24-h integrated GH level has normalized *(64,71)*. Although some have found that a persistent paradoxical GH response to thyrotropin-releasing hormone indicative of residual tumor and a higher risk for biochemical recurrence *(71)*, others have questioned the prognostic merits of this test and the necessity of its inclusion in the definition of p/o remission *(69,72)*.

Reported Rates of Endocrine Remission Despite of the difficulties in defining p/o endocrinologic remission in acrome-

galy and the variations in remission criteria used by different investigators, a large body of data does exist for evaluating the results of operative therapy for somatotroph adenomas. Using a p/o GH level of <5 ng/mL as the remission criterion, Ross and Wilson *(73)* analyzed the results of 30 published surgical series, and identified an overall endocrine remission rate of 60% in 771 patients. Similar results were reported by Zervas in a multicenter survey *(74)*. Of 1256 acromegalic patients in whom the minimum of several remission criteria included basal GH level <5 ng/mL, an overall rate of endocrine remission was 66%. These composite data also compare with the results of individual series from the literature *(62,66,69,72,73,75–81)*. When surgery is used as the sole primary therapy, and in the absence of any prior therapy, endocrine remission can be expected in 42–84% of patients (Table 5). Understandably, with the application of more rigorous remission criteria, such as those outline above, rates of surgical success are lower. This is illustrated in the 222 patient series of Fahlbusch et al. *(69)* wherein a 71% remission rate was observed when the GH <5 ng/mL was used, but which dropped to 57% when remission was defined on the basis of suppressibility of GH to <2 ng/mL on an oral glucose tolerance test (OGTT). Similarly, Losa et al. *(79)* reported a remission rate of 55% when GH <1 ng/mL and normal IGF-I levels were used to define remission.

As discussed below, tumor size and invasion status have a clear influence on surgical outcome. Understandably, remission rates will be highest for microadenomas, tending to drop somewhat for diffuse macroadenomas, and dropping very significantly for invasive macroadenomas and those with extrasellar extension. For microadenomas, p/o endocrine remission has been variably reported in 66–100% of somatotroph microadenomas (Table 5). When all

Table 6
Rates Of Somatotroph Adenoma Recurrence after Prior Successful Surgery

Series	No. of patients in remission	Recurrence rate %	Mean follow-up (yr)	Original remission criteria
Serri et al., 1985 (76)	21	14.3	8.9	GH <2.5 ng/mL during OGTT
Grisoli et al., 1985 (62)	60	10.0	N/A	GH <5 ng/mL
Ross et al., 1988 (73)	117	4.3	6.3	GH <5 ng/mL
Landolt et al., 1988 (82)	169	2.4	4.1	GH <5 ng/mL
van't Verlaat et al., 1988 (78)	14	0.0	3.5	GH <2 ng/mL during OGTT
Losa et al., 1989 (79)	16	0.0	2.9	GH <1 ng/mL during OGTT and normal IGF-I level
Buchfelder et al., 1991 (83)	61	6.6	6.0	GH <5 ng/mL
Buchfelder et al., 1991 (83)	63	0.0	6.5	GH <2 ng/mL during OGTT
Davis et al., 1993 (81)	90[a]	17.8	5.8	GH <2 ng/mL (fasting or on OGTT)
Sheaves et al., 1996 (66)	32[b]	3.1	3.8	GH <2.5 ng/mL

[a]25% of patients in this series had p/o radiation therapy.
[b]Includes only those patients in whom surgery was the only treatment.

macroadenomas are considered, including all grades of invasion and extrasellar extension, p/o remission has been reported in 49–77% of patients. When remission rates of diffuse (i.e., grade II) and invasive (i.e., grade III–IV) macroadenomas are separated, however, the outcome among the latter is considerable less favorable. Among grades II, III, and IV tumors, Tindall et al. (80) reported remission rates of 60, 23.1, and 0%, respectively. A relationship between tumor size/grade and outcome was less obvious in the series of Ross and Wilson (73): Aside from grade IV tumors, which had a remission rate of 23%, the remission rates for grade II and III tumors in that series were similar (57%). In the authors' series of 445 acromegalic patients, using GH less than 2 ng/mL as the remission criterion, remission rates for microadenomas, diffuse macroadenomas, and invasive macroadenomas were 65, 55, and 52%, respectively.

Tumor Recurrence   In considering the problem of recurrence, an initial distinction should be made between the genuine recurrence of a previously removed tumor and the regrowth of a persistent, incompletely excised tumor. In this context, the authors strictly adopt the former definition and consider recurrence as new tumor growth after gross total removal and/or the relapse of active acromegaly after a sustained and well-documented period of endocrine remission. Understandably, the rate of recurrence in acromegaly will depend on the stringency of the criteria with which remission was originally defined, as well as the period of follow-up. When strict criteria are used to define remission, such a suppression of GH levels to <1 ng/mL on an OGTT and normalization of IGF-I levels, a durable remission is usually achieved, and recurrence tends to be infrequent. The rate of recurrence in several large series has ranged from 0 to 18% during mean follow-up periods of 2.9–8.9 yr; in aggregate, the rate of recurrence in these nine series was approx 6% (Table 6; 62,66,73,76,78,81–83). Of surgically treated acromegalic patients in whom endocrine remission had been achieved, the authors have encountered an 8% recurrence rate during a 10-yr follow-up period (51). The series of Davis et al. (81) emphasizes the importance of long-term follow-up and the tendency of recurrences to increase with time. In that report, an overall recurrence rate of 18% was noted.

CORTICOTROPH ADENOMAS   Once it has been established that the etiology for hypercortisolism is a corticotroph adenoma, surgery remains the undisputed therapy of first choice (34,51,84–90). In fact, the merits of transsphenoidal surgery are

particularly well illustrated in the treatment of corticotroph adenomas, in which selective removal of the adenoma, cure of hypercortisolemia, and preservation of normal glandular function are all reasonable therapeutic expectations of the procedure. With most adenomas being only a few millimeters in size, together with their frequent deep location within the gland, simply finding the adenoma is perhaps the biggest operative challenge. This is especially true when the tumor is not visualized on preoperative imaging studies. What is generally required is a careful and systematic dissection of the sellar contents. If a tumor is not evident upon opening the dura, or after examining all glandular surfaces, the gland must be incised and systematically explored. To the experienced surgeon, subtle changes in tissue color and texture will aid in the identification of an adenoma, and in distinguishing it from the normal gland. If no adenoma is found, excisional biopsies from within the substance of the gland are obtained, beginning with the central mucoid wedge. If an adenoma is not evident in the resected material, the lateral wings of the gland are carefully inspected and resected as necessary. In the adult patient in whom an adenoma cannot be identified by this stage, and for whom fertility is not an issue, a subtotal hypophysectomy is generously performed, leaving only a stump of residual anterior lobe tissue attached to the stalk. If careful examination of the resected tissues still fails to reveal an adenoma, both cavernous sinuses must be evaluated, as well as the posterior lobe; the latter has, on rare occasion, been known to harbor a minute adenomatous nodule. Failing to see an adenoma by now, the surgeon must at least consider the possibility of a supradiaphragmatic tumor nodule. Given the additional operative risks of a diaphragmatic breach, one would not ordinarily contemplate transdiaphragmatic exploration without clear imaging evidence pointing to such a possibility.

In the authors' experience of some 380 patients with Cushing's disease, curative resections can be achieved in more than 90% of microadenomas and in 60% of macroadenomas. Comparable results have been reported by others (see Table 7). Whether or not surgical cure has been achieved is generally evident by the second or third p/o day. Morning cortisol levels should be less than 5 μg/dL, and serum ACTH levels should be undetectable, if the procedure is to be considered curative. In the occasional patient in whom a curative result has also been obtained, the decline in cortisol levels may be less precipitous, with subnormal cortisol levels

Table 7
Results of Primary Transsphenoidal Surgery for Cushing's Disease

Series	No. of patients	Remission rates						
		Micro	Macro	Other pathology	Remission rate		Recurrence rate		Follow-up period
Chandler et al., 1987 (85)	34	21	3	10[a]	25/34	(74%)	Not stated		Not stated
Nakane et al., 1987 (86)	100	76	17	7[b]	86/100	(86%)	8/86	(9%)	3.2 yr (mean)
Guilhaume et al., 1988 (87)	64	36	4	24[c]	42/64	(66%)	6/42	(14%)	2 yr (median)
Mampalam et al., 1988 (88)	216	135	36	45[d]	171/216	(79%)	9/171	(5%)	3.9 yr (mean)
Tindall et al., 1990 (89)	53	37	7	9[e]	45/53	(85%)	1/45	(2%)	4.8 yr (mean)
Bochicchio et al., 1995 (84)	668[f]	Not stated	Not stated		510/668	(76%)	65/510	(8%)	3.8 yr (mean)
Petrusen et al., 1997 (34)	31	28	3		24/31	(77%)	1/24	(4%)	4.5 yr (median)
Blevins et al., 1998 (90)	21[g]		21		14/21	(67%)	5/14	(36%)	5.2 yr (mean)

[a]Ectopic ACTH syndrome (2 cases); presumed adenoma, but not histologically verified (4 cases); unknown pathology (4 cases).
[b]Nontumorous pituitary gland (7 cases).
[c]Nontumorous pituitary gland (22 cases); no surgical tissue (2 cases).
[d]No abnormal tissue (38 cases); ectopic ACTH syndrome (5 cases); hyperplasia (2 cases).
[e]No abnormal tissue (7 cases); hyperplasia (2 cases).
[f]Data based on a multicenter retrospective survey of the European Cushing's Disease Survey Group.
[g]Series consisted of macroadenomas only.

being evident only after several days. As a rule, a p/o AM cortisol level that persists within the normal range, even if it represents a dramatic decrease from the pretreatment level, almost always indicates incomplete removal and persistent disease. For those patients successfully treated, regression of Cushingoid features and restitution of the pituitary–adrenal axis occur within months. Patients routinely relate feelings of full rejuvenation, both physically and emotionally. Depending on the extent of glandular resection, hormonal replacement may be required, although this will be a long-term requirement for only a minority of patients. Once remission has been achieved, biochemical or radiologic recurrence is uncommon; approx 12% of patients can be expected to recur, although some do so many years after successful surgery (34,51,84–90).

In patients not initially cured by surgery, four options remain: repeat transsphenoidal exploration, medical therapy, radiation therapy, and bilateral adrenalectomy. The latter three modalities are discussed below. When confronted with such a situation, the surgeon must first ascertain the cause of failed surgery. In some situations, such as with laterally extending invasive adenomas, complete excision is not a reasonable expectation of the procedure, thus the issue of repeat exploration does not arise. A more common scenario, however, relates to an inability to definitively find and remove the tumor, which is either the result of technical issues or because of a diagnostic error (i.e., the cause of hypercortisolemia is not a pituitary tumor). At this point, all preoperative diagnostic studies should be carefully reevaluated, and the diagnosis of pituitary dependent disease should be reaffirmed. If bilateral inferior petrosal sinus (IPS) sampling was not performed preoperatively, it would clearly be indicated at this time. Assuming all studies continue to point to a pituitary tumor, some consideration of sellar re-exploration should be given, although the viability and effectiveness of this option will depend on the surgeon's impression of the completeness of the initial resection.

Nelson-Salassa Syndrome Transsphenoidal surgery for corticotroph adenomas in the context of Nelson's syndrome remains primarily a palliative procedure. Surgical resection and re-resections are, however, sometimes necessary to control mass

effect among the larger tumors. The authors' surgical experience with Nelson's syndrome includes approx 60 patients. In approximately one-half of these, surgical resection was followed by lessening of hyperpigmentation and significant reductions in serum ACTH levels. In only 27% of patients, however, was a curative result achieved, as evidenced by normalization of the initial ACTH level. For patients not controlled by surgery, and in those not previously irradiated RT is recommended. Because of the adenoma's aggressive nature, and in spite of all therapeutic interventions possible, as many as 20% of patients will eventually succumb to uncontrolled local tumor growth.

THYROTROPH ADENOMAS Accounting for less than 1% of all pituitary adenomas, the thyrotroph adenoma is the rarest functional pituitary tumor type. Beck-Peccoz et al. (91) in a comprehensive literature review of thyrotroph adenomas, identified some 280 examples. Most thyrotroph adenomas will present with the classic signs and symptoms of hyperthyroidism. Ordinarily, a diffusely enlarged thyroid gland will be demonstrable. Because these tumors can also co-secrete GH, a small proportion of patients will present with true acromegaly. Depending on the tumor size and degree of glandular and/or stalk compression, hypopituitarism and moderate hyperprolactinemia may be additional features of an endocrine presentation. Neurologic symptomatology is also common, particularly in those having undergone prior thyroidectomy, in whom it may be the dominant mode of presentation. In one literature review (92), more than one-half of all patients had demonstrable visual field defects at presentation. Of cases cited in the literature, approx one-third were confined to the sella, one-third extended beyond the sella, and one-third exhibited gross invasion of parasellar structures (91).

Surgical resection, RT and medical therapy with somatostatin analogs are all therapeutic options for thyrotroph adenomas. Surgery is the clear first choice and should be initially considered in all patients in whom a thyrotroph adenoma is suspected. Because the majority of cases reported to date have been large and/or invasive lesions that had often been subject to considerable diagnostic delay and possible disinhibiting effects of thyroidectomy, biochemical remission can be achieved in only the minority of patients. Of 177 cases reviewed by Beck-Peccoz et al. *(91)* surgery alone was curative in only 33%. The majority of patients, however, required postoperative adjuvant radiotherapy to control thyrotropin hypersecretion. Similarly, in the single-institution study reported by the National Institutes of Health, involving the treatment and follow-up of 22 surgically treated patients, a 35% surgical remission rate was achieved *(93)*. Of patients in whom surgery does not induce remission, somatostatin analogs and radiation alone or in combination represent important adjuvants.

CLINICALLY NONFUNCTIONING PITUITARY TUMORS

Included in the class of clinically nonfunctional pituitary adenomas are the null cell adenoma, oncocytoma, and silent adenomas (subtypes 1–3) *(19)*. It is customary and convenient to also include the gonadotroph adenoma in this class. The latter are hormonally active lesions that may secrete gonadotrophic hormones in measurable excess, but such secretion is unassociated with a clinically evident hypersecretory state. Accordingly, clinically nonfunctioning tumors present with the neurologic, visual, and endocrine sequelae of progressive intrasellar mass.

Surgery is the primary treatment of choice for this class of tumors. Surgical objectives involve the elimination of mass effect, restoration of neurologic and visual function, and preservation/restoration of pituitary function. Although gross total removal remains an intuitive surgical goal for all pituitary tumors, and should certainly be attempted to the extent that is safely possible, it will not be a realistic expectation nor will it be an absolute necessity for many nonfunctioning adenomas. For example, in the elderly patient in whom progressive visual loss is the only presenting feature, a radical procedure that attempts total surgical resection may be less prudent than a satisfactory but less radical and less dangerous decompression. Because of the relatively slow growth of these tumors and their usual occurrence among elderly patients, symptomatic recurrence is generally a less serious and a less frequent threat than it is for most functioning adenomas. Guided by these principles, the surgical outcome in the authors' series of over 850 nonfunctioning tumors has been quite satisfactory. Among a cohort of 100 patients systematically analyzed and followed for 10 yr or more, the operative mortality was 2%; both patients had undergone prior therapy for large tumors *(94)*. Symptoms referable to mass effect, such as headache and cavernous sinus compression, were almost always relieved. Among all patients presenting with progressive visual field and acuity deficits, p/o improvement occurred in 87%, stabilization was achieved in 9%, and only 4% suffered further visual deterioration *(61,95)*.

Preservation of pituitary function can be routinely achieved, but restoration of established deficits is far more difficult. Among patients without preoperative hypopituitarism, 97% retained normal pituitary function postoperatively. Of patients with established preoperative endocrine deficits, partial or complete restoration was achieved in only 16%. The experience of Arafah et al. *(96)* was somewhat more optimistic, with some 60% of patients experiencing improvement in one or more hormonal axes. Permanent DI occurred in 3–5% of patients *(94,97)*.

Symptomatic recurrence develops in relatively few patients. In the authors' experience, recurrence was documented in 16/100 patients, only six of whom were symptomatic and in need of subsequent therapy *(94)*. During the 10-yr follow-up period, the overall outcome was quite favorable, with 76% of patients enjoying symptom-free and/or progression-free survival. Comparable results were reported by Bradley et al. *(98)*, who documented a 90% recurrence free survival over a 5-yr period. A somewhat higher symptomatic recurrence rate was reported by Comtois et al. *(97)*. In a cohort of 71 patients, all of whom had gross total tumor resection, and were followed for a mean period of more than 6 yr, symptomatic recurrence occurred in 15 (21%).

Although it was once common practice to administer p/o RT to all incompletely excised tumors, this has generally been abandoned as a routine strategy. Nowadays, RT is employed in a far more selective fashion, generally being reserved for those patients in whom rapid progression can be documented. For the more indolent and slow-growing lesions, when years may pass before symptomatic recurrence, repeat resection is generally preferable to RT. Among the more aggressive variants that appear destined for prompt regrowth, adjuvant RT is recommended. Stereotactic radiosurgery may be useful in such circumstances.

CONCLUSION

Surgical management of pituitary adenomas continues to be a safe and effective method for treating many patients with these lesions. The goal of overall management should be to provide the patient with the most effective means of long-term control of this benign but potentially disabling disease. Currently, surgery has an important role. As understanding of pituitary pathophysiology continues to advance and new pharmacologic adjuvants and primary therapies are developed, it is expected that surgical management of these lesions will become even more focused, more precise, and more effective over time.

REFERENCES

1. Caton R, Paul F. Notes on a case of acromegaly treated by operation. Br Med J 1893;2:1421–1423.
2. Horsely V. On operative technique of operations on the central nervous system. Br Med J 1906;2:411–423.
3. Schloffer H. Erfolgreiche Operation eines Hypophysentumors auf nasalem Wege. Wiener klinische Wochenschrift 1907;20:621–624.
4. von Eisenberg A. Operations upon the hypophysis. Ann Surg 1910;52:1–14.
5. Hochenegg J. Operative cure of acromegaly by removal of a hypophysial tumor. Ann Surg 1908;??:781–784.
6. Halstead A. Remarks on the operative treatment of tumors of the hypophysis: with the report of two cases operated on by an oro-nasal method. Trans Am Surg Assoc 1910;28:73–93.
7. Cushing H. Partial hypophysectomy for acromegaly. Ann Surg 1909;50:1002–1017.
8. Kanavel A. The removal of tumors of the pituitary body. JAMA 1909;53:1704–1707.
9. Hirsch O. Endonasal method of removal of hypophyseal tumors: with report of two cases. JAMA 1910;55:772–774.
10. Guiot G, Arfel G, Brion S, et al. Adenomes Hypophysaires. Masson, Paris, 1958, pp. 276.
11. Hardy J. Transsphenoidal surgery of the normal and pathological pituitary. Clin Neurosurg 1969;16:185–217.
12. Thapar K, Kovacs K, Muller P. Clinical-pathologic correlations of pituitary tumors. Bailliére Clin Endocrinol Metab 1995;9:243–270.
13. Thorner MO, Vance ML, Horvath E, Kovacs K. The anterior pituitary. In: Wilson JD, Foster DW, eds. Williams Textbook of Endocrinology. W.B. Saunders, Philadelphia, 1992, pp. 221–310.
14. Molitch M. Incidental pituitary adenomas. Am J Med Sci 1993;306: 264–264.
15. Chong B, Kucharczyk W, Singer W, et al. Pituitary gland MR: a comparative study of healthy volunteers and patients with microadenomas. AJNR 1994;15:675–679.
16. Laws ER Jr. Surgical management of pituitary apoplexy. In: Welch K, Caplan L, Reis D, et al., eds. Primer on Cerebrovascular Diseases. Academic, New York, 1997, pp. 508–510.

17. Ebersold MJ, Laws ER Jr, Scheithauer BW, Randall RV. Pituitary apoplexy treated by transsphenoidal surgery: a clinicopathological and immunocytochemical study. J Neurosurg 1983;58: 315–320.

18. Bills D, Meyer F, Laws E, Davis D, Ebersold M, Scheithauer B, Ilstrup D, Abboud C. Retrospective analysis of pituitary apoplexy. Neurosurgery 1993;33:602–609.

19. Thapar K, Kovacs K. Tumors of the sellar region. In: Bigner DD, McLendon RE, Bruner JM, eds. Russel and Rubinstein's pathology of tumors of the nervous system. 6th ed. Williams & Wilkins, Baltimore, 1998, pp. 561–677.

20. Barrow D, Tindall G, Tindall S. Combined simultaneous transsphenoidal transcranial operative approach to selected sellar tumors. Perspect Neurol Surg 1992;3:49–57.

21. Laws ER Jr. Transsphenoidal approach to pituitary tumors. In: Schmidek HH, Sweet WH, eds. Operative Neurosurgical Techniques, vol. 1, 3rd ed. W.B. Saunders, Philadelphia, 1995, pp. 283–292.

22. Laws ER Jr. Transsphenoidal surgery. In: Apuzzo MLJ, ed. Brain Surgery: Complication Avoidance and Management, vol. 1. Churchill Livingstone, New York, 1993, pp. 357–362.

23. Messick JM, Laws ER Jr, Abboud CF. Anesthesia for transsphenoidal surgery of the hypophyseal region. Anesth Analg 1978;57:206–210.

24. Wilson WR, Laws ER. Transnasal septal displacement approach for secondary transsphenoidal pituitary surgery. Laryngoscope 1992; 102:951–953.

25. Jho HD, Carrau RL. Endoscopic endonasal transsphenoidal surgery: experience with 50 patients. J Neurosurg 1997;87:44–51.

26. Zervas NT. Surgical results for pituitary adenomas: results of an international survey. In: Black PM, Zervas NT, Ridgeway EC, Martin J, eds. Secretory Tumors of the Pituitary Gland. Raven, New York, 1984, pp. 377–385.

27. Laws ER Jr, Kern EB. Complications of transsphenoidal surgery. In: Laws ER, Randall RV, Kern EB, Abboud CF, eds. Management of pituitary adenomas and related lesions with emphasis on transsphenoidal microsurgery. Appleton Century Crofts, New York, 1982, pp. 329–346.

28. Laws ER, Fode NC, Redmond MJ. Transsphenoidal surgery following unsuccessful prior therapy: An assessment of benefits and risks in 158 patients. J Neurosurg 1985;63:823–829.

29. Laws ER Jr, Thapar K. Pituitary Surgery. Endocrinol Metab Clin N Am 1999;28:119–131.

30. Laws ER. Pituitary Tumors. In: Little JR, Awad IA, eds. Reoperative Neurosurgery. Williams and Wilkins, Baltimore, 1992, pp. 106–112.

31. Rand R. Transfrontal transsphenoidal craniotomy in pituitary and related tumors. In: Rand R, ed. Microneurosurgery, vol. 1. Mosby, St. Louis, 1978, pp. 93–104.

32. Fahlbusch R, Honegger J. Extended transsphenoidal approach to the pituitary region and upper clivus. In: Torrens M, Al-Mefty O, Kobayashi S, eds. Operative skull base surgery. Churchill Livingstone, New York, 1997, pp. 69–88.

33. Laws E. Clivus chordomas. In: Sekhar L, Janecka I, eds. Surgery of cranial base tumors. Raven, New York, 1993, pp. 679–686.

34. Petruson K, Jakobsson K, Oetryseib B, Lindstedt G, Bengtsson B. Transsphenoidal adenomectomy in Cushing's disease via a lateral rhinotomy approach. Surg Neurol 1997;48:37–45.

35. Torrens M, Kazanas S. Alternative endonasal and paranasal approaches. In: Torrens M, Al-Mefty O, Kobayashi S, eds. Operative Skull Base Surgery. Churchill Livingstone, New York, 1997, pp. 89–105.

36. Hoyt TE, Turnbull FM, Kusske JA. Transantral transsphenoidal approach to the pituitary. J Neurosurg 1983;59:1102–1104.

37. Fujitsu K. Cranio-orbito-zygomatic approach to the skull base. In: Torrens M, Al-Mefty O, Kobayashi S, eds. Operative Skull Base Surgery. Churchill Livingstone, New York, 1997, pp. 189–205.

38. Sekhar L, Nanda A, Sen C, et al. Extended frontal approach to tumors of the anterior, middle, and posterior skull base. J Neurosurg 1992;76:198–206.

39. Derome P, Akerman M, Anquez L. Les tumeurs spheno-ethmoidales. Possibilities d'exerese et de reparation chirurgicales. Neurochirurgie 1972;18(Suppl):1–164.

40. Thapar K, Laws E. Current management of prolactin-secreting tumors. In: Salcman M, ed. Current Techniques in Neurosurgery. Current Medicine, Philadelphia, 1998, pp. 175–190.

41. Randall RV, Laws ER, Jr, Abboud CF, et al. Transsphenoidal microsurgical treatment of prolactin-producing pituitary adenomas: results in 100 patients. Mayo Clin Proc 1983;58:108–121.

42. Landolt AM. Surgical treatment of pituitary prolactinomas: postoperative prolactin and fertility in seventy patients. Fert Steril 1981;36:620–625.

43. Molitch ME. Pathologic hyperprolactinemia. Endocrinol Metab Clin N Am 1992;21:877–901.

44. Randall RV, Scheithauer BW, Laws ER Jr, et al. Pituitary adenomas associated with hyperprolactinemia: a clinical and immunohistochemical study of 97 patients operated on transsphenoidally. Mayo Clin Proc 1985;53:24–28.

45. Serri O, Rasio E, Beauregard H, Hardy J, Somma M. Recurrence of hyperprolactinemia after selective transsphenoidal adenomectomy in women with prolactinoma. N Engl J Med 1983;309:280–283.

46. Perrin G, Treluyer C, Trouillas J, et al. Surgical outcome and pathological effects of bromocriptine pretreatment in prolactinomas. Pathol Res Prac 1991;187:587–592.

46a. Weiss MH, Teal J, Goss P, et al. Natural history of microprolactinomas: six-year followup. Neurosurgery 12:640–642.

47. Hubbard J, Scheithauer B, Abboud C, Laws E. Prolactin-secreting adenomas: the preoperative response to bromocriptine treatment and surgical outcomes. J Neurosurg 1987;67:816–821.

48. Wilson C. A decade of pituitary microsurgery: the Herbert Olivecrona Lecture. J Neurosurg 1984;61:814–833.

49. Laws ER, Thapar K. Recurrent pituitary adenomas. In: Landolt A, Vance M, Reilly P, eds. Pituitary Adenomas. Churchill Livingstone, Edinburgh, 1996, pp. 385–394.

50. Post K, Habas JE. Comparison of long term results between prolactin secreting adenomas and ACTH secreting adenomas. Can J Neurol Sci 1990;17:74–77.

51. Laws ER, Chenelle AG, Thapar K. Recurrence after transsphenoidal surgery for pituitary adenomas: clinical and basic science aspects. In: von Werder K, Fahlbusch R, eds. Pituitary Adenomas: From Basic Research to Diagnosis and Therapy. Elsevier, Amsterdam, 1996, pp. 3–9.

52. Massoud F, Serri O, Hardy J, Somma M, Beauregard H. Transsphenoidal adenomectomy for microprolactinomas: 10 to 20 years of follow-up. Surg Neurol 1996;45:341–346.

53. Molitch M. Pregnancy in the hyperprolactinemic woman. N Engl J Med 1985;312:1365–1370.

54. Brodsky J, Cohen E, Brown B, Wu M, Whichter C. Surgery during pregnancy and fetal outcome. Am J Obstet Gynecol 1980;138: 1165–1167.

55. Laws ER. Neurosurgical management of acromegaly. In: Cooper PR, ed. Contemporary Diagnosis and Management of Pituitary Adenomas. American Association of Neurological Surgeons, Park Ridge, IL, 1990, pp. 53–59.

56. Balagura S, Derome P, Guiot G. Acromegaly: analysis of 132 cases treated surgically. Neurosurgery 1981;8:413–416.

57. Tucker H, Grubb S, Wigand J, Watlington C, Blackard W, Becker D. Treatment of acromegaly by transsphenoidal surgery. Arch Intern Med 1980;140:795–802.

58. Nabarro JDN. Acromegaly. J Clin Endocrinol 1987;26:481–512.

59. Laws E, Piepgras D, Randall R, Abboud C. Neurosurgical management of acromegaly. J Neurosurg 1979;50:454–461.

60. Arafah B, Brodkey J, Kaufman B, Velasco M, Manni A, Pearson O. Transsphenoidal microsurgery in the treatment of acromegaly and gigantism. J Clin Endocrinol Metab 1980;50:578–585.

61. Laws ER Jr, Trautmann JC, Hollenhorst RW Jr. Transsphenoidal decompression of the optic nerve and chiasm: visual results in 62 patients. J Neurosurg 1977;46:717–722.

62. Grisoli F, Leclercq T, Jaquet P, Guibout M, Winteler JP, Hassoun J, Vincentelli F. Transsphenoidal surgery for acromegaly: Long-term results in 100 patients. Surg Neurol 1985;23:513–519.

63. Melmed S. Acromegaly. N Engl J Med 1990;322:966–977.
64. Melmed S. Acromegaly. In: Melmed S, ed. The Pituitary. Blackwell, Cambridge, 1995, pp. 413–442.
65. Newman C, Kleinberg D. Acromegaly: How do you define cure? In: Cooper P, ed. Contemporary Diagnosis and Management of Pituitary Adenomas. American Association of Neurological Surgeons, Park Ridge, IL, 1990, pp. 47–52.
66. Sheaves R, Jenkins P, Blackburn P, Huneidi A, Afshart F, Medbak S, et al. Outcome of transsphenoidal surgery for acromegaly using strict criteria for surgical cure. Clin Endocrinol 1996;45:407–413.
67. Lindholm J, Giwercman B, A G, Astrup J, Bjerre P, Skakkebaek N. Investigation of the criteria for assessing the outcome of treatment in acromegaly. Clin Endocrinol 1987;27:553–562.
68. Klibanski A, Zervas NT. Diagnosis and management of hormone-secreting pituitary adenomas. N Engl J Med 1991;324:822–831.
69. Fahlbusch R, Honegger J, Buchfelder M. Surgical management of acromegaly. Endocrinol Metab Clin N Am 1992;21:669–692.
70. Bates A, Van't Hoff W, Jones J, Clayton R. Audit on the outcome of acromegaly. Q J Med 1993;86:293–299.
71. Arafah B, Rosenzweig J, Fenstermaker R, Salazar R, McBride C, Selman W. Value of growth hormone dynamics and somatostatin C (insulin-like growth factor 1) levels in predicting the long-term benefit after transsphenoidal surgery for acromegaly. J Lab Clin Med 1987;109:346–354.
72. Valdemarsson S, Bramnert M, Cronquist S, Elner A, Eneroth C, Hedner P, et al. Early postoperative basal serum GH level and the GH response to TRH in relation to the long-term outcome of surgical treatment for acromegaly: a report on 39 patients. J Intern Med 1991;230:49–54.
73. Ross DA, Wilson CB. Results of transsphenoidal microsurgery for growth hormone-secreting pituitary adenoma in a series of 214 patients. J Neurosurg 1988;68:854–867.
74. Zervas N. Multicenter surgical results in acromegaly. In: Lüdecke D, Tolis G, eds. Growth hormone, growth factors, and acromegaly. Raven, New York, 1987, pp. 253–257.
75. Teasdale G, Hay I, Beasttall G, McCruden D, Thomson J, Davies D, Grossart K, Ratcliffe J. Cryosurgery or microsurgery in the management of acromegaly. JAMA 1982;247:1289–1291.
76. Serri O, Somma M, Comtois R, Rasio E, Beauregard H, Jilwan N, Hardy J. Acromegaly: biochemical assessment of cure after long term follow-up of transsphenoidal selective adenomectomy. J Clin Endocrinol Metab 1985;61:1185–1189.
77. Roelfsema F, van Dulken H, Frölich M. Long-term results of transsphenoidal pituitary microsurgery in 60 acromegalic patients. Clin Endocrinol 1985;23:555–565.
78. van't Verlaat J, Nortier J, Hendriks M, Bosma N, Graamans K, Lubsen H, et al. Transsphenoidal microsurgery as primary treatment in 25 acromegalic patients: results and follow-up. Acta Endocrinologica (Copenh) 1988;117:154–158.
79. Losa M, Oeckler R, Schopohl J, Muller O, Alba-Lopez J, von Werder K. Evaluation of selective transsphenoidal adenomectomy by endocrinological testing and somatostatin-C measurement in acromegaly. J Neurosurg 1989;70:561–567.
80. Tindall G, Oyesiku N, Watts N, Clark R, Christy J, Adams D. Transsphenoidal adenomectomy for growth hormone secreting pituitary adenomas in acromegaly: outcome analysis and determinants of failure. J Neurosurg 1993;78:205–215.
81. Davis D, Laws EJ, Ilstrup D, Speed J, Caruso M, Shaw E, et al. Results of surgical treatment for growth hormone-secreting pituitary adenomas. J Neurosurg 1993;79:70–75.
82. Landolt AM, Illig R, Zapf J. Surgical treatment of acromegaly. In: Lamberts SWJ, ed. Sandostatin in the Treatment of Acromegaly. Springer-Verlag, Berlin, 1988, pp. 23–35.
83. Buchfelder M, Brockmeier S, Fahlbusch R, et al. Recurrence following transsphenoidal surgery for acromegaly. Horm Res 1991;35:113–118.
84. Bochicchio D, Losa M, Buchfelder M. Factors influencing the immediate and late outcome of Cushing's disease treated by transsphenoidal surgery: a retrospective study by the European Cushing's disease survey group. J Clin Endocrinol Metab 1995;80:3114–3120.
85. Chandler W, Schteingart D, Lloyd R, McKeever P, Ibarra-Perez G. Surgical treatment of Cushing's disease. J Neurosurg 1987;66:204–212.
86. Nakane T, Kuwayama A, Watanabe M, Takahashi T, Katoi T, Ichihara K, Kageyama N. Long term results of transsphenoidal adenomectomy in patients with Cushing's Disease. Neurosurgery 1987;21:218–222.
87. Guilhaume B, Bertagna X, Thomsen M, et al. Transsphenoidal pituitary surgery for the treatment of Cushing's Disease: results in 64 patients and long term follow-up studies. J Clin Endocrinol Metab 1988;66:1056–1064.
88. Mampalam TJ, Tyrell JB, Wilson CB. Transsphenoidal microsurgery for Cushing's Disease. A report of 216 cases. Ann Intern Med 1988;109:487–493.
89. Tindall GT, Herring CJ, Clark RV, Adams DA, Watts NB. Cushing's disease: results of transsphenoidal microsurgery with emphasis on surgical failures. J Neurosurg 1990;72:363–369.
90. Blevins L, Christy J, Khajavi M, Tindall G. Outcomes of therapy for Cushing's disease due to adrenocorticotropin-secreting pituitary macroadenomas. J Clin Endocrinol Metab 1998;83:63–67.
91. Beck-Peccoz P, Brucker-Davis F, Persani L, et al. Thyrotropin-secreting pituitary tumors. Endocr Rev 1996;17:610–638.
92. Greenman Y, Melmed S. Thyrotropin-secreting pituitary tumors. In: Melmed S, ed. The Pituitary. Blackwell, Cambridge MA, 1995, pp. 546–558.
93. Brucker-Davis F, Oldfield E, Skarulis M, Doppman J, Weintraub B. Thyrotropin-secreting pituitary tumors: Diagnositc criteria, thyroid hormone sensitivity, and treatment outcome in 25 patients followed at the National Institutes of Health. J Clinc Endocrinol Metab 1999;84:476–486.
94. Ebersold MJ, Quast LM, Laws ERJ, Scheithauer B, Randall RV. Longterm results in transsphenoidal removal of nonfunctioning pituitary adenomas. J Neurosurg 1986;64:713–719.
95. Trautmann JC, Laws ER Jr. Visual status after transsphenoidal surgery at the Mayo Clinic, 1971–1982. Am J Ophthalmol 1983;96:200–208.
96. Arafah B, Brodkey J, Manni A, Velasco M, Kaufman B, Pearson O. Recovery of pituitary function following removal of large nonfunctioning pituitary adenomas. Clin Endocrinol 1982;17:213–222.
97. Comtois R, Beauregard H, Somma M, Serri O, Aris-Jilwan N, Hardy J. Clinical and endocrine outcome to trans-sphenoidal microsurgery of nonsecreting pituitary adenomas. Cancer 1991;68:860–868.
98. Bradley K, Adams C, Potter C, Wheeler D, Anslow P, Burke C. Audit of selected patients with non-functioning pituitary adenoma treated by transsphenoidal surgery without irradiation. Clin Endocrinol 1994;41:655–659.

14 Medical Therapy of Pituitary Tumors

MARK E. MOLITCH, MD

INTRODUCTION

Tremendous progress has been made in medical therapy of pituitary tumors over the past 20 years, developing in an orderly fashion from information gained from basic physiology and pathophysiology. Thus, tumor-specific medications have been developed based on knowledge about the releasing and inhibiting hormones regulating pituitary hormone secretion and the receptors on pituitary cells that respond to such hormones.

Although medical therapy has traditionally been regarded as being adjunctive to surgery, in some types of tumors, viz, prolactinomas, empirically derived data from clinical trials has shown that medical therapy should, in fact, be regarded as primary, rather than secondary or adjunctive. This chapter will review the efficacy and pharmacology of the medications used to treat various types of pituitary tumors. In subsequent chapters, the place of medical therapy vs other modes of treatment will be discussed in more detail. The discussion in this chapter, for clinical relevance, is organized around tumor type, although clearly some medications can be used for different tumor types.

PROLACTINOMAS

BROMOCRIPTINE **Introduction** Bromocriptine (2-bromo-α-ergocryptine mesylate) is an ergot derivative (Figure 1) developed by Flückiger and colleagues at Sandoz Pharmaceuticals in the late 1960s for the purpose of inhibiting prolactin (PRL) secretion without the uterotonic, vasospastic properties of other ergots *(1)*. The development of this drug was a logical progression from work done years earlier by Shelesnyak *(2)*, which documented the effect of a variety of ergot alkaloids on inhibiting the formation of deciduomas in rats, which is a PRL-mediated response. Bromocriptine was initially shown by Lutterbeck et al. *(3)* to be clinically useful in suppressing nonpuerperal galactorrhea, and shortly thereafter, Besser et al. *(4)* showed that this beneficial effect was accompanied by a reduction in serum PRL levels. A great number of subsequent animal and clinical studies have confirmed this beneficial effect on galactorrhea and amenorrhea owing to hyperprolactinemia as well as on the manifestations of hyperprolactinemia in men, and it became recognized that these effects were the result of its activity as a long-acting dopamine (DA) receptor agonist *(5,6)*.

From: *Diagnosis and Management of Pituitary Tumors* (K. Thapar, K. Kovacs, B. W. Scheithauer, and R. V. Lloyd, eds.), ©Humana Press Inc., Totowa, NJ.

Pharmacology During the initial period of demonstration of the efficacy of bromocriptine in reducing PRL levels, more basic studies elucidated the mechanism of action. Although L-DOPA was found to increase PRL inhibitory activity in the hypothalamus of rats *(7)*, it was also found to decrease PRL secretion in pituitary cell cultures after decarboxylation to DA *(8,9)*. A wealth of evidence has subsequently documented that DA is the primary physiologic PRL inhibitory factor *(10)*. Bromocriptine stimulates hypothalamic DA receptors *(11)*, but ergocryptine and bromocriptine also decrease PRL synthesis by pituitary cells in vitro *(12–14)*. Dopamine (D_2) receptors have been demonstrated on normal and adenomatous lactotroph cells *(15)*, and bromocriptine has been found to bind reversibly to this receptor with high affinity *(16)*.

Bromocriptine pharmacokinetic studies show that after a single oral dose of 2.5 mg, serum levels peak after 3 h, and the nadir is observed at 7 h with very little bromocriptine detectable in the circulation after 11–14 h *(17)*. The biologic activity parallels the serum levels, but there is a continued biologic effect even with undetectable serum levels. The absorption rate from the GI tract is 25–30% with a linear relationship between peak plasma levels and dose. Only the native compound is bioactive and metabolites are inactive. There is a very high first-pass effect, with 93.6% of a dose being metabolized and only 6.5% of an absorbed dose reaching the systemic circulation unchanged *(17)*. Total urinary excretion is only 2% with virtually all of the remainder of the drug excreted via the biliary route into the feces. More than 20 metabolites have been identified in the bile, representing the products of isomerization and hydrolysis of the lysergic acid moiety, as well as oxidative attack on the proline fragment of the peptide moiety.

In rats, measurable tissue levels of bromocriptine can be found in almost all organs 2 h after an oral dose (17). Highest levels are found in liver, lung, kidney, and pituitary. Despite its very low solubility in water, bromocriptine seems to penetrate most areas of the brain. Studies in pregnant rats show low, but significant transfer of bromocriptine across the placenta, with levels in the fetus about one-fourth of that found in maternal blood *(17)*. Levels in the placenta are higher than levels in the fetus, suggesting that the placenta may act as a partial barrier to the transfer of bromocriptine.

In humans, there is little intraindividual variability in the absorption and peak blood levels achieved, but there is considerable interindividual variability *(17)*. There is also considerable variability in the PRL lowering effects of a given dose of bromocriptine that does not correlate with serum bromocriptine levels, implying differences in sensitivity to the drug *(18)*. Decreased response to bromocriptine in vivo has been shown to correspond

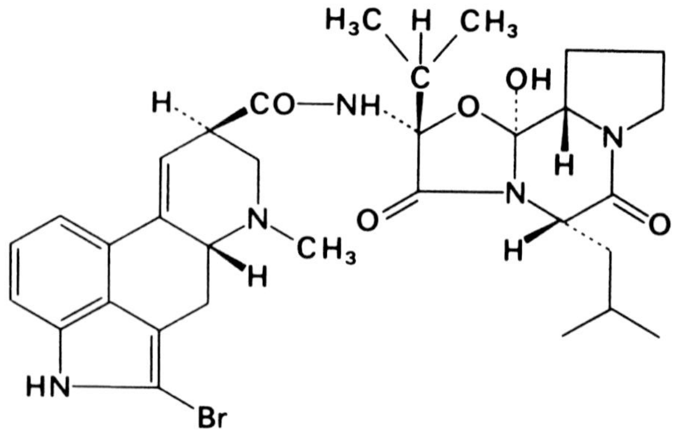

Figure 14-1 Structure of bromocriptine.

to decreased numbers of DA receptors on lactotroph cell membranes and decreased inhibition of adenyl cyclase when the same tumors are studied in vitro following surgery (19).

In vitro studies have found that bromocriptine not only decreases PRL synthesis, but also DNA synthesis, cell multiplication and tumor growth (12,13,20). Studies using DNA flow cytometry demonstrated that bromocriptine causes a decrease in cellular growth rate, an increase in the relative proportion of cells in the S-phase, and a reduced portion of cells in the G_1-phase (21). In 1971, Quadri et al. (22) also found that bromocriptine was able to decrease prolactinoma size in vivo, paving the way for human studies.

The mechanism by which bromocriptine causes tumor size reduction is essentially a turning off of the intracellular PRL-synthesizing machinery, i.e., an inhibition of transcription of PRL mRNA and PRL synthesis (14). Bergström et al. (23), using positron emission tomography (PET) scanning and ^{11}C-methionine to monitor amino acid incorporation into protein, have shown that within the first few hours of bromocriptine administration, tumor amino acid metabolism decreases by 40%, and by 7–9 d, this decreases by 70%, accompanied by marked tumor shrinkage. Morphologically, within the first 6 wk, there is a decrease in the number of exocytoses, an initial increase and later decrease in the number of PRL secretory granules, involution of the rough endoplasmic reticulum and Golgi, and a decrease in cytoplasmic volume (24–26). By 6 mo, there is a paucity of cellular organelles with numerous vacuoles, fragmented rough endoplasmic reticulum, many lysosomes, and lipofuscin granules along with aggregated chromatin in the nucleus. At that point, there is considerable breakdown of tumor cells with cytoplasmic fragmentation, macrophage infiltration, and an increase in stromal tissue and collagen fibers between cells (24–30). When bromocriptine is stopped for 1 wk before surgery after 2 wk of therapy, regrowth of tumor cells occurs with development of the rough endoplasmic reticulum and Golgi, and a decrease in the number of secretory granules (25,29). However, with longer periods of treatment, stopping bromocriptine may not result in a reversal of cell atrophy, and tumor regrowth does not always occur (30). Prolactinomas that do not regress in size, but still respond to bromocriptine with a normalization of serum PRL levels retain a considerably more normal tumor morphology (27).

Treatment to Reduce Hyperprolactinemia In several large, early studies in the literature (reviewed in ref. 31) totaling more than 400 hyperprolactinemic patients treated with bromocriptine, normoprolactinemia or return of ovulatory menses

occurred in 80–90% of patients. When both PRL levels and return of menses were studied in the same patients, it was found that substantial reductions in PRL levels to still slightly elevated levels often were enough to restore ovulation and menses, despite the fact that normal PRL levels were achieved in only 70–80% of treated patients. Patients without roentgenographic evidence of tumor responded somewhat better (88.6%) than patients with such evidence of tumor (80.7%). In other reviews of these early studies, similar response rates of 80–85% were found (6).

Treatment to Reduce Prolactinoma Size Subsequent to the initial report by Corenblum et al. (32), several individual case reports documented bromocriptine-induced tumor size reduction and a number of series of patients have now been reported. Table 1 reports the tumor size responses to bromocriptine from 19 different series of patients, totaling 236 patients with macroadenomas (24,33–50). Each series was examined carefully so that patients with combined growth hormone- (GH) and PRL-secreting tumors and those who had prior radiotherapy were excluded. In almost all of the patients, documentation of size reduction was by computed tomography (CT) scan, although in a few of the patients in earlier studies, pneumoencephalography was used; data from ordinary hypocycloidal polytomography and visual fields without these other studies were not considered acceptable for this data analysis. For some series, it appeared that patients had also been reported in earlier, less complete compilations. Only the latest publication was used, on the assumption that it represented the most complete collection of data and would prevent duplication of patients. It is possible that some of those earlier series represented different patients, but that was not clear from the publications. In some series, estimates of the amount of size change were given, whereas in others, only the fact that some response occurred was noted. Of these 236 patients analyzed (51), 77% had some tumor size decrease in response to bromocriptine with periods of observation ranging from 6 wk to over 10 yr. In their review of the literature, Bevan et al. found that 79% of subjects had >25% tumor shrinkage and 89% shrank to some degree (52).

In the large, multicenter trial conducted in the US (33), 27 patients were followed prospectively for at least 12 mo on varying doses of bromocriptine, CT scans being done at 6 wk, 6 mo, and 12 mo. Of these 27 patients, 13 (48%) had a much >50% reduction in size of their tumors (Figure 2), 5 (18.5%) had a 25–50% reduction in tumor size, and 9 (33.3%) had a <25% reduction in tumor size. In no patient was there no change. Seven other series quantitated their tumor size reductions as well (24,34,35,39,41,44,48). Including our series, this gave a total of 106 patients, out of whom 45 (42.5%) had a >50% reduction in tumor size, 30 (28.3%) had a 25–50% reduction in tumor size, 12 (11.3%) had a <25% reduction, and 19 (17.9%) had no evidence of any reduction in tumor size.

Two studies used high-resolution CT scans to determine whether bromocriptine could also reduce the size of microadenomas. Bonneville et al. (53) found that of 15 such patients, 6 tumors disappeared completely, 5 decreased approx 50% in volume, and 4 remained unchanged with treatment of 3–12 mo. Demura et al. (54) reported a reduction in size in all patients.

The time-course of tumor size reduction is variable. Some patients may experience extremely rapid decrease in tumor size, significant changes in visual fields being noted within 24–72 h, and significant changes noted on scan within 2 wk (55). In others, little change may be noted at 6 wk, but scanning again at 6 mo may show significant changes (33). In the multicenter trial cited above

Table 1
Macroadenoma Size Responses to Bromocriptine[a]

Series	Total	\>50%	25–50%	0–25%	Not quantified	No change	Duration of treatment, mo
			Tumor size reduction				
Molitch et al. (173)[b]	27	13	5	9	—	0	12
Bevan et al. (177)	7	5	2	0	—	0	1.5
Wang et al. (228)	3	3	0	0	—	0	24–144
McGregor et al. (261)	5	—	—	—	5	0	3
Sobrino et al. (262)	12	—	—	—	9	3	6
Spark et al. (263)	10	—	—	—	8	2	8–27
Nissim et al. (264)	7	4	—	—	—	3	1.5
Wass et al. (265)	14	—	—	—	9	5	3–22
Wollesen et al. (266)	4	4	—	—	—	0	15–45
Horowitz et al. (267)	6	—	—	—	3	3	6
Corenblum et al. (268)	16	—	—	—	11	5	60–108
Weiss et al. (269)	19	—	10	0	—	9	1.5
Johnston et al. (270)	14	—	—	—	10	4	18–84
Warfield et al. (271)	6	—	—	—	4	2	6
Barrow et al. (272)	11	3	2	0	—	6	1.6
Liuzzi et al. (273)	38				29	9	30–88
Pullan et al. (274)	5	4	0	1	—	0	6–24
Gasser et al. (275)	9	—	—	—	6	3	
Fahlbusch et al. (276)	23	9	11	2	—	1	0.5–1.5
Total	236	45	30	12	94	55	

[a]Reproduced with permission from Molitch ME. Prolactinoma. In: Melmed S, ed. The Pituitary. Blackwell Scientific, Boston, 1995, pp. 443–477.
[b]Numbers in parentheses are reference numbers in source.

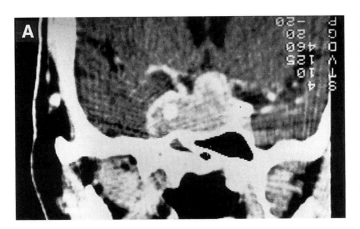

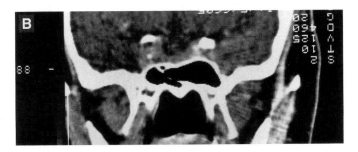

Figure 14-2 Coronal CT scans demonstrating **(A)** large pituitary tumor arising out of the sella turcica and extending in suprasellar and parasellar fashion before starting bromocriptine, and **(B)** this tumor now confined to the sella turcica after 6 mo of bromocriptine therapy. Arrows denote tumor extension. (From King LW, Molitch ME, Gittinger JW, Wolpert SM, Stern J. Cavernous sinus syndrome due to prolactinoma: resolution with bromocriptine. Surg Neurol 1983;19:280–284. Reproduced with permission.)

(33), 19 patients had a tumor size reduction noted by 6 wk, but in 8 others, improvement was not noted until the 6-mo scans. A progressive decrease was often noted between 6 mo and 1 yr. In many patients followed subsequently, and in other reports noted above, continued tumor size decreases were noted progressively after 1 yr for up to several years.

In the multicenter study *(33)*, visual field improvement occurred in 9 of the 10 patients with significant visual field abnormalities; 80–90% of patients have had substantial improvement in other studies as well *(34,36,38,39,44,46,47,48,50)*. Visual field improvement generally parallels and often precedes the changes seen on scan *(33,48)*. It is often difficult to determine before treatment whether visual defects are temporary or permanent, and only the response to therapy provides a final answer. These studies with medical therapy are reassuring in that a relatively slow chiasmal decompression over several weeks provides excellent restoration of visual fields and that immediate surgical decompression is not necessary. Usually, when there is no significant change in visual fields despite significant evidence of tumor reduction on scan, subsequent surgery also does not improve these fields *(50)*.

Analysis of data in the multicenter study *(33)* showed that the extent of tumor size reduction did not correlate with basal PRL levels, nadir PRL levels achieved, the percent fall in PRL, or whether PRL levels reached normal. Some patients had excellent reduction in PRL levels into the normal range, but only modest changes in tumor size, whereas others had persistent hyperprolactinemia (although >88% suppression from basal values) with almost complete disappearance of tumor. A reduction in PRL levels always preceded any detectable change in tumor size, and PRL nonresponders are also tumor size nonresponders. As Liuzzi et al. *(47)* have noted, once maximum size reduction is achieved, the dose of bromocriptine can often be substantially reduced, gradually.

The reduction in tumor size is usually not only accompanied by improved visual fields and reduction of hyperprolactinemia, but also by improvement in other pituitary function. In the multicenter study *(33)*, estradiol levels improved markedly in 13/15 premenopausal women, and menses returned in all except these two. Testosterone levels were low in 11 men and increased in 9 during treatment, but returned to normal in only 4. Peak testosterone levels occurred between 6 and 12 mo for most men. Warfield et al. *(46)* noted that two patients who were hypothyroid before bromocriptine treatment became euthyroid, and one patient who was hypoadrenal became euadrenal. When the prolactinoma is present prepubertally, improved pituitary function allows resumption of normal growth and pubertal development *(56)*.

Long-Term Considerations With long-term treatment, perivascular fibrosis develops in some tumors, and this has implications for possible subsequent surgery. Landolt et al. called attention to this phenomenon in 1982 *(57)*, stating that their surgical results were much poorer in patients who had received bromocriptine. Landolt and Osterwalder subsequently showed an increase in perivascular fibrosis in treated patients *(58)*. Esiri et al. *(59)* demonstrated a striking, time-dependent increase in tumor fibrosis with bromocriptine, finding the fibrosis to be specific to prolactinomas, since it did not occur in similarly treated nonsecreting adenomas. The development of this fibrosis may be important with regard to the ability of a surgeon to cure a patient surgically after bromocriptine treatment and also with regard to tumor re-expansion once bromocriptine is stopped.

Landolt et al. found that for their patients with microadenomas, bromocriptine resulted in a decrease in his surgical cure rate from 81 to 33% *(57)*. Other series have not corroborated this experience for microadenomas, however. Faglia et al. *(60)* reported that they had a 69% surgical cure rate for 29 patients with microadenomas that had never received bromocriptine and a 65% cure for 20 patients that had previously received bromocriptine. Fahlbusch et al. *(61)* found an 80% surgical cure rate for microadenoma patients with PRL levels <200 ng/mL not treated with bromocriptine and an 85% cure rate for such patients who had been treated with bromocriptine. On the other hand, the cure rate for 12 patients not treated with bromocriptine, but with PRL levels >200 ng/mL was 58% and only 33% for 12 such patients treated with bromocriptine *(61)*. Hubbard et al. *(62)* compared the results in their bromocriptine-treated patients with historical controls, finding that the surgical cure rates from the bromocriptine-treated patients were 68, 17, and 17% for microadenomas, diffuse expansive adenomas, and invasive adenomas compared to 72, 47, and 17% in the corresponding groups of patients not having been treated with bromocriptine. Bevan et al. *(34)* also found no significant difference in surgical cure rates for microadenomas between patients previously treated with bromocriptine (6/10 patients) and those not receiving bromocriptine (8/14). On the other hand, Bevan et al. *(34)* found that the fibrosis that developed in the macroadenoma patients produced a tough tumor consistency, making surgical removal extremely difficult. For such patients, the cure rate was only 1/8, whereas in such patients who had not been treated with bromocriptine, it was 7/20. Furthermore, these patients with fibrotic tumors had a much greater rate of surgical complications. Weiss et al. *(44)*, however, pretreated all of their macroadenoma patients with bromocriptine for 6–12 wk, and found that of the 10 tumors that had >30% reduction in tumor size, the cure rate was 70%, and of the 9 tumors that did not respond with a significant

size change, the cure rate was 22%. Thus, most series suggest that bromocriptine has little or no effect on later surgical results for microadenomas. For macroadenomas, there may be a problem with bromocriptine treatment longer than 6–12 wk, at which point fibrosis becomes limiting to complete tumor removal.

An alternative to late surgical treatment is continued bromocriptine. Prolonged bromocriptine treatment for up to 10 yr appears to be well tolerated *(35,43,45,46,63,64)* and the dose can often be reduced considerably *(47,65)*. Thorner et al. *(66)* pointed out that when bromocriptine is discontinued in a patient with a macroadenoma that has become reduced in size, the tumor can re-expand within 2 wk. In the multicenter study *(33)*, bromocriptine withdrawal after 1 yr resulted in tumor re-expansion in 3/4 patients. In one of those, placement back on bromocriptine and withdrawal again after 4 yr showed a similar re-expansion of tumor. Johnston et al. *(67)* systematically examined 15 patients treated with either bromocriptine or pergolide *(see below)* for 3.7 yr for recurrence after stopping therapy. Hyperprolactinemia recurred in 14, symptoms related to hyperprolactinemia recurred in 13, but tumor size increased in only 2. The PRL levels after bromocriptine withdrawal were lower than pretreatment in 12/13 cases. Van't Verlaat and Croughs *(68)* found that of 12 patients with macroprolactinomas whose bromocriptine was withdrawn, 11 had a recurrence of hyperprolactinemia, but tumor re-expansion occurred only in 1. Wang et al. *(35)* found that of 24 patients treated solely with bromocriptine for over 3.4 ± 2.3 yr, in 5 (24%) serum PRL levels remained normal with no clinical symptoms after drug withdrawal. Only one patient with a macroadenoma had drug withdrawn, and this patient had normal PRL levels and no evidence of tumor recurrence after 2 yr. Ho et al. *(64)* found that 4/15 patients with prolactinomas maintained normal PRL levels off bromocriptine after 5.5 ± 0.6 yr of treatment. Rasmussen et al. *(69)* found PRL levels to remain normal in 4 of 75 hyperprolactinemic women (mixed idiopathic and tumor) after a median of 24 mo of therapy. Thus, 10–20% of patients can maintain normal PRL levels after stopping treatment, although 70–80% with marked tumor size reduction may not experience tumor re-expansion with stopping of therapy. With patients with very large tumors who have excellent tumor size reduction, stopping therapy must be done very cautiously, if at all. The best approach is probably to reduce the dose gradually, following PRL levels, and only discontinue the drug if there are no increases in PRL levels or tumor size on just 2.5 mg/d. Those with tumors that extend along the clivus and midbrain that have had substantial size reduction probably should never have their drug stopped, as a sudden enlargement could prove lethal.

Side Effects of Bromocriptine Treatment Bromocriptine is, in general, well tolerated. The most common side effects are nausea and sometimes vomiting; these are usually transient, but may recur with each dose increase. Orthostatic hypotension usually is only a problem when initiating therapy, and rarely recurs with dose increases. Limiting nausea and vomiting occurs in 3–5% of patients, and digital vasospasm, nasal congestion, and depression occur in rare patients when doses <7.5 mg/d are used *(5,6)*. Side effects can be minimized by starting with 1.25 mg daily with a snack at bedtime. The dose is gradually increased to 2.5 mg twice daily with meals over 7–10 d and PRL levels checked after 1–2 mo. Most patients respond within 1–2 mo if they are going to respond. Doses higher than 7.5 mg/d are usually not necessary, except in some patients with very large tumors.

One notable additional side effect is a psychotic reaction. Turner et al. *(70)* noted psychotic reactions in 8 of 600 patients receiving either bromocriptine or lisuride *(see below)* for treatment of hyperprolactinemia or acromegaly. Symptoms included auditory hallucinations, delusional ideas, and changes in mood. Rare reports of exacerbation of pre-existing schizophrenia also exist, and the drug should be given cautiously to such patients *(71,72)*. However, in a careful trial when bromocriptine was given to psychiatric patients who had been stabilized on neuroleptic agents, no exacerbation of psychosis was observed *(73)*. It should be noted that phenothiazines given to prolactinoma patients may blunt the action of bromocriptine on the prolactinomas *(33)*.

Reversible pleuropulmonary changes consisting of pleural effusions, pleural thickening, and parenchymal lung changes have been reported in patients treated with high doses of bromocriptine for Parkinson's disease *(74)*. Retroperitoneal fibrosis has been found with very high doses of bromocriptine (30–140 mg daily) used to treat Parkinson's disease *(75,76)*. These findings have not been reported with doses used for patients treated for hyperprolactinemia, although the authors has heard anecdotally about such cases.

Single case reports have suggested other potential side effects that may be observed, including leukopenia and thrombocytopenia *(77)*, hepatitis *(78)*, edema *(79)*, worsening of headache *(80,81)*, myocardial infarction *(82)*, and supraventricular tachycardia *(83)*. Rarely, the prolactinoma serves as a "cork," and tumor size reduction with bromocriptine may cause cerebrospinal fluid (CSF) rhinorrhea *(84,85)*.

Bromocriptine Resistance   Between 5 and 10% of patients either do not respond to bromocriptine or have only minimal responses. Decreased response to bromocriptine in vivo has been shown to correspond to decreased numbers of DA receptors on lactotroph cell membranes *(19)*. Because resistance is associated with a decrease in the relative proportion of the short receptor isoform, it has been postulated that resistance may not only involve defects in receptor expression but also in posttranscriptional splicing *(85a)*. Brue et al. *(86)* found that 27 of the 288 patients they treated with prolactinomas were resistant to bromocriptine; about half subsequently responded to quinagolide (CV 205-502, *see below*).

One troubling problem is the tumor that initially shrinks in response to bromocriptine and then enlarges. This is usually owing to noncompliance, which is further worsened by the tendency for the patient and physician to resume the full dose instead of gradually restarting. This tends to make side effects worse, further exacerbating the noncompliance. Dallabonzana reported two such patients; one had a concomitant rise in PRL but the other did not *(87)*. Although a similar patient was reported by Crosignani et al. *(88)*, a 6-wk period of treatment elapsed before the repeat radiologic evaluation. A patient reported by Schwarzstein et al. *(89)* initially demonstrated a PRL response to bromocriptine but subsequently both PRL levels and tumor size continued to increase despite maximal doses of bromocriptine, quinagolide, and lisuride. Although extremely rare, tumors that continue to enlarge while being treated with bromocriptine may turn out to be carcinomas *(90)*.

New Bromocriptine Routes and Preparations   Two new methods of giving bromocriptine have been tried recently. Vermesh et al. *(91)* reported that similar reductions in PRL levels are achieved with oral and intravaginal administration of oral bromocriptine tablets. Bromocriptine levels rise more slowly, but to eventually higher levels with the intravaginal compared to the oral route *(92)*. With vaginal administration, the drug effect lasts for up to 24 h with a single dose, and gastrointestinal side effects are much less than with the oral route *(93)*. Jasonni et al. *(93)* reported normalization of PRL levels in all 15 women with hyperprolactinemia with bromocriptine given as 2.5–5 mg in a single dose intravaginally, and Katz et al. *(94)* reported a woman intolerant of oral bromocriptine with a macroadenoma who responded well with tumor shrinkage to intravaginal bromocriptine. The author has now treated a few women with intravaginal bromocriptine with similar results, although one developed local irritation at the site of tablet placement. Jasonni et al. *(93)* also found that three women experienced vaginal burning with this treatment. Thus, the GI side effects appear to be caused by local effects rather than being mediated centrally.

A new, long-acting, injectable, depot preparation of bromocriptine (Parlodel-LAR®) causes high blood levels of bromocriptine within 5 h with only minimal side effects and PRL levels fall to 10–20% of basal levels within 12–24 h *(95–97)*. PRL levels stay down for 2–6 wk, and tumor shrinkage occurs rapidly, although there are no prospective studies comparing the rapidity of tumor reduction with this preparation to the oral route. Despite the obvious efficacy and appeal of this preparation, at present there are no plans to market this preparation in the USA.

Pregnancy and Bromocriptine   Hyperprolactinemia is usually associated with anovulation and infertility and correction of the hyperprolactinemia with DA agonists restores ovulation in about 90% of cases. When a woman harbors a prolactinoma as the cause of the hyperprolactinemia, two major issues arise when ovulation and fertility are restored: (1) the effects of the DA agonist on early fetal development occurring before a pregnancy is diagnosed; and (2) the effect of the pregnancy itself on the prolactinoma.

As a general principle, it is advised that fetal exposure to bromocriptine be limited to as short a period as possible. Most advise that mechanical contraception be used until the first two to three cycles have occurred, so that an intermenstrual interval can be established. In this way, a woman will know when she has missed a menstrual period, a pregnancy test can be performed quickly, and bromocriptine can be stopped. Thus, bromocriptine will have been given for only about 3–4 wk of the gestation. When used in this fashion, bromocriptine has not been found to cause any increase in spontaneous abortions, ectopic pregnancies, trophoblastic disease, multiple pregnancies, or congenital malformations (Table 2) *(98,99)*. Long-term follow-up studies of 64 children between the ages of 6 mo and 9 yr whose mothers took bromocriptine in this fashion have shown no ill effects *(100)*. Little data are available on the safety during pregnancy of pergolide or any of the experimental medications used to treat hyperprolactinemia at this point.

Estrogens have a marked stimulatory effect on PRL synthesis and secretion, and the hormonal milieu of pregnancy can stimulate lactotroph cell hyperplasia and prolactinoma growth *(101)*. Microadenomas and macroadenomas carry risks of significant tumor enlargement during pregnancy of 1.6 and 15.5%, respectively *(101)*. About 25–50% of the cases of symptomatic tumor enlargement required surgery before it was known that bromocriptine could reduce tumor size. However, bromocriptine has been used successfully during pregnancy to reduce symptomatic tumor enlargement in a number of cases *(102,103)*. No ill effects on the infant were observed in these cases.

Table 2
Effect of Bromocriptine on Pregnancies[a]

	Bromocriptine		Normal population,
	n	%	%
Pregnancies	6239	100.0	100.0
Spontaneous abortion	620	9.9	10–15
Terminations	75	1.25	
Ectopic	31	0.5	0.5–1.0
Hydatidiform moles	11	0.2	0.05–0.7
Deliveries (known duration)	4139	100.0	100.0
At term (>38 wk)	3620	87.5	85
Preterm (<38 wk)	519	12.5	15
Deliveries (known outcome)	5120	100.0	100.0
Single births	5031	98.3	98.7
Multiple births	89	1.7	1.3
Babies (known details)	5213	100.0	100.0
Normal	5030	96.5	95.0
With malformations	93	1.8	3–4
With perinatal disorders	90	1.7	>2

[a]Adapted from Molitch ME. N Engl J Med 1985;312:1364–1360.

As stated above, no teratogenic or other untoward effects of bromocriptine on pregnancy have been noted when bromocriptine was stopped within a few weeks of conception. Experience is limited, however, with the use of bromocriptine throughout the gestation. Studies have been reported with just over 100 women who took bromocriptine during 20–41 wk of gestation; no abnormalities were noted in the infants except one with an undescended testicle and one with a talipes deformity (98,104–106). In two studies in which bromocriptine was given before elective therapeutic abortions at 6–9 wk (107) or 20 wk (108) of gestation, there were no effects on amniotic fluid levels of estradiol, estriol, progesterone, testosterone, dehydroepiandrosterone, dehydroepiandrosterone sulfate, androstenedione, cortisol, or human placental lactogen. In all studies, maternal and fetal PRL levels were suppressed, but in the three cases in which amniotic fluid PRL was measured, it was suppressed in two (108) and normal in the third (104). Thus, these few studies of bromocriptine treatment late in gestation suggest that such use is probably safe, but there have been no large-scale or long-term studies. The use of prophylactic bromocriptine throughout the pregnancy likely prevents tumor regrowth during the pregnancy in most cases.

OTHER DOPAMINE AGONISTS A number of other DA agonists have been developed to treat hyperprolactinemia over the years. Although efficacy has been found for a number of these medications (lergotrile, lisuride, metergoline, mesulergine, dihydroergocristine, dihydroergocriptine, hydergine, terguride, and CQP 201-403), they have not been approved, and do not appear to be near such approval for clinical use in the USA for a variety of reasons.

Pergolide Another dopamine agonist that went through early trials demonstrating efficacy in the treatment of prolactinomas is pergolide (Permax®), which has been approved by the US Food and Drug Administration for the treatment of Parkinson's disease. Although such approval for the treatment of hyperprolactinemia is lacking, there is considerable experience with its use in prolactinoma patients, and such use is well documented in the literature. Initial studies demonstrated its specificity for PRL (109) and showed that hyperprolactinemia could be controlled with single daily doses of 50–150 μg (110). Several studies have shown comparability to bromocriptine with respect to tolerance and efficacy, including tumor size reduction (42,111–115). Experience has shown that some patients who do not respond to bromocriptine may do so to pergolide (116,117) and vice versa. Recently, outcome data were reported for 22 patients with macroadenomas treated with pergolide for a mean of 27.4 mo (range 9–64 mo), with the findings that 15 (68%) achieved normal PRL levels and two additional patients achieved near normal levels (< 30 ng/mL) (117a). Tumor shrinkage was 23% or greater in all patients, 50% or greater in 19 patients, and 75% or greater in 9 patients (117a).

Quinagolide Quinagolide (CV 205-502) is a nonergot dopamine agonist again with similar tolerance and efficacy to bromocriptine and pergolide, and can also can be given once daily (118–121). About 50% of patients who are resistant to bromocriptine respond to quinagolide (120,121). Although side effects are similar, some patients appear to tolerate quinagolide better than bromocriptine (118–121). The status of this drug in the US is uncertain.

Cabergoline Cabergoline (1-ethyl-3,3-[3'-dimethylaminopropyl]3-[6'allylergoline-8β-carbonyl]urea diphosphate) is different from the other drugs in that it has a very long half-life and can be given orally once weekly. The long duration of action stems from its slow elimination from pituitary tissue (122), its high-affinity binding to pituitary dopamine receptors (123), and extensive enterohepatic recycling (124). After oral administration, PRL-lowering effects are initially detectable at 3 h, and gradually increase so that there is a plateau of effect between 48 and 120 h (124–126), and with weekly doses, there is a sustained reduction of PRL (126). There is a linear dose–serum PRL level response (124). A number of studies have now shown that cabergoline is at least as effective as bromocriptine in lowering PRL levels and reducing tumor size, but with a substantial reduction in side effects (127–130). In the multicenter European collaborative study, in which bromocriptine and cabergoline were administered in a double-blind fashion for 8 wk, normoprolactinemia was achieved in 83% of the cabergoline- and 59% of the bromocriptine-treated women, whereas 3% of the women stopped taking cabergoline

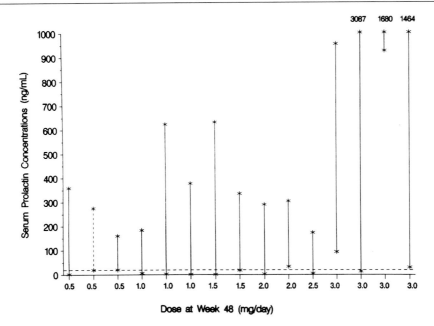

Figure 14-3 Individual PRL levels at baseline and 48 wk according to final dose in macroprolactinoma patients treated with cabergoline. The dotted horizontal line indicates normal serum prolactin (<20 ng/mL). The dotted vertical line refers to a patient who normalized prolactin at week 6, but did not complete 48 wk because of a complication (pituitary hemorrhage). (From Biller et al. *[130]*. Reproduced by permission. ©The Endocrine Society.)

and 12% stopped taking bromocriptine because of side effects *(129)*. In our studies of 15 patients with macroadenomas *(130)*, normal PRL levels were achieved in 73% of patients at doses of 0.5–3.0 mg/wk (Figure 3). Three of 5 patients who had failed to normalize PRL on prior dopamine agonists achieved normal levels with cabergoline. Gonadal function was restored in all hypogonadal men and in 75% of premenopausal women with amenorrhea. Tumor size decreased in 11 of the 15 patients. Of the five patients who had experienced side effects on prior dopamine agonists, four had none on cabergoline and the fifth had milder symptoms.

Several studies have assessed the effect of cabergoline on macroadenoma size, but in most of these series many of the patients had been previously treated with other DA agonists, some being intolerant and others resistant *(125,127,130,130a,130b,130c)*. In the study of Colao et al. *(130a)*, only 8 of the 23 macroadenoma patients had received short courses of bromocriptine previously and were only intolerant and not resistant to bromocriptine; of the total of 23, 12 (52%) had a <50% reduction in tumor size, 9 (39%) had a 25–50% reduction in tumor size, and 2 (9%) had a <25% reduction in tumor size. In a series of 27 patients, who had all been previously shown to be resistant to bromocriptine or quinagolide (CV205-502), Colao et al. *(130b)* showed that cabergoline was able to normalize PRL levels in 15 of 19 patients with macroadenomas and all 8 patients with microadenomas. Tumor shrinkage was documented in 9 of the 19 macroadenomas and 4 of the 8 microadenomas *(130b)*. In a recent report of 455 patients treated in Belgium with cabergoline under compassionate use, of whom 292 had previously received bromocriptine with 140 being intolerant and 58 being resistant to bromocriptine, Verhelst et al. *(130c)* reported that in 86% PRL levels normalized and tumor shrinkage occurred in 67% of cases.

Outcome data available on 290 pregnancies in which cabergoline was administered to facilitate ovulation do not show increased risks of preterm, ectopic, or multiple birth deliveries or malforma-

tions *(130c,130d,130e)*. However, this data is relatively sparse compared to the data in over 6000 pregnancies with bromocriptine, so that at the moment bromocriptine use is favored when fertility is the major reason for treatment. On the other hand, this data is encouraging and the mother may be reassured if she gets pregnant while taking cabergoline. Over the next few years we will likely gain a sufficient amount of data so as to be able to recommend cabergoline for fertility without reservation.

ACROMEGALY

DOPAMINE AGONISTS Liuzzi and colleagues *(131)* demonstrated that l-DOPA, a dopamine and norepinephrine precursor, was capable of suppressing GH secretion in patients with acromegaly, unlike its previously demonstrated stimulating effect on GH in normal subjects *(132)*. High-affinity dopamine receptors have been shown to be present on human GH-secreting pituitary adenoma cell membranes *(133)*.

The acute GH-lowering effect of bromocriptine, a long-acting dopamine agonist was demonstrated by Liuzzi et al. *(134)*. Many studies have subsequently documented the efficacy of bromocriptine in the treatment of acromegaly. In 1992, Jaffe and Barkan *(135)* reviewed data from 31 series published to that point totaling 549 patients with acromegaly treated with bromocriptine, finding that although about 70–75% of patients respond with some decrease in GH levels, only 20% achieve a GH of <5 ng/mL and only 10% achieve a normal insulin-like growth factor-1 (IGF-1) level. When a satisfactory response is achieved, however, it can be maintained for many years *(136)*. Doses, in general, are higher than those used to treat prolactinomas, although doses higher than 30 mg/d are rarely needed. Although some have suggested that the presence of elevated PRL levels (indicating a GH/PRL-secreting tumor) predicts a good GH response to bromocriptine *(137)*, a good response may also be seen in patients without hyperprolactinemia *(138)*, so PRL levels should not be used prospectively to screen out potential candidates for therapy.

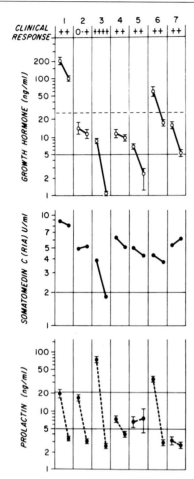

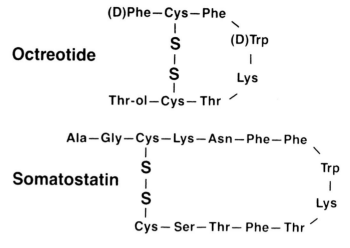

Figure 14-5 Structures of octreotide and somatostatin.

Figure 14-4 The association of clinical response with changing levels of GH, somatomedin C (SM-C), and PRL. Hormone levels were determined before and during bromocriptine therapy for each patient. Hormone values before bromocriptine are to the left, and values during bromocriptine are to the right for each patient. Each point represents the mean ± SEM of 3–25 determinations. The upper limits of normal for each hormone are shown by the horizontal lines. Clinical response is indicated from 0 to ++++. (From Moses et al. *(142)*. Reproduced by permission. ©The Endocrine Society.)

In many studies, the subjective and objective clinical improvement of the acromegaly appeared to be greater than would be predicted from the degree of decrease of the GH levels. A clear explanation for this is still lacking. In some *(139)*, but not other *(140,141)* studies, bromocriptine appeared to reduce the level of monomeric GH more than those of the GH dimer and higher-mol-wt species. Furthermore, Hizuka et al. *(141)* found that bromocriptine does not alter the radioreceptor-assayable to radio-immunoassayable ratio of GH, and does not alter the affinity or concentration of GH receptors on IM-9 lymphocytes. IGF-1 levels have also been used to assess changes in the bioactivity of GH during bromocriptine therapy. We showed no correlation between changes in IGF-1 levels and the clinical response to bromocriptine (Figure 4), and also showed that GH levels had to be reduced to <2 ng/mL before IGF-1 levels would be normalized *(142)*. Although Wass et al. *(143)* found a good correlation of clinical improvement and decreased IGF-1 levels in their patients, Carlson et al. *(140)* and Nortier et al. *(144)* did not find such a correlation in their patients. Recently, it was also found that IGF-1 binding protein 1 (IGF-BP1) levels, found to be elevated by octreotide,

were not elevated by bromocriptine *(145)*. From a practical, therapeutic point of view, these findings suggest that not only should GH and IGF-1 levels be monitored, but also objective indices of clinical activity, such as serial facial photographs, ring size, hand volume, heel pad thickness, left ventricular mass, and insulin resistance.

In contrast to its documented high efficacy in shrinking tumor size in PRL-secreting macroadenomas *(51)*, bromocriptine has been found to be much less efficacious in shrinking GH-secreting tumors. In their summary, Jaffe and Barkan *(135)* found that in 9 studies totaling 62 patients, only 18 (29%) had a decrease in tumor size and few decreased substantially, as may be seen in PRL-secreting macroadenomas.

Depot injectable forms of bromocriptine have been found to be similar to oral bromocriptine in efficacy, with perhaps less side effects *(146)*. In addition, pergolide *(147,148)* and quinagolide (CV 205-502) *(149)* have efficacies similar to that of bromocriptine, but do not appear to offer significant advantages. On the other hand, one-third of patients had a normalization of IGF-1 levels with cabergoline in a recent study *(149a)*, suggesting that it may be the DA agonist of choice.

OCTREOTIDE Introduction Somatostatin was initially isolated and characterized on the basis of its ability to inhibit GH secretion *(150,151)*. Shortly after it was shown to decrease GH secretion in humans *(152)*, it was demonstrated to decrease GH levels in patients with acromegaly *(153,154)*. Its very short plasma half-life of 2–3 min precluded clinical use, however. It was subsequently determined that the 4 amino acid sequence phe-trp-lys-thr corresponding to amino acids 7–10 of native somatostatin was essential for bioactivity *(155)*, and a variety of derivatives of somatostatin were developed to increase the therapeutic ratio as well as prolong the bioactive half-life. Of these, only octreotide (Figure 5) has achieved widespread clinical use in the treatment of acromegaly.

Pharmacology Octreotide has a 40-fold greater activity in suppressing GH compared with insulin levels *(155)*. The metabolic clearance rate is much slower than that of somatostatin, the half-life in plasma being 113 min following sc injection in normal persons *(156)*. Unlike native somatostatin, octreotide withdrawal does not cause GH hypersecretion *(157)*. Single sc injections of 50–100 μg of octreotide result in peak plasma concentrations within 1 h that are proportionate to the dose administered *(156)* and that suppress GH levels for 6–12 h, the nadir occurring at 2–3 h (157). Plasma clearance is reduced in patients with severe renal insufficiency, and dosages may need to be reduced (158). Only two patients have been reported who developed specific IgG antibodies against octreotide after 2–3 yr of treatment of acromegaly (159). These antibodies reduced the plasma disappearance rate, but did not impair biological activity (159). When antibodies were looked for in a systematic study of 13 patients receiving octreotide for 1–36 mo, however, no evidence of antibody formation was found (160).

Studies in animals in doses up to 30 times the highest human dose have not shown any teratogenicity (161). Only three patients treated with octreotide during pregnancy (one for a TSH-secreting tumor) have been reported, and no malformations were found in these children (162–164). In the patient with a TSH-secreting tumor (164), octreotide was reinstituted near term because of tumor enlargement; cord blood octreotide levels were found to be about 40% of maternal levels and declined following delivery with an estimated half-life in the infant of 350 min. Because of such limited safety data, it is recommended that octreotide be discontinued if pregnancy is considered, and contraception should be used when octreotide is administered.

The GH responses to octreotide are partially determined by adenoma somatostatin receptor status, the best clinical responses correlating with the density of receptors on the adenomas (165). Five subtypes of the somatostatin receptor have been characterized and cloned, and are identical in 42–60% of their amino acid sequences (166). The receptors belong to the receptor class that has seven transmembrane domains and are linked to adenylyl cyclase through guanine nucleotide binding proteins (166). Octreotide binds with high affinity to somatostatin receptor subtypes 2 and 5 and with moderate affinity to subtype 3, but does not bind to subtypes 1 and 4. Subtypes 2 and 5 are the primary somatostatin receptors in the normal pituitary, but subtypes 1, 2, 3, and 5 have been found in adenomas (167,168). Because of differences in binding affinities to the different receptor subtypes, it appears that most of the clinical activity of octreotide in GH-secreting adenomas occurs through receptor subtype 2 (169).

Although the predominant clinical effect of octreotide in patients with acromegaly is at the pituitary somatostatin receptor to decrease pituitary GH secretion, there is evidence that it may have other beneficial modes of action as well. Flyvbjerg et al. (170) have shown that octreotide partially inhibits GH-induced IGF-1 generation by liver, kidney, heart, and lung with resulting decreased plasma IGF-1 levels. Serri et al. (171) also showed that octreotide administered simultaneously with GH to hypophysectomized rats blocked GH-induced IGF-1 mRNA expression. This may account for the fact that IGF-1 normalization is seen in a greater number of patients than is GH normalization with octreotide treatment (see below). In addition, octreotide simulates IGF-BP1 expression (172) and serum levels (173) independently of effects on insulin or GH (174). Since IGF-BP1 inhibits IGF-1 action, this effect may provide a further beneficial effect on clinical activity of IGF-1 in acromegaly. Interestingly, in the rare patients with acromegaly owing to GH-releasing hormone (GHRH)-secreting carcinoid tumors, octreotide has been shown to reduce GHRH release by these carcinoid tumors in addition to reducing GH levels, providing control of hormone secretion at yet another level (175,176).

The tumor morphologic response to octreotide is highly variable. Some tumors appear to be unaltered by such treatment, and none show necrotic changes after 4 mo (177). Most tumors show a mild, but not marked decrease in cell and cytoplasmic size, and some show an increase in hormone granule number and size (177). Many tumors also display increased perivascular and interstitial fibrosis (177). The absence of a marked effect on cell size corresponds with the generally modest effect octreotide has on tumor size in vivo (178). Interestingly, studies using the reverse, hemolytic plaque assay show that at any one point in time, only a small proportion of the cells in an adenoma are secreting GH in large amounts, but it is these cells that seem to be preferentially inhibited by octreotide (179).

Treatment of Acromegaly   A number of studies have documented the efficacy of octreotide in treating acromegaly (reviewed previously in ref. 180). Subsequent to these smaller studies, four large, multicenter studies have been reported. The International Multicenter Acromegaly Study Group reported data on 189 patients treated with octreotide for a median of 24.2 (range 1–231) wk at a median daily dose of 300 μg (range 100–1500 μg) (181). They reported that GH levels decreased in 94% of subjects and to <5 ng/mL in 45%. Suppression of IGF-1 levels to normal occurred in 45%. Tumor size decreased by more than 20% in 44% of subjects evaluated prospectively. Clinical improvement was significant, headaches decreasing in 84%, hyperhidrosis decreasing in 65%, and ring size decreasing in 55% (181).

Data from 58 patients treated for 12–26 mo in doses of 300–1500 μg/d were reported by the French SMS-201-995 Acromegaly Study Group (182). In this study, some improvement in GH levels was seen in 78%, with 22% actually obtaining GH levels <2 ng/nL; IGF-1 levels were not measured. Facial features improved in 50%, hyperhidrosis improved in 60%, and headache improved in 75%. A reduction of tumor size of ≥50% occurred in 25% and of 20–50% in 20% of patients with macroadenomas.

In the US multicenter study, 115 patients were randomized to treatment with 300 or 750 μg/d in 3 doses for 6 mo (178). Integrated mean GH levels were reduced to <5 ng/mL in 53 and 49%, and IGF-1 levels were normalized in 68 and 55% of patients receiving the low and high doses, respectively. Headache and hyperhidrosis were reduced in about 2/3 of patients. Nineteen percent of the low-dose and 37% of the higher-dose group experienced significant tumor size reduction (178). One hundred three of these patients enrolled in a long-term (mean of 24 additional months) open-label study, in which the doses could be adjusted to achieve maximal lowering of GH levels, up to a maximum dose of 1500 μg daily (183). In this follow-up study 64% of patients treated for 12–30 mo achieved plasma IGF-1 levels that remained in the normal range for at least half of the treatment visits. The lower the baseline GH level, the greater the chance of achieving normal IGF-1 levels (Figure 6). There was no evidence of drug tachyphylaxis in patients. There were many patients who required doses larger than 300 μg daily to achieve maximal lowering of GH and IGF-1 levels.

Most recently, the Italian Multicenter Octreotide Study reported data on 68 patients treated with 100 μg tid for 1 yr (184). On this dose, GH levels were lowered to <2.5 ng/mL in 25% of patients, and IGF-1 levels were normalized in 40% of patients. Tumor shrinkage was noted in 50% of patients (184).

Some additional studies have focused on the effect of octreotide on specific complications and other selected aspects of acromegaly. Van der Lely et al. (185) found that elderly male patients appear to respond better to octreotide compared to other categories of patients. In the multicenter studies, glucose tolerance usually

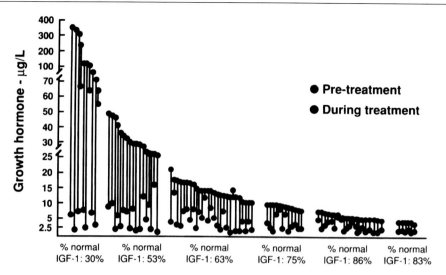

Figure 14-6   GH concentrations are shown before treatment (shaded circles) and after 12 mo of octreotide (closed circles). GH levels were measured 2 h after octreotide injection. The patients were divided into six groups based on the initial GH level. The percentage of patients with normal IGF-1 levels at the 12-mo visit is shown below the horizontal axis. Patients with the highest initial GH concentrations were less likely to achieve normal IGF-1 levels during treatment. (From Newman et al. *[183]*. Reproduced by permission. ©The Endocrine Society.)

did not change substantially, although in some patients, there was a worsening, and in others there was an improvement *(178,181,182,184)*. On the other hand, Koop et al. *(186)* found that 20 and 29% of patients with normal glucose tolerance developed impaired glucose tolerance and NIDDM, respectively. However, of those with pre-existing diabetes, 18% became normal and 9% improved to impaired glucose tolerance *(186)*. In general, it has been observed that the decrease in insulin secretion caused by the octreotide is largely balanced by the decrease in insulin resistance caused by the reduction in GH levels.

Sleep apnea, common in acromegalic patients *(187)*, is markedly improved with octreotide, with a 40% decrease in total apnea time, and similar improvements in oxygen desaturation, sleep quality, and subjective sleepiness *(188)*. This improvement took place regardless of whether the apnea was obstructive or central, implying CNS effects as well as reduction of obstructive soft tissue volume *(188)*. Cardiac changes may also improve, since 6–12 mo of octreotide have been shown to cause a reduction in left ventricular wall mass and thickness along with a decrease in stroke volume and cardiac index *(189,190)*. In patients with overt heart failure, a dramatic clinical improvement may be associated with an increase in stroke volume, a decrease in filling pressures, and pulmonary wedge pressures with a normalization of the cardiac index *(190)*.

The beneficial effects of reducing headache occur within 5 min of injection in many individuals, suggesting a mechanism of action different from binding to pituitary somatostatin receptors. Some patients develop what appears to be tolerance for this analgesic effect, experiencing shorter periods of analgesia and requiring an increasing dose. On acute cessation, restlessness, irritability, blood pressure elevation, nausea, and yawning may occur, suggesting narcotic withdrawal *(191)*. Although the analgesic effect is not influenced by naloxone *(192)*, the clinical observations certainly suggest that there is some interaction with opioid peptide receptors.

The fact that tumor size reduction occurs led to the concept of using octreotide preoperatively to determine whether that would improve surgical cure rates. Stevenaert and Beckers *(193)* compared their surgical results in 48 patients pretreated with octreotide for 3–39 mo to those in 107 operated on without pretreatment.

Cure rates (normal IGF-1 levels, postglucose GH <1 ng/mL) were significantly higher in pretreated patients for patients with enclosed adenomas (88.9 vs 68.8%) or tumors <16 mm in height (77.8 vs 63.4%), but not in invasive adenomas (28.6 vs 30.5%) or tumors ≥16 mm in height (16.7 vs 37.9%). Thus, benefit was not seen in the group in whom it was most hoped for, i.e. the larger, more invasive tumors for which surgical success is less assured.

A long-acting preparation of octreotide has been developed called Sandostatin-LAR, which has incorporated the octreotide into microspheres of the biodegradable polymer, poly (DL-lactidecoglycolide) *(194,195)*. After im injection, octreotide concentrations initially peak at 60 min, decrease to low levels for the next 7 d, and then gradually increase, remaining high for the subsequent 3 wk *(194,195)*. GH levels are a mirror image of this pattern, remaining suppressed for up to 28 d *(194,195)*. The results with 20–30 mg every 4 wk is sustained GH and IGF-1 suppression with no accumulation of octreotide *(194,195)*. Recent data from a European multicenter 12-mo study of 151 acromegalic patients showed that in 69.8% of patients mean serum GH levels could be suppressed to <2.5 µg/L, and in 63.1% IGF-1 could be normalized *(196)*. Symptoms of headache, fatigue, perspiration, joint pains, and paresthesias all improved significantly *(196)*.

Lanreotide (also known as somatuline) is a different, cyclic analogue of somatostatin with a longer half-life than octreotide but a shorter half-life than octreotide-LAR and is given im at 7–14 d intervals *(197,198)*. In a summary of four studies of 61 patients given lanreotide *(199)*, it was found that 59% achieved normal IGF-1 levels. A longer-acting formulation of lanreotide, lanreotide-autogel, is currently being evaluated.

Adverse Effects   The primary adverse effects of octreotide have been on the gastrointestinal tract. Loose stools, abdominal bloating, nausea, and flatulence occur in 53–88% of patients in the first 2 wk, but such symptoms persist past the first 1–2 wk of treatment in only 3–25% of patients in the above-cited multicenter studies *(178,180–184)*. Carotene levels decrease significantly with octreotide *(178)* and stay low for the duration of treatment *(183)*. Fecal fat excretion often increases modestly, although there is no change in d-xylose absorption *(200)*. Rarely, the induced malabsorption may be clinically significant, and vitamin K deficiency causing an abnormal prothrombin time has been reported (183). Active gastritis has also been reported in 9 of 10 patients studied prospectively by Plöckinger et al. (201) with damage to the superficial and deeper layers of the mucosa and focal atrophy. However, in another study by Anderson et al. (202), 10 of 33 (30%) patients had gastritis before any therapy with octreotide, 17 of 36 (47%) patients had gastritis while taking octreotide, and 3 of 21 (14%) patients developed gastritis during treatment; only 2 of the 48 patients in the whole group spontaneously complained of dyspepsia. In these studies, there was a highly significant association between the presence of gastritis and the presence of *Helicobacter pylori* (201,202). Although Plöckinger et al. (201) found a decrease in serum vitamin B-12 concentrations in all of their patients and abnormally low levels in four, Anderson et al. (202) found that only 4 of 33 tested patients had parietal cell antibodies and two of these had no gastritis on gastroscopy. At present, it would appear to be prudent to check serum vitamin B-12 concentrations and prothrombin times periodically, and to consider that gastritis may be present in patients with dyspepsia. Specific treatment of the *H. pylori*, if found, may then prove useful.

The multicenter studies have also documented that gallstones are present in 4–15% of patients before starting octreotide, and asymptomatic gallstones develop over 6–12 mo in another 10–15% (178,180–184). Over the course of more prolonged treatment, Newman et al. (183) noted the development of sludge in 36% and gallstones in 24% of patients, with resolution occurring without stopping treatment in 36.1% of the patients with sludge and 29.2% of the patients with stones. Of those patients initially with sludge, only 16.7% went on to develop stones. The development of sludge and gallstones was not related to dosage of octreotide (183). In this series of Newman et al. (183), most patients had little or no symptoms. Of three patients who had elective cholecystectomies because of vague abdominal symptoms, the symptoms persisted postoperatively. One patient had a cholecystectomy because of an episode consistent with biliary colic. Other smaller series have shown similar results (203–208). The mechanism involves an octreotide-induced inhibition of cholecystokinin release with resulting inhibition of gallbladder contraction following a meal (203,205,206). The inhibition of postprandial gallbladder contractility by octreotide lasts for at least 4 h following injection and contractility reverts to normal by 8 h (203,206). Because most patients who develop stones are asymptomatic and rarely develop cholecystitis, the finding of asymptomatic gallstones is not an indication to stop treatment. There are some data to suggest that ursodeoxycholic acid may cause dissolution of stones, and this may be worth trying in the rare, symptomatic patient. Furthermore, given the low morbidity of laparascopic cholecystectomy now, that procedure would appear warranted in the symptomatic patient rather than stopping octreotide, if the octreotide treatment is effecting a good clinical and biochemical response. Because of the normal contractility that occurs by 8 h after stopping octreotide, it has been suggested that the morning dose be withheld until 1–2 h after breakfast to allow at least one good contraction per day; long-term studies showing benefit of this approach have not been reported as yet.

Use with Bromocriptine In patients who have been tried on both bromocriptine and octreotide, a better response is usually seen with octreotide (209,210). Some studies have shown that some patients respond acutely to a combination of bromocriptine and octreotide who do not respond to either drug alone (211) and chronic use also shows synergy between these two drugs (210). Part of this synergistic effect may be owing to altered pharmacokinetics; although the pharmacokinetics of octreotide are unchanged by coadministration of bromocriptine, the bioavailability of bromocriptine is increased by 40% when octreotide is coadministered (210).

GH-RECEPTOR ANTAGONISTS A new approach to the medical treatment of acromegaly is the development of an antagonist that inhibits the binding of GH to its receptor. Normally, GH initially causes a dimerization of the extracellular domain of the receptor with binding of the single GH molecule. One antagonist of this binding, termed "pegvisomant," blocks this dimerization and binding, resulting in a decrease in GH action. In a preliminary study of its efficacy over 12 wk in 112 acromegalic patients, IGF-1 levels were normalized in 89.3% of patients treated with the highest dose, 20 mg/d, with significant improvements in the symptoms of soft tissue swelling, excessive perspiration, and fatigue (211a). In one patient serum transaminase levels increased to normal after the drug was stopped but no other adverse effects were seen other than local irritation at the site of injection (211a). Longer studies must be completed before it can be seen how this medication fits into the overall therapeutic armamentarium for acromegaly.

CUSHING'S DISEASE

The medical therapy of Cushing's disease has been less successful than that of PRL- and GH-secreting tumors. A number of medications have been used over the past 20 years with varying success. At present, the most useful drug appears to be ketoconazole, which combines efficacy with tolerability. Clearly, some patients respond to the other drugs as well, but because of lower efficacy rates, their use is limited to the occasional patient who does not respond to other modalities.

KETOCONAZOLE Pharmacology Ketoconazole is an imidazole derivative with broad-spectrum antifungal properties that has been found to interfere with steroid synthesis. Ketoconazole inhibits several cytochrome P-450 enzymes in this pathway, including the cholesterol side-chain cleavage 17,20 lyase and 11 β-hydroxylase steps (212). The drug also binds to glucocorticosteroid receptors and serves as a competitive inhibitor to cortisol. Unfortunately, ketoconazole also blocks the 17,20 lyase step in the testes, which is necessary for converting 17-hydroxyprogesterone to androstenedione, which ultimately is converted to testosterone (212). The inhibition of other P-450 enzyme systems results in altered metabolism of a number of drugs, including rifampin, phenytoin, cyclosporin, and warfarin.

In addition to its effects on adrenal steroid synthesis and action, ketoconazole has also been shown to inhibit ACTH secretion by corticotrophs in a dose-dependent action (213). It inhibits basal and corticotropin-releasing hormone (CRH)-stimulated cAMP content and release, and ACTH mRNA transcription and ACTH release (213) via a direct effect on the catalytic subunit of adenylyl cyclase (214). In two patients with Nelson's syndrome whose tumors were studied in short-term cultures in vitro, the addition of ketoconazole to the medium resulted in decreased ACTH secretion accompanied by cellular involution with reduction in endoplasmic reticulum surface density, granule size, and lysosomal size (215).

The hormonal changes caused by a single dose of ketoconazole are reversible, recovery occurring between 8 and 16 h after an oral dose (216). Peak serum concentrations occur at 2 h, and the plasma half-life is between 1 and 3.3 h for an initial phase and 8 h for a second phase *(216)*. Gastric acidity is required for absorption, and antacids and acid-reducing drugs should be avoided near the time of taking the drug *(216)*. Ketoconazole undergoes extensive hepatic metabolism to inactive products, and both metabolites and unchanged drug are excreted into the feces. Hepatic insufficiency is a contraindication to use, but renal impairment does not cause accumulation of the drug *(216)*. The doses used for clinical effect, 600–1200 mg/d, are generally two- to threefold higher than the doses used for antifungal activity *(216)*.

Clinical Effects of Ketoconazole   Several small studies have shown the efficacy of ketoconazole in the treatment of patients with Cushing's disease *(217,218)*. In one large series of 28 patients with Cushing's disease *(219)*, all had normalization of urinary free cortisol levels at one point or another in follow-up, but in two control was only partial and/or transient. In none did ACTH levels rise. Treatment in these patients ranged from 1 to 36 mo, and many received concomitant pituitary irradiation. In another series of 178 patients with Cushing's disease treated either before surgery, after surgical failure or relapse, or in association with pituitary irradiation, ketoconazole brought about a normalization of urinary free-cortisol levels in 43% of patients and a reduction in another 42% *(219a)*. During treatment, complications, such as diabetes, hypertension, and hypokalemia, generally resolved or improved substantially. However, adrenal function needs to be monitored and the dose adjusted to avoid adrenal insufficiency. Although minor, asymptomatic transaminase elevations are common, but more severe abnormalities require drug discontinuation and it is recommended that along with measurements of urinary free cortisol, liver function tests be carried out at 1, 2, and 4 wk and then monthly *(219b)*.

Adverse Effects   Because of the effects on testicular steroidogenesis, depression of testosterone levels with loss of libido, impotence, and gynecomastia is common *(216)*. Other side effects include skin rash, edema, nausea, bloating, diarrhea, pruritus, alterations in hepatic function (usually transient), liver damage, and anaphylaxis.

OTHER MEDICATIONS   Cyproheptadine   The hypothesis that ACTH-secreting tumors might arise because of underlying hypothalamic dysregulation, perhaps increased serotoninergic tone in the hypothalamus, led to the concept of interfering with serotonin action by the use of cyproheptadine, a serotonin antagonist. Although early reports showed the benefit of high-dose (24 mg daily) cyproheptadine in a number of patients with Cushing's disease and Nelson's syndrome *(220–223)*, subsequent reports did not show similar success *(224,225)*. Although there were never any larger, randomized, placebo-controlled studies proving or disproving its efficacy, cyproheptadine is not currently being used for the treatment of Cushing's disease.

Bromocriptine   Because ergotamine had been shown to inhibit corticotroph tumor growth in rats and because bromocriptine had proved successful in the treatment of prolactinomas and acromegaly, it was tried in Cushing's disease. Some studies showed acute effects in lowering ACTH levels *(226)*, but case reports of more prolonged use have shown variable results *(227–230)*. Bromocriptine is generally not used for the treatment of Cushing's disease, at present.

Metyrapone   Metyrapone blocks the conversion of 11-deoxycortisol to cortisol and has been used in the treatment of Cushing's disease either as primary or adjunctive treatment following surgery or irradiation. In most cases, the enzyme block is only partial, and with decreased feedback of cortisol, ACTH levels rise further, eventually overcoming the block *(231)*. Nonetheless, there are some case reports of prolonged remission with metyrapone as the sole therapeutic agent, and in these cases, ACTH levels did not rise *(232,233)*. The only extensive experience using metyrapone has been reported from St. Bartholomew's Hospital *(234)*, where 57 patients with Cushing's disease were treated. They treated 53 patients for 1–16 wk, finding excellent responses in all with no escape despite an increase in ACTH levels of 76%. Twenty-four patients were treated for a median of 27 mo following pituitary irradiation and cortisol levels were well controlled in 20. After 6 yr of treatment, six patients were still on metyrapone, nine had gone into remission and five patients were treated by other means. Thus, metyrapone may well play a role in the management of patients who have had irradiation while awaiting full effects of the irradiation. Side effects include hypoadrenalism, hypokalemia, edema, rash, nausea, and hirsutism.

Sodium Valproate   γ-Amino butyric acid (GABA) is thought to be an inhibitory neurotransmitter and there is experimental evidence that it may inhibit CRH secretion *(235)*. Sodium valproate, an anticonvulsant, inhibits GABA-transaminase, resulting in increased levels of GABA in synapses. Thus, by increasing GABA, sodium valproate might be able to decrease CRH secretion and possibly ACTH secretion. Several studies have tried sodium valproate in the treatment of patients with Cushing's disease or Nelson's syndrome, but early reports of success *(236–239)* were not repeated when larger numbers of patients were studied *(240,241)*. However, one study has found synergistic effects between sodium valproate and metyrapone in the management of Cushing's disease *(242)*.

Mitotane (*o,p*'DDD)   Mitotane (1,1-dichloro-2-[*o*-chlorophenyl]-2-[*p*-chlorophenyl]-ethane or *o,p*'DDD) is an adrenolytic agent used primarily in the treatment of adrenal cancer. It causes selective damage and eventual atrophy to the zona fasciculata and zona reticularis with sparing of the zona glomerulosa. Low-dose mitotane (3 g/d) has been used in some patients with Cushing's disease with considerable success *(243,244)*, but there is considerable neurologic and gastrointestinal toxicity even at these low doses, and patients generally do not tolerate it well.

Octreotide   Octreotide has been given to a small number of patients with mostly negative results, although a few patients have responded *(245,246)*.

CLINICALLY NONFUNCTIONING ADENOMAS

As discussed in Chapter 19, more than three-quarters of clinically nonfunctioning adenomas are, in fact, gonadotroph adenomas. Measurement of basal or thyrotropin-releasing hormone (TRH)-stimulated, luteinizing hormone (LH), follicle-stimulating hormone (FSH), α-subunit, or the β-subunit of LH and FSH will often allow this diagnosis to be made preoperatively (*see* Chapter 19). Many of the earlier studies that attempted to show beneficial effect of medical treatment on clinically nonfunctioning tumors did not make this distinction. The discussion to follow will try to sort out data based on whether the studies were of tumors in which the gonadotroph status had or had not been defined. In general, medical therapy for this group of tumors has been quite unsatisfactory.

BROMOCRIPTINE   High-affinity dopamine binding sites have been found on the membranes of nonfunctioning adenomas but the number of binding sites was lower in nonfunctioning adenomas, compared to prolactinomas and normal pituitaries *(52)*. A number of case reports *(247–249)* and anecdotal information suggested that some patients with clinically nonfunctioning tumors do indeed respond with tumor size reduction to bromocriptine. However, Barrow et al. *(24)* found that of six such patients treated with bromocriptine, none experienced tumor shrinkage, and Grossman et al. *(250)* found that of 15 patients treated with bromocriptine, mesulergine, or pergolide, none experienced tumor size reduction. In this latter study, at surgery, one patient was found to have an epidermoid cyst and another a Rathke's pouch cyst, indicating the lack of specificity of radiologic identification of these tumors. In a review by Bevan et al. *(52)*, 84 cases of nonsecreting macroadenomas treated with bromocriptine reported in 7 series were reviewed, and they concluded that only 8% responded with a significant size change by 1 yr and 15.4% responded in this fashion for a longer period of time.

When patients with clinically nonfunctioning adenomas were further characterized as having gonadotroph adenomas, similar results have been found. Glycoprotein hormone or subunit concentrations were often able to be reduced with bromocriptine and other dopamine agonist *(251–259)*. However, actual tumor size reduction has been reported only in a small number of patients *(255,258,259)*.

GONADOTROPIN-RELEASING HORMONE (GnRH) ANALOGS AND ANTAGONISTS

Gonadotropins normally are stimulated by the pulsatile secretion of GnRH, but are inhibited by continuous high levels of GnRH because of densensitization *(260)*. Long-acting GnRH analogs similarly will inhibit gonadotropin secretion in normal humans *(261)*. This fact led to the attempt to control gonadotroph adenomas with long-acting GnRH agonists. Unfortunately, although such agonists did indeed reduce gonadotropin and glycoprotein subunit levels in some tumors, they did not result in shrinkage of any tumors *(262–267)*. Similarly, a potent GnRH antagonist, Nal-Glu, was effective in reducing gonadotropin and glycoprotein subunit levels in some patients with gonadotroph adenomas, but did not result in tumor shrinkage (Figure 7) *(268,269)*.

OCTREOTIDE

Somatostatin receptors have been identified on the cell membranes of gonadotroph adenomas *(270)*. In vitro, Klibanski et al. *(271)* found that somatostatin could suppress intact gonadotropin or gonadotropin subunit production from most such tumors. In subsequent studies, DeBruin et al. *(272)* found that octreotide reduced FSH slightly in two of four patients with gonadotroph adenomas, improved visual field defects in three of the four, but did not result in any changes in CT scan appearance. Katznelson et al. *(273)* showed that octreotide reduced α-subunit secretion in three of six patients, the tumor mass in two patients by MRI scan, and visual fields without radiologic improvement into two additional patients. Similarly, Warnet et al. *(273a)* showed that in 24 patients, visual improvement was noted in 60% and in 7 patients who had been treated for up to 2 mo, three had substantial reductions in tumor size (26%, 55%, and 73%), three had no change, and one had an increase in tumor size.

CONCLUSIONS

In summary, despite theoretical reasons why they should work, GnRH agonist and antagonists have thus far not been successful in reducing tumor size. When medical therapy is indicated, it seems to be useful to try bromocriptine first because of its ease of use, realizing the relatively poor chance of

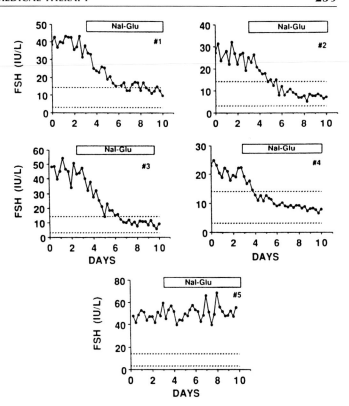

Figure 14-7 Serum FSH concentrations of five patients with gonadotroph adenomas for the 3 d before and 7 d during administration of Nal-Glu GnRH (5 mg/h, sc). (From McGrath et al. *[269]*. Reproduced by permission. ©The Endocrine Society.)

success. On the other hand, there is only limited experience with octreotide, but it does appear to offer a higher rate of success, although with a higher cost in both dollars and convenience.

THYROTROPIN-SECRETING ADENOMAS

Somatostatin is the primary thyroid-stimulating hormone (TSH) inhibitory hormone, and early studies showed that it inhibits TSH in normal humans *(274)* and those with TSH-secreting pituitary adenomas *(275)*. Thus, it was only logical to try octreotide for the medical treatment of TSH-secreting adenomas, and it has proven to be quite successful. The first report of this use was by Comi et al. *(276)*, who found that octreotide decreased TSH levels substantially in four of five patients and corrected the hyperthyroidism in both clinically hyperthyroid patients. Although dopamine also suppresses TSH and bromocriptine has been successful in reducing TSH secretion in a small number of patients with TSH-secreting adenomas *(277)*, the tremendous success with octreotide has rendered use of bromocriptine beneficial to those patients not responding to octreotide.

In 1993, Chanson et al. *(278)* reviewed not only all of the original case reports from the literature, but also information supplied by Sandoz on additional cases, so that a comprehensive picture of the effect of octreotide on these tumors was provided based on data from 52 patients from 24 medical centers in 9 countries. Thirty-three patients were treated for 1–2 wk with octreotide (50–100 μg 2–3 times/d); in 88% TSH levels were reduced to <50% of baseline, and in 72%, TSH levels returned to normal (Figure 8). In the three patients whose TSH levels did not normalize, thyroid hormone levels did return to normal after 1 wk. Two patients appeared to

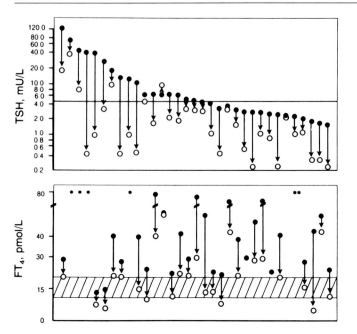

Figure 14-8 Individual levels of TSH and free thyroxine (FT₄) during short-term (1–2 wk) octreotide therapy in patients with TSH-secreting adenomas. Closed circles denote basal levels, and open circles denote levels at the end of the short-term study. In patients who also received levothyroxine (indicated by single asterisk) or antithyroid drug (indicated by double asterisk) treatment, interpretation of FT₄ course was impossible. The unbroken horizontal line in upper panel indicates the upper limit of normal for TSH. The horizontal hatched area in lower panel indicates the normal range for FT₄. (Reproduced from Chanson et al. *[278]* with copyright permission from the American College of Physicians.)

escape, thyroid hormone levels increasing despite increasing octreotide dosage. Octreotide was continued for 3–61 mo in 25 of these patients, and normal thyroid hormone levels were maintained in 84%. Tachyphylaxis was observed in 5 of these 21 patients, requiring a doubling of the octreotide dose. Three of the 25 showed true escape, thyroid hormone levels increasing despite incremental doses of octreotide. In all patients in whom the drug was stopped, TSH and thyroid hormone levels returned to pretreatment levels. However, the dose could be decreased slightly in 5 of the 25, but in others, the dose had to be maintained. MRI or CT scans showed that tumor volume decreased in 10 of the 25 patients, the amount of shrinkage being 30–70%. Side effects of treatment were similar to those observed in patients with acromegaly treated with octreotide, i.e., bloating, diarrhea, and gallstones. In a later review of the literature and their own experience, Beck-Peccoz et al. *(279)* found that of 73 patients, octreotide caused a normalization of the thyroid state in 95% with vision improvement in 75% and tumor shrinkage in 52%. They also found tachyphylaxis in 22% of patients with true escape occurring in 10%. Lanreotide has also been shown to be effective in these tumors *(280)*.

REFERENCES

1. Flückiger, Wagner HR. 2-Br-α-ergokryptin: beeinflussung von fertilität und laktation bei der ratte. Experientia 1968;24:1130,1131.
2. Shelesnyak MC. Ergotoxine inhibition of deciduoma formation and its reversal by progesterone. Am J Physiol 1954;179:301–304.
3. Lutterbeck PM, Pryor JS, Varga L, Wenner R. Treatment of non-puerperal galactorrhoea with an ergot alkaloid. Br Med J 1971;3:228,229.
4. Besser GM, Parke L, Edwards CRW, Forsyth IA, McNeilly AS. Galactorrhoea: successful treatment with reduction of plasma prolactin levels by Brom-ergocryptine. Br Med J 1972;3:669–672.
5. Molitch ME, Reichlin S. Hyperprolactinemic disorders. Disease-a-Month 1982;28(9):1–58.
6. Vance ML, Evans WS, Thorner MO. Bromocriptine. Ann Intern Med 1984;100:78–91.
7. Lu K-H, Meites J. Effects of L-DOPA on serum prolactin and PIF in intact and hypophysectomized, pituitary-grafted rats. Endocrinology 1972;91:868–872.
8. Birge CA, Jacobs LS, Hammer CT, Daughaday WH. Catecholamine inhibition of prolactin secretion by isolated rat adenohypophyses. Endocrinology 1970;86:120–130.
9. MacLeod RM, Fontham EH, Lehmeyer JE. Prolactin and growth hormone production as influenced by catecholamines and agents that affect brain catecholamines. Neuroendocrinology 1970;6:283–294.
10. Molitch ME. Prolactin. In: Melmed S, ed. The Pituitary. Blackwell Scientific, Boston, 1995, 136–186.
11. Corrodi H, Fuxe K, Hökfelt T, Lidbrink P, Ungerstedt U. Effect of ergot drugs on central catecholamine neurons: evidence for a stimulation of central dopamine neurons. J Pharm Pharmacol 1973;25:409–411.
12. MacLeod RM, Lehmeyer JE. Suppression of pituitary tumor growth and function by ergot alkaloids. Cancer Res 1973;33:849–855.
13. Davies C, Jacobi J, Lloyd HM, Meares JD. DNA synthesis and the secretion of prolactin and growth hormone by the pituitary gland of the male rat effects of diethylstilbestrol and 2-bromo-α-ergocryptine methanesulphonate. J Endocrinol 1974;61:411–417.
14. Maurer RA. Dopaminergic inhibition of prolactin synthesis and prolactin messenger RNA accumulation in cultured pituitary cells. J Biol Chem 1980;255:8092–8097.
15. Cronin MJ, Cheung CY, Wilson CB, Jaffe RB, Weiner RI. [³H]Spiperone binding to human anterior pituitaries and pituitary adenomas secreting prolactin, growth hormone, and adrenocorticotropic hormone. J Clin Endocrinol Metab 1980;50:387–391.
16. Sibley DR, Creese I. Interactions of ergot alkaloids with anterior pituitary D-2 dopamine receptors. Mol Pharmacol 1983;23:585–593.
17. Schran HR, Bhuta SI, Schwarz HJ, Thorner MO. The pharmacokinetics of bromocriptine in man. In: Goldstein M, Calne D, Lieberman A, Thorner M, eds. Ergot Compounds and Brain Function: Neuroendocrine and Neuropsychiatric Aspects. Raven, NY, 1980, pp. 125–189.
18. Thorner MO, Schran HF, Evans WS, Rogol AD, Morris JL, MacLeod RM. A broad spectrum of prolactin suppression by bromocriptine in hyperprolactinemic women: a study of serum prolactin and bromocriptine levels after acute and chronic administration of bromocriptine. J Clin Endocrinol Metab 1980;50:1026–1033.
19. Pellegrini I, Rasolonjanahary R, Gunz G, Bertrand P, Delivet S, Jedynak CP, et al. Resistance to bromocriptine in prolactinomas. J Clin Endocrinol Metab 1989;69:500–509.
20. Lloyd HM, Meares JD, Jacobi J. Effects of oestrogen and bromocryptine on in vivo secretion and mitosis in prolactin cells. Nature 1975;255:497–498.
21. Johansen PW, Clausen OPF, Haug E, Fossum S, Gautvik KM. Effects of bromocriptine on cell cycle distribution and cell morphology in cultured rat pituitary adenoma cells. Acta Endocrinol 1985;110:319–328.
22. Quadri SK, Meites KH, Lu J. Ergot-induced inhibition of pituitary tumor growth in rats. Science 1972;176:417,418.
23. Bergström M, Muhr C, Lundberg PO, Bergstrom K, Gee AD, Fasth K-J, et al. Rapid decrease in amino acid metabolism in prolactin-secreting pituitary adenomas after bromocriptine treatment: A PET study. J Comp Asst Tomography 1987;11:815–819.

24. Barrow DL, Tindall GT, Kovacs K, Thorner MO, Horvath E, Hoffman JC Jr. Clinical and pathological effects of bromocriptine on prolactin-secreting and other pituitary tumors. J Neurosurg 1984;60:1–7.

25. Tindall GT, Kovacs K, Horvath E, Thorner MO. Human prolactin-producing adenomas and bromocriptine: a histological, immuno-cytochemical, ultrastructural, and morphometric study. J Clin Endocrinol Metab 1982;55:1178–1183.

26. Niwa J, Minase T, Mori M, Hashi K. Immunohistochemical, electron microscopic, and morphometric studies of human prolactinomas after short-term bromocriptine treatment. Surg Neurol 1987;28:339–344.

27. Anniko M, Wersäll J. Clinical and morphological findings in two cases of bromocriptine-treated prolactinomas. Acta Pathol Microbiol Scand 1981;89:41–47.

28. Bassetti M, Spada A, Pezzo G, Giannattasio G. Bromocriptine treatment reduces the cell size in human macroprolactinomas: a morphometric study. J Clin Endocrinol Metab 1984;58:268–273.

29. Mori H, Mori S, Saitoh Y, Arita N, Aono T, Uozumi T, et al. Effects of bromocriptine on prolactin-secreting pituitary adenomas. Cancer 1985;56:230–238.

30. Kovacs K, Stefaneanu L, Horvath E, Lloyd RV, Lancranjan I, Buchfelder M, et al. Effect of dopamine agonist medication on prolactin producing pituitary adenomas. A morphological study including immunocytochemistry, electron microscopy and in situ hybridization. Virch Arch A Pathol Anat 1991;418:439–446.

31. Molitch ME, Reichlin S. The amenorrhea, galactorrhea and hyperprolactinemia syndromes. In: Stollerman GD, ed. Advances in Internal Medicine, vol. 26. Year Book Medical Publishers, Chicago, 1980, pp. 37–65.

32. Corenblum B, Webster BR, Mortimer CB, Ezrin C. Possible anti-tumour effect of 2 patients with large prolactin-secreting pituitary adenomas. Clin Res 1975;23: 614A.

33. Molitch ME, Elton RL, Blackwell RE, Caldwell B, Chang RJ, Jaffe R, et al. Bromocriptine as primary therapy for prolactin-secreting macroadenomas: results of a prospective multicenter study. J Clin Endocrinol Metab 1985;60:698–705.

34. Bevan JS, Adams CBT, Burke CW, Morton KE, Molyneux AJ, Moore RA, et al. Factors in the outcome of trans-sphenoidal surgery for prolactinoma and non-functioning pituitary tumour, including pre-operative bromocriptine therapy. Clin Endocrinol 1987;26:541–556.

35. Wang C, Lam KSL, Ma JTC, Chan T, Liu MY Yeung RTT. Long-term treatment of hyperprolactinaemia with bromocriptine: effect of drug withdrawal. Clin Endocrinol 1987;27:363–371.

36. McGregor AM, Scanlon MF, Hall R, Hall K. Effects of bromocriptine on pituitary tumour size. Br Med J 1979;2: 700–703.

37. Sobrinho LG, Nunes MC, Jorge-Calhaz C, Mauricio JC, Santos MA. Effect of treatment with bromocriptine on the size and activity of prolactin producing pituitary tumours. Acta Endocrinol 1981;96:24–29.

38. Spark RF, Baker R, Bienfang DC, Bergland R. Bromocriptine reduces pituitary tumor size and hypersecretion. JAMA 1982; 247:311–316.

39. Nissim M, Ambrosi B, Bernasconi V, et al. Bromocriptine treatment of macroprolactinomas: studies on the time course of tumor shrinkage and morphology. J Endocrinol 1982;5:409–415.

40. Wass JAH, Williams J, Charlesworth M, et al. Bromocriptine in management of large pituitary tumours. Br Med J 1982;284: 1908–1911.

41. Wollesen F, Andersen T, Karle A. Size reduction of extrasellar pituitary tumours during bromocriptine treatment. Ann Intern Med 1982;96:281–286.

42. Horowitz BL, Hamilton DJ, Sommers CJ, Bryan RN, Boyd AE III. Effect of bromocriptine and pergolide on pituitary tumor size and serum prolactin. AJNR 1983;4:415–417.

43. Corenblum B, Taylor PJ. Long-term follow-up of hyperprolactinemic women treated with bromocriptine. Fertil Steril 1983;40:596–599.

44. Weiss MH, Wycoff RR, Yadley R, Gott P, Feldon S. Bromocriptine treatment of prolactin-secreting tumors: surgical implications. Neurosurgery 1983;12:640–642.

45. Johnston DG, Hall K, Kendall-Taylor P, Patrick D, Watson M, Cook DB. Effect of dopamine agonist withdrawal after long-term therapy in prolactinomas. Lancet 1984;2:187–192.

46. Warfield A, Finkel DM, Schatz NJ, Savino PJ, Snyder PJ. Bromocriptine treatment of prolactin-secreting pituitary adenomas may restore pituitary function. Ann Intern Med 1984;101:783–785.

47. Liuzzi A, Dallabonzana D, Oppizzi G, Verde GG, Cozzi R, Chiodini P, et al. Low doses of dopamine agonist in the long-term treatment of macroprolactinomas. N Engl J Med 1985;313:656–659.

48. Pullan PT, Carroll WM, Chakera TMH, Khangure MS, Vaughan RJ. Management of extra-sellar pituitary tumours with bromocriptine: comparison of prolactin secreting and non-functioning tumours using half-field visual evoked potentials and computerised tomography. Aust NZ J Med 1985;15:203–208.

49. Gasser RW, Holzner-Mueller E, Skrabal F, Finkenstedt G, Mayr U, Tabarelli M, et al. Macroprolactinomas and functionless pituitary tumours. Immunostaining and effect of dopamine agonist therapy. Acta Endocrinol 1987;116:253–259.

50. Fahlbusch R, Buchfelder M, Schrell U. Short-term preoperative treatment of macroprolactinomas by dopamine agonists. J Neurosurg 1987;67:807–815.

51. Molitch ME. Prolactinoma. In: Melmed S, ed. The Pituitary. Blackwell Scientific, Boston, 1995, 443–477.

52. Bevan JS, Webster J, Burke CW, Scanlon MF. Dopamine agonists and pituitary tumor shrinkage. Endocr Rev 1992;13:220–240.

53. Bonneville JF, Poulignot D, Cattin F, Couturier M, Mollet E, Dietemann JL. Computed tomographic demonstration of the effects of bromocriptine on pituitary microadenoma size. Radiology 1982;143:451–455.

54. Demura R, Kubo O, Demura H, Shizume K, Kitamura K. Changes in computed tomographic findings in microprolactinomas before and after bromocriptine. Acta Endocrinol 1985;110:308–312.

55. Thorner MO, Martin WH, Rogol AD, Morris JL, Perryman RL, Conway BP, et al. Rapid regression of pituitary prolactinomas during bromocriptine treatment. J Clin Endocrinol Metab 1980; 51:438–445.

56. Dalzell GW, Atkinson AB, Carson DJ, Sheridan B. Normal growth and pubertal development during bromocriptine treatment for a prolactin-secreting pituitary macroadenoma. Clin Endocrinol 1987;169–172.

57. Landolt AM, Keller PJ, Froesch ER, Mueller J. Bromocriptine: does it jeopardize the result of later surgery for prolactinomas? Lancet 1982;2:657–658.

58. Landolt AM, Osterwalder V. Perivascular fibrosis in prolactinomas: is it increased by bromocriptine? J Clin Endocrinol Metab 1984;58:1179–1183.

59. Esiri MM, Bevan JS, Burke CW, Adams CBT. Effect of bromocriptine treatment on the fibrous tissue content of prolactin-secreting and nonfunctioning macroadenomas of the pituitary gland. J Clin Endocrinol Metab 1986;63:383–388.

60. Faglia G, Moriondo P, Travaglini P, Giovanelli MA. Influence of previous bromocriptine therapy on surgery for microprolactinoma. Lancet 1983;1:133–134.

61. Fahlbusch R, Buchfelder M. Influence of preoperative bromocriptine therapy on success of surgery for microprolactinoma. Lancet 1984;2:519–520.

62. Hubbard JL, Bernd MD, Scheithauer W, Abboud CF, Laws ER Jr. Prolactin-secreting adenomas: the preoperative response to bromocriptine treatment and surgical outcome. J Neurosurg 1987;67:816–821.

63. Johnston DG, Prescott RWG, Kendall-Taylor P, Hall K, Crombie AL, Hall R, et al. Hyperprolactinemia: long-term effects of bromocriptine. Am J Med 1983;75:868–874.

64. Ho KY, Smythe GA, Compton PJ, Lazarus L. Long-term bromocriptine therapy may restore the inhibitory control of prolactin release in some patients with pathological hyperprolactinemia. Aust NZ J Med 1985;15:213–219.

65. Soto-Albors CE, Randolph JF, Ying YK, Riddick DH. Medical management of hyperprolactinemia: a lower dose of bromocriptine may be effective. Fertil Steril 1987;48:213–217.

66. Thorner MO, Perryman RL, Rogol AD, Conway BP, MacLeod RM, Login IS, et al. Rapid changes of prolactinoma volume after withdrawal and reinstitution of bromocriptine. J Clin Endocrinol Metab 1981;53:480–483.

67. Johnston DG, Hall K, Kendall-Taylor P, Patrick D, Watson M, Cook DB. Effect of dopamine agonist withdrawal after long-term therapy in prolactinomas. Lancet 1984;ii:187–192.

68. Van't Verlaat JW, Croughs RJM. Withdrawal of bromocriptine after long-term therapy for macroprolactinomas; effect on plasma prolactin and tumour size. Clin Endocrinol 1991;34:175–178.

69. Rasmussen C, Bergh T, Wide L. Prolactin secretion and menstrual function after long-term bromocriptine treatment. Fertil Steril 1987;48:550–554.

70. Turner TH, Cookson JC, Wass JAH, Drury PL, Price PA, Besser GM. Psychotic reactions during treatment of pituitary tumours with dopamine agonist. Br Med J 1984;289:1101–1103.

71. Le Feuvre CM, Isaacs AJ, Frank OS. Bromocriptine-induced psychosis in acromegaly. Br Med J 1982;285:1315.

72. Procter AW, Littlewood R, Fry AH. Bromocriptine induced psychosis in acromegaly. Br Med J 1983;286:50,51.

73. Perovich RM, Lieberman JA, Fleischhacker WW, Alvir J: The behavioral toxicity of bromocriptine in patients with psychiatric illness. J Clin Psychopharmacol 1989;9:417–422.

74. McElvaney NG, Wilcox PG, Churg A, Fleetham JA. Pleuropulmonary disease during bromocriptine treatment of Parkinson's disease. Arch Intern Med 1988;148:2231–2236.

75. Demonet JF, Rostin M, Dueymes JM, Ioualalen A, Montrastruc JL, Rascol A. Retroperitoneal fibrosis and treatment of Parkinson's disease with high doses of bromocriptine. Clin Neuropharmacol 1986;9:200,201.

76. Bowler JV, Ormerod IE, Legg NJ. Retroperitoneal fibrosis and bromocriptine. Lancet 1986;2:466.

77. Giampietro O, Ferdghini M, Petrini M. Severe leukopenia and mild thrombocytopenia after chronic bromocriptine (CB-154) administration. Am J Clin Sci 1981;281:169–172.

78. Liberato NL, Poli M, Bollati P, Chiofalo F, Filipponi M. Bromocriptine-induced acute hepatitis. Lancet 1992;340:969–970.

79. Blackard WG. Edema—an infrequently recognized complication of bromocriptine and other ergot dopaminergic drugs. Am J Med 1993;94:445.

80. Ferrari MD, Haan J, van Seters AP. Bromocriptine-induced trigeminal neuralgia attacks in a patient with a pituitary tumor. Neurology 1988;38:1482–1484.

81. Kulig K, Moore LL, Kirk M, Smith D, Stallworth J, Rumack B. Bromocriptine-associated headache: possible life-threatening sympathomimetic interaction. Obstet Gynecol 1991;78:941–943.

82. Larrazet F, Spaulding C, Lobreau HJ, Weber S, Guerin F. Possible bromocriptine-induced myocardial infarction. Ann Intern Med 1993;118:199,200.

83. Nickels D, Poth M. SVT and bromocriptine: a case report. The Endocrinologist 1995;5:238–239.

84. Afshar F, Thomas A. Bromocriptine-induced cerebrospinal fluid rhinorrhea. Surg Neurol 1982;18:61–63.

85. Kok JG, Bartelink AKM, Schulte BPM, et al. Cerebrospinal fluid rhinorrhea during treatment with bromocriptine for prolactinoma. Neurology 1985;35:1193–1195.

85a. Caccavelli L, Feron F, Morange I, et al. Decreased expression of the two D_2 dopamine receptor isoforms in bromocriptine-resistant prolactinomas. Neuroendocrinology 1994;60:314–322.

86. Brue T, Pellegrini I, Priou A, Morange I, Jaquet P. Prolactinomas and resistance to dopamine agonist. Horm Res 1992;38:84–89.

87. Dallabonzana D, Spelta B, Oppizzi G, Tonon C, Luccarelli G, Chiodini PH, et al. Reenlargement of macropro-lactinomas during bromocriptine treatment: report of two cases. J Endocrinol Invest 1983;6:47–50.

88. Crosignani PG, Mattei A, Ferrari C, Giovanelli MA. Enlargement of a prolactin-secreting pituitary microadenoma during bromocriptine treatment. Br J Obstet Gynecol 1982;89:169–170.

89. Schwarzstein D, Garcia-Patterson A, Giménez G, Calaf J, Puig-Domingo M, Caixàs A, et al. Dopaminergic resistance in a case of invasive macroprolactinoma. J Endocrinol Invest 1993;16:443–447.

90. Martin NA, Hales M, Wilson CB. Cerebellar metastasis from a prolactinoma during treatment with bromocriptine. J Neurosurg 1981;55:615–619.

91. Vermesh M, Fossum GT, Kletzky OA. Vaginal bromocriptine: pharmacology and effect on serum prolactin in normal women. Obstet Gynecol 1988;72:693–698.

92. Katz E, Scharan JF, Weiss BE, Adashi EY, Hassell A. Increased circulating levels of bromocriptine after vaginal compared with oral administration. Fertil Steril 1991;55:882–884.

93. Jasonni VM, Raffelli R, de March A, Frank G, Flamigni C. Vaginal bromocriptine in hyperprolactinemic patients and puerperal women. Acta Obstet Gynecol Scand 1991;70:493–495.

94. Katz E, Schran HF, Adashi EY. Successful treatment of a prolactin-producing pituitary macroadenoma with intravaginal bromocriptine mesylate: a novel approach to intolerance of oral therapy. Obstet Gynecol 1989;73:517–520.

95. Montini M, Pagani G, Gianola D, Pagani MD, Salmoiraghi L, Ferrari L, et al. Long-lasting suppression of prolactin secretion and rapid shrinkage of prolactinomas after a long-acting, injectable form of bromocriptine. J Clin Endocrinol Metab 1986;63:266–268.

96. Grossman A, Ross R, Wass JAH, Besser GM. Depot-bromocriptine treatment for prolactinomas and acromegaly. Clin Endocrinol 1986;24:231–238.

97. Ciccarelli E, Miola C, Grottoli S, Avataneo T, Lancranjan I, Camanni F. Long term therapy of patients with macroprolactinoma using repeatable injectable bromocriptine. J Clin Endocrinol Metab 1993;76:484–488.

98. Krupp P, Monka C. Bromocriptine in pregnancy: safety aspects. Klin Wochenschr 1987;65:823–827.

99. Krupp P, Monka C, Richter K. The safety aspects of infertility treatments. Program of the Second World Congress of Gynecology and Obstetrics, Rio de Janeiro, October, 1988.

100. Raymond JP, Goldstein E, Konopka P, Leleu MF, Merceron RE, Loria Y. Follow-up of children born of bromocriptine-treated mothers. Hormone Res 1985;22:239–246.

101. Molitch ME. Pregnancy and the hyperprolactinemic woman. N Engl J Med 1985;312:1365–1370.

102. Van Roon E, van der Vijver JCM, Gerretsen G, Hekster REM, Wattendorff RA. Rapid regression of a suprasellar extending prolactinoma after bromocriptine treatment during pregnancy. Fertil Steril 1981;36:173–177.

103. Maeda T, Ushiroyama T, Okuda K, Fujimoto A, Ueki M, Sugimoto O. Effective bromocriptine treatment of a pituitary macroadenoma during pregnancy. Obstet Gynecol 1983;61:117–121.

104. Bigazzi M, Ronga R, Lancranjan I, Ferrado S, Branconi F, Buzzoni P, et al. A pregnancy in an acromegalic woman during bromocriptine treatment: effects on growth hormone and prolactin in the maternal, fetal, and amniotic compartments. J Clin Endocrinol Metab 1979;48:9–12.

105. Canales ES, García IC, Ruíz JE, Zàrate A. Bromocriptine as prophylactic therapy in prolactinoma during pregnancy. Fertil Steril 1981;36:524–526.

106. Ruiz-Velasco V, Tolis G. Pregnancy in hyperprolactinemic women. Fertil Steril 1984;41:793–805.

107. Ylikorkala O, Kivinen S, Rönnberg L. Bromocriptine treatment during early human pregnancy: effect on the levels of prolactin, sex steroids and placenta lactogen. Acta Endocrinol 1980;95:412–415.

108. Lehmann WD, Musch K, Wolf AS. Influence of bromocriptine on plasma levels of prolactin and steroid hormones in the 20th week of pregnancy. J Endocrinol Invest 1979;2:251–255.

109. Lemberger L, Crabtree R, Callaghan JT. Pergolide, a potent long-acting dopamine-receptor agonist. Clin Pharmacol Ther 1980;27:642–651.

110. Franks S, Lynch SS, Horrocks PM, Butt WR. Treatment of hyperprolactinaemia with pergolide mesylate: acute effects and preliminary evaluation of long-term treatment. Lancet 1981; 2:659–661.

111. Blackwell RE, Bradley EL, Kline LB, Duvall JJ, DeVane GW, Change RJ. Comparison of dopamine agonist in the treatment of hyperprolactinemic syndromes: a multicenter study. Fertil Steril 1983;39:744–748.

112. Grossman A, Bouloux P-MG, Loneragan R, Rees LH, Wass JAH, Besser GM. Comparison of the clinical activity of mesulergine and pergolide in the treatment of hyperprolactinaemia. Clin Endocrinol 1985;22:611–616.

113. Mattox JH, Bernstein J, Buckman MT. Control of hyperprolactinemia with pergolide. Int J Fertil 1986;30:39–43.

114. Kletzky OA, Borenstein R, Mileikowsky GN. Pergolide and bromocriptine for the treatment of patients with hyperprolactinemia. Am J Obstet Gynecol 1986;154:431–435.

115. Lamberts SWJ, Quik RFP. A comparison of the efficacy and safety of pergolide and bromocriptine in the treatment of hyperprolactinemia. J Clin Endocrinol Metab 1991;72:635–6341.

116. Ahmed SR, Shalet SM. Discordant responses of prolactinoma to two different dopamine agonist. Clin Endocrinol 1986;24:421–426.

117. Berezin M, Avidan D, Baron E. Long-term pergolide treatment of hyperprolactinemic patients previously unsuccessfully treated with dopaminergic drugs. Isr J Med Sci 1991;27:375–379.

117a. Freda PU, Andreadis CI, Khandji AG, et al. Long-term treatment of prolactin-secreting macroadenomas with pergolide. J Clin Endocrinol Metab 2000;85:8–13.

118. Vance ML, Cragun JR, Reimnitz C, Chang RJ, Rashef E, Blackwell RE, et al. CV 205-502 treatment of hyperpro-lactinemia. J Clin Endocrinol Metab 1989;68:336–339.

119. Vance ML, Lipper M, Klibanski A, Biller BMK, Samaan NA, Molitch ME. Treatment of prolactin-secreting pituitary macroadenomas with the long-acting non-ergot dopamine agonist CV 205-502. Ann Intern Med 1990;112:668–673.

120. Duranteau L, Chanson P, Lavoinne A, Horlait S, Lubetzki J, Kuhn JM. Effect of the new dopaminergic agonist CV 205-502 on plasma prolactin levels and tumour size in bromocriptine-resistant prolactinomas. Clin Endocrinol 1991;34:25–29.

121. Brue T, Pellegrini I, Gunz G, Morange I, DeWailly D, Brownell J, et al. Effects of the dopamine agonist CV 205-502 in human prolactinomas resistant to bromocriptine. J Clin Endocrinol Metab 1992;74:577–584.

122. DiSalle E, Ornati G, Giudici D. A comparison of the *in vivo* and *in vitro* duration of prolactin lowering effect in rats of FCE 21336, pergolide and bromocriptine. J Endocrinol Invest 1984;7 (Suppl 1):32.

123. Strolin Benedetti M, Doster P, Barone D, Efthymiopoulos C, Peretti G, Roncucci R. *In vivo* interaction of CAB with rat brain dopamine receptors labelled with 3H-*N*-*n*-propylinorapomorphine. Eur J Pharmacol 1990;187:399–408.

124. Andreotti AC, Pianezzola E, Persiani S, Pacciarini MS, Strolin Benedetti M, Pontiroli AE. Pharmacokinetics, pharmacodynamics, and tolerability of cabergoline, a prolactin-lowering drug after administration of increasing oral doses (0.5, 1.0, and 1.5 milligrams) in healthy male volunteers. J Clin Endocrinol Metab 1995;80:841.

125. Ferrari C, Barbieri C, Caldara R, Mucci M, Codecasa F, Parachhi A, et al. Long-lasting prolactin-lowering effect of cabergoline, a new dopamine agonist, in hyperprolactinemic patients. J Clin Endocrinol Metab 1986;63:941–945.

126. Melis GB, Gambacciani M, Paoletti AM, Beneventi F, Mais V, Baroldi P, et al. Dose-related prolactin inhibitory effect of the new long-acting dopamine receptor agonist cabergoline in normal cycling, puerperal, and hyperprolactinemic women. J Clin Endocrinol Metab 1987;65:541–545.

127. Ciccarelli E, Giusti M, Miola C, Potenzoni F, Sgheoni D, Camanni F, et al. Effectiveness and tolerability of long term treatment with cabergoline, a new long-lasting ergoline derivative, in hyperprolactinemic patients. J Clin Endocrinol 1989;69:725–728.

128. Ferrari C, Mattei A, Melis GB, Paracchi A, Muratori M, Faglia G, et al. Cabergoline: long-acting oral treatment of hyperprolactinemic disorders. J Clin Endocrinol Metab 1989;68:1201–1206.

129. Webster J, Piscitelli G, Polli A, Ferrari CI, Ismail I, Scanlon MF for the Cabergoline Comparative Study Group. A comparison of cabergoline and bromocriptine in the treatment of hyperprolactinemic amenorrhea. N Engl J Med 1994;331:904–909.

130. Biller BMK, Molitch ME, Vance ML, Cannistraro KB, Davis KR, Simons JA, et al. Treatment of prolactin-secreting macroadenomas with the once-weekly dopamine agonist cabergoline. J Clin Endocrinol Metab 1996;81:2338–2343.

130a. Colao A, DeSarno A, Landi ML, et al. Long-term and low-dose treatment with cabergoline induces macroprolactinoma shrinkage. J Clin Endocrinol Metab 1997;82:3574–3579.

130b. Colao A, DiSarno A, Sarnacchiaro S, et al. Prolactinomas resistant to standard dopamine-agonists respond to chronic cabergoline treatment. J Clin Endocrinol Metab. 1997;82:876–883.

130c. Verhelst J, Abs R, Maiter D, et al. Cabergoline in the treatment of hyperprolactinemia: a study in 455 patients. J Clin Endocrinol Metab 1999;84:2518–2522.

130d. Robert E, Musatti L, Piscitelli G, Ferrari CI. Pregnancy outcome after treatment with the ergot derivative, cabergoline. Reprod Toxicol 1996;10:333–337.

130e. Pharmacia and Upjohn, Inc. Data on File, June, 1999.

131. Liuzzi A, Chiodini PG, Botalia L, Cremascoli G, Silverstrini F. Inhibitory effect of l-dopa on GH release in acromegalic patients. J Clin Endocrinol Metab 1972;35:941–943.

132. Boyd AE III, Lebovitz HE, Pfeiffer JB. Stimulation of human-growth-hormone secretion by L-dopa. N Engl J Med 1970;283: 1425–1429.

133. Bression D, Brandt AM, Nousbaum A, Le Dafniet M, Racadot J, Peillon F. Evidence of dopamine receptors in human growth hormone (GH)-secreting adenomas with concomitant study of dopamine inhibition of GH secretion in a perifusion system. J Clin Endocrinol Metab 1982;55:589–593.

134. Liuzzi A, Chiodini PG, Botalla L, Cremascoli G, Müller EE, SIlvestrini F. Decreased plasma growth hormone (GH) levels in acromegalics following CB 154 (2-Br-α-ergocryptine) administration. J Clin Endocrinol Metab 1974;38:910–912.

135. Jaffe CA, Barkan AL. Treatment of acromegaly with dopamine agonist. Endocrinol Metab Clin N Am 1992;21:713–735.

136. Rau H, Althoff P-H, Schmidt K, Usadel KH. Bromocriptine treatment over 12 years in acromegaly: effect on growth hormone and prolactin secretion. Acta Endocrinol 1992;126:247–252.

137. Lamberts SWJ, Klijn JGM, Kwa HG, Birkenhager JC. The dynamics of growth hormone and prolactin secretion in acromegalic patients with "mixed" pituitary tumours. Acta Endocrinol 1979; 90:198–210.

138. Nortier JW, Croughs RJ, Donker GH. Changes in plasma GH levels and clinical activity during bromocriptine therapy in acromegaly: effects. The value of predictive tests. Acta Endocrinol 1984;106:175–183.

139. Benker G, Sandmann K, Tharandt L, Hackenburg K, Reinwein D. Gel filtration studies of serum growth hormone in acromegaly following bromocriptine administration. Horm Res 1979;11: 151–160.

140. Carlson HE, Levin SR, Braunstein GD, Spencer EM, Wilson SE, Hershman JM. Effect of bromocriptine on serum hormones in acromegaly. Horm Res 1984;19:142–152.

141. Hizuka N, Hendricks CM, Roth J, Gorden P. Failure of bromocriptine to alter the qualitative characteristics of human growth hormone in acromegaly. Metabolism 1984;33:582–584.

142. Moses AC, Molitch ME, Sawin CT, Jackson IMD, Biller MJ, Furlanetto R, et al. Bromocriptine therapy in acromegaly: use in patients resistant to conventional therapy and effect on serum levels of somatomedin C. J Clin Endocrinol Metab 1981;53:752–758.

143. Wass JAH, Clemmons DR, Underwood LE, Barrow I, Besser GM, Van Wyk JJ. Changes in circulating somatomedin-C levels in bromocriptine-treated acromegaly. Clin Endocrinol 1982;17: 369–377.

144. Nortier JWR, Croughs RJM, Thijssen JHH, Schwarz F. Bromo-criptine therapy in acromegaly: effects on plasma GH levels, Somatomedin-C levels and clinical activity. Clin Endocrinol 1985;22:209–217.

145. De Herder WW, Uitterlinden P, van der Lely AJ, Hofland LJ, Lamberts SW. Octreotide, but not bromocriptine, increases circu-lating insulin-like growth factor binding protein 1 levels in acromegaly. Eur J Endocrinol 1995 133:195–199.

146. Jaspers C, Haase R, Pfingsten H, Benker G, Reinwein D. Long-term treatment of acromegalic patients with repeatable parenteral depot-bromocriptine. Clin Invest 1993;71:547–551.

147. Kleinberg DL, Boyd AE III, Wardlaw S, Frantz AG, George A, Bryan N, et al. Pergolide for the treatment of pituitary tumors secreting prolactin or growth hormone. N Engl J Med 1983; 309:704–709.

148. Kendall-Taylor P, Upstill-Goddard G, Cook D. Long term pergolide treatment of acromegaly. Clin Endocrinol 1983;19:711–719.

149. Chiodini PG, Attanasio R, Cozzi R, Dallabonzana D, Oppizzi G, Orlandi P, et al. CV 205-502 in acromegaly. Acta Endocrinol 1993;128:389–393.

149a. Abs R, Verhelst J, Maiter D, et al. Cabergoline in the treatment of acromegaly: a study in 64 patients. J Clin Endocrinol Metab 1998;83:375–378.

150. Krulich l, Dhariwal PS, McCann SM. Stimulatory and inhibitory effects of purified hypothalamic extracts on growth hormone release from rat pituitary in vitro. Endocrinology 1968;83:783–790.

151. Brazeau P, Vale W, Burgus R Ling N, Butcher M, Rivier J, et al. Hypothalamic polypeptide that inhibits the secretion of immu-noreactive pituitary growth hormone. Science 1973;179:77–79.

152. Siler TM, VandenBerg G, Yen SSC, Brazeau P, Vale W, Guillemin R. Inhibition of growth hormone release in humans by somatosta-tin. J Clin Endocrinol Metab 1973;37:632–634.

153. Besser GM, Mortimer CH, Carr D, Schally AV, Coy DJ, Evered D, et al. Growth hormone release inhibiting hormone in acromegaly. Br Med J 1974;1:352–355.

154. Yen SSC, Siler TM, DeVane GW. Effect of somatostatin in patients with acromegaly. Suppression of growth hormone, prolactin, insu-lin and glucose levels. N Engl J Med 1974;290:935–938.

155. Bauer W, Briner U, Doepfner W, Hall R, Huguenin R, Marbach P, et al. SMS 201-995: a very potent and selective octapeptide ana-logue of somatostatin with prolonged action. Life Sci 1982;31:1133–1140.

156. Del Pozo E, Neufeld M, Schlüter K, Tortosa F, Clarenbach P, Bieder E, et al. Endocrine profile of a long-acting somatostatin derivative SMS 201-995. Study in normal volunteers following subcutaneous administration. Acta Endocrinol 1986;111:433–439.

157. Lamberts SWJ, Oosterom R, Neufeld M, del Pozo A. The soma-tostatin analog SMS 201-995 induces long-acting inhibition of growth hormone secretion without rebound hypersecretion in acromegalic patients. J Clin Endocrinol Metab 1985;60:1161–1165.

158. Kallivretakis N, Yolis A, del Pozo E, et al. Pharmacokinetics of SMS 201-995 in normal subjects and in patients with severe renal failure. Neuroendocrinol Lett 1985;7:92.

159. Ørskov H, Christensen SE, Weeke J, Kaal A, Harris AG. Effects of antibodies against octreotide in two patients with acromegaly. Clin Endocrinol 1991;34:395–398.

160. Van Liessum PA, Swinkels LM, Pieters GF, Ross AA, Smals AG, Benraad TJ, et al. Lack of antibody formation during long-term subcutaneous treatment with the somatostatin analogue octreotide in acromegaly. Acta Endocrinol 1990;12:309–312.

161. Sandoz Pharmaceuticals, information on file

162. Landolt AM, Schmid J, Wimpfheimer C, Karlsson ERC, Boerlin V. Successful pregnancy in a previously infertile woman treated with SMS 201-995 for acromegaly. N Engl J Med 1989;320:671–672.

163. Montini M, Pagani G, Gianola D, Pagani MD, Piolini R, Camboni MG. Acromegaly and primary amenorrhea: ovulation and preg-nancy induced by SMS 201-995 and bromocriptine. J Endocrinol Invest 1990;13:193.

164. Caron P, Gerbeau C, Pradayrol L. Maternal-fetal transfer of octreotide. N Engl J Med 1995;333:601,602.

165. Reubi JC, Landolt AM. The growth hormone responses to octreotide in acromegaly correlate with adenoma stomatostatin receptor status. J Clin Endocrinol Metab 1989;68:844–850.

166. Lamberts SWJ, van der Lely A-J, de Herder WW, Hofland LJ. Octreotide. N Engl J Med 1996;334:246–254.

167. Greenman Y, Melmed S. Heterogeneous expression of two soma-tostatin receptor subtypes in pituitary tumors. J Clin Endocrinol Metab 1994;78:398–403.

168. Greenman Y, Melmed S. Expression of three somatostatin recep-tor subtypes in pituitary adenomas: evidence for preferential SSTR5 expression in the mammosomatotroph lineage. J Clin Endocrinol Metab 1994;79:724–729.

169. James RA, Weightman DR. Somatostatin receptors: types and clas-sification in the pituitary. The Endocrinologist 1995;5:55–60.

170. Flyvberg A, Jørgensen KD, Marshall SM, Ørskov H. Inhibitory effect of octreotide on growth hormone-induced IGF-I generation and organ growth in hypophysectomized rats. Am J Physiol 1991;260 (Endocrinol Metab 23): E568–574.

171. Serri O, Brazeau P, Kachra Z, Posner B. Octreotide inhibits insu-lin-like growth factor-I hepatic gene expression in the hypophy-sectomized rat: evidence of a direct and indirect mechanism of action,. Endocrinology 1992;130:1816–1821.

172. Ren S-G, Ezzat S, Melmed S, Braunstein GD. Somatostatin analog induces insulin-like growth factor binding protein-1 (IGFBP-1) expression in human hepatoma cells. Endocrinology 1992;131:2479–2481.

173. Ezzat S, Ren S-Q, Braunstein GD, Melmed S. Octreotide stimu-lates insulin-like growth factor binding protein-1 (IGFBP-1) lev-els in acromegaly. J Clin Endocrinol Metab 1991;73:441–443.

174. Ezzat S, Ren S-G, Braunstein GD, Melmed S. Octreotide stimu-lates insulin-like growth factor-binding protein-1: a potential pitu-itary-independent mechanism for drug action. J Clin Endocrinol Metab 1992;75:1459–1463.

175. Melmed S, Ziel FJ, Braunstein GD, Downs T, Frohman LA. Medi-cal management of acromegaly due to ectopic production of growth hormone-releasing hormone by a carcinoid tumor. J Clin Endocrinol Metab 1988;67:395–399.

176. Moller DE, Moses AC, Jones K, Thorner MO, Vance ML. Octreotide suppresses both growth hormone (GH) and GH-releas-ing hormone (GHRH) in acromegaly due to ectopic GHRH secre-tion. J Clin Endocrinol Metab 1989;68:499–504.

177. Ezzat S, Horvath E, Harris AG, Kovacs K. Morphological effects of octreotide on growth hormone-producing pituitary adenomas. J Clin Endocrinol Metab 1994;79:113–118.

178. Ezzat S, Snyder PJ, Young WF, Boyajy LD, Newman C, Klibanski A, et al. Octreotide treatment of acromegaly. A randomized, multicenter study. Ann Intern Med 1992;117:711–718.

179. Hofland LJ, van Koetsveld PM, van Vroonhoven CCJ, Stefanko SZ, Lamberts SWJ. Heterogeneity of growth hormone (GH) release by individual pituitary adenoma cells from acromegalic patients, as determined by the reverse hemolytic plaque assay: effects of SMS 201-995, GH-releasing hormone, and thyrotropin-releasing hormone. J Clin Endocrinol Metab 1989;68:613–620.

180. Lamberts SWJ. The role of somatostatin in the regulation of ante-rior pituitary hormone secretion and the use of its analogs in the treatment of human pituitary tumors. Endocr Rev 1988;9:417–436.

181. Vance ML, Harris AG. Long-term treatment of 189 acromegalic patients with the somatostatin analog octreotide. Results of the International Multicenter Acromegaly Study Group. Arch Intern Med 1991;151:1573–1578.

182. Sassolas G, Harris AG, James-Deidier A and the French SMS 201-995 Acromegaly Study Group: Long term effect of incremental doses of the somatostatin analog SMS 201-995 in 58 acromegalic patients. J Clin Endocrinol Metab 1990;71:391–397.

183. Newman CB, Melmed S, Snyder PJ, Young WF, Boyajy LD, Levy R, et al. Safety and efficacy of long term octreotide therapy of acromegaly: results of a multicenter trial in 103 patients—a clini-cal research center study. J Clin Endocrinol Metab 1995;80:2768–2775.

184. Arosio M, Macchelli S, Rossi CM, Casati G, Biella O, Faglia G and the Italian Multicenter Octreotide Study Group. Effect of treatment with octreotide in acromegalic patients—a multicenter Italian study. Eur J Endocrinol 1995;133:430–439.

185. Van der Lely AJ, Harris AG, Lamberts SWJ. The sensitivity of growth hormone secretion to medical treatment in acromegalic patients: influence of age and sex. Clin Endocrinol 1992;37:181–185.

186. Koop BL, Harris AG, Ezzat S. Effect of octreotide on glucose tolerance in acromegaly. Eur J Endocrinol 1994;130:581–586.

187. Grunstein RR, Ho KKY, Sullivan CE. Sleep apnea in acromegaly. Ann Intern Med 1991;115:527–532.

188. Grunstein RR, Ho KKY, Sullivan CE. Effect of octreotide, a somatostatin analog, on sleep apnea in patients with acromegaly. Ann Intern Med 1994;121:478–483.

189. Thuesen L, Christensen SE, Weeke J, Orskov H, Henningsen P. The cardiovascular effects of octreotide treatment in acromegaly: an echocardiographic study. Clin Endocrinol 1989;30:619–625.

190. Chanson P, Timsit J, Masquet C, et al. Cardiovascular effects of the somatostatin analog octreotide in acromegaly. Ann Intern Med 1990;113:921–925.

191. Paunović VR, Popović V. The development of dependence to an octapeptide somatostatin analog: contribution of the study of somatostatin analgesia. Biol Psychiatry 1989;26:97–101.

192. Pascual J, Freijanes J, Berciano J, Pesquera C. Analgesic effect of octreotide in headache associated with acromegaly is not mediated by opioid mechanisms. Case report. Pain 1991;46:341–344.

193. Stevenaert A, Beckers A. Presurgical octreotide treatment in acromegaly. Acta Endocrinol 1993;129 (Suppl 1):18–20.

194. Stewart PM, Kane KF, Stewart SE, Lancranjan I, Sheppard MC. Depot long-acting somatostatin analog (Sandostatin-LAR) is an effective treatment for acromegaly. J Clin Endocrinol Metab 1995;80:3267–3272.

195. Grass P, Marbach P, Bruns C, et al. Sandostatin LAR (microencapsulated octreotide acetate) in acromegaly: pharmacokinetics and pharmacodynamics relationships. Metabolism 1996; 45(suppl 1):27–30.

196. Lancranjan I, Atkinson AB, and the Sandostatin LAR Group. Results of a European Multicentre Study with Sandostatin LAR in acromegalic patients. Pituitary 1999;1:105–114.

197. Heron I, Thomas F, Dero M, Gancel A, Ruiz JM, Schatz B, et al. Pharmacokinetics and efficacy of a long-acting formulation of the new somatostatin analog BIM 23014 in patients with acromegaly. J Clin Endocrinol Metab 1993;76:721–727.

198. Motange I, De Boisvilliers F, Chanson P, Lucas B, Dewailly D, Catus F, et al. Slow release lanreotide treatment in acromegalic patients previously normalized by octreotide. J Clin Endocrinol Metab 1994;79:145–151.

199. Newman CB. Medical therapy for acromegaly. Endocrinol Metab Clin N Amer 1999;28:171–190.

200. Ho PJ, Boyajy LD, Greenstein E, Barkan AL. Effect of chronic octreotide treatment on intestinal absorption in patients with acromegaly. Dig Dis Sci 1993;38:309–315.

201. Plöckinger U, Dinemann D, Quabbe H-J. Gastrointestinal side-effects of octreotide during long term treatment of acromegaly. J Clin Endocrinol Metab 1990;71:1658–1662.

202. Anderson JV, Catnach S, Lowe DG, Fairclough PD, Besser GM, Wass JAH. Prevalence of gastritis in patients with acromegaly: untreated and during treatment with octreotide. Clin Endocrinol 1992;37:227–232.

203. Hopman WPM, van Liessum PA, Pieters GFFM, Jansen JBMJ, Lamers CBHW, Smals AGH, et al. Postprandial gallbladder motility and plasma cholecystokinin at regular time intervals after injection of octreotide in acromegalics on long-term treatment. Dig Dis Sci 1992;37:1685–1690.

204. Eastman RC, Arakaki RF, Shawker T, Schock R, Roach P, Comi RJ, et al. A prospective examination of octreotide-induced gall-bladder changes in acromegaly. Clin Endocrinol 1992;36:265–269.

205. Catnach SM, Anderson JV, Fairclough PD, Trembath RC, Wilson PAJ, Parker E, et al. Effect of octreotide on gall stone prevalence and gall bladder motility in acromegaly. Gut 1993;34:270–273.

206. Stolk MFJ, van Erpecum KJ, Koppeschaar JPF, de Bruin WI, Jansen JBMJ, Lamers CBHW, et al. Postprandial gall bladder motility and hormone release during intermittent and continuous subcutaneous octreotide treatment in acromegaly. Gut 1993;34: 808–813.

207. Shi Y-F, Zhu X-F, Harris AG, Zhang J-X, Dai Q. Prospective study of the long-term effects of somatostatin analog (octreotide) on gallbladder function and gallstone formation in chinese acromegalic patients. J Clin Endocrinol Metab 1993;76:32–37.

208. Tauber JP, Poncet MF, Harris AG, Barthel HR, Simonetta-Chateauneuf C, Buscail L, et al. The impact of continuous subcutaneous infusion of octreotide on gallstone formation in acromegalic patients. J Clin Endocrinol Metab 1995;80:3262–3266.

209. Chiodini PG, Cozzi R, Dallabonzana D, Oppizzi G, Verde G, Petroncini M, et al. Medical treatment of acromegaly with SMS 201-995, a somatostatin analog: a comparison with bromocriptine. J Clin Endocrinol Metab 1987;64:447–453.

210. Fløgstad AK, Halse J, Grass P, Abisch E, Djøseland O, Kutz K, et al. A comparison of octreotide, bromocriptine, or a combination of both drugs in acromegaly. J Clin Endocrinol Metab 1994;79: 462–466.

211. Lamberts SWJ, Zeens M, Verschoor L, del Pozo E. A comparison among the growth hormone-lowering effects in acromegaly of the somatostatin analog SMS 201–995, bromocriptine, and the combination of both drugs. J Clin Endocrinol Metab 1986;63:16–19.

211a. Trainer PJ, Drake WM, Katznelson L, et al. Treatment of acromegaly with pegvisomant, a genetically-engineered human growth hormone receptor antagonist. N Engl J Med. In Press.

212. Feldman D. Ketoconazole and other imidazole derivatives as inhibitors of steroidogenesis. Endocr Rev 1986;7:409–420.

213. Stalla GK, Stalla J, Huber M, Loeffler J-P, Hollt V, van Werder K, et al. Ketoconazole inhibits corticotropic cell function in vitro. Endocrinology 1988;122:618–623.

214. Stalla GK, Stalla J, von Werder K, Müller OA, Gerzer R, Höllt V, et al. Nitroimidazole derivatives inhibit anterior pituitary cell function apparently by a direct effect on the catalytic subunit of the adenylate cyclase holoenzyme. Endocrinology 1989;125:699–706.

215. Reina LJ, Leal-Cerro A, Garcia J, Garcia-Luna PP, Astorga R, Bernal G. In vitro effects of ketoconazole on corticotrope cell morphology and ACTH secretion of two pituitary adenomas removed from patients with Nelson's syndrome. Acta Endocrinol 1989;121:185–190.

216. Sonino N. The use of ketoconazole as an inhibitor of steroid production. N Engl J Med 1987;317:812–818.

217. Cerdas S, Billaud L, Guilhaume B, Laudat MH, Bertagna X, Luton JP. Effects a court terme due ketoconazole dans les syndromes de Cushing. Ann d'Endocrinologie 1989;50;489–496.

218. Tabarin A, Navarranne A, Guérin J, Corcuff J-B, Parneix M, Roger P. Use of ketoconazole in the treatment of Cushing's disease and ectopic ACTH syndrome. Clin Endocrinol 1991;34:63–69.

219. Sonino N, Boscaro M, Paoletta A, Manetero F, Ziliotto D. Ketoconazole treatment in Cushing's syndrome: experience in 34 patients. Clin Endocrinol 1991;35:347–352.

219a. Invitti C, Giraldi P, de Martin M, Cavagnini F, and The Study Group of the Italian Society of Endocrinology on the Pathophysiology of the Hypothalamic-Pituitary-Adrenal Axis. Diagnosis and management of Cushing's syndrome: results of an Italian Multicenter Study. J Clin Endocrinol Metab 1999;84:440–448.

219b. Sonino N, Boscaro M. Medical therapy for Cushing's disease. Endocrinol Metab Clin N Amer 1999;28:211–222.

220. Krieger DT, Amorosa L, Linick F. Cyproheptadine-induced remission of Cushing's disease. N Engl J Med 1975;293:893–896.

221. Middler SA. Cyproheptadine for pituitary disorders. N Engl J Med 1976;295:394.

222. Barnes P, Shaw K, Ross E. Cushing's disease: successful treatment with cyproheptadine. Lancet 1977;1:1148–1149.

223. Krieger DT, Condon EM. Cyproheptadine treatment of Nelson's syndrome: restoration of plasma ACTH circadian periodicity and reversal of response to TRF. J Clin Endocrinol Metab 198;46: 349–352.

224. Tyrrell JB, Brooks RM, Forsham PH. More on cyproheptadine. N Engl J Med 1976;295:1137–1138.

225. Pearce CJ, Isaacs AJ, Gomez J. Treatment of Cushing's disease with cyproheptadine. Lancet 1977;1:1368–1369.

226. Lamberts SWJ, Birkenhager JC. Effect of bromocriptine in pituitary-dependent Cushing's syndrome. J Endocr 1976;70:315–316.

227. Del Arbol JL, Lopez-Luque A, Jimenez J, Escobar F, Pena A, Arcelus I, et al. Lack of responsiveness to bromocriptine of Cushing's disease elevated ACTH. Arch Pharmacol Toxicol 1977;3:171–176.

228. Kennedy J, Montgomery DAD. Bromocriptine for Cushing's disease. Br Med J 1977;1:1083–1084.

229. Hale AC, Coates PJ, Doniach I, Howlett TA, Grossman A, Rees LH, et al. A bromocriptine responsive corticotroph adenoma secreting alpha-MSH in a patient with Cushing's disease. Clin Endocrinol 1988;28:215–223.

230. Croughs RJM, Koppeschaar HPF, van't Verlaat JW, McNicol AM. Bromocriptine-responsive Cushing's disease associated with anterior pituitary corticotroph hyperplasia or normal pituitary gland. J Clin Endocrinol Metab 1989;68:495–498.

231. Orth DN. Metyrapone is useful only as adjunctive therapy in Cushing's disease. Ann Intern Med 1978;89:128–130.

232. Beardwell CG, Adamson AR, Shalet SM. Prolonged remission in florid Cushing's syndrome following metyrapone treatment. Clin Endocrinol 1981;14:485–492.

233. Dickstein G, Lahav M, Shen-Orr Z, Edoute Y, Barzilai D. Primary therapy for Cushing's disease with metyrapone. JAMA 1986;255:1167–1169.

234. Verhelst JA, Trainer PJ, Howlett TA, Perry L, Rees LH, Grossman AB, et al. Short and long-term responses to metyrapone in the medical management of 91 patients with Cushing's syndrome. Clin Endocrinol 1991;35:169–178.

235. Jones MT, Hillhouse EW. Neurotransmitter regulation of corticotropin-releasing factor in vitro. Ann N Y Acad Sci 1977;297:536–560.

236. Jones MT, Gillham B, Beckford U, Dornhorst A, Abraham RR, Seed M, et al. Effect of treatment with sodium valproate and diazepam on plasma corticotropin in Nelson's syndrome. Lancet 1981;1:1179–1181.

237. Elias AN, Gwinup G, Valenta LJ. Effects of valproic acid, naloxone and hydrocortisone in Nelson's syndrome and Cushing's disease. Clin Endocrinol 1981;15:151–154.

238. Cavagnini F, Invitti C, Polli EE. Sodium valproate in Cushing's disease. Lancet 1984;2:162,163.

239. Glaser B, Kahana L, Elias V, Sheinfeld M. Sodium valproate and metyrapone for pituitary-dependent Cushing's disease. Lancet 1984;2:640.

240. Reincke M, Allolio B, Kaulen D, Jaursch-Hancke C, Winkelmann W. The effect of sodium valproate in Cushing's disease, Nelson's syndrome and Addison's disease. Klin Wochenschr 1988;66:686–689.

241. Kelly W, Adams JE, Laing I, Longson D, Davies D. Long-term treatment of Nelson's syndrome with sodium valproate. Clin Endocrinol 1988;28:195–204.

242. Nusey SS, Price P, Jenkins JS, Altaher ARH, Gillham B, Jones MT. The combined use of sodium valproate and metyrapone in the treatment of Cushing's syndrome. Clin Endocrinol 1988;28:33–380.

243. Temple TE Jr, Jones DJ Jr, Liddle GW, Denter RN. Treatment of Cushing's disease. Correction of hypercortisolism by o,p'DDD without induction of aldosterone deficiency. N Engl J Med 1969;281:801–805.

244. Luton JP, Mahoudreau JA, Bouchard P, Thieblot P, Hautecourverture M, Simon D, et al. Treatment of Cushing's disease by o,p'-DDD. Survey of 62 cases. N Engl J Med 1979;300:459–464.

245. Invitti C, de Martin M, Brunani A, Piolini M, Cavagnini F. Treatment of Cushing's syndrome with the long-acting somatostatin analogue SMS 201-995 (Sandostatin). Clin Endocrinol 1990;32:275–387.

246. Woodhouse NJY, Dagogo-Jack S, Ahmed M, Judzewitsch R. Acute and long-term effects of octreotide in patients with ACTH-dependent Cushing's syndrome. Am J Med 1993;95:305–308.

247. Johnston DG, Hall K, McGregor A, Ross WM, Kendall-Taylor P, Hall R. Bromocriptine therapy for 'non-functioning' pituitary tumors. Am J Med 1981;71:1059–1061.

248. D'Emden MC, Harrison LC. Rapid improvement in visual field defects following bromocriptine treatment of patients with nonfunctioning adenomas. Clin Endocrinol 1986;25:697–702.

249. Garcia-Luna PP, Leal-Cerro A, Pereira JL, Monero C, Acosta D, Trujillo F, et al. Rapid improvement of visual defects with parenteral depot-bromocriptine in a patient with a non-functioning pituitary adenoma. Horm Res 1989;32:183–187.

250. Grossman A, Ross R, Charlesworth M, Adams CBT, Wass JAH, Doniach I, et al. The effect of dopamine agonist therapy on large functionless pituitary tumours. Clin Endocrinol 1985;22:679–686.

251. MacFarlane IA, Beardwell CG, Shalet SM, Ainslie G, Rankin E. Glycoprotein hormone alpha-subunit secretion in patients with pituitary adenomas: influence of TRH, LRH and bromocriptine. Acta Endocrinol 1982;99:487–492.

252. Berezin M, Olchovsky D, Pines A, Tadmor R, Lunenfeld B. Reduction of follicle-stimulating hormone (FSH) secretion in FSH-producing pituitary adenoma by bromocriptine. J Clin Endocrinol Metab 1984;59:1220–1223.

253. Vance ML, Ridgway EC, Thorner MO. Follicle-stimulating hormone- and alpha-subunit-secreting pituitary tumor treated with bromocriptine. J Clin Endocrinol Metab 1985;61:580–584.

254. Lamberts SWJ, Verleun T, Oosterom R, Hofland L, van Ginkel LA, Loeber JG, et al. The effects of bromocriptine, thyrotropin-releasing hormone, and gonadotropin-releasing hormone on hormone secretion by gonadotropin-secreting pituitary adenomas in vivo and in vitro. J Clin Endocrinol Metab 1987;64:524–530.

255. Klibanski A, Shupnik MA, Bikkal HA, Black PM, Kliman B, Zervas NT. Dopaminergic regulation of alpha-subunit secretion and messenger ribonucleic acid levels in alpha-secreting pituitary tumors. J Clin Endocrinol Metab 1988;65:96–102.

256. Comtois R, Bouchard J, Robert F. Hypersecretion of gonadotropins by a pituitary adenoma: pituitary dynamic studies and treatment with bromocriptine in one patient. Fertil Steril 1989;52:569–573.

257. Kwekkeboom DJ, de Jong FH, Lamberts SWJ. Gonadotropin release by clinically nonfunctioning and gonadotroph pituitary adenomas in vivo and in vitro: relation to sex and effects of thyrotropin-releasing hormone, gonadotropin-releasing hormone, and bromocriptine. J Clin Endocrinol Metab 1989;68:1128–1133.

258. Abs R, Parizel PM, Beckers A. Acute effects of Parlodel-LAR and response to long-term treatment with bromocriptine in a patient with a follicle stimulating hormone-secreting pituitary adenoma. J Endocrinol Invest 1991;14:135–138.

259. Kwekkeboom DJ, Lamberts SWJ. Long-term treatment with the dopamine agonist CV 205-502 of patients with a clinically nonfunctioning, gonadotroph, or alpha-subunit secreting pituitary adenoma. Clin Endocrinol 1992;36:171–176.

260. Belchetz PE, Plant TM, Nakai Y, Keogh EJ, Knobil E. Hypophyseal response to continuous and intermittent delivery of hypothalamic gonadotropin releasing hormone (GnRH). Science 1978;202:631–633.

261. Conn PM, Crowley WF Jr. Gonadotropin-releasing hormone and its analogues. N Engl J Med 1991;324:93–103.

262. Roman SH, Goldstein M, Kourides IA, Comite F, Bardin CW, Krieger DT. The luteinizing hormone-releasing hormone (LHRH) agonist [D-Trp^6-Pro^9-Net]LHRH increased rather than lowered LH and alpha-subunit levels in a patient with an LH-secreting pituitary tumor. J Clin Endocrinol Metab 1984;58:313–319.

263. Zarate A, Fonseca M, Mason M, Tapia R, Miranda R, Kovacs K, et al. Gonadotropin-secreting pituitary adenoma with concomitant hypersecretion of testosterone and elevated sperm count. Treatment with LRH agonist. Acta Endocrinol 1986;113:29–34.

264. Daniels M, Newland P, Dunn J, Kendall-Taylor P, White MC. Long-term effects of a gonadotrophin-releasing hormone agonist ([D-Ser(Bu^t)^6] GnRH(1-9)nonapeptide-ethylamide) on gonadotrophin secretion from human pituitary gonadotroph cell adenomas *in vitro*. J Endocr 1988;118:491–496.

265. Sassolas G, Lejeune H, Trouillas J, et al. Gonadotropin releasing hormone agonist are unsuccessful in reducing tumoral gonadotropin secretion in two patients with gonadotropin-secreting pituitary adenomas. J Clin Endocrinol Metab 1988;67:180–185.

266. Klibanski A, Jameson JL, Biller BMK, Crowley WF Jr, Zervas NT, Rivier J, et al. Gonadotropin and alpha-subunit responses to chronic gonadotropin-releasing hormone analog administration in patients with glycoprotein hormone-secreting pituitary tumors. J Clin Endocrinol Metab 1989;68:81–86.

267. Columbo P, Ambrosi B, Saccomanno K, Tassetti M, Cortelazzi D, Faglia G. Effects of long-term treatment with the gonadotropin-releasing hormone analog nafarelin in patients with non-functioning pituitary adenomas. Eur J Endocrinol 1994;130:339–345.

268. Daneshdoost L, Pavlou SN, Molitch ME, Gennarelli TA, Savino PJ, Sergott RC, et al. Inhibition of follicle-stimulating hormone secretion from gonadotroph adenomas by repetitive administration of a gonadotropin-releasing hormone antagonist. J Clin Endocrinol Metab 1990;71:92–97.

269. McGrath GA, Goncalves RJ, Udupa JK, Grossman RI, Pavlou SN, Molitch ME, et al. New technique for quantitation of pituitary adenoma size: use in evaluating treatment of gonadotroph adenomas with a gonadotropin-releasing hormone antagonist. J Clin Endocrinol Metab 1993;76:1363–1368.

270. Reubi JC, Heitz PU, Landolt AM. Visualization of somatostatin receptors and correlation with immunoreactive growth hormone and prolactin in human pituitary adenomas: evidence for different tumor subclasses. J Clin Endocrinol Metab 1987;65:65–73.

271. Klibanski A, Alexander JM, Bikkal HA, Hsu DW, Swearingen B, Zervas NT. Somatostatin regulation of glycoprotein hormone and free subunit secretion in clinically nonfunctioning and somatotroph adenomas in vitro. J Clin Endocrinol Metab 1991;73:1248–1255.

272. DeBruin TWA, Kwekkeboom DJ, van't Verlaat JW, Reubi J-C, Krenning EP, Lamberts SWJ, et al. Clinically nonfunctioning pituitary adenoma and octreotide response to long term high dose treatment, and studies *in vitro*. J Clin Endocrinol Metab 1992;75:1310–1317.

273. Katznelson L, Oppenheim DS, Coughlin JF, Kliman B, Schoenfeld DA, Klibanski A. Chronic somatostatin analog administration in patients with alpha-subunit-secreting pituitary tumors. J Clin Endocrinol Metab 1992;75:1318–1325.

273a. Warnet A, Harris AG, Renard E, Martin D, James-Deidier A, Chaumet-Riffaud P, and the French Multicenter Octreotide Study Group: A prospective multicenter trial of octreotide in 24 patients with visual defects caused by nonfunctioning and gonadotropin-secreting pituitary adenomas. Neurosurgery 1997;41:786–796.

274. Siler TM, Yen SSC, Vale W, Guillemin R. Inhibition by somatostatin on the release of TSH induced in man by thyrotropin-releasing factor. J Clin Endocrinol Metab 1974;38:742–745.

275. Reschini E, Giustina G, Cantalamessa Lperrachi M. Hyperthyroidism with elevated plasma TSH levels and pituitary tumor: study with somatostatin. J Clin Endocrinol Metab 1976;46:924–927.

276. Comi RJ, Gesundheit N, Murray L, Gorden P, Weintraub BD. Response of thyrotropin-secreting pituitary adenomas to a long-acting somatostatin analogue. N Engl J Me 1987;317:12–17.

277. Smallridge RC. Thyrotropin-secreting pituitary tumors. Endocrinol Metab Clin N Am 1987; 16:765–792.

278. Chanson P, Weintraub BD, Harris AG. Octreotide therapy for thyroid-stimulating hormone-secreting pituitary adenomas. A follow-up of 52 patients. Ann Intern Med 1993;119:236–240.

279. Beck-Peccoz P, Brucker-Davis F, Persani L, Smallridge RC, Weintraub BD. Thyrotropin-secreting pituitary tumors. Endocr Rev 1996;17:610–638.

280. Gancel A, Vuillermet P, Legrand A, Catus F, Thomas F, Kuhn JM. Effects of a slow-release formulation of the new somatostatin analogue lanreotide in TSH-secreting pituitary adenomas. Clin Endocrinol 1994;40:421–428.

15 Radiation Therapy of Pituitary Tumors

Including Stereotactic Radiosurgery

B. Dawn Moose, md and Edward G. Shaw, md

INTRODUCTION

Pituitary adenomas comprise approximately 12% of all intracranial tumors *(1)*. In autopsy series, unsuspected adenomas have been identified in as many as 25% of patients *(2)*. Although these lesions are histologically benign, they can result in morbidity and mortality owing to local extension and/or hormonal effects. Mass effects caused by pituitary adenomas can produce headaches, visual field deficits, and decreased visual acuity. Secretory adenomas can cause elevated levels of growth hormone (GH), prolactin, adrenocorticotrophin hormone (ACTH), or a combination of these. The hormonal effects of these secretory tumors can result in debilitating side effects and life-threatening conditions, including hypertension and cardiomyopathy (GH); amenorrhea, galactorrhea, infertility, and libido changes (prolactin); and truncal obesity, hypertension, striae, edema, glucosuria, and osteoporosis (ACTH).

The goals of treatment of patients with pituitary adenomas are control of hypersecretion, removal of the tumor mass, reversal of functional deficits, such as impaired vision, and prevention of recurrences *(3)*. Historically, radiotherapy has been reserved for patients with incompletely excised or recurrent tumors, for patients medically unfit for surgical intervention, and for secretory tumors uncontrolled by other therapy. The acceptance of radiotherapy as an effective treatment for pituitary adenomas is based on numerous retrospective reports, which span four to five decades over which the radiotherapy equipment and techniques have evolved, imaging capabilities have improved, and immunohistochemical and hormonal assays have emerged.

PROLACTINOMAS

The majority of women with prolactin-secreting pituitary adenomas present with galactorrhea and/or menstrual irregularities, such as amenorrhea, oligo-ovulation, anovulation, or luteal-phase defect. Galactorrhea is present in 35–80% of patients at presentation *(4,5)*. In men, impaired sexual function and symptoms resulting from mass effect are the predominate presenting complaints.

A variety of therapeutic modalities have been used in the management of hyperprolactinemia associated with a prolactin-secreting pituitary adenoma. These include surgical resection, dopamine agonist therapy, radiation therapy, or some combination of these.

From: *Diagnosis and Management of Pituitary Tumors* (K. Thapar, K. Kovacs, B. W. Scheithauer, and R. V. Lloyd, eds.), ©Humana Press Inc., Totowa, NJ.

Although surgery can result in a rapid decline in serum prolactin levels, numerous series have reported high recurrence rates, especially for macroadenomas *(6–10)*. Serri et al. reported the results of long-term follow-up of women with micro- and macroprolactinomas undergoing transsphenoidal hypophysectomy *(11)*. Although 85% of the patients with microadenomas achieved initial normalization of their serum prolactin levels following surgery, 50% ultimately developed recurrent hyperprolactinemia within 5 yr. Only 31% of the patients with macroadenomas had reduction in their prolactin levels to the normal range and 80% ultimately developed recurrence of their hyperprolactinemia.

In 1979, Keye and associates reported restoration of menstrual function in 34 of 41 women and elimination of lactation in 30 of 40 women following microsurgical removal of the prolactin-producing adenoma *(12)*. The most important prognostic factors identified in this series were tumor size and preoperative serum prolactin level. Women with tumors >2 cm in diameter or prolactin levels exceeding 200 ng/mL were significantly less likely to respond favorably to surgical resection. Similar results were reported by Halberg and Sheline at UCSF *(13)*. In their experience, 93% of patients with microadenomas and 88% of patients with tumors lacking significant suprasellar extension were controlled with transsphenoidal resection. Of the patients with significant extrasellar extension, only 37% of women and 12% of men achieved control with surgery alone. In addition to tumor size, the preoperative prolactin level also appeared to be an important prognostic factor. The overall remission rate for women with preoperative prolactin levels of <200 ng/mL was 88 vs 37% for those with levels exceeding 200 ng/mL. Surgical resection alone appears to be successful only in patients with microadenomas and low serum prolactin levels.

Dopamine agonist therapy, most commonly bromocriptine, has been shown to normalize the prolactin level rapidly in 80–95% of women with microadenomas and in 50–66% of women with macroadenomas *(5,14–16)*. Significant reductions in tumor size have also been reported with dopamine agonist therapy *(14,16)*. In a large multicenter, prospective trial for patients with macroadenomas with suprasellar extension, bromocriptine therapy reduced the prolactin levels in all patients with two-thirds achieving normal levels *(14)*. A reduction in tumor size was noted in 50% of the patients. Bassetti et al. performed a microscopic analysis of macroadenomas removed from patients following bromocriptine therapy and compared them to glands removed from untreated patients (17). They found shrinkage of both the cytoplasm and nucleus in patients who received bromocriptine, but no reduction in the number of tumor cells. Re-expansion of the tumor cells and recurrence of hyperprolactinemia are seen in over 90% of patients following the discontinuation of the bromocriptine (5,14,15,18). Surgical resection or radiation therapy is ultimately necessary in order to avoid the need for lifelong bromocriptine administration.

The traditional role of radiation therapy in the management of hyperprolactinemia appeared to be limited to reducing the serum prolactin levels in patients who were medically inoperable. In these early reports, the serum prolactin levels rarely returned to the normal range following radiotherapy (19–24). In the majority of these older studies, follow-up did not exceed 5 yr, and the details of ovulatory function, pituitary status, and complications were generally not reported. More recent radiation therapy series with long-term follow-up have shown reduction in prolactin levels to the normal range in 36–70% of patients (5,24–27). Sheline and colleagues reported the results of conventional radiation following transsphenoidal resection in 14 patients with invasive prolactin-secreting adenomas (23). The mean prolactin values were 10,500 ng/mL before surgery, 4700 ng/mL after surgery and before radiotherapy, and 820 ng/mL after radiotherapy (3–61 mo). The prolactin levels returned to normal in 5 of the 14 patients. In a separate series of 14 patients with macroprolactinomas, 9 of which underwent transfrontal surgery for decompression of the optic chiasm prior to radiotherapy, 43% had reduction in their prolactin levels to the normal range following irradiation (5). Of the four women who presented with galactorrhea and menstrual irregularities, three had resolution of the galactorrhea and one had normal menstrual cycles return.

Although the numbers of patients are small, several recent series with long-term follow-up have reported excellent results with radiation therapy alone or in combination with bromocriptine. Clark and coworkers recently reported the results of radiation therapy in the management of 44 patients with functional pituitary adenomas, 19 of whom had prolactin-secreting tumors (27). Patients received radiotherapy alone, postoperative radiotherapy, or radiotherapy as salvage. The median tumor dose was 45 Gy with a median dose per fraction of 225 cGy. With a median follow-up of 89 mo, 71% of patients had reached normal prolactin levels, and another 14% had a reduction in prolactin levels of at least 50%. In one of the largest reported series, 36 women with prolactinomas, all of whom had macroadenomas with radiologic abnormalities of the pituitary fossa, received pituitary radiation consisting of 45 Gy in 25 fractions over 35 elapsed days (26). The mean follow-up after completion of irradiation was 8.7 yr and ranged from 3 to 14 yr. Shortly before or during the radiotherapy, treatment with dopamine agonists was started in all patients. At 1- to 2-yr intervals, dopamine agonist therapy was withheld and not reinstituted if the serum prolactin level was within the normal range or had substantially decreased, and the patient was menstruating regularly. At the latest follow-up, 50% of the patients had normal prolactin levels, and another 28% had levels slightly above the normal range. Sixty-one percent of the patients resumed regular menses. Of 29 patients who wished to conceive, 25 (86%) were successful within the first 5 yr. During their pregnancies, none of the patients developed signs or symptoms of tumor expansion.

Mehta et al. reported the results of radiotherapy alone for eight women who presented with amenorrhea and galactorrhea (24).

The pituitary fossa was enlarged in six patients, whereas two patients had a normal size fossa but localized erosion or double fossa. The patients received 44–50 Gy in 20–28 fractions through six portals on a Co60 unit. Normal prolactin levels were achieved in five patients (62.5%). Of the remaining three patients, two patients continue to have stable hyperprolactinemia with no evidence of tumor progression on CT scans, and one patient underwent surgery owing to worsening hyperprolactinemia. Galactorrhea resolved in all eight patients 6 mo to 4 yr after radiotherapy. Ovulatory menses resumed in four of the five patients who had reached normal prolactin levels.

In patients achieving normal prolactin levels following radiation, the normal levels are reached up to 13 yr after completion of therapy. In the series of 36 patients reported by Tsagarakis et al., the mean time to reach normal levels was 7.3 yr with a range of 2–13 yr (26). Mehta and coworkers also noted a variable time-course of reduction in the prolactin levels (24). In the 5 patients who had prolactin levels return to the normal range, they did so in 2, 9, 10, 12, and 13 yr following irradiation. There appears to be an initial phase of a rapid fall in prolactin levels during the first 2–3 yr after radiotherapy. This is followed by a more gradual decline during the ensuing years (24,26).

Similar to the time-course for normalization of prolactin levels after radiation therapy, most pituitary adenomas regress slowly over numerous years (5,25). The majority of prolactinomas show little if any change over the first 3–5 yr following treatment. Johnston et al. reported the first observed radiological evidence of a decrease in tumor size at a mean of 5 yr (1–9 yr) after radiotherapy (5). There is very little if any role for radiotherapy in the management of microprolactinomas, since surgical resection and dopamine agonist therapy are both highly successful and rapidly effective. For macroprolactinomas, however, postoperative radiotherapy should be considered, given the high recurrence rates following surgical resection alone, especially for large invasive tumors and those that are incompletely resected. The combined approach of using dopamine agonist therapy to shrink the tumor initially and reduce the prolactin levels rapidly followed by radiation therapy is a viable, though infrequently utilized, alternative to surgical resection or dopamine agonist therapy alone. With this treatment approach, dopamine agonist therapy should be continued after the completion of radiation, and periodically reduced and eventually stopped once the prolactin levels remain within the normal range of therapy.

ACROMEGALY

The signs and symptoms of acromegaly are the result of the effects of excess growth hormone secretion, mass effects of the tumor, and hypopituitarism. Excess circulating levels of growth hormone can cause coarsening of facial features, acral hypertrophy, fatigue, sweating, arthropathy, neuropathy, metabolic disturbances such as diabetes, nephrolithiasis, and cardiovascular and pulmonary disease (28–30). These systemic effects lead to increased rates of mortality in patients suffering from acromegaly. In a large retrospective study of all acromegalic patients admitted to five hospitals in England and Wales between 1939 and 1967, the number of deaths in the acromegalic group was almost twice that in individuals of similar age and sex in the general population (30). Deaths were the result of cardiovascular and respiratory disease in the men, and cerebrovascular and respiratory disease in women. Among acromegalic patients who had been treated for their disease, the mortality rate was significantly lower than in those who had not received treatment. In patients who are medically operable, an attempt at surgical resection is generally the first therapeutic intervention. Baskin et al. reported the results of 102 patients who underwent transsphenoidal surgery for GH-secreting pituitary adenomas at UCSF (31). A remission was defined as clinical improvement, restoration of fasting GH levels to normal, and maintenance of normal GH levels. A partial response was defined as clinical improvement and reduction of the GH level to <50% of the preoperative value. Remission was achieved in 78% of patients with transsphenoidal surgery alone, and in an additional 16% of patients after postoperative radiation, for an overall remission rate of 94%. The factors most closely associated with treatment failure or only a partial response were a high preoperative GH level and the presence of suprasellar extension of tumor. In patients with either diffuse destruction of the sellar floor or extensive suprasellar or parasellar extension, the rate of remission was 82%, which was lower than the overall remission rate of 94%. Of the patients with preoperative GH levels exceeding 50 ng/mL, only 15% achieved a partial response. These results suggest that patients with preoperative GH levels in excess of 50 ng/mL and those with extensive extrasellar spread are unlikely to be controlled with transsphenoidal resection alone and may benefit from postoperative radiation.

The efficacy of radiotherapy on GH hypersecretion has been demonstrated in numerous series. By 10 yr after treatment, 62–100% of patients have GH levels below 10 ng/mL (32–36). As noted previously, control by transsphenoidal surgery as primary management failed in 22 of 102 patients at UCSF (31). Following radiotherapy, 16 of these 22 patients (73%) subsequently obtained normal GH levels. Trampe and colleagues reported the results of radiotherapy in 56 patients who had persistent postoperative GH hypersecretion and clinical manifestations of the disease (37). The majority of patients received 50 Gy at 180 cGy/fraction to the tumor volume. Following radiotherapy, the GH levels fell in all patients. Preirradiation GH levels were reduced by 50% within an average of 2 yr and by 75% within another 2 yr. There was a tendency toward a more pronounced GH reduction in patients with concomitant hyperprolactinemia. Several other studies have reported similar response rates following radiotherapy for surgical failures, suggesting that prior surgical intervention is not generally associated with future unresponsiveness to radiotherapy (33,36,38–40).

In addition to its efficacy in surgical failures, radiotherapy has also been shown to be effective as initial therapy. Eastman et al. reported the results of conventional radiotherapy in 47 acromegalic patients followed up at 2, 5, and 10 yr (39). At 5 yr, 73% of patients had GH levels of 10 ng/mL or less and 42% had levels of 5 ng/mL or less. In the 16 patients followed for at least 10 yr, the corresponding values were 81 and 69%. These results at 5 and 10 yr are comparable to those achieved with surgery. The fall in plasma GH levels was accompanied by an improvement in the metabolic and skeletal abnormalities associated with acromegaly. These results were recently updated with longer follow-up (41). At 15 yr, 83% of patients had GH levels below 10 ng/mL and 92% of patients followed for longer than 15 yr had levels below 10 ng/mL. Pistenma and colleagues reported the results of radiotherapy in 22 patients with signs and symptoms of acromegaly (42). Nineteen patients received radiotherapy alone and three postoperative radiotherapy. Of the eight who had abnormal visual fields before

treatment, four had return to normal after treatment. Either subjective or objective improvement in the physical manifestations of acromegaly was observed in 36.4% of patients. There appears to be a highly positive correlation between preirradiation and final GH levels, which is in agreement with numerous reports of a higher frequency and earlier appearance of normal GH levels after radiotherapy in patients with lower pretherapy GH levels (36,38,43,44). In 17 patients with initial GH levels <50 ng/mL, Sheline and Wara reported that all patients achieved normal GH levels within 3 yr following radiotherapy (36). Only 5/7 patients with initial GH levels of 50 ng/mL or more were controlled at 3 yr or longer. Similar findings were reported by Chang (45). In his series, 6/6 patients with initial GH levels <50 ng/mL and 2/3 patients with initial levels exceeding 50 ng/mL achieved normal GH levels by 6 yr. Bloom and Kramer reported that all nine of their patients with pretreatment GH levels of 40 ng/mL or less returned to normal GH levels by 6 mo to 2 yr (43). Only 5/8 patients with levels >40 ng/mL obtained normal levels after radiotherapy. In a separate series of 24 patients with GH levels <30 ng/mL prior to radiation, 83% achieved normal levels by 2 yr, whereas only 21% of patients with initial GH levels in excess of 30 ng/mL achieved normal levels (44).

In the series reported by Eastman et al., the percent fall in GH was dependent on the initial GH elevation (41). Therefore, patients with higher GH levels at the time of radiation were less likely to achieve GH levels below 5 ng/mL after radiotherapy. Patients with GH levels exceeding 100 ng/mL were significantly less likely to achieve a GH level below 5 ng/mL during long-term follow-up. These studies are consistent in that normalization of GH levels took 2–3 yr and that the probability of control was related to the pretreatment GH level.

Caruso et al. reported the results of radiotherapy in 74 patients with GH secreting pituitary tumors at the Mayo Clinic (46). Fifty-three patients underwent radiation therapy following transsphenoidal resection, and 21 received radiation therapy alone. The median radiation doses were 48 and 50 Gy for the surgery plus radiotherapy group and the radiotherapy alone group, respectively. Cure was defined as a fasting or suppressed GH level ≤2 ng/mL and control as ≤5 ng/mL. The overall survivals at 2, 5, and 10 yr were 100, 92, and 86% in the surgery plus radiotherapy group vs 89, 79, and 56% in the radiotherapy only group. At 6 yr follow-up, the cure and control rates were 62 and 84% for the surgery plus radiotherapy group vs 32 and 43% for the radiotherapy alone group, respectively. There was no significant difference in cure or control rates in patients receiving doses <48–50 Gy vs more. In this series, which used a strict definition of cure (GH ≤2), patients who received surgery plus postoperative radiotherapy were more likely to achieve biochemical cure or control than patients treated primarily with radiotherapy.

In patients with microadenomas, transsphenoidal resection results in rapid reductions in circulating GH levels and provides excellent long-term control. For those patients who have persistent elevations of serum GH levels postoperatively, radiotherapy should be considered. In patients with large GH-secreting tumors with extrasellar extension, radiation is usually indicated postoperatively in order to reduce the likelihood of tumor recurrence. If complete surgical resection is not possible without producing significant complications, transsphenoidal debulking followed by postoperative radiotherapy should be considered. Radiotherapy is also indicated in patients who are considered medically inoperable.

CUSHING'S SYNDROME

Cushing's syndrome is an endocrinopathy caused by hypercortisolism, which results in distinctive clinical features and associated systemic changes (47). This syndrome is characterized by truncal obesity, hypertension, fatigability and weakness, amenorrhea, hirsutism, purplish abdominal striae, edema, glucosuria, and osteoporosis. When this disorder is caused by a pituitary source, usually an ACTH-secreting microadenoma, it is referred to as "Cushing's disease." A variety of therapeutic modalities have been used in the management of Cushing's disease since it was first described by Cushing in 1932 (48). Owing to the development of effective adrenal replacement therapy, management for this disorder was directed toward the target organ with bilateral adrenalectomy serving as the treatment of choice in the 1950s through the 1970s (49). Following the development of pituitary microsurgical techniques, transsphenoidal microsurgical resection became the primary treatment of choice for Cushing's disease.

Because of the early clinical manifestations of the disease, the majority of patients with ACTH-secreting pituitary adenomas have small, localized adenomas at the time of presentation. In a review of several large series encompassing over 1200 patients with ACTH-secreting pituitary tumors, the pituitary adenomas were localized in 70–94% of patients (50). Approximately 10% of patients with Cushing's disease have macroadenomas at presentation.

Transsphenoidal microsurgical exploration of the sella is considered the surgical approach of choice for patients with Cushing's disease. This approach results in excellent remission rates and offers the chance of selective resection of the secretory tumor while preserving normal pituitary tissue and its function. In a retrospective review of 216 patients treated with transsphenoidal microsurgery for Cushing's disease at UCSF, 173 patients underwent selective adenomectomy, 25 had total hypophysectomy, 6 had partial hypophysectomy, and 12 had exploration only (51). Remission was defined as the resolution of the presenting features of Cushing's disease, and persistence of normal plasma cortisol levels, plasma ACTH levels, and cortisol suppression at the most recent testing. Of the 166 patients (95.9%) with adenomas confined to the sella turcica at the time of surgery, 86% achieved remission. Of the 46 patients who were thought to have extrasellar extension of the adenoma on the basis of intraoperative observations, 46% had remission of their disease.

Robert and Hardy reported the results of transsphenoidal microsurgery in 78 patients with ACTH-secreting pituitary adenomas (52). Of the adenomas pathologically evaluated, 89% were microadenomas with 20% of these measuring <1 mm in diameter. The remission rates following surgery were 82% for microadenomas and 81% for all intrasellar tumors. Similar results were reported by Tindall and colleagues (53). In their series, 56 patients underwent transsphenoidal microsurgical exploration of the pituitary gland for the preoperative diagnosis of Cushing's disease. Sustained remission was achieved in 85% of patients with only 8 patients experiencing a therapeutic failure. The causes for failure were invasion by the tumor (one patient), hyperplasia mistaken for an adenoma (two patients), misdiagnosis (one patient), atypical tumor (one patient), and recurrence of disease following remission (one patient).

At UCSF, 15 children and adolescents with Cushing's disease were treated by transsphenoidal exploration and microadenomectomy (54). Hypercortisolism corrected in 14 patients, all of whom lost weight and cushingoid stigmata, and had normal or catch-up growth and progression of puberty. The low morbidity and failure rate of the procedure, the low recurrence rate, the rapid amelioration of signs of hypercortisolism, and the preservation of pituitary function in this study support transsphenoidal resection as a low-risk approach to the initial treatment of Cushing's disease in childhood and adolescence.

In a review of several large series, Tyrrell and Wilson noted initial remission rates of 80–90% in patients with microadenomas based on correction of hypercortisolism in the immediate postoperative period (50). Only approx 50% of patients with macroadenomas achieved remission after initial pituitary microsurgery. Larger tumors may be adherent to adjacent structures, and local invasion of the dura is the most common reason for residual disease and surgical failure.

Given the low rate of remission after initial pituitary microsurgery in patients with macroadenomas, additional therapy, such as radiotherapy, should be considered. Numerous series have confirmed the efficacy of radiotherapy in the management of patients with Cushing's disease (55–57). Aristizabal et al. reported the results of radiotherapy in 45 patients with Cushing's disease treated between 1952 and 1970 at Vanderbilt (55). With follow-up ranging from 2 to 15 yr, complete clinical and laboratory regression of Cushing's disease occurred in 25% of the patients. An additional 28% of patients exhibited enough improvement that they did not require any further therapy, except, in some cases, aminoglutethemide. When the results of treatment were compared against total doses of radiation, the control rate was unsatisfactory at doses of below 40 Gy. In those patients receiving <40 Gy, only 25% were believed to be cured or improved after radiotherapy, whereas 57% of patients who received 40 Gy or more were cured or improved. The maximum benefits of radiation were evident in the 45- to 50-Gy dose range with 70% of patients achieving cure or having improvement. At the University of Michigan, 36 patients with Cushing's disease were treated with external beam radiotherapy. Mitotane was given concurrently or after radiation (58). Clinical and biochemical remission occurred in 29 patients (80%) with 17 patients responding within 4 mo. In 17 of the 29 patients who responded to treatment, drug therapy has been discontinued, and they remain in remission. Jennings et al. reported the results of radiotherapy in 15 children with Cushing's disease (59). Twelve patients were cured within 18 mo and 10 were cured within 9 mo of completing the radiotherapy. Sexual development proceeded normally in all 15 patients.

Since the development of pituitary microsurgical techniques, there have been few patients treated with initial radiotherapy. Following transsphenoidal resection, patients should be assessed endocrinologically in the first few weeks, and those with persistent elevations of cortisol should be considered for additional therapy. For patients with microadenomas that invaded the dura of the cavernous sinus or sellar floor at the first operation, further surgery is rarely beneficial and radiotherapy and medical management are indicated. Since macroadenomas commonly exhibit extrasellar extension, patients with persisting hypercortisolism following resection usually do not achieve remission with reoperation. Postoperative radiotherapy is generally indicated for these patients. With conventional radiotherapy, long-term remission rates of 56–80% in patients with persisting hypercortisolism following initial pituitary microsurgery can be achieved (55–58). For patients who are medically unfit for surgery, radiotherapy should be used as the primary therapy. The reported remission rates are as high as 55–59% in this setting (3,57,60).

NELSON'S SYNDROME

Nelson's syndrome is the development of progressive cutaneous melanosis and a pituitary tumor after bilateral adrenalectomy for Cushing's syndrome *(61)*. These patients present with hyperpigmentation, elevated ACTH levels, and a progressive pituitary lesion on MRI. The reported incidence of Nelson's syndrome in adrenalectomized patients ranges from 0 to 20% *(62–64)*. There are conflicting reports in the literature regarding the effectiveness of radiotherapy in preventing the development of Nelson's syndrome in adrenalectomized patients. Some authors have suggested that pituitary irradiation may prevent its development *(59,63)*. In 120 patients who were adrenalectomized for bilateral adrenal hyperplasia, 20 underwent pituitary irradiation as the initial treatment *(62)*. With follow-up ranging from 2 to 20 yr, 2 of these 20 (10%) patients subsequently developed pituitary tumors. This was not significantly different from the incidence in patients not receiving pituitary radiation (8%).

The majority of patients with Nelson's syndrome have macroadenomas and at least 50% are found to be locally invasive at the time of surgery *(65–67)*. Invasion of the cavernous sinus, visual impairment, and pituitary apoplexy are common. These tumors are usually aggressive. Death in patient's with Nelson's syndrome have been reported in up to 22% of patients *(60,64,65,66–68)*. Derome et al. reported the results of transsphenoidal surgical resection in 19 patients with Nelson's syndrome *(68)*. Postoperative radiotherapy was given in five patients. The tumors were controlled locally in 37% of patients with 21% of patients ultimately succumbing to their disease. These results confirm the poor prognosis in patients with Nelson's syndrome.

There are few reports in the literature regarding the management of patients with Nelson's syndrome. Radiotherapy has been used as an adjunct to surgery as well as primary therapy. The number of patients is small. Therefore, it is difficult to draw firm conclusions regarding the benefit of radiation. Given the local invasiveness of these tumors, complete surgical resection is usually not possible. Halberg and Sheline recommend resecting the primary lesion initially and adding postoperative radiotherapy if the resection is incomplete or the ACTH level remains elevated *(13)*.

NONFUNCTIONING PITUITARY ADENOMAS

In contrast to functioning pituitary adenomas, which are generally detected when the adenomas are small, clinically nonfunctioning adenomas are typically silent until they cause symptoms owing to mass effect. At the time of diagnosis, they have usually extended beyond the sella into the suprasellar region and have sometimes invaded the sphenoid sinus or cavernous sinus(es). The most common presenting symptoms are decreased visual acuity or visual field defects, hypopituitarism owing to pressure-induced atrophy, and headaches. Because of tumor extension and invasion, these tumors are often not completely removed at the time of surgery and frequently recur.

Brada et al. reported the results of conservative surgery followed by radiotherapy in 411 patients with pituitary adenomas treated at the Royal Marsden Hospital *(69)*. Of these 411 patients, 252 had clinically nonfunctioning pituitary adenomas. All patients received postoperative radiotherapy or radiotherapy alone to 45–50 Gy. In patients with nonfunctioning adenomas, tumor progression was defined as tumor enlargement detected clinically and by imaging. The 10-yr and 20-yr progression-free survivals for nonsecretory adenomas were 97% and 92%, respectively. Visual field defects were present in 257 patients following surgery and prior to starting radiotherapy. Vision improved in 167 (55%) patients following radiotherapy. The only significant prognostic factor for progression-free survival identified on univariate analysis was the secretory state of the adenoma. The 10-yr and 20-yr progression-free survivals for secretory adenomas were 89 and 69%, respectively, vs 97 and 92% for nonsecretory adenomas. For patients with nonfunctioning pituitary adenomas, progression-free survival at 10 yr was 94% following primary radiotherapy and 97% following surgery plus radiotherapy.

Halberg and Sheline reported the UCSF experience with treatment of 140 patients with large, nonsecretory pituitary adenomas *(13)*. Ninety-seven percent of patients had grossly enlarged sella, 92% had visual field deficits, and 10% had direct invasion of the brain or nasopharynx. Radiotherapy alone was used in 23 patients who were predominantly poor surgical candidates or had minimal visual field deficits. Of the remaining 117 patients, 37 underwent surgery alone and 80 underwent surgery followed by radiotherapy. At 10 yr, 100% of patients who received radiotherapy were recurrence-free compared to 14% with surgery only and 73% with surgery plus radiotherapy. With 15–20 yr follow-up, 100% of patients treated with radiotherapy were recurrence-free as were 73% of patients treated with surgery and postoperative radiotherapy. When visual field loss was limited to one quadrant, two-thirds of the patients in both the radiotherapy and the surgery groups regained normal visual fields. In patients with loss of more than one visual field, only one-third of the surgery patients and none of the radiotherapy only patients achieved normal vision.

Urdaneta et al. reported the results of radiotherapy alone or following surgery in 66 patients with nonfunctioning pituitary adenomas *(70)*. Thirty-two patients received radiotherapy alone, and 34 were treated with surgery and postoperative radiotherapy. Of the patients followed for 10 yr, 55% were disease-free in the radiotherapy alone group vs 75% in the surgery plus radiotherapy group. The overall survival rates were the same in both groups owing to a significant number of the radiotherapy failures being salvaged with surgery.

Flickinger and associates reported the results of radiotherapy in 112 patients with nonsecretory pituitary adenomas *(71)*. Twenty-five patients received radiotherapy alone, and 87 were treated with surgical resection followed by postoperative irradiation. Tumor recurrence was defined as an increase in tumor size found on radiologic studies and was accompanied in all patients by decreased vision. The progression-free survival rates for all patients at 5, 10, 15, and 20 yr were 97, 89, 87, and 76%, respectively. Although the number of patients is small, there was no difference in progression-free survival rates between those patients receiving radiotherapy alone vs surgery and postoperative radiation. The radiotherapy field size was significantly associated with outcome. The 10-yr progression-free survival rate for patients treated with field sizes <30 cm^2 was 97 vs 71% for field sizes exceeding 30 cm^2. This finding is not surprising, since larger field sizes are used in patients with larger tumors, which are more difficult to control with radiotherapy.

At UCLA, radiotherapy alone was successful in controlling nonfunctioning pituitary adenomas in 3 out of 4 patients, whereas surgery followed by postoperative radiation resulted in tumor control in 27 out of 32 patients (84%) *(72)*. Grigsby et al. reported a 79.6% disease-free survival rate at 10 yr in 19 patients who received radiotherapy alone for nonfunctioning pituitary adenomas *(73)*.

For patients with large nonfunctioning pituitary macro-adenomas presenting with symptoms owing to mass effect, surgical resection should be attempted, especially if visual field deficits are present. Postoperative radiotherapy should be given for most patients since surgical resection alone results in high recurrence rates. Radiotherapy alone is effective in selected patients.

STEREOTACTIC RADIOSURGERY

Stereotactic radiosurgery (SRS) is a highly precise technique of localization and radiation of small intracranial lesions. Currently, there are three methodologies for radiosurgery, including charged-particle beams, gamma-ray-based technologies (Gamma Knife, Elekta Instruments, Inc., Atlanta, GA, and Rotating Gamma System, OUR Scientific, Inc., New York, NY), and linear accelerators (74–82).

Irrespective of the technique used, successful SRS requires precise localization of the lesion and its relationship to surrounding critical structures. In treating patients with pituitary adenomas, the critical surrounding structures include the optic chiasm, the cranial nerves in the cavernous sinus, and the uninvolved pituitary tissue. The goal of SRS is to cause tumor cell death or necrosis without resulting in damage to the adjacent normal brain tissues. In radiosurgery, a single large fraction of radiation is delivered to the target. Although single-fraction radiosurgery may be more effective than fractionated radiotherapy in treating pituitary adenomas, normal tissues may be at increased risk of radiation damage, emphasizing the need for precise target localization and treatment delivery.

Gamma-Knife stereotactic radiosurgery was first used in the treatment of patients with pituitary adenomas in Sweden during the 1970s (83). Thorén et al. first reported the results of Gamma-Knife radiosurgery in the treatment of four patients with pituitary-dependent Cushing's syndrome in 1978 (83). Single-fraction doses varied between 70 and 100 Gy. A gradual improvement of the clinical symptoms occurred in all four patients within 7 mo after treatment, with three patients achieving a complete clinical remission. One patient developed ACTH insufficiency and required cortisol replacement therapy.

The most recent report from Stockholm included 77 adult patients with Cushing's disease (84). Fifty-nine patients were followed for 2–15 yr. Localization using pneumocisternography/CT was performed in 51 patients. In this group, complete remission was achieved in 82%, whereas all eight patients who underwent MRI localization obtained remission.

Gamma-Knife radiosurgery was used to treat eight children and adolescents with Cushing's disease, 6–18 yr of age, at the Karolinska Hospital in Stockholm, Sweden (85). The target doses were 50–70 Gy. With follow-up ranging from 12 to 40 mo, seven patients reached full clinical remission, and there have been no recurrences 2.6–6.6 yr following treatment. All patients developed GH deficiency, two hypothyroidism, and three hypogonadism.

Twenty-one patients with GH-secreting pituitary adenomas were treated with Gamma-Knife stereotactic radiosurgery at the Karolinska (86). Twenty of the 21 patients had locally invasive macroadenomas with parasellar growth present in most. Seven patients underwent SRS as their initial treatment, whereas the remaining 14 patients had prior surgery, 8 of which also failed conventional external beam radiotherapy. The target doses ranged from 40 to 70 Gy in each of one to three sessions in the 13 patients who had not previously received radiation. In the patients who had undergone previous external beam radiotherapy, the doses were slightly lower (30–50 Gy in each of one or two sessions). The periphery of the tumor usually received 50% of the maximum dose, and the optic pathways received <5 Gy. With a mean follow-up of 5.4 yr, GH levels returned to the normal range in 10 of the 21 patients (48%), whereas the remaining 10 patients had minor or no effects from the treatment. Of the seven patients who were treated solely with radiosurgery, only three achieved normal growth hormone levels following irradiation. There were no complications from the radiosurgery, except the development of pituitary insufficiency in 2 of 13 patients who had not received previous conventional external beam radiation.

Ganz et al. reported the results of Gamma-Knife radiosurgery in 15 patients with pituitary adenomas (87). Four patients had Cushing's disease, four had acromegaly, three had Nelson's syndrome, three had prolactinomas, and one had a nonsecretory adenoma. In 12 patients, radiosurgery was the primary treatment method. CT scans were used for tumor localization. The central doses were 30–83 Gy, but doses to the tumor periphery were 6–25 Gy. The dose to the optic chiasm was ≤10 Gy, except in two patients in whom the doses were 12 and 15 Gy. The adenomas associated with Cushing's disease (mean maximum diameter 8.5 mm) were significantly smaller than those associated with acromegaly (mean maximum diameter 16.25 mm), which were significantly smaller than the prolactinomas (mean maximum diameter 29 mm). With the exception of one patient who was retreated for Nelson's syndrome, all patients showed an improvement in their endocrinopathy. There was a poor correlation between changes on CT scan and endocrinologic improvement, with 5 of 14 patients showing no radiographic change. Complete remission was achieved in 2/4 Cushing's patients, 1/4 acromegalics, and none of the patients with prolactinomas or Nelson's syndrome. These results are relatively poor when compared to those reported from Stockholm, perhaps reflecting the lower doses used (to limit optic chiasm dose) and the larger size of many of the tumors.

Pollock et al. recently updated the Gamma-Knife radiosurgery experience from the University of Pittsburgh (88). Thirty-five patients with imaging, endocrinological, or surgical evidence of a pituitary adenoma underwent SRS. Prior microsurgical removal of the adenomas had been attempted in 30 patients. Stereotactic localization of the tumor was performed using either CT or MRI. Selective beam blocking, small beam diameters, and multiple isocenters were used to limit the dose to the optic apparatus to ≤8 Gy. Radiation dose to the tumor margin varied from 10 to 30 Gy, usually to the 50% isodose line, with 27 patients receiving ≥18 Gy. Of the 35 patients irradiated, 30 had clinical and radiological follow-up at least 6 mo after radiosurgery. Eight of 11 (73%) evaluable patients with Cushing's disease achieved normalization of the hypothalamic–pituitary–adrenal axis with 5 patients requiring continued cortisol suppression. Of the eight evaluable patients with GH-secreting adenomas, three (38%) had GH levels return to the normal range after radiosurgery. None of the patients have developed pituitary insufficiency. Tumor growth control was achieved in 28 of the 30 patients (93%) with the adenomas decreasing in size in 14 patients and remaining unchanged in the other 14 patients. Visual function remained normal in 27 patients and improved in 2 patients following radiosurgery.

Rocher et al. reported the results of linac-based radiosurgery in 36 patients with pituitary adenomas <30–35 mm in maximum diameter *(89)*. All patients were treated either for a residual tumor after surgery or a recurrence. The tumor dose was 20 Gy delivered to the 70% isodose line. Twenty-two of the 36 patients had adenomas larger than 2 cm. Thirty-one patients had a complete endocrine, radiographic, and visual evaluation 12–18 mo after radiosurgery. Radiographically, 9 tumors regressed, 12 remained stable, and 4 showed tumor density modifications. Imaging was not informative in the remaining six patients. Of the six patients with GH-secreting adenomas, two were stabilized and three improved. Of the four patients with ACTH-producing adenomas, two achieved a complete remission and two improved. Of the 16 patients who had either a partial or no pituitary deficit prior to radiosurgery, 4 developed panhypopituitarism, 1 GH deficit, 1 TRH-GH deficit, and 1 ACTH deficit following the radiosurgery.

In summary, the precise role of radiosurgery in the management of patients with pituitary adenomas remains ill-defined. In reviewing the published data, it is difficult to draw conclusions regarding the efficacy and morbidity of radiosurgery owing to the time frame over which the studies were conducted, diversity of indications, and ranges of doses used. A general consensus is that the dose to the optic apparatus should be kept as low as possible, not to exceed 8 Gy *(77,88)*. For large tumors that encroach on the optic chiasm, this significantly limits the dose that can be safely delivered to the entirety of the tumor. MRI localization and the use of fractionated stereotactic radiosurgery are both proposed ways of reducing the incidence of hypopituitarism and visual complications *(90,91)*.

COMPLICATIONS

The most frequently observed sequelae following radiation therapy for pituitary tumors is the development of hypopituitarism. The incidence appears to increase with time following radiation. In a series of 25 patients with acromegaly who were treated following surgery, 24% had thyroid hormone deficiency, 28% cortisol insufficiency, and 44% gonadal deficiency prior to radiation *(40)*. Following radiation, the incidence of hypothyroidism increased from 32% at 2 yr to 42 and 64% at 3 and 5 yr, respectively. Cortisol insufficiency was evident in 36% of the patients at 2 yr, 42% at 3 yr, and 55% at 5 yr. The incidence of gonadal deficiency at 2, 3, and 5 yr follow-up was 56, 58, and 73%, respectively. Prior surgical intervention appears to increase significantly the incidence of radiation-induced hypopituitarism *(92)*. Pituitary function was evaluated before and after irradiation in 35 patients with pituitary adenomas. Twenty-two of the patients had undergone prior surgical intervention and the remaining 13 had no previous surgery. During a mean observation period of 4.2 yr, deficiencies of adrenal, thyroid, and gonadal function developed in 67, 55, and 67% of patients who had previously undergone surgery and 55, 15, and 50% of patients who did not have prior surgery. The authors compared these results with the those of 10 patients who underwent surgical resection, but did not receive irradiation. The corresponding deficiencies developed in 13, 13, and 0% of patients.

Radiation-induced CNS necrosis, optic neuropathy, auditory complications, cerebral infarctions, and second malignancies have been reported following radiation therapy for pituitary adenomas *(93–107)*. In the majority of cases of CNS necrosis, the daily radiation doses exceeded 200 cGy and/or the total radiation doses exceeded 50 Gy *(93–97)*. With total doses around 50 Gy and daily fraction sizes not exceeding 200 cGy, radiation-induced CNS necrosis should rarely be a complication of treatment. Optic neuropathy following irradiation of pituitary tumors is an uncommon complication of radiation with radiation doses of 45–50 Gy given in fractions of 200 cGy or less per day *(41,98–101)*. Although exceedingly rare, case reports of meningiomas, malignant gliomas, and sarcomas following pituitary radiation can also be found in the literature *(102–106)*.

REFERENCES

1. Grigsby PW, Sheline GE. Pituitary. In: Perez CA, Brady LW, eds. Principles and Practice of Radiation Oncology, 2nd ed. JB Lippincott, Philadelphia, 1992, pp. 564–581.
2. Burrow GN, Wortzman B, Rewcastle NB, Holgate RC, Kovacs K. Microadenomas of the pituitary and abnormal sellar tomograms in an unselected autopsy series. N Engl J Med 1981;304:156–158.
3. Hughes MN, Llamas KJ, Yelland ME, Obst D, Tripcony LB. Pituitary adenomas: long-term results for radiotherapy alone and postoperative radiotherapy. Int J Radiat Oncol Biol Phys 1993; 27:1035–1043.
4. Davajan V, Kletzky O, March CM, Roy S, Mishell DR Jr. The significance of galactorrhea in patients with normal menses, oligomenorrhea, and secondary amenorrhea. Am J Obstet Gynecol 1978;130:894–904.
5. Johnston DG, Hall K, Kendall-Taylor P, Ross WM, Crombie AL, Cook DB, et al. The long-term effects of megavoltage radiotherapy as sole or combined therapy for large prolactinomas:studies with high definition computerized tomography. Clin Endocrinol 1986;24:675–685.
6. Buchfelder M, Lierheimer A, Schreel U, VonWerder K, Fahlbusch R. Recurrence of hyperprolactinemia detected in long-term followup of surgically normalized microprolactinomas (abstract 24). In: Proceedings of the International Symposium on Prolactinomas, Graz, Austria, 1984, p. 73.
7. Faglia G, Moriondo P, Travaglini P, Giovanelli MA. Influence of previous bromocriptine therapy on surgery for microprolactinoma. Lancet 1983;1:133–134.
8. Fahlbusch R. Transsphenoidal operation for prolactinomas (abstract 27). In: Proceedings of the International Symposium on Prolactinomas, Graz, Austria, 1984, p. 79.
9. Rodman EF, Molitch ME, Post KD, Biller BJ, Reichlin S. Longterm follow-up of transsphenoidal selective adenomectomy for prolactinoma. JAMA 1984;252:921–924.
10. Schlecthe JA, Sherman BM, Chapler FK, VanGilder J. Long-term follow-up of women with surgically treated prolactin-secreting pituitary tumors. J Clin Endocrinol Metab 1986;62:1296–1301.
11. Serri O, Rasio E, Beauregard H, Hardy J, Somma M. Recurrence of hyperprolactinemia after selective transsphenoidal adenomectomy in women with prolactinoma. N Engl J Med 1983;309:280–283.
12. Keye WR Jr, Chang RJ, Monroe SE, Wilson CB, Jaffe RB. Prolactin-secreting pituitary adenomas in women. II. Menstrual function, pituitary reserves, and prolactin production following microsurgical removal. Am J Obstet Gynecol 1979;134:360–365.
13. Halberg FE, Sheline GE. Radiotherapy of pituitary tumors. Endocrinol Metab Clin 1987;16(3):667–684.
14. Molitch ME, Elton RL, Blackwell RE, Caldwell B, Chang RJ, Jaffe R, et al. Bromocriptine as primary therapy for prolactin-secreting macroadenomas: results of a prospective multicenter study. J Clin Endocrin Metab 1985;60:698–705.
15. Thorner MO, Evans WS, Vance ML. Medical management of prolactinomas: I. In: Black McL P, Zervas NT, Ridgway EC, Martin JB, eds. Secretory Tumors of the Pituitary Gland. Raven, New York, 1984, pp. 53–63.
16. Wollesen F, Bendsen BB. Effect rates of different modalities for treatment of prolactin adenomas. Am J Med 1985;78:114–122.
17. Bassetti M, Spada A, Pezzo G, Giannattasio G. Bromocriptine treatment reduces the cell size in human macroprolactinomas: a morphometric study. J Clin Endocrinol Metab 1984;58:268–273.
18. Antunes JL, Housepian EM, Frantz AG, Holub DA, Hui RM, Carmel PW, et al. Prolactin-secreting pituitary tumors. Ann Neurol 1977;2:148–153.

19. Gomez F, Reyes FI, Faiman C. Nonpuerperal galactorrhea and hyperprolactinemia. Clinical findings, endocrine features and therapeutic responses in 56 cases. Am J Med 1977;62:648–660.

20. Grossman A, Cohen BL, Charlesworth M, Plowman PN, Rees LH, Wass JAH, et al. Treatment of prolactinomas with megavoltage radiotherapy. Br Med J 1984;288:1105–1109.

21. Kleinberg DL, Noel GL, Frantz AG. Galactorrhea: a study of 235 cases, including 48 with pituitary tumors. N Engl J Med 1977;296:589–600.

22. Nabarro JDN. Pituitary prolactinomas. Clin Endocrinol 1982;17:129–155.

23. Sheline GE, Grossman A, Jones AE, Besser GM. Radiation therapy for prolactinomas. In: Black McL P, Zervas NT, Ridgway EC, Martin JB, eds. Secretory Tumors of the Pituitary Gland. Raven, New York, 1984, pp. 93–108.

24. Mehta AE, Reyes FI, Faiman C. Primary radiotherapy of prolactinomas: eight to 15 year follow-up. Am J Med 1987;83:49–58.

25. Rush SC, Newall J. Pituitary adenoma: the efficacy of radiotherapy as the sole treatment. Int J Radiat Oncol Biol Phys 1989;17:165–169.

26. Tsagarakis S, Grossman A, Plowman PN, Jones AE, Touzel R, Rees LH, et al. Megavoltage pituitary irradiation in the management of prolactinomas: long-term follow-up. Clin Endocrinol 1991;34:399–406.

27. Clark SD, Woo SY, Butler EB, Dennis WS, Lu H, Carpenter LS, et al. Treatment of secretory pituitary adenoma with radiation therapy. Radiology 1993;188:759–763.

28. Baldwin A, Cundy T, Butler J, Timmis AD. Progression of cardiovascular disease in acromegalic patients treated by external pituitary irradiation. Acta Endocrinol 1985;108:26–30.

29. Krishna AY, Phillips LS. Management of acromegaly: a review. Am J Med Sci 1994;308(6):370–375.

30. Wright AD, Hill DM, Lowy C, Fraser TR. Mortality in acromegaly. Q J Med 1970;39:1–16.

31. Baskin DS, Boggan JE, Wilson CB. Transsphenoidal microsurgical removal of growth hormone-secreting pituitary adenomas. J Neurosurg 1982;56:634–641.

32. Dowsett RJ, Fowble B, Sergott RC, Savino PJ, Bosley TM, Snyder PJ, et al. Results of radiotherapy in the treatment of acromegaly: Lack of ophthalmologic complications. Int J Radiat Oncol Biol Phys 1990;19:453–459.

33. Feek CM, McLelland J, Seth J, Toft AD, Irvine WJ, Padfield PL, et al. How effective is external pituitary irradiation for growth hormone-secreting pituitary tumours? Clin Endocrinol 1984;20:401–408.

34. Lamberg BA, Kivikangas V, Vartiainen J, Raitta C, Pelkonen R. Conventional pituitary irradiation in acromegaly. Acta Endocrinol 1976;82:267–281.

35. Macleod AF, Clarke DG, Pambakian M, Lowy C, Sonksen PH, Collins CD: Treatment of acromegaly by external irradiation. Clin Endocrinol 1989;30:303–314.

36. Sheline GE, Wara WM. Radiation therapy of acromegaly and nonsecretory chromophobe adenomas of the pituitary. In: Seydel HG, ed. Tumours of the Nervous System. John Wiley, New York, 1975, pp. 119–131.

37. Trampe EA, Lundell G, Lax I, Werner S. External irradiation of growth hormone producing pituitary adenomas: prolactin as a marker of hypothalamic and pituitary effects. Int J Radiat Oncol Biol Phys 1991;20:655–660.

38. Ciccarelli E, Valetto MR, Vasario E, Avataneo T, Grottoli S, Camanni F. Hormonal and radiological effects of megavoltage radiotherapy in patients with growth hormone-secreting pituitary adenoma. J Endocrinol Invest 1993;16:565–572.

39. Eastman RC, Gorden P, Roth J. Conventional supervoltage irradiation is an effective treatment for acromegaly. J Clin Endocrinol Metab 1979;48(6):931–940.

40. Werner S, Trampe EA, Palacios P, Lax I, Hall K. Growth hormone producing pituitary adenomas with concomitant hypersecretion of prolactin are particularly sensitive to photon irradiation. Int J Radiat Oncol Biol Phys 1985;11:1713–1720.

41. Eastman RC, Gorden P, Glatstein E, Roth J. Radiation therapy of acromegaly. Endocrinol Metab Clin North Am 1992;21(3):693–712.

42. Pistenma DA, Goffinet DR, Bagshaw MA, Hanbery JW, Eltringham JR. Treatment of acromegaly with megavoltage radiation therapy. Int J Radiat Oncol Biol Phys 1976;1:885–893.

43. Bloom B, Kramer S. Conventional radiation therapy in the management of acromegaly. In: Black McL P, Zervas NT, Ridgway EC, Martin JB, eds. Secretory Tumors of the Pituitary Gland. Raven, New York, 1984, pp. 179–190.

44. Wass JAH, Laws ER Jr, Randall RV, Sheline GE. The treatment of acromegaly. Clin Endocrinol Metab 1986;15:683–707.

45. Chang CH. Radiotherapy of secretory and nonsecretory pituitary adenomas. In: Tumors of the Central Nervous System: Modern Radiotherapy in Multidisciplinary Management. Masson, New York, 1982, pp. 201–213.

46. Caruso M, Shaw E, Davis D, Scheithauer B, Abboud C, Speed J, et al. Radiation treatment of growth hormone secreting pituitary adenomas. Int J Radiat Oncol Biol Phys 1991;21(Suppl):121–122.

47. Williams GH, Dluhy RG. Diseases of the adrenal cortex. In: Braunwald E, Isselbacher KJ, Petersdorf RG, Wilson JD, Martin JB, Fauci AS, eds. Harrison's Principles of Internal Medicine, 11th ed. McGraw-Hill, New York, 1987, pp. 1760–1767.

48. Cushing H. The basophilic adenomas of the pituitary body and their clinical manifestations. Bull Johns Hopkins Hosp 1932;50:137–195.

49. Melby JC. Therapy of Cushing disease: a consensus for pituitary microsurgery. Ann Int Med 1988;109(6):445,446.

50. Tyrrell JB, Wilson CB. Cushing's disease:therapy of pituitary adenomas. Endocrinol Metab Clin North Am 1994;23(4):925–938.

51. Mampalam TJ, Tyrrell JB, Wilson CB. Transsphenoidal microsurgery for Cushing disease:a report of 216 cases. Ann Int Med 1988;109:487–493.

52. Robert F, Hardy J. Cushing's disease: a correlation of radiological, surgical and pathological findings with therapeutic results. Pathol Res Pract 1991;187:617–621.

53. Tindall GT, Herring CJ, Clark RV, Adams DA, Watts NB. Cushing's disease: results of transsphenoidal microsurgery with emphasis on surgical failures. J Neurosurg 1990;72:363–369.

54. Styne DM, Grumbach MM, Kaplan SL, Wilson CB, Conte FA. Treatment of Cushing's disease in childhood and adolescence by transsphenoidal microadenectomy. N Engl J Med 1984;310:889–893.

55. Aristizabal S, Caldwell WL, Avila J, Mayer EG. Relationship of time dose factors to tumor control and complications in the treatment of Cushing's disease by irradiation. Int J Radiat Oncol Biol Phys 1977;2:47–54.

56. Littley MD, Shalet SM, Beardwell CG, Ahmed SR, Sutton ML. Long-term follow-up of low-dose external pituitary irradiation for Cushing's disease. Clin Endocrinol 1990;33:445–455.

57. Murayama M, Yasuda K, Minamori Y, Mercado-asis LB, Yamakita N, Miura K. Long term follow-up of Cushing's disease treated with reserpine and pituitary irradiation. J Clin Endocrinol Metab 1992;75:935–942.

58. Schteingart DE, Tsao HS, Taylor CI, McKenzie A, Victoria R, Therrien BA. Sustained remission of Cushing's disease with mitotane and pituitary irradiation. Ann Int Med 1980;92:613–619.

59. Jennings AS, Liddle GW, Orth DN. Results of treating childhood Cushing's disease with pituitary irradiation. N Engl J Med 1977;297:957–962.

60. Howlett TA, Plowman PN, Wass JAH, Rees LH, Jones AE, Besser GM. Megavoltage pituitary irradiation in the management of Cushing's disease and Nelson's syndrome: long-term follow-up. Clin Endocrinol 1989;31:309–323.

61. Nelson DH, Meakin JW, Dealy JB Jr, Matson DD, Emerson K, Thorn GW. ACTH-producing tumor of the pituitary gland. N Engl J Med 1958;259:161–164.

62. Moore TJ, Dluhy RG, Williams GH, Cain JP. Nelson's syndrome: frequency, prognosis, and effect of prior pituitary irradiation. Ann Int Med 1976;85:731–734.

63. Orth DN, Liddle GW. Results of treatment in 108 patients with Cushing's syndrome. N Engl J Med 1971;285:243–247.

64. Kasperlik-Zaluska AA, Nielubowicz J, Wislawski J, Hartwig W, Zaluska J, Jeske W, et al. Nelson's syndrome: incidence and prognosis. Clin Endocrinol 1983;19:693–698.

65. Buchfelder M, Fahlbusch R, Schrell U, Stalla GK, Müller OA. Evaluation of the efficacy of a treatment regimen for ACTH-secreting pituitary adenomas associated with Nelson's syndrome. Adv Biosci 1988;69:383–384.

66. Scanarini M. Transsphenoidal surgery in Cushing's disease and Nelson's syndrome. J Endocrinol Invest 1990;15:230.

67. Scheithauer BW, Kovacs KT, Laws ER Jr, Randall RV. Pathology of invasive pituitary tumors with special reference to functional classification. J Neurosurg 1986;65:733–744.

68. Derome PJ, Delalande O, Visot A, Jedynak CP, Dupuy M. Short and long term results after transsphenoidal surgery for Cushing's disease; incidence of recurrences. Adv Biosci 1988;69:375–379.

69. Brada M, Rajan B, Traish D, Ashley S, Holmes-Sellors PJ, Nussey S, et al. The long-term efficacy of conservative surgery and radiotherapy in the control of pituitary adenomas. Clin Endocrinol 1993;38:571–578.

70. Urdaneta N, Chessin H, Fischer JJ. Pituitary adenomas and craniopharyngiomas: analysis of 99 cases treated with radiation therapy. Int J Radiat Oncol Biol Phys 1976;1:895–902.

71. Flickinger JC, Nelson PB, Martinez AJ, Deutsch M, Taylor F. Radiotherapy of nonfunctional adenomas of the pituitary gland: results of long-term follow-up. Cancer 1989;63:2409–2414.

72. Tran LM, Blount L, Horton D, Sadeghi A, Parker RG. Radiation therapy of pituitary tumors: results in 95 cases. Am J Clin Oncol 1991;14(1):25–29.

73. Grigsby PW, Stokes S, Marks JE, Simpson JR. Prognostic factors and results of radiotherapy alone in the management of pituitary adenomas. Int J Radiat Oncol Biol Phys 1988;15:1103–1110.

74. Spiegel EA, Wycis HT, Marks M, Lee AJ. Stereotactic apparatus for operations on the human brain. Science 1947;106:349–350.

75. Mehta MP. The physical, biologic, and clinical basis of radiosurgery. Curr Problems Cancer 1995;19(5):267–328.

76. Leksell L. Stereotactic radiosurgery. J Neurol Neurosurg Psychol 1983;46:797–803.

77. Stephanian E, Lunsford LD, Coffey RJ, Bissonette DJ, Flickinger JC. Gamma knife surgery for sellar and suprasellar tumors. Neurosurg Clin North Am 1992;3:207–218.

78. Lunsford LD, Kondziolka D, Flickinger JC. Stereotactic radiosurgery for benign intracranial tumors. Clin Neurosurg 1993;40:475–497.

79. Fabrikant JI, Levy RP, Steinberg GK, Phillips MH, Frankel KA, Silverberg GD. Stereotactic charged-particle radiosurgery:clinical results of treatment of 1200 patients with intracranial arteriovenous malformations and pituitary disorders. Clin Neurosurg 1992;38:472–492.

80. Ganz JC. Gamma knife treatment of pituitary adenomas. Stereotact Funct Neurosurg 1995;64(Suppl):3–10.

81. Ostertag ChB. Stereotactic radiation therapy and radiosurgery. Stereotact Funct Neurosurg 1994;63:220–232.

82. Kjellberg RN, Masamitsu A. Stereotactic Bragg peak proton beam therapy. In: Lunsford LD, ed. Modern Stereotactic Neurosurgery. Martinus Nijhoff, Boston, 1988, pp. 463–470.

83. Thorén M, Rähn T, Hall K, Backlund EO. Treatment of pituitary dependent Cushing's syndrome with closed stereotactic radiosurgery by means of ^{60}Co gamma radiation. Acta Endocrinol 1978;88:7–17.

84. Steiner, et al. Radiosurgery. Adv Tech Stand Neurosurg 1992; 19:21–97.

85. Thorén M, Rähn T, Hallengren B, Kaad PH, Nilsson O, Ravn H, et al. Treatment of Cushing's disease in childhood and adolescence by stereotactic pituitary irradiation. Acta Pœdiatr Scand 1986;75:388–395.

86. Thorén M, Rähn T, Guo W-Y, Werner S. Stereotactic radiosurgery with the cobalt-60 gamma unit in the treatment of growth hormone-producing pituitary tumors. Neurosurgery 1991;29:663–667.

87. Ganz JC, Backlund E-O, Thorsen FA. The effects of gamma knife surgery of pituitary adenomas on tumor growth and endocrinopathies. Stereotact Funct Neurosurg 1993;6(Suppl):30–37.

88. Pollock BE, Kondziolka D, Lunsford LD, Flickinger JC. Stereotactic radiosurgery for pituitary adenomas: imaging, visual and endocrine results. Acta Neurochir 1994;62(Suppl):33–38.

89. Rocher FP, Sentenac I, Berger C, Marquis I, Romestaing P, Gerard JP. Stereotactic radiosurgery: the Lyon experience. Acta Neurochir 1995;63(Suppl):109–114.

90. Dunbar SF, Tarbell NJ, Kooy HM, Alexander E III, Black McL P, Barnes PD, et al. Stereotactic radiotherapy for pediatric and adult brain tumors: preliminary report. Int J Radiat Oncol Biol Phys 1994;30(3):531–539.

91. Shrieve DC, Tarbell NJ, Alexander E III, Kooy HM, Black McL P, Dunbar S, et al. Stereotactic radiotherapy: a technique for dose optimization and escalation for intracranial tumors. Acta Neurochir 1994;62(Suppl):118–123.

92. Snyder PJ, Fowble BF, Schatz NJ, Savino PJ, Gennarelli TA. Hypopituitarism following radiation therapy of pituitary adenomas. Am J Med 1985;81:457–462.

93. Sheline GE, Wara WM, Smith V. Therapeutic irradiation and brain injury. Int J Radiat Oncol Biol Phys 1980;6:1215–1228.

94. Harris JR, Levene MB. Visual complications following irradiation for pituitary adenomas and craniopharyngiomas. Radiology 1976; 120:167–171.

95. Marks JE, Baglan RJ, Prassad SC, Blank WF. Cerebral radionecrosis: incidence and risk in relation to dose, time, fractionation and volume. Int J Radiat Oncol Biol Phys 1981;7:243–252.

96. Aristizabal S, Caldwell WL, Avila J. The relationship of time-dose fractionation factors to complications in the treatment of pituitary tumors by irradiation. Int J Radiat Oncol Biol Phys 1977; 2:667–673.

97. Grattan-Smith PJ, Morris JG, Langlands AO. Delayed radiation necrosis of the central nervous system in patients irradiated for pituitary tumours. J Neurol Neurosurg Psychiatry 1992;55:949–955.

98. Blount L, Horton D, Sadeghi A, Parker RG. Radiation therapy of pituitary tumors: results in 95 cases. Am J Clin Oncol 1991;14:25–29.

99. Fisher BJ, Gaspar LE, Noone B. Radiation therapy of pituitary adenoma: delayed sequelae. Radiology 1993;187:843–846.

100. Kline LB, Kim JY, Ceballos R. Radiation optic neuropathy. Ophthamology 1985;92(8):1118–1126.

101. Millar JL, Spry NA, Lamb DS, Delahurt J. Blindness in patients after external beam irradiation for pituitary adenomas: two cases occurring after small daily fractional doses. Clin Oncol 1991;3:291–294.

102. Hufnagel TJ, Kim JH, Lesser R, Miller JM, Abrahams JJ, Piepmeier J, et al. Malignant glioma of the optic chiasm eight years after radiotherapy for prolactinoma. Arch Ophthalmol 1988;106:1701–1705.

103. Marus G, Levin CV, Rutherfoord GS. Malignant glioma following radiotherapy for unrelated primary tumors. Cancer 1986;58:886–894.

104. Partington MD, Davis DH. Radiation-induced meningioma after treatment for pituitary adenoma: case report and literature review. Neurosurgery 1990;26(2):329–331.

105. Romero FJ, Ortega A, Ibarra B, Piqueras J, Rovira M. Post-radiation cranial malignant fibrous histiocytoma studied by CT. Comput Med Imaging Graphics 1989;13(2):191–194.

106. Sridhar K, Ramamurthi B. Intracranial meningioma subsequent to radiation for a pituitary tumor: case report. Neurosurgery 1989; 25(4):643–645.

107. Flickinger JC, Nelson PB, Taylor FH, Robinson A. Incidence of cerebral infarction after radiotherapy for pituitary adenoma. Cancer 1989;63:2404–2408.

16 Prolactinomas

CHARLES F. ABBOUD, MD AND MICHAEL J. EBERSOLD, MD

INTRODUCTION

Prolactinomas are the most commonly occurring pituitary adenomas, accounting for 40–60% of clinically recognizable hyperfunctioning pituitary tumors. Our understanding of their pathogenesis, presentations, and therapy is continually evolving. Prolactinomas pose significant challenges to the diagnostic and therapeutic acumen of the physician. The diagnostic process is taxing, because the clinical presentations, and the laboratory and radiologic features, are varied and nonspecific. Although an optimal therapeutic option is not universally accepted or applied at present, there are available to the physician effective pharmacologic, surgical, and radiotherapeutic ablative treatment options. The choice of the appropriate therapeutic option for a given patient demands considerable therapeutic and considerable skills. The purpose of this chapter is to bring to the clinician up-to-date information that is relevant to meeting these diagnostic and therapeutic challenges.

PATHOLOGY

Prolactinomas are usually sparsely granulated, monohormonal, lactotroph adenomas (1,2). Rarely, they are found to be acidophil stem or mammosomatroph plurihormonal adenomas composed of one cell line secreting prolactin as well as growth hormone, or are mixed plurihormonal adenomas consisting of two cell lines.

The precise incidence of prolactinomas is largely unknown. The reported incidence of pituitary microadenomas in unselected autopsy series ranged from 6 to 23%; 40% of these microadenomas were positive for prolactin with immunoperoxidase stain (3). The incidence of macroprolactinomas is not known, but in clinical practice, these tumors occur less frequently than do microprolactinomas. A higher proportion of prolactinomas in women are microadenomas, whereas in men a higher proportion are macroadenomas; the difference is likely related to a certain extent to the earlier diagnosis in women owing to the heightened awareness of gonadal dysfunction (1,4,5).

Based on distinctive clinical and therapeutic implications, prolactinomas are usually classified into microprolactinomas (<10 mm) or macroprolactinomas (>10 mm). Microprolactinomas are usually located in the lateral wings of the pituitary gland, and although some tumors are well demarcated, many do not have a

From: *Diagnosis and Management of Pituitary Tumors* (K. Thapar, K. Kovacs, B. W. Scheithauer, and R. V. Lloyd, eds.), ©Humana Press Inc., Totowa, NJ.

well-defined capsule and show microscopic invasive properties. In one study, 69% of microprolactinomas, compared to 88% of macroprolactinomas, showed histologic evidence of dural invasion (6). Macroprolactinomas can be intrasellar or can extend, to a variable extent, into the extrasellar neighborhood and invade the dura, sphenoid bone, cavernous sinuses, the suprasellar cisterns, and the adjoining parts of the brain. Prolactinomas may exhibit cystic or hemorrhagic degeneration (7), or dystrophic calcification (8); very rarely, the tumor may be ossified (9).

The most commonly encountered tumors are the sparsely granulated prolactinomas (1,4). Light microscopy shows that these tumors are usually chromophobic and have a diffuse pattern, occasionally exhibiting abundant hyaline stroma or amyloid deposits. Immunohistochemical studies reveal intense prolactin positivity in a juxtanuclear location corresponding to the Golgi apparatus. Ultrastructural features are characteristic of lactotroph hyperactivity:

1. The cells are similar to stimulated nontumorous lactotrophs and show large nuclei, prominent rough endoplasmic reticulum, and Golgi apparatus.
2. Storage granules are sparse, spherical, and vary in diameter from 150 to 300 nm.
3. Diagnostic pattern of granule extrusion is evident, with the granules being extruded along the lateral borders of the cell, the so-called misplaced exocytosis.

The rare densely granulated prolactinomas (1,4) are acidophilic tumors. The cells resemble the resting nontumorous lactotroph. Immunostaining studies show diffuse intense positivity for prolactin throughout the cytoplasm. Ultrastructural studies reveal findings of a "resting" lactotroph: a less prominent endoplasmic reticulum, and numerous spherical and electron-dense secretory granules measuring up to 1200 nm with some "misplaced exocytosis."

Acidophil stem-cell adenomas (10) are a rare chromophobic monocellular bihormonal tumors that possess the immunohistochemical and ultrastructural features common to somatotrophs and lactotrophs. The ultrastructural features are diagnostic: the cells are irregular and elongated, the nuclei are irregular and ovoid, the mitochondria are enlarged and numerous and often harbor tubular structures, the rough endoplasmic reticulum and Golgi apparatus are well developed, and the secretory granules are sparse and small, measuring 150–200 nm, and often showing "misplaced exocytosis." These tumors, usually macroadenomas at presentation, cosecrete prolactin and growth hormone (GH). The clinical presentations are those of the hyperprolactinemic syndrome, the acromegalic features being few or subtle.

Mixed pituitary tumors are acidophilic or chromophobic tumors composed of two adenohypophyseal cell lines. Most commonly, these tumors are mixed somatotroph–lactotroph tumors *(11–13)*; very rarely they may be mixed lactotroph/corticotroph *(14)* lactotroph/thyrotrophs *(15)*, or lactotroph/gonadotrophs *(16,17)* tumors. Immunohistochemical and ultrastructural studies show the features of the two cell lines; the neoplastic lactotrophs are either of the sparsely or densely granulated variants.

True malignant prolactinomas with metastates distant from the pituitary region are exceedingly rare *(1,19)*.

The factors that impact on the pathogenesis, the initiation, and development of the neoplastic process are unknown. Present evidence supports the hypothesis that for the majority of prolactinomas, the neoplasm is a primary pituitary disorder *(19)*, the result of a monoclonal process involving expansion of a single somatically mutated or transformed cell *(20,21)*. A role for hypothalamic dysregulation in the genesis or development of some prolactinomas has not been excluded *(19)*.

The role of estrogen in the genesis and development of human prolactinomas is largely undefined. In experimental animals, estrogens increase mitosis and growth of prolactinomas. Estrogens cause hypertrophy and hyperplasia of normal *(22)* and neoplastic *(22)* lactotrophs. Rising levels of estrogen in normal pregnancy are responsible for lactotroph hypertrophy and hyperplasia, and the progressive increase in prolactin secretion, as well as the increase in size of the pituitary gland *(23)*. They are also believed to be responsible for the enlargement of prolactinomas during pregnancy *(see below)*. Case-controlled studies have shown that prolactinomas are not more frequent in user of oral contraceptives users vs nonusers *(24)*, and prospective studies have shown that the use of oral contraceptives does not increase the risk of development of prolactinomas *(25)*. The use of estrogen-replacement therapy in prolactinomas, in the short term, is not associated with tumor growth *(26)*. In idiopathic hyperprolactinemia, the use of estrogens, over a period of 4 yr, has not been shown to increase the risk of clinical appearance of prolactinomas *(26)*.

CLINICAL FEATURES

The clinical features of prolactinomas are composed of the clinical expressions of the hyperprolactinemic state, the endocrine syndrome, and those of tumor-mass effects, the neuroendocrine syndrome *(see* Table 1).

THE HYPERPROLACTINEMIC ENDOCRINE SYNDROME
Hyperprolactinemic Manifestations   The endocrine presentations result from the biologic effects of hyperprolactinemia on prolactin-target tissues, dominantly on the gonadal/reproductive axis and on the breasts. Adult patients with prolactinoma, who are in their reproductive years, manifest gonadal axis impairment, infertility, and hypogonadism, which result primarily from the central inhibitory effects of hyperprolactinemia on hypothalamic–gonadotropin-releasing hormone (GnRH) production and cyclicity. In children and postmenopausal women, who normally have inoperative reproductive axes, the gonadal manifestations of hyperprolactinemia are absent. In adolescents, the suppressed gonadal axis is expressed in failure of sexual/reproductive development. In the hormonally adequately prepared breast, usually that of the adult female, galactorrhea is a common expression. This is usually not seen in the breast of the male or prepubertal female.

Table 1
Clinical Manifestations of Prolactinomas

Endocrine (or hyperprolactinemic) syndrome:
  Adult female: reproductive life:
    Galactorrhea
    Ovulatory dysfunction
      Short luteal phase
      Anovulation
      Infertility
    Menstrual dysfunction—oligo/amenorrhea
    Hypogonadism
      Osteopenia
    Hyperandrogenic manifestations
      Hirsutism; acne
    Decreased libido and mood effects (related to hypoestrogenism plus direct effects of hyperprolactinemia)
  Adult female—postmenopausal
    All of the above with the exception of ovulatory and menstrual dysfunction
  Adult male
    Decreased libido
    Potency impairment
    Oligospermia/infertility
    Other manifestations of adult hypogonadism
    Galactorrhea—rare
  Adolescents
    Delayed puberty
Neuroendocrine (or mass effects) syndrome
  Chronic presentation:
    Neurologic:
      Headaches
      Effects of superior extension
        Chiasmal syndrome
          Impaired visual acuity and fields
          Hypothalamic syndrome
          Disturbances of thirst, appetite, satiety, sleep and temperature regulation
        Diabetes insipidus
        Inappropriate antidiuretic (ADH) syndrome
        Obstructive hydrocephalus
        Frontal lobe syndrome
      Effects of lateral extension
        Cranial III, IV, VI, and V impairment
          Diplopia, ptosis, or facial pain
        Temporal lobe syndrome
      Effects of inferior extension
        Nasopharyngeal mass
      CSF rhinorrhoea
    Endocrine:
      Hypopituitarism
        Unihormonal
        Multihormonal
  Acute presentation
    Neurologic
      Pituitary apoplexy
    Endocrine
      Hyponatremic syndrome
      Adrenocortical crisis
      Hypoglycemic syndrome
  Asymptomatic Presentation
    The pituitary "incidentaloma"
Associated endocrinopathies
  MEN I
    Primary hyperparathyroidism
    Tumors of the endocrine pancreas
    Lipomas
    Other endocrine tumors (thyroid, adrenal)
  "Mixed pituitary tumors"
    Acromegaly
    Cushing's disease
    TSH hyperthyroidism

In the adult female in her reproductive years, a spectrum of gonadal and reproductive disorders occurs, depending largely on the degree and the duration of the hyperprolactinemic state (5,27–32). The disorders may include decreased libido, a short luteal phase or anovulation with regular periods, or oligo/amenorrhea; the composite expression is that of infertility or hypoestrogenic state. It has been estimated that 20–40% of women with oligo/amenorrhea, whether primary or secondary, have hyperprolactinemia, with prolactinomas being the most frequent cause of the hyperprolactinemic state (33,34). The incidence rises to 70–80% of women in whom the amenorrhea is associated with galactorrhea. Decreased libido and hypoestrogenic symptoms of mood changes, decreased vaginal secretions and dyspareunia, and osteopenia are common. Osteopenia, which affects trabecular and cortical bone, and predominantly the former, is seen in both hyperprolactinemic hypogonadal women (35) and men (36), and is believed to be related to hypogonadism and not to the hyperprolactinemia per se (37,38). Patients with hyperprolactinemia and normal gonadal function do not have osteopenia. The osteopenia is progressive and correlates with the duration of the hypogonadal state (39); the progression may be more prominent in a subset of women with low body fat and lower androgen levels (38). Restoration of the eugonadal state halts bone loss and increases bone mass; bone density, however, remains lower than normal (40).

Galactorrhea is a common symptom, being present in 50–80% of hyperprolactinemic women. The presence and degree of galactorrhea do not correlate with serum prolactin levels. Galactorrhea may be clinical or subclinical, unilateral or bilateral, spontaneous or expressed, and scanty or copious in quantity. The presence of galactorrhea does not always indicate hyperprolactinemia; in the absence of menstrual dysfunction, it may be present in about 25% of normal multiparous women in whom it is usually expressible and of small quantity. Galactorrhea in nulliparous women is always abnormal.

The order of appearance of menstrual/ovulatory disorder and of galactorrhea may vary, with either of the two symptoms preceding the other, often by a period of months or years.

In some patients, a hyperandrogenic state with hirsutism and acne may be seen, and is thought to be the result, in part, of a prolactin-induced, adrenocorticotropic hormone (ACTH)-dependent, increased dihydroepiandrosterone (DHEA) production by the adrenal cortices (41). There is an infrequent association between prolactinomas and the polycystic ovarian syndrome (42,43).

In the postmenopausal patient, the only clinical expressions of the hyperprolactinemic state may be decreased libido and galactorrhea.

In the adult male, the most common clinical expressions of hyperprolactinemia are decreased libido and potency impairment (44–46). Decreased spermatogenesis and poor semen quality may result in infertility. Other features of male hypogonadism may appear in time. Gynecomastia is unusual, and galactorrhea is exceedingly rare.

In the adolescent, hyperprolactinemic hypogonadism presents itself as failure of sexual maturation (47,48).

Associations Clinical features of the hormone(s) cosecreted with prolactin may be apparent in patients with acidophil stem-cell tumors (GH) or mixed pituitary tumors (GH, ACTH, thyroid-stimulating hormone [TSH], or gonadotropins). Prolactinomas may occur in the context of multiple endocrine neoplasia type 1

(MEN 1) (49,50) and the patient may also have clinical manifestations of primary hyperparathyroidism, gastrinoma, insulinoma, or other syndromes of tumors of the endocrine pancreas.

THE MASS EFFECTS OF NEUROENDOCRINE SYNDROME Mass effects are caused by the impact of the expanding tumor mass on the normal pituitary gland and the extrasellar structures, and are expressed most commonly with symptoms of a chronic slowly evolving process. Acute presentations are rare.

The Chronic Mass Effects Hypopituitarism may be partial or complete (51). Diabetes insipidus occurs only in patients with prolactinomas with significant suprasellar extension and impingement on the median eminence and upper stalk (28,51).

The extrasellar effects, which result from compression/invasion of the adjacent structures, depend on the direction and extent of growth of the macroprolactinoma. Suprasellar extension is common and results usually in the chiasmal syndrome and rarely in the hypothalamic syndrome (5,28). Parasellar extension is macroscopically and radiologically common, but the parasellar syndrome, which may result from cranial nerve III, IV, VI, and V dysfunction, and from temporal lobe dysfunction, is rare (52). Sphenoidal extension is usually asymptomatic; occasionally it manifests as a nasopharyngeal mass, and in those patients with a degenerating cystic prolactinoma, particularly with DA agonist therapy (see later), it may manifest as cerebrospinal (CSF) rhinorrhea.

The Acute Mass Effects These effects include (1) pituitary apoplexy (7) or (2) the acute endocrine presentations of adrenocortical crisis, hyponatremia, and hypoglycemia seen in the patients with hypopituitarism (51).

THE "UNSUSPECTED" PROLACTINOMA Prolactinomas may be asymptomatic and found during the evaluation of a pituitary mass lesion detected incidentally on imaging studies performed for nonendocrine reasons, the so-called pituitary incidentaloma (3,53). This may be the presentation in some adult males or postmenopausal females. Adult females in their reproductive years, and most men with macroprolactinomas, are predominantly symptomatic. Occasionally prolactinomas are first detected during the evaluation of patients with MEN 1 or during screening of their immediate family members.

DIAGNOSIS

The diagnosis of prolactinomas depends on (1) the consideration of the various other causes of the hyperprolactinemic syndrome and of the other mass lesions in the pituitary–hypothalamic area, and (2) on the pursuit of a disciplined organized diagnostic approach.

DIFFERENTIAL DIAGNOSIS Hyperprolactinemia can be either physiologic or pathologic in origin. The etiology of hyperprolactinemia is outlined in Table 2. Physiologic hyperprolactinemia occurs in stressful situations, such as surgery, anesthesia, exercise, and hypoglycemia. Pregnancy and the postpartum state are the most important causes of physiologic hyperprolactinemia. In pregnancy, prolactin levels start to rise early between the first and second months, reaching peak levels of several hundred nanograms per milliliter during the third trimester (23). The increased production is owing to the hypertrophy and hyperplasia of the lactotroph cell resulting from the rising estrogen levels and the hormonal milieu during pregnancy. After delivery and in those women who do not breast-feed, prolactin levels decrease rapidly, returning to normal in 1–2 wk. In those who do breast-feed, basal

Table 2
The Etiology of Hyperprolactinemia

Physiologic
    Pregnancy
    Postpartum state
    Suckling
    Stress
    Neonate
Pathologic
    Eutopic
        Organic pituitary disorder
          Prolactinomas
          "Mixed" pituitary tumors
          Lymphocytic hypophysitis
          Primary empty sella
          Nonfunctioning tumor with "stalk effect"
          "Idiopathic"
        Organic hypothalamic/stalk disorder
          Traumatic
             Radiotherapy
          Inflammatory
             Sarcoidosis
             Histiocytosis
             Autoimmune
             Other granulomatous disorders
          Vascular
             Aneurysms
          Neoplastic
             Primary
                Craniopharyngiomas
                Meningiomas
                Dysgerminomas
                Giomas, and so forth
             Secondary
                Metastatic
        "Idiopathic"
        Functional hypothalamic disease
          Drugs
             Neuroleptics (phenothiazines, haloperidol, and so on)
             Antidepressants (tricyclic, MAO-inhibitors, fluoxetine, and so forth)
             Antihypertensives (α-methyldopa, reserpine)
             Metoclopramide
             Opiates/cocaine
             H_2 receptor blockers (cimetidine, ranitidine)
             Calcium channel blockers (verapamil)
          Primary hypothyroidism
          Neurogenic
             Chest wall disorders
             Spinal nerves or cord disorders
          Chronic renal failure
          Cirrhosis
          Pseudocyesis
    Ectopic
        Hypernephroma
        Gonadoblastoma
        Ovarian teratomas

serum prolactin levels remain high for the first few weeks, with sharp surges in prolactin secretion occurring during suckling. Despite continued lactation, basal levels and post suckling surges decrease, and prolactin levels return to normal in a few months. It is critical to rule out pregnancy in any patient presenting with recent development of amenorrhea and hyperprolactinemia.

Pathologic hyperprolactinemia (27,28,54) can be eutopic or ectopic in origin. Eutopic hyperprolactinemia results from hypersecretion of prolactin by the anterior pituitary lactotrophs; this may be primary and caused by pituitary disease or secondary, and resulting from hypothalamic/stalk disease and loss of the dominant inhibitory regulation by hypothalamic dopamine. Very rarely, hyperprolactinemia results from the ectopic prolactin hypersecretion by an extrapituitary tumor.

Eutopic Hyperprolactinemia In addition to prolactinoma, other pituitary tumors can be associated with hyperprolactinemia. As mentioned previously, functioning "mixed" pituitary tumors may produce more than one pituitary hormone, and hyperprolactinemia has been noted in 20–30% of patients with acromegaly (12,13), and rarely in patients with Cushing's disease (14), or TSH tumors (15). A "nonfunctioning" pituitary tumor may be associated with a modest degree of hyperprolactinemia if it has a suprasellar extension impinging on the pituitary stalk or hypothalamus, and interfering with the access of the hypothalamic inhibitor dopamine to the normal anterior pituitary lactotrophs, the so-called stalk effect (56). Mild hyperprolactinemia has been reported in association with <15% of patients with primary empty sella (57); in such patients, a search for coexistent microprolactinoma is in order. Other pituitary masses, such as developmental cysts, e.g., Rathke's cleft cyst, can be associated with hyperprolactinemia. Lymphocytic hypophysitis (58), a presumed autoimmune disease, affects women preferentially, and usually occurs in temporal relationship to pregnancy and the postpartum state. It presents clinically with hyperprolactinemia, unitropic or multitropic pituitary failure, and a mass lesion, occasionally with extrasellar compressive effects. Frequently there may be clinical or laboratory evidence of autoimmune involvement of the other endocrine glands. Organic hypothalamic and infundibular disorders can be associated with hyperprolactinemia because of interruption of hypothalamic dopamine-inhibitory regulation, another expression of the stalk effect (56,59) mentioned above.

Craniopharyngiomas (60) are the most common extrapituitary tumors associated with hyperprolactinemia. Other hypothalamic tumors, whether primary or metastatic (28), tumors of adjacent structures, such as optic glioma or suprasellar meningioma, infiltrative disorders, such as sarcoidosis (61) or histiocytosis X (62), hypothalamic radiation (63), or stalk section can be associated with hyperprolactinemia. In such disorders, hyperprolactinemia may be the only demonstrable endocrine abnormality. However, these disorders are also frequently associated with diabetes insipidus, hypopituitarism, and vegetative hypothalamic dysfunction, which may include disturbances of sleep, temperature, appetite, and thirst.

Functional hypothalamic disorders can cause hyperprolactinemia by interference with secretion or action of dopamine, and/or other hypothalamic inhibitory regulators, or direct stimulation of the pituitary lactotroph. Drugs (54,64) are the most common cause of the hyperprolactinemic syndrome. Among the offending drugs are dopamine depletors, such as alphamethyldopa, dopamine receptor antagonists, such as phenothiazines, opiates, cocaine, H_2 receptor blockers, and the calcium channel blocker verapamil. Drug-induced hyperprolactinemia usually resolves in a few days to weeks following the discontinuation of the offending drug. Hyperprolactinemia is estimated to occur in 20–30% of patients with primary hypothyroidism (65,66), and may be related to dopamine dysregulation or decreased prolactin clearance. It resolves in few weeks or months with thyroid hormone replacement therapy and restitution of the euthyroid state. It is important to remember that in addition to hyperprolactinemia, primary hypothyroidism can lead to thyrotroph hypertrophy and hyperplasia, a TSH-pituitary mass lesion and be frequently misdiagnosed as "prolactinoma" *(67)*. Chest wall lesions, including trauma *(68)*, thoracotomy *(69)*, radical mastectomy, herpes zoster, and other lesions involving the fourth to sixth intercostal nerves or thoracic spinal segments, can cause hyperprolactinemia by activation of the afferent sensory mechanisms of the suckling reflex *(70)*. Hyperprolactinemia occurs in 20–40% of patients with chronic renal failure and in nearly all patients requiring hemodialysis *(71,72)*. The cause is indeterminate, but may be related to decreased prolactin clearance or impaired prolactin secretion control; hyperprolactinemia is only reversed by successful renal transplantation *(73)*. Alcoholic and nonalcoholic liver cirrhosis *(70)*, and liver failure *(74)*, especially with hepatic encephalopathy, can also be associated with hyperprolactinemia, which is also probably owing to a decreased prolactin clearance or altered hypothalamic prolactin secretion control.

Ectopic Hyperprolactinemia   This rare entity has been described in patients with hypernephroma *(75)*, gonadoblastoma *(76)*, or ovarian teratomas *(77)*. The clinical effects of hyperprolactinemia are usually overshadowed by those of the underlying neoplasm. At the time of detection of hyperprolactinemia, the ectopic neoplasm is usually evident.

LABORATORY AND RADIOLOGIC EVALUATION
Serum Prolactin   Serum prolactin levels in patients with prolactinomas vary from just above the upper limit of normal to values >10,000 ng/mL (normal 0–23 ng/mL in females, 0–20 ng/mL in males) *(33,78,79)*. The levels in a given patient show considerable variation, suggesting intermittent hormone secretion by the tumor, but in general, they parallel the size of the prolactinomas *(80)*. Prolactin levels >250 ng/mL are almost always indicative of a prolactinoma. It is important to remember that the secretion of prolactin in the normal individual may be episodic and labile, and that prolactin is a stress-responsive hormone; in patients with marginal hyperprolactinemia, it is prudent to obtain two or three separate samples on different days (or to perform multiple samplings over 1–2 h and measure prolactin in the pooled sample) to confirm the presence of pathologic hyperprolactinemia.

Prolactin-Provocative Tests   Many prolactin-stimulation and prolactin-suppression tests are available. They demonstrate differences between prolactin secretion in normal individuals and in patients with pathologic hyperprolactinemia. Unfortunately none of these tests has proven to be reliable in the differential diagnosis between tumorous and nontumorous hyperprolactinemia *(81,82)*. Abnormal responses, such as the blunted or absent prolactin response to thyrotropin-releasing hormone (TRH), the inhibitory effect of dopamine or L-dopa, the attenuation of the dopaminergic effect of L-dopa by carbidopa, the lack of suppressive effect by the dopamine reuptake inhibitor nomifensine, the lack of stimulatory effect by dopamine receptor blockade by sulpiride or chlorpromazine, and the absence of stimulation by the histamine-H2 receptor uptake cimetidine, are common to prolactinomas, idiopathic hyperprolactinemia, and other causes of hyperprolactinemia associated with hypothalamic–pituitary disease.

RADIOLOGIC EVALUATION   An ideal radiologic tool would have the following capabilities:

1. To outline the normal pituitary gland and its boundaries.

2. To outline the extrasellar structures whether bony or soft tissue.
3. To delineate pituitary tumors irrespective of their size.
4. To define the extent of the pituitary tumors, and, when present, their extrasellar extension and potential encroachment on vital structures.
5. To identify cystic, hemorrhagic, and calcific degeneration in the tumor.
6. To differentiate pituitary tumors from other masses in the area.
7. To show the response of the tumors to therapy.
8. To avoid exposure of the patients to ionizing radiation.
9. To be safe and inexpensive.

There is no radiologic tool available at present that meets all these characteristics. Most importantly, radiologic study cannot differentiate prolactinomas or other pituitary tumors from other masses in the region *(82)*.

Magnetic resonance imaging (MRI) with gadolinium (Gd)-DTPA enhancement comes closest to meeting most of these characteristics and is, therefore, the radiologic tool of choice in the evaluation of disorders of the pituitary–hypothalamic region *(82)*. However, its present sensitivity renders it incapable of detection of microadenomas <3 mm in diameter. Its other limitations include its inability to visualize adjacent bones or tumor calcification and its expense.

Dynamic computerized tomography (CT) scanning *(82)* after the iv administration of contrast media, with direct coronal scanning, is an adequate alternative. Its advantages include its ability to detect focal bony changes and tumor calcification, and its lesser expense. Its disadvantages include the exposure to ionizing radiation and, unfortunately in prolactinomas, the contraindication of its use in pregnancy.

There is a strong correlation between the serum prolactin level and the presence and size of a prolactinoma *(78,79)*. As mentioned, patients with serum prolactin >250 ng/mL almost always have a radiologically demonstrable tumor, and patients with macroprolactinomas usually have prolactin levels in excess of 500 ng/mL.

DIAGNOSTIC APPROACH   The diagnostic approach to a patient with suspected prolactinoma is based on the history, physical examination, consideration of the level of hyperprolactinemia, and neuroradiologic studies *(5,27,28,32)*. Additional studies are done, when appropriate, to assess pituitary function, and to evaluate for suspected MEN 1. The diagnostic approach to hyperprolactinemia is outlined in Figure 1.

The diagnostic steps should include:

1. The exclusion of pregnancy.
2. The exclusion of offending drugs by a careful drug history.
3. The exclusion of other functional causes, such as a chest wall lesion, renal or hepatic failure, or systemic or metastatic disease, by a careful history and physical examination, and standard laboratory and radiologic studies.
4. The exclusion of primary hypothyroidism by a TSH assay.

If a reversible cause of hyperprolactinemia is found, such as drug use or primary hypothyroidism, its discontinuation or treatment should allow resolution of the hyperprolactinemia. If the cause cannot be removed or managed, or if the hyper-

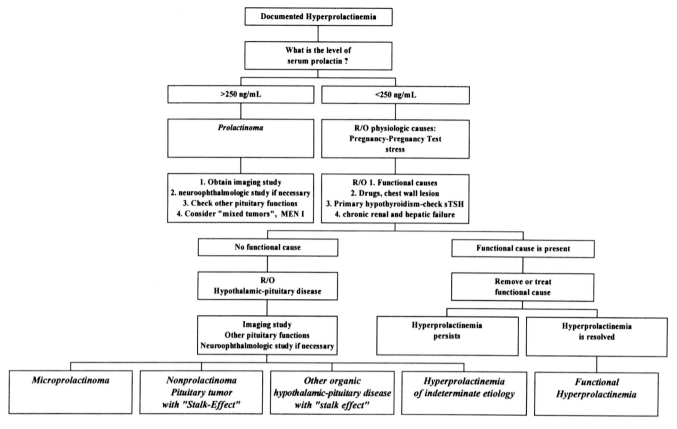

Figure 16-1 Diagnostic approach to hyperprolactinemia.

prolactinemia persists despite adequate management of the reversible cause, a search for other causes of hyperprolactinemia should be made.

The diagnosis of a prolactinoma is based on the consideration of the level of serum prolactin and the radiologic findings. As mentioned earlier, most patients with serum prolactin of >100 ng/mL and almost all patients with prolactin >250 ng/mL harbor a prolactinoma. Marginal or modest levels of hyperprolactinemia do not rule out a microprolactinoma, and radiologic studies become crucial for diagnosis; the finding of a pituitary sellar mass in these circumstances is compatible with a provisional diagnosis of microprolactinoma. Modest levels of hyperprolactinemia, usually <100 ng/mL, in the presence of a sellar mass with suprasellar extension point away from a diagnosis of macroprolactinoma (where a prolactin level >250 ng/mL is expected) and point to nonprolactinoma mass lesions with stalk effect hyperprolactinemia.

The diagnostic evaluation should also include:

1. Other pituitary function tests to assess the presence of other pituitary hypersecretory states or of hypopituitarism.
2. A neuroophthalmologic assessment if the mass lesion is seen to be impinging on the suprasellar space.
3. Appropriate studies, when applicable, to search for other evidences of MEN 1.

If after a thorough clinical, laboratory, and radiologic evaluation, no discernible cause is found, the hyperprolactinemia is labeled as "idiopathic," or preferably "of indeterminate etiology" *(83)*. Followup of these patients is important *(83)*, because some of them may harbor microadenomas or other hypothalamic–pitu-

itary organic disease too small to be detected by our present radiologic tools.

THERAPY

The goals of optimal therapy should be:

1. To remove the tumor completely and preserve normal pituitary function.
2. To achieve normalization of prolactin secretion and to reverse the clinical manifestations of hyperprolactinemia.
3. To prevent tumor recurrence.
4. To achieve all the above goals without mortality or morbidity.

It is safe to say that, at this time, we do not have any therapeutic modality that meets these objectives in all patients.

The treatment options that are available at present include dopamine (DA) agonist drug therapy, surgical adenomectomy, and radiation therapy

A number of factors enter into the therapeutic decision-making *(5,32)*: (1) There is no universally accepted therapeutic modality of choice. The options of medical therapy with DA agonists and transphenoidal adenomectomy are well established, effective, and reasonably safe. Radiation therapy is reserved, in most instances, for the special circumstances where DA agonists and/or surgery have failed to meet the therapeutic objectives. Therapeutic decisions vary from one center to the other, and depend on experiences and biases that are, to some extent, engendered by availability of expertise in the delivery of the preferred option of therapy. (2) The natural history of microprolactinomas: Untreated microprolactinomas have a benign history, at least over the short term of up to 8 yr *(84–87)*. Most microprolactinomas remain stable in size; <10% progress into macroprolactinomas, and up to 10% may actually regress. Based on these short-term findings, some authorities regard the untreated mass lesion in microprolactinomas as devoid of any significant potential threat to pituitary functions and to the extrasellar structures, at least for the first decade of observation, and believe that treatment in patients with micro-prolactinomas should therefore be directed dominantly at the hyperprolactinemic syndrome. Should hyperprolactinemic effects be minimal, or should they be easily managed with other hormonal therapies, then active treatment is believed to be unnecessary, and the option of "observation and follow-up" is pursued.

The natural history of macroprolactinomas is unknown, princi-pally because macroprolactinomas are treated expeditiously, as soon as the diagnosis is made because of their mass effects and the threat to the integrity of the extrasellar structures.

DRUG THERAPY

Medical therapy is based on the use of DA agonists *(5,32,88,89)*. These drugs bind to the D2-receptors on the cell membranes of the normal, as well as the neoplastic, lactotroph *(89)*. Binding of the drug to the receptor leads to intracellular responses consisting of a decrease in adenylate cyclase activity, in generation of cyclic AMP, and in levels of intracellular calcium. The cellular expres-sions of these drug effects are the decrease in synthesis and release of prolactin, and the anatomical regression of the cytoplasmic hormone synthesis machinery. In humans, these drugs do not have significant antimitotic activity. Therefore, DA agonist therapy is largely temporizing and, in most cases, effective only while the drug is being administered. Discontinuation of drug therapy (with some exceptions outlined below) results in resumption of the endocrine and neoplastic tumor activity.

The DA agonists used in therapy are of two classes *(32)*: (1) ergot alkaloids, which are devoid of the uterotonic and vascular effects of the parent compound. These include the lysergic acid amides (e.g., bromocriptine), the aminoergolines (e.g., lisuride), the clavine alkaloids (e.g., pergolide), and the ergoline derivatives (e.g., cabergoline), and (2) the nonergot compounds, such as CV 205-502 or quinagolide.

In the US, the only DA agonist approved for management of prolactinomas is bromocriptine *(90,91)*. Pergolide is also avail-able in the US market, but approved only for use in the manage-ment of Parkinson's disease. Worldwide, the most experience has been with bromocriptine (>25 yr). Lisuride *(92,93)* has also been used extensively over the years. The other newer compounds have only been recently introduced into the therapeutic armamentarium outside the US.

BROMOCRIPTINE At present, oral bromocriptine is con-sidered the "gold standard" of DA agonist therapy *(5,32,88,91,94)*. About 25–30% of the drug is absorbed. It is rapidly and effectively removed by the liver and undergoes hepatic degradation into bio-logically inactive metabolites. Only <7% of an absorbed dose reaches the systemic circulation. The drug easily traverses the blood–brain barrier, and the placenta serum bromocriptine level peaks in 3 h and reaches nadir in about 7 h *(95)*. The biologic half-life is similar to the plasma half-life. It is excreted dominantly in bile; only 2–6% is excreted unchanged in the urine. There is con-siderable interindividual variability in the absorption, and peak blood levels are attained.

Ultrastructurally, the use of DA agonist therapy in prolac-tinomas has been shown to induce rapid involution of the rough endoplasmic reticulum and Golgi apparatus, and decreased extru-sion of secretory granules *(96)*.

In hyperprolactinemic patients, and irrespective of the cause of hyperprolactinemia, bromocriptine therapy restores normopro-lactinemia in 80–90% of patients, and reverses the reproductive and galactogenic effects of the hyperprolactinemic syndrome in 70–80% of treated patients (experience reviewed in *30*). In addition, its use in patients with prolactinomas leads, in many patients, to a reduction in lactotroph size and to tumor-size regression *(93,97,98)* *(see below)*. The variation in the biologic responses to bromocriptine in terms of prolactin-inhibitory and tumor regression effects is in all likelihood the result of variation in the number of D₂ receptors on lactotroph cell membranes and in the intracellular responses to the drug *(99)*. The onset of bromocriptine effect is rapid and usually occurs in 1–2 h; it lasts for 6–8 h. The greatest decrease in prolactin levels occurs at the initiation of therapy; the achievement of normal-ization of prolactin levels may take weeks to months.

In the hyperprolactinemic woman, galactorrhea ceases in a few weeks and, in those patients with an intact, but suppressed gonadal axis, ovulatory cycles are restored within the first 2–3 mo. For patients desiring fertility, pregnancy may occur with the first ovu-latory cycle and prior to the resumption of menstrual function *(see below)*. In the hyperprolactinemic man, and in those patients with an intact but suppressed gonadal axis, the normalization of prolac-tin and restoration of normal sexual/reproductive functions may take 3–6 mo. It is to be remembered that the restoration of the sexual and reproductive functions does not require normalization of serum prolactin levels; it may occur in the face of persistent, but improved prolactin levels.

Bromocriptine-induced suppression of prolactin hypersecre-tion is typically associated with reduction in tumor size *(97,100)*. This subject is discussed below under specific therapy for microprolactinomas and macroprolactinomas.

LIMITATIONS OF BROMOCRIPTINE THERAPY Side Effects and Drug Intolerance In general, bromocriptine therapy is effective and well tolerated *(5,32,101,102)*. The most common encountered side effects *(90,91)* are nausea (50%) and occasional vomiting (10–15%); these symptoms usually occur with initiation of therapy and are believed to be caused principally by local gastrointestinal drug effects, and not by central effects. Although they are usually transient, they may recur with each increase in dosage. They are significant enough to have the patient become reluctant to continue the use of bromocriptine in <10% of cases. Other side effects that occur early in therapy and are usually self-limiting, include headaches (20%), orthostatism (20%), nasal congestion, and constipation (5%).

There are other side effects that are rare and only seen in patients who require high-dose chronic therapy, i.e., patients with acrome-galy or Parkinson's disease, but they have not been reported with the doses usually used in the therapy of prolactinomas *(5,90,91)*. Such rare side effects include (1) cold-sensitive painless digital vasospasm (30%) and (2) alcohol intolerance (10%). Very rarely, other side effects may appear:

1. Dyskinesias, erythromelalgia, psychotic reactions, which may include auditory hallucinations and delusional ideas, and exacerbations of schizophrenia.
2. Reversible pleuropulmonary changes *(103)*.
3. Retroperitoneal fibrosis *(104)*.

Rarely, bromocriptine therapy is complicated in patients with macroprolactinomas, particularly those with cystic degeneration and intrasphenoidal extension, by the occurrence of CSF rhinor-rhea, owing to tumor regression and loss of the "tumor-plug or cork" effects *(105,106)*.

Bromocriptine Resistance   Drug resistance *(5,32,107)* is encountered in <10% of treated patients, and has been shown to be related in great measure to a decrease in drug binding to cell membranes because of a decrease in D_2 receptors *(99)*. No correlation has been found between bromocriptine resistance and tumor size or the height of the prolactin levels. It is more commonly a relative resistance where prolactin levels are decreased, but not normalized, and the tumor-suppressive effects are absent *(108)*. Absolute resistance to prolactin-suppressive effects and progression in tumor growth despite drug therapy are very rarely observed. It is important to remember that a "resistant macroprolactinoma" may indeed be a prolactin cell carcinoma.

Dosage and Administration   The side effects of bromocriptine therapy can be minimized by starting with a small dose of 1.25 mg once daily, taken with food to delay absorption, and at bedtime to avoid orthostatic hypotensive symptoms *(90,91)*. The dose is gradually increased by 1.25 mg every 4–5 d, and according to individual tolerance, to a dose of 2.5 mg bid always taken with meals. Serum prolactin levels are checked in 1–2 mo, and the dosage is adjusted to achieve normalization of serum prolactin levels. The usual effective dose, in the management of prolactinomas, is 5–7.5 mg daily and in divided doses. Doses higher than 7.5 mg are rarely necessary, except in patients with extensive macroprolactinomas. When side effects occur, they can be managed by temporary reduction of dosage. If bromocriptine therapy is interrupted, the side effects often recur when the drug is reintroduced.

ALTERNATIVES TO ORAL BROMOCRIPTINE   The widespread appeal of bromocriptine therapy in the management of prolactinomas is faced with three challenges: drug intolerance, drug resistance, and drug reluctance by the treated patients. These challenges are seen in 10–20% of the treated patients. An alternative option of therapy is needed for these patients. Several such options may be available.

Use of Another Route of Bromocriptine Administration
The only option available in the US at this time is the use of intravaginal bromocriptine, which has been found to have the same effectiveness as oral bromocriptine and to be associated with much less pronounced local gastrointestinal side effects *(37,109)*. An intravaginal bromocriptine tablet of 2.5 mg has a 24-h duration of effect.

Long-acting injectable depot bromocriptine (Parlodel LAR) is effective within hours of administration and for a duration of 2–6 wk. Its efficacy in prolactin suppression and tumor size reduction is equivalent to that of bromocriptine, and it has only minimal side effects *(110,111)*.

Use of an Alternative DA Agonist *(94,112)*

1. Cabergoline is an ergoline derivative with selective and potent long-acting DA agonist properties *(113–115)*. It has been found to be highly effective in the management of hyperprolactinemia and in inducing tumor mass regression in microprolactinomas and macroprolactinomas *(115,116)*. Its advantages include ease of administration (once or twice weekly) and an improved side effects profile relative to bromocriptine *(113,115)*. Cabergoline is now available under compassionate use in the US.
2. CV 205-502 or Quinagolide is a nonergot long-acting DA agonist. Compared to bromocriptine, it appears to have

heightened D_2 receptor binding properties, and therefore, it may be particularly helpful in patients with bromocriptine resistance *(117–120)*. Its efficacy is comparable to that of bromocriptine, and its side effects are less common.

3. Pergolide has been approved in the US only for the management of Parkinson's disease. It has been found to be effective in the management of hyperprolactinemia and tumor mass in patients with prolactinomas *(121,122)*. Compared to bromocriptine therapy, pergolide has a comparable efficacy and side effects profile Hyperprolactinemia can usually be controlled with a single daily dose of 25–150 µg. Some patients who do not respond to bromocriptine respond to pergolide and vice versa.

The Use of Alternative Medical Therapy   As mentioned earlier, there is no major threat, in the short term at least, of mass effects in patients with microprolactinomas. The indications for therapy are mostly infertility and the hypogonadal state. When bromocriptine use is not possible, one can use other ovulation-induction agents for fertility, such as clomiphene *(123)*, pulsatile GnRH *(124,125)*, or exogenous gonadotropins *(126)*. The hypogonadal woman not desiring fertility may be safely treated with estrogen replacement. Short-term studies have shown no untoward effects from the use of oral contraceptives or other forms of estrogen/progestin supplementation *(26)*. It is prudent, however, to follow these patients with more frequent serial prolactin levels and MRI scanning than would have been otherwise indicated to monitor for tumor expansion, particularly with chronic therapy.

Use of Alternative Tumor Ablative Therapy   In many centers, the options of surgical and radiotherapeutic treatment of prolactinomas are reserved for the bromocriptine-intolerant or the bromocriptine-resistant patient, or for the patient who is reluctant to embark on long-term drug therapy.

SURGERY

Surgery provides the option of tumor removal, and therefore, the potential of restoration of normoprolactinemia and reversal of the hyperprolactinemic syndrome. The challenges of surgery *(127–133)* are:

1. The completeness of tumor excision.
2. The success of control of hyperprolactinemia
3. The potential persistence/recurrence of the hyperprolactinemic state or tumor mass.
4. The morbidity and mortality of the procedure
5. Consideration of the available options for the management of the patients with postoperative persistent or recurrent disease.

The surgical results, which are discussed later, are dependent to a large degree on the expertise of the neurosurgical team, and on the size and extent of the tumor *(79,128,129)*.

Transphenoidal surgery is the surgical procedure of choice for all patients with microprolactinomas and the vast majority of patients with macroprolactinoma. Transcranial surgery is reserved for those patients with macroprolactinoma with extensive extrasellar extension. The effect on prolactin hypersecretion is prompt and appears postoperatively within the first few hours. Transphenoidal surgery can be employed as a primary therapy. In most centers, however, it is used as an adjunctive therapy reserved for the patients who refuse, are intolerant of, or are resistant to DA agonist therapy *(see below)*.

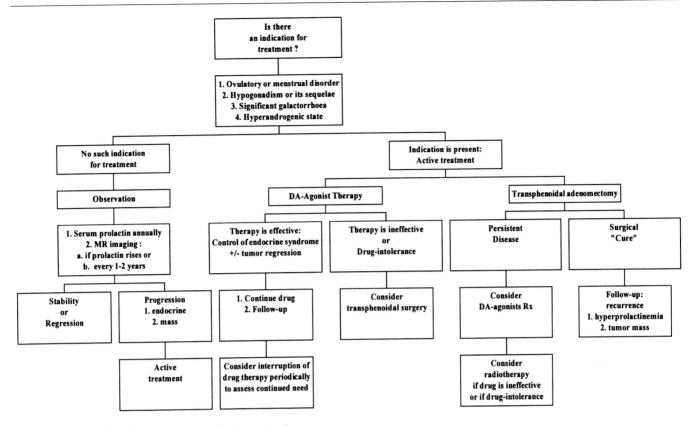

Figure 16-2 Options for management of microprolactinoma.

RADIOTHERAPY

Radiotherapy may be used as primary therapy in the management of prolactinomas *(13,133–136)*. Compared to the two other therapy alternatives, experience with radiotherapy has been limited. It appears that only a small number of patients achieve normoprolactinemia and only after a latent period, which may extend to few years. Postradiotherapy hypopituitarism is a significant side effect occurring in at least a third of the treated patients, but with incidence varying from 5.5 *(57)* to 93.3% *(1)*. Because of these limitations, most authorities regard radiotherapy as an adjunctive therapy *(134,135,137)* which is mainly used in those patients who are unsuitable for, or who have failed to respond to, medical or surgical therapy.

THERAPEUTIC CONSIDERATIONS IN THE MANAGEMENT OF MICROPROLACTINOMAS
The available options for the management of microprolactinomas are outlined in Figure 2. The two critical issues in the management of microprolactinomas are (1) to determine whether or not therapy is indicated and (2) to decide on the best option of therapy.

Is Therapy Indicated? The clinical presentations of microprolactinomas are dominated by the clinical effects of the hyperprolactinemic syndrome, and mass effects are practically absent. As mentioned earlier, microprolactinomas have a benign course, over the short term at least, and tumor growth over a period <10 yr is seen only in about 10% of patients. Therapy is therefore directed at the effects of the hyperprolactinemic syndrome, which impact significantly on the patient's health or on fertility needs.

Indications for therapy *(5,32,78)* include:

1. The hypogonadotrophic hypogonadal state, which encompasses the issues of fertility, hypoestrogenic state in women

and the hypoandrogenic state in men, failure of sexual maturation in adolescents, and their potential sequelae.
2. Hyperandrogenic state in women.
3. Significant galactorrhea (rare).
4. Documented progression in size of the microprolactinoma.

In the absence of these indications, active treatment may be withheld, and observation and careful follow-up are pursued. Since only few of microprolactinomas progress in size, and since such progression is not always accompanied by an increase in serum prolactin levels, prudent observation and follow up include yearly serum prolactin levels, and MRI every 2–3 yr or whenever prolactin levels rise.

What is the Best Therapeutic Option? Several considerations have made DA-agonist therapy the preferred primary therapy, in many centers, for microprolactinomas:

1. The absence of experienced surgical teams in many centers.
2. The disenchantment with the relatively high incidence of postoperative persistent or recurrent hyperprolactinemia.
3. The benign natural history of microprolactinomas.
4. The effectiveness, ease of administration, and safety of DA agonist therapy.

DA Agonist Therapy The use of DA agonist has been discussed earlier. Bromocriptine therapy is very effective in normalization of prolactin secretion (80–90%) and in restoration of sexual/gonadal/and reproductive functions (70–80%) *(5,90,91,105)*. The restoration of eugonadism halts the progression of osteopenia and partially restores bone density. Bromocriptine can also induce tumor mass regression in patients with a microprolactinoma *(98,138)*. Issue relating to bromocriptine intolerance and resistance are detailed above. Since spontaneous tumor regression does

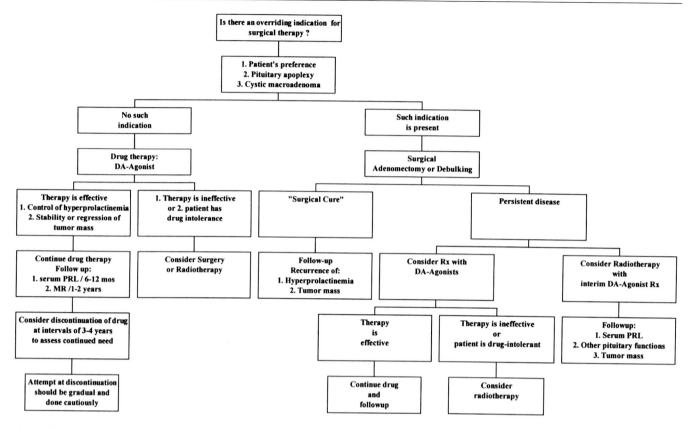

Figure 16-3 Options for management of macroprolactinoma.

occur in some patients with microprolactinomas (10%), it is prudent to discontinue bromocriptine therapy periodically to assess the need for continued therapy.

Surgery In transphenoidal surgery, the tumor mass is removed successfully in almost all patients. The main therapeutic challenge is that of persistent/recurrent hyperprolactinemia, postoperative recurrence of the tumor mass being distinctly unlikely *(79,127–129,132).* Transphenoidal microadenomectomy can normalize serum prolactin in 50–80% of patients *(31;* published series were reviewed in ref. *5* showing a cure rate of 71.2%). The clinical manifestations of hyperprolactinemia may resolve even in patients who have persistent, but improved hyperprolactinemia. In the reported surgical series, the mortality rate is 0.27%, and morbidity which is related to injury to surrounding structures, bleeding, infection, or CSF rhinorrhea is <1%. In almost all patients, normal anterior pituitary functions are preserved, and postoperative diabetes insipidus occurs only transiently.

Early persistent hyperprolactinemia is seen in about 10–30% of patients; in an additional 15–25% of patients, hyperprolactinemia reappears within the first 12 mo postoperatively, after an initial period of normalization *(127–129,132,139).* "Recurrence" is believed to be related to persistent tumor microscopic remnants rather than "true recurrence." This opinion is based on consideration of the natural history of microprolactinoma, and pathologic studies of microprolactinomas and their surrounding tissues. Pathologic studies have shown invasiveness of surrounding tissues in 69% of microprolactinomas. True recurrence of prolactinomas is distinctly rare.

Management of Postoperative Persistent Disease Persistent hyperprolactinemia is usually associated with persistence of

the hyperprolactinemic clinical syndrome and the potential, though low, for future tumor recurrence. DA agonist therapy is usually administered to correct the hyperprolactinemic syndrome *(140) (see above).* Long-term follow-up is necessary. Serum prolactin levels are checked on a yearly basis. MRI is done when serum prolactin levels rise or every 2–3 yr to exclude the unlikely possibility that tumor growth has occurred without concomitant increase in the serum prolactin levels.

THERAPEUTIC CONSIDERATIONS IN THE MANAGEMENT OF MACROPROLACTINOMAS Therapy for macroprolactinoma is directed at the hyperprolactinemic syndrome as well as the tumor mass effects. Macroprolactinomas have already documented their propensity to grow, and because of the risk of further growth, all patients with macroprolactinomas are candidates for therapy. The available options for the management of macroprolactinomas are outlined in Figure 3.

DA Agonist Therapy For the same reasons discussed under therapy for microprolactinomas, and in view of the suboptimal surgical results, morbidity, and mortality, and of the effectiveness and safety of DA agonist therapy, most centers regard DA agonist therapy with bromocriptine as the therapeutic option of choice *(141,142).* It is effective in normalization of prolactin hypersecretion (60–80%) and in inducing tumor-size regression (80%), and is easily administered and safe. Studies have raised the possibility that in some patients, drug-associated tumor fibrosis may lead to long-term "cure."

The majority of bromocriptine- treated patients experience a significant reduction in tumor size *(5,97,141–143),* with >50% of patients experiencing a >50% tumor size reduction. The extent of tumor size reduction does not correlate with baseline prolactin levels, or with the degree of prolactin suppression (80). The prolactin-suppressive effects uniformly precede any demonstrable regression in tumor size. Although prolactin suppression can take place without tumor regression, tumor regression does not occur in those patients who do not experience prolactin suppression.

The time-course of tumor size reduction is variable (144); in some patients, it may occur in a few days; in most, however, it may take up to 6 mo. In few patients, maximum size reduction may take one to a few years.

Improvement in mass effects accompanies the tumor regression; recovery in visual functions may appear dramatically and early, whereas recovery of other extrasellar functions and of tumor mass-associated hypopituitarism may take weeks to months.

Effectiveness of bromocriptine occurs initially with relatively high doses. In many patients on chronic therapy, however, it is often possible to maintain drug effectiveness with a substantially lower dose.

Long-term administration of bromocriptine is associated with fibrosis within the tumor (145), This carries two implications: (1) fibrosis may be significant enough potentially to limit tumor resectability and the effectiveness of surgical therapy, should surgery be needed at a later date; whether or not this is borne out in practice is controversial (120,145,146), and (2) tumor fibrosis may lead to permanent tumor mass regression allowing discontinuation of therapy, in some patients, without resumption of the neoplastic activity. Ten to 20% of patients remain normoprolactinemic and do not show tumor regrowth over one to a few years after drug discontinuation (147). A longer period of observation and controlled studies are necessary before a definitive statement can be made regarding possible bromocriptine-induced "cure."

Discontinuation of therapy, however, is followed in most patients by recurrence of hyperprolactinemia and re-expansion of the tumor, usually over a few weeks to a few months, but in some patients, re-expansion occurs more rapidly (147,148). If discontinuation of drug therapy is deemed appropriate, it should be done gradually and cautiously.

Surgery Macroadenomectomy is usually performed via the transphenoidal route; only rarely is the transcranial approach necessary. Tumor excision may be complete, but usually, and because of surgical limitations, the excision is subtotal "tumor debulking" (79,128,129). Surgery is prompt in its effects (79,128).

As mentioned earlier, in most centers, DA-agonist therapy is the primary treatment modality in the management of macroprolactinoma, and surgery is reserved for the drug-intolerant or drug-resistant patients, and when the patient has concerns about the use of long-term drug therapy.

In some circumstances, however, surgery is preferred as the primary therapy (79,128,129). Such preference occurs when the tumor is: (1) largely cystic and medical therapy is less effective, or (2) accompanied by significant intrasphenoidal extension (when medical therapy may be complicated by CSF rhinorrhea as a result of regression of the tumor mass between the CSF pathways and the nasopharynx, the so-called tumor-cork effect." Surgery is indicated for the management of pituitary apoplexy. Surgery may also be preferred for young women with macroprolactinoma seeking fertility in an attempt to minimize the risk of tumor enlargement during a subsequent pregnancy.

Surgical extirpation of the tumor mass leads to rapid improvement in headaches and visual dysfunction (128,129,148). Transient diabetes insipidus is the rule. Normal preoperative anterior pituitary function is usually preserved, and those with preoperative hypopituitarism do not show recovery (79,128,129,150). In those patients with visual failure preoperatively, visual function is improved in 1/3 of patient, stabilized in another 1/3, and worsened in 1/3 of patients (149). Worsening of visual functions (151) may occur as a result of inadvertent trauma to the optic chiasm or impairment of its blood supply, and occurrence of postoperative herniation of the chiasm into the sella. The mortality rate in macroprolactinoma treated by an expert neurosurgical team is <1%; the morbidity is <4% (5,79,127–129).

Restoration of normoprolactinemia is seen in <20–30% of patients (5 for review). Persistent disease is a persistence of macroscopic tumor remnant, in addition to the persistence of the hyperprolactinemic state. The options of management of the persistent disease include DA agonist therapy or radiation. DA agonist therapy can be used as sole therapy or as an interim therapy while awaiting the full effects of radiation.

Postoperative follow-up consists of (1) endocrine assessment of the serum prolactin levels and the anterior/posterior pituitary function, and (2) MRI assessment of the tumor mass. Serum prolactin is checked every 6–12 mo and an MRI is repeated at 6-mo intervals in the first year and then annually thereafter.

PREGNANCY AND PROLACTINOMAS

Prolactinomas pose three major challenges to normal reproductive functions:

1. Infertility: The vast majority of patients who harbor prolactinomas and are in their reproductive years are infertile. Infertility is related to: (a) functional anovulation caused by the inhibitory effects of hyperprolactinemia; this can be seen in patients with prolactinomas of any size; in this circumstance, the normalization of prolactin by medical or ablative means leads to restoration of ovulatory function and the potential for fertility (152,153), and (2) hypogonadotropism, in the context of hypopituitarism, owing to loss of the gonadotroph cell population. This may occur in patients with extensive macroprolactinomas or in those who have had previous surgical or radiotherapeutic tumor ablation. In such patients, normalization of prolactin secretion with the use of DA agonist therapy will not restore ovulatory function, and ovulation can only be induced by the provision of exogenous gonadotropin therapy.

2. The risk of tumor enlargement during pregnancy (152,154, 155): The rising estrogen levels and the hormonal milieu of pregnancy have a marked stimulatory effect on the normal lactotrophs resulting in hypertrophy, hyperplasia, and increased prolactin synthesis and secretion; the normal pituitary shows a 1- to 1.5-fold increase in size during normal pregnancy (2). Neoplastic lactotrophs also have estrogen receptors (155); they respond to estrogen also with hypertrophy and hyperplasia, which may result in tumor enlargement; the enlargement occurs mostly in the second and third trimesters. In most patients, bromocriptine therapy is used to restore fertility and is stopped at the first sign of pregnancy. In such bromocriptine-induced pregnancies, the risk of tumor enlargement is <5% in microprolactinomas (152,156) and between 15 and 30% in macroprolactinomas (152,154,156). Such tumor enlargement may be asymptomatic; when symptomatic, the usual symptoms are headaches and visual disturbances. The risk

of tumor enlargement in patients with macroprolactinomas is considerably less (<5%) if there was prior tumor ablation with surgery or radiation therapy.

3. The effects on fetal and postnatal development of the treatment modalities used to restore fertility, or to prevent or treat tumor enlargement during pregnancy *(152,155)*. Experience has shown that bromocriptine therapy, when used to normalize prolactin secretion and restore ovulation, and when it is discontinued at the first sign of pregnancy, is not associated with an increased risk of spontaneous abortions, ectopic pregnancies, trophoblastic disease, multiple pregnancies, or congenital malformations *(126,156,157)*. Long-term follow-up of children born from such bromocriptine-induced pregnancies has shown no ill effects. Unfortunately, no such reassuring data are available for the other DA agonists.

   Surgery during pregnancy carries the risk of fetal loss *(158)*. This has been estimated to be increased 1.5-fold in the first trimester and fivefold in the latter part of pregnancy. Surgery does not increase the risk of congenital malformations.

PREGNANCY IN THE PATIENT WITH A MICROPRO-LACTINOMA In the patient with a microprolactinoma, the infertility is usually owing to the suppressive effects of hyperprolactinemia on the gonadotropin axis *(152)*. Fertility can be restored by the normalization or near-normalization of prolactin secretion with either bromocriptine *(152,153)* or transphenoidal surgery *(159,160)*.

Bromocriptine is used as primary therapy in most centers. It is highly effective in normalization of prolactin secretion and in restoration of ovulatory function *(see above)*. Extensive experience, as mentioned earlier, has demonstrated its safety. The standard mode of therapy is to ask the patient to use barrier contraceptives until regular menstrual function is established for two to three cycles. The patient is then allowed to discontinue the contraceptive and pursue unprotected intercourse. As soon as a period is missed, the drug is stopped and a pregnancy test is done. Used in this standard fashion, the risk of enlargement of the microprolactinoma during pregnancy is 1–5%.

Transphenoidal surgery can be used as primary therapy, or in those patients who prove intolerant of or resistant to bromocriptine. Surgery has two goals: to normalize prolactin levels and restore fertility potential, and to reduce the risk of tumor enlargement during pregnancy. Transphenoidal surgery is safe when it is performed by an experienced neurosurgical team. It is rapidly effective in restoring normoprolactinemia in about 70% of patients. If hyperprolactinemia persists in the postoperative state, bromocriptine therapy can be used to normalize serum prolactin levels. Transphenoidal surgery is effective in removing the risk of tumor enlargement during pregnancy, but that risk is low to start with. The disadvantages of transphenoidal surgery have been alluded to earlier and include:

1. Morbidity and mortality: these are very low in experienced hands, but still present.
2. Greater than 30% of patients have persistent hyperprolactinemia postoperatively and will need bromocriptine therapy to normalize prolactin.
3. Development of hypopituitarism and loss of gonadotropin function if the surgery is done by inexperienced hands; this

will necessitate gonadotropin therapy for the induction of ovulation.

Radiation therapy, because of the limitations mentioned earlier, is not considered a practical and safe therapy for the management of microprolactinomas in preparation for fertility objectives.

Follow-up during and after pregnancy consists of:

1. Periodic follow-up of serum prolactin levels, and periodic visual field testing during pregnancy, in a patient with microprolactinoma, are not recommended. An increase in serum prolactin levels does not mean tumor growth, and stability of serum prolactin levels does not mean that tumor size is stable *(161)*. After stopping bromocriptine therapy at the first diagnosis of pregnancy, serum prolactin levels rise over 6–10 wk, and then stabilize and do not rise further. Because of low risk of tumor enlargement, periodic visual field testing is not cost-effective.
2. The patient is instructed in potential symptoms of tumor enlargement. If the patient becomes symptomatic, perimetry and MRI is done.
3. In the early postpartum period, an MRI scan is done to detect any asymptomatic tumor growth that may have occurred during pregnancy.

Pregnancy in the Patient with a Macroprolactinoma
Restoration of Fertility Anovulatory infertility is usually caused by the effects of hyperprolactinemia, but in some patients, the infertility is owing to hypopituitarism induced by the expanding tumor mass. Bromocriptine may be used as primary therapy for the hyperprolactinemic anovulatory state, and this is the therapy of choice in most centers. It is highly effective in normalization of prolactin secretion and in restoration of ovulatory function (60–70%). If used in the standard recommended fashion, and discontinued at the first sign of pregnancy, the risk of tumor expansion during pregnancy is 20–30%.

In the patient with hypopituitarism, gonadotropin therapy is needed to achieve ovulation. Provision of adequate thyroid and glucocorticoid hormonal replacement of thyroid, if needed, is important for fertility.

Therapeutic Options for Reducing the Risk of Tumor Enlargement During Pregnancy Tumor ablation, before pregnancy is attempted, reduces the risk of subsequent tumor expansion during pregnancy to <5%. Ablative treatment can be accomplished by: (1) transphenoidal surgical macroadenomectomy; bromocriptine therapy is added to those who have persistent postoperative hyperprolactinemia; or (2) radiation therapy: bromocriptine can be used as interim therapy until effects of radiation become evident.

Bromocriptine can be used as primary therapy to restore fertility. Its use can then be continued throughout pregnancy to prevent tumor enlargement *(126,161)*. Although this option has been reported to be effective and safe, it is not recommended in the authors' opinion because it has not be tested adequately for safety to the developing fetus and to the children born to these pregnancies.

Follow-up During and After Pregnancy Careful follow-up during pregnancy is important, because the risk of tumor enlargement is significant. Visual field testing is done every month and whenever the patient becomes symptomatic. MRI is done when symptoms develop and/or visual field abnormalities appear. MRI scan is done in early postpartum state to detect any asymptomatic tumor enlargement. In some individuals, tumor size and prolactin levels are reduced postpartum when compared to prepregnancy levels *(163)*.

Options of Management of the Expanding Tumor Mass

1. Early delivery is considered if the tumor enlargement occurs late in the third trimester and the fetus is viable.
2. Transphenoidal macroadenomectomy is promptly effective in reversing the extrasellar effects of the pituitary mass.
3. Reinstitution of bromocriptine therapy is effective in most patients in causing tumor mass regression and resolution of symptoms *(143)*. No ill effects on the fetus or the infant have been observed. The only issue is potential ineffectiveness in some patients. Close follow-up is essential; surgery is recommended if bromocriptine proves ineffective.

REFERENCES

1. Horvath E, Kovacs K. The adenohypophysis. In Kovacs K, Asa SL, eds. Functional Endocrine Pathology. Blackwell Scientific, Boston, 1991, p. 245.
2. Gonzalez JG, Elizondo G, Saldivar D, et al. Pituitary gland growth during normal pregnancy: an in vivo study using magnetic resonance images. Am J Med 1988;85:217–220.
3. Molitch ME, Russell EJ. The pituitary "incidentaloma." Ann Intern Med 1990;112:925–931.
4. Scheithauer BW. Surgical pathology of the pituitary: the adenomas. Pathol Annu 1980;19:317–374.
5. Molitch ME. Prolactinoma. In: Melmed S, ed. The Pituitary. Blackwell Science, Cambridge, MA, 1995, p. 443–477.
6. Selman WR, Laws ER, Scheithauer BW, et al. The occurrence of dural invasion in pituitary adenomas. J Neurosurg 1986;64:402–407.
7. Bills DC, Meyer FB, Laws ER Jr, et al. A retrospective analysis of pituitary apoplexy. Neurosurgery 1993;33:602–608.
8. Guay AT, Freeman R, Rish BL, et al. Calcified pituitary tumor with hyperprolactinemia : selective removal by transphenoidal adenomectomy. Fertil Steril 1978;29:585–588.
9. Mukada K, Ohta M, Uozumi, et al. Ossified prolactinoma: case report. Neurosurgery 1987;20:473–475.
10. Horvath E, Kovacs K, Singer W, et al. Acidophil stem cell adenoma of the human pituitary: clinicopathologic analysis of 15 cases. Cancer 1981;47:761–771.
11. Corenblum B, Sirek AMT, Horvath E, et al. Human mixed somatotrophic and lactotrophic pituitary adenomas. J Clin Endocrinol Metab 1976;42:857–863.
12. Lloyd RV, Gikas PW, Chandler WF. Prolactin and growth hormone-producing adenomas. Am J Surg Pathol 1983;7:251–260.
13. Melmed S, Braunstein GD, Chang RJ, et al. Pituitary tumors secreting growth hormone and prolactin. Ann Int Med 1986;105:238–253.
14. Yamaji T, Ishibashi M, Teramoto A, et al. Hyperprolactinemia in Cushing's disease and Nelson's syndrome. J Clin Endocrinol Metab 1984;58:790–795.
15. Duello TM, Halmi NS. Pituitary adenoma producing thyrotropin and prolactin. Virchows Arch Pathol Anat Histol 1977;376:255–265.
16. Cunningham GR, Huskins C. An FSH and prolactin-secreting pituitary tumor: pituitary dynamics and testicular histology. J Clin Endocrinol Metab 1977;44:248–253.
17. Spertini F, Deruaz JP, Perentes E, et al. Luteinizing hormone (LH) and prolactin-releasing pituitary tumor: possible malignant transformation of the LH cell line. J Clin Endocrinol Metab 1986;62:849–854.
18. Scheithauer BW, Randall RV, Laws ER Jr, et al. Prolactin cell carcinoma of the pituitary. Cancer 1985;55:598–604.
19. Molitch ME. Pathogenesis of pituitary tumors. Endocrinol Metab Clin North Am 1987;16:503–527.
20. Herman V, Fagin J, Gonsky R, et al. Clonal origin of pituitary adenomas. J Clin Endocrinol Metab 1990;71:1427–1433.
21. Jacoby LB Hedley-Whyte ET, Pulaaski K, et al. Clonal origin in pituitary adenomas. J Neurosurg 1990;73:731–735.
22. Pichon MF, Bresson D, Peillon F, et al. Estrogen receptors in human pituitary adenomas. J Clin Endocrinol Metab 1980;51:897–902.
23. Rigg LA, Lein A, Yen SS. Pattern of increase in circulating prolactin levels during human gestation. Am J Obstet Gynecol 1977;129:454–456.
24. Molitch ME. Manifestations, epidemiology and pathogenesis of prolactinomas in women. In: Olefsky JM, Robbins RJ, eds. Prolactinomas. Churchill Livingstone, New York, 1986, p. 78.
25. Wingrave SJ, Kay CR, Vessey MP. Oral contraceptives and pituitary adenomas. Br Med J 1980;1:685–686.
26. Corenblum B, Donovan L. The safety of physiological estrogen plus progestin replacement therapy with oral contraceptive therapy in women with pathological hyperprolactinemia. Fertil Steril 1993;59:671–673.
27. Abboud CF. Hyperprolactinemia and galactorrhoea. In: Samiy AH, Gordon Douglas R Jr, Barondess JA, eds. Textbook of Diagnostic Medicine. Lea & Febiger, Philadelphia, Samiy AH, Gordon Douglas R Jr, Barondess JA (eds). 1987, p. 362–366.
28. Abboud CF, Laws ER Jr. Diagnosis of pituitary tumors. Endocrinol Metab Clin North Am 1988;17:241–280.
29. Jacobs HS, Franks S, Murray MA, et al. Clinical and endocrine features of hyperprolactinemic amenorrhoea. Clin Endocrinol 1976;5:437–454.
30. Molitch ME, Reichlin S. The amenorrhoea, galactorrhoea and hyperprolactinemic syndromes. In: Stollerman GD, ed. Advances in Internal Medicine, vol 26. Year Book Medical, Chicago, 1980, pp. 37–65.
31. Schlecte J, Sherman B, Halmi N, et al. Prolactin-secreting pituitary tumors in amenorrhoeic women; a comprehensive study. Endocrinol Rev 1986;1:295–308.
32. von Werder K, Muller OA, Fink U, Jurgen Graf K. Diagnosis and treatment of hyperprolactinemia. In: Imura H, ed. The Pituitary Gland, Raven, New York, 1994, pp. 453–489.
33. Bergh T, Nilius SJ, Wide L. Hyperprolactinemia in amenorrhoea-incidence and clinical significance. Acta Endocrinol 1977;86:683–694.
34. Franks S Murray MAF, Jequier AM, et al. Incidence and significance of hyperprolactinemia in women with amenorrhoea. Clin Endocrinol 1975;4:597–607.
35. Klibanski A, Neer RM, Beitins IZ, et al. Decreased bone density in hyperprolactinemic women. N Engl J Med 1980;303:1511–1514.
36. Greenspan SL, et al. Osteoporosis in men with hyperprolactinemic hypogonadism. Ann Int Med 1986;104:777–782.
37. Klibanski A, Biller BMK, Rosenthal DI, et al. Effects of prolactin and estrogen deficiency in amenorrhoeic bone loss. J Clin Endocrinol Metab 1988;67:124–130.
38. Schlechte J, Walkner L, Kathol M. A longitudinal analysis of premenopausal bone loss in healthy women and women with hyperprolactinemia. J Clin Endocrinol Metab 1992;75:698–703.
39. Biller BM, Baum HB, Rosenthal DI, et al. Progressive trabecular osteopenia in women with hyperprolactinemic amenorrhoea. J Clin Endocrinol Metab 1992;75:692–697.
40. Klibanski A, Greenspan SL. Increased bone mass in treated hyperprolactinemic amenorrhoeic women. NEJM 1986;315:542–546.
41. Glickman SP, Rosenfeld RL, Bergenstal RM, et al. Multiple androgenic abnormalities, including elevated free testosterone, in hyperprolactinemic women. J Clin Endocrinol Metab 1982;55:251–257.
42. Corenblum B, Taylor PJ. The hyperprolactinemic polycystic ovarian syndrome may not be a distinct entity. Fertil Steril 1982;38:549–552.
43. Futterweit W, Krieger DT. Pituitary tumors associated with hyperprolactinemia and polycystic ovarian disease. Fertil Steril 1979;31:608–613.
44. Berezin M, Shimon I, Hadani M. Prolactinoma in 53 men: clinical characteristics and modes of treatment (male prolactinoma). J Endocrinol Invest 1995;18:436–441.
45. Carter JN, Tyson JE, Tolis G, et al. Prolactin-secreting tumors and hypogonadism in 22 men. N Engl J Med 1978;299:847–852.

46. Grisoli F, Vincentelli F, Jacquet P, et al. Prolactin-secreting adenoma in 22 men. Surg Neurol 1980;13:241–247.

47. Mindermann T, Wilson CB. Pituitary adenomas in childhood and adolescence [Review]. J Pediatr Endocrinol Metab 1995;8:79–83.

48. Partington M, Davis D, Laws E, et al. Pituitary adenomas in childhood and adolescence. J Neurosurg 1994;80:209–216.

49. Burgess JR, Shepherd JJ, Parameswaran V, et al. Spectrum of pituitary disease in multiple endocrine neoplasia type 1 (MEN I): clinical, biochemical and radiologic features of pituitary disease in a large MEN I kindred. J Clin Endocrin Metab 1996;81:2642–2646.

50. Scheithauer BW, Laws ER Jr, Kovacs K, et al. Pituitary adenomas of the multiple endocrine neoplasia type I syndrome. Semin Diagn Pathol 1987;4:205–211.

51. Abboud CF. Anterior pituitary failure. In: Melmed S, ed. The Pituitary. Blackwell Science, Cambridge, MA, 1995, p. 341.

52. Thomas JE, Yoss RE. The parasellar syndrome: problems in determining etiology. Mayo Clin Proc 1970;45:617–623.

53. Molitch ME. Evaluation and treatment of the patient with a pituitary incidentaloma. J Clin Endocrinol Metab 1995;80:3–6.

54. Molitch ME. Prolactin. In Melmed S (ed). The Pituitary. Blackwell Science, Cambridge, MA, 1995, pp. 136–186.

55. Franks S, Jacobs HS, Nabarro JDN. Prolactin concentrations in patients with acromegaly-clinical significance and response to surgery. Clin Endocrinol 1976;5:63–69.

56. Bevan JS, Burke CW, Esiri MM, et al. Misinterpretation of prolactin levels leading to management errors in patients with sellar enlargement. Am J Med 1987;82:29–32.

57. Gharib H, Frey HM, Laws ER Jr, et al. 1983. Coexistent primary empty sella syndrome and hyperprolactinemia. Arch Intern Med 1983, p. 143.

58. Josse R. Autoimmune hypophysitis. In: Volpe R ed. Autoimmune Diseases of the Endocrine System. CRC, Boca Raton, FL, 1990, p. 331.

59. Freda PU, Wardlaw SL, Post KD, et al. Incidence and significance of hyperprolactinemia in women with amenorrhea. Clin Endocrinol 1975;4:597–607.

60. Kapcala LP, Molitsch ME, Post KD, et al. Galactorrhoea, oligo/amenorrhoea, and hyperprolactinemia in patients with craniopharyngioma. J Clin Endocrinol Metab 1980;51:798–800.

61. Munt PW, Marshall RN, Underwood LE. Hyperprolactinemia in sarcoidosis. Incidence and utility in predicting hypothalamic involvement. Ann Rev Respir Dis 1975;112:269–272.

62. Tabarin A, Corcuff JB, Dautheribes M, et al. Histiocytosis X of the hypothalamus. J Endocrinol Invest 1991;14:139–145.

63. Tang LCH, Ma H. Hyperprolactinemic amenorrhoea after external irradiation for nasopharyngeal carcinoma. Fertil Steril 1983; 40:118–119.

64. Carson HE. Drugs and pituitary function. In: Melmed S, ed. The Pituitary. Blackwell Science, Boston, 1995, pp. 645–660.

65. Edwards CRW, Forsyth IA, Besser GM. Amenorrhoea, galactorrhoea and primary hypothyroidism with high circulating levels of prolactin. Br Med J 1971;3:462–464.

66. Honbo KS, Herle AJV, Kellett KA. Serum prolactin levels in untreated primary hypothyroidism. Am J Med 1978;64:782–787.

67. Smallridge RC. Thyrotropin-secreting pituitary tumors. Endocrinol Metab Clin North Am 1987;16:765–792.

68. Morley JE, Dawson M., Hodgkinson H, et al. Galactorrhoea and hyperprolactinemia associated with chest wall injury. J Clin Endocrinol Metab 1977;45:931–935.

69. Herman VS, Kalk WJ. Neurogenic prolactin release: effects of mastectomy and thoracotomy. Prog Reprod Biol 1980;6:83.

70. Borzio M, Caldara R, Ferrari C. Growth hormone and prolactin secretion in liver cirrhosis; evidence for dopaminergic dysfunction. Acta Endocrinol 1981;97:441–447.

71. Cowden EA, et al. Hyperprolactinemia in renal disease Clin Endocrinol 1978;9:241–248.

72. Hou SH, Grossman S, Molitch ME. Hyperprolactinemia in patients with renal insufficiency and chronic renal failure requiring hemodialysis or chronic ambulatory peritoneal dialysis. Am J Kidney Dis 1985;6:245–249.

73. Lim VS, Kathpalia S, Frohman LA. Hyperprolactinemia and impaired pituitary responses to suppression and stimulation in chronic renal failure. Reversal following transplantation. J Clin Endocrinol Metab 1979;48:101–107.

74. Morgan MY, Jacobovitz AW, Gore MB, et al. Serum prolactin in liver disease and its relationship to gynecomastia. Gut 1978;19: 170–174.

75. Stanisic TH, Donova J. Prolactin secreting renal cell carcinoma. J Urol 1986;136:85–86.

76. Hoffman WH, Gala RR, Kovacs K, et al. Ectopic prolactin secretion from a gonadoblastoma. Cancer 1987;60:2690–2695.

77. Kallenberg GA, Pesce CM, Norman B, et al. Ectopic hyperprolactinemia resulting from an ovarian teratoma. JAMA 1990;263: 2472–2474.

78. Nabarro JD. Pituitary prolactinomas. Clin Endocrinol 1982;17: 129–155.

79. Randall RV, Laws ER Jr, Abboud CF, et al. Transphenoidal microsurgical treatment of prolactin-producing pituitary adenomas. Mayo Clin Proc 1983;58:108–121.

80. Klijn JGM, Lamberts SWJ, DeJong FH, et al. The importance of pituitary tumor size in patients with hyperprolactinemia in relation to hormonal variables and extrasellar extension of tumor. Clin Endocrinol 1980;12:341–355.

81. Molitch ME, Reichlin S. Neuroendocrine studies of prolactin secretion in hyperprolactinemic states. In: Mena F, Valverde-Rodriguez C, eds. Prolactin Secretion: A Multidisciplinary Approach. Academic, New York, 1984, p. 393.

82. Oehler M, Chakeres D. Diagnostic imaging of the sellar region. In: Becker KL, ed. Principles and Practice of Endocrinology and Metabolism. 2nd ed. Lippincott JB, Philadelphia, 1995, pp. 207–223.

83. Martin TL, Kim M, Malarkey WB. The natural history of idiopathic hyperprolactinemia. J Clin Endocrinol Metab 1985;60:855–858.

84. March DM, Kletzky OA, Davajan V, et al. Longitudinal evaluation of patients with untreated prolactin-secreting pituitary adenomas. Am J Obstet Gynecol 1981;139:835–844.

85. Schlecte J, Dolan K, Sherman B, et al. The natural history of untreated hyperprolactinemia: A prospective analysis. J Clin Endocrinol Metab 1989;68:412–418.

86. Sisam DA, Sheehan JP, Sheeler LR. The natural history of untreated microprolactinoma. Fertil Steril 1987;48:67–71.

87. Weiss MH, Teal J, Gott P, et al. Natural history of microprolactinomas: six-year follow-up. Neurosurgery 1983;12:180–183.

88. Jacquet P. Medical therapy of prolactinomas. Acta Endocrinol 1993;129(S1):31–33.

89. Sibley DR, Creese I. Interactions of ergot alkaloids with anterior pituitary D-2 dopamine receptors. Mol Pharmacol 1983;23: 585–593.

90. Thorner MO, Fluckiger E, Calne DB. Bromocriptine: A Clinical and Pharmacological Review. Raven, New York, 1980.

91. Vance ML, Evans WS, Thorner MO. Bromocriptine. Ann Intern Med 1984;100:78–91.

92. Bouloux PMJ, Besser GM, Grossman A. Clinical evaluation of lysuride in the management of hyperprolactinemia. Br Med J 1987;294:1323–1324.

93. Chidini P, Liuzzi A, Cozzi R, et al. Size reduction of macroprolactinoma by bromocriptine or lisuride treatment. J Clin Endocrinol Metab 1981;53:737–743.

94. Ciccarelli E, Camanni F. Diagnosis and drug therapy of prolactinoma. Drugs 1996;51(6):954–965.

95. Schran HR, Bhuta SI, Schwarz HJ, et al. The pharmacokinetics of bromocriptine in man. In: Goldstein M, Calne D, Lieberman A, Thorner M, eds. Ergot Compounds and Brain Function: Neuroendocrine and Neuropsychiatric Aspects. Raven, New York, 1980, pp. 125–139.

96. Tindall GT, Kovacs L, Horvath E, et al. Human prolactin-producing adenomas and bromocriptine; a histologic, immunocytochemical, ultrastructural and morphometric study. J Clin Endocrinol Metab 1982;55:1178–1183.

97. Bevan JS, Webster J, Burke CW, et al. Dopamine agonists and pituitary tumor shrinkage. Endocr Rev 1992;13:220–240.

98. Bonneville JF, Poulignot D, Cattin F et al. Computed tomographic demonstration of the effects of bromocriptine on pituitary microadenoma size. Radiology 1982;143:451–455.

99. Pelligrini I, Rasolonjanahary R, Gunz G, et al. Resistance to bromocriptine in prolactinomas. J Clin Endocrinol Metab 1989; 69:500–509.

100. McGregor AM, et al. Effects of bromocriptine on pituitary tumor size. Br Med J 1979;2:700–703.

101. Corenblum B, Taylor PJ. Long term follow-up of hyperprolactinemic women treated with bromocriptine. Fertil Steril 1983;40:596–599.

102. Johnston DG, Prescott RWG, Kendall-Taylor P, et al. Hyperprolactinemia: long term effects of bromocriptine. Am J Med 1983;75:868–874.

103. McElvaney NG, Wilcox PG, Churg A, et al. Pleuropulmonary disease during bromocriptine treatment of Parkinson's disease. Arch Intern Med 1988;148:2231–2236.

104. Bowler JV, Ormerod IE, Legg NJ. Retroperitoneal fibrosis and bromocriptine. Lancet 1986, ii:466.

105. Davis JRE, Sheppard MC, Heath D A. Giant invasive prolactinoma. Q J Med 1990;74:227–238.

106. Kok JG, Bartelink AKM, Schulte BPM, et al. Cerebrospinal fluid rhinorrhoea during treatment with bromocriptine for prolactinoma. Neurology 1985;35:1193–1195.

107. Boulanger CM, Mashechak CA, Chang RJ. Lack of tumor reduction in hyperprolactinemic women with extrasellar macroadenomas treated with bromocriptine. Fertil Steril 1985;44:532–535.

108. Dallabonzana D, Spella B, Oppizzi G, et al. Reenlargement of macroprolactinomas during bromocriptine treatment: report of two cases. J Endocrinol Invest 1983;6:47–50.

109. Katz E, Schran HF, Adashi EY. Successful treatment of a prolactin-producing pituitary macroadenoma with intravaginal bromocriptine mesylate: a novel approach to intolerance of oral therapy Obstet Gynecol 1989;73:517–520.

110. Espinos JJ, Rodriquez-Espinosa J, Webb SM, et al. Long-acting repeatable bromocriptine in the treatment of patients with microprolactinoma intolerant or resistant to oral dopaminergics. Fertil Steril 1994;62:926–931.

111. Haase R, Jaspers C, Schulte HM, et al. Control of prolactin-secreting macroadenomas with parenteral, longacting bromocriptine in 30 patients treated for up to 3 years. Clin Endocrinol 1993;38:165–176.

112. Colao A, Merola B, Sarnacchiaro F, et al. Comparison among different dopamine-agonists of new formulation in the clinical management of macroprolactinomas. Horm Res 1995;44:222–228.

113. Ferrari C, Parrachi A, Mattei AM, et al. Cabergoline in the long-term therapy of hyperprolactinemic disorders. Acta Endocrinol 1992;126:489–494.

114. Webster J, Piscetelli G, Polli A, et al. Dose-dependent suppression of serum prolactin by cabergoline in hyperprolactinemia: a placebo-controlled, double-blind, multicenter study. Clin Endocrinol 1992;37:534–541.

115. Webster J, Piscitelli G, Polli A, et al. A comparison of cabergoline and bromocriptine in the treatment of hyperprolactinemic amenorrhoea. N Engl J Med 1994;331:904–909.

116. Ciccarelli E, Giusti M, Miola C, et al. Effectiveness and tolerability of long term treatment with cabergoline: a new long-lasting ergoline derivative, in hyperprolactinemic women. J Clin Endocrinol Metab 1989;69:725–728.

117. Brue T. Pelligrini Lancet. Gunz G, et al. Effects of the dopamine agonist CV205-502 in human prolactinomas resistant to bromocriptine. J Clin Endocrinol Metab 1992;74:577–584.

118. Serri O, Beauregard H, Lesage J, et al. Long-term treatment with CV 205-502 in patients with prolactin- secreting pituitary macroadenomas. J Clin Endocrinol Metab 1990;71:682–687.

119. Vance ML, Lipper M, Klibanski A, et al. Treatment of prolactin-secreting pituitary macroadenomas with the long-acting non-ergot dopamine agonist CV205-502. Ann Int Med 1990;112:668–673.

120. Van-der-Lely AJ, Brownell J, Lamberts SW. The efficacy and tolerability of CV205-502 (a nonergot dopaminergic drug) in macroprolactinoma patients and in prolactinoma patients intolerant of bromocriptine. J Clin Endocrinol Metab 1991;72:1136–1141.

121. Klezky OA, Borenstein R, Mileilkowsky GN. Pergolide and bromocriptine for the treatment of patients with hyperprolactinemia. Am J Obstet Gynecol 1986;15:431–435.

122. Lambert SWJ, Quick RFP. A comparison of the efficacy and safety of pergolide and bromocriptine in the treatment of hyperprolactinemia. J Clin Endocrinol Metab 1991;72:635–641.

123. Radwanska E, McGarrigle HHG, Little V, et al. Induction of ovulation in women with hyperprolactinemic amenorrhoea using clomiphene and human chorionic gonadotropin or bromocriptine. Fertil Steril 1979;32:187–192.

124. Bergh T, Skarin G, Nilius SJ, et al. Pulsatile GnRH therapy—an alternative successful therapy for induction of ovulation in infertile normo- and hyperprolactinemic amenorrhoeic women with pituitary tumors. Acta Endocrinol 1985;110:440–444.

125. Polson DW, Sagle M, Mason HD, et al. Ovulation and normal luteal function during LHRH treatment of women with hyperprolactinemic amenorrhoea. Clin Endocrinol 1986;24:531–537.

126. Krupp P, Monka C, Richter K. The safety aspects of infertility treatments. Program of the Second World Congress of Gynecology and Obstetrics, Rio de Janeiro, October 1988:9.

127. Feigenbaum SL, Downey DE, Wilson CB, et al. Transphenoidal pituitary resection for preoperative diagnosis of a prolactin-secreting pituitary adenoma in women: long term follow-up. J Clin Endocrinol Metab 1996;81:1171–1179.

128. Laws ER Jr. Pituitary surgery. Endocrinol Metab Clin North Am 1987;16:647–665.

129. Laws ER Jr, Ebersold MJ, Piepgras DG, et al. The role of surgery in the management of prolactinoma. In: Macleod RM, Thorner MO, Scapagnini U, eds. Prolactin, Basic and Clinical Correlates. Springer-Verlag, New York, 1985, p. 849.

130. Schlecte JA, Sherman BM, Chapler FK, et al. Long-term follow-up of women with surgically-treated prolactin-secreting tumors. J Clin Endocrinol Metab 1986;62:1296–1301.

131. Soule SG, Farhi J, Conway GS, et al. The outcome of hypophysectomy for prolactinomas in the era of dopamine agonist therapy. Clin Endocrinol 1996;44:711–716.

132. Thomson JA, Davies DL, McLaren EH, et al. Ten year follow-up of microprolactinoma treated by transphenoidal surgery. Br Med J 1994;309:1409–1416.

133. Grossman A, Cohen BL, Charlesworth M, et al. Treatment of prolactinomas with megavoltage radiotherapy. Br Med J 1984;288:1105–1109.

134. Johnston D, Hall K, Kendall-Taylor P, et al. The long-term effects of megavoltage radiotherapy as a sole or combined therapy for large prolactinomas: studies with high-definition computerized tomography. Clin Endocrinol 1986;24:675–685.

135. Tran LM, Blount L, Horton D, et al. Radiation therapy of pituitary tumors: results in 95 cases. Am J Clin Oncol 1991;14:25–29.

136. Zierhut D, Flentje M, Adolph J, et al. External radiotherapy for pituitary adenomas. Int J Radiat Oncol Biol Phys 1995;33:307–314.

137. Mehta MP, Rozental JM. Radiotherapy of pituitary–hypothalamic tumors. In: Becker KL, ed. Principles and Practice of Endocrinology and Metabolism, 2nd ed. Lippincott JB, Philadelphia, 1995, pp. 229–238.

138. Demura R, Kubo O, Demura H, et al. Changes in computed tomographic findings in microprolactinomas before and after bromocriptine. Acta Endocrinol 1985;110:308–312.

139. Serri O, Rasio E, Beauregard H, et al. Recurrence of hyperprolactinemia after selective transphenoidal adenomectomy in women with prolactinoma. N Engl J Med 1983;309:280–283.

140. Pelkonen R, Grahne B, Hirvonen E, et al. Pituitary function in prolactinoma. Effect of surgery and postoperative bromocriptine therapy Clin Endocrinol 1981;14:335–348.

141. Molitch ME, Elton RL, Blackwell RE, et al. Bromocriptine as primary therapy for prolactin-secreting macroadenomas: Result of a prospective multicenter study. J Clin Endocrinol Metab 1985;60:698–705.

142. Wass JAH, et al. Bromocriptine in the management of large pituitary tumors. Br Med J 1982;284:1908–1911.

143. Crosignani PG, Ferrari C, Mattei AM. Visual field defects and reduced visual acuity during pregnancy in two patients with prolactinoma: rapid regression of symptoms under bromocriptine; Case reports. Br J Obstet Gynecol 1984;91:821–823.

144. Nissim M, Ambrosi B, Bernasconi V, et al. Bromocriptine treatment of macroprolactinomas: studies on the time course of tumor shrinkage and morphology. J Endocrinol 1982;5:409–415.

145. Landolt AM, Osterwalder V. Perivascular fibrosis in prolactinomas: is it increased by bromocriptine? J Clin Endocrinol Metab 1984; 58:1179–1183.

146. Bevan JS, Adams CBT, Burke CW, et al. Factors in the outcome of transphenoidal surgery for prolactinoma and non-functioning pituitary tumor, including pre-operative bromocriptine therapy. Clin Endocrinol 1987;26:541–556.

147. Wang C, Lam KSL, Ma JTC, et al. Long-term treatment of hyperprolactinemia with bromocriptine: effect of drug withdrawal. Clin Endocrinol 1987;27:363–371.

148. Thorner MO, Perryman RL, Rogol AD, et al. Rapid changes of prolactinoma volume after withdrawal and reinstitution of bromocriptine. J Clin Endocrinol Metab 1981;53:480–483.

149. Trautman JC, Laws ER. Visual status after transphenoidal surgery at the Mayo Clinic. Am J Ophthalmol 1983;96:200–208.

150. Nelson AT Jr, Tucker HSG Jr, Becker DP. Residual anterior pituitary function following transphenoidal resection of pituitary macroadenomas. J Neurosurg 1984;61:557–580.

151. Barrow DL, Tindall GT. Loss of vision after transphenoidal surgery Neurosurgery 1990;27:60–68.

152. Molitch ME. Pregnancy and the hyperprolactinemic women. N Engl J Med 1985;312:1364–1370.

153. Ruiz-Velasco V, Tolis G. Pregnancy in hyperprolactinemic women. Fertil Steril 1984;41:793–805.

154. Gemzell C, Wang CF. Outcome of pregnancy in women with pituitary adenoma. Fertil Steril 1979;31:363–372.

155. Pragor D, Braunstein GD. Pituitary disorders during pregnancy. Endocrinol Metab Clin North Am 1995;24(1):1–14.

156. Bergh T, Nilius SJ, Wide L. Clinical course and outcome of pregnancies in amenorrhoeic women with hyperprolactinemia and pituitary tumors. Br Med J 1978;1:875–880.

157. Turkalj I, Braum P, Krupp P. Surveillance of bromocriptine in pregnancy. JAMA 1982;247:1589–1591.

158. Brodsky JB, Cohen EN, Brown BW, et al. Surgery during pregnancy and fetal outcome. Am J Obstet Gynecol 1980;138:1165–1167.

159. Laws ER Jr, Fode NC, Randall RV, et al. Pregnancy following transphenoidal resection of prolactin-secreting pituitary tumors. J Neurosurg 1983;58:685–688.

160. Samaan NA, Schultz PN, Leavens TA, et al. Pregnancy after treatment in patients with prolactinoma: operation vs bromocriptine. Am J Obstet Gynecol 1986;155:1300–1305.

161. Yen SSC, Divers WA Jr. Prolactin-producing microadenomas in pregnancy. Obstet Gynecol 1983;61:425–429.

162. Konopka P, et al. Continuous administration of bromocriptine in the prevention of neurological complications in pregnant women with prolactinomas. Am J Obstet Gynecol 1983;146:935–938.

163. Crosignani PG, Mattei AM, Scarduelli C, et al. Is pregnancy the best treatment for hyperprolactinemia. Hum Reprod 1989;4:910–912.

17 Somatotroph Adenomas
Acromegaly and Gigantism

HANS-JÜRGEN QUABBE, MD AND URSULA PLÖCKINGER, MD

INTRODUCTION

The prevalence of acromegaly is approx 40–70 patients/1 million, and the incidence 3–4/yr/million (1–4). In most patients, the disease probably begins early in life, but the diagnosis is often made belatedly in the fourth, fifth, or even sixth decade. In our series of 114 patients, the diagnosis was made before the age of 20 yr in 2–3%—in patients with pituitary gigantism—and after the age of 70 yr in 3–4% of the patients. The sex ratio (female-to-male) is close to 1, with possibly a slight preponderance of females, and ranges from 0.7 to 1.8 in different series (5). Untreated or insufficiently treated acromegaly not only increases morbidity, but also shortens life expectancy (4–8).

The diagnosis of acromegaly is based on the unmistakable clinical picture and the demonstration of nonsuppressibility of growth hormone (GH) secretion by glucose. Usually a space-occupying lesion can also be identified in the sella turcica.

Advances in microsurgical techniques, irradiation procedures, and medical treatment have greatly improved the outlook for patients with acromegaly. Unfortunately, however, in many cases, the disease still cannot be cured or must be treated at the expense of considerable side effects.

PHYSIOLOGY OF GH SECRETION

REGULATION OF SECRETION GH release from the pituitary gland is regulated by the interaction of the hypothalamic hormones, GH release-inhibiting hormone (somatostatin), and GH-releasing hormone (GHRH). The release is pulsatile, and thus, the GH concentration in the blood is characterized by a succession of peaks and troughs throughout the 24-h day (9,10). The hypothalamic release mechanism in turn is subject to influences from higher brain centers—notably the limbic system and the sleep–wake-regulating mechanisms. Slow-wave sleep (SWS) and daytime napping stimulate, but rapid-eye-movement sleep (REM) and daytime activity stages inhibit GH secretion (9,10). The physiological significance of this link to the sleep–wake cycle is still not clear. Together with the pituitary hormones ACTH and prolactin (PRL), GH increases in response to stress. The 191 amino acid, single-chain GH molecule circulates in the blood bound to a carrier protein (GH binding protein [GHBP]), which—in humans—consists of the extracellular part of the GH receptor (11).

It follows from the pulsatile pattern of GH secretion that a "normal" fasting concentration cannot be defined. Normal values can only be given for the range of nadir and peak concentrations. Ultrasensitive assays place the nadir GH concentration at approx 0.02 µg/L (12). Peak concentrations—which are approx 30 µg/L in young women, but may sometimes be much higher—decrease with advancing age, are lower in obesity, and increase during prolonged fasting. Nadir concentrations as well as the pattern of episodic secretion are also influenced by age, gender, and obesity (13–16).

FEEDBACK MECHANISMS, METABOLIC MODULATION, AND METABOLIC ACTION Feedback mechanisms arise from peripheral GH and the GH-dependent insulin-like growth factor-1 (IGF-1). Other hormones (e.g., gonadal and thyroid hormones) and metabolic influences further modulate the secretion of GH (17–19). Metabolic factors acutely modify GH secretion, and nutritional factors have long-term influences. Hyperglycemia and elevation of free fatty acids (FFA) both suppress GH release, whereas hypoglycemia and lack of FFA as well as protein/amino acids stimulate GH secretion (17). After a meal, GH and insulin undergo opposite changes: In the early postprandial period, insulin increases and promotes glucose uptake into muscle and inhibits lipolysis, whereas the GH concentration is low. In the late postprandial period, insulin secretion is low and GH increases. GH then mobilizes FFA from the adipose tissue and inhibits glucose uptake. The cooperative action of both hormones favors protein synthesis (20).

GH RECEPTOR GH binds to a specific cell membrane receptor, a member of the cytokine/hematopoietin superfamily of receptors. The GH molecule has two binding sites, each of which reacts—in series—with one receptor molecule, thus inducing receptor dimerization (21). At very high concentrations, the GH excess may prevent dimerization. When the site-1 binding sites of GH have occupied all receptor molecules, no spare receptors for binding with site-2 of the GH molecules would be left over. Thus, no receptor activation would occur. Whether this has clinical implications in acromegaly is unknown. However, the mechanism provided for the development of a GH antagonist that may be useful for the treatment of acromegaly. The antagonist binds to the receptor, but blocks receptor dimerization (22,22a,22b).

From: *Diagnosis and Management of Pituitary Tumors* (K. Thapar, K. Kovacs, B. W. Scheithauer, and R. V. Lloyd, eds.), ©Humana Press Inc., Totowa, NJ.

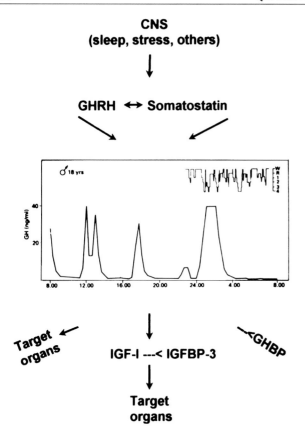

Figure 17-1 Physiology of GH secretion. Hypothalamo→pituitary→end-organ axis. The basic 24-h profile (inset) is mainly determined by the GHRH-somatostatin interplay and the influence of the sleep–wake cycle/sleep-stage pattern. Metabolic influences and feedback routes are not shown. —< indicates binding. For details, *see text*.

INSULIN-LIKE GROWTH FACTOR-1 (IGF-1) AND INSULIN-LIKE GROWTH FACTOR-1 BINDING PROTEIN (IGF-BP)

In many tissues, including the liver and the growth plate of the longitudinal bones, but also, e.g., in the ovary, GH induces the synthesis of IGF-1 *(19)*. IGF-1 is responsible for many—though not all—effects of GH and is also part of the feedback loop, which regulates GH secretion from the pituitary gland *(23–25)*. Circulating IGF-1 is mainly produced in the liver. Locally produced IGF-1 in other tissues probably acts as a paracrine or autocrine factor *(25)*. The molecule has a high degree of homology with the proinsulin/insulin molecule. The circulating IGF-1 concentration is influenced by the nutritional status. Diabetes mellitus and malnutrition cause low IGF-1 concentrations *(26,27)*. Although tissue-specific IGF-1 production is influenced by circulating GH, other factors are also important, but are as yet poorly defined.

Less than 10% of the circulating IGF-1 is in the free form, but most of it is bound to a carrier protein, IGF-1 binding protein 3 (IGF-BP3), a member of the group of six different IGF binding proteins *(28)*. IGF-BP3 is considered to serve as a reservoir for IGF-1, prolonging its half-life in the blood and influencing its availability to the tissues. The concentration of IGF-BP3 is in turn influenced by GH. The physiological importance of the other IGF binding proteins is not very well understood. All may be involved in modulation of the GH–IGF-BP3 axis systemically or in an organ-specific manner *(29)*. *See* Figure 1 for a schematic outline of the hypothalamo–pituitary–target organ axis.

ACROMEGALY—CLINICAL ASPECTS

PHYSIOGNOMY The symptoms of acromegaly develop insidiously, and early changes are suspicious only to the experienced endocrinologist. The mean delay between the onset of symptoms and the final diagnosis is estimated to be approx 7–9 yr *(1,7,30)*. However, a patient with full-blown acromegaly cannot be overlooked (Figure 2). There is a typical change in the facial appearance. Growth of the mandible results in an elongation of the face, malocclusion, and tooth gaps in the lower jaw. The large tongue and similar changes in the larynx cause snoring, sleep apnea, and hence, increased daytime sleepiness. The frontal and mastoid sinuses are bulging, the nose is large, and the lips are thick. Hands and feet are large, plump, and pudgy. In some patients, the diagnosis is made in the course of workup for a carpal tunnel syndrome, and in others, because of a visual field defect. A pituitary space-occupying lesion owing to a pituitary adenoma is also increasingly diagnosed in a computer tomography (CT) or in magnetic resonance imaging (MRI) of the head, done for unrelated reasons, e.g., following an accident or for headaches unrelated to the pituitary tumor "pituitary incidentaloma."

The skin of acromegalic patients is thick and coarse, and is wrinkled at the face and the skull. Body hair becomes thick, and patients complain of increased sweating. Small fibromas and skin tags may appear. The changes are owing to a direct action of GH, which promotes connective tissue proliferation and increases fluid capture by hyaluronates. Skin accessory organs, hair follicles, and eccrine sweat glands have specific GH receptors *(31)*.

GH SECRETORY DYNAMICS IN ACROMEGALY Physiological GH secretion is pulsatile. The pulsatility is preserved in many acromegalic patients, but the pattern is different from that in healthy subjects. A refined analysis reveals that there is significantly elevated basal GH secretion—i.e., absence of very low trough values—and that secretion is irregular and "disorderly," with an increased pulse frequency *(32–35)*. The irregularity of the pulsatile pattern persists following surgical "cure," as defined by "normal" basal or mean 24-h GH concentrations. This has been used as an argument for the role of an intrinsic hypothalamic abnormality in acromegaly. However, many such patients probably have persistently detectable GH trough concentrations in a frequent-sampling 24-h profile and are thus not cured in a strict sense *(33)*.

Patients in whom the diagnosis of acromegaly has been made belatedly in older age often have relatively low GH concentrations. They commonly harbor an adenoma with a moderate growth potential. Most GH-secreting adenomas probably develop around the third decade of age. Aggressive adenomas will then cause symptoms after only a short period of time, but slowly growing, low-secreting adenomas cause symptoms insidiously and therefore are diagnosed only in higher age.

BONE AND JOINTS In acromegaly, bone growth is by apposition, i.e., cortical thickening. In addition, there is muscle hypertrophy and soft tissue swelling. Therefore, acromegalic patients appear strong and sturdy at first sight. However, although bone mass is increased, the quality of bone is poor. Urinary collagen crosslinks, markers of bone collagen turnover and serum osteocalcin, a marker of osteoblastic activity, are both elevated. Thus, osteoclastic as well as osteoblastic activity is increased and bone turnover is high. In vitro studies have shown that GH stimulates osteoclast formation and differentiation as well as osteoclast activity *(36)*. Moreover, although cortical bone is thick, trabecular

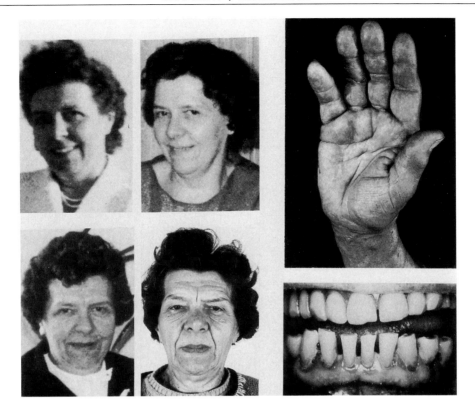

Figure 17-2 Physiognomy of acromegalic patient. Slow development of acromegalic features. Slight signs are already present in the second photograph. The development spans approx 25 yr. Large, pudgy hands and tooth gaps in the lower jaw are also shown.

bone density tends to be lower than normal *(37,38)*. Although the increased cortical bone density is owing to the elevated GH/IGF-1 concentration, the decrease of vertebral bone density is a result of hypogonadism, which often accompanies GH-secreting macroadenomas *(39)*. Intestinal calcium absorption is increased, but urinary calcium excretion exceeds intestinal absorption and the calcium balance is therefore negative *(40)*, which promotes calcium mobilization from bone and osteoporosis. Nevertheless, serum parathyroid hormone and serum calcium concentrations are usually normal *(37)*, but vitamin D concentrations have been variously described as being normal *(37)*, or elevated *(41,42)*. Under the influence of GH and IGF-1, cartilage and osteophytic proliferation is increased, and causes osteoarthrosis and later severe osteoarthritis *(43)*.

CARDIOVASCULAR AND PULMONARY SYSTEMS
Cardiovascular and respiratory disease are causes of increased mortality in acromegaly *(44,45)*. Acromegalic patients have an increased risk of cardiac failure as compared with healthy subjects of the same age *(46)*. The heart is enlarged (cardiomegaly), and left ventricular muscle hypertrophy is frequently found. Diastolic rather than systolic function is impaired in most patients at rest, but systolic function is inadequate during exercise *(46,47)*. Right ventricular function may also be compromised *(48)*. Blood pressure elevation is apparently not an important factor in these changes *(48–51)*, although mild hypertension is often found in acromegaly. Acromegalic patients have an increased plasma volume *(52)*, which is probably owing to the antinatriuretic effect of GH and an activation of the renin-angiotensin-aldosterone system *(53,54)*. The cardiac changes seem to be at least partially reversible *(55,56)*, although there is only a poor correlation with GH or IGF-1 concentrations *(57)*. However, the presence of interstitial fibrosis *(58)*

makes a total restitution questionable even following complete normalization of the GH concentration.

Adults with childhood-onset GH deficiency have diminished lung volume and respiratory muscle strength *(59)*, pointing to an important influence of GH and/or IGF-1 in pulmonary development. However, the effect of GH excess on the lung and pulmonary function have not been well studied. In vitro studies with human lung fibroblasts and with human airway epithelial cells document stimulation of collagen formation and fibroblast proliferation by IGF-1. These cells also produce IGF-1 and probably express the IGF-1 receptor *(60,61)*. It is therefore conceivable that changes of the elastic properties of the lung may occur. Further studies may well reveal hitherto unknown changes of pulmonary function in acromegaly. In long-standing acromegaly kyphoscoliosis and arthropathy of the lumbo-costal joints may diminish thoracic excursions. A large tongue and hypertrophy of lymphoid tissue cause upper airflow obstruction, especially during sleep position with the consequence of snoring and a nocturnal oxygen deficit *(62)*.

GASTROINTESTINAL AND GENITOURINARY SYSTEMS
Visceromegaly is always present in acromegaly. The gut is elongated. Gallbladder emptying is decreased, but the incidence of gallstones apparently is not different from that in the general population *(63)*. The kidneys are large owing to an increase in the size of both the glomerula and the tubules. There is renal hyperfiltration associated with afferent glomerular vasodilatation. Tubular reabsorption of phosphate, calcium excretion and albumin excretion are increased *(64,65)*. These changes are reversible when the GH concentration is normalized. Prostate volume is often increased, but the incidence of prostate cancer is not elevated *(65a)*.

PERIPHERAL AND CENTRAL NERVOUS SYSTEMS, AND NEUROMUSCULAR SYSTEM
Despite their elevated GH

secretion, acromegalic patients can suffer from remarkable muscle weakness owing to neuropathic changes and also to a specific acromegalic myopathy *(66,67)*. The acromegalic myopathy may result from a differential effect of GH on type-1 and type-2 muscle fibers. In a rat model with excessive GH secretion, type-1 fibers were hypertrophic, but type-2 fibers were either unchanged or atrophic *(68)*. When the effect of long-term GH elevation was studied in transgenic mice model with high-GH production, grip strength was found to be inadequate for the increase in muscle mass *(69)*.

In peripheral nerves, the GH excess causes peri- and endoneural thickening with neuronal damage owing to demyelination and hypertrophic formations affecting the Schwann cell system. This causes peripheral neuropathy of motor and sensory nerves with muscular atrophy, distal sensory symptoms, neuropathic joints, and other sequelae of nerve dysfunction. The presence of neuropathy is apparently independent of coexisting diabetes mellitus or hypothyroidism. Once nerve damage has occurred, it is probably not reversible, even following normalization of the GH concentration *(70–72)*. The carpal tunnel syndrome, in contrast, is owing to the mechanical factor of median nerve compression by soft tissue swelling in the carpal tunnel.

Effects of acromegaly on the brain have not been studied. There is some evidence, however, of an effect on sleep regulation. REM and SWS have been found to be reduced, and this was not related to sleep apnea. As a consequence, acromegalic patients have increased daytime sleepiness. The disappearance of these changes following GH normalization suggests a central origin *(73)*. In another study, however, a nocturnal breathing abnormality, periodic breathing, was found several years after treatment (although incomplete in some of the patients) of acromegaly *(74)*. Sleep apnea is frequent in acromegalic patients *(75,75a)*. Often it is of central rather than peripheral origin *(75)*. In contrast to these effects of chronic GH excess on sleep, acute nighttime elevation of GH in healthy subjects does not alter the sleep pattern *(76)*. At the present time, the influence of chronic GH elevation on the brain remains insufficiently known.

Having acromegaly has important psychological consequences *(77)*. The emotional disturbance may be secondary to the somatic disfigurement and to psychosocial problems associated with the disease. Whether they also include a disease-specific *a priori* trait is speculative. It is of interest, however, that the limbic system is an important modulator of GH regulation in experimental animals (including nonhuman primates). GH secretion can be stimulated or inhibited by electrical stimulation of different areas of the limbic system *(78,79,* our own unpublished results in the Rhesus monkey), which, on the other hand, expresses GH receptors *(80)*. The significance of these findings for the acromegalic patient remains to be investigated. The psychological aspects of acromegaly have recently been discussed, and the reader is referred to this review *(77)*.

ENDOCRINE ORGANS   The influence of acromegaly on peripheral endocrine glands is potentially twofold: On the one hand, GH excess causes an enlargement of possibly all glands, probably mediated by elevated IGF-1 concentrations. Goiter is common in acromegaly, but thyroid function is usually normal *(17,30,44,44a)*. The basal metabolic rate may be slightly elevated, but this is a direct effect of the GH excess rather than a symptom of hyperthyroidism. The parathyroid glands are often enlarged, but PTH secretion is normal *(37)*. The pancreatic B-cell mass is

increased. Whether this is owing to an effect of GH/IGF-1 or to the effect of GH-induced peripheral insulin resistance with concomitant hyperinsulinism has not been determined, but probably both mechanisms are involved.

On the other hand, growth of the pituitary tumor to a macroadenoma may cause partial or complete anterior pituitary insufficiency, followed by atrophy of the respective peripheral endocrine glands. The clinical picture of these secondary insufficiencies is similar to that of primary failure of the glands. In accordance with the sequence of pituitary hormone insufficiency, hypogonadism occurs more often than adrenocortical deficiency, and secondary hypothyroidism is rare. Hyperprolactinemia is often seen in acromegaly and may either be owing to PRL secretion by the tumor or to functional stalk section by a macroadenoma. If ovarian function is preserved, pregnancy is possible in women with active acromegaly.

IMMUNE SYSTEM   Changes in immunocompetence are not a clinically obvious feature in acromegaly. However, recent studies suggest a stimulatory role for GH as well as GHRH and IGF-1 in the immune system. All three hormones as well as their respective receptors are produced by immunocompetent cells. GH stimulates proliferation of lymphocytes and their specific functions. GH and also IGF-1 promote proliferation of erythroid progenitor cells and stimulate erythropoiesis. Conversely, the immune system modulates the secretion of GH via the brain and also directly at the pituitary gland *(81,82)*. Many of the studies on the GH–immune system relationship have been performed in vitro and in experimental animals, and their physiological and pathophysiological significance in humans has yet to be ascertained. There is evidence, however, that GH treatment of GH-deficient children can restore impaired function of immunocompetent cells to normal. More recently, several observations were made that suggest a possible effect of the augmented GH secretion on the immune system in acromegalic patients. Decreased polymorphonuclear chemotaxis, elevated phagocytic activity of lymphocytes, and enhanced T-cell activity have been reported *(83,84)*. These observations deserve confirmation from further studies.

PITUITARY GIGANTISM

If a GH-secreting pituitary adenoma develops before or during puberty, i.e., before the epiphyseal growth plates are fused, children may grow in excess before the correct diagnosis of pituitary gigantism is made. Usually secondary hypogonadism is also present, since these tumors tend to be large, grow invasively, and compromise the secretion of gonadotropins. Therefore, these adolescents continue to grow long after the age of normal growth arrest and develop eunuchoid body proportions. Acromegalic features usually develop in addition, if the GH excess is not remedied in very young age. Although gigantism is usually owing to a GH-secreting pituitary adenoma, it has also been observed in cases of ectopic GHRH secretion, e.g., by a pancreatic carcinoma or a carcinoid tumor *(85)*. In one patient, no source of ectopic GHRH secretion could be identified, and "idiopathic" hypothalamic hypersecretion of GHRH was suspected *(86)*. Gigantism owing to a pituitary somatotroph adenoma in both of a pair of siblings has also been reported *(87)*. One out of five patients with gigantism may have the McCune-Albright syndrome *(85)*. Because of their large body weight combined with muscular weakness, neuropathy, and osteoarthropathy, such patients often have foot problems and a risk of foot ulcerations *(67,88)*. Attention to these problems, pedography, and adequate orthopedic care are mandatory. Modalities of diagnosis and treatment are similar to those in adult patients with acromegaly. The differential diagnosis of gigantism has recently been reviewed *(85)*.

METABOLIC CHANGES IN ACROMEGALY

GH excess induces a number of characteristic metabolic changes. These are owing to the insulin-antagonistic, lipolytic, and protein-anabolic actions of the hormone *(17,20)*. In acromegaly, GH causes increased lipolysis and reduced glucose uptake into muscle tissue. The resulting insulin resistance is compensated for by a concomitant increase in insulin secretion. However, when the pancreatic B-cells become exhausted, impaired glucose tolerance, and eventually, frank diabetes mellitus of the counterregulatory type develops in approx 20–50% of the patients *(30,44)*. In most, but not all patients, normalization of the GH concentration also reverts glucose metabolism to normal. A genetic background of diabetes mellitus, the duration of the GH excess, the degree of hypersomatotropism, and other factors (e.g., obesity) are important variables that determine whether or not diabetes develops *(89,90)*. The influence of GH excess on lipid metabolism is difficult to dissect, because of the concomitant stimulation of insulin and IGF-1, which both have effects opposite to those of GH. Thus, although GH is lipolytic, lipid oxidation was unexpectedly found to be reduced, rather than increased *(91)*. The adipocyte hormone leptin is low in patients with acromegaly, probably owing to a decreased body fat mass. It rises to normal concentrations following successful treatment *(91a,91b)*.

GH induces amino acid retention and stimulates protein synthesis *(20)*. In acromegaly, the GH excess facilitates protein anabolism and increases lean body mass *(92–95)*. However, muscle strength is not increased, as has already been discussed (*see* Peripheral and Central Nervous Systems, and Neuromuscular System Section.)

ACROMEGALY AND MALIGNANCIES

Acromegaly probably carries an increased risk of malignancy, although published surveys vary greatly in their findings and interpretation *(96,96a,96b)*. An increased prevalence of colonic polyps has been found by several groups *(3,96–100,100a,100b, 100c)*. Adenomatous colonic polyps are considered a precancerous condition. In a group of 13 acromegalic patients *(101)*, three patients had colonic cancer, and three additional patients (out of eight who had a colonoscopy) had colonic polyps. Since colonic adenomas may be associated with multiple skin tags *(102)*, it has been proposed that such patients should be offered colonoscopy *(100b,103,104)*.

However, in several other studies, no increased prevalence of colonic polyps *(105)* or colon cancer *(2,4,30)* was evident. A US study of 87 acromegalic patients reported no excess of colonic cancer, but described a risk for thyroid cancer, not noticed in any other publication *(106)*. A Swedish survey of 166 acromegalic patients found an increased number of deaths owing to various malignancies (15 compared to 5.6 expected), but no single type of cancer was responsible for the overall increase in cancer mortality. In this study, there was no case of colonic cancer that caused death *(2)*. In a group of 131 patients in Northern Ireland, the overall rate of malignancies was increased and 4 patients had died from colonic cancer, but the number was considered to be too small for statistical evaluation *(3)*. An evaluation of computer-based data of 1041

acromegalic patients (US veterans administration, all male) revealed an increased rate of digestive tract cancers, including colonic cancers. The number of colonic polyps, however, was not significantly increased *(107)*. In all these studies, no correlation was seen between colonic polyps and either the known duration of acromegaly or the degree of GH elevation *(100,108,109)*. Thus, colonic polyps in acromegaly may be a trait that is independent of GH and IGF-1 and polyps may not necessarily tend to degenerate into cancer. The different findings in these reports are probably owing to the relatively small number of patients in most investigations and to differences in the study protocols. They may also relate to a different genetic background between the populations. Taken together, these studies indicate that regular checks for colonic polyps and cancer, as well as heightened attention to the possibility of malignant disease of other organs are indicated in acromegalic patients.

RARE CAUSES OF ACROMEGALY

Acromegaly owing to causes other than a pituitary GH-secreting adenoma is rare. However, ectopic secretion of GHRH or—exceptionally—ectopic production and secretion of GH itself, a GH-secreting pituitary adenoma in the setting of the multiple-endocrine-neoplasia syndrome type 1 (MEN 1) or the McCune-Albright syndrome must all be considered.

ECTOPIC GHRH SECRETION GHRH can be produced in tumors outside the hypothalamus and the pituitary *(110,111)*, e.g., by a pulmonary or gastrointestinal carcinoid or a pancreatic islet cell tumor *(111–113)*. In most cases, not enough GHRH is apparently secreted to cause acromegaly. Less than 2% of all cases of acromegaly are owing to ectopic GHRH secretion *(114)*. Ectopic GHRH secretion with elevated circulating GHRH concentrations usually causes diffuse or nodular pituitary somatotroph hyperplasia and not a pituitary adenoma *(115,116)*. Exceptionally, a eutopic GHRH-secreting tumor, i.e., an intra- or suprasellar hamartoma or gangliocytoma, gives rise to a true pituitary GH-secreting adenoma, possibly owing to the direct contact between GHRH-secreting cells and the pituitary somatotrophs *(117–120)*. The latter concept, however, has recently been challenged. The coexistence of a neuronal choristoma and a pituitary adenoma was explained as the "result of neuronal differentiation within sparsely granulated GH cell adenomas" *(121)*. It remains to be explained, why such neuronal choristomas develop in some GH-secreting pituitary adenomas and not in others. Could differences in paracrine actions of the adenomatous somatotrophs be responsible? Unusual cases of GHRH-secreting tumors causing acromegaly include pheochromocytomas producing GHRH or a GHRH-like substance *(122,123)*, an intrasellar gangliocytoma producing not only GHRH, but also gastrin *(124)* and an intrasellar metastasis of a GHRH-secreting neuroendocrine pancreatic malignoma *(125)*.

Endocrine testing in acromegaly does not distinguish between ectopic GHRH secretion and a primary pituitary adenoma. GH is not suppressible by glucose, paradoxical responses to thyrotropin-releasing hormone (TRH) and glucose do occur, and an increased PRL concentration may also be present. A paradoxical GH response to TRH as well as absence of response to GHRH are more often found in ectopic than in classical acromegaly, but these tests cannot differentiate the two conditions in an individual patient *(111)*. Somatostatin and its analogs suppress GHRH secretion from the tumor as well as GH secretion from the hyperplastic pituitary gland. The diagnosis should be suspected in a patient with acromegaly in whom a clearly delineated lesion cannot be identified in the cranial MRI or when acromegaly occurs in the presence of another tumor disease. Confirmation should be based on the measurement of the plasma GHRH concentration. Measurable concentrations (usually >200 ng/L) confirm secretion by an ectopic neuroendocrine tumor *(114)*. GHRH-producing tumors may also secrete other hormonal polypeptides, such as gastrin-releasing peptide, vasoactive inhibitory peptide, glucagon, or insulin. Removal of the GHRH secreting tumor is followed by regression of acromegaly *(126)*.

ECTOPIC GH SECRETION   GH production in nonpituitary tumors is not rare *(127)*. However, secretion of GH by such tumors is exceptional, at least in amounts that would cause elevated circulating GH concentrations and acromegaly *(111)*. There are only two well-documented cases in the literature in whom ectopic GH production and secretion has been convincingly proved, including GH production and secretion in vitro as well as GH mRNA expression. The secreting tissue was a pancreatic islet cell tumor in one patient and a non-Hodgkin's lymphoma in the other patient *(128,128a)*. Several other less well documented cases of acromegalic patients with alleged ectopic GH secretion have been reported *(111,129,130)*. Ectopic GH secretion might be considered in an acromegalic patient with a normal sized homogenous pituitary gland in the MRI (since the pituitary is not the source of the GH excess). The plasma GHRH concentration should be unmeasurably low.

MCCUNE-ALBRIGHT SYNDROME   Acromegaly may occur as part of the McCune-Albright syndrome *(131,132)*, which, in addition to an endocrinopathy, includes osteitis fibrosa disseminata and café au lait spots. Patients with the McCune-Albright syndrome have an activating mutation of the α-subunit of the G_s-protein in the affected tissues *(133)*. A similar mutation occurs in the somatotrophs of approx 40% of Caucasian acromegalic patients unrelated to the McCune-Albright syndrome *(134)*.

MULTIPLE ENDOCRINE NEOPLASIA TYPE 1 (MEN 1) SYNDROME AND FAMILIAL ACROMEGALY   MEN 1 is an autosomal genetic disease with dominant inheritance. These patients develop parathyroid, pancreatic islet, and pituitary hyperplasia or neoplasias. Pituitary adenomas are of the somatotroph type causing acromegaly in approximately one-quarter of the cases *(135)*. Ectopic GHRH secretion causing acromegaly (e.g., by a pancreatic tumor) may also occur *(126)*. Familial acromegaly, not related to the MEN 1 syndrome, has been described in a few families *(136–138,138a)*. The genetic basis in these latter cases is unknown.

DIAGNOSTIC WORKUP

The diagnostic workup of a patient with acromegaly must confirm the autonomy of GH secretion, look for possible concomitant hyperprolactinemia, and document the space-occupying lesion and its extension. Furthermore, it must search for possible complications, e.g., anterior pituitary insufficiency, visual impairment, carpal tunnel syndrome, and so forth. A schematic outline of the procedure is given in Figure 3.

"BASAL" GH CONCENTRATION AND ORAL GLUCOSE TEST   GH secretion in healthy subjects occurs episodically throughout the 24-h day. Therefore, very low as well as high GH concentrations are not diagnostic of GH insufficiency or of acromegaly, respectively. GH concentrations of 30 µg/L or higher can often be measured at the height of a spontaneous secretory peak in young healthy subjects, especially in women. Moreover, although the diagnosis of acromegaly requires elevated baseline

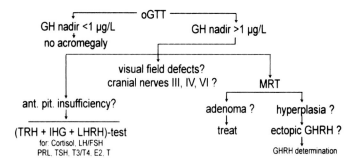

Figure 17-3   Diagnostic work-up of acromegaly. With rare exceptions, a GH nadir >1.0 µg/L in the oGTT is diagnostic of acromegaly. Anterior pituitary function and adenoma size (by MRI) must be determined. Ophthalmologic and neurologic examinations need not be done if MRI reveals a microadenoma. The extent of pituitary testing depends on the clinical situation (normal menstruation renders LH/FSH determinations unnecessary). If the pituitary is enlarged, but delineation of an adenoma is not possible in MRI, ectopic GHRH secretion may be suspected and confirmed by an elevated serum GHRH concentration.

GH concentration (i.e., absence of very low values), very high GH concentrations are not seen in all patients. It follows that single "basal" GH values are of limited value for the diagnostic confirmation of acromegaly. Moreover, IGF-1 concentrations and even mean 24-h GH concentrations overlap between patients with mild acromegaly and normal subjects *(33,139,139a)*. For confirmation of acromegaly, it is therefore necessary to document autonomy of GH secretion. This is achieved by the demonstration of nonsuppressibility by an oral glucose load. In healthy subjects, but not in acromegaly, the GH concentration falls to below 1.0 µg/L during an oral glucose tolerance test *(139a,139b,139c)*. Workup of a patient suspected to have acromegaly is schematically depicted in Figure 3.

ANTERIOR PITUITARY FUNCTION   Small pituitary adenomas usually do not compromise normal pituitary function. However, macroadenomas may cause partial or complete pituitary insufficiency. The proper secretion of the different pituitary hormones must therefore be ascertained. This is done by a battery of tests, which stimulate the secretion of the different pituitary hormones. Often a cocktail of releasing hormones is used ("combined releasing hormone test") or a combination of insulin hypoglycemia, gonadotropin-releasing hormone (GnRH), and TRH ("combined pituitary function test"), which allow evaluation of all anterior pituitary functions in a single 90-min test. Diabetes insipidus is exceptionally rare. Details of the test procedures, as used in our department, are outlined in Table 1.

RADIOLOGICAL, OPHTHALMOLOGICAL, AND NEUROLOGICAL EXAMINATION   In more than 98% of all patients acromegaly is owing to a somatotroph adenoma of the pituitary gland *(114)*. The size of the tumor and its expansion must be documented by magnetic resonance tomography (MRT). Coronal and sagittal views in 2-mm slices, gadolinium-enhanced will give optimal results. If the tumor extends into the suprasellar space and/or laterally beyond the cavernous sinus, an ophthalmological examination must determine the outline of the visual fields and proper function of the oculomotor nerves. If clinical symptoms suggest a carpal tunnel syndrome or peripheral neuropathy, an appropriate neurological examination is necessary. Details of these procedures are discussed in Chapters 10 and 11.

Table 1
Clinical Testing for Acromegaly and Evaluation of Pituitary Function: Outline of Test Conditions as Used in the Authors' Department

Test	Test substance	Timing of samples	Hormone determination	Normal value
oGTT	Glucose 100 g orally	0, 30, 60, 90, 120 min	GH	GH nadir <1 µg/L
LHRH/TRH	LHRH 100 µg +TRH 200 µg iv	0, 30, 60, 90 min	LH/FSH, PRL, TSH, GH[e]	Normal LH/FSH, PRL, and TSH increase, no GH increase
Insulin hypoglycemia	Insulin 0.1 IU/kg iv[c]	0, 30, 60, 90, 120 min	ACTH/cortisol, GH	Basal cortisol ≥200 nmol/L Δ Cortisol ≥190 nmol/L
Metyrapone[a]	Metyrapone 30 mg/kg orally at 24.00 h	08.00 h	Desoxy-cortisol	>200 nmol/L
GH profile[b]	Spontaneous secretion	08.00–14.00 h (half-) hourly samples	GH	At least one value <1 µg/L
IGF-1 determination	Morning basal value[d]	08.00 h	IGF-1	IGF-1 normal for age and sex

[a]Alternative testing of the hypothalamo–pituitary–adrenal axis if insulin-hypoglycemia is contraindicated
[b]Alternative for oGTT in patients with diabetes mellitus, gastric surgery, and so on.
[c]Use less insulin if there is suspicion of adrenal insufficiency/hypopituitarism.
[d]IGF-1 is elevated for several days following depot-testosterone injection for substitution therapy.
[e]GH measurement for determination of a paradoxical increase.

OTHER TOOLS FOR DIAGNOSIS AND FOLLOW-UP

IGF-1, IGF-BP3, AND GHBP The GH-dependent IGF-1 can serve as a measure of disease activity in acromegaly. Its serum concentration is relatively stable (because of its being bound to the carrier protein IGF-BP3), and a single specimen may be used for its determination. However, certain limitations must be considered. The correlation between GH and IGF-1 is linear only up to GH concentrations of approx 10 µg/L, and a GH increase beyond 20–30 µg/L has little effect on the IGF-1 concentration (140). Moreover, there is an overlap with normal concentrations in cases of borderline acromegalic activity. In a recent survey (141) of 500 acromegalic patients, 4% had a normal IGF-1 value, although their mean 8-h (or longer) profile GH concentrations were between 5 and 29 µg/L. In our own experience, the IGF-1 concentration may be in the upper normal range in patients with clinically active acromegaly and GH concentrations below 5 µg/L. IGF-1 concentrations vary with developmental stage in children and adolescents and advancing age in adults. Therefore, age- and gender-specific values must be used. Furthermore, IGF-1 concentrations are influenced by metabolic and nutritional factors. In malnutrition and in poorly controlled diabetes mellitus, GH is elevated, but IGF-1 concentrations are low, owing to a decreased response of the liver to GH (142–144).

IGF-BP3 is under the direct influence of circulating GH. Its serum concentration correlates with that of IGF-1 and is elevated in acromegaly (145–147). IGF-BP3 measurement has therefore been proposed for use as a biochemical marker of acromegaly in diagnosis and follow-up (147). There is evidence, however, that the GH dependence of IGF-BP3 is mediated via IGF-1 (148). Effects independent of GH may therefore alter the IGF-BP3 concentration. In the opposite situation, diagnosis of GH deficiency, IGF-BP3 has not been found to be a reliable screening test (149). Its usefulness for the diagnosis and follow-up of acromegaly must await further validation.

GHBP is identical in humans to the extracellular part of the GH receptor. GH excess in acromegaly should lead to downregulation of its receptor in tissues, and hence, the concentration of circulating GHBP would decrease. The GHBP serum concentration is indeed low in acromegaly (150,151). Since a negative correlation between GH and the GHBP concentration was found in patients with acromegaly (152), GHBP determination has been proposed as an indicator of GH oversecretion in acromegaly (150). These observations need confirmation before they can possibly be used in clinical practice.

URINARY EXCRETION OF GH GH is filtered in the kidney glomerula, reabsorbed in the tubules, and partly excreted in the urine (153–155). Therefore, measurement of urinary GH has been proposed for determination of the GH secretory status. However, its clinical usefulness has been debated. Normal values in overnight or 24-h urine samples vary widely inter- and intraindividually, both in children and in adults. Less than 0.01% of circulating GH finally appears in the urine, requiring very sensitive assays for determination. Furthermore, rigid standardization of assay conditions is necessary to compensate for variations in ionic composition, pH, and overall salt concentration of the urine samples, which may all influence the antigen/antibody reaction in any immunoassay (156). Nevertheless, a close correlation between plasma and urinary GH has been reported for normal subjects and in acromegalic patients by some authors (157–159). Others have noted not only the large intraindividual variation, but also an overlap of the values between normal subjects and patients with acromegaly (160–164). Infradian rhythms of urinary GH excretion have been observed in children (165), but have not been investigated in the adult. Overall, at the present time, the determination of urinary GH excretion seems to offer no advantage for the diagnosis of acromegaly, determination of disease activity, and treatment results.

PARADOXICAL GH RESPONSES Between 30 and 80% of acromegalic patients respond with a GH increase to the injection of the hypothalamic TSH-releasing hormone, TRH. A response to the hypothalamic GnRH occurs less frequently (166–168). The responses to TRH and GnRH are not always concordant, and therefore, a combined test (simultaneous injection of both TRH and GnRH) has also been used (169,170). The GH response in these tests is called "paradoxical," since these releasing hormones do not usually induce a GH rise in healthy subjects. Paradoxical GH response to other substances, e.g., vasoactive intestinal polypeptide

(VIP) *(171)* or peptide histidine-methionine *(172)*, and even to glucose *(173)*, as well as paradoxical suppression by stimulatory agents, dexamethason *(174)* and galanin *(175)*, have also been reported. However, the paradoxical GH response is not specific for acromegaly. It may also occur in diabetes mellitus, hepatic or renal failure, hypothyroidism, and other diseases unrelated to acromegaly, e.g., schizophrenia *(166,167,176)*. Paradoxical GH responses are not a diagnostic tool for acromegaly.

On the other hand, it has been proposed that the GH response to TRH predicts the GH-suppressive effect of bromocriptine treatment and that the GH increase following VIP or GnRH administration predicts a smaller GH response to bromocriptine *(171)*. However, the predictive value for individual patients is low, and the response to dopamine-agonist treatment can be better tested by acute administration of the drug.

The GH response to TRH has also been evaluated as a possible prognostic parameter following surgery. A preoperative paradoxical GH response as well as its disappearance following surgery have been suggested to predict a good prognosis *(168,177)*. However, the correlation has not been confirmed by others *(169,178)*. It has also been postulated that the TRH response is more often positive in patients with PRL-cosecreting somatotropinomas than in those with pure GH-secreting adenomas *(179,180)*, but this has not been confirmed by others *(181)*. Some of the differences may be owing to the lack of strict criteria for a specific response in terms of both its magnitude and its timing. These are important in view of the occurrence of spontaneous secretory GH episodes in many patients *(182)*.

The mechanism responsible for the paradoxical response is at present unknown. Removal of the hypothalamic influence on the pituitary gland (e.g., by autotransplantation of the pituitary gland under the kidney capsule in experimental animals) induces a permanent paradoxical response to TRH *(183)*. Alternatively, the paradoxical response may be owing to the (pathological) expression of specific receptors for TRH and/or GnRH on the somatotroph adenoma *(184)*.

GHRH TEST The GH response to the hypothalamic GHRH is preserved to some degree in patients with acromegaly. Attempts have been made to use this response for prognostic purposes. Thus, an exaggerated GH response to GHRH correlated with a nonsuppressible or paradoxically increasing GH during an oral glucose tolerance test (oGTT). It was suggested that this was indicative of a more active disease *(185)*. In other studies, the predictive value of the GH response to GHRH for the success of bromocriptine treatment was evaluated. The response to bromocriptine was better in patients with a smaller GH reaction to GHRH *(180,186)*. However, partly in view of large interindividual variations, these observations have not found a place in the treatment decisions for patients with acromegaly.

The synthetic GH-releasing peptide (GHRP, a hexapeptide) and related compounds stimulate GH secretion in most patients with acromegaly *(187–189)*. However, although the synthetic GHRPs hold promise for the treatment of patients with GH deficiency of hypothalamic origin, at present they have no diagnostic or prognostic value for patients with acromegaly.

SCINTIGRAPHIC TUMOR VISUALIZATION

Scintigraphic methods for in vivo visualization of somatostatin receptors are now available. Somatostatin receptors have been demonstrated in surgical specimens of GH-secreting adenomas by autoradiography *(190)* and also in vivo *(191–193)*. Early experience was gained with ^{123}I-Tyr^3-octreotide *(191,192)*. Subsequently, the ^{111}Indium-labeled derivative of the octreotide analog, ^{111}In-DTPA-D-Phe-octreotide (Octreoscan®), became commercially available. A good correlation between scintigraphic demonstration of somatostatin receptors on the adenoma and subsequent response to octreotide treatment was reported with the ^{123}I-Tyr^3-octreotide preparations *(191,192)*. Our own experience with the Octreoscan procedure is less encouraging. Since ^{111}In-DTPA-D-Phe-octreotide visualizes the normal pituitary gland more frequently than ^{123}I-Tyr^3-octreotide *(193)*, it becomes difficult to distinguish an adenoma with a low number of receptors from a normal gland *(194)*. Moreover, in our experience, the scintigraphic results were not correlated with the GH response to octreotide treatment, nor did they predict a volume reduction in response to preoperative octreotide therapy *(194)*. Thus, although the Octreoscan is apparently of great help in the localization of gastroenteropancreatic tumors *(195)*, its value for the diagnosis of a GH-secreting pituitary adenoma and for treatment decision is at present questionable. The Octreoscan procedure delivers a relatively high radiation dose of approx 16 mSV *(193)*.

Other radioactively labeled octreotide derivatives are being developed with the use of gallium isotopes for gamma-scintigraphy and also for positron emission tomography (PET; *196,197*). Technetium-99m-pentavalent-dimercaptosuccinic acid (99mTc[V]DSMA) imaging has also been used to visualize pituitary tumors, independent of their hormonal activity or their somatostatin receptor status *(198)*. A PET study has been performed with fluorine-18-2-fluorodeoxyglucose (FDG; *199*). This procedure measures the metabolic activity of a pituitary adenoma and not its hormonal activity. PET has also been used for demonstration of dopamine receptors on pituitary tumors, including somatotroph adenomas. Two different dopamine D$_2$ receptor ligands were used in an attempt to correlate receptor demonstration with the result of dopamine agonist treatment *(200)*. Dopamine D$_2$ receptors have also been visualized scintigraphically in prolactinoma patients using iodobenzamide in order to predict treatment response to dopamine agonist drugs *(201)*. Patients with somatotroph tumors and their response to dopamine agonists have yet to be studied. The clinical importance of these developments for the diagnosis and prognostic predictions in patients with acromegaly awaits further investigation. PET, in particular, is not widely available and remains largely a research tool at the present time.

HYPERPROLACTINEMIA, AND MULTIHORMONAL ADENOMAS

Elevated PRL concentrations are somewhat common in acromegaly and occur in about one third of the patients *(202,203)*. Hyperprolactinemia may be owing to cosecretion of PRL from the tumor or to pituitary stalk compression by a macroadenoma. Stalk compression interrupts the dopamine flow from the hypothalamus that inhibits PRL secretion from the nonadenomatous pituitary gland. PRL concentrations in such patients usually remain below approx 200 µg/L. In other patients, hyperprolactinemia is owing to PRL secretion from the pituitary adenoma. PRL is then either secreted from the same cell that produces GH, or each hormone is secreted from its own cell (mammosomatotroph cell and mixed GH/PRL adenoma, respectively *[115]*). Cosecretion of TSH with GH resulting in acromegaly with concomitant secondary hyperthyroidism does occur, but is a very rare combination *(115,204,205)*.

In histological specimens of GH-secreting tumors, other hormones can often be documented immunohistochemically or by *in situ* hybridization. Usually, these hormones are either not secreted at all or only in amounts which cause no clinical symptoms *(115)*. Almost all GH-secreting adenomas, with the exception of densely granulated somatotroph adenomas, contain cells that express PRL, TSH, LH, FSH, α-subunit, and rarely, ACTH *(194,206,207)*.

Patients with concomitant PRL secretion have been reported to suppress their GH concentration better in response to the dopamine agonist bromocriptine *(202,208)*. However, in another series, the GH response to a dopamine infusion was similar in patients with and without PRL-positive cells in their adenoma *(209)*. Operative results have been reported to be worse in patients with a PRL component in their adenoma. The surgical outcome was not related to the invasiveness of the adenoma. It was suggested that the higher postoperative GH concentration in these patients might indicate a risk for a higher recurrence rate *(203)*. The clinical relevance of these observation is at present uncertain.

PITUITARY INSUFFICIENCY

Normal pituitary function is usually preserved when the GH-secreting adenoma is small. Even in patients with a macroadenoma, there is often surprisingly little impairment of pituitary function. The contrast-enhanced MRI visualizes a displaced, more or less deformed pituitary gland adjacent to the adenoma in most patients with a macroadenoma. Often, the tumor displaces the normal pituitary gland upward or laterally, rather than pressing it against the bones of the sellar cavity *(210)*. If hormonal insufficiency occurs, gonadotropin deficiency is more common than ACTH deficiency, but TSH insufficiency is rare *(170,211)*. The incidence of damage to the PRL cells of the nonadenomatous gland is difficult to determine because of cosecretion of PRL from many adenomas and disinhibition of PRL secretion by stalk compression. Secondary insufficiency of the respective peripheral glands ensues, and must be diagnosed and treated appropriately. We define as "partial insufficiency" of a pituitary hormone the combination of a normal basal value with insufficient response in a stimulation test. This is often compatible with a normal secretion of the peripheral target gland. However, partial insufficiency of a pituitary hormone should arouse attention for incipient or manifest secondary insufficiency of the target gland. In the case of partial ACTH insufficiency, patients should be provided a health card and carry appropriate medication (e.g., parenteral prednisone) for use in an emergency. Following surgery or during drug-induced tumor shrinkage, partial insufficiency of any pituitary function may improve or even normalize.

TREATMENT OF ACROMEGALY

CRITERIA FOR TREATMENT SUCCESS Criteria for success in treating patients with acromegaly have become progressively more ambitious, based on new insights into the normal physiology of GH secretion and also on the long-term follow-up of patients operated since the (re)-introduction of transsphenoidal pituitary surgery. The aim of treatment is of course to cure the patient from acromegaly and also to preserve or restore anterior pituitary function. However, it is important to distinguish "remission" from "cure" of acromegaly. The former may be defined as a postoperative GH nadir in the oGTT—or occurring spontaneously during a profile—of less than 2 µg/L *(212,213,213a)* and an IGF-I concentration in the normal (age- and sex-corrected) range. Others use

a concentration of 2.5 µg/L in a random sample or as the mean of a day profile *(213b)*. While this indicates absence of "active disease" at the time of testing, it does not exclude a late recurrence. In contrast, "cure of acromegaly" requires GH suppression to concentrations below 1.0 µg/L by oral glucose administration and a normal IGF-I concentration *(139c,214–216)*. However, even these criteria do not exclude late recurrences. There is mounting evidence that the required GH concentration during oGTT may be even lower than these limits *(139c,216a)*. "Cure of acromegaly" does not exclude GH insufficiency caused by damage to the normal pituitary somatotrophs. Finally, "normal GH secretion" as a treatment result requires restitution of feedback-regulated somatotroph function, which includes a normal GH response in a stimulation test. Strictly speaking, it also includes the physiological pattern of pulsatile secretion *(217)*. In clinical practice, the spontaneous GH concentration during a "profile," the GH nadir during oral glucose loading, and the IGF-I concentration are usually accepted as criteria for treatment success.

A refined analysis of the pulsatile pattern of GH secretion in patients with acromegaly, using 24-h frequent blood sampling, revealed an increase in the pulse frequency (17 pulses vs 6.7 in healthy controls). Treated patients with a GH nadir <1.0 µg/L had a normal pulse frequency *(139)*. However, when analyzed with a new statistical tool (calculation of "approximate entropy"), the secretory pattern of patients in remission following surgery (GH nadir <1.0 µg/L) remained nevertheless more "disorderly" than that of control subjects *(32)*. In two other series, the increased pulse frequency was not normalized postoperatively *(34,35)*. The discrepancies may in part relate to different criteria for treatment success in acromegaly. Whether the persistence of some—though subtle—pathology of the secretory pattern of GH in patients with very low GH concentrations following surgery is attributable to an intrinsic alteration of the hypothalamic GH release mechanisms is at present not clear. However, these observations underline that for treatment success, "remission" and "cure" must be defined differently.

SURGERY

Selective transsphenoidal adenomectomy is the treatment of choice for all pituitary tumors, including GH-secreting micro- and macroadenomas. Adenomas with invasive growth and those presenting with a high basal GH concentration are candidates for poor surgical results *(212)*. Very large tumors may require a primary or secondary transcranial approach. Transsphenoidal surgery achieves GH concentrations below 2 µg/L in approx 50–70% of the patients *(178,212,213,213a,213c)*. It is important that difficult cases always be operated on in a specialized center *(213d,213e)*. Details of the surgical treatment will be discussed in Chapter 12.

Any patient who is referred to the neurosurgeon should have had a complete workup of his or her pituitary function and—in all cases with a macroadenoma—visual field determination, neurological examination (oculomotor nerves and—possibly—carpal tunnel syndrome), and MRI for determination of tumor size and invasiveness. If pituitary insufficiency is detected, substitution therapy will be initiated prior to surgery. The pituitary–adrenal axis and the thyroid status are of special importance for the stress of anesthesia and surgery. For the pituitary–adrenal axis, basal serum cortisol or plasma ACTH concentrations are not sufficient, since these values may be within normal limits in the presence of partial insufficiency. For thyroid function, on the other hand,

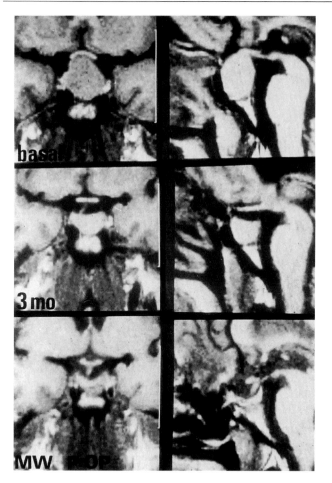

Figure 17-4 *Octreotide-induced preoperative tumor shrinkage. Cranial MRI (coronal [left] and sagital [right] of 28-yr old patient with GH-secreting macroadenoma. Compression of optic chiasm and bilateral invasion of cavernous sinus are clearly visible before treatment. After 3 mo of octreotide treatment (3 × 100 μg/d sc) the tumor size is considerably reduced, and the optic chiasm is no longer compressed. The pituitary stalk is now visible, deviating to the right. The operative result is also shown. GH concentration before octreotide: "basal" (mean of 6 values) 94.3 μg/L, nadir in oGTT 68.4 μg/L. During octreotide treatment: "basal" 6.4 μg/L; nadir in oGTT 2.0 μg/L. Postoperative: "basal" 1.5 μg/L; nadir in oGTT 1.1 μg/L.*

peripheral thyroid hormone concentrations are more important than the TSH basal value or response to TRH. Further preoperative testing depends on the interest of specialized centers and the desire of the neurosurgeon to document deterioration or improvement of partial pituitary function as caused by the surgical intervention.

PREOPERATIVE OCTREOTIDE TREATMENT FOR TUMOR SHRINKAGE AND HORMONE SUPPRESSION Attempts have been made to reduce the size of GH-secreting macroadenomas and suppress GH concentrations prior to surgery in order to achieve better surgical results. The long-acting somatostatin analog octreotide has been most widely used. Tumor shrinkage has been achieved in approx 50% of patients with macroadenomas. Most of the shrinkage occurs within the first 2–3 wk of treatment *(194,218–221)*. An example is shown in Figure 4. There is some indication that improvement of surgical results may be obtained *(219,222, 223,223a)*. However, the impact on the recurrence rate—rather than immediate operative results—cannot yet be judged. Perioperative improvements—e.g., of glucose tolerance/diabetes

mellitus, cardiac function, easier intubation for surgery, easier suction of adenoma tissue by the surgeon, etc.—have been described *(223a,223b)*. Whether they justify the preoperative use of somatostatin analogues should there be no long-term improvement of the surgical results, remains uncertain. The final verdict on this type of treatment must await larger numbers of treated patients and longer postoperative observation periods. Details of the treatment modalities are discussed in Chapter 13.

Therapy with a dopamine agonist drug may induce tumor shrinkage in a few patients *(224)*. However, in view of the much higher efficacy of octreotide, dopamine agonists are no longer in use for preoperative tumor shrinkage.

IRRADIATION Irradiation is a secondary treatment choice for somatotroph adenomas. It is indicated when surgery has failed to induce a complete remission and a second operation does not promise a better result, or when surgery is contraindicated or refused *(225–228)*. The main disadvantages of conventional irradiation therapy are a long delay before maximal GH decline is reached and a high rate of secondary pituitary insufficiency *(225,229,230)*. Late damage to sensitive structures (optic nerve, third cranial nerve, hypothalamus, temporal lobes, delayed cerebral radiation necrosis) have occurred. The indication for pituitary irradiation should therefore be considered with caution in patients in the reproductive age and in patients with pre-existing damage of the optic or the oculomotor nerves. However, irradiation techniques have been improved, and these complications have become increasingly rare.

Conventional multiple-port irradiation uses fractionated doses of 1.8 gy for a total of 45–48 gy. Recently, a much lower total dose of 20 gy given in 8 fractions over 11 d was reported to be as effective as a higher dose to suppress the GH concentration in acromegalic patients and to cause less pituitary insufficiency *(231)*.

Following conventional supervoltage irradiation, GH falls by about 50% within 2 yr and 75% within 5 yr. The average percent fall of GH/yr is approx 20%. It is independent of tumor size and initial GH concentration. Therefore, patients with a high initial GH concentrations will reach low GH concentrations only very belatedly, if at all. They should therefore undergo surgical tumor debulking prior to radiation therapy if possible *(225,225a,225b)*. It has been suggested that conventional irradiation may be ineffective in normalizing the IGF-I concentration even in the presence of a low GH concentration *(225b)*, but this needs confirmation. Pituitary insufficiency develops in a substantial number of patients and increases with time: 5 yr after irradiation, secondary gonadal, adrenal, and thyroid insufficiency develop in approx 20–40% of patients in whom these functions were normal before treatment. The rate of insufficiencies continues to increase thereafter. The order of appearance is gonads > adrenal > thyroid. PRL may slightly increase in patients who had normal concentrations before irradiation, probably owing to a loss of dopaminergic inhibition caused by hypothalamic irradiation damage *(225)*.

Stereotactic radiosurgery with the so-called Gamma-Knife (a multiple cobalt-60 source) allows delivery of a high-radiation dose to well defined, small target areas ("focused irradiation"). Similar precision delivery of radiation is now possible from a linear accelerator (Linac) using rotational techniques. High-quality MRI imaging of the tumor tissue is a prerequisite for optimal targeting. Although optimal treatment modalities for focussed irradiation have yet to be defined, there is evidence that GH concentrations can be reduced more quickly than by conventional irradiation *(225c,225d,225e,225f,232,233)*.

Table 2
Dopamine Agonist Drugs for Treatment of Acromegaly

Drug	Dose	Dose schedule	Administration
Bromocriptine	1.25–30 mg/24 h	Thrice daily	Orally
Lisuride	0.2–2.0 mg/24 h	Thrice daily	Orally
Cabergoline	0.25–4.5 mg/week	Once or twice/week	Orally
Quinagolide	0.025–0.6 mg/24 h	Once daily	Orally

MEDICAL THERAPY Dopamine Agonist Drugs Dopamine agonist drugs suppress GH secretion in a number of patients with acromegaly *(234,235)*. This is a "paradoxical" effect, since dopamine stimulates GH secretion in healthy subjects. The mechanism is still unclear. The first dopamine agonist drug, bromocriptine, is still widely used. Newer drugs have essentially similar effects, but their longer half-life makes less frequent ingestion possible. Although their side effects overlap, individual patients may tolerate one drug better than the other one in either direction. The currently available preparations are listed in Table 2.

In contrast to their great value in patients with prolactinomas, the dopamine agonist drugs are less effective in patients with acromegaly. The largest experience has accumulated with bromocriptine. Although this drug lowers GH concentrations in more than 50% of the patients, values below 5 µg/L are obtained in only approx 20% patients, and concentrations below 2 µg/L are rarely achieved. GH concentrations return to pretreatment values after cessation of therapy. IGF-1 concentrations are normalized in only 10% of the patients *(224)*.

A long-acting depot preparation of bromocriptine for monthly intramuscular injection has been studied in only a small number of acromegalic patients. From these reports, it seems to be equally as effective as oral dopamine agonists, but may be more tolerable in terms of gastrointestinal and circulatory side effects when treatment is begun with a low dose of 50 mg *(236–238)*. However, this preparation is no longer marketed.

Two recently introduced dopamine agonist drugs, cabergoline and quinagolide, are longer-acting and allow administration only once daily (quinagolide) or once or twice weekly (cabergoline). While bromocriptine, lisuride, and cabergoline are ergot derivatives, quinagolide is a nonergot dopamine agonist. Although there is some controversy in the comparison of these drugs, they both seem to be more efficient than bromocriptine in reducing GH concentrations and may also be better tolerated *(239,240a,240b,240c)*.

Somatostatin Analogs Octreotide is a long-acting analog of the hypothalamic GH release-inhibiting hormone somatostatin *(241)*. More recently another preparation, lanreotide, has become available. Octreotide lowers the GH concentration to <2–5 µg/L in up to 50% of the patients and considerably reduces GH in another 20–30% *(220,242)*. GH concentrations are reduced to <5 µg/L in 50% or more of the patients. IGF-1 apparently is normalized more often than the GH concentration. Treatment with a somatostatin analog is indicated when surgery is not possible or has failed to achieve a GH concentration of 2 µg/L or less. It is also used following radiation therapy to reduce GH concentrations until the effect of irradiation becomes fully established. Its use for preoperative tumor shrinkage has already been discussed.

Octreotide must be self-injected subcutaneously by the patient and is usually administered thrice daily in single doses of 100 µg. In some patients higher doses (up to 3 × 1000 µg) may achieve

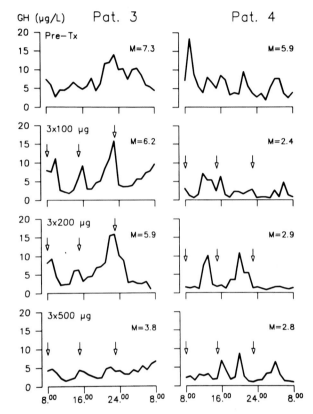

Figure 17-5 Effect of increasing doses of octreotide on 24-h GH profile in acromegaly. One patient (left) responds to increasing doses of octreotide with a progressive decrease of his 24-h GH concentration. The other patient (right) responds to a dose of 3 × 100 µg/d, but no further decrease is obtained by the higher doses. M = mean concentration of the 24-h profile. Note that the intrinsic temporal pattern of episodic secretion persists during treatment at least in patient (4): the GH decrease from peak values clearly begins before the second and third injections (on 3 × 200 µg/d) and before the third injection (on 3 × 500 µg/d). (From ref. *242*. Copyright The Endocrine Society. Used with permission.)

somewhat better results (Fig. 5). Continuous subcutaneous infusion has been reported to yield better suppression with a lower dose *(243–245)*. Octreotide and lanreotide are now available as depot preparations which need to be injected only every 4 or 2 wk respectively *(246–249,249a,249b,249c,249d)*. There is mounting evidence that these preparations are more efficient than the shorter acting formulations. They are presently discussed as primary therapy for some patients with acromegaly *(249e)*.

Approximately 10% of the patients are resistant to octreotide therapy *(221,242,250)*. On cessation of octreotide administration, GH concentrations quickly return to pretreatment values *(250,251)*. On the other hand, there is no loss of the GH-suppressive effect even after 10 yr of therapy *(252)*. In patients with acromegaly owing to ectopic GHRH secretion, octreotide suppresses both GHRH from the ectopic source and GH from the hyperplastic pituitary gland *(253)*.

Inhibition of GH secretion and tumor size reduction are poorly correlated during octreotide therapy *(194)*. This may be partly owing to a marked heterogeneity of the individual cells in somatotroph adenomas. Cells differ in their GH secretory activity. Actively secreting cells respond to octreotide with a larger reduction of hormone secretion *(254)*. Therefore, an important GH decrease may be owing to an octreotide effect on only a minority of cells, which could explain the absence of tumor volume reduction. Minor effects of octreotide on PRL (suppression) and the pituitary–thyroid axis have been reported *(207,255)*, but have no clinical importance.

Beneficial clinical effects—reduction of headaches, sweating, joint pain, snoring, and sleep apnea—are sometimes more pronounced than the degree of GH suppression would suggest. This may be owing to a direct suppressive effect of octreotide on IGF-1 generation *(256)* and to stimulation of the IGF-1 binding protein 1 (IGF-BP1 *[257,258]*). Increased IGF-1 binding to IGF-BP1 would decrease the availability of free IGF-1. General improved well-being may also result from a direct central nervous effect. Some somatostatin analogs have been shown to bind to brain opioid receptors *(259)*. The rapid reduction of headaches—sometimes within minutes of sc injection—also suggests a central effect *(260)*.

Octreotide—like its mother substance, somatostatin—has many other actions in addition to its GH-lowering effect (for a recent review, *see 261*). Inhibition of insulin secretion may induce carbohydrate intolerance. The insulin-releasing intestinal incretin, glucagon-like peptide (7-36) amide (GLP-1), is also suppressed *(261a)*. On the other hand, octreotide-induced GH suppression tends to improve carbohydrate tolerance *(262,263)*. The net outcome depends on the relative importance of these opposing effects for the individual patient (e.g., pre-existing insulin resistance owing to obesity, genetic predisposition for diabetes mellitus and so forth). In clinical experience, both development of carbohydrate intolerance as well as amelioration do occur.

Side effects of octreotide treatment include gastrointestinal discomfort and diarrhea, which usually subside within days or weeks, and the development of gallstones. Gallstones usually remain silent owing to the inhibition of gallbladder motility by the drug. However, complications may arise, when octreotide is discontinued, necessitating in some cases acute cholecystectomy *(264)*. Gallbladder hypermotility has been described to occur within 24–96 h after cessation of octreotide therapy. Therefore, a drug-free period each week has been proposed for patients on chronic octreotide therapy in order to flush the gallbladder from sludge *(265,266)*. However, GH concentrations also rise after cessation of octreotide *(251)*, although this may occur more slowly than the restoration of gallbladder motility. The development of gallstones can be prevented and existing cholesterol gallstones can be dissolved with cheno/ursodeoxycholic acid preparations *(267,268)*. Long-term octreotide treatment also predisposes to chronic gastritis *(251,269,270)* and vitamin B-12 deficiency *(269)*. Reversible loss of scalp hair in four of seven women has been described during long-term octreotide treatment in a single report *(271)*. Antibody formation against octreotide has been detected in a few patients, but does not seem to diminish the GH-suppressive effect of the drug *(272–274)*.

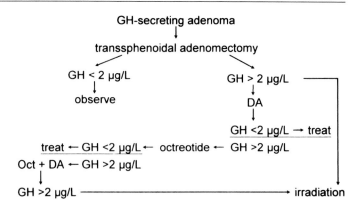

Figure 17-6   Treatment scheme for acromegaly. Simplified treatment scheme for acromegaly. Individual treatment choices depend on additional considerations (e.g., age, risk factors for surgery, patient's preferences, and so forth). A GH value of 2 µg/L (others use 2.5 µg/L) indicates "normalization of GH concentration" and, hence, no need for further treatment. It does not assure "cure of disease." For details, *see text.*

COMBINATION TREATMENT   When octreotide treatment alone fails to normalize the GH concentration, combination of octreotide and bromocriptine (or probably any other dopamine agonist drug) has been suggested to give more favorable results in some patients. When either 50 µg of octreotide, 2.5 mg bromocriptine, or a combination of both drugs was given acutely to acromegalic patients, the combination was slightly, but significantly better than either drug alone to suppress GH *(275)*. This was also seen in a subacute study on 12 patients in which octreotide alone (200 µ twice daily) was compared with bromocriptine alone (5 mg twice daily) and the combination of both drugs *(276)*. However, in a third study, when treatment conditions more closely resembled the pattern usually applied in clinical practice (octreotide 3×100 µg/d plus bromocriptine 2×5 mg/d), no difference was found between the two regimens *(277)*. Thus, the value of combination therapy as compared with octreotide alone is at present uncertain and marginal at best. A schematic outline of the decision tree for the treatment of a patient with acromegaly is shown in Figure 6.

GROWTH HORMONE RECEPTOR ANTAGONIST   A growth hormone receptor antagonist, pegvisomant, has recently been developed by molecular engineering of the human growth hormone molecule. Eight amino acid substitutions at the first binding site increase its affinity to the receptor and one amino acid substitution at the second binding site abolishes binding to a second receptor. In normal subjects the antagonist lowered serum IGF-1 concentrations in a 12 wk trial without causing a (rebound) GH increase *(22a)*. In 112 patients with acromegaly the antagonist normalized serum IGF-1 concentrations in almost 90% of the patients *(22b)*. Since IGF-1 exerts a negative feedback on the pituitary somatotroph, a GH increase and growth of the GH-secreting adenoma are potential unwanted effects (prior radiation therapy would probably prevent tumor regrowth). A significant, dose-dependent GH elevation did indeed occur. Although an increase in the size of the pituitary adenoma has recently been observed in one patient on long-term treatment *(277a)*, this antagonist will probably be a valuable additional tool in the spectrum of treatment strategies.

FOLLOW-UP   Patients with acromegaly who have been treated by surgery, irradiation, or who are under medical therapy must be followed regularly in order to determine treatment success, decide on secondary intervention, and rule out relapse or worsening of persisting disease. Following surgery, the patient should undergo evaluation similar to the preoperative scheme. An MRI must determine the completeness of the operation and also serves as a baseline for later checkups looking for possible recurrence. Pituitary function must be determined for hormonal substitution therapy to be inaugurated—or modified—should normal secretion be compromised. Diagnostic workup and criteria in the decision tree are similar to those used preoperatively. It is now suggested that GH deficiency also be treated by substitution therapy with recombinant human GH not only in children, but also in the adult *(278)*. The risks and benefits of such GH-replacement therapy for patients who previously had acromegaly have not been studied. Should it be inaugurated in such a patient, it must of course be controlled meticulously. Following irradiation therapy, lifelong care and control are mandatory in view of the slow development of anterior pituitary insufficiency. A word of caution is necessary not to dismiss any patient with acromegaly from continuing control. We have seen recurrence of the disease more than 10 yr after surgery and after irradiation treatment in patients who had postoperative or postirradiation GH concentrations below 1.0 µg/L.

REFERENCES

1. Alexander L, Appleton D, Hall R, Ross WM, Wilkinson R. Epidemiology of acromegaly in the Newcastle region. Clin Endocrinol 1980;12:71–79.
2. Bengtsson B-Å, Edén S, Ernest I, Odén A, Sjögren B. Epidemiology and long-term survival in acromegaly. Acta Med Scand 1988;223:327–335.
3. Ritchie CM, Atkinson AB, Kennedy AL, Lyons AR, Gordon DS, Fannin T, et al. Ascertainment and natural history of treated acromegaly in Northern Ireland. The Ulster Med J 1990;59:55–62.
4. Etxabe J, Gaztambide S, Latorre P, Vazquez JA. Acromegaly: An epidemiological study. J Endocrinol Invest 1993;16:181–187.
5. Quabbe H-J, Plöckinger U. Acromegaly: clinical findings and endocrinology. In: Landolt AM, Vance M-L, Reilly P, eds. Pituitary Adenomas—Biology, Diagnosis and Treatment. Churchill-Livingstone, Edinburgh, 1996, pp. 85–100.
6. Bates AS, Van't Hoff W, Jones JM, Clayton RN. An audit of outcome of treatment in acromegaly. Q J Med 1993;86:293–299.
7. Rajasoorya C, Holdaway IM, Wrightson P, Scott DJ, Ibbertson HK. Determinants of clinical outcome and survival in acromegaly. Clin Endocrinol 1994;41:95–102.
8. Bates AS, Van't Hoff W, Jones JM, Clayton RN. Does treatment of acromegaly affect life expectancy? Metabolism 1995;44 (Suppl 1):1–5.
9. Quabbe H-J, Schilling E, Helge H. Pattern of growth hormone secretion during a 24-h fast in normal adults. J Clin Endocrinol Metab 1966;26:1173–1177.
10. Takahashi Y, Kipnis DM, Daughaday WH. Growth hormone secretion during sleep. J Clin Invest 1968;47:2079–2090.
11. Baumann G, Amburn K, Shaw MA. The circulating growth hormone (GH)-binding protein complex: a major constituent of plasma GH in man. Endocrinology 1988;122:976–984.
12. Iranmanesh A, Grisso B, Veldhuis JD. Low basal and persistent pulsatile growth hormone secretion are revealed in normal and hyposomatotropic men studied with a new ultrasensitive chemiluminescence assay. J Clin Endocrinol Metab 1994;78:526–535.
13. Chapman IM, Hartman ML, Straume M, Johnson ML, Veldhuis JD, Thorner MO. Enhanced sensitivity growth hormone (GH) chemiluminescence assay reveals lower postglucose nadir GH concentrations in men than women. J Clin Endocrinol Metab 1994;78:1312–1319.
14. Veldhuis JD, Liem AY, South S, Weltman A, Weltman J, Clemmons DA, et al. Differential impact of age, sex steroid hormones, and obesity on basal versus pulsatile growth hormone secretion in men as assessed in an ultrasensitive chemiluminescence assay. J Clin Endocrinol Metab 1995;80:3209–3222.
15. Veldhuis JD. Gender differences in secretory activity of the human somatotropic (growth hormone) axis. Eur J Endocrinol 1996;134:287–295.
16. Pincus SM, Gevers EF, Robinson ICAF, Van Den Berg G, Roelfsema F, Hartman ML, et al. Females secrete growth hormone with more process irregularity than males in both humans and rats. Am J Physiol Endocrinol Metab 1996;270:E107–E115.
17. Quabbe H-J. Growth hormone. In: Lightman SL, Everitt BJ, eds. Neuroendocrinology. Blackwell, Oxford, 1986, pp. 409–449.
18. Ceda GP. IGFs in the feedback control of GH secretion: hypothalamic and/or pituitary action. J Endocrinol Invest 1995;18:734–737.
19. Strobl JS, Thomas MJ. Human growth hormone. Pharmacol Rev 1994;46:1–34.
20. Weil R. Pituitary growth hormone and intermediary metabolism. I. The hormonal effect on the metabolism of fat and carbohydrate. Acta Endocrinol (Copenh) 1965;49(Suppl 98):7–92.
21. Cunningham BC, Ultsch M, de Vos AM, Mulkerrin MG, Clauser KR, Wells JA. Dimerization of the extracellular domain of the human growth hormone receptor by a single hormone molecule. Science 1991;254:821–825.
22. Fuh G, Cunningham BC, Fukunaga R, Nagata S, Goeddel DV, Wells JA. Rational design of potent antagonists to the human growth hormone receptor. Science 1992;256:1677–1680.
22a. Thorner MO, Strasburger CJ, Wu Z, Straume M, Bidlingmaier M, Pezzoli SS, Zib K, Scarlett JC, Bennett WF. Growth hormone (GH) receptor blockade with a PEG-modified GH (B2036-PEG) lowers serum insulin-like growth factor-I but does not acutely stimulate serum GH. J Clin Endocrinol Metab 1999;84:2098–2103.
22b. Trainer PJ, Drake WM, Katznelson L, Freda PU, Herman-Bonert V, van der Lely AJ, Dimaraki EV, Stewart PM, Friend KE, Vance ML, Besser GM, Scarlett JA. Treatment of acromegaly with the growth hormone-receptor antagonist pegvisomant. New England Journal of Medicine 2000;342:1171–1177.
23. Hartman ML, Clayton PE, Johnson ME, Celniker A, Perlman AJ, Alberti KGMM, et al. A low dose euglycemic infusion of recombinant human insulin-like growth factor I rapidly suppresses fasting-enhanced pulsatile growth hormone secretion in humans. J Clin Invest 1993;91:2453–2462.
24. Bermann M, Jaffe CA, Tsai W, DeMott-Friberg R, Barkan AL. Negative feedback regulation of pulsatile growth hormone secretion by insulin-like growth factor I. Involvement of hypothalamic somatostatin. J Clin Invest 1994;94:138–145.
25. Isaksson OGP, Lindahl A, Nilsson A, Isgaard J. Mechanism of the stimulatory effect of growth hormone on longitudinal bone growth. Endocr Rev 1987;8:426–438.
26. Counts DR, Gwirtsman H, Carlsson LMS, Lesem M, Cutler Jr. GB. The effect of anorexia nervosa and refeeding on growth hormone-binding protein, the insulin-like growth factors (IGFs), and the IGF-binding proteins. J Clin Endocrinol Metab 1992;75:762–767.
27. Flyvbjerg A. Growth factors and diabetic complications. Diabetic Med 1990;7:387–389.
28. Ketelslegers JM, Maiter D, Maes M, Underwood LE, Thissen JP. Nutritional regulation of the growth hormone and insulin-like growth factor-binding proteins. Horm Res 1996;45:252–257.
29. Casanueva FF. Acromegaly. Physiology of growth hormone secretion and action. In: Melmed S, ed. Acromegaly, Endocrinology and Metabolism Clinics of North America. WB Saunders, Philadelphia, 1992, vol. 21, pp. 483–517.
30. Nabarro JDN. Acromegaly. Clin Endocrinol 1987;26:481–512.
31. Lobie PE, Breipohl W, Lincoln DT, García-Aragón J, Waters MJ. Localization of the growth hormone receptor/binding protein in skin. J Endocrinol 1990;126:467–472.
32. Hartman ML, Pincus SM, Johnson ML, Matthews DH, Faunt LM, Vance ML, et al. Enhanced basal and disorderly growth hormone secretion distinguish acromegalic from normal pulsatile growth hormone release. J Clin Invest 1994;94:1277–1288.

33. Ho KKY, Weissberger AJ. Characterization of 24-hour growth hormone secretion in acromegaly: implications for diagnosis and therapy. Clin Endocrinol 1994;41:75–83.

34. Ho PJ, Jaffe CA, Demott Friberg R, Chandler WF, Barkan AL. Persistence of rapid growth hormone (GH) pulsatility after successful removal of GH-producing pituitary tumors. J Clin Endocrinol Metab 1994;78:1403–1410.

35. Semer M, Faria ACS, Nery M, Salgado LR, Knoepfelmacher M, Wajchenberg BL, et al. Growth hormone pulsatility in active and cured acromegalic subjects. J Clin Endocrinol Metab 1995; 80:3767–3770.

36. Nishiyama K, Sugimoto T, Kaji H, Kanatani M, Kobayashi T, Chihara K. Stimulatory effect of growth hormone on bone resorption and osteoclast differentiation. Endocrinology 1996; 137:35–41.

37. Ezzat S, Melmed S, Endres D, Eyre DR, Singer FR. Biochemical assessment of bone formation and resorption in acromegaly. J Clin Endocrinol Metab 1993;76:1452–1457.

38. Piovesan A, Terzolo M, Reimondo G, Pia A, Codegone A, Osella G, et al. Biochemical markers of bone and collagen turnover in acromegaly or Cushing's Syndrome. Horm Metab Res 1994; 26:234–237.

39. Diamond T, Nery L, Posen S. Spinal and peripheral bone mineral densities in acromegaly: the effects of excess growth hormone and hypogonadism. Ann Intern Med 1989;111:567–573.

40. Haymovitz A, Horwith M. The miscible calcium pool in metabolic bone disease - in particular, acromegaly. J Clin Endocrinol Metab 1964;24:4–14.

41. Takamoto S, Tsuchiya H, Onishi T, Morimoto S, Imanaka S, Mori S, et al. Changes in calcium homeostasis in acromegaly treated by pituitary adenomectomy. J Clin Endocrinol Metab 1985;61:7–11.

42. Eskildsen PC, Lund Bj, Sorensen OH, Lund Bi, Bishop JE, Norman AW. Acromegaly and vitamin D metabolism: effect of bromocriptine treatment. J Clin Endocrinol Metab 1979;49: 484–486.

43. Lieberman SA, Björkengren AG, Hoffman AR. Rheumatologic and skeletal changes in acromegaly. In: Melmed S, ed. Acromegaly. Endocrinology and Metabolism Clinics of North America. WB Saunders, Philadelphia, 1992, vol. 21, pp. 615–631.

44. Molitch ME. Clinical manifestations of acromegaly. In: Melmed S, ed. Acromegaly, vol. 21, Endocrinology and Metabolism Clinics of North America. WB Saunders, Philadelphia, 1992, vol. 21, pp. 597–614.

44a. Kasagi K, Shimatsu A, Miyamoto S, Misaki T, Sakahara H, Konishi J. Goiter associated with acromegaly: Sonographic and scintigraphic findings of the thyroid gland. Thyroid 1999;9: 791–796.

45. Wright AD, Hill DM, Lowy C, Fraser TR. Mortality in acromegaly. Q J Med 1970;153:1–16.

46. Saccà L, Cittadini A, Fazio S. Growth hormone and the heart. Endocrine Reviews 1994;15:555–573.

47. Giustina A, Boni E, Romanelli G, Grassi V, Giustina G. Cardiopulmonary performance during exercise in acromegaly, and the effects of acute suppression of growth hormone hypersecretion with octreotide. Am J Cardiol 1995;75:1042–1047.

48. Fazio S, Cittadini A, Cuocolo A, Merola B, Sabatini D, Colao A, et al. Impaired cardiac performance is a distinct feature of uncomplicated acromegaly. J Clin Endocrinol Metab 1994;79:441–446.

49. Savage DD, Henry WL, Eastman RC, Borer JS, Gorden P. Echocardiographic assessment of cardiac anatomy and function in acromegalic patients. Am J Med 1979;67:823–829.

50. Cuocolo A, Nicolai E, Fazio S, Pace L, Maurea S, Cittadini A, et al. Impaired left ventricular diastolic filling in patients with acromegaly: Assessment with radionuclide angiography. J Nuclear Med 1995;36:196–201.

51. Terzolo M, Avonto L, Matrella C, Pozzi R, Luceri S, Borretta G, et al. Doppler echocardiographic patterns in patients with acromegaly. J Endocrinol Invest 1995;18:613–620.

52. Hirsch EZ, Sloman JG, Martin FIR. Cardiac function in acromegaly. Am J Med Sci 1969;257:1–8.

53. Kraatz C, Benker G, Weber F. Lüdecke D, Hirche H, Reinwein D. Acromegaly and hypertension: prevalence and relationship to the renin-angiotensin-aldosterone system. Klinische Wochenschrift 1990;68:583–587.

54. Ho KY, Weissberger AJ. The antinatriuretic action of biosynthetic human growth hormone in man involves activation of the renin-angiotensin system. Metabolism 1990;39:133–137.

55. Lim MJ, Barkan AL, Buda AJ. Rapid reduction of left ventricular hypertrophy in acromegaly after suppression of growth hormone hypersecretion. Ann Intern Med 1992;117:719–726.

56. Merola B, Cittadini A, Colao A, Ferone D, Fazio S, Sabatini D, et al. Chronic treatment with the somatostatin analog octreotide improves cardiac abnormalities in acromegaly. J Clin Endocrinol Metab 1993;77:790–793.

57. Lacka K, Piszczek I, Kosowicz J, Gembicki M. Echocardiographic abnormalities in acromegalic patients. Exp Clin Endocrinol 1988;91:212–216.

58. Lie TJ, Grossman SJ. Pathology of the heart in acromegaly: anatomic findings in 27 autopsied patients. Am Heart J 1980;100: 41–52.

59. Merola B, Sofia M, Longobardi S, Fazio S, Micco A, Esposito V, et al. Impairment of lung volumes and respiratory muscle strength in adult patients with growth hormone deficiency. Eur J Endocrinol 1995;133:680–685.

60. Cambrey AD, Kwon OJ, Gray AJ, Harrison NK, Yacoub M, Barnes PJ, Laurent GJ, et al. Insulin-like growth factor I is a major fibroblast mitogen produced by primary cultures of human airway epithelial cells. Clin Sci 1995;89:611–617.

61. Goldstein RH, Poliks CF, Pilch PF, Smith BD, Fine A. Stimulation of collagen formation by insulin and insulin-like growth factor I in cultures of human lung fibroblasts. Endocrinology 1989;124: 964–970.

62. Trotman-Dickenson B, Weetman AP, Hughes JMB. Upper airflow obstruction and pulmonary function in acromegaly: relationship to disease activity. Q J Med 1991;79:527–538.

63. Catnach SM, Anderson JV, Fairclough PD, Trembath RC, Wilson PAJ, Parker E, et al. Effect of octreotide on gall stone prevalence and gall bladder motility in acromegaly. Gut 1993;34:270–273.

64. Dullaart RPF, Meijer S, Marbach P, Sluiter WJ. Effect of a somatostatin analogue, octreotide, on renal haemodynamics and albuminuria in acromegalic patients. Eur J Clin Invest 1992;22: 494–502.

65. Hoogenberg K, Sluiter WJ, Dullaart RPF. Effect of growth hormone and insulin-like growth factor I on urinary albumin excretion: Studies in acromegaly and growth hormone deficiency. Acta Endocrinol (Copenh) 1993;129:151–157.

65a. Colao A, Marzullo P, Spiezia S, Ferone D, Giaccio A, Cerbone G, Pivonello R, Di Somma C, Lombardi G. Effect of growth hormone (GH) and insulin-like growth factor I on prostate diseases: An ultrasonographic and endocrine study in acromegaly, GH deficiency, and healthy subjects. J Clin Endocrinol Metab 1999;84: 1986–1991.

66. Lewis PD. Neuromuscular involvement in pituitary gigantism. Br Med J 1972;2:499–500.

67. Nagulesparen M, Trickey R, Davies MJ, Jenkins JS. Muscle changes in acromegaly. Br Med J 1976;2:914,915.

68. Prysor-Jones RA, Jenkins JS. Effect of excessive secretion of growth hormone on tissues of the rat, with particular reference to the heart and skeletal muscle. J Endocrinol 1980;85:75–82.

69. Wolf E, Wanke R, Schenck E, Hermanns W, Brem G. Effects of growth hormone overproduction on grip strength of transgenic mice. Eur J Endocrinol 1995;133:735–740.

70. Low PA, McLeod JG, Turtle JR, Donelly P, Wright RG. Peripheral neuropathy in acromegaly. Brain 1974;97:139–152.

71. Dinn JJ, Dinn EI. Natural history of acromegalic peripheral neuropathy. Q J Med 1985;224:833–842.

72. Jamal GA, Kerr DJ, McLellan AR, Weir AI, Davies DL. Generalized peripheral nerve dysfunction in acromegaly: a study by conventional and novel neurophysiological techniques. J Neurol, Neurosurg, Psychiatry 1987;50:886–894.

73. Åström C, Christensen L, Gjerris F, Trojaborg W. Sleep in acromegaly before and after treatment with adenomectomy. Neuroendocrinology 1991;53:328–331.

74. Pelttari L, Polo O, Rauhala E, Vuoriluoto J, Aitasalo K, Hyyppä MT, et al. Nocturnal breathing abnormalities in acromegaly after adenomectomy. Clin Endocrinol 1995;43:175–182.

75. Grunstein RR, Ho KY, Sullivan CE. Sleep apnea in acromegaly. Ann Intern Med 1991;115:527–532.

75a. Rosenow F, Reuter S, Deuss U, Szelies B, Hilgers RD, Winkelmann W, Heiss WD. Sleep apnoea in treated acromegaly: Relative frequency and predisposing factors. Clin Endocrinol 1996;45:563–569.

76. Kern W, Halder R, Al-Reda S, Späth-Schwalbe E, Fehm HL, Born J. Systemic growth hormone does not affect human sleep. J Clin Endocrinol Metab 1993;76:1428–1432.

77. Ezzat S. Living with acromegaly. In: Melmed S, ed. Acromegaly, vol. 21, Endocrinology and Metabolism Clinics of North America. WB Saunders, Philadelphia, 1992, vol. 21, pp. 753–760.

78. Martin JB. Plasma growth hormone (GH) response to hypothalamic or extrahypothalamic electrical stimulation. Endocrinology 1972;91:107–115.

79. Koibuchi N, Kagegawa T, Suzuki M. Electrical stimulation of the basolateral amygdala elicits only growth hormone secretion among six anterior pituitary hormones in the pentobarbital-anesthetized male rat. J Neuroendocrinol 1991;3:685–687.

80. Burton KA, Kabigting EB, Clifton DK, Steiner RA. Growth hormone receptor messenger ribonucleic acid distribution in the adult male rat brain and its colocalization in hypothalamic somatostatin neurons. Endocrinology 1992;131:958–963.

81. Gelato MC. Growth hormone-insulinlike growth factor I and immune function. Trends Endocrinol Metab 1993;4:106–110.

82. Auernhammer CJ, Strasburger CJ. Effects of growth hormone and insulin-like growth factor I on the immune system. Eur J Endocrinol 1995;133:635–645.

83. Fornari MC, Palacios MF, Diez RA, Intebi AD. Decreased chemotaxis of neutrophils in acromegaly and hyperprolactinemia. Eur J Endocrinol 1994;130:463–468.

84. Kotzmann H, Köller M, Czernin S, Clodi M, Svoboda T, Riedl M, et al. Effect of elevated growth hormone concentrations on the phenotype and functions of human lymphocytes and natural killer cells. Neuroendocrinology 1994;60:618–625.

85. Daughaday WH. Pituitary gigantism. In: Melmed S, ed. Acromegaly, Endocrinology and Metabolism Clinics of North America. WB Saunders, Philadelphia, 1992, vol. 21, pp. 633–647.

86. Zimmerman D, Young WF Jr, Ebersold MJ, Scheithauer BW, Kovacs K, Horvath E, et al. Congenital gigantism due to growth hormone-releasing hormone excess and pituitary hyperplasia with adenomatous transformation. J Clin Endocrinol Metab 1993;76:216–222.

87. Matsuno A, Teramoto A, Yamada S, Kitanaka S, Tanaka T, Sanno N, et al. Gigantism in sibling unrelated to multiple endocrine neoplasia: case report. Neurosurgery 1994;35:952–956.

88. Jennings AM, Robinson A, Kandler RH, Betts RP, Ryder REJ, Cullen DR. Severe peripheral neuropathy and elevated plantar pressures causing foot ulceration in pituitary gigantism. Clin Endocrinol 1993;39:113–118.

89. Foss MC, Saad MJA, Paccola GMGF, Paula FJA, Piccinato CE, Moreira AC. Peripheral glucose metabolism in acromegaly. J Clin Endocrinol Metab 1991;72:1048–1053.

90. Møller N, Schmitz O, Jørgensen JOL, Astrup J, Bak JF, Christensen SE, et al. Basal- and insulin-stimulated substrate metabolism in patients with active acromegaly before and after adenomectomy. J Clin Endocrinol Metab 1992;74:1012–1019.

91. O'Sullivan AJ, Kelly JJ, Hoffman DM, Baxter RC, Ho KKY. Energy metabolism and substrate oxidation in acromegaly. J Clin Endocrinol Metab 1995;80:486–491.

91a. Miyakawa M, Tsushima T, Murakami H, Isozaki O, Demura H, Tanaka T. Effect of growth hormone (GH) on serum concentrations of leptin: Study in patients with acromegaly and GH deficiency. J Clin Endocrinol Metab 1998;83:3476–3479.

91b. Damjanovic SS, Petakov MS, Raicevic S, Micic D, Marinkovic J, Dieguez C, Casanueva FF, Popovic V. Serum leptin levels in patients with acromegaly before and after correction of hypersomatotropism by trans-sphenoidal surgery. J Clin Endocrinol Metab 2000;85:147–154.

92. Fryburg DA, Gelfand RA, Barrett EJ. Growth hormone acutely stimulates forearm muscle protein synthesis in normal humans. Am J Physiol 1991;260:E499–E504.

93. Del Barrio AS, Martínez JA, Larralde J. Homeorhetic actions on tissue protein metabolism after the administration of rat growth hormone to normal rats. Endocr Res 1993;19:163–173.

94. Russell-Jones DL, Weissberger AJ, Bowes SB, Kelly JM, Thomason M, Umpleby AM, et al. The effects of growth hormone on protein metabolism in adult growth hormone deficient patients. Clin Endocrinol 1993;38:427–431.

95. Salomon F, Cuneo RC, Hesp R, Morris JF, Poston L, Sönksen PH. Basal metabolic rate in adults with growth hormone deficiency and in patients with acromegaly: relationship with lean body mass, plasma insulin level and leucocyte sodium pump activity. Clin Sci 1992;83:325–330.

96. Ezzat S, Melmed S. Are patients with acromegaly at increased risk for neoplasia? J Clin Endocrinol Metab 1991;72:245–249.

96a. Cheung NW, Boyages SC. Increased incidence of neoplasia in females with acromegaly. Clin Endocrinol 1997;47:323–327.

96b. Renehan AG, O'Dwyer ST, Shalet SM. Colorectal neoplasia in acromegaly: The reported increased prevalence is overestimated. Gut 2000;46:440.

97. Klein I. Acromegaly and cancer. Ann Intern Med 1984;101:706,707.

98. Brunner JE, Johnson CC, Zafar S, Peterson EL, Brunner JF, Mellinger RC. Colon cancer and polyps in acromegaly: increased risk associated with family history of colon cancer. Clin Endocrinol 1990;32:65–71.

99. Vasen HFA, van Erpecum KJ, Roelfsema F, Raue F, Koppeschaar H, Griffioen G, et al. Increased prevalence of colonic adenomas in patients with acromegaly. Eur J Endocrinol 1994;131:235–237.

100. Delhougne B, Deneux C, Abs R, Chanson P, Fierens H, Laurent-Puig P, et al. The prevalence of colonic polyps in acromegaly: a colonoscopic and pathological study in 103 patients. J Clin Endocrinol Metab 1995;80:3223–3226.

100a. Terzolo M, Boccuzzi A. The prevalence of colonic polyps in acromegaly: A colonoscopic and pathological study in 103 patients. J Clin Endocrinol Metab 1996;81:2406,2407.

100b. Jenkins PJ, Fairclough PD, Richards T, Lowe DG, Monson J, Grossman A, Wass JAH, Besser M. Acromegaly, colonic polyps and carcinoma. Clin Endocrinol 1997;47:17–22.

100c. Orme SM, McNally RJQ, Cartwright RA, Belchetz PE. Mortality and cancer incidence in acromegaly: A retrospective cohort study. J Clin Endocrinol Metab 1998;83:2730–2734.

101. Ituarte EA, Petrini J, Hershman JM. Acromegaly and colon cancer. Ann Intern Med 1984;101:627,628.

102. Leavitt J, Klein I, Kendricks F, Gavaler J, VanThiel DH. Skin tags: a cutaneous marker for colonic polyps. Ann Intern Med 1983;98:928–930.

103. Klein I, Parveen G, Gavaler JS, Vanthiel DH. Colonic polyps in patients with acromegaly. Ann Intern Med 1982;97:27–30.

104. Ezzat S, Strom C, Melmed S. Colon polyps in acromegaly. Ann Intern Med 1991;114:754,755.

105. Ortego J, Vega B, Sampedro J, Escalada J, Boixeda D, Varela C. Neoplastic colonic polyps in acromegaly. Horm Metab Res 1994;26:609,610.

106. Barzilay J, Heatley GJ, Cushing GW. Benign and malignant tumors in patients with acromegaly. Arch Intern Med 1991;151:1629–1632.

107. Ron E, Gridley G, Hrubec Z, Page W, Arora S, Fraumeni JF Jr. Acromegaly and gastrointestinal cancer. Cancer 1991;68:1673–1677.

108. Terzolo M, Tappero G, Borretta G, Asnaghi G, Pia A, Reimondo G, et al. High prevalence of colonic polyps in patients with acromegaly. Arch Intern Med 1994;154:1272–1276.

109. Ladas SD, Thalassinos NC, Ioannides G, Raptis SA. Does acromegaly really predispose to an increased prevalence of gastrointestinal tumours? Clin Endocrinol 1994;41:597–601.

110. Losa M, Wolfram G, Mojto J, Schopohl J, Spiess Y, Huber R, et al. Presence of growth hormone-releasing hormone-like immunoreactivity in human tumors: characterization and immunological and biological properties. J Clin Endocrinol Metab 1990;70: 62–68.

111. Faglia G, Arosio M, Bazzoni N. Ectopic acromegaly. In: Melmed S, ed. Acromegaly, Endocrinology and Metabolism Clinics of North America. WB Saunders, Philadelphia, 1992, vol. 21, pp. 575–595.

112. Barkan A L, Shenker Y, Grekin R J, Vale W W, LLoyd R V, Beals T F. Acromegaly due to ectopic growth hormone (GH)-releasing hormone (GHRH) production: Dynamic studies of GH and ectopic GHRH secretion. J Clin Endocrinol Metab 1986;63:1057–1064.

113. Melmed S, Ziel FH, Braunstein GD, Downs T, Frohman LA. Medical management of acromegaly due to ectopic production of growth hormone-releasing hormone by a carcinoid tumor. J Clin Endocrinol Metab 1988;67:395–399.

114. Thorner MO, Frohman LA, Leong DA, Thominet J, Downs T, Hellmann P, et al. Extrahypothalamic growth-hormone-releasing factor (GRF) secretion is a rare cause of acromegaly: plasma GRH levels in 177 acromegalic patients. J Clin Endocrinol Metab 1984;59:846–849.

115. Asa SL, Kovacs K. Pituitary pathology in acromegaly. In: Melmed S, ed. Acromegaly. Endocrinology and Metabolism Clinics of North America. WB Saunders, Philadelphia, 1992, vol. 21, pp. 553–574.

116. Ezzat S, Asa SL, Stefaneanu L, Whittom R, Smyth HS, Horvath E, et al. Somatotroph hyperplasia without pituitary adenoma associated with a long standing growth hormone-releasing hormone-producing bronchial carcinoid. J Clin Endocrinol Metab 1994;78: 555–560.

117. Scheithauer BW, Kovacs K, Randall RV, Horvath E, Okazaki H, Laws ER Jr. Hypothalamic neuronal hamartoma and adenohypophyseal neuronal choristoma: their association with growth hormone adenoma of the pituitary gland. J Neuropathol Exp Neurol 1983;42:648–663.

118. Asa SL, Scheithauer BW, Bilbao JM, Horvath E, Ryan N, Kovacs K, et al. A case for hypothalamic acromegaly: a clinicopathological study of six patients with hypothalamic gangliocytomas producing growth hormone-releasing factor. J Clin Endocrinol Metab 1984;58:796–803.

119. Saeger W, Puchner MJA, Lüdecke DK. Combined sellar gangliocytoma and pituitary adenoma in acromegaly or Cushing's disease. A report of 3 cases. Virchows Arch Int J Pathol 1994;425:93–99.

120. Puchner MJA, Lüdecke DK, Saeger W, Riedel M, Asa SL. Gangliocytomas of the sellar region—a review. Exp Clin Endocrinol 1995;103:129–149.

121. Horvath E, Kovacs K, Scheithauer BW, Lloyd RV, Smyth HS. Pituitary adenoma with neuronal choristoma (PANCH): composite lesion or lineage infidelity? Ultrastruct Pathol 1994;18:565–574.

122. Roth KA, Wilson DM, Eberwine J, Dorin RI, Kovacs K, Bensch KG, et al. Acromegaly and phaeochromocytoma: a multiple endocrine syndrome caused by a plurihormonal adrenal medullary tumor. J Clin Endocrinol Metab 1986;63:1421–1426.

123. Saito H, Sano T, Yamasaki R, Mitsuhashi S, Hosoi E, Saito S. Demonstration of biological activity of a growth hormone-releasing hormone-like substance produced by a pheochromocytoma. Acta Endocrinol (Copenh) 1993;129:246–250.

124. Bevan JS, Asa SL, Rossi ML, Esiri MM, Adams CBT, Burke CW. Intrasellar gangliocytoma containing gastrin and growth hormone-releasing hormone associated with a growth hormone-secreting pituitary adenoma. Clin Endocrinol 1989;30:213–224.

125. Genka S, Soeda H, Takahashi M, Katakami H, Sanno N, Osamura Y, et al. Acromegaly, diabetes insipidus, and visual loss caused by metastatic growth hormone-releasing hormone-producing malignant pancreatic endocrine tumor in the pituitary gland—Case report. J Neurosurg 1995;83:719–723.

126. Sano T, Asa SL, Kovacs K. Growth hormone-releasing hormone-producing tumors: clinical, biochemical, and morphological manifestations. Endocr Rev 1988;9:357–373.

127. Beck C, Burger HG. Evidence for the presence of immunoreactive growth hormone in cancers of the lung and stomach. Cancer 1972;30:75–79.

128. Melmed S, Ezrin C, Kovacs K, Goodman RS, Frohman LA. Acromegaly due to secretion of growth hormone by an ectopic pancreatic islet-cell tumor. N Engl J Med 1985;312:9–17.

128a. Beuschlein F, Strasburger CJ, Siegerstetter V, Moradpour D, Lichter P, Bidlingmaier M, Blum HE, Reincke M. Acromegaly caused by secretion of growth hormone by a Non-Hodgkin's lymphoma. New Engl J Med 2000;342:1871–1876.

129. Steiner H, Dahlbäck O, Waldenström J. Ectopic growth-hormone production and osteoarthropathy in carcinoma of the bronchus. Lancet i,1968;783–785.

130. Greenberg PB, Martin TJ, Beck C, Burger HG. Synthesis and release of human growth hormone from lung carcinoma in cell culture. The Lancet i,1972;350–352.

131. Pun KK, Chan G, Kung A, Lam K, Chan FL, Wang C. McCune-Albright syndrome with acromegaly. Horm Metab Res 1989;21: 527,528.

132. Chanson P, Dib A, Visot A, Derome PJ. McCune-Albright syndrome and acromegaly: clinical studies and responses to treatment in five cases. Eur J Endocrinol (Copenh.) 1994;131:229–234.

133. Weinstein LS, Shenker A, Gejman PV, Merino MJ, Friedman E, Spiegel AM. Activating mutations of the stimulatory G protein in the McCune-Albright syndrome. N Engl J Med 1991;325:1688–1695.

134. Spada A, Bassetti M, Gil-del-Alamo P, Saccomanno K, Lania A. Etiology of acromegaly: a molecular biological approach. Metabolism 1995;44(Suppl 1):31–33.

135. Brandi ML, Marx SJ, Aurbach GD, Fitzpatrick LA. Familial multiple endocrine neoplasia type I: a new look at pathophysiology. Endocr Rev 1987;8:391–405.

136. Pestell RG, Alford FP, Best JD. Familial acromegaly. Acta Endocrinologica (Copenh) 1989;121:286–289.

137. McCarthy MI, Noonan K, Wass JAH, Monson JP. Familial acromegaly: studies in three families. Clin Endocrinol 1990;32:719–728.

138. Benlian P, Giraud S, Lahlou N, Roger M, Blin C, Holler C, et al. Familial acromegaly: a specific clinical entity—further evidence from the genetic study of a three-generation family. Eur J Endocrinol 1995;133:451–456.

138a. Ackermann F, Krohn K, Windgassen M, Buchfelder M, Fahlbusch R, Paschke R. Acromegaly in a family without a mutation in the menin gene. Exp Clin Endocrinol Diabetes 1999;107:93–96.

139. Hartman ML, Veldhuis JD, Vance ML, Faria ACS, Furlanetto RW, Thorner MO. Somatotropin pulse frequency and basal concentrations are increased in acromegaly and are reduced by successful therapy. J Clin Endocrinol Metab 1990;70:1375–1384.

139a. Wass JAH. Growth hormone, insulin-like growth factor-I and its binding proteins in the follow-up of acromegaly. J Endocrinol 1997;155:517–519.

139b. Stoffel-Wagner B, Springer W, Bidlingmaier F, Klingmüller D. A comparison of different methods for diagnosing acromegaly. Clin Endocrinol 1997;46:531–537.

139c. Giustina A, Barkan A, Casanueva FF, Cavagnini F, Frohman L, Ho K, Veldhuis J, Wass J, von Werder K, Melmed S. Criteria for cure of acromegaly: A consensus statement. J Clin Endocrinol Metab 2000;85:526–529.

140. Barkan AL, Beitins IZ, Kelch RP. Plasma insulin-like growth factor-I/somatomedin-C in acromegaly: correlation with the degree of growth hormone hypersecretion. J Clin Endocrinol Metab 1988;67:69–73.

141. Ezzat S, Forster MJ, Berchtold P, Redelmeier DA, Boerlin V, Harris AG. Acromegaly. Clinical and biochemical features in 500 patients. Medicine 1994;73:233–240.

142. Fagin JA, Roberts CT Jr, Le Roith D, Brown AT. Coordinate decreases of tissue insulinlike growth factor I posttranscriptional alternative mRNA transcripts in diabetes mellitus. Diabetes 1989;38:428–434.

143. VandeHaar MJ, Moats-Staats BM, Davenport ML, Walker JL, Ketelslegers JM, Sharma BK, et al. Reduced serum concentrations of insulin-like growth factor-I (IGF-I) in protein-restricted growing rats are accompanied by reduced IGF-I mRNA levels in liver and skeletal muscle. J Endocrinol 1991;130:305–312.

144. LeRoith D, Roberts CT Jr. Insulin-like growth factors and their receptors in normal physiology and pathological states. J Pediat Endocrinol 1993;6:251–255.

145. Baxter RC, Martin JL. Radioimmunoassay of growth hormone-dependent insulinlike growth factor binding protein in human plasma. J Clin Invest 1986;78:1504–1512.

146. Blum WF, Ranke MB, Kietzmann K, Gauggel E, Zeisel HJ, Bierich JR. A specific radioimmunoassay for the growth hormone (GH)-dependent somatomedin-binding protein: its use for diagnosis of GH deficiency. J Clin Endocrinol Metab 1990;70:1292–1298.

147. Grinspoon S, Clemmons D, Swearingen B, Klibanski A. Serum insulin-like growth factor-binding protein-3 levels in the diagnosis of acromegaly. J Clin Endocrinol Metab 1995;80:927–932.

148. Clemmons DR, Thissen JP, Maes M, Ketelslegers JM, Underwood LE. Insulin-like growth factor-I (IGF-I) infusion into hypophysectomized or protein-deprived rats induces specific IGF-binding proteins in serum. Endocrinology 1989;125:2967–2972.

149. Sklar C, Sarafoglou K, Whittam E. Efficacy of insulin-like growth factor binding protein 3 in predicting the growth hormone response to provocative testing in children treated with cranial irradiation. Acta Endocrinol (Copenh) 1993;129:511–515.

150. Roelen CAM, Donker GH, Thijssen JHH, Koppeschaar HPF, Blankenstein MA. High affinity growth hormone binding protein in plasma of patients with acromegaly and the effect of octreotide treatment. Clin Endocrinol 1991;37:373–378.

151. Amit T, Ish-Shalom S, Glaser B, Youdim MBH, Hochberg Z. Growth-hormone-binding protein in patients with acromegaly. Horm Res 1992;37:205–211.

152. Kratzsch J, Blum WF, Ventz M, Selisko T, Birkenmeyer G, Keller E. Growth hormone-binding protein-related immunoreactivity in the serum of patients with acromegaly is regulated inversely by growth hormone concentration. Eur J Endocrinol 1995;132:306–312.

153. Haffner D, Schaefer F, Girard J, Ritz E, Mehis O. Metabolic clearance of recombinant human growth hormone in health and chronic renal failure. J Clin Invest 1994;93:1163–1171.

154. Hattori N, Kato Y, Murakami Y, Hashida S, Ishikawa E, Mohri Z, et al. Urinary growth hormone levels measured by ultrasensitive enzyme immunoassay in patients with renal insufficiency. J Clin Endocrinol Metab 1988;66:727–732.

155. Sukegawa I, Hizuka N, Takano K, Asakawa K, Horikawa R, Hashida S, et al. Urinary growth hormone (GH) measurements are useful for evaluating endogenous GH secretion. J Clin Endocrinol Metab 1988;66:1119–1123.

156. Hourd P, Edwards R. Current methods for the measurement of growth hormone in urine. Clin Endocrinol 1994;40:155–170.

157. Hattori N, Shimatsu A, Kato Y, Koshiyama H, Ishikawa Y, Tanoh T, et al. Urinary excretion of human growth hormone: daily variation and relationship with albumin and α_1-microglobulin in urine. Acta Endocrinol (Copenh) 1989;121:533–537.

158. Evans AJ, Willis DS, Wood PJ. The assay of urinary growth hormone in normal and acromegalic adults. Clin Endocrinol 1991;35:413–418.

159. Sukegawa I, Hizuka N, Takano K, Asakawa K, Horikawa R, Hashida S, et al. Measurement of nocturnal urinary growth hormone values. Acta Endocrinol (Copenh) 1989;121:290–296.

160. Winer LM, Shaw MA, Baumann G. Urinary growth hormone excretion rates in normal and acromegalic man: a critical appraisal of its potential clinical utility. J Endocrinol Invest 1989;12:461–467.

161. Lunt H, Tucker AJ, Bullen H, Gibbs C, Wilkin TJ. Overnight urinary growth hormone measurement in the diagnosis of acromegaly. Clin Endocrinol 1990;33:205–212.

162. Fredstorp L, Werner S. Growth hormone and insulin-like growth factor-1 in blood and urine as response markers during treatment of acromegaly with octreotide: a double-blind placebo-controlled study. J Endocrinol Invest 1993;16:253–258.

163. Weissberger AJ, Ho KY, Stuart MC. Quantification of urinary growth hormone (GH) excretion by centrifugal ultrafiltration and radioimmunoassay: appraisal of the relationship between 24 h urinary GH and mean 24 h serum GH levels in normal and abnormal states of GH secretion. Clin Endocrinol 1989;30:687–698.

164. Main KM, Lindholm J, Vandeweghe M, Skakkebaek NE. Urinary growth hormone excretion in acromegaly: diagnostic value in mild disease activity. Acta Endocrinol (Copenh) 1993;129:409–413.

165. Thalange NKS, Gill MS, Gill L, Whatmore AJ, Addison GM, Price DA, et al. Infradian rhythms in urinary growth hormone excretion. J Clin Endocrinol Metab 1996;81:100–106.

166. Chang-DeMoranville BM, Jackson IMD. Diagnosis and endocrine testing in acromegaly. In: Melmed S, ed. Acromegaly, Endocrinology and Metabolism Clinics of North America. WB Saunders, Philadelphia, 1992, vol. 21, pp. 649–668.

167. Harvey S. Thyrotrophin-releasing hormone: a growth hormone-releasing factor. J Endocrinol 1990;125:345–358.

168. De Marinis L, Mancini A, Zuppi P, Anile C, Maira G. Paradoxical growth hormone response to thyrotropin-releasing hormone in acromegaly. Clinical correlations and prognostic value. Acta Endocrinol (Copenh) 1990;122:443–449.

169. Brockmeier SJ, Buchfelder M, Fahlbusch R. TRH/GnRH test in acromegaly—Long-term follow-up experience with successfully treated patients. Horm Metab Res 1993;25:275–277.

170. Quabbe H-J. Treatment of acromegaly by trans-sphenoidal operation, 90-yttrium implantation and bromocriptine: results in 230 patients. Clin Endocrinol 1982;16:107–119.

171. Watanobe H, Tamura T. Clinical significance of the growth hormone response to vasoactive intestinal peptide and gonadotropin-releasing hormone in acromegaly. Neuropeptides 1995;28:115–124.

172. Watanobe H, Sasaki S, Sone K, Takebe K. Paradoxical response of growth hormone to peptide histidine methionine in acromegaly: comparison with the effects of thyrotropin-releasing hormone and vasoactive intestinal peptide. J Clin Endocrinol Metab 1991;72:982–985.

173. Lawrence AM, Goldfine ID, Kirsteins L. Growth hormone dynamics in acromegaly. J Clin Endocrinol 1970;31:239–247.

174. Popovic V, Damjanovic S, Micic D, Manojlovic D, Micic J, Casanueva FF. Modulation by glucocorticoids of growth hormone secretion in patients with different pituitary tumors. Neuroendocrinology 1993;58:465–472.

175. Giustina A, Bresciani E, Bussi AR, Bollati A, Bonfanti C, Bugari G, et al. Characterization of the paradoxical growth hormone inhibitory effect of galanin in acromegaly. J Clin Endocrinol Metab 1995;80:1333–1340.

176. Sirota P, Gil-Ad I, Hermesh H, Munitz H, Laron Z, Weizman R. Growth hormone response to TRH in families multiply affected with schizophrenia. Biol Psychiatry 1992;31:1241–1244.

177. Faglia G, Paracchi A, Ferrari C, Beck-Peccoz P. Evaluation of the results of trans-sphenoidal surgery in acromegaly by assessment of the growth hormone response to thyrotrophin-releasing hormone. Clin Endocrinol 1978;8:373–380.

178. Osman IA, James RA, Chatterjee S, Mathias D, Kendall-Taylor P. Factors determining the long-term outcome of surgery for acromegaly. Q J Med 1994;87:617–623.

179. Smals AEM, Pieters GFFM, Smals AGH, Hermus ARMM, Benraad TJ, Kloppenborg PWC. Growth hormone responses to the releasing hormones GHRH and GnRH and the inhibitors somatostatin and bromocriptine in TRH-responsive and non-responsive acromegalics. Acta Endocrinol (Copenh) 1987;116:53–58.

180. Smals AEM, Pieters GFFM, Smals AGH, Hermus ARMM, Benraad TJ, Kloppenborg PWC. The higher the growth hormone response to growth hormone releasing hormone the lower the response to bromocriptine and thyrotrophin releasing hormone in acromegaly. Clin Endocrinol 1987;27:43–47.

181. Villabona CM, Soler J, Virgili N, Gómez JM, Montaña E, Navarro MA. Growth hormone response to thyrotropin-releasing hormone in acromegalic patients: reproducibility and dose-response study. Horm Res 1992;37:14–17.

182. Valentini U, Cimino A, Rotondi A, Rocca L, Pelizzari R, Giustina A, et al. Growth hormone response to thyrotropin releasing hormone and placebo in a group of insulin dependent diabetic patients. J Endocrinol Invest 1989;12:643–646.

183. Udeschini G, Cocchi D, Panerai AE, Gil-Ad I, Rossi GL, Chiodini PG, et al. Stimulation of growth hormone release by thyrotropin-releasing hormone in the hypophysectomized rat bearing an ectopic pituitary. Endocrinology 1976;98:807–814.

184. Le Dafniet M, Garnier P, Bression D, Brandi AM, Racadot J, Peillon F. Correlative studies between the presence of thyrotropin-releasing hormone (TRH) receptors and the in vitro stimulation of growth hormone (GH) secretion in human GH-secreting adenomas. Horm Metab Res 1985;17:476–479.

185. Wood SM, Ch'ng JLC, Adams EF, Webster JD, Joplin GF, Mashiter K, et al. Abnormalities of growth hormone release in response to human pancreatic growth hormone releasing factor (GRF (1-44) in acromegaly and hypopituitarism. Br Med J 1983;286:1687–1691.

186. Chiodini PG, Liuzzi A, Dallabonzana D, Oppizzi G, Verde GG. Changes in growth hormone (GH) secretion induced by human pancreatic GH releasing hormone-44 in acromegaly: a comparison with thyrotropin-releasing hormone and bromocriptine. J Clin Endocrinol Metab 1985;60:48–52.

187. Alster DK, Bowers CY, Jaffe CA, Ho PJ, Barkan AL. The growth hormone (GH) response to GH-releasing peptide (His-DTrp-Ala-Trp-DPhe-Lys-NH₂), GH-releasing hormone, and thyrotropin-releasing hormone in acromegaly. J Clin Endocrinol Metab 1993;77: 842–845.

188. Hanew K, Utsumi A, Sugawara A, Shimizu Y, Abe K. Enhanced GH responses to combined administration of GHRP and GHRH in patients with acromegaly. J Clin Endocrinol Metab 1994;78: 509–512.

189. Popovic V, Damjanovic S, Micic D, Petakov M, Dieguez C, Casanueva FF. Growth hormone (GH) secretion in active acromegaly after the combined administration of GH-releasing hormone and GH-releasing peptide-6. J Clin Endocrinol Metab 1994;79: 456–460.

190. Reubi JC, Heitz PU, Landolt AM. Visualization of somatostatin receptors and correlation with immunoreactive growth hormone and prolactin in human pituitary adenomas: evidence for different tumor subclasses. J Clin Endocrinol Metab 1987;65:65–73.

191. Faglia G, Bazzoni N, Spada A, Arosio M, Ambrosi B, Spinelli F, et al. In vivo detection of somatostatin receptors in patients with functionless pituitary adenomas by means of a radioiodinated analog of somatostatin ([¹²³I]SDZ 204-090). J Clin Endocrinol Metab 1991;73:850–856.

192. Ur E, Mather SJ, Bomanji J, Ellison D, Britton KE, Grossman AB, et al. Pituitary imaging using labeled somatostatin analogue in acromegaly. Clin Endocrinol 1992;36:147–150.

193. Krenning EP, Bakker WH, Kooij PPM, Breeman WAP, Oei HY, de Jong M, et al. Somatostatin receptor scintigraphy with Indium-111-DTPA-D-Phe-1-octreotide in man: metabolism, dosimetry and comparison with Iodine-123-Tyr-3-octreotide. J Nuclear Med 1992;33:652–658.

194. Plöckinger U, Reichel M, Fett U, Saeger W, Quabbe H-J. Preoperative octreotide treatment of growth hormone-secreting and clinically nonfunctioning pituitary macroadenomas: effect on tumor volume and lack of correlation with immunohistochemistry and somatostatin receptor scintigraphy. J Clin Endocrinol Metab 1994;79:1416–1423.

195. Krenning EP, Kwekkeboom DJ, Bakker WH, Breeman WAP, Kooij PPM, Oei HY, et al. Somatostatin receptor scintigraphy with [¹¹¹In-DTPA-D-Phe¹]- and [¹²³J-Tyr³]-octreotide: the Rotterdam experience with more than 1000 patients. Eur J Nuclear Med 1993;20:1–16.

196. Stolz B, Smith-Jones PM, Albert R, Reist H, Mäcke H, Bruns C. Biological characterisation of [⁶⁷Ga] or [⁶⁸Ga] labelled DFO-octreotide (SDZ 216-927) for PET studies of somatostatin receptor positive tumors. Horm Metabolic Res 1994;26:453–459.

197. Mäcke HR, Smith-Jones P, Maina T, Stolz B, Albert R, Bruns Ch, et al. New octreotide derivatives for in vivo targeting of somatostatin receptor-positive tumors for single photon emission computed tomography (SPECT) and positron emission tomography (PET). Horm Metab Res 1993;27:12–17.

198. Lastoria S, Colao A, Vergara E, Ferone D, Varrella P, Merola B, et al. Technetium-99m pentavalent dimercaptosuccinic acid imaging in patients with pituitary adenomas. Eur J Endocrinol 1995;133:38–47.

199. De Souza B, Brunetti A, Fulham MJ, Brooks RA, DeMichele D, Cook P, et al. Pituitary microadenomas: a PET study. Radiology 1990;177:39–44.

200. Bergström M, Muhr C, Lundberg PO, Långström B. PET as a tool in the clinical evaluation of pituitary adenomas. J Nuclear Med 1991;32:610–615.

201. Scillitani A, Dicembrino F, Di Fazio P, Paleani Vettori P, D´Angelo V, Scarabino T, et al. In vivo visualization of pituitary dopaminergic receptors by iodine-123 methoxybenzamide (IBZM) correlates with sensitivity to dopamine agonists in two patients with macroprolactinomas. J Clin Endocrinol Metab 1995;80: 2523–2525.

202. Lamberts SWJ, Klijn JGM, van Vroonhoven CCJ, Stefanko SZ, Liuzzi A. The role of prolactin in the inhibitory action of bromocriptine on growth hormone secretion in acromegaly. Acta Endocrinol (Copenh) 1983;103:446–450.

203. Nyquist P, Laws ER Jr, Elliott E. Novel features of tumors that secrete both growth hormone and prolactin in acromegaly. Neurosurgery 1994;35:179–184.

204. Malarkey WB, Kovacs K, O'Dorisio TM. Response of a GH- and TSH-secreting pituitary adenoma to a somatostatin analogue (SMS 201-995): evidence that GH and TSH coexist in the same cell and secretory granules. Neuroendocrinology 1989;49:267–274.

205. Wémeau JL, Dewailly D, Leroy R, D'Herbomez M, Mazzuca M, Decoulx M, et al. Long term treatment with the somatostatin analog SMS 201-995 in a patient with a thyrotropin- and growth hormone-secreting pituitary adenoma. J Clin Endocrinol Metab 1988;66:636–639.

206. Tallen G, Fehr S, Saeger W, Uhlig H, Lüdecke DK. Detection of growth hormone, prolactin and human β-chorionic gonadotropin mRNA in growth hormone-secreting pituitary adenomas and in prolactin-secreting pituitary adenomas by in situ hybridization using a non-isotopic detection method. Acta Endocrinol (Copenh) 1993;128:411–417.

207. Saeger W, Uhlig H, Bäz E, Fehr S, Lüdecke DK. In situ hybridization for different mRNA in GH-secreting and in inactive pituitary adenomas. Pathol Res Prac 1991;187:559–563.

208. Lamberts SWJ, Klijn JGM, van Vroonhoven CCJ, Stefanko SZ. Different responses of growth hormone secretion to guanfacine, bromocriptine, and thyrotropin-releasing hormone in acromegalic patients with pure growth hormone (GH)-containing and mixed GH/prolactin-containing pituitary adenomas. J Clin Endocrinol Metab 1985;60:1148–1153.

209. Bassetti M, Arosio M, Spada A, Brina M, Bazzoni N, Faglia G, et al. Growth hormone and prolactin secretion in acromegaly: correlations between hormonal dynamics and immunocytochemical findings. J Clin Endocrinol Metab 1988;67:1195–1204.

210. Steiner E, Math G, Knosp E, Mostbeck G, Kramer J, Herold CJ. MR-appearance of the pituitary gland before and after resection of pituitary macroadenomas. Clin Radiol 1994;49:524–530.

211. Vance ML. Hypopituitarism. N Engl J Med 1994;330:1651–1662.

212. Fahlbusch R, Honegger J, Buchfelder M. Surgical management of acromegaly. In: Melmed S, ed. Acromegaly. Endocrinology and Metabolism Clinics of North America. WB Saunders, Philadelphia, 1992, vol. 21, pp. 669–692.

213. Davis DH, Laws ER Jr, Ilstrup DM, Speed JK, Caruso M, Shaw EG, et al. Results of surgical treatment for growth hormone-secreting pituitary adenomas. J Neurosurg 1993;79:70–75.

213a. Swearingen B, Barker FI, Katznelson L, Biller BMK, Grinspoon S, Klibanski A, Moayeri N, Black PMCL, Zervas NT. Long-term mortality after transsphenoidal surgery and adjunctive therapy for acromegaly. J Clin Endocrinol Metab 1998;83:3419–3426.

213b. Sheaves R, Jenkins P, Blackburn P, Huneidi AH, Afshar F, Medbak S, Grossman AB, Besser GM, Was JAH. Outcome of transsphenoidal surgery for acromegaly using strict criteria for surgical cure. Clin Endocrinol 1996;45:407–413.

213c. Freda PU, Wardlaw SL, Post K. Long-term endocrinological follow-up evaluation in 115 patients who underwent transsphenoidal surgery for acromegaly. J Neurosurg 1998;89:353–358.

213d. Yamada S, Aiba T, Takada K, Ozawa Y, Shimizu T, Sawano S, Shishiba Y, Sano T. Retrospective analysis of long-term surgical results in acromegaly: Preoperative and postoperative factors predicting outcome. Clin Endocrinol 1996;45:291–298.

213e. Lissett CA, Peacey SR, Laing I, Tetlow L, Davis JRE, Shalet SM. The outcome of surgery for acromegaly: The need for a specialist pituitary surgeon for all types of growth hormone (GH) secreting adenomas. Clin Endocrinol 1998;49:653–657.

214. Quabbe H-J. Clinical aspects of growth hormone excess: achievements and problems. J Pediatr Endocrinol 1993;6:333–338.

215. Melmed S, Ho K, Klibanski A, Reichlin S, Thorner M. Recent advances in pathogenesis, diagnosis, and management of acromegaly. J Clin Endocrinol Metab 1995;80:3395–3402.

216. Levitt NS, Ratanjee BD, Abrahamson MJ. Do "so-called" normal growth hormone concentrations (2–5 μg/L) indicate cure in acromegaly? Horm Metab Res 1995;27:185–188.

216a. Freda PU, Post KD, Powell JS, Wardlaw SL. Evaluation of disease status with sensitive measures of growth hormone secretion in 60 postoperative patients with acromegaly. J Clin Endocrinol Metab 1998;83:3808–3816.

217. Hulting AL, Werner S, Wersäll J, Tribukait B, Anniko M. Normal growth hormone secretion is rare after microsurgical normalization of growth hormone levels in acromegaly. Acta Med Scand 1982;212:401–405.

218. Shi YF, Harris AG, Zhu XF, Deng JY. Clinical and biochemical effects of incremental doses of the long-acting somatostatin analogue SMS 201-995 in ten acromegalic patients. Clin Endocrinol 1990;32:695–705.

219. Stevenaert A, Beckers A. Presurgical octreotide treatment in acromegaly. Acta Endocrinol 1993;129(Suppl 1):18–20.

220. Lamberts SWJ, Reubi J-C, Krenning EP. Somatostatin analogs in the treatment of acromegaly. In: Melmed S, ed. Acromegaly. Endocrinology and Metabolism Clinics of North America, WB Saunders, Philadelphia, 1992, vol. 21, pp. 737–752.

221. Ezzat S, Snyder PJ, Young WF, Boyajy LD, Newman C, Klibanski A, et al. Octreotide treatment of acromegaly. A randomized, multicenter study. Ann Intern Med 1992;117:711–718.

222. Lucas-Morante T, García-Uría J, Estrada J, Saucedo G, Cabello A, Alcaniz J, et al. Treatment of invasive growth hormone pituitary adenomas with long-acting somatostatin analog SMS 201-995 before transsphenoidal surgery. J Neurosurg 1994; 81:10–14.

223. Barkan AL, Lloyd RV, Chandler WF, Hatfield MK, Gebarski SS, Kelch RP, et al. Preoperative treatment of acromegaly with long-acting somatostatin analog SMS 201-995: shrinkage of invasive pituitary macroadenomas and improved surgical remission rate. J Clin Endocrinol Metab 1988;67:1040–1048.

223a. Colao A, Ferone D, Cappabianca P, De CM, Marzullo P, Monticelli A, Alfieri A, Merola B, Cali A, De DE, Lombardi G. Effect of octreotide pretreatment on surgical outcome in acromegaly. J Clin Endocrinol Metab 1997;82:3308–3314.

223b. Wasko R, Ruchala M, Sawicka J, Kotwicka M, Liebert W, Sowinski J. Short-term pre-surgical treatment with somatostatin analogues, octreotide and lanreotide, in acromegaly. J Endocrinol Invest 1999;23:12–18.

224. Jaffe CA, Barkan AL. Treatment of acromegaly with dopamine agonists. In: Melmed S, ed. Acromegaly. Endocrinology and Metabolism Clinics of North America. WB Saunders, Philadelphia, 1992, pp. 713–735.

225. Eastman RC, Gorden P, Glatstein E, Roth J. Radiation therapy of acromegaly. In: Melmed S, ed. Acromegaly. Endocrinology and Metabolism Clinics of North America, WB Saunders, Philadelphia, 1992, vol. 21, pp. 693–712.

225a. Thalassinos NC, Tsagarakis S, Ioannides G, Tzavara I, Papavasiliou C. Megavoltage pituitary irradiation lowers but seldom leads to safe GH levels in acromegaly: A long-term follow-up study. Eur J Endocrinol 1998;138:160–163.

225b. Barkan AL, Halasz I, Dornfeld KJ, Jaffe CA, Friberg RD, Chandler WF, Sandler HM. Pituitary irradiation is ineffective in normalizing plasma insulin-like growth factor I in patients with acromegaly. J Clin Endocrinol Metab 1997;82:3187–3191.

225c. Landolt AM, Haller D, Lomax N, Scheib S, Schubiger O, Siegfried J, Wellis G. Stereotactic radiosurgery for recurrent surgically treated acromegaly: Comparison with fractionated radiotherapy. J Neurosurg 1998;88:1002–1008.

225d. Voges J, Sturm V, Deuss U, Traud C, Treuer H, Schlegel W, Winkelmann W, Müller RP, LINAC-radiosurgery (LINAC-RS) in pituitary adenomas – preliminary results. Acta Neurochir Suppl 1996;65:41–43.

225e. Morange-Ramos I, Regis J, Dufour H, Andrieu JM, Grisoli F, Jaquet P, Peragut JC. Gamma-knife surgery for secreting pituitary adenomas. Acta Neurochir 1998;140:437–443.

225f. Jackson IMD, Noren G. Role of gamma knife therapy in the management of pituitary tumors. In: Molitch ME, ed. Advances in the management of pituitary tumors. Endocrinology and Metabolism Clinics of North America, WB Saunders,Philadelphia 1999, vol. 28, pp. 133–142.

226. af Trampe E, Lundell G, Lax I, Werner S. External irradiation of growth hormone producing pituitary adenomas: prolactin as a marker of hypothalamic and pituitary effects. Int J Radiat Oncol Biol Phys 1991;20:655–660.

227. Ciccarelli E, Valetto MR, Vasario E, Avataneo T, Grottoli S, Camanni F. Hormonal and radiological effects of megavoltage radiotherapy in patients with growth hormone-secreting pituitary adenoma. J Endocrinol Invest 1993;16:565–572.

228. Zaugg M, Adaman O, Pescia R, Landolt AM. External irradiation of macroinvasive pituitary adenomas with telecobalt: a retrospective study with long-term follow-up in patients irradiated with doses mostly of between 40-45 Gy. Int J Radiat Oncol Biol Phys 1995;32:671–680.

229. Littley MD, Shalet SM, Beardwell CG, Ahmed SR, Applegate G, Sutton ML. Hypopituitarism following external radiotherapy for pituitary tumours in adults. Q J Med 1989;70:145–160.

230. Littley MD, Shalet SM, Beardwell CG, Robinson EL, Sutton ML. Radiation-induced hypopituitarism is dose-dependent. Clin Endocrinol 1989;31:363–373.

231. Littley MD, Shalet SM, Swindell R, Beardwell CG, Sutton ML. Low-dose pituitary irradiation for acromegaly. Clin Endocrinol 1990;32:261–270.

232. Thorén M, Rähn T, Guo WY, Werner S. Stereotactic radiosurgery with the cobalt-60 gamma unit in the treatment of growth hormone-producing pituitary tumors. Neurosurgery 1991;29:663–668.

233. Ganz JC. Gamma knife treatment of pituitary adenomas. Stereotactic Funct Neurosurg 1995;64(Suppl 1):3–10.

234. Liuzzi A, Chiodini PG, Botalla L, Cremascoli G, Silvestrini F. Inhibitory effect of L-DOPA on GH release in acromegalic patients. J Clin Endocrinol Metab 1972;35:941–943.

235. Chiodini PG, Liuzzi A, Botalla L, Cremascoli G, Silvestrini F. Inhibitory effect of dopaminergic stimulation on GH release in acromegaly. J Clin Endocrinol Metab 1974;38:200–206.

236. Plöckinger U, Quabbe H-J. Evaluation of a repeatable depot-bromocriptine preparation (Parlodel LAR®) for the treatment of acromegaly. J Endocrinol Invest 1991;14:943–948.

237. Jaspers C, Haase R, Pfingsten H, Benker G, Reinwein D. Long-term treatment of acromegalic patients with repeatable parenteral depot-bromocriptine. Clin Invest 1993;71:547–551.

238. Tsagarakis S, Tsiganou E, Tzavara I, Nikolou H, Thalassinos N. Effectiveness of a long-acting injectable form of bromocriptine in patients with prolactin and growth hormone secreting macroadenomas. Clin Endocrinol 1995;42:593–599.

239. Lombardi G, Colao A, Ferone D, Sarnacchiaro F, Marzullo P, Di Sarno A, et al. CV 205-502 treatment in therapy-resistant acromegalic patients. Eur J Endocrinol 1995;132:559–564.

240. Chiodini PG, Attanasio R, Cozzi R, Dallabonzana D, Oppizzi G, Orlandi P, et al. CV 205-502 in acromegaly. Acta Endocrinologica (Copenh) 1993;128:389–393.

240a. Colao A, Ferone D, Marzullo P, Di SA, Cerbone G, Sarnacchiaro F, Cirillo S, Merola B, Lombardi G. Effect of different dopaminergic agents in the treatment of acromegaly. J Clin Endocrinol Metab 1997;82:518–523.

240b. Abs R, Verhelst J, Maiter D, Van AK, Nobels F, Coolens JL, Mahler C, Beckers A. Cabergoline in the treatment of acromegaly: A study in 64 patients. J Clin Endocrinol. Metab 1998; 83:374–378.

240c. Cozzi R, Attanasio R, Barausse M, Dallabonzana D, Orlandi P, Da RN, Branca V, Oppizzi G, Gelli G. Cabergoline in acromegaly: A renewed role for dopamine agonist treatment? Eur J Endocrinol 1998;139:516–521.

241. Bauer W, Briner U, Doepfner W, Haller R, Huguenin R, Marbach P, et al. SMS 201-995: a very potent and selective octapeptide analogue of somatostatin with prolonged action. Life Sci 1982;31: 1133–1140.

242. Quabbe H-J, Plöckinger U. Dose–response study and long term effect of the somatostatin analog octreotide in patients with therapy-resistant acromegaly. J Clin Endocrinol Metab 1989; 68:873–881.

243. Christensen SE, Weeke J, Ørskov H, Moller N, Flyvbjerg A, Harris AG, et al. Continuous subcutaneous pump infusion of somatostatin analogue SMS 201-995 versus subcutaneous injection schedule in acromegalic patients. Clin Endocrinol 1987; 27:297–306.

244. Tauber JP, Babin Th, Tauber MT, Vigoni F, Bonafe A, Ducasse M, et al. Long term effects of continuous subcutaneous infusion of the somatostatin analog octreotide in the treatment of acromegaly. J Clin Endocrinol Metab 1989;68:917–924.

245. Harris AG, Kokoris SP, Ezzat S. Continuous versus intermittent subcutaneous infusion of octreotide in the treatment of acromegaly. J Clin Pharmacol 1995;35:59–71.

246. Fløgstad AK, Halse J, Haldorsen T, Lancranjan I, Marbach P, Bruns C, et al. Sandostatin LAR in acromegalic patients: a dose-range study. J Clin Endocrinol Metab 1995;80: 3601–3607.

247. Stewart PM, Kane KF, Stewart SE, Lancranjan I, Sheppard MC. Depot long-acting somatostatin analog (Sandostatin LAR) is an effective treatment for acromegaly. J Clin Endocrinol Metab 1995;80:3267–3272.

248. Kaal A, Frystyk J, Skjaerbaek C, Nielsen S, Jorgensen JOL, Bruns C, et al. Effects of intramuscular microsphere-encapsulated octreotide on serum growth hormone, insulin-like growth factors (IGFs), free IGFs, and IGF-binding proteins in acromegalic patients. Metabolism 1995;44(Suppl 1):6–14.

249. Caron P, Cogne M, Gusthiot-Joudet B, Wakim S, Catus F, Bayard F. Intramuscular injections of slow-release lanreotide (BIM 23014) in acromegalic patients previously treated with continuous subcutaneous infusion of octreotide (SMS 201-995). Eur J Endocrinol 1995;132:320–325.

249a. Al Maskari M, Gebbie J, Kendall-Taylor P. The effect of a new slow-release, long-acting somatostatin analogue, lanreotide, in acromegaly. Clin Endocrinol 1996;45:415–421.

249b. Giusti M, Ciccarelli E, Dallabonzana D, Delitala G, Faglia G, Liuzzi A, Gussoni G, Disem GG. Clinical results of long-term slow-release lanreotide treatment of acromegaly. Eur J Clin Invest 1997;27:277–284.

249c. Davies PH, Stewart SE, Lancranjan I, Sheppard MC, Stewart PM. Long-term therapy with long-acting octreotide (Sandostatin-LAR®) for the management of acromegaly. Clin Endocrinol 1998;48:311–316.

249d. Hunter SJ, Shaw JAM, Lee KO, Wood PJ, Atkinson AB, Bevan JS. Comparison of monthly intramuscular injections of Sandostatin LAR with multiple subcutaneous injections of octreotide in the treatment of acromegaly: Effects on growth hormone and other markers of growth hormone secretion. Clin Endocrinol 1999; 50:245–251.

249e. Newman CB, Melmed S, George A, Torigian D, Duhaney M, Snyder P, Young W, Klibanski A, Molitch ME, Gagel R, Sheeler L, Cook D, Malarkey W, Jackson I, Vance ML, Barkan A, Frohman L, Kleinberg DL. Octreotide as primary therapy for acromegaly. J Clin Endocrinol Metab 1998;83:3034–3040.

250. Newman CB, Melmed S, Snyder PJ, Young WF, Boyajy LD, Levy R, et al. Safety and efficacy of long term octreotide therapy of acromegaly: results of a multicenter trial in 103 patients—a clinical research center study. J Clin Endocrinol Metab 1995;80: 2768–2775.

251. Plöckinger U, Liehr R-M, Quabbe H-J. Octreotide long-term treatment of acromegaly: effect of drug withdrawal on serum growth hormone/insulin like growth factor-I concentrations and on serum gastrin/24-hour intragastric pH values. J Clin Endocrinol Metab 1993;77:157–162.

252. Melmed S. Consensus statement: benefits versus risks of medical therapy for acromegaly. Am J Med 1994;97:468–473.

253. Moller DE, Moses AC, Jones K, Thorner MO, Vance ML. Octreotide suppresses both growth hormone (GH) and GH-releasing hormone (GHRH) in acromegaly due to ectopic GHRH secretion. J Clin Endocrinol Metab 1989;68:499–504.

254. Hofland LJ, van Koetsveld PM, van Vroonhoven CCJ, Stefanko SZ, Lamberts SWJ. Heterogeneity of growth hormone (GH) release by individual pituitary adenoma cells from acromegalic patients, as determined by the reverse hemolytic plaque assay: effects of SMS 201-995, GH-releasing hormone and thyrotropin-releasing hormone. J Clin Endocrinol Metab 1989;68:613–620.

255. Andersen M, Hansen TB, Bollerslev J, Bjerre P, Schroder HD, Hagen C. Effect of 4 weeks of octreotide treatment on prolactin, thyroid stimulating hormone and thyroid hormones in acromegalic patients. A double blind placebo-controlled cross-over study. J Endocrinol Invest 1995;18:840–846.

256. Flyvbjerg A, Jørgensen KD, Marshall SM, Ørskov H. Inhibitory effect of octreotide on growth hormone-induced IGF-I generation and organ growth in hypophysectomized rats. Am J Physiol (Endocrinol Metab 23) 1991;260:E568–E574.

257. Ezzat S, Ren S-G, Braunstein GD, Melmed S. Octreotide stimulates insulin-like growth factor-binding protein-1: a potential pituitary-independent mechanism for drug action. J Clin Endocrinol Metab 1992;75:1459–1463.

258. De Herder WW, Uitterlinden P, Van der Lely A-J, Hofland LJ, Lamberts SWJ. Octreotide, but not bromocriptine, increases circulating insulin-like growth factor binding protein 1 levels in acromegaly. Eur J Endocrinol 1995;133:195–199.

259. Gulya K, Pelton JT, Hruby VJ, Yamamura HI. Cyclic somatostatin analogues with high affinity and selectivity toward mu opioid receptors. Life Sci 1986;38:2221–2229.

260. Williams G, Ball JA, Lawson RA, Joplin GF, Bloom SR, Maskill MR. Analgesic effect of somatostatin analogue (octreotide) in headache associated with pituitary tumours. Br Med J 1987;295: 247,248.

261. Lamberts SWJ, van der Lely AJ, de Herder WW, Hofland LJ. Octreotide. N Engl J Med 1996;334:246–254.

261a. Plöckinger U, Holst JJ, Messerschmidt D, Hopfenmüller W, Quabbe H-J. Octreotide suppresses the incretin glucagon-like peptide (7-36) amide in patients with acromegaly or clinically nonfunctioning pituitary tumors and in healthy subjects. Eur J Endocrinol 1999;140:538–544.

262. Koop BL, Harris AG, Ezzat S. Effect of octreotide on glucose tolerance in acromegaly. Eur J Endocrinol 1994;130:581–586.

263. Ho KKY, Jenkins AB, Furler SM, Borkman M, Chisholm DJ. Impact of octreotide, a long-acting somatostatin analogue, on glucose tolerance and insulin sensitivity in acromegaly. Endocrinology 1992;36:271–279.

264. James RA, Rhodes M, Rose P, Kendall-Taylor P. Biliary colic on abrupt withdrawal of octreotide. The Lancet 1991;338:1527.

265. Rhodes M, James RA, Bird M, Clayton B, Kendall-Taylor P, Lennard TWJ. Gallbladder function in acromegalic patients taking long-term octreotide: evidence of rebound hypermotility on cessation of treatment. Scand J Gastroenterol 1992;27:115–118.

266. Shi Y-F, Zhu X-F, Harris AG, Zhang J-X, Deng J-Y. Restoration of gallbladder contractility after withdrawal of long-term octreotide therapy in acromegalic patients. Acta Endocrinol (Copenh.) 1993;129:207–212.

267. Montini M, Gianola D, Pagani MD, Pedroncelli A, Caldara R, Gherardi F, et al. Cholelithiasis and acromegaly: therapeutic strategies. Clin Endocrinol 1994;40:401–406.

268. Hussaini SH, Pereira SP, Murphy GM, Kennedy C, Wass JAH, Besser GM, et al. Composition of gall bladder stones associated with octreotide: response to oral ursodeoxycholic acid. Gut 1995;36:126–132.

269. Plöckinger U, Dienemann D, Quabbe H-J. Gastrointestinal side-effects of octreotide during long term treatment of acromegaly. J Clin Endocrinol Metab 1990;71:1658–1662.

270. Anderson JV, Catnach S, Lowe DG, Fairclough PD, Besser GM, Wass JAH. Prevalence of gastritis in patients with acromegaly: untreated and during treatment with octreotide. Clin Endocrinol (Oxford) 1992;37:227–232.

270a. Plöckinger U, Perez-Canto A, Emde C, Liehr R-M, Hopfenmüller W, Quabbe H-J. Effect of the somatostatin analog octreotide on gastric mucosal function and histology during 3 months of preoperative treatment in patients with acromegaly. Eur J Endocrinol 1998;139:387–394.

271. Jönsson A, Manhem P. Octreotide and loss of scalp hair. Ann Intern Med 1991;115:913.

272. Kendall-Taylor P, Chatterjee S, White MC, Harris MM, Davidson K, Besser GM, et al. Octreotide. The Lancet ii,1989;859–860.

273. Kwekkeboom DJ, Assies J, Hofland LJ, Reubi JC, Lamberts SWJ, Krenning EP. A case of antibody formation against octreotide visualized with ^{111}In-octreotide scintigraphy. Clin Endocrinol 1993;39:239–243.

274. Ørskov H, Christensen SE, Weeke J, Kaal A, Harris AG. Effects of antibodies against octreotide in two patients with acromegaly. Clin Endocrinol 1991;34:395–398.

275. Wagenaar AH, Harris AG, van der Lely AJ, Lamberts SWJ. Dynamics of the acute effects of octreotide, bromocriptine and both drugs in combination on growth hormone secretion in acromegaly. Acta Endocrinol (Copenh) 1991;125:637–642.

276. Fløgstad AK, Halse J, Grass P, Abisch E, Djoseland O, Kutz K, et al. A comparison of octreotide, bromocriptine, or a combination of both drugs in acromegaly. J Clin Endocrinol Metab 1994;79:461–465.

277. Fredstorp L, Kutz K, Werner S. Treatment with octreotide and bromocriptine in patients with acromegaly: an open pharmacodynamic interaction study. Clin Endocrinol 1994;41:103–108.

277a. van der Lely AJ, Lamberts SWJ. GH antagonists. Acromegaly treatment consensus workshop. Monte Carlo, 23–25 May 2000, page 11 (abstract).

278. Cuneo RC, Salomon F, McGauley GA, Sönksen PH. The growth hormone deficiency syndrome in adults. Clin Endocrinol 1992;37:387–397.

18 Corticotroph Adenomas

Cushing's Disease and Nelson's Syndrome

JOAN C. LO, MD, J. BLAKE TYRRELL, MD, AND CHARLES B. WILSON, MD

CUSHING'S DISEASE

BACKGROUND In 1932, Harvey Cushing published a report of 12 cases in which he described the metabolic derangements associated with pituitary basophilic adenomas, characterizing the syndrome that was later to bear his name *(1)*. The term Cushing's syndrome refers to the clinical manifestations of glucocorticoid excess regardless of specific etiology, whereas Cushing's disease refers to those cases of Cushing's syndrome secondary to pituitary adrenocorticotropic hormone (ACTH) hypersecretion. In the adult population, Cushing's disease accounts for approx 70% of patients with endogenous Cushing's syndrome, whereas the remaining 30% are attributable to the ectopic ACTH syndrome and primary adrenal tumors *(2)*.

Cushing's disease generally presents between the second to sixth decade of life, with a peak incidence at 30–40 yr of age *(3)*. There is a clear female predominance, with an overall female to male ratio of 4:1, which increases to 8:1 at peak incidence *(3,4)*. Untreated Cushing's syndrome has an extremely poor prognosis, and historical observations indicate a 50% mortality rate at 5 yr *(5)*. Over the last 30 yr, however, significant advances in the diagnosis, therapy, and surgical management of Cushing's disease have dramatically improved patient outcome, leading to successful cure in the majority of cases.

ETIOLOGY AND PATHOGENESIS The etiology and pathogenesis of corticotroph adenomas will only be briefly discussed here, since this subject is covered more extensively in other chapters. Since Cushing's initial report, the etiology of Cushing's disease has been a subject of controversy. Over the last 30 years, there has been some debate concerning whether the primary defect is at the level of the hypothalamus or pituitary gland *(6,7)*. The former hypothesis postulates that hypothalamic dysfunction gives rise to excessive corticotropin-releasing hormone (CRH), which leads to chronic overstimulation of pituitary corticotrophs, resulting in hyperplasia and adenoma formation. This theory has been supported by the observation of corticotroph hyperplasia in a small subset of patients with Cushing's disease *(8)*. In rare cases, an ectopic source of CRH secretion has been found, substantiating the role of CRH in the development of Cushing's syndrome *(9–11)*. In addition, the response to treatment with centrally acting agents

cyproheptadine and sodium valproate, which diminish ACTH secretion in patients with Cushing's disease, is consistent with a hypothalamic etiology *(7,12)*. Current evidence, however, supports a primary pituitary defect in the pathogenesis of Cushing's disease for nearly all cases. The high curative rate of selective adenomectomy, with overall remission rates of 75–85%, provides strong evidence for a pituitary origin *(13)*. This theory is further strengthened by the observation of prolonged secondary hypoadrenalism following successful transsphenoidal resection with eventual recovery of normal corticotroph function *(14,15)*. Molecular studies indicate that these adenomas are monoclonal in nature, emphasizing that a genetic defect at the level of the pituitary plays a major role in tumorigenesis *(16–18)*.

CLINICAL AND LABORATORY FEATURES The clinical features of Cushing's disease are the result of glucocorticoid and androgen excess, and are often insidious in onset. The most common finding is obesity, with a central distribution, leading to fat accumulation in the face (moon faces), neck, trunk, and abdomen, with relative sparing of the limbs *(19,20)*. Dorsocervical (buffalo hump) and supraclavicular fat pad enlargement are also seen. Centripetal obesity can be documented by an elevated waist-to-hip circumference or central obesity index *(21,22)*. (Table 1 and Figure 1.)

The skin changes reflect connective tissue atrophy, leading to thin fragile skin, easy bruisability, and violaceous striae *(22a)*. Facial telangiectasia contributes to the facial plethora characteristic of these patients. Hirsutism frequently occurs with increased lanugo hair on the face and arms resulting from cortisol excess, whereas an increase in terminal hair reflects relative androgen excess. A variable degree of acne can also be seen, and is comedogenic in nature if androgen levels are increased. Recurrent superficial fungal infections are secondary to the immunosuppression caused by hypercortisolism. Acanthosis nigricans can be seen in some patients and is associated with the insulin resistance caused by glucocorticoid excess. Patients tend not to be hyperpigmented, since ACTH levels are often only mildly elevated, in contrast to those with ectopic ACTH hypersecretion.

Muscle weakness occurs in many patients, because cortisol is known to cause muscular atrophy. Proximal myopathy is characteristic, generally more prominent in the lower extremities, although all muscle fibers can be affected. Patients typically first note difficulty in climbing stairs and in more severe cases may have difficulty arising from a chair.

From: *Diagnosis and Management of Pituitary Tumors* (K. Thapar, K. Kovacs, B. W. Scheithauer, and R. V. Lloyd, eds.), ©Humana Press Inc., Totowa, NJ.

Table 1
Clinical Features of Cushing's Disease

Features	% Incidence
General	
Obesity	85
Hypertension	75
Headache	10
Skin	
Facial plethora	80
Hirsutism	75
Superficial fungal infections	50
Striae	50
Acne	35
Bruising	35
Hyperpigmentation	5
Neuropsychiatric	85
Gonadal dysfunction	
Menstrual disorders	75
Impotence/decreased libido	65
Musculoskeletal	
Osteopenia	80
Back pain	65
Weakness	50
Metabolic	
Glucose intolerance/diabetes	75/20
Kidney stones	15
Polyuria	10

From Findling JW, Aron DC, Tyrrell JB. Cushing's Disease. In: Imura H, ed. The Pituitary Gland. New York, Raven Press, 1985, pp. 441–446; with permission.

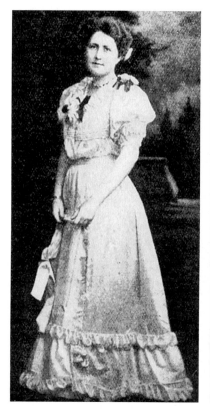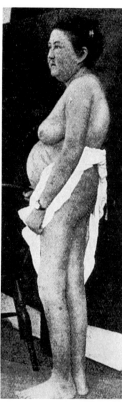

Figure 18-1 A patient from Cushing's initial series before (left) and 3 yr after (right) the development of clinical features. (From Cushing H. The basophil adenomas of the pituitary body and their clinical manifestations [pituitary basophilism]. Bull Johns Hopkins Hosp 1932;50:137–195, with permission of Johns Hopkins University Press.)

Diastolic hypertension occurs frequently, and cardiovascular compromise can develop with long-standing disease. Peripheral edema is occasionally seen and is believed to be secondary to mineralocorticoid excess, leading to salt retention and volume expansion. Hypokalemia and metabolic alkalosis, however, are infrequent, and if present, suggest the ectopic ACTH syndrome or an adrenal carcinoma.

Metabolic abnormalities are common in patients with Cushing's disease and occasionally are the presenting clinical features leading to diagnosis. Impaired glucose tolerance and hyperglycemia reflect hyperinsulinemia and increased insulin resistance from cortisol excess. Approximately 10% of these patients progress to frank diabetes. In the renal tubule, cortisol inhibition of calcium reabsorption leads to hypercalciuria, and an increased incidence of renal calculi is evident in patients with hypercortisolism. Glucocorticoid-induced osteopenia can also be seen with long-standing Cushing's disease and is associated with significant fracture risk.

A broad spectrum of psychiatric manifestations can be seen in Cushing's disease, which include emotional lability, irritability, anxiety, and depression. Occasionally, patients present with mania or acute psychosis. Cognitive deficits can be more subtle, with memory loss, poor concentration, and impaired mental ability.

Gonadal dysfunction is extremely common and is attributable to cortisol suppression of gonadotropin release, as well as androgen excess in females. Amenorrhea occurs in the majority of premenopausal patients and is usually associated with infertility *(20)*. In males, decreased libido, sexual dysfunction, and diminished testicular size are often evident.

Ophthalmologic complications in Cushing's disease include cataracts and glaucoma. The steroid-associated lens changes clas-sically lead to posterior subcapsular cataracts, although the exact pathogenesis is not fully known *(23)*. Chronic glucocorticoid excess also causes an increase in intraocular pressure and subsequent glaucoma.

Glucocorticoid-mediated hematologic changes include an elevation in white blood cell count, secondary to demargination and increased leukocyte release from the bone marrow. Lymphotoxic effects, however, lead to diminished numbers of lymphocytes, eosinophils, and monocytes. A relatively hypercoagulable state can also be seen, the mechanism of which is unclear, and thromboembolic complications are known to occur with a higher frequency in patients with Cushing's syndrome.

DIAGNOSIS AND TUMOR LOCALIZATION Biochemical confirmation of Cushing's disease is based on the establishment of cortisol excess secondary to pituitary ACTH hypersecretion. For the most part, ACTH-dependent hypercortisolism is easily established with current methods of cortisol measurement and highly sensitive immunoradiometric ACTH assays. Occasionally, however, equivocal results necessitate more extensive biochemical investigation. Once ACTH-dependent Cushing's syndrome has been confirmed, localizing the source of ACTH hypersecretion is often the greatest challenge. High-resolution pituitary magnetic resonance imaging (MRI) and especially accurate petrosal and cavernous sinus sampling have enhanced the ability to diagnose Cushing's disease considerably, and the diagnostic approach to Cushing's disease can now be much more direct. Generally, there is little need for extensive biochemical maneuvers.

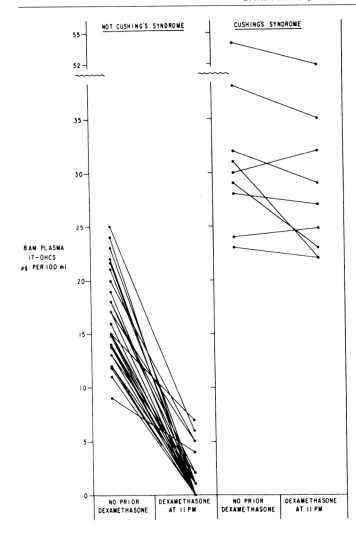

Figure 18-2 Plasma cortisol (8 AM plasma 17-OHCS) response to the low-dose overnight dexamethasone suppression test in control subjects and patients with Cushing's syndrome. (From Nugent CA, Nichols T, Tyler FH. Diagnosis of Cushing's syndrome. Arch Intern Med 1965;116:172–176, with permission, copyright 1965, American Medical Association.)

Diagnosis of Cushing's Syndrome The overnight low-dose dexamethasone suppression test (DST), which demonstrates autonomy of the hypothalamic–pituitary–adrenal (HPA) axis, is a convenient and reliable outpatient screening test for patients suspected of having Cushing's syndrome. Dexamethasone (1 mg) is administered orally at 11 PM, with plasma cortisol measurement the following morning at 8 AM to assess suppressibility of the HPA axis (24; Figure 2). In normal patients, plasma cortisol typically suppresses to <138 nmol/L (5 µg/dL), excluding the diagnosis of Cushing's syndrome in most cases (24,25). However, because false-negative results have been reported, many investigators recommend using a more stringent cortisol level of 50–70 nmol/L (1.8–2.5 µg/dL) or less (26,26a,26b). Using these criteria, the overnight low dose DST has a sensitivity greater than 95%, although the specificity may be as low as 88%. Individuals with Cushing's syndrome usually have plasma cortisol levels >275 nmol/L (10 µg/dL) following low-dose dexamethasone administration. False-positive results can be seen in patients with acute illness, depression, alcoholism, and extreme obesity, in which cortisol

secretion is increased, and high estrogen states in which corticosteroid binding globulin levels are raised. Lack of cortisol suppression may also be seen with administration of drugs that accelerate dexamethasone metabolism, such as phenytoin, phenobarbital, primidone, and rifampin. False-negative results are rare using the criteria of 50–70 nmol/L (1.8–2.5 µg/dL), but can occur in patients with episodic Cushing's syndrome or delayed clearance of dexamethasone.

Confirmation of hypercortisolism is established by documenting elevated 24-h urine free cortisol excretion, which is increased in over 90% of individuals with Cushing's syndrome (27–29). False-positive results may also be seen during acute illness, depression, and alcoholism. Although obesity and high estrogen states increase total cortisol levels and may lead to abnormal dexamethasone suppression, they do not affect urinary free cortisol excretion to a significant degree and are therefore the preferred approach in these situations. The current method of choice is measurement of urine free cortisol by HPLC, which is not interfered with by drugs, medications, or synthetic steroids other than cortisol (30). The normal range for this assay in most laboratories is 14–138 nmol/d (5–50 µg/d); patients with Cushing's syndrome usually have levels >276 nmol/d (100 µg/d) (28,29). Occasionally, multiple urine measurements will be needed if biochemistry does not corroborate clinical suspicion, and either incomplete urine collection or episodic Cushing's is suspected.

The biochemical diagnosis of Cushing's syndrome is established if both tests are abnormal, after excluding pertinent false positives. In patients with equivocal or borderline results, the 2-d low-dose DST (Liddle test) can be performed. Patients are given dexamethasone 0.5 mg orally every 6 h for 2 d, with measurement of urinary 17-hydroxycorticosteroids; levels >11 µmol/d (4 mg/d) or urine free cortisol >69 nmol/d (25 µg/d) are consistent with Cushing's syndrome (27,31). Some centers prefer measurement of plasma cortisol six hours after the last dose of dexamethasone; for instance, if the 2-d low dose DST is initiated at 0900 h, plasma cortisol is measured 48 h later at 0900 h (31a). Using a plasma cortisol criteria of 50 nmol/L (1.8 µg/dL) or less, the Liddle test has a sensitivity and specificity greater than 95% (26,31a,31b). Thus, it would appear that the 2-d low-dose DST is as sensitive as the 1 mg overnight low-dose DST and perhaps more specific. However, because the 2-d test can be cumbersome to perform accurately in the outpatient setting, its application in many centers is limited to those patients in whom the diagnosis is equivocal or borderline.

Late-night (2300 h) salivary cortisol measurement has recently been introduced as a simple and potentially reliable screening test for endogenous Cushing's syndrome (31b). Because salivary cortisol concentration is in equilibrium with free plasma cortisol, it is independent of salivary production rate, and patients need only chew on a cotton tube for a few minutes to obtain the sample (31c). In a preliminary study of 78 patients with suspected Cushing's syndrome (of whom 39 had proven Cushing's syndrome) and 73 normal subjects, a salivary cortisol greater than 3.6 nmol/L yielded a diagnostic sensitivity of 92% (31c). A single sleeping midnight plasma cortisol level > 50 nmol/L (1.8 µg/dL) under nonstressed conditions, in the absence of acute illness, and after hospitalization for 48 h has also been shown to have 100% sensitivity for the diagnosis of Cushing's syndrome; however, this approach would not be practical in the outpatient setting (31b).

Pseudo-Cushing States In some instances, it may be difficult to distinguish mild Cushing's syndrome from pseudo-Cushing

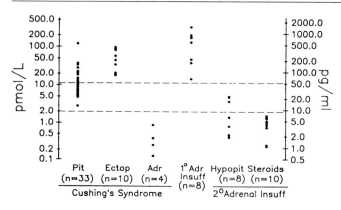

Figure 18-3 Plasma ACTH-IRMA (pmol/L or pg/mL) of patients with pituitary adrenal disorders. Dashed horizontal lines indicate normal range. (From Findling JW. Clinical application of a new immunoradiometric assay for ACTH. The Endocrinologist 1992; 2:360–365, with permission of Williams & Wilkins.)

states, as both are associated with hypercortisolism and incomplete dexamethasone suppressibility, although the latter condition is not associated with the development of Cushing's syndrome. Alcoholism, ethanol withdrawal, severe stress, illness, renal failure, anorexia nervosa, depression, glucocorticoid resistance, and severe obesity are among some of the conditions associated with the pseudo-Cushing's syndrome. In these situations, hypercortisolism presumably arises from increased hypothalamic secretion of CRH, which in Cushing's syndrome is suppressed *(32)*. In such cases where the suspicion for pseudo-Cushing's is high, the dexamethasone-CRH test has been proposed as a more accurate means to distinguish Cushing's syndrome from pseudo-Cushing's states and is particularly useful for identifying patients with Cushing's disease *(28,32)*. In patients with Cushing's syndrome, CRH administration following the 2-d low-dose DST leads to cortisol levels >38 nmol/L (1.4 µg/dL) when measured 15 min after CRH injection, reflecting diminished suppression by exogenous glucocorticoids *(32)*. In contrast, patients with pseudo-Cushing's states show reduced responsiveness to CRH, secondary to greater inhibition by dexamethasone. The dexamethasone-CRH test has been reported to achieve a diagnostic accuracy close to 100% when particularly sensitive cortisol assays are used *(32)* and can be helpful in cases where the diagnosis of pseudo-Cushing is unclear. A single midnight cortisol measurement >207 nmol/L (7.5 µg/dL) has also been used to differentiate Cushing's syndrome from pseudo-Cushing states with a sensitivity of 96% at 100% specificity *(32a)*.

Differential Diagnosis of Cushing's Syndrome *Establishing ACTH Dependency* Once the diagnosis of Cushing's syndrome has been established, the specific etiology must be determined. In particular, it is important to distinguish Cushing's syndrome caused by pituitary ACTH hypersecretion from ectopic ACTH secretion and primary adrenal tumors. Previously, ACTH radioimmunoassays were hampered by limited sensitivity and specificity, with lack of precision at the lower ranges of detection. However, current measurement of plasma ACTH using immunoradiometric assays (IRMA), which are highly sensitive and specific, allows reliable and accurate distinction of corticotropin-dependent and corticotropin-independent disorders *(28,33,33a;* Figure 3). A suppressed ACTH level <1.1 pmol/L (5 pg/mL) by IRMA is consistent with an ACTH-independent process, and in

these patients, adrenal imaging by computed tomography (CT) should be obtained to look for a primary adrenocortical tumor. Normal to elevated ACTH levels are consistent with ACTH-dependent hypercortisolism, and the differentiation of pituitary vs ectopic corticotropin hypersecretion should then be pursued. Generally, ectopic tumors tend to demonstrate more marked elevations in plasma ACTH, in contrast to levels more frequently seen with Cushing's disease, although much overlap exists. In the rare situation of low–normal ACTH levels of 1.1–2.2 pmol/L (5–10 pg/mL), the assay should be repeated with confirmation of ACTH dependency by dexamethasone testing and CRH stimulation, as described below. This should be followed by an adrenal CT to rule out a solitary adrenal tumor. In most cases, the CT will show bilateral nodularity or hyperplasia.

Biochemical Tests Distinguishing between pituitary ACTH hypersecretion and ectopic ACTH secretion continues to be a diagnostic challenge. Prior to the routine availability of MRI and petrosal sinus sampling, various diagnostic tests were designed based on the observation that ACTH-secreting adenomas were partially responsive to alterations in the HPA axis, in contrast to ectopic ACTH syndromes and primary adrenal tumors which generally were not.

The high-dose overnight DST, a convenient and reliable alternative to the standard 2-d high-dose (Liddle) test, involves the administration of dexamethasone (8 mg) orally at 11 PM, with measurement of plasma cortisol the following morning at 8–9 AM *(34,35)*. Most cases of Cushing's disease show cortisol suppression to <50% of baseline values, in contrast to patients with ectopic ACTH production and adrenocorticotropic tumors *(34,36)*. However, 10–20% of patients with Cushing's disease will fail to suppress with high-dose dexamethasone, whereas 50% of ACTH-secreting bronchial carcinoids will demonstrate cortisol suppression, and thus, the initially reported diagnostic accuracy of 93% can fall much lower when a greater number of patients with ACTH-secreting carcinoid tumors are included in the analysis *(37–39)*. Therefore, high-dose dexamethasone testing adds little to existing clinical information *(40)*, although it continues to be used by many clinicians in the workup of Cushing's disease.

The CRH stimulation test has also been used to distinguish corticotropin-producing pituitary adenomas from ectopic ACTH syndromes and primary adrenal tumors based on responsiveness of pituitary adenomas to CRH infusion, as measured by ACTH and cortisol increase. Differentiation may be difficult, however, since up to 10% of patients with Cushing's disease do not respond to CRH stimulation as expected, whereas a few ectopic ACTH-producing tumors do *(41–43)*. Modifications in the timing of ACTH and cortisol measurements with CRH stimulation may yield a diagnostic accuracy >90% *(42)*, although the need for precise methodology can be tedious and clinical experience remains limited. Moreover, interpretation of CRH responsiveness requires suppression of normal corticotroph function; therefore, the results may be biased by the degree of endogenous hypercortisolism at the time of study *(28,42)*. Desmopressin administration in conjunction with CRH may improve the discrimination of Cushing's disease, although further confirmatory studies need to be done *(44,45)*.

Metyrapone, an inhibitor of 11β-hydroxylase, has occasionally been used to identify individuals with Cushing's disease, based on the dramatic ACTH-mediated increase in 11-deoxycortisol seen in these patients when cortisol feedback is removed. Unfortunately, there is considerable overlap with ectopic ACTH tumors, which show some responsiveness to manipulations in the HPA axis, and thus the overall accuracy of the metyrapone test is low, ranging from 40 to 70% (46).

Various combinations of the high-dose DST, CRH stimulation test and the metyrapone test have been proposed to improve the sensitivity and specificity in differentiating pituitary from ectopic ACTH secretion (38,46,47). Although each successive biochemical test does contribute additional information, their overall diagnostic accuracy remains limited, even with the application of more stringent criteria. Furthermore, extensive evaluation can be tedious, and in many cases, the information obtained may be no better than the pretest probability of disease.

As discussed earlier, the authors currently recommend high-dose dexamethasone testing and CRH stimulation only in those cases where the diagnosis of ACTH dependency remains equivocal, as in the rare patient with low-normal ACTH values. These tests are less useful in differentiating eutopic from ectopic ACTH hypersecretion (48). In situations where ACTH dependency is clear and the pretest probability of Cushing's disease is >90%, further biochemical testing may be of marginal benefit. Therefore, the authors generally proceed directly to pituitary MRI for tumor localization. In patients with an equivocal or normal pituitary MRI, petrosal sinus sampling now provides the most direct and reliable method of establishing the diagnosis of Cushing's disease. Lack of a central to peripheral ACTH gradient should prompt a search for an ectopic corticotropin-producing tumor.

Tumor Localization *Pituitary Imaging* Over the last 30 years, pituitary imaging technology has changed dramatically, and MRI is now the primary imaging modality for detection of pituitary adenomas. Earlier methods of sellar visualization, which include skull radiography, hypocycloidal sellar tomography, and pneumoencephalography, were limited by poor anatomic detail, low sensitivity, and the inability to detect small adenomas, necessitating transsphenoidal pituitary exploration in patients suspected of having Cushing's disease. With the advent of CT, which provided thin-section images in the axial plane, the ability to visualize pituitary adenomas improved significantly. The sensitivity for pituitary CT detection of ACTH-producing microadenomas ranged from 30 to 58% in the reported series, whereas for macroadenomas, the detection rate was nearly 100% (49–51). These low sensitivities reflected the limited ability of CT to detect adenomas <4–6 mm in diameter. With the introduction of high-field (1.5 T) MRI, however, thin-section coronal T1-weighted images enhanced with gadolinium have been shown to provide superior resolution and detection of pituitary tumors. Current MRI series of ACTH-producing microadenomas report a sensitivity of 65–71% and specificity of 87–88% on precontrast studies, with the sensitivity increasing up to 70–75% postgadolinium injection for the detection of microadenomas as small as 2–3 mm (52–54). On immediate T1-weighted postcontrast images, the microadenoma generally appears hypointense with diminished gadolinium enhancement when compared to the normal surrounding pituitary. Overall detection rates of ACTH-secreting adenomas, however, are as low as 50% in some series, largely owing to the small size of these tumors (49,55).

The incidence of asymptomatic pituitary adenomas in the general population ranges from 3 to 27% in published autopsy series, with most of these lesions found to be microadenomas and over two-thirds <3 mm at pathologic examination (56,57). In current MRI series, the incidence of pituitary incidentalomas detected by MRI is estimated at 10% in the general population, and lesions range from 3 to 6 mm in diameter (58). Considering that the average diameter of an ACTH-secreting adenoma is 4–5 mm (4,59), it is conceivable that in a few rare cases, patients with the ectopic ACTH syndrome may inappropriately undergo pituitary microsurgery based on MRI findings of an incidentaloma. To address this potential issue, the authors recommend using a minimum diameter of 5 mm to define a distinct adenoma, since the majority of incidentalomas are <5 mm. In patients with a clinical presentation highly suggestive of Cushing's disease, who have documented hypercortisolism, a normal to elevated ACTH level, and a pituitary adenoma of at least 5 mm in diameter, transsphenoidal surgery with complete sellar exploration and selective adenomectomy is the procedure of choice. In the authors' experience, approx 50% of pituitary ACTH-secreting adenomas are localized in this way. The remaining patients with either normal to equivocal MRI scans (<5 mm) or those with presentations atypical for Cushing's disease (male sex, markedly elevated ACTH and cortisol levels, or hypokalemia) should undergo venous sampling to confirm a pituitary source before proceeding to surgery.

Venous Sampling The venous drainage from the anterior pituitary empties through plexiform networks into ipsilateral hypophyseal veins. These pituitary veins drain directly into the cavernous sinuses, trabeculated venous structures, which also receive tributaries from the ophthalmic veins, and the sphenoparietal sinus. The cavernous sinuses lie on both sides of the sphenoid body and are connected by various communicating channels, although there appears to be little intercavernous mixing (60). The cavernous sinus drains posteriorly into the inferior petrosal sinus, which ultimately becomes a vein as it exits the jugular foramen and joins the internal jugular vein. Bilateral venous sampling of the inferior petrosal or the cavernous sinuses allows accurate determination of pituitary ACTH hypersecretion and thus provides critical information in the diagnosis of Cushing's disease (Figure 4). Precise catheter positioning, sampling technique, and anatomical considerations, however, are crucial to avoid erroneous results (61,62). Complication rates are generally low in the hands of experienced radiologists, with a reported 0.2% incidence of major neurological complications (63). The most common complication is a groin hematoma at the site of venipuncture (3–4%), and patients often complain of a transient discomfort in the ear (61).

The role of inferior petrosal sinus sampling (IPSS) in the evaluation of Cushing's disease was first reported in 1977 (64), and has since become a critical diagnostic tool in confirming pituitary ACTH hypersecretion in situations where the MRI findings are normal or equivocal (65,66,66a; Figure 5). In early studies from experienced centers, simultaneous bilateral petrosal sinus sampling demonstrating a central (IPS) to peripheral (venous) gradient of >2:1 reportedly distinguished patients with Cushing's disease from ectopic ACTH secretion with a sensitivity of 95% and specificity of 100% (65,67), although somewhat lower sensitivity using basal IPS values has been reported in a recent series, likely attributable to the intermittent nature of ACTH hypersecretion in Cushing's disease (67a). In contrast, most patients with ectopic ACTH secretion have a gradient <1.6:1 (65,67,68). With administration of CRH at the time of sampling to augment central ACTH hypersecretion, the sensitivity for Cushing's disease exceeds 95%; hence, a basal or CRH-stimulated IPS to peripheral ACTH gradient greater than 2.0 or 3.0 will reliably indicate the presence of Cushing's disease (43,67,67a,68,68a). In rare cases

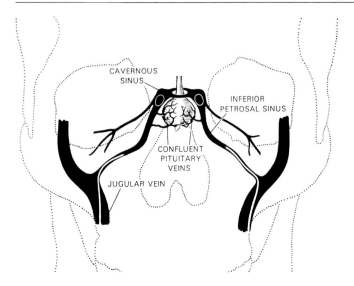

Figure 18-4 Catheter placement for bilateral simultaneous blood sampling of the inferior petrosal sinuses. Confluent pituitary veins empty laterally into the cavernous sinuses, which drain into the inferior petrosal sinuses. (From Oldfield EH, Chrousos GP, Schulte HM, et al. Preoperative lateralization of ACTH-secreting pituitary microadenomas by bilateral and simultaneous inferior petrosal venous sinus sampling. N Engl J Med 1985;312:100–103, with permission of the Massachusetts Medical Society. All rights reserved.)

(less than 1% of patients with surgically proven Cushing's disease), the presence of a hypoplastic inferior petrosal sinus will lead to a false-negative result with IPSS (68b).

Although the diagnostic accuracy of IPSS in the identification of pituitary ACTH hypersecretion is >95%, tumor lateralization based on sampling results is correct in only 50–70% of cases owing to variable patterns of venous drainage, which can lead to dilution and/or mixing (43,69,70). Furthermore, CRH stimulation does not significantly improve preoperative localization of pituitary microadenomas by IPSS (43,67,69,70). Presampling venography to delineate the cavernous to inferior petrosal sinus drainage pattern (designated as symmetric or asymmetric) was performed at one center and revealed that lateralizing data was correct in 86% of cases with symmetric venous drainage in contrast to 44% of patients with asymmetric drainage (69). Thus, venography data can significantly impact on the surgeon's decision to proceed with partial hypophysectomy if an adenoma is not identified intraoperatively. In the authors' experience, routine venography in all patients undergoing inferior petrosal sinus sampling allows more accurate interpretation of lateralizing ACTH gradients and thereby improves preoperative tumor localization. On one occasion, the venogram has also identified an entirely intracavernous adenoma, which was the source of ACTH hypersecretion (71).

Superselective catheterization of the cavernous sinuses has also been performed at some centers with equally low morbidity, although theoretically there is a slightly increased risk of neurologic complications (69). In general, unstimulated ACTH levels from the cavernous sinuses are higher than those obtained from the inferior petrosal sinuses, increasing the test sensitivity of cavernous sinus sampling (CSS) in the diagnosis of Cushing's disease (69,72,73). However, there have been isolated reports in which the diagnosis of Cushing's disease was established by IPSS and not CSS (74). Therefore, sampling from both sites should increase

diagnostic accuracy (69). Whether CSS is superior to IPSS for tumor lateralization is debatable although preliminary data suggest that CSS may be more accurate in predicting a lateral tumor (73,74,75). On the other hand, CRH-stimulated CSS appeared less accurate than basal CSS for tumor lateralization (73). Overall, however, it is likely that the effects of venous drainage asymmetry predominate, providing further support for presampling venography prior to interpreting lateralization results (69,74).

Although the role of cavernous sinus sampling is still being defined, the procedure is relatively safe, easily performed, and highly accurate. Moreover, the cavernous sinuses are already accessed at the time of venography. Thus, in patients with ACTH-dependent hypercortisolism and equivocal MRI findings, the authors recommend routine presampling venography followed by both CSS and IPSS with CRH stimulation, thereby maximizing the yield of diagnostic information. Venous sampling should also be considered in cases that appear atypical for Cushing's disease, even if the pituitary MRI shows a clear adenoma.

PITUITARY SURGERY Transsphenoidal pituitary microsurgery is the initial procedure of choice for patients with Cushing's disease. Developed as early as 1907, the transsphenoidal approach was refined in the late 1960s with the introduction of new microscopic techniques for the selective removal of pituitary adenomas (76). Adenomas causing Cushing's disease average 4–5 mm in diameter and only 10% are macroadenomas (4,59). Because of their small size, surgical localization is often challenging, and operative results vary widely among different institutions (77). Therefore, the authors recommend that patients with Cushing's disease be referred to centers with extensive experience in treating this disorder.

Macroadenomas Surgical exploration and resection of macroadenomas are almost always approached via the transsphenoidal route, even if there is suprasellar or sphenoidal extension. The transcranial approach is very rarely used and is only indicated when tumors have significant lateral parasellar extension, massive suprasellar extension, or dumbbell-shaped configuration with constriction at the diaphragma sella (78,79). After intraoperative localization, the adenoma is exposed and dissected away from the normal anterior pituitary and dura lining the sella turcica. Local invasion of the dura is the most common reason for residual disease, and larger tumors may be adherent to adjacent structures with evidence of local extension. After removal of the mass, the tumor bed is treated with absolute ethanol to destroy any residual tumor cells, and the cavity is packed as needed with subcutaneous fat to achieve hemostasis and prevent CSF rhinorrhea (78,79).

Microadenomas The surgical approach to microadenomas with abnormal MRI is straightforward, although false radiologic localization can occur in a small number of patients. After opening the dura of the anterior sellar wall, the pituitary surface is carefully inspected for an adenoma corresponding to the abnormality on the MR image. Tumors <5 mm may not be visible on the surface of the gland, in which case a vertical incision will frequently reveal the lesion (78). After careful tumor excision, the superficial (1 mm in thickness) layer of the anterior pituitary adjacent to the adenoma is frequently removed to reduce the possibility of regrowth, particularly in cases where a clear surgical margin is not defined (13). Absolute ethanol is then instilled into the tumor cavity, followed by subcutaneous fat packing and closure (78,80). The authors recommend careful inspection of the entire sella and cavernous

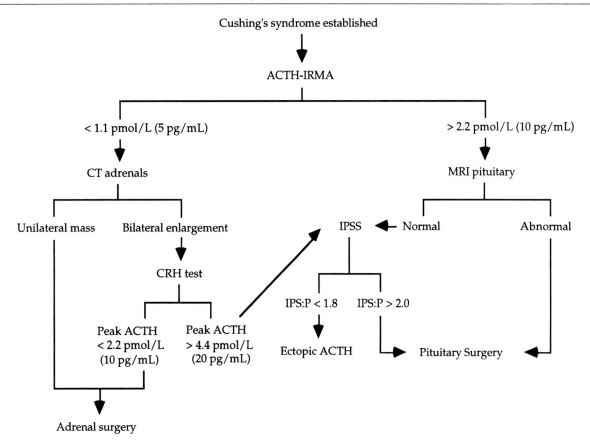

Figure 18-5 The differential diagnosis of Cushing's syndrome. (IRMA, immunoradiometric assay; IPSS, inferior petrosal sinus sampling; IPS:P, inferior petrosal sinus:peripheral ACTH ratio; CRH, corticotropin-releasing hormone). (From Findling JW, Aron DC, Tyrrell JB. Glucocorticoid and adrenal androgens. In: Greenspan FS, Strewler GJ, eds. Basic and Clinical Endocrinology. Stamford, Connecticut, Appleton & Lange, 1997, pp. 317–358; with permission.)

sinuses to exclude previously nonvisualized extension of the adenoma or the rare presence of multiple or incidental adenomas.

In most current series, 50% of adenomas are not visualized with pituitary MRI *(55,80,81)*. In these cases, cavernous or petrosal sinus sampling will usually exclude the ectopic ACTH syndrome, and lateralization data can often assist the surgeon in pituitary exploration.

In patients where presampling venography confirms symmetric venous drainage and a lateralizing gradient >2:1 is documented, the surgeon should first explore the appropriate lobe and excise the adenoma if found. If no adenoma is discovered, the entire sellar contents should be explored meticulously before removal of any anterior pituitary tissue. This is essential because false lateralization by venous sampling has been reported *(69)*. Rarely, an entirely intracavernous adenoma has been found and should be considered if no intrasellar tumor is identified despite definite lateralization by venous sampling *(71)*. Cavernous sinus adenomas large enough to resect are generally visualized by venography; therefore, for patients without a preoperative venogram, cavernous sinus exploration is recommended prior to partial hypophysectomy *(71)*. If no adenoma is confirmed after a thorough exploration of the sellar and parasellar contents, a hemihypophysectomy is performed, removing the lobe identified by ACTH gradient. This will result in surgical remission in the great majority of patients.

In patients with an obvious central to peripheral ACTH gradient but without lateralization of ACTH secretion or lateralization with asymmetric venous drainage, the entire anterior and posterior lobes should be explored with a series of horizontal and vertical excisions as described previously in early surgical series prior to CT, MRI, and venous sampling data *(79,82)*. Multiple incisions into the anterior lobe have not been shown to produce detectable impairment in function, and in most cases, an adenoma will be localized by an experienced surgeon *(79)*. A minority of cases involve tumors that may be extrapituitary, extrasellar, or extremely small, leading to negative exploratory findings. In these few patients where reproductive capacity is not desired, a total hypophysectomy can be considered, provided that an intracavernous adenoma has not been identified and an extrapituitary source has otherwise been excluded by venous sampling data. This latter approach is contraindicated in children and young adults.

Postoperative Evaluation and Follow-up At the present time, there is no clear consensus regarding postoperative endocrine evaluation and the criteria predicting long-term remission. In general, the operative and pathologic findings may not correlate closely with the final outcome, and thus, biochemical evaluation is essential in the postoperative period *(83)*. An undetectable morning cortisol level within the first 2 wk of surgery (after withdrawal of glucocorticoid therapy) has been shown to predict long-term cure accurately *(83–85)*, although a significant number of patients with long-term remission may have normal cortisol levels in the immediate postsurgical period *(86,87)*. This has led some groups to assess for subnormal cortisol levels 6–12 wk after surgery, resulting in better discrimination of recurrent or persistent disease *(14,88)*. Alternatively, suppression of urinary cortisol excretion with maintenance doses of dexamethasone (0.5–0.75 mg daily) has been used to predict remission *(89)*. Demonstration of postoperative low dose (1 mg) dexamethasone suppressibility has also been useful, although results should be interpreted carefully, since rare false-positives have been reported *(83,86,90)*. Other predictors of remission include deficient responses with CRH stimulation or insulin-induced hypoglycemia and lack of adrenal responsiveness to ACTH *(14,91)*. In fact, patients who require prolonged glucocorticoid therapy appear to have the lowest risk of relapse *(85)*.

The authors routinely measure plasma cortisol days 2–5 after surgery while patients are maintained on dexamethasone 1 mg twice daily to prevent hypoadrenalism. A plasma cortisol level <138 nmol/L (5 µg/dL) has been shown to predict long-term remission. Patients are then tapered to a maintenance dose of hydrocortisone (30 mg/d) over a few days. Individuals with significant cortisol excess prior to surgery are at risk for the steroid withdrawal syndrome and are generally maintained on 40 mg/d of hydrocortisone for 2–4 wk before tapering to 30 mg/d. Because most patients subsequently develop prolonged but temporary secondary hypoadrenalism averaging 12–14 mo, a Cosyntropin (0.25 mg) stimulation test is performed 1–2 mo after surgery to confirm adrenal unresponsiveness, followed by repeat adrenal function studies at 3-mo intervals until the HPA axis recovers *(14,92)*. Normalization of cortisol secretion, diurnal rhythm, dexamethasone suppressibility, and hypoglycemia responsiveness have been shown to return eventually *(93)*. Early adrenal recovery or lack of hypoadrenalism may suggest recurrent or persistent Cushing's disease, and these individuals should be followed closely. Long-term evaluation of all patients can be conveniently assessed with urinary free cortisol measurements.

Surgical Outcome Current large series from surgeons experienced in the management of Cushing's disease demonstrate that adenomas are successfully localized in 70–94% of cases *(13)*. In these series, a total of 1201 patients with Cushing's disease underwent pituitary surgery, and 957 (80%) achieved initial remission of hypercortisolism, regardless of tumor size or the type of operation performed *(13)*. Features more likely to result in successful surgery include accurate radiographic visualization of a pituitary lesion, intraoperative tumor localization, selective adenomectomy, and histologic confirmation *(4,94,95)*. The major reasons for surgical failure consists of the following *(4,94,96)*:

1. Failure to identify or localize the adenoma surgically.
2. Local extension of the adenoma into adjacent normal pituitary.
3. Extension of the adenoma into the dura of the lateral sellar wall or perforation of the sellar floor.

Overall long-term remission rates after pituitary surgery range from 75 to 80% with recurrence rates of approx 11% *(80)*. It is also important to realize that therapeutic failures reflect the misdiagnosis of ectopic ACTH syndromes in a very small subset of patients.

For microadenomas, initial remission rates approach 80–90% based on correction of hypercortisolism in the immediate postop-erative period *(4,59,97)*. In the majority of cases, selective adenoma excision is successful; however, approx 5–15% of patients will require partial or total hypophysectomy *(4,96,97)*. Late recurrences are seen in 3–20% of patients in current series, resulting in long-term remission rates of 75–85% *(4,15,96–98)*. Surgical success with macroadenomas is limited; only 50–70% of patients achieve remission after initial pituitary surgery, and recurrence rates are higher *(4,15,97)*. Invasion of the dura, cavernous sinus, and adjacent structures are common reasons for persistent disease, and postoperative radiation therapy is generally warranted. Repeat surgery or more radical resection often does not improve therapeutic outcome to a significant degree, and recommendations for further treatment include pituitary irradiation, medical therapy, and bilateral adrenalectomy.

Complications Transsphenoidal pituitary microsurgery has proven to be a relatively safe and effective approach in the treatment of Cushing's disease. Perioperative mortality ranges between 1 and 2% with the major causes of death related to myocardial infarction or pulmonary embolism *(4,85)*. A few patients have also died of subsequent meningitis *(59,96)*. The most frequent complications reported include transient hyponatremia (5–20%), transient diabetes insipidus (10–15%), and CSF rhinorrhea (2–5%), with approximately half requiring surgical correction *(4,99)*. Permanent diabetes insipidus is seen in <3% and generally occurs in patients undergoing radical surgery or total hypophysectomy *(4,85)*. Meningitis occurs in a small subset of patients who develop a CSF leak and is generally treatable. Other rare complications include opthalmopathy, severe hemorrhage, and hypopituitarism, which occur in <2% of patients *(4,59)*.

Residual Disease Patients with residual Cushing's disease demonstrate either persistent hypercortisolism following transsphenoidal surgery or occasionally a transient reduction in cortisol secretion. Assuming that dural invasion and ectopic ACTH secretion were definitely excluded during the initial investigation, a second transsphenoidal operation with selective adenomectomy may be considered, although a higher incidence of hypopituitarism has been seen *(94,100)*. Reoperation is also indicated if the initial operation was performed by an inexperienced surgeon or if technical difficulties were encountered. In adult patients in whom no tumor was localized at the first surgery and in those with persisting disease despite adenoma localization, partial or total hypophysectomy may be considered, provided the ectopic ACTH syndrome has been excluded. Patients with evidence of dural invasion are not candidates for reoperation, and instead should be referred for radiation and medical therapy. In refractory cases, bilateral adrenalectomy may be considered.

Recurrent Disease Recurrence of Cushing's disease after successful transsphenoidal surgery is defined as the return of hypercortisolism after a period of adrenal insufficiency followed by a period of normal HPA axis function *(93)*. Although low, recurrence rates are appreciable, and with extended follow-up can be as high as 20% *(98)*. Management of recurrent Cushing's disease is highly dependent on the clinical situation. Reoperation with attempted selective adenomectomy is indicated if the initial operation was performed by an inexperienced surgeon. In adult patients, total hypophysectomy can be considered if no tumor is localized and may be curative if the tumor is intrasellar. Patients with initially invasive tumors will not be cured at reoperation; however, surgical debulking of the lesion can induce a temporary remission and may improve outcome with subsequent radiotherapy. In certain situations where a second transsphenoidal procedure is contraindicated, medical adrenal inhibition and bilateral adrenalectomy provide direct removal of cortisol excess.

RADIOTHERAPY The first case of Cushing's disease with improvement after pituitary radiotherapy was among the 12 patients in Cushing's original 1932 report *(1,101)*. Over the next 30 yr, radiation therapy alone was frequently used in the management of Cushing's disease *(101)*. In a landmark paper published in 1971 on the treatment of Cushing's syndrome, Orth and Liddle reported that primary radiotherapy was curative in 20% of adult patients, whereas improvement was seen in another 25% *(102)*. With the introduction of pituitary microsurgery in the 1970s, transsphenoidal resection became the treatment of choice for microadenomas, yielding cure rates of up to 90%. Radiation therapy, however, still remains an important second-line agent, especially in situations where surgery is contraindicated or unsuccessful, and macroadenomas often require a combined approach for residual disease. Remission rates for pituitary radiotherapy range from 50 to 70%, although there is considerable variability in the definition of cure and not all patients demonstrate a return of diurnal cortisol secretion and responsiveness to insulin-induced hypoglycemia *(103)*. More importantly, many of these patients were treated prior to the availability of sophisticated pituitary imaging.

Conventional pituitary radiotherapy for Cushing's disease most commonly involves external beam irradiation from a high-energy linear accelerator. Patients generally receive 4500–5000 cgy (rads), administered in daily fractions of 180 rad. A few centers have used high-voltage cobalt-60 particle irradiation with a similar dose fractionation, although the beam edge is more precisely defined with a modern linear accelerator *(101,104)*. Some centers are also experienced in more sophisticated methods of radiation delivery, including heavy particle beam radiotherapy and stereotactic radiosurgery, although these latter methods have not yet gained widespread use.

Primary Radiotherapy Since the demonstration of the effectiveness of pituitary microsurgery, relatively few patients have been treated with primary radiotherapy. Current retrospective series indicate that primary radiation treatment with doses ranging from 4500 to 5000 rad results in remission of Cushing's disease in only 55–59% of patients *(105,106)*. However, the response may be delayed by 2–4 yr before hypercortisolism is corrected. Lower-dose pituitary irradiation (2000 cgy) has been associated with higher relapse rates, achieving long-term remission in only 25–37% of patients *(107,108)*.

Postoperative Radiotherapy The major role of radiotherapy is in patients who have persistent or recurrent disease after pituitary microsurgery. However, only a few published studies are available. One series reported a 61% remission rate at 1 yr and 70% at 2 yr in patients with persistent or recurrent Cushing's disease after unsuccessful transsphenoidal surgery *(109)*. A much larger study from the same group indicated that 83% of patients achieved remission with a median of 3.5 yr *(110)*. In another series, 56% of patients were in remission at a median of 3 yr *(105)*. The majority of these patients studied had microadenomas; limited data available on postoperative radiotherapy of macroadenomas indicate that the response is less favorable *(103,105,111)*.

Combination Therapy Because remission of hypercortisolism in Cushing's disease may not occur until several years after radiotherapy, other treatment modalities have been used in the interim to reduce cortisol levels while awaiting the delayed effect of pituitary irradiation. These include medical therapy, targeting either the pituitary or the adrenal gland, and the more historical approach of unilateral adrenalectomy. Pituitary irradiation in combination with reserpine, metyrapone, aminoglutethimide, or mitotane (o,p'-DDD) demonstrates remission rates of 56–60%, not significantly improved from radiotherapy alone *(105,112,113)*. Therefore, there is no current evidence that additional treatment modalities improve the long-term outcome in patients treated with primary radiotherapy. The authors recommend pituitary radiotherapy only in those patients who have had unsuccessful pituitary microsurgery. Concurrent medical therapy can be used in the first few years to correct hypercortisolism while radiation treatment takes effect *(105,108)*.

Complications The major long-term complication of conventional radiotherapy is hypopituitarism, which can occur up to 5–10 yr after treatment. Most series reviewing pituitary adenomas of all types report hypopituitarism in at least 50% of patients with a higher incidence when radiation and surgery are combined *(101,114)*. In a large series of patients followed for up to 10 yr, the incidence of deficiencies in growth hormone, gonadotropins, ACTH, and TSH was 100, 96, 84, and 49%, respectively, by 8 yr *(115)*. Radiation-induced hyperprolactinemia also developed in 44% of this group with peak values at 2 yr followed by a decline toward basal levels, suggesting some degree of hypothalamic dysfunction *(115)*. Data specific to patients with Cushing's disease are limited to small series, although there is little reason to believe that the incidence of hypopituitarism should be much different.

Rare complications of pituitary irradiation include optic nerve or optic chiasm injury, brain necrosis, and carcinogenesis, which occur in fewer than 1–2% of patients *(101,103,106)*. One series suggested mild cognitive-memory deficits in 11% as assessed by clinical impression, although formal psychometric testing was not done *(111)*. A number of these patients had also undergone craniotomy or multiple surgeries.

Other Forms of Radiotherapy Particle beam irradiation has been successfully used at a few centers in the management of ACTH-secreting pituitary adenomas. The principle of treatment is based on large doses of radiation delivered to a highly restricted (intrasellar) target volume *(101)*. Specifically, proton beam pituitary radiotherapy with dosages ranging from 12,000 to 14,000 rad results in remission rates as high as 85% *(116)*. With this technique, the hypothalamus is exposed to less than 500 rad, likely accounting for the lower incidence (15–30%) of anterior pituitary insufficiency as defined by cortisol or thyroid hormone deficiency, when compared to other radiation techniques *(116)*. A 4% incidence of ophthalmopathy has been noted, however, with an increased risk in patients treated with prior X-ray therapy *(116)*. Complication rates may also be higher with larger target fields, limiting this approach in postoperative therapy. Currently, high-dose particle beam radiotherapy is available only at two centers.

γ-Irradiation from cobalt-60 administered with stereotactic technique in a single dose (γ-knife radiosurgery) has been used in the treatment of Cushing's disease at one center, with reported long-term remission rates of 48% after a single treatment and 76% after multiple treatments in a total of 29 cases *(117)*. Although local complications were not seen, pituitary insufficiency developed in 55% of patients. A more recent review by the same group indicated that clinical remission was achieved in up to 82% of patients, with only 20% requiring hormone replacement therapy

(118). Of the small number of patients who were treated based on MRI, the remission rate was 100% with no evidence of pituitary insufficiency during a brief follow-up period of 2–4 yr *(118)*. With the availability of sophisticated sellar imaging, γ-knife radiosurgery may prove superior to conventional radiotherapy, especially for intrasellar lesions, providing there is no evidence of chiasmal involvement *(119)*. Larger and more extensive parasellar tumors may also be suitable if care is taken to avoid injury to the optic nerves.

For historical interest, interstitial radiation with needle implantation of yttrium-90 or gold-198 has also been investigated in the treatment of Cushing's disease. One study reported remission rates of 77% at 1 yr with no subsequent relapse after a mean follow-up of 10 yr *(120)*. Hypopituitarism was seen in only 37% (Y-90) and 47% (G-198) of this group. Disadvantages of interstitial radiation included variable dose distribution and a higher incidence of local complications, such as CSF rhinorrhea and meningitis from the implant itself *(101,121)*.

Management and Follow-up Patients need lifelong follow-up after radiation treatment, with routine endocrinologic tests to exclude hypopituitarism or recurrent disease *(103)*. Periodic MRI should be considered to document reduction in tumor size, and routine visual field testing is recommended in the subsequent evaluation of patients who initially present with visual acuity or visual field impairment *(103)*.

MEDICAL THERAPY **Inhibition of Cortisol Production** A variety of drugs that inhibit adrenal steroidogenesis have been used in the treatment of Cushing's disease not amenable to surgical or radiation therapy. Medical therapy is a useful adjunct to pituitary irradiation, since the therapeutic effects of radiotherapy may be delayed for several years. Occasionally, adrenal inhibition is used to control hypercortisolism in patients awaiting surgery, with the hope of minimizing complications associated with glucocorticoid excess. Of the various agents that block adrenal steroid synthesis, the authors have the most experience with ketoconazole as effective first-line therapy; in more severe cases, metyrapone is often added to achieve better control of hypercortisolism.

Ketoconazole was noted to cause gynecomastia in some patients, which led to the discovery that multiple sites in the steroidogenic pathways were inhibited by this antifungal agent *(122)*. Cholesterol side-chain cleavage, 17α-hydroxylase, 11β-hydroxylase, 18-hydroxylase, and especially 17,20-lyase enzymes are all blocked by ketoconazole, resulting in diminished glucocorticoid and androgen levels *(123,124)*. In Cushing's disease, doses of 400–1200 mg/d (average 800 mg/d) are usually required to control hypercortisolism and are effective in up to 70% of cases, although a 15% incidence of liver toxicity has been reported *(125,126)*. Most cases of transaminase elevation usually resolve with cessation of therapy; however, rare cases of fatal hepatotoxicity have been reported *(126,127)*. Ketoconazole has also been used successfully in combination with metyrapone for more resistant cases.

Metyrapone, a selective inhibitor of 11β-hydroxylase, was initially introduced to test pituitary adrenal reserve and subsequently used to distinguish Cushing's disease from other entities of hypercortisolism *(128)*. Later applied in the treatment of Cushing's syndrome, metyrapone also demonstrated effectiveness in the control of Cushing's disease (50–75%), although monotherapy was limited by virilization and salt retention from 11β-hydroxylase inhibition and consequent ACTH elevation *(126,129,130)*. Combination with either aminoglutethamide or ketoconazole has

thus been more effective, and these regimens are a useful adjunct to radiotherapy *(131,132)*.

Aminoglutethimide, formerly marketed as an anticonvulsant, inhibits the first step in cortisol biosynthesis (cholesterol → pregnenolone) by interfering with the side-chain cleavage system. Because its inhibition occurs early in steroidogenesis, aminoglutethimide leads to diminished levels of all adrenal and gonadal steroids. Its efficacy in Cushing's disease is limited as monotherapy, although improved results are seen in combination with metyrapone or pituitary irradiation *(131–133)*. The main side effects include sedation, nausea and a transient rash *(133)*.

The adrenolytic agent mitotane (o,p'-DDD) was developed after investigators observed that the insecticide DDD, a related isomer, caused selective necrosis of the zona fasciculata and zona reticularis of the adrenal cortex in dogs *(134)*. Introduced in the late 1950s for the treatment of metastatic adrenal carcinoma, mitotane was also shown to suppress hypercortisolism in Cushing's syndrome *(135)*. The mechanism of action involves both adrenocorticolytic effects and direct inhibition of steroid synthesis *(126,136)*. In Cushing's disease, short-term remission is obtained in 83% of patients, although over half relapse when therapy is discontinued *(137)*. The relative frequency of gastrointestinal side effects and elevation of serum cholesterol have been problematic, and low rates of long-term remission necessitate longer duration of therapy *(126,137)*.

Newer investigational agents have also been studied, although experience is limited, and the effectiveness of these drugs is not well established. The anesthetic agent etomidate is an imidazole derivative that inhibits 11β-hydroxylase action, thereby reducing cortisol levels with relatively safe low doses *(138,139)*. The need for intravenous administration does limit its role in chronic therapy, although the rapid decrease of cortisol levels may be advantageous in the acute treatment of severe hypercortisolism *(138)*. Trilostane, an inhibitor of the 3β-hydroxysteroid dehydrogenase:4-5 isomerase enzyme system, has been shown to lower cortisol levels, although responses among patients with Cushing's syndrome can be quite variable *(140,141)*. Overall, trilostane is believed to be less effective than other agents.

Antagonism of Cortisol Action RU 486, a competitive glucocorticoid antagonist, has been used successfully in one patient with Cushing's syndrome owing to ectopic ACTH secretion, leading to improvement in all the somatic features of cortisol excess *(142)*. Its role in Cushing's disease, however, will likely be limited by subsequent ACTH elevation leading to further cortisol increase *(142)*. There are currently little data on treatment of patients with Cushing's disease.

Inhibition of ACTH Secretion Pharmacologic inhibition of ACTH secretion, mediated by neurotransmitter activity, received much attention in the past, although the effectiveness of these agents has proved disappointing. Cyproheptadine (serotonin antagonist), bromocriptine (dopamine agonist), and valproic acid (GABA-transaminase inhibitor) have all been used in the therapy of Cushing's disease with the aim of controlling ACTH hypersecretion *(12,133)*. However, remission is achieved in only a few cases, and relapse frequently occurs after cessation of treatment. Octreotide has also been tried with mixed results *(133)*, although in a few patients, combination therapy with ketoconazole has been somewhat effective *(142a)*. Currently, there does not appear to be a major role for neuropharmacologic inhibition of ACTH secretion in the medical treatment of Cushing's disease, in light of more effective therapy.

BILATERAL ADRENALECTOMY Prior to the widespread availability of pituitary surgery, bilateral adrenalectomy was recommended as the treatment of choice for severe Cushing's disease, with external pituitary irradiation reserved for milder cases (143,144). This afforded immediate removal of cortisol excess, although patients were then committed to lifelong replacement therapy. However, the operative mortality from bilateral adrenalectomy ranged from 4 to 12%, and only over the last 20 yr has this has improved considerably with advances in anesthetic and surgical care, preoperative medical therapy, and the use of the posterior incisional approach (126,145). Two current series report an operative mortality of 0% in a total of 82 patients, with perioperative morbidity ranging from 15 to 32% (145,146). The most frequent perioperative events include infection, hemorrhage, pulmonary embolism, and cardiovascular complications (144,145,147). More recently with the introduction of laparoscopic adrenalectomy, perioperative morbidity has decreased even further, and laparoscopic surgery is now the preferred approach at institutions with surgeons experienced in this technique (148,149). Patients are subsequently at risk for Addisonian crises and Nelson's syndrome, both of which contribute to an increase in long-term morbidity and mortality (150).

The complete removal of all functioning adrenal tissue can be difficult, and excision of the right adrenal gland is often technically challenging (126,151). Even in experienced hands, persistence of pituitary-dependent Cushing's syndrome has been reported to be as high as 7–10% (144,152). More current series indicate recurrence rates of <3% following bilateral adrenalectomy, although up to 24% of patients may still demonstrate residual adrenocortical function with biochemical testing (146,153). These findings are presumably the result of residual or ectopic adrenal tissue.

In summary, bilateral adrenalectomy is an important alternative in patients who have failed pituitary surgery, particularly in situations where radiotherapy and medical treatment have proven insufficient in controlling hypercortisolism. Laparoscopic adrenalectomy should be considered at centers with sufficient surgical experience, since this approach results in lower complication rates. Postoperatively, patients require lifelong glucocorticoid and mineralocorticoid replacement, although investigation for persistent adrenocortical function should be performed to rule out residual or ectopic tissue. Patients should also be followed closely for the development of Nelson's syndrome, which can occur as late as 12 yr postadrenalectomy (92,154,155).

NELSON'S SYNDROME

PRESENTATION Nelson's syndrome, first reported in 1958 by Nelson and colleagues, describes the rapid enlargement of ACTH-secreting pituitary adenomas after bilateral adrenalectomy for Cushing's disease (156,157). The mechanism is believed to be related to the accelerated growth of a pre-existing pituitary microadenoma after correction of hypercortisolism, although at a molecular level, the exact pathogenesis is not clear (158,159). Diagnosis has historically been established by the classic criteria of hyperpigmentation and radiologic evidence of pituitary enlargement (160,161). The incidence of Nelson's syndrome ranges from 5 to 78% in reported series, with increasing detection utilizing immunoreactive plasma ACTH assays and more sophisticated imaging techniques (162). In a more recent series, the incidence ranges from 28 to 38% of adrenalectomized patients (146,152,

154,163). Currently, Nelson's syndrome is seldom encountered, since bilateral adrenalectomy is performed only in those patients who have failed transsphenoidal surgery. Among patients undergoing bilateral adrenalectomy as primary therapy for Cushing's disease, it is estimated that up to 30% may later present with classic Nelson's syndrome, another 50% develop evidence of microadenomas that do not show marked progression, whereas the remaining 20% show no evidence of an adenoma (92).

Despite this marked clinical variability, not much is known about the factors that predispose patients to Nelson's syndrome. There appears to be little correlation with duration of Cushing's disease or preoperative ACTH values, and only one study supports an association with pretreatment urinary cortisol levels (95,164,165). The presence of a pre-existing pituitary adenoma may be a significant marker, and evidence suggests that ACTH rise following adrenal surgery may discriminate patients prone to developing Nelson's syndrome, with the most predictive levels obtained after the first postoperative year (159,165,166). Age is also a significant factor, and it has long been known that children have a higher incidence of Nelson's syndrome (167,168). A recent retrospective study indicates that age <35 yr at the time of adrenalectomy may be an important predictive factor (164). At the present time, recommendations for long-term evaluation of all adrenalectomized patients include periodic visual field testing, sellar imaging, and plasma ACTH assays, since patients can present with pituitary enlargement up to 12 yr after surgery (154). The beneficial role of prophylactic pituitary irradiation prior to adrenalectomy remains unresolved and has not been routinely practiced (145,160,169,170).

Nelson's syndrome presents with aggressive and rapidly growing tumors, hyperpigmentation, and elevated ACTH levels (frequently >1000 pg/mL), often accompanied by headaches and visual fields defects (92,154). Patients generally manifest symptoms within the first few years after adrenalectomy. The majority of tumors are macroadenomas, and up to 50% are invasive at surgical examination (171). Cavernous sinus invasion, pituitary apoplexy, and malignant transformation can also be seen (154,159, 160,163). Occasionally, the continuous stimulation of excessive ACTH levels leads to hyperplasia of adrenal rests in the testes and more rarely in the ovaries, leading to recurrent hypercortisolism and androgen excess (172–174).

TREATMENT Aggressive treatment of Nelson's syndrome is indicated because of its high morbidity and mortality. Pituitary surgery with complete tumor excision is the treatment of choice, and the transsphenoidal route is preferred unless massive extrasellar extension necessitates a craniotomy approach. MRI is currently used to define the extent of tumor growth and response to therapy. Patients with macroadenomas may require more radical excision of sellar contents, and evidence of dural or cavernous sinus invasion warrants postoperative radiotherapy (155). In general, therapy is more successful with microadenomas, whereas large macroadenomas with extrasellar extension may be unresectable at surgery by either transsphenoidal or craniotomy approaches. Pituitary irradiation remains an important second-line therapy in Nelson's syndrome (105). There is not much of a role for medical therapy except in cases where surgery and pituitary irradiation have failed or are contraindicated. Unfortunately, treatment with bromocriptine, cyproheptidine, and valproate has provided mixed results, and only a few cases of octreotide efficacy have been reported (159).

REFERENCES

1. Cushing H. The basophil adenomas of the pituitary body and their clinical manifestations (pituitary basophilism). Bull Johns Hopkins Hosp 1932;50:137–195.

2. Huff TA. Clinical syndromes related to disorders of adrenocorticotrophic hormone. In: Allen MB, Mahesh VB, eds. The Pituitary: A Current Review. Academic, New York, 1977, p. 154.

3. Mindermann T, Wilson CB. Age-related and gender-related occurrence of pituitary adenomas. Clin Endocrinol (Oxford) 1994;41:359–364.

4. Mampalam TJ, Tyrrell JB, Wilson CB. Transsphenoidal microsurgery for Cushing disease: A report of 216 cases. Ann Intern Med 1988;109:487–493.

5. Plotz CM, Knowlton AI, Ragan C. The natural history of Cushing's syndrome. Am J Med 1952;13:597–614.

6. Krieger DT. Physiopathology of Cushing's disease. Endocr Rev 1983;4:22–43.

7. Biller BMK. Pathogenesis of pituitary Cushing's syndrome: Pituitary versus hypothalamic. Endocrinol Metab Clin North Am 1994;23(3):547–554.

8. Saeger W, Ludecke DK. Pituitary hyperplasia. Virchows Arch 1983;399:277–287.

9. Gertz BJ, Contreras LN, McComb DJ, Kovacs K, Tyrrell JB, Dallman MF. Chronic administration of corticotropin-releasing factor increases pituitary corticotroph number. Endocrinology 1987;120:381–388.

10. Carey RM, Varma SK, Drake CR, Thorner MO, Kovacs K, Rivier J, et al. Ectopic secretion of corticotropin-releasing factor as a cause of Cushing's syndrome. N Engl J Med 1984;311:13–20.

11. Belsky JL, Cuello B, Swanson W, Simmons DM, Jarrett RM, Braza F. Cushing's syndrome due to ectopic production of corticotropin-releasing factor. J Clin Endocrinol Metab 1985;60:496–500.

12. Krieger DT. Medical management of Cushing's disease. In: Black PM, Zervas NT, Ridgway EC, Martin JB, eds. Secretory Tumors of the Pituitary Gland. Raven, New York, 1984, pp. 273–285.

13. Tyrrell JB, Wilson CB. Cushing's disease: Therapy of pituitary adenomas. Endocrinol Metab Clin North Am 1994;23(4):925–938.

14. Fitzgerald PA, Aron DC, Findling JW, Brooks RM, Wilson CB, Forsham PH, et al. Cushing's disease: Transient secondary adrenal insufficiency after selective removal of pituitary microadenomas; Evidence for a pituitary origin. J Clin Endocrinol Metab 1982; 54:413–422.

15. Nakane T, Kuwayama A, Watanabe M, Takahashi T, Kato T, Ichihara K, et al. Long term results of transsphenoidal adenomectomy in patients with Cushing's disease. Neurosurgery 1987;21:218–222.

16. Gicquel C, Le Bouc Y, Luton J, Girard F, Bertagna X. Monoclonality of corticotroph macroadenomas in Cushing's disease. J Clin Endocrinol Metab 1992;75:472–475.

17. Herman V, Fagin J, Gonsky R, Kovacs K, Melmed S. Clonal origin of pituitary adenomas. J Clin Endocrinol Metab 1990;71:1427–1433.

18. Biller BMK, Alexander JM, Zervas NT, Hedley-Whyte ET, Arnold A, Klibanski A. Clonal origins of adrenocorticotropin-secreting pituitary tissue in Cushing's disease. J Clin Endocrinol Metab 1992;75:1303–1309.

19. Nugent CA, Warner HR, Dunn JT, Tyler FH. Probability theory in the diagnosis of Cushing's syndrome. J Clin Endocrinol 1964;24: 621–627.

20. Ross EJ, Linch DC. Cushing's syndrome—killing disease: Discriminatory value of signs and symptoms aiding early diagnosis. Lancet 1982;2:646–649.

21. Hiramatsu R, Yoshida K, Sato T. A body measurement to evaluate the pattern of fat distribution in central obesity. JAMA 1983;250: 3174–3178.

22. Yanovski JA, Cutler GB. Glucocorticoid action and the clinical features of Cushing's syndrome. Endocrinol Metab Clin North Am 1994;23(3):487–509.

22a. Findling JW, Aron DC, Tyrrell JB. Cushing's Disease. In: Imura H, ed. The Pituitary Gland. Raven, New York, 1985, pp. 441–446.

23. Bouzas EA, Mastorakos G, Friedman TC, Scott MH, Chrousos GP, Kaiser-Kupfer MI. Posterior subcapsular cataract in endogenous Cushing syndrome: An uncommon manifestation. Invest Ophthalmol Vis Sci 1993;34:3497–3500.

24. Nugent CA, Nichols T, Tyler FH. Diagnosis of Cushing's syndrome. Arch Intern Med 1965;116:172–176.

25. Pavlatos FC, Smilo RP, Forsham PH. A rapid screening test for Cushing's syndrome. 1965 JAMA 1965;193:96–99.

26. Fok ACK, Tan KT, Jacob E, Sum CF. Overnight (1 mg) dexamethasone suppression testing reliably distinguishes non-cushingoid obesity from Cushing's syndrome. Steroids 1991;56:549–551.

26a. Wood PJ, Barth JH, Freedman DB, Perry L, Sheridan B. Evidence for the low dose dexamethasone suppression test to screen for Cushing's syndrome–recommendations for a protocol for biochemistry laboratories. Ann Clin Biochem 1997;34: 222–229.

26b. Cronin C, Igoe D, Duffy MJ, Cunningham SK, McKenna TJ. Clin Endocrinol (Oxford) 1990;33:27–33.

27. Crapo L. Cushing's syndrome: A review of diagnostic tests. Metabolism 1979;28:955–977.

28. Findling JW, Doppman JL. Biochemical and radiologic diagnosis of Cushing's syndrome. Endocrinol Metab Clin North Am 1994;23:511–537.

29. Mengden T, Hubmann P, Muller J, Greminger P, Vetter W. Urinary free cortisol versus 17-hydroxycorticosteroids: A comparative study of their diagnostic value in Cushing's syndrome. Clin Invest 1992;70:545–548.

30. Schoneshofer M, Fenner A, Altinok G, Dulce HJ. Specific and practicable assessment of urinary free cortisol by combination of automatic high-pressure liquid chromatography and radioimmunoassay. Clin Chim Acta 1980;106:63–73.

31. Liddle GW. Tests of pituitary-adrenal suppressibility in the diagnosis of Cushing's syndrome. J Clin Endocrinol Metab 1960;20: 1539–1560.

31a. Newell-Price J, Trainer P, Besser M, Grossman A. The diagnosis and differential diagnosis of Cushing's syndrome and pseudo-Cushing's states. Endocr Rev 1998; 19:647–672.

31b. Newell-Price J, Trainer P, Perry L, Wass J, Grossman A, Besser M. A single sleeping midnight cortisol has 100% sensitivity for the diagnosis of Cushing's syndrome. Clin Endocrinol (Oxford) 1995;43:545–550.

31c. Raff H, Raff JL, Findling JW. Late-night salivary cortisol as a screening test for Cushing's syndrome. J Clin Endocrinol Metab 1998;83 :2681–2686.

32. Yanovski JA, Cutler GB, Chrousos GP, Nieman LK. Corticotropin-releasing hormone stimulation following low-dose dexamethasone administration. JAMA 1993;269:2232–2238.

32a. Papanicolaou DA, Yanovski JA, Cutler GB, Chrousos GP, Nieman LK. A single midnight serum cortisol measurement distinguishes Cushing's syndrome from pseudo-Cushing states. J Clin Endocrinol Metab 1998;83:1163–1167.

33. Raff H, Findling JW. A new immunoradiometric assay for corticotropin evaluated in normal subjects and patients with Cushing's syndrome. Clin Chem 1989;35:596–600.

33a. Findling JW. Clinical application of a new immunoradiometric assay for ACTH. Endocrinologist 1992;2:360–365.

34. Tyrrell JB, Findling JW, Aron DC, Fitzgerald PA, Forsham PH. An overnight high-dose dexamethasone suppression test for rapid differential diagnosis of Cushing's syndrome. Ann Intern Med 1986;104:180–186.

35. Dichek HL, Nieman LK, Oldfield EH, Pass HI, Malley JD, Cutler GB. A comparison of the standard high dose dexamethasone suppression test and the overnight 8 mg dexamethasone suppression test for the differential diagnosis of adrenocorticotropin-dependent Cushing's syndrome. J Clin Endocrinol Metab 1994;78: 418–422.

36. Bruno OD, Rossi MA, Contreras LN, Gomez RM, Galparsoro G, Cazado E, et al. Nocturnal high-dose dexamethasone suppression test in the aetiological diagnosis of Cushing's syndrome. Acta Endocrinol (Copenh) 1985;109:158–162.

37. Limper AH, Carpenter PC, Scheithauer B, Staats BA. The Cushing syndrome induced by bronchial carcinoid tumors. Ann Intern Med 1992;117:209–214.

38. Grossman AB, Howlett TA, Perry L, Coy DH, Savage MO, Lavender P, et al. CRF in the differential diagnosis of Cushing's syndrome: A comparison with the dexamethasone suppression test. Clin Endocrinol (Oxford) 1988;29:167–178.

39. Findling JW, Tyrrell JB. Occult ectopic secretion of corticotropin. Arch Intern Med 1986;146:929–933.

40. Aron DC, Raff H, Findling JW. Effectiveness versus efficacy: The limited value in clinical practice of high dose dexamethasone suppression testing in the differential diagnosis of adrenocorticotropin-dependent Cushing's syndrome. J Clin Endocrinol Metab 1997;82:1780–1785.

41. Loriaux DL, Nieman L. Corticotropin-releasing hormone testing in pituitary disease. Endocrinol Metab Clin North Am 1991;20(2): 363–369.

42. Nieman LK, Oldfield EH, Wesley R, Chrousos GP, Loriaux DL, Cutler GB. A simplified morning ovine corticotropin-releasing hormone stimulation test for the differential diagnosis of adrenocorticotropin-dependent Cushing's syndrome. J Clin Endocrinol Metab 1993;77:1308–1312.

43. Tabarin A, Greselle JF, San-Galli F, Leprat F, Caille JM, Latapie JL, et al. Usefulness of the corticotropin-releasing hormone test during bilateral inferior petrosal sinus sampling for the diagnosis of Cushing's disease. J Clin Endocrinol Metab 1991;73:53–59.

44. Newell-Price J, Perry L, Medbak S, Monson J, Savage M, Besser M, et al. A combined test using desmopressin and corticotropin-releasing hormone in the differential diagnosis of Cushing's syndrome. J Clin Endocrinol Metab 1997;82:176–181.

45. Dickstein G, DeBold CR, Gaitan D, DeCherney GS, Jackson RV, Sheldon WR, et al. Plasma corticotropin and cortisol responses to ovine corticotropin-releasing hormone (CRH), arginine vasopressin (AVP), CRH plus AVP, and CRH plus metyrapone in patients with Cushing's disease. J Clin Endocrinol Metab 1996; 81:2934–2941.

46. Avgerinos PC, Yanovski JA, Oldfield EH, Nieman LK, Cutler GB. The metyrapone and dexamethasone suppression tests for the differential diagnosis of the adrenocorticotropin-dependent Cushing's syndrome: A comparison. Ann Intern Med 1994;121: 318–327.

47. Nieman LK, Chrousos GP, Oldfield EH, Avgerinos PC, Cutler GB, Loriaux DL. The ovine corticotropin-releasing hormone stimulation test and the dexamethasone suppression test in the differential diagnosis of Cushing's syndrome. Ann Intern Med 1986;105:862–867.

48. Findling JW. Eutopic or ectopic adrenocorticotropic hormone-dependent Cushing's syndrome? A diagnostic dilemma. Mayo Clin Proc 1990;65:1377–1380.

49. Buchfelder M, Nistor R, Fahlbusch R, Huk WJ. The accuracy of CT and MR evaluation of the sella turcica for detection of adrenocorticotropic hormone-secreting adenomas in Cushing disease. Am J Neuroradiol 1993;14:1183–1190.

50. Marcovitz S, Wee R, Chan J, Hardy J. The diagnostic accuracy of preoperative CT scanning in the evaluation of pituitary ACTH-secreting adenomas. Am J Neuroradiol 1987;8:641–644.

51. Saris SC, Patronas NJ, Doppman JL, Loriaux DL, Cutler GB, Nieman LK, et al. Cushing syndrome: Pituitary CT scanning. Radiology 1987;162:775–777.

52. Colombo N, Loli P, Vignati F, Scialfa G. MR of corticotropin-secreting pituitary microadenomas. Am J Neuroradiol 1994;15: 1591–1595.

53. Peck WW, Dillon WP, Norman D, Newton TH, Wilson CB. High-resolution MR imaging of microadenomas at 1.5 T: Experience with Cushing disease. Am J Neuroradiol 1988;9:1085–1091.

54. de Herder WW, Uitterlinden P, Pieterman H, Tanghe HLJ, Kwekkeboom DJ, Pois HAP, et al. Pituitary tumor localization in patients with Cushing's disease by magnetic resonance imaging. Is there a place for petrosal sinus sampling? Clin Endocrinol (Oxford) 1994;40:87–92.

55. Scanarini M. Transsphenoidal surgery in Cushing's disease and Nelson's syndrome. J Endocrinol Invest 1992;15:230–231.

56. Burrow GN, Wortzman G, Rewcastle NB, Holgate RC, Kovacs K. Microadenomas of the pituitary and abnormal sellar tomograms in an unselected autopsy series. N Engl J Med 1981;304:156–158.

57. Parent AD, Bebin J, Smith RR. Incidental pituitary adenomas. J Neurosurg 1981;54:228–231.

58. Hall WA, Luciano MG, Doppman JL, Patronas NJ, Oldfield EH. Pituitary magnetic resonance imaging in normal human volunteers: Occult adenomas in the general population. Ann Intern Med 1994;120:817–820.

59. Ludecke DK. Transnasal microsurgery of Cushing's disease 1990. Pathol Res Pract 1991;187:608–612.

60. Oldfield EH, Girton ME, Doppman JL. Absence of intercavernous venous mixing: Evidence supporting lateralization of pituitary microadenomas by venous sampling. J Clin Endocrinol Metab 1985;61:644–647.

61. Miller DL, Doppman JL. Petrosal sinus sampling: Technique and rationale. Radiology 1991;178:37–47.

62. Doppman JL, Oldfield E, Krudy AG, Chrousos GP, Schulte HM, Schaaf M, et al. Petrosal sinus sampling for Cushing syndrome: Anatomical and technical considerations. Radiology 1984;150: 99–103.

63. Miller DL, Doppman JL, Peterman SB, Nieman LK, Oldfield EH, Chang R. Neurologic complications of petrosal sinus sampling. Radiology 1992;185:143–147.

64. Corrigan DF, Schaaf M, Whaley RA, Czerwinski CL, Earll JM. Selective venous sampling to differentiate ectopic ACTH secretion from pituitary Cushing's syndrome. N Engl J Med 1977; 296:861–862.

65. Findling JW, Aron DC, Tyrrell JB, Shinsako JH, Fitzgerald PA, Norman D, et al. Selective venous sampling for ACTH in Cushing's syndrome: Differentiation between Cushing's disease and the ectopic ACTH syndrome. Ann Intern Med 1981;94:647–652.

66. Oldfield EH, Chrousos GP, Schulte HM, Schaaf M, McKeever PE, Krudy AG, et al. Preoperative lateralization of ACTH-secreting pituitary microadenomas by bilateral and simultaneous inferior petrosal venous sinus sampling. N Engl J Med 1985;312: 100–103.

66a. Findling JW, Aron DC, Tyrrell JB. Glucocorticoid and adrenal androgens. In: Greenspan FS, Strewler GJ, eds. Basic and Clinical Endocrinology. Stamford, CT, Appleton & Lange, 1997, pp. 317–358.

67. Oldfield EH, Doppman JL, Nieman LK, Chrousos GP, Miller DL, Katz DA, et al. Petrosal sinus sampling with and without corticotropin-releasing hormone for the differential diagnosis of Cushing's syndrome. N Engl J Med 1991;325:897–905.

67a. Kaltsas GA, Giannulis MG, Newell-Price JDC, Dacie JE, Thakkar C, Afshar F, Monson JP, Grossman AB, Besser GM, Trainer PJ. A critical analysis of the value of simultaneous inferior petrosal sinus sampling in Cushing's disease and the occult ectopic adrenocorticotropin syndrome. J Clin Endocrinol Metab 1999;84:487–492.

68. Findling JW, Kehoe ME, Shaker JL, Raff H. Routine inferior petrosal sinus sampling in the differential diagnosis of adrenocorticotropin (ACTH)-dependent Cushing's syndrome: Early recognition of the occult ectopic ACTH syndrome. J Clin Endocrinol Metab 1991;73:408–413.

68a. Findling JW, Raff H. Newer diagnostic techniques and problems in Cushing's disease. Endocrinol Metab Clin North Am 1999; 28(1):191–210.

68b. Doppman JL, Chang R, Oldfield EH, Chrousos G, Stratakis CA, Nieman LK. The hypoplastic inferior petrosal sinus: A potential source of false-negative results in petrosal sampling for Cushing's disease. J Clin Endocrinol Metab 1999;84:533–540.

69. Mamelak AN, Dowd CF, Tyrrell JB, McDonald JF, Wilson CB. Venous angiography is needed to interpret inferior petrosal sinus and cavernous sinus sampling data for lateralizing adrenocorticotropin-secreting adenomas. J Clin Endocrinol Metab 1996;81: 475–481.

70. Miller DL, Doppman JL, Nieman LK, Cutler GB, Chrousos G, Loriaux DL, et al. Petrosal sinus sampling: Discordant lateralization of ACTH-secreting pituitary microadenomas before and after stimulation with corticotropin-releasing hormone. Radiology 1990;176:429–431.

71. Wilson CB, Mindermann T, Tyrrell JB. Extrasellar, intracavernous sinus adrenocorticotropin-releasing adenoma causing Cushing's disease. J Clin Endocrinol Metab 1995;80:1774–1777.

72. Teramoto A, Nemoto S, Takakura K, Sasaki Y, Machida T. Selective venous sampling directly from cavernous sinus in Cushing's syndrome. J Clin Endocrinol Metab 1993;76:637–641.

73. Graham KE, Samuels MH, Nesbit GM, Cook DM, O'Neill OR, Barnwell SL, Loriaux DL. Cavernous sinus sampling is highly accurate in distinguishing Cushing's disease from the ectopic adrenocorticotropin syndrome and in predicting intrapituitary tumor location. J Clin Endocrinol Metab 1999; 84:1602–1610.

74. Doppman JL, Nieman LK, Chang R, Yanovski J, Cutler GB, Chrousos GP, et al. Selective venous sampling from the cavernous sinuses is not a more reliable technique than sampling from the inferior petrosal sinuses in Cushing's syndrome. J Clin Endocrinol Metab 1995;80:2485–2489.

75. Samuels MH, Cook DM, O'Neill O, Nesbitt G, Barnwell S, Loriaux DL. Cavernous sinus sampling (CSS) is superior to inferior petrosal sinus sampling (IPSS) in the evaluation of Cushing's syndrome. Presented at the 10th International Congress of Endocrinology, Abstract OR49-3. San Francisco, June 1996.

76. Hardy J. Transphenoidal microsurgery of the normal and pathological pituitary. Clin Neurosurg 1969;16:185–217.

77. Burch W. A survey of results with transsphenoidal surgery in Cushing's disease. N Engl J Med 1983;308:103–104.

78. Wilson CB. A decade of pituitary microsurgery. J Neurosurg 1984;61:814–833.

79. Wilson CB, Dempsey LC. Transsphenoidal microsurgical removal of 250 pituitary adenomas. J Neurosurg 1978;48:13–22.

80. Wilson CB. The long-term results following pituitary surgery for Cushing's disease and Nelson's syndrome. In: Black PM, Zervas NT, Ridgway EC, Martin JB, eds. Secretory Tumors of the Pituitary Gland. Raven, New York, 1984, pp. 287–294.

81. Landolt AM, Schubiger O, Maurer, Girard J. The value of inferior petrosal sinus sampling in diagnosis and treatment of Cushing's disease. Clin Endocrinol (Oxford) 1994;40:485–492.

82. Wilson CB, Tyrrell JB, Fitzgerald PA, Pitts LH. Cushing's disease and Nelson's syndrome. Clin Neurosurg 1980;27:19–30.

83. McCance DR, Besser M, Atkinson AB. Assessment of cure after transsphenoidal surgery for Cushing's disease. Clin Endocrinol (Oxford) 1996;44:1–6.

84. Trainer PJ, Lawrie HS, Verhelst J, Howlett TA, Lowe DG, Grossman AB, Savage MO, et al. Transsphenoidal resection in Cushing's disease: Undetectable serum cortisol as the definition of successful treatment. Clin Endocrinol (Oxford) 1993;38:73–78.

85. Bochicchio D, Losa M, Buchfelder M, et al. Factors influencing the immediate and late outcome of Cushing's disease treated by transsphenoidal surgery: A retrospective study by the European Cushing's Disease Survey Group. J Clin Endocrinol Metab 1995;80:3114–3120.

86. McCance DR, Gordon DS, Fannin TF, Hadden DR, Kennedy L, Sheridan B, et al. Assessment of endocrine function after transsphenoidal surgery for Cushing's disease. Clin Endocrinol (Oxford) 1993;38:79–86.

87. Friedman TC, Chrousos GP. Transsphenoidal resection in Cushing's disease: Definition of success. Clin Endocrinol (Oxford) 1993; 39:701.

88. Toms GC, McCarthy MI, Niven MJ, Orteu CH, King TT, Monson JP. Predicting relapse after transsphenoidal surgery for Cushing's disease. J Clin Endocrinol Metab 1993;76:291–294.

89. Arnott RD, Pestell RG, McKelvie PA, Henderson JK, McNeill PM, Alford FP. A critical evaluation of transsphenoidal pituitary surgery in the treatment of Cushing's disease: Prediction of outcome. Acta Endocrinol (Copenh) 1990;123:423–430.

90. Jeffcoate WJ, Dauncey S, Selby C. Restoration of dexamethasone suppression by incomplete adenomectomy in Cushing's disease. Clin Endocrinol (Oxford) 1985;23:193–199.

91. Avgerinos PC, Chrousos GP, Nieman LK, Oldfield EH, Loriaux DL, Cutler GB. The corticotropin-releasing hormone test in the postoperative evaluation of patients with Cushing's syndrome. J Clin Endocrinol Metab 1987;65:906–913.

92. Aron DC, Findling JW, Tyrrell JB. Cushing's disease. Endocrinol Metab Clin North Am 1987;16(3):705–730.

93. Lamberts SWJ, Klijn JGM, deJong FH. The definition of true recurrence of pituitary-dependent Cushing's syndrome after transsphenoidal operation. Clin Endocrinol (Oxford) 1987;26:707–712.

94. Ram Z, Nieman LK, Cutler GB, Chrousos GP, Doppman JL, Oldfield EH. Early repeat surgery for persistent Cushing's disease. J Neurosurg 1994;80:37–45.

95. Sonino N, Zielezny M, Fava GA, Fallo F, Boscaro M. Risk factors and long-term outcome in pituitary-dependent Cushing's disease. J Clin Endocrinol Metab 1996;81:2647–2652.

96. Tindall GT, Herring CJ, Clark RV, Adams DA, Watts NB. Cushing's disease: Results of transsphenoidal microsurgery with emphasis on surgical failures. J Neurosurg 1990;72:363–369.

97. Robert F, Hardy J. Cushing's disease: A correlation of radiological, surgical and pathological findings with therapeutic results. Pathol Res Pract 1991;187:617–621.

98. Tahir AH, Sheeler LR. Recurrent Cushing's disease after transsphenoidal surgery. Arch Intern Med 1992;152:977–981.

99. Olson BR, Rubino D, Gumowski J, Oldfield EH. Isolated hyponatremia after transsphenoidal pituitary surgery. J Clin Endocrinol Metab 1995;80:85–91.

100. Friedman RB, Oldfield EH, Nieman LK, Chrousos GP, Doppman JL, Cutler GB, et al. Repeat transsphenoidal surgery for Cushing's disease. J Neurosurg 1989;71:520–527.

101. Halberg FE, Sheline GE. Radiotherapy of pituitary tumors. Endocrinol Metab Clin North Am 1987;16(3):667–684.

102. Orth DN, Liddle GW. Results of treatment in 108 patients with Cushing's syndrome. N Engl J Med 1971;285:243–247.

103. Larson DA. Radiation therapy of pituitary tumors. In: Youmans JR, ed. Neurological Surgery. W.B. Saunders, Philadelphia, 1996, pp. 2970–2979.

104. Flickinger JC, Rush SC. Linear accelerator therapy of pituitary adenomas. In: Landolt AM, Vance ML, Reilly PL, eds. Pituitary Adenomas. Churchill-Livingstone, New Jersey, 1996, pp. 475–483.

105. Howlett TA, Plowman PN, Wass JAH, Rees LH, Jones AE, Besser GM. Megavoltage pituitary irradiation in the management of Cushing's disease and Nelson's syndrome: Long-term follow-up. Clin Endocrinol (Oxford) 1989;31:309–323.

106. Hughes MN, Llamas KJ, Yelland ME, Tripcony LB. Pituitary adenomas: Long-term results for radiotherapy alone and post-operative radiotherapy. Int J Radiat Oncol Biol Phys 1993;27:1035–1043.

107. Littley MD, Shalet SM, Beardwell CG, Ahmed SR, Sutton ML. Long-term follow-up of low-dose external pituitary irradiation for Cushing's disease. Clin Endocrinol (Oxford) 1990;33:445–455.

108. Ahmed SR, Shalet SM, Beardwell CG, Sutton ML. Treatment of Cushing's disease with low dose radiation therapy. Br Med J 1984;289:643–646.

109. Vincente A, Estrada J, de la Cuerda C, Astigarraga B, Marazuela M, Blanco C, et al. Results of external pituitary irradiation after unsuccessful transsphenoidal surgery in Cushing's disease. Acta Endocrinol (Copenh) 1991;125:470–474.

110. Estrada J, Boronat M, Mielgo M, Magallon R, Millan I, Diez S, et al. The long-term outcome of pituitary irradiation after unsuccessful transsphenoidal surgery in Cushing's disease. N Engl J Med 1997;336:172–177.

111. Clarke SD, Woo SY, Butler EB, Dennis WS, Lu H, Carpenter LS, et al. Treatment of secretory pituitary adenoma with radiation therapy. Radiology 1993;188:759–763.

112. Murayama M, Yasuda K, Minamori Y, Mercado-Asis LB, Yamakita N, Miura K. Long term follow-up of Cushing's disease treated with reserpine and pituitary irradiation. J Clin Endocrinol Metab 1992;75:935–942.

113. Ross WM, Evered DC, Hunter P, Benaim M, Cook D, Hall R. Treatment of Cushing's disease with adrenal blocking drugs and megavoltage therapy to the pituitary. Clin Radiol 1979;30: 149–153.

114. Snyder PJ, Fowble BF, Schatz NJ, Savino PJ, Gennarelli TA. Hypopituitarism following radiation therapy of pituitary adenomas. Am J Med 1986;81:457–462.

115. Littley MD, Shalet SM, Beardwell CG, Ahmed SR, Applegate G, Sutton ML. Hypopituitarism following external radiotherapy for pituitary tumors in adults. Q J Med 1989;(70)262:145–160.

116. Kjellberg RN, Kliman B, Swisher B, Butler W. Proton beam therapy of Cushing's disease and Nelson's syndrome. In: Black PM, Zervas NT, Ridgway EC, Martin JB, eds. Secretory Tumors of the Pituitary Gland. Raven, New York, 1984, pp. 294–307.

117. Degerblad M, Rahn T, Bergstrand G, Thoren M. Long-term results of stereotactic radiosurgery to the pituitary gland in Cushing's disease. Acta Endocrinol (Copenh) 1986;112:310–314.

118. Rahn T, Thoren M, Werner S. Stereotactic radiosurgery in pituitary adenomas. In: Faglia G, Beck-Peccoz P, Ambrosi B, Travaglini P, Spada A, eds. Pituitary Adenomas: New Trends in Basic and Clinical Research. Elsevier Science, New York, 1991 pp. 303–312.

119. Ganz JC. Gamma knife treatment of pituitary adenomas. In Landolt AM, Vance ML, Reilly PL, eds. Pituitary Adenomas. Churchill-Livingstone, New Jersey, 1996, pp. 461–474.

120. Sandler LM, Richards NT, Carr DH, Mashiter K, Joplin GF. Long term follow-up of patients with Cushing's disease treated by interstitial irradiation. J Clin Endocrinol Metab 1987;65:441–447.

121. Burke CW, Doyle FH, Joplin GF, Arnot RN, Macerlean DP, Fraser TR. Cushing's disease: Treatment by pituitary implantation of radioactive gold or yttrium seeds. Q J Med 1973;42(168):693–714.

122. Pont A, Williams PL, Loose DS, Feldman D, Reitz RE, Bochra C, et al. Ketoconazole blocks adrenal steroid synthesis. Ann Intern Med 1982;97:370–372.

123. Sonino N. The use of ketoconazole as an inhibitor of steroid production. N Eng J Med 1987;317:812–818.

124. Sonino N, Boscaro M, Merola G, Mantero F. Prolonged treatment of Cushing's disease by ketoconazole. J Clin Endocrinol Metab 1985;61:718–722.

125. Engelhardt D, Weber MM. Therapy of Cushing's syndrome with steroid biosynthesis inhibitors. J Steroid Biochem Mol Biol 1994;49:261–267.

126. Trainer PJ, Besser M. Cushing's syndrome: Therapy directed at the adrenal glands. Endocrinol Metab Clin North Am 1994;23(3): 571–584.

127. Duarte PA, Chow CC, Simmons F, Ruskin J. Fatal hepatitis associated with ketoconazole therapy. Arch Intern Med 1984;144: 1069–1070.

128. Liddle GW, Estep HL, Kendall JW, Williams WC, Townes AW. Clinical application of a new test of pituitary reserve. J Clin Endocrinol Metab 1959;19:875–894.

129. Jeffcoate WJ, Rees LH, Tomlin S, Jones AE, Edwards CRW, Besser GM. Metyrapone in long-term management of Cushing's disease. Br Med J 1977;2:215–217.

130. Verhelst JA, Trainer PJ, Howlett TA, Perry L, Rees LH, Grossman AB, et al. Short and long-term responses to metyrapone in the medical management of 91 patients with Cushing's syndrome. Clin Endocrinol (Oxford) 1991;35:169–178.

131. Thoren M, Adamson U, Sjoberg HE. Aminoglutethimide and metyrapone in the management of Cushing's syndrome. Acta Endocrinol (Copenh) 1985;109:451–457.

132. Sonino N, Boscaro M, Ambroso G, Merola G, Mantero F. Prolonged treatment of Cushing's disease with metyrapone and aminoglutethimide. IRCS Med Sci 1986;14:485–486.

133. Miller JW, Crapo L. The medical treatment of Cushing's syndrome. Endocr Rev 1993;14:443–458.

134. Nelson AA, Woodard G. Severe adrenal cortical atrophy (cytotoxic) and hepatic damage produced in dogs by feeding 2,2-bis(parachlorophenyl)-1,1-dichloroethane (DDD or TDE). Arch Pathol 1949;48:387–394.

135. Southren AL, Weisenfeld S, Laufer A, Goldner MG. Effect of o,p'DDD in a patient with Cushing's syndrome. J Clin Endocrinol Metab 1961;21:201–208.

136. Sonino N. Medical treatment: Inhibitors of adrenal steroid production. J Endocrinol Invest 1992;15:234–235.

137. Luton JP, Mahoudeau JA, Bouchard P, Thieblot P, Hautecouverture M, Simon D, et al. Treatment of Cushing's disease by o,p'DDD: Survey of 62 cases. N Engl J Med 1979;300:459–464.

138. Schulte HM, Benker G, Reinwein D, Sippell WG, Allolio B. Infusion of low dose etomidate: Correction of hypercortisolemia in patients with Cushing's syndrome and dose-response relationship in normal subjects. J Clin Endocrinol Metab 1990;70:1426–1430.

139. Wagner RL, White PF, Kan PB, Rosenthal MH, Feldman D. Inhibition of adrenal steroidogenesis by the anesthetic etomidate. N Engl J Med 1984;310:1415–1421.

140. Dewis P, Anderson DC, Bu'lock DE, Earnshaw R, Kelly WF. Experience with trilostane in the treatment of Cushing's syndrome. Clin Endocrinol (Oxford) 1983;18:533–540.

141. Komanicky P, Spark RF, Melby JC. Treatment of Cushing's syndrome with trilostane (WIN 24,540), an inhibitor of adrenal steroid biosynthesis. J Clin Endocrinol Metab 1978;47:1042–1051.

142. Nieman LK, Chrousos GP, Kellner C, Spitz IM, Nisula BC, Cutler GB, et al. Successful treatment of Cushing's syndrome with the glucocorticoid antagonist RU 486. J Clin Endocrinol Metab 1985;61:536–540.

142a. Vignati F, Loli P. Additive effect of ketoconazole and octreotide in the treatment of severe adrenocorticotropin-dependent hypercortisolism. J Clin Endocrinol Metab 1999;81:2885–2890.

143. Besser GM, Edwards CRW. Cushing's syndrome. Clin Endocrinol Metab 1972;1:451–490.

144. Scott HW, Liddle GW, Mulherin JL, McKenna TJ, Stroup SL, Rhamy RK. Surgical experience with Cushing's disease. Ann Surg 1977;185:524–534.

145. Jenkins PJ, Trainer PJ, Plowman PN, Shand WS, Grossman AB, Wass JAH, et al. The long term outcome after adrenalectomy and prophylactic pituitary radiotherapy in adrenocorticotropin-dependent Cushing's syndrome. J Clin Endocrinol Metab 1995;80:165–171.

146. McCance DR, Russell CFJ, Kennedy TL, Hadden DR, Kennedy L, Atkinson AB. Bilateral adrenalectomy: low mortality and morbidity in Cushing's disease. Clin Endocrinol (Oxford) 1993;39:315–321.

147. Welbourn RB. Survival and causes of death after adrenalectomy for Cushing's disease. Surgery 1985;97:16–20.

148. Bax TW, Marcus DR, Galloway GQ, Swanstrom LL, Sheppard BC. Laparoscopic bilateral adrenalectomy following failed hypophysectomy. Surg Endosc 1996;10:1150–1153.

149. Gagner M. Laparoscopic adrenalectomy. Surg Clin North Am 1996;76(3):523–537.

150. O'Riordain DS, Farley DR, Young WF, Grand CS, van Heerdan JA. Long-term outcome of bilateral adrenalectomy in patients with Cushing's syndrome. Surgery 1994;116:1088–1094.

151. Schteingart DE, Conn JW, Lieberman LM, Beierwaltes WH. Persistent or recurrent Cushing's syndrome after "total" adrenalectomy. Arch Intern Med 1972;130:384–387.

152. Kelly WF, MacFarlane IA, Longson D, Davies D, Sutcliffe H. Cushing's disease treated by total adrenalectomy: Long-term observations of 43 patients. Q J Med 1983;52(206):224–231.

153. Kemink L, Hermus A, Pieters G, Benraad T, Smals A, Kloppenborg P. Residual adrenocortical function after bilateral adrenalectomy for pituitary-dependent Cushing's syndrome. J Clin Endocrinol Metab 1992;75:1211–1214.

154. Kasperlik-Zaluska AA, Nielubowicz J, Wislawski J, Hartwig W, Zaluska J, Jeske W, et al. Nelson's syndrome: incidence and prognosis. Clin Endocrinol (Oxford) 1983;19:693–698.

155. Wislawski J, Kasperlik-Zaluska AA, Jeske W, Migdalska B, Janik J, Zaluska J, et al. Results of neurosurgical treatment by a transsphenoidal approach in 10 patients with Nelson's syndrome. J Neurosurg 1985;62:68–71.

156. Nelson DH, Meakin JW, Dealy JB, Matson DD, Emerson K, Thorn GW. ACTH-producing tumor of the pituitary gland. New Engl J Med 1958;259:161–164.

157. Nelson DH, Meakin JW, Thorn GW. ACTH-producing pituitary tumors following adrenalectomy for Cushing's syndrome. Ann Intern Med 1960;52:560–569.

158. Karl M, von Wichert G, Kempter E, Katz DA, Reincke M, Monig H, et al. Nelson's syndrome associated with a somatic frame shift mutation in the glucocorticoid receptor gene. J Clin Endocrinol Metab 1996;81:124–129.

159. Grua JR, Nelson DH. ACTH-producing pituitary tumors. Endocrinol Metab Clin North Am 1991;20(2):319–362.

160. Moore TJ, Dluhy RG, Williams GH, Caine JP. Nelson's syndrome: Frequency, prognosis, and effect of prior pituitary irradiation. Ann Intern Med 1976;85:731–734.

161. Weinstein M, Tyrrell B, Newton TH. The sella turcica in Nelson's syndrome. Radiology 1976;118:363–365.

162. Miller WM, Tyrrell JB. The adrenal cortex. In: Felig P, Baxter JD, Frohman LA, eds. Endocrinology and Metabolism. McGraw-Hill, New York, 1995, pp. 555–711.

163. Cohen KL, Noth RH, Pechinski T. Incidence of pituitary tumors following adrenalectomy. Arch Intern Med 1978;138:575–579.

164. Kemink L, Pieters G, Hermus A, Smals A, Kloppenborg P. Patient's age is a simple predictive factor for the development of Nelson's syndrome after total adrenalectomy for Cushing's disease. J Clin Endocrinol Metab 1994;79:887–889.

165. Barnett AH, Livesey JH, Friday K, Donald RA, Espiner EA. Comparison of preoperative ACTH concentrations after bilateral adrenalectomy in Cushing's disease. Clin Endocrinol (Oxford) 1983;18:301–305.

166. Moreira AC, Castro M, Machado HR. Longitudinal evaluation of adrenocorticotrophin and β-lipotrophin plasma levels following bilateral adrenalectomy in patients with Cushing's disease. Clin Endocrinol (Oxford) 1993;39:91–96.

167. Hopwood NJ, Kenny FM. Incidence of Nelson's syndrome after adrenalectomy for Cushing's disease in children. Am J Dis Child 1977;131:1353–1356.

168. Thomas CG, Smith AT, Benson M, Griffith J. Nelson's syndrome after Cushing's disease in childhood: A continuing problem. Surgery 1984;96:1067–1077.

169. Cassar J, Doyle FH, Lewis PD, Mashiter K, Noorden SV, Joplin GH. Treatment of Nelson's syndrome by pituitary implantation of yttrium-90 or gold-198. Br Med J 1976;2:269–272.

170. Wild W, Nicolis GL, Gabrilove JL. Appearance of Nelson's syndrome despite pituitary irradiation prior to bilateral adrenalectomy for Cushing's syndrome. Mt. Sinai J Med 1972;40:68–71.

171. Scheithauer BW, Kovacs KT, Laws ER, Randall RV. Pathology of invasive pituitary tumors with special reference to functional classification. J Neurosurg 1986;65:733–744.

172. Verdonk C, Guerin C, Lufkin E, Hodgson SF. Activation of virilizing adrenal rest tissues by excessive ACTH production. Am J Med 1982;73:455–459.

173. Baranetsky NG, Zipser RD, Goebelsmann U, Kurman RJ, March CM, Morimoto I, et al. Adrenocorticotropin-dependent virilizing paraovarian tumors in Nelson's syndrome. J Clin Endocrinol Metab 1979;49:381–386.

174. Hamwi GJ, Gwinup G, Mostow JH, Besch PK. Activation of testicular adrenal rest tissue by prolonged excessive ACTH production. J Clin Endocrinol Metab 1963;23:861–869.

19   Thyrotroph Adenomas

MICHAEL BUCHFELDER, MD AND RUDOLF FAHLBUSCH, MD

INTRODUCTION

Physiological thyroid function is intricately controlled by an elegant interplay between stimulatory hypothalamic influences and a negative feedback system. The major stimulatory influence is hypothalamic thyrotrophin-releasing hormone (TRH), which induces thyroid-stimulating hormone (TSH) secretion by pituitary thyrotrophs. TSH, in turn, is transported by the bloodstream to the thyroid gland, where it promotes synthesis and release of the thyroid hormones, tri-iodotyronine (T3) and thyroxine (T4). T3 is the most important physiological inhibitor of TSH secretion whereby its elevated circulating serum levels act at the hypothalamus and pituitary to downregulate the hypothalamo–pituitary–thyroid axis. In addition to these major influences, dopamine, somatostatin, and corticosteroids have been shown to possess TSH secretion-inhibiting properties, whereas epinephrine and estrogens contribute to stimulatory control *(1)*. Modern immunoassay techniques allow the clear differentiation between normal and subnormal serum TSH levels. Hyperthyroidism is most usually because of primary thyroid disease, such as autonomous hyperfunctioning nodular goiter or overstimulation by immunoglobulins (Graves' disease). In these conditions, TSH secretion is clearly suppressed to subnormal levels. However, a small group of patients with hyperthyroidism have normal or even elevated TSH levels, and in these conditions, it is TSH itself that is responsible for thyroid hyperstimulation. A normal or elevated level of TSH observed in the presence of elevated serum thyroid hormone indicates a disruption of feedback regulation and is termed "inappropriate secretion of TSH," *(2,3)*, "TSH-induced hyperthyroidism," or "central hyperthyroidism" *(4)*. Inappropriate secretion of TSH may result either from a thyrotroph pituitary adenoma (TSH-secreting pituitary adenoma, thyrotropinoma) or from a selective resistance to thyroid hormone in which defective, but nonneoplastic pituitary thyrotrophs are not sufficiently suppressed by elevated circulating T3 levels. Careful radiological, laboratory, and clinical studies are required to differentiate between these two forms of inappropriate TSH secretion, i.e., neoplastic and nonneoplastic disease. It is also important to distinguish these conditions from pituitary thyrotroph hyperplasia resulting from longstanding severe hypothyroidism, for example, after thyroid ablation for cancer. In such cases, the lack of adequate thyroid hormone feedback results in excess TSH secretion, and the consequent thyrotroph hyperplasia is a condition that may also result in a space-occupying pituitary lesion. The latter, however, is usually differentiated from adenoma, since in most cases, hyperplasia will regress following regular substitution therapy with thyroid hormones.

Although this chapter is mainly concerned with thyrotroph adenomas, the authors consider it necessary to describe briefly the nonneoplastic conditions, since these require different managements than those for thyrotropinomas. Differential diagnosis is therefore imperative. The terms thyrotroph adenoma, TSH-secreting pituitary adenoma, thyrotropinoma, and TSHoma are used synonymously.

INAPPROPRIATE SECRETION OF TSH WITH PITUITARY TUMOR

INCIDENCE   Originally, pituitary tumors producing TSH were considered very exceptional rarities. Only when specific sensitive assays for TSH became available could this condition be diagnosed. Hamilton et al. *(5)* were the first to describe a case of hyperthyroidism secondary to a TSH-secreting pituitary adenoma diagnosed by modern radioimmunoassay techniques in 1970. Subsequently, other cases were reported. Thyrotroph adenomas may arise from a *de novo* somatic mutation of a thyrotroph cell or may be owing to thyrotroph hyperplasia following hypothyroidism. Their incidence is low. The authors *(6)* have encountered 7 such cases in a series of 1224 pituitary adenomas (0.65%). Beckers et al. *(7)* found 7 cases among 800 pituitary adenomas, and Wilson *(8)* had only 2 thyrotropinomas among 1000 pituitary adenomas in his surgical series. To date, however, there have been more than 300 well-reported cases, mostly in small series as anecdotal findings. The majority of cases of inappropriate secretion of TSH are caused by a thyrotropinoma.

CLINICAL PRESENTATION   The patient with a thyrotroph adenoma of the pituitary gland usually presents with signs of hormonal oversecretion. Goiter and clinical signs of hyperthyroidism are the most frequent initial complaints. Many of these patients then undergo therapies targeted primarily to the thyroid, since the underlying cause of the disease remains unrecognized at this stage. Frequently, goiter had recurred after subtotal surgical thyroidectomy or radioiodine therapy, when the diagnosis of a thyrotropinoma was established *(4,9)*. Later, with progression of adenoma size, such symptoms as headache, visual disturbances, and other disturbances associated with a pituitary mass lesion such as third nerve palsy, become apparent and direct the clinical attention to the sellar region. Since most of these tumors are medium-

From: *Diagnosis and Management of Pituitary Tumors* (K. Thapar, K. Kovacs, B. W. Scheithauer, and R. V. Lloyd, eds.), ©Humana Press Inc., Totowa, NJ.

sized or large, some degree of hypopituitarism is commonly encountered. The patients lack stigmata of Graves' disease, such as ophthalmopathy, pretibial edema, and acropachy. A unilateral exophthalmus, observed in the case reported by Yovos et al. *(10)*, was the result of invasion of the orbit and certainly not the result of an autoimmune reaction. Some patients who harbor pluri-hormonal adenomas present with acromegaly or symptoms consistent with the diagnosis of prolactinoma. The age of the patients thus far reported ranged from 13 *(11)* to 84 *(7)* yr. The most common age range of those coming to clinical attention is between 30 and 60 yr *(12)*. In contrast to autoimmune hyperthyroidism, there is no sex predilection for thyrotroph adenomas. In a total of 4 cases was there an association between MEA type 1 and a thyrotropinoma *(13,13a)*.

ENDOCRINE TESTING It is characteristic of these tumors that the TSH level is not completely suppressed, although circulating levels of T3 and T4 are elevated. Patients may have TSH levels that are either elevated or within the normal range for euthyroid individuals, despite the presence of hyperthyroidism. A specific and sufficiently sensitive immunoassay needs to be employed to document inappropriate secretion of TSH and, thus, central hyperthyroidism *(4,12,14)*. The presence of a pituitary mass lesion and the laboratory feature of inappropriate secretion of TSH are diagnostic. Theoretically, a hormonally inactive pituitary adenoma could coincide with thyrotoxicosis, resulting from a primary thyroid origin. In the latter case, completely suppressed TSH levels, which would exclude the presence of a TSH-secreting adenoma, would be expected. The magnitude of TSH elevation has been reported to range from 1.1 to 568 µU/mL *(7,15)*. The mean serum TSH levels were found to be significantly higher in the patients with a treated thyroid as compared to those with an intact thyroid *(15a)*. The biological activity of the TSH produced by thyrotroph adenoma cells may vary considerably. Beck-Peccoz et al. *(16,17)* demonstrated that immunoreactive TSH synthesized by a thyrotroph adenoma when partially purified by immunoaffinity chromatography showed a higher activity in stimulating adenylate cyclase from a human thyroid membrane preparation than normal TSH. Gel-filtration studies revealed that this biologically hyperactive TSH had a smaller apparent molecular weight than normal TSH. Similarly, Bevan et al. *(18)* found a much higher activity of their tumor TSH by utilizing a cytochemical bioassay. Additionally, Kourides et al. *(26)* demonstrated that patients with TSH-secreting adenomas usually produce excess amounts of the common glycoprotein α-subunit (α-TSH). This should result in a molar ratio of greater than unity in such cases. Although all 27 patients compiled by Smallridge *(29)* fulfilled this criterion, a few patients with unequivocally documented thyrotropinomas have levels below 1.0 *(4,7,11,13,21,22)*. Furthermore, a few cases of thyrotropinomas with undetectable α-subunit levels have been reported *(6,7,15,23)*. In the authors' series, there was one of seven cases with an undetectable serum α-subunit. However, in two further cases with normal α-subunit levels, the α-subunit/TSH ratio was below 1.0. Furthermore, the presence of molar α-subunit/TSH ratios was as high as 5.7 in controls with normal levels of TSH and gonadotropins, respectively, and 29.1 in euthyroid postmenopausal women, indicates the need to compare the individual values with those of controls matched for the TSH and gonadotropin levels before drawing any diagnostic conclusions *(13a)*. Thus, although generally helpful, some caution is certainly required regarding this test. β-TSH levels are normal in patients

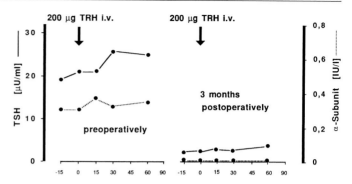

Figure 19-1 Pre- and postoperative response of TSH and α-TSH to TRH in a patient successfully treated by transsphenoidal surgery.

with thyrotropinomas. Thyrotroph microadenomas may pose a much greater diagnostic problem, since they might escape direct depiction at the first instance by their minute size. Sophisticated magnetic resonance imaging (MRI) utilizing thin-section techniques and gadolinium-enhanced images is required to document even these lesions that carry an excellent prognosis if submitted to transsphenoidal pituitary microsurgery. Whether a lateralization gradient obtained during simultaneous bilateral petrosal sinus catheterization performed in radiologically negative cases is helpful to differentiate neoplastic and nonneoplastic cases of inappropriate TSH secretion *(12)* has as yet not been convincingly demonstrated.

During the past 20 years, many patients with TSH-secreting pituitary adenomas underwent a variety of provocative and suppressive tests. The TRH test is generally believed to be the most important of them, and it was originally attributed major importance in the discrimination of tumorous and nontumorous inappropriate TSH secretion. Although basal TSH levels were measurable with thyrotropinomas, only 25% of these patients exhibit at least a 100% increase in basal values after intravenous TRH *(4,14,15)*. However, 39% had a significant response of TSH after TRH administration *(24)*. Thus, a negative test strongly accounts for a TSH-secreting adenoma, but a positive test does not exclude neoplastic TSH secretion from a thyrotroph adenoma. The majority of patients with tumors have at least some response of TSH following TRH administration. Despite the variable response of TSH to TRH in these cases, α-TSH usually parallels the TSH response *(21,25–28)*.

The influence of basal thyroid hormones on TSH secretion can indirectly be deducted from the response of TSH to thyrostatic medical treatment. In 70% of cases, an increase in TSH levels occurs when antithyroid medical treatment is instituted in order to control hyperthyroidism *(29)*. It is not yet clearly elucidated whether this increase in serum TSH after thyrostatic drug administration is owing to increased secretion by the normal or adenomatous thyrotrophs. Low basal TSH levels that lack stimulation after TRH administration, however, support the concept that normal thyrotrophs are suppressed in this condition (Figure 1) and that they only regain function some time after resection of the TSH-secreting adenoma. We have not found a case in the medical literature in which ectopic TRH secretion was reported. Testing for antithyroglobulin and antimicrosomal antibodies yields negative results in thyrotroph adenomas, unless there is a coexisting thyroid immunopathy.

Despite the fact that the vast majority of patients with TSH-secreting adenomas only exhibit an oversecretion of TSH (and α-subunit), several patients with thyrotropinomas were found to have a cosecretion of TSH and other pituitary hormones *(13a,15a)*. Frequently, this multihormonal potency is expressed by concomitant excessive growth hormone and prolactin secretion. There are many instances of TSH hypersecretion associated with acromegaly reported *(15,17,30,30a)*. The combination was found in 13 cases in the review by Smallridge *(29)* and in 7 cases in the review by Faglia et al. *(4)*. Acromegaly may frequently be the cardinal clinical feature at presentation of these patients. Other patients have hyperprolactinemia concomitant to TSH hypersecretion and the highest incidence of this combination in a single series was reported by Gesundheit et al. *(15)* in whose material seven of nine patients exhibited this feature.

IN VITRO STUDIES Because of their rarity, there have been relatively few studies on the behavior of thyrotroph adenomas in vitro. Nevertheless, during the past decade or so, a number of reports have appeared in the literature from various groups demonstrating consistent findings and from which some conclusions can be drawn concerning the in vitro characteristics of thyrotropinomas. In one of the earliest reports, pituitary tumor material from a 36-yr-old female who presented with elevated serum TSH and T4 levels was found to secrete only TSH in explant culture *(31)*. The rate of secretion declined with time in culture, and this pattern was confirmed in a later report *(28)*. This latter group also demonstrated stimulatory effects of both TRH and luteinizing hormone releasing hormone (LHRH) on TSH secretion. Interestingly, in this tumour, T3 and dopamine were ineffective in inhibiting TSH secretion, suggesting resistance to these factors. In another in vitro study using cultures of a single TSH-secreting pituitary adenoma, TRH was found to increase powerfully the rate of membrane phosphatidylinositol hydrolysis *(32)*, although the effects on TSH secretion were not reported.

Because of its potential clinical importance in treating thyrotroph adenomas, a few in vitro studies have concentrated on examining the effects of the long-acting somatostatin analog, octreotide. As well as decreasing TSH secretion in vitro, octreotide also inhibits adenylyl cyclase activity *(33)* and reduces the stimulation of phosphatidylinositol hydrolysis exerted by TRH *(32)*. Consistent with these findings, thyrotroph adenomas possess receptors for somatostatin, although at less density than found in GH-secreting pituitary cells *(33)*.

In culture, some thyrotroph adenomas have been shown to contain and secrete other pituitary hormones, most usually GH *(28,34)*. Additionally, α-subunit secretion by cultured thyrotropinomas is a very consistent finding *(28,33,34)*. In our own studies, six pituitary tumors removed from hyperthyroid patients were all found to secrete high levels of α-subunit as well as TSH *(6,35)*. Confirming other findings, TSH secretion was stimulated by TRH and LHRH in three cases, and TRH also increased the rate of phosphatidylinositol hydrolysis. Octreotide dose-dependently inhibited TSH secretion in these same three tumors (Figure 2). Interestingly, however, these factors had no effect in three other cultured thyrotroph adenomas in our series, supporting the above-mentioned findings that some tumors may be inherently resistant to normal control mechanisms, including inhibitory influences. It is worth mentioning that none of these six tumors contained gsp oncogenes, indicating that these specific defects, commonly present in GH-secreting tumors and some functionless tumors, are unlikely to be a common etiological factor in thyrotropinomas.

More recently, some studies have been directed at examining the molecular characteristics of thyrotroph adenomas *(36)*. These

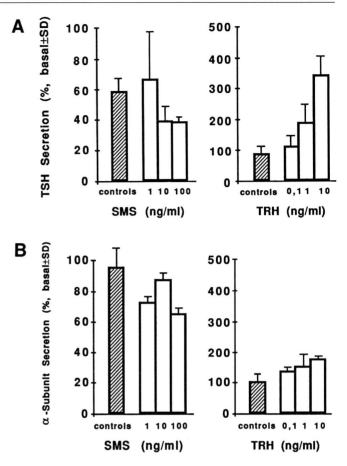

Figure 19-2 In vitro studies on the influence of TRH and octreotide on TSH and α-TSH secretion of a thyrotroph pituitary adenoma in dispersed cell cultures.

studies have demonstrated the presence of the transcription factor, Pit-1, in TSH-secreting tumor cells, and thus raise the possibility that this factor plays a pivotal role in controlling TSH secretion and perhaps tumorigenesis. A recent study screening candidate oncogenes in thyrotroph adenomas also could not identify a responsible somatic mutation. It revealed the absence of activating mutations in the $G\alpha_q$, $G\alpha_{11}$, and thyrotropin-releasing hormone receptor genes *(37)*.

MORPHOLOGICAL STUDIES Thyrotrophinomas originate from thyrotroph cells of the anterior pituitary. Although mostly benign, they have a tendency to invade adjacent structures more than other pituitary adenomas *(38–40)*. In this respect, they are comparable to ACTH-secreting adenomas associated with Nelson's syndrome whose growth is also promoted by a deficient negative feedback system *(38)*. Only recently have Mixons et al. *(40)* reported the first case of a thyrotropin-secreting pituitary carcinoma. A 40-yr-old woman developed a sacral metastasis 5 yr after incomplete transsphenoidal and transcranial surgery followed by external megavoltage radiotherapy. She later died from generalized metastatic disease.

On light microscopy, thyrotroph adenoma cells are chromophobic and contain a few small PAS-positive cytoplasmatic granules or, less frequently, large PAS-positive lysosomal globules. Immunohistochemistry reveals the presence of TSH and α-TSH in most, but not all tumors, in a variable percentage of cells *(36,41)*. Frequently, the plurihormonality of these tumors is also reflected by immunohistochemistry, which most frequently documents growth hormone and prolactin, but occasionally also gonadotropins. Investigations using the double-staining method showed that β-TSH and α-TSH were frequently colocalized in the same cell, but some cells were found only to stain for α-TSH or β-TSH *(36).* Terzolo et al. *(42)* could immunohistochemically detect α-TSH in all cells of their tumor. Using a double gold immunolabeling, they found that only a few cells stained positively for both α-TSH and β-TSH. They concluded that their tumor was composed of two different cell types.

Ultrastructurally, many of these adenomas are monomorphic and consist of cells with the characteristics of thyrotrophs *(41,43).* Electron microscopy reveals that the tumors are composed of middle-sized or large, well-differentiated cells. Their cytoplasm contains a well-developed rough endoplasmatic reticulum. The Golgi complexes are represented in a variable degree. The secretory granules are mostly spherical and usually small, measuring 100–200 nm in their largest diameter. Occasionally, such adenomas have larger secretory granules that measure up to 400 nm in diameter.

SURGERY   A most radical but selective neurosurgical operation today is considered the treatment of choice for TSH-secreting adenomas. The criteria applied to define "remission" and "success" vary considerably and still are matters of controversy *(6,15a,29,39,44a,46).* In the earlier literature, a success rate of only 31% (19 of 62 patients) was reported for a compiled series *(4).* Once postoperative irradiation was added, the normalization rate increased to 42%. Grisoli et al. *(39)* found only 5 normalizations achieved by transcranial surgery in 16 patients, when they reviewed the literature a decade ago. Early reports on surgical treatment were not only discouraging for their unfavorable results with respect to normalization of the hormone excess and their failure to eradicate all the tumor mass. McCutcheon et al. *(31)* report on a 50% mortality (2 of 4) from surgical treatment of large and invasive thyrotroph adenomas. The clinical outcome of these patients was adversely influenced by the delay in establishing the correct diagnosis and improper first-line treatments. In the earlier NIH series compiled by Gesundheit et al. *(15),* the average delay between documentation of clinical hyperthyroidism and the diagnosis of a thyrotrophinoma was 6.2 ± 4.8 (SD) yr. Four of their patients who developed invasive macroadenomas and who had a poor surgical outcome had erroneously been treated for a period as long as 18 yr for primary hyperthyroidism. More recent series *(6,7,15a,36,44a)* report much more promising figures for normalization with transsphenoidal surgery with normalization rates of 75–100% being achieved, depending on the criteria for normalization applied. Subnormal serum TSH levels are indicative of successful surgery, at least in patients with an intact thyroid. In successfully operated patients, TSH and α-TSH levels normalize quickly, as demonstrated by peri- and postoperative measurements (Figure 3). In the authors' series, normal values for both serum parameters were achieved within 500 min after tumor resection in the patients who underwent successful transsphenoidal surgery for thyrotropinoma *(35).* However, this time interval is clearly dependent on the absolute height of the TSH excess prior to surgery. Beckers et al. *(7)* observed the reincrease of serum TSH and thyroid hormones as early as 10 d after initial normalization of these parameters following surgery of an invasive macroadenoma. The plasma clearance rates may, however, vary owing to different glycosylation rates of α-TSH and TSH secreted by thyrotroph

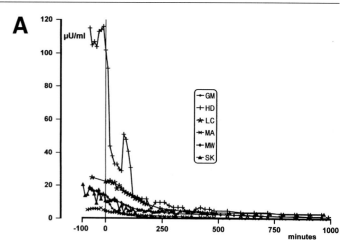

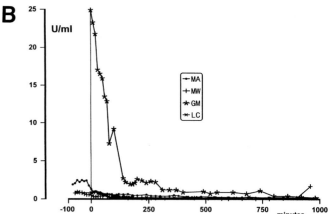

Figure 19-3   Perioperative measurements of TSH **(A)** and α-TSH **(B)** in 6 and 4 patients, respectively, treated successfully by transsphenoidal microsurgery.

tumors from normal values, which are 40–60 mL/min for the metabolic clearance rate and 50–80 min for the plasma half-life *(44).* It is important to perform the postoperative assessment when the patient is in a steady-state condition. Losa et al. *(44a)* favor the T_3-suppression test as the most stringent criterion for a complete postoperative remission. The results of transsphenoidal surgery are particularly favorable in thyrotroph microadenomas (<10 mm) of which unfortunately only a few cases have been diagnosed *(11,13,13a,15a,19,31,44a,45–47).* However, there is no doubt that many of these tumors carry unfavorable prognostic factors, namely large size and a high rate of invasion into surrounding structures. The biological behavior of the neoplasms in terms of their invasive nature has been closely related to whether or not they were previously treated by thyroid ablation *(13a,44a).* A primary therapy targeted against the thyroid gland seems to increase the proportion of large and invasive adenomas. In these, the main goal of surgery, whether via the transsphenoidal or transcranial approach, is to debulk the tumor in order to obtain a more promising outcome after subsequent irradiation.

RADIOTHERAPY   Conventional external irradiation of the adenoma utilizing a fractionation scheme that delivers some 45 gy over 4–5 wk to the tumor has mostly been used to supplement surgery in patients in whom the operation has failed to eradicate the tumor mass and to normalize TSH secretion *(29).* Rarely, it has been employed as the primary treatment *(48).* One would expect

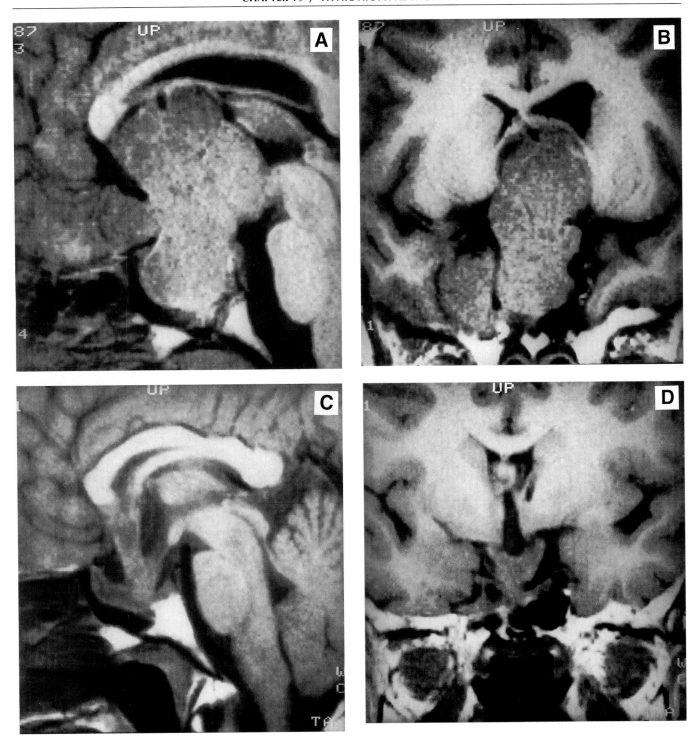

Figure 19-4 Effect of postoperative radiotherapy on the large residual tumor mass in a 11-yr-old girl with a giant invasive thyrotroph adenoma who had persistent inappropriate secretion of TSH after transcranial surgery. The tumor is depicted in sagittal (**A,C**) and coronal (**B,D**) sections both before surgery (**A,B**) and 8 yr after the completion of a course of external radiotherapy (**C,D**). When the repeat MRI investigation was performed, TSH secretion was normal in the presence of euthyroidism.

that similarly to other hormone oversecretion syndromes associated with pituitary tumors, irradiation would cause a slowly progressive effect on excessive hormone secretion, although there is little documentation of such courses in thyrotroph adenomas. The authors have observed the normalization of TSH secretion in an 11-yr-old girl with an invasive giant thyrotropinoma who had incomplete transcranial surgery followed by a course of external

radiotherapy (Figure 4). In this patient, persistently elevated TSH levels in the presence of euthyroidism were achieved after 8 yr. In a previous compilation of therapy results *(29)*, patients treated by external irradiation of the tumor were curative in only 1 of 8 patients, whereas 11 out of 24 patients (46%) who underwent both surgery and postoperative irradiation were treated successfully with the follow-up interval ranging between 3 and 36 mo. Thus,

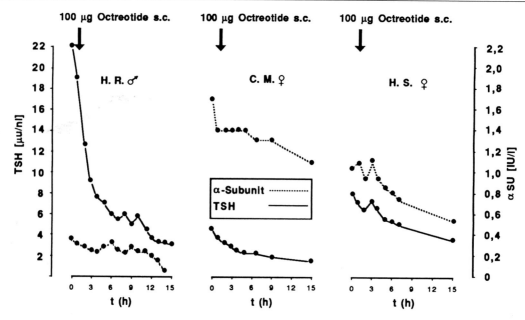

Figure 19-5   Acute effect of 100 μg octreotide subcutaneously on TSH and α-TSH levels.

irradiation of residual tumor is recommended once surgery fails to eradicate the tumor mass completely or if the inappropriate secretion of TSH persists postoperatively. No conclusive data are to date available about the efficacy of focused radiotherapy in this group of adenomas.

MEDICAL THERAPY   Since the patients with thyrotropinomas mostly present with hyperthyroidism, some kind of medical therapy is usually required to achieve euthyroidism before they can undergo pituitary surgery. This medical therapy can be directed toward either the thyroid or the pituitary gland. The conventional approach was to administer inhibitors of thyroid hormone synthesis, namely thioamines or potassium iodide as a short-term medical treatment in order to prepare the patient for surgery (12). Sometimes, the symptoms can be controlled by β-blockers alone. Since decreasing thyroid hormones may promote tumor growth in these lesions, a long-term administration of antithyroid drugs should be avoided as should be surgical or radioiodine-induced thyroid ablation. Therapies directed at the thyroid may not only cause an increase in circulating TSH levels, but also increase the proliferative potential of these tumors. In addition, they impede the proper follow-up of the patient after pituitary surgery, since recurrence of the thyrotropinoma can no longer be recognized by a return of hyperthyroidism (12). Medical therapy with dopamine agonists has proved to be generally unsuccessful in these tumors (29,49).

In contrast, octreotide, a long-acting somatostatin analog has been shown to be a valuable medical treatment option for TSH-secreting pituitary adenomas, which possess somatostatin receptors (33). A rapid suppression of TSH and α-TSH levels occurs and, subsequently, by prolonged therapy also a decrease in elevated thyroid hormones (50). Administration of a single dose of 50–100 μg of octreotide subcutaneously led to a significant decrease in TSH levels in all but one of the 21 patients tested by Chanson and Warnet (49). The authors observed a dramatic decrease in both TSH and α-TSH levels in all eight patients studied in this respect (Figure 5). Fischler and Reinhart (43a) have documented rapid tumor shrinkage and recovery from hyperthy-

roidism within 3 wk of octreotide treatment of a large macroadenoma. Long-term treatment with octreotide has been shown to normalize TSH secretion in 78% of patients (49). In some cases, octreotide also produces a reduction in tumor size, which leads to an improvement in visual function (23,51) and to a radiologically detectable regression of the tumor mass (7,51–54), possibly reflecting its direct mode of action. However, this therapy is also associated with side effects, and at least initially, most patients complain of some abdominal discomfort and diarrhea after initiation of octreotide. Many patients develop gallstones during long-term treatment. Since the drugs have the property to restore euthyroidism, they should be considered first in either the preoperative (54a) or postoperative (54b) period. The development of long acting formulations of somatostatin analogs has helped to reduce side effects with efficient treatments. This has been shown also for lanreotide (54b). Occasionally, an escape from this treatment is observed (55). Furthermore, there may be an individual patient who does not respond to somatostatin analogs. Karlsson et al. (56) report on such a case who was insensitive to treatment with octreotide, but responded to D-thyroxine and dopamine agonists.

INAPPROPRIATE SECRETION OF TSH WITHOUT PITUITARY TUMOR

Hyperthyroidism resulting from inappropriate secretion of TSH has also been described in several patients without evidence of a pituitary tumor. In these, it is thought to be caused by a selective resistance of the pituitary to thyroid hormones. A selective pituitary resistance to thyroid hormone is mandatory for a clinical manifestation, since hyperthyroidism only results if the pituitary gland is more resistant to thyroid hormone than peripheral tissues (24). This group comprises approx 25% of patients with inappropriate secretion of TSH and is thus the minority. In 1975, Gershengorn and Weintraub (2) reported the first case of such a nonneoplastic secretion of TSH. Meanwhile, the number of case reports of patients suffering from this condition exceeds 50. In their review, Refetoff et al. (24) found 51 well-documented cases published in the medical literature until 1993. Selective pituitary resistance to thyroid hormone is less frequent than generalized resistance of all tissues to thyroid hormone. The latter, however, does not produce clinical symptoms. It is of paramount importance to differentiate nonneoplastic inappropriate secretion of TSH from thyrotroph adenoma, since their ideal therapies are completely different (4,56a). Clinically, hyperthyroidism is a consistent finding in these patients. They lack ophthalmopathy and pretibial edema as do patients with a pituitary tumor. High-resolution imaging of the sella turcica region is probably the most important and most reliable single diagnostic tool. Poor-quality imaging in the past has somewhat obscured a clear-cut differentiation of the pathogenetic entities and led to a misinterpretation of data in a few cases. Tests for thyroid antibodies and thyroid-stimulating antibodies are usually negative. During endocrine testing, these patients exhibit a suppression of TSH by thyroid hormones, by somatostatin, and by dopamine agonists (4,12,24). In response to TRH stimulation, an exaggerated response is usually found, which is clearly different in most patients with thyrotropinomas. However, the suppression of TSH after high doses of exogenous glucocorticoids is a similar response that is observed in both the tumorous and the nontumorous groups. The α-subunit level is usually normal as well as the α-subunit/TSH ratio, which is <1.0. Primary therapy should be aimed at pharmacologically suppressing the TSH hypersecretion. The ideal agent would have a strong TSH-suppressive effect, yet no thyromimetic activity. Octreotide has been shown to be variably effective. Although an intravenous infusion readily suppressed TSH secretion, the effects of prolonged subcutaneous injection were weak and short-lasting (57). 3,5,3'-Triiodoacetic acid (TRIAC), a T3 analog that binds to nuclear receptors with higher affinity than T3 and has negligible metabolic effects, has been employed successfully to inhibit TSH secretion (58). Both T3 and T4 are known to suppress TSH secretion, but a normalization of TSH is rarely achieved. Furthermore, they cause hyperthyroidism. Long term therapy with glucocorticoids is also not recommended for their side effects, although they have the ability to suppress TSH secretion effectively.

There are a few other conditions that can be confused with TSH-induced hyperthyroidism. However, these result from abnormalities in pituitary and thyroid physiology and misinterpretations of laboratory values: Laboratory artifacts, inhibition of T_4 to T_3 conversion, abnormal thyroid hormone binding by serum proteins, and disequilibration (nonsteady state) of thyroid hormones and TSH (4,12).

HYPOTHYROIDISM AND PITUITARY TUMOR

In long-standing hypothyroidism, pituitary mass lesions may eventually result from the lack of thyroid hormone feedback. In this context, it does not matter whether hypothyroidism is owing to congenital aplasia of the thyroid gland or induced by iatrogenic thyroid ablation, antithyroid drugs, or X-ray exposure of the thyroid. As early as 1851, Niepce (59) observed enlargement of the sellar content during autopsies of several cretins. More recently, Scheithauer et al. (60) investigated the pituitary glands of 64 patients with long-standing hypothyroidism. They found thyrotroph hyperplasia in 94% of the glands, although without significant mass effect. Hyperplasia was diffuse in 69% of cases. However, in 25% of the species, they detected nodular thyrotroph hyperplasia. They even found five tiny microadenomas staining for TSH. In addition, in 20% of these pituitaries, lactotroph hyperplasia was present.

Pituitary mass lesions in the presence of hypothyroidism have important clinical implications, since their management also differs completely from that of thyrotrophin-secreting adenomas. Furthermore, there is experimental evidence for the possible induction of a thyrotrophinoma by producing hypothyroidism (20,61).

The diagnostic basis is the detection of hypothyroidism. This occurs more commonly in females than in males and is frequently a result of autoimmune thyroiditis. Thus, thyroid antibodies will commonly be found in the serum. Congenital hypothyroidism and missing compliance with thyroid hormone substitution are other common causes. Hypothyroidism is mostly symptomatic once it causes thyrotroph hyperplasia of the pituitary. An occasional patient may present for symptoms of hyperprolactinemia resulting from mixed thyrotroph and lactotroph hyperplasia (34). However, sometimes an individual patient appears to be completely asymptomatic. Unexplained weight gain, cold intolerance, fatigue, and headache are frequent among the presenting symptoms. In children, thyrotroph hyperplasia from hypothyroidism has occasionally been reported in association with precocious puberty. Hypogonadism and galactorrhea are important findings in adults. Decreased libido and potency in males and menstrual abnormalities in females most likely result from concomitant hyperprolactinemia. Radiologically detectable sellar mass lesions and elevated prolactin levels occasionally lead to the erroneous diagnosis of prolactinoma in such cases. The underlying pathophysiological mechanism is the effect of an increased action of TRH, which stimulates both TSH and prolactin secretion. A few women who developed their pituitary enlargement as a result of postpartum thyroiditis have been reported (62).

On laboratory investigation, virtually all of these patients reveal the combination of hypothyroidism and clearly elevated TSH levels. Baseline TSH levels and their response to TRH mainly depend on the levels of serum thyroid hormones (Figure 6). They almost uniquely show an exaggerated response of TSH. Today, measurements of free T4, TSH, and prolactin are recommended once this diagnosis is suspected. Hyperprolactinemia was present in up to 78% of cases in a cumulative series (29). A deficiency of the hypothalamic–pituitary–adrenal axis, of gonadal regulation, and of growth hormone secretion were also occasionally found during dynamic endocrine testing. MRI and thin collimation computerized tomography may reveal a pituitary mass lesion of variable size. This may be difficult to distinguish from a pituitary adenoma if it has a size of around 10 mm or more. However, with hyperplasia, there is usually no distinct intrasellar circumscribed low-intensity region visible, in contrast to microadenomas. Even when plain skull X-rays only are obtained, these consistently show some sellar enlargement in these cases. Yamada et al. (63) deducted a close correlation between the sella turcica and serum TSH levels from these.

To recognize the fact that the pituitary mass lesion in this condition usually represents pituitary hyperplasia is essential and leads to the institution of proper treatment, i.e., substitution therapy with thyroxine. Once the underlying lack of thyroid hormone is corrected, these pituitaries usually have the potential to return to their former normal size. The process of involution of such a "tumor" has frequently been documented, historically by plain skull X-rays, and more recently by computerized tomography (CT) (64,65) and MRI (66,67,67a). The authors have observed a patient who became severely hypothyroid after total thyroidectomy and irradiation for thyroid cancer when she failed to comply with her substitution scheme. She had a regression of her enlarged gland when she

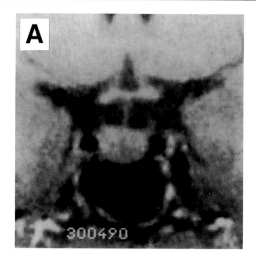
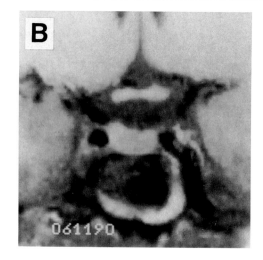
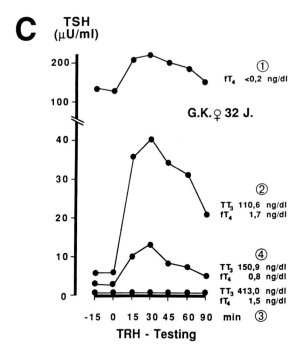

Figure 19-6 Pituitary hyperplasia in a 32-yr-old woman with hypothyroidism following thyroidectomy and radiotherapy for thyroid cancer. The patient was incompliant with her thyroid hormone substitution therapy and had severe hyperthyroidism. The MRI documented pituitary hyperplasia (**A**), which showed considerable size reduction on appropriate substitution therapy half a year later (**B**). Basal and TRH-induced TSH levels in the same case of pituitary thyrotroph hyperplasia (**C**) before (1) and during induction of a consequent substitution therapy with thyroid hormone. In contrast to thyrotroph adenomas, iatrogenic induction of hyperthyroidism leads to a complete suppression of both basal and TRH-induced TSH-secretion (4). The laboratory findings in the euthyroid status, half a year after institution of therapy, correspond to the MRI findings in B.

finally reached euthyroidism on regular medication as documented by repeat MRI (Figure 6). Katevuo et al. *(68)* documented a decrease of lesion density in enhanced CT scans in seven of eight patients following proper substitution therapy with thyroxine. A complete resolution of the pituitary mass lesion has been observed as early as 1 wk after replacement was commenced *(67a)*. It may, however, take up to 1 yr to achieve a satisfactory result. The radiologically detectable regression of the mass is mostly paralleled by an impressive clinical improvement. In patients with long-standing hypothyroidism, it is advisable to start with a rather small dose of thyroxine and gradually increase this until normal levels of T4 and T3 are achieved. In the past, some of these patients have been submitted to pituitary surgery, and the diagnosis of hyperplasia

has consequently been made by the pathologist. Retrospectively, these patients would probably have done just as well had they been placed on proper replacement therapy.

In a few cases, however, replacement therapy with thyroxine is not able to decrease the size of the lesion even if high normal values of thyroid hormones are reached. An occasional patient may even exhibit an increase in the size of the lesion despite adequate substitution therapy *(69)*. Therefore, such patients need to be closely monitored.

REFERENCES

1. Jackson IMD. Regulation of thyrotropin secretion. In: Imura H, ed. The Pituitary Gland. Raven, New York 1994, pp. 179–216.

2. Gershengorn MC, Weintraub BD. Thyrotropin-induced hyperthyroidism caused by selective pituitary resistance to thyroid hormone: a new syndrome of inappropriate secretion of TSH. J Clin Invest 1975;56:633–642.

3. Weintraub BD, Gershengorn MC, Kourides IA, Fein H. Inappropriate secretion of thyroid-stimulating hormone. Ann Int Med 1981; 95:339–351.

4. Faglia G, Beck-Peccoz P, Piscitelli G, Medri G. Inappropriate secretion of thyrotropin by the pituitary. Horm Res 1987;26:79–99.

5. Hamilton CR, Adams LC, Maloof F. Hyperthyroidism due to thyrotropin-producing pituitary chromophobe adenomas. N Engl J Med 1970;283:1077–1080.

6. Buchfelder M, Fahlbusch R, Becker W, Mann K. TSH-sezernierende Hypophysenadenome. Med Welt 1991;42:1033–1037.

7. Beckers A, Abs R, Mahler C, Vandalem JL, Pirens G, Hennen G, et al. Thyrotropin-secreting pituitary adenomas: Report of seven cases. J Clin Endocrinol Metab 1991;72:477–483.

8. Wilson CB. A decade of pituitary microsurgery. The Herbert Olivecrona Lecture. J Neurosurg 1984;61:814–833.

9. Horn K, Erhardt F, Fahlbusch R, Pickardt CR, von Werder K, Scriba PC. Recurrent goiter, hyperthyroidism, galactorrhea and amenorrhea due to a thyrotropin and prolactin-producing pituitary tumor. J Clin Endocrinol Metab 1976;43:137–143.

10. Yovos SJG, Falko JM, O'Dorisio TM, Malarkey WB, Cataland S, Capen CC. Thyrotoxicosis and a thyrotropin-secreting pituitary tumor causing unilateral exophthalmus. J Clin Endocrinol Metab 1981;53:338–343.

11. Korn EA, Gaich G, Brines M, Carpenter TO. Thyrotropin-secreting adenoma in an adolescent girl without increased serum thyrotropin-alpha. Horm Res 1994;42:120–123.

12. Gesundheit N. Thyrotropin-induced hyperthyroidism. In: Braverman LE, Utiger RD, eds. The Thyroid. J.B. Lippincott, Philadelphia, 1991, pp. 682–691.

13. Wolansky LJ, Leavitt GD, Elias BJ, Lee HJ, Dasmahapatra A, Byrne W. MRI of pituitary hyperplasia in hypothyroidism. Neuroradiology 1996;38:50–52.

13a. Beck-Peccoz P, Persani L, Asteria C, Romoli R. In: von Werder K, Fahlbusch R, eds. Pituitary Adenomas: From Basic Research to Diagnosis and Therapy. Elsevier, Amsterdam, 1996, pp. 277–290.

14. Gharib H, Carpenter PC, Scheithauer BW, Service FJ. The spectrum of inappropriate pituitary thyrotropin secretion associated with hyperthyroidism. Mayo Clin Proc 1982;57:556–563.

15. Gesundheit N, Petrick PA, Nissim M, Dahlberg A, Doppman JL, Emerson CH, et al. Thyrotropin-secreting pituitary adenomas: Clinical and biochemical heterogeneity. Ann Int Med 1989;111:827–835.

15a. Bruckner-Davis F, Oldfield EH, Skarulis MC, Doppman JL, Weintraub BD. Thyrotropin-secreting pituitary tumors: Diagnostic criteria, thyroid hormone sensitivity, and treatment outcome in 25 patients followed at the National Institutes of Health. J Clin Endocrinol Metab 1999;84:476–486.

16. Beck-Peccoz P, Persani L. Variable biological activity of thyroid-stimulating hormone. Eur J Endocrinol 1994;131:331–340.

17. Beck-Peccoz P, Piscitelli G, Amr S, Ballabio M, Bassetti M, Giannattasio G, et al. Endocrine, biochemical and morphological studies of a pituitary adenoma secreting growth hormone, thyreotropin (TSH) and α-subunit: Evidence for secretion of TSH with increase of bioactivity. J Clin Endocrinol Metab 1986;62:704–711.

18. Bevan JS, Esiri MM, Loveridge N, Faglia G, Burke CW. TSH secreting pituitary adenoma: case report, characterization of TSH and tumor cell perifusion. J Endocrinol 1985; 104, Suppl.:51.

19. Jackson JA, Smigiel M, Green JF. Hyperthyroidism due to a thyrotropin-secreting pituitary microadenoma. Henry Ford Hosp Med J 1987;35:198–200.

20. Moore GE, Brackney EL, Bock FG. Production of pituitary tumors in mice by chronic administration of a thiouracil derivative. Proc Soc Exp Biol Med 1953;82:643–645.

21. Chanson P, Orgiazzi J, Derome PJ, Bression D, Jedynac CP, et al. Paradoxical response of thyrotropin to L-dopa and presence of dopaminergic receptors in a thyrotropin-secreting pituitary adenoma. J Clin Endocrinol Metab 1984;59:542–546.

22. Koide Y, Kugai N, Kimura S, Fujita T, Kameya T, Azukizawa M, et al. A case of pituitary adenoma with possible simultaneous secretion of thyrotropin and follicle-stimulating hormone. J Clin Endocrinol Metab 1982;54:397–403.

23. Caron P, Gerbeau C, Prodagrol L, Simonetta C, Bayard F. Successful pregnancy in an infertile woman with a thyrotropin-secreting macroadenoma treated with somatostatin analog (octreotide). J Clin Endocrinol Metab 1996;81:1164–1168.

24. Refetoff S, Weiss RE, Usala SJ. The syndromes of resistance to thyroid hormone. Endocr Rev 1993;14:348–399.

25. Chanson P, Li JY, Le Dafniet M, Derome P, Kujas M, Murat A, et al. Absence of receptors for thyrotropin (TSH)-releasing hormone in human TSH-secreting pituitary adenomas associated with hyperthyroidism. J Clin Endocrinol Metab 1988;66:447–450.

26. Kourides IA, Ridgway EC, Weintraub BD, Bigos ST, Gershengorn MC, Maloof F. Thyrotropin-induced hyperthyroidism: Use of α- and β-subunit levels to identify patients with pituitary tumors. J Clin Endocrinol Metab 1977;45:534–543.

27. Samuels MH, Wood WM, Gordon DF, Kleinschmidt-DeMasters BK, Lillehei K, Ridgway EC. Clinical and molecular studies of a thyrotropin-secreting pituitary adenoma. J Clin Endocrinol Metab 1989;68:1211–1215.

28. Simard M, Mirell CJ, Pekary AE, Drexler J, Kovacs K, Hershman JM. Hormonal control of thyrotropin and growth hormone secretion in a human thyrotrop pituitary adenoma studied in vitro. Acta Endocrinol 1988;119:283–290.

29. Smallridge RC. Thyrotropin-secreting pituitary tumors. Diagnostic and therapeutic considerations. Endocrinol Metabol Clin North Am 1987;16:765–792.

30. Meinders AE, Willekens FLA, Bardens CAE, Seevinck J, Nieuwenhuijzen Kruseman AC. Acromegaly and thyrotoxicosis induced by a GH- and TSH-producing pituitary tumour which also contained prolactin. Neth J Med 1981;24:136–144.

30a. Patrick AW, Atkin SL, MacKenzie J, Foy PM, White MC, MacFarlane IA. Hyperthyroidism secondary to a pituitary adenoma secreting TSH, FSH, alpha-subunit and GH. Clin Endocrinol 1994;40:275–278.

31. Mashiter K, van Noorden S, Fahlbusch R, Skrabal K. Hyperthyroidism due to a TSH secreting pituitary adenoma: Case report, treatment and evidence for adenoma TSH by morphological and cell culture studies. Clin Endocrinol 1983;18:473–483.

32. Levy A, Eckland DJA, Gurney AM, Reubi JC, Lightman SL. Somatostatin and thyrotropin-releasing hormone response and receptor status of a thyrotropin-secreting pituitary adenoma: clinical and in vitro studies. J Neuroendocrinol 1989;1:321–326.

33. Bertherat J, Brue T, Enjalbert A, Gunz G, Rasolonjanahary R, Warnet A, et al. Somatostatin receptors on thyrotropin-secreting pituitary adenomas: comparison with the inhibitory effects of octreotide upon in vivo and in vitro hormonal secretion. J Clin Endocrinol Metab 1992;75:540–546.

34. Pioro EP, Scheithauer BW, Laws ER, Randall RV, Kovacs KT, Horvath E. Combined thyrotroph and lactotroph cell hyperplasia simulating prolactin-secreting pituitary adenoma in longstanding hypothyroidism. Surg Neurol 1988;29:218–226.

35. Buchfelder M, Fahlbusch R, Becker W, Berger P, Schwarz S, Mann K. Concomitant TSH and alpha-subunit secretion in 2 cases of successfully operated thyreotropinomas. Acta Endocrinol 1990; 122, Suppl. 1:70.

36. Sanno N, Teramoto A, Matsuno A, Inada K, Itoh J, Osamura RY. Clinical and immunohistochemical studies on TSH-secreting pituitary adenomas: Its multihormonality and expression of Pit-1. Mod Pathol 1994;7:893–899.

37. Dong Q, Brucker-Davis F, Weintraub BD, Smallridge RC, Carr FE, Battey J, et al. Screening of candidate oncogenes in human thyrotroph tumors: absence of activating mutations of the Gαq, Gα11, Gαs or thyrotropin-releasing hormone receptor gene. J Clin Endocrinol Metab 1996;81:1134–1140.

38. Buchfelder M, Fahlbusch R, Adams EF, Kiesewetter F, Thierauf P. Proliferation parameters for pituitary adenomas. Acta Neurochir 1996; 65, Suppl: 18–21.

39. Grisoli F, Leclerq T, Winteler JP, Jaquet P, Diaz-Vasquez P, Hassoun J, et al. Thyroid-stimulating hormone pituitary adenomas and hyperthyroidism. Surg Neurol 1986;25:361–368.

40. Mixons AJ, Friedman IC, Katz DA, Feuerstein IM, Taubenberger JM, Colandrea JM, et al. Thyrotropin-secreting pituitary carcinoma. J Clin Endocrinol Metab 1993;76:529–533.

41. Kovacs K, Horvath E, Stefaneanu L. Anatomy and pathology of the thyrotrophs. In: Braverman LE, Utiger RD, eds. The Thyroid. J.B. Lippincott, Philadelphia, 1991, pp. 40–50.

42. Terzolo M, Orlandi F, Bassetti M, Medri G, Paccotti P, Cortelazzi D, et al. Hyperthyroidism due to a pituitary adenoma composed of two different cell types, one secreting alpha-subunit alone and another cosecreting alpha-subunit and thyrotropin. J Clin Endocrinol Metab 1991;72:415–421.

43. Saeger W, Lüdecke DK. Pituitary adenomas with hyperfunction of TSH. Frequency, histological classification, immunocytochemistry and ultrastructure. Virchows Arch [Pathol Anat] 1982;394:255–267.

43a. Fischler MP, Reinhart WH. TSH-secreting pituitary macroadenoma: Rapid tumor shrinkage and recovery from hyperthyroidism with octreotide. J Endocrinol Invest 1999;22:64–65.

44. Kourides IA, Re RN, Weintraub BD, Ridgway EC, Maloof F. Metabolic clearance and secretion rates of subunits of human thyrotropin. J Clin Invest 1977;59:508–516.

44a. Losa M, Giovanelli M, Persani L, Mortini F, Faglia G, Beck-Peccoz P. Criteria of cure and follow-up of central hyperthyroidism due to thyrotropin-secreting pituitary adenomas. J Clin Endocrinol Metab 1996;81:3084–3090.

45. Kellett HA, Wyllie AH, Dale BAB, Best JJK, Toft AD. Hyperthyroidism due to a thyrotrophin-secreting microadenoma. Clin Endocrinol 1983;19:57–65.

46. McCutcheon IE, Weintraub BD, Oldfield EH. Surgical treatment of thyrotropin-secreting pituitary adenomas. J Neurosurg 1990;73:674–683.

47. Ridgway EC, Weintraub BD, Maloof F. Metabolic clearance and production rates of human thyrotropin. J Clin Invest 1974;53:895–903.

48. McLellan AR, Connell JMC, Alexander WD, Davies DL. Clinical response of thyrotropin-secreting macroadenoma to bromocriptine and radiotherapy. Acta Endocrinol 1988;119:189–194.

49. Chanson P, Warnet A. Treatment of thyroid-stimulating hormone-secreting adenomas with octreotide. Metabolism 1992; 41, Suppl 2:62–65.

50. Comi RJ, Gesundheit N, Murray L, Gorden P, Weintraub B. Response of thyrotropin-secreting pituitary adenomas to a long-acting somatostatin analogue. N Engl J Med 1987;317:12–17.

51. Allyn GSR, Bernstein R, Chynn KY, Kourides IA. Reduction in size of a thyrotropin- and gonadotropin-secreting pituitary adenoma treated with octreotide acetate (somatostatin analog). J Clin Endocrinol Metab 1992;74:690–694.

52. Lee EJ, Kyung RK, Sung KL, Hyun CL, Dong IK, Sun HK, et al. Reduction in size of a thyrotropin-secreting pituitary adenoma treated with octreotide acetate (somatostatin analog). Eur J Endocrinol 1994;131:109–112.

53. Shaker JL, Brickner RC, Sirus SR, Cerletty JM. Ocreotide acetate-induced size reduction of a large thyrotropin (TSH) secreting pituitary tumor with correction of hyperthyroidism and hypopituitarism. 73rd Annual Meeting of the Endocrine Society, Washington 1991 [abstract No. 1138].

54. Sy RAG, Bernstein R, Chynn KY, Kourides IA. Reduction in size of a thyrotropin- and gonadotropin secreting pituitary adenoma treated with octreotide acetate (somatostatin analog). J Clin Endocrinol Metab 1992;74:690–694.

54a. Iglesias P, Diez JJ. Long-term preoperative management of thyrotropin-secreting pituitary adenoma with octreotide. J Endocrinol Invest 1998;21:775–778.

54b. Kuhn JM, Arlot S, Levebre H, Caron P, Cortet-Rudelli C, Archambaud F, et al. Evaluation of the treatment of thyrotropin-secreting pituitary adenomas with a slow release formulation of the somatostatin analog lanreotide. J Clin Endocrinol Metab 2000;85:1487–1491.

55. Wémeau JL, Dewailly D, Leroy R, D'Herbomz M, Mazzuca M, Decoulx M, et al. Long-term treatment with the somatostatin analog SMS 201-995 in a patient with a thyrotropin- and growth hormone secreting tumor. J Clin Endocrinol Metab 1988;66:636–639.

56. Karlsson FA, Burman P, Kämpe O, Westlin JE, Wide L. Large somatostatin-insensitive thyrotropin-secreting pituitary tumour responsive to D-thyroxine and dopamine agonists. Acta Endocrinol 1991;129:291–295.

56a. Chatterjee VKK. Resistance to thyroid hormone. Horm Res 1997;48 (suppl 4):43–46.

57. Beck-Peccoz P, Mariotti S, Guillausseau PJ, Medri G, Piscitelli G, Bertli A, et al. Treatment of hyperthyroidism due to inappropriate secretion of thyrotropin with the somatostatin analog SMS 201-995. J Clin Endocrinol Metab 1989;68:208–214.

58. Dulgeroff AJ, Geffner ME, Koyal SN, Wong M, Hershman JM. Bromocriptine and Triac therapy for hyperthyroidism due to pituitary resistance to thyroid hormone. J Clin Endocrinol Metab 1992;75:1071–1075.

59. Niepce B. Traité du Goitre et du Crétinism. J.B. Ballière, Paris, 1851.

60. Scheithauer BW, Kovacs K, Randall RV, Ryan N. Pituitary gland in hypothyroidism: histologic and immunocytologic study. Arch Pathol Lab Med 1985;109:499–503.

61. Furth J, Dent JN, Burnett WT, Gadsden EL. The mechanism of induction and the characteristics of pituitary tumors induced by thyroidectomy. J Clin Endocrinol Metab 1955;15:81–91.

62. Valenta LJ, Tamkin JRS, Elias AN, Eisenberg H. Regression of a pituitary adenoma following levothyroxine therapy of primary hypothyroidism. Fertil Steril 1983;40:389–392.

63. Yamada T, Tsukui T, Ikejiri K, Yukimura Y, Kotani M. Volume of sella turcica in normal subjects and in patients with primary hypothyroidism and in hyperthyroidism. J Clin Endocrinol Metab 1976;42:817–822.

64. Okuno T, Sudo M, Momoi T, Takao T, Ito M, Konishi Y, et al. Pituitary hyperplasia due to hypothyroidism. J Comput Assist Tomogr 1980;4:600–602.

65. Pita JC, Shafey S, Pina R. Diminution of large pituitary tumor after replacement therapy for primary hypothyroidism. Neurology 1979;29:1169–1172.

66. Hutchins WW, Crues JV, Miya P, Pojunas KW. MR demonstration of pituitary hyperplasia and regression after therapy for hypothyroidism. AJNR 1990;11:410.

67. Wynne AG, Gharib H, Scheithauer BW, Davis DH, Freeman SL. Hyperthyroidism due to inappropriate secretion of Thyrotropin in 10 patients. Am J Med 1992;92:15–24.

67a. Sarlis NJ, Brucker-Davis F, Doppman JL, Skarulis MC. MRI-demonstrable regression of a pituitary mass in a case of primary hypothyroidism after a week of acute thyroid hormone therapy. J Clin Endocrinol Metab 1997;82:808–811.

68. Katevuo K, Välimäki M, Ketonen L, Lamberg BA, Pelkonen R. Computed tomography of the pituitary fossa in primary hypothyroidism. Effect of thyroxine treatment. Clin Endocrinol 1985;22:617–621.

69. Gup RS, Sheeler LR, Maeder MC, Tew JM. Pituitary enlargement and primary hypothyroidism: a report of two cases with sharply contrasting outcomes. Neurosurgery 1982;11:792–794.

20 Clinically Nonfunctioning Pituitary Adenomas

WILLIAM F. YOUNG, JR., MD

INTRODUCTION

Clinically nonfunctioning pituitary tumors are benign neoplasms that fail to cause a clinically recognizable syndrome. Although hormonal hypersecretion-determined clinical syndromes herald most pituitary adenomas, clinically "nonfunctioning" tumors represent approximately one-third of all discovered pituitary tumors. Despite their often chromophobic appearance, all are granule-containing and presumably hormone-producing *(1)*. Four types of tumors are included in the clinically nonfunctioning category:

1. Neoplasms that hypersecrete a hormone to such a minor degree that no symptoms result.
2. Neoplasms that hypersecrete a biologically active hormone that does not result in clinical symptomatology.
3. Neoplasms that hypersecrete an abnormal, biologically inactive version of hormone that fails to cause an endocrine syndrome.
4. Neoplasms that fail to secrete any hormone at all.

Clinically nonfunctioning tumors are derived from one of five cell types: corticotroph, gonadotroph, lactotroph, somatotroph, or thyrotroph. Most gonadotroph pituitary adenomas present as clinically nonfunctioning tumors because only 19% hypersecrete luteinizing hormone (LH) or follicle-stimulating hormone (FSH) *(2)*, and even when LH or FSH are hypersecreted, a clinically recognizable syndrome is not produced *(3)*. In a recent study, the clinical symptoms and factors leading to a diagnosis of pituitary tumor included: visual loss (43%), symptoms of hypopituitarism (22%), no symptoms (incidental diagnosis, 17%), headache (8%), and a combination of visual loss, hypopituitarism, and headache (10%) *(2)*.

The silent corticotroph adenoma is an uncommon type of nonfunctioning pituitary tumor. In a patient series of functioning and nonfunctioning pituitary tumors, 9% were silent corticotroph adenomas *(4)*. Among corticotroph adenomas, the frequency of the silent subtype may be as high as 43% *(5)*, but in those corticotroph adenomas removed at surgery, the frequency of the silent subtype is closer to 6% (author's personal observation). Owing to the lack of clinical symptomatology, this tumor is usually not recognized until immunohistochemical analyses on the adenomatous tissue are completed. In some cases, the increased

serum levels of bioinactive corticotropin precursors have been documented preoperatively *(6)*.

Although lactotroph adenomas cause amenorrhea and galactorrhea in premenopausal women, they are usually "silent" in postmenopausal women. In addition, the symptoms of hypogonadism and impotence in men caused by lactotroph adenomas may go unrecognized or unreported. Silent somatotroph and thyrotroph adenomas also occur, but are less frequent than the other subtypes.

CLINICAL PRESENTATION

Clinically nonfunctioning pituitary tumors are usually discovered in one of the following three clinical settings:

1. Local mass-effect symptoms from the tumor.
2. Symptoms related to various degrees of hypopituitarism.
3. Incidental discovery on computerized imaging of the head performed for reasons unrelated to pituitary disorders (Table 1).

Most pituitary tumors are slow-growing, and the mass-effect-related symptoms have an insidious onset over years. The suprasellar extension of the tumor compresses the optic chiasm, and visual field defects progress from superior temporal quadrantopsia to bitemporal hemianopsia, and eventually, blindness. The cause for the associated headaches is not always clear, but may be related to local traction effects. Rarely, the clinically nonfunctioning pituitary tumor patient may present with diplopia owing to oculomotor nerve compression, sudden hemorrhage into the adenoma (pituitary apoplexy), or cerebrospinal fluid rhinorrhea.

Table 1
Clinically Nonfunctioning Pituitary Tumors—
Clinical Presentations

Mass effects of the pituitary tumor
    Visual field loss
    Headaches
    Diplopia owing to oculomotor nerve compression
    Pituitary apoplexy
    Amenorrhea and galactorrhea
    Cerebrospinal fluid rhinorrhea
Hypopituitarism
    Hypogonadism
    Hypoadrenalism
    Hypothyroidism
    Diabetes insipidus (rare)
Incidental finding on computerized imaging

From: *Diagnosis and Management of Pituitary Tumors* (K. Thapar, K. Kovacs, B. W. Scheithauer, and R. V. Lloyd, eds.), ©Humana Press Inc., Totowa, NJ.

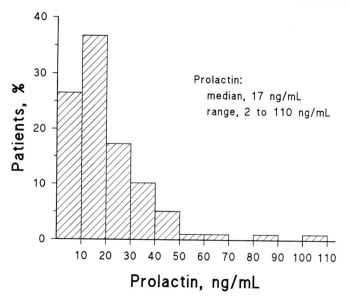

Figure 20-1 Serum prolactin levels from 97 patients with gonadotroph pituitary adenomas. Hyperprolactinemia was found in 32% of patients. The upper limit of normal for prolactin was 20 ng/mL and 23 ng/mL in men and women, respectively. (Reprinted with permission from ref. *2*. Copyright 1996 by Mayo Foundation for Medical Education and Research.)

The majority of clinically nonfunctioning pituitary tumors are macroadenomas when discovered, and frequently various degrees of pituitary hypofunction are present. Although these deficiencies may be recognized by the clinician at the time of diagnosis of a macroadenoma, they usually are not the primary reason for the patient to seek medical attention. Gonadal axis deficiency in patients with clinical nonfunctioning pituitary macroadenomas is relatively common. In men, the low testosterone levels usually result in decreased libido and energy; in premenopausal women, the lack of normal gonadotropin secretion may result in amenorrhea. Symptoms owing to deficiency of other pituitary-dependent target gland hormones (e.g., thyroid hormone, cortisol, growth hormone) or increased serum prolactin (PRL) concentrations may dominate the clinical presentation. Very rarely, the clinically nonfunctioning pituitary tumor may cause diabetes insipidus; when diabetes insipidus is part of the presentation, it should raise the suspicion of a nonpituitary tumor (e.g., metastatic disease) or a granulomatous process.

Because of pituitary stalk compression and interruption of dopamine transport, serum PRL concentrations are frequently increased in patients with nonfunctioning pituitary macroadenomas (Figure 1). It is important to emphasize that the combination of serum PRL concentration <200 ng/mL and a pituitary mass with a largest lesional diameter >10 mm is not consistent with a PRL-secreting pituitary tumor, but rather reflects PRL secretion by normal lactotrophs. Although treatment with dopamine agonists will normalize the serum PRL in such a patient, the pituitary mass will not change in size.

See Nonfunctioning Pituitary Adenoma Presenting as a Pituitary Incidentaloma for further discussion.

CLINICAL DIAGNOSIS

HORMONAL EVALUATION   Despite the apparent lack of clinical function based on the patient interview and physical examination, the possibility of subclinical hormonal excess should be evaluated. Typical studies to be considered include serum concentrations of PRL, total or free serum thyroxine, cortisol, gonadotropins, α-subunit, and insulin-like growth factor 1 (IGF-1). If abnormalities in any of these baseline values are found, then further specific studies are indicated. Although preoperative dynamic hormonal testing to detect gonadotroph pituitary adenomas has been advocated (*7*), this information is of limited utility and does not change the treatment or follow-up plans (*2*).

Pituitary-dependent hormonal deficiencies also should be assessed. Secondary thyroid or adrenal insufficiency may be detected in 81 and 62% of patients, respectively (*8*). Growth hormone deficiency is also demonstrable in the majority of patients (*8*). Variable degrees of hypogonadism are present in more than 90% of patients with clinically nonfunctioning pituitary macroadenomas (*8,9*).

IMAGING   The clinically nonfunctioning pituitary tumor is usually found in the process of evaluating the cause of vision loss or hypopituitarism. Occasionally, this tumor is found serendipitously on computerized imaging performed for other reasons. Magnetic resonance imaging (MRI) is the optimal diagnostic imaging technique to demonstrate small and large sellar lesions (Figure 2). Another advantage of MRI is the ability to distinguish other sellar abnormalities, such as carotid artery aneurysm (Figure 3) or hemorrhage into a pituitary tumor (Figure 4). Occasionally, the apparent nonfunctioning pituitary tumor may represent meningioma, craniopharyngioma, granulomatous diseases, gliomas, chordomas, Rathke's cleft cyst, or metastatic disease. The key features on pituitary computerized imaging are the degree of suprasellar extension, the proximity to the optic chiasm, and the presence of parasellar extension with cavernous sinus invasion. These findings help determine the optimal treatment plan.

VISUAL ABNORMALITIES   All patients with pituitary macroadenomas should have visual fields performed by quantitative perimetry. One or both eyes may be affected. A superior bitemporal quandrantopsia is a relatively common finding in patients with nonfunctioning pituitary tumors that extend into the suprasellar space (Figure 5). A primary goal of treatment is to relieve chiasmal pressure and correction of visual field deficits.

TREATMENT

Treatment options are limited and listed in Table 2. The specific cell type of the clinically nonfunctioning pituitary tumor does not impact on treatment recommendations. Because most of these patients present with mass-effect symptoms (e.g., vision loss), surgical debulking is usually indicated. Typically when a pituitary tumor is large enough to cause chiasmal compression, there is also cavernous sinus, bone, or dural invasion, which makes a surgical cure unlikely. However, the immediate and most urgent goal of transsphenoidal surgery is to relieve the pressure on the optic chiasm or cavernous sinus (cranial nerve palsy) (Figure 6). When we reviewed our experience with 100 patients with gonadotroph pituitary tumors, 68% had visual defects and 69% of those patients had improvement in the defects with transsphenoidal surgery (*2*). We usually repeat the visual fields by quantitative perimetry, hormonal function tests, and computerized head imaging at 3 and 12 mo after surgery. Patients with apparent surgical cure are followed with computerized head imaging annually for 5 yr and then every 2 yr for a total of 9 or 11 yr. We also follow patients with residual tumor on an annual basis to determine the rate and site(s)

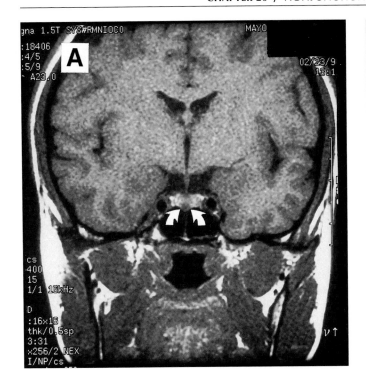
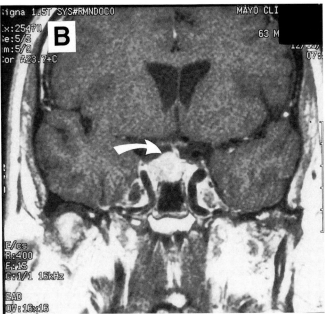

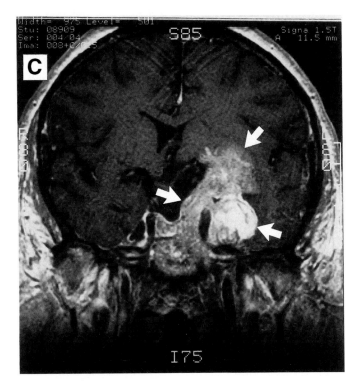

Figure 20-2 Computerized imaging of pituitary tumors. **(A)** Microadenoma—computed axial tomographic scan showing 0.5-cm pituitary microadenoma (arrow) in a 32-yr-old woman with headaches. **(B)** Macroadenoma—MRI showing a 1.2-cm homogeneous enhancing right-sided sellar gonadotroph pituitary macroadenoma (arrow) in a 63-yr-old man with secondary hypogonadism. **(C)** Giant macroadenoma—MRI showing a $7.0 \times 4.0 \times 4.5$ cm gonadotroph pituitary macroadenoma (arrows) in a 55-yr-old woman with symptoms owing to obstructive hydrocephalus.

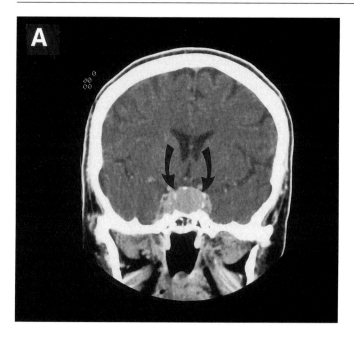

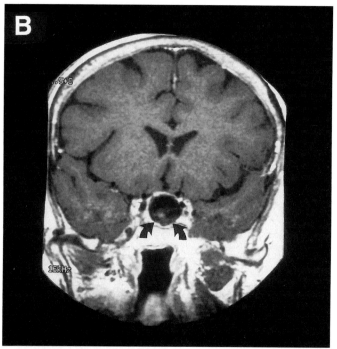

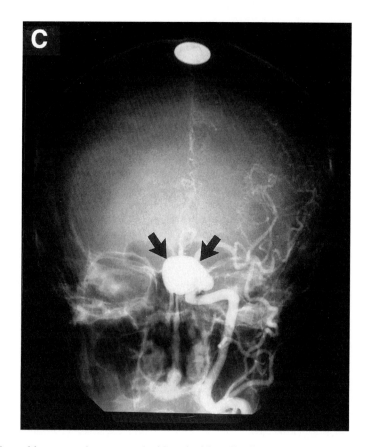

Figure 20-3   Images from a 60-yr-old woman who presented with an incidentally discovered sellar mass. **(A)** Computed tomographic scan shows a 1.8-cm contrast-enhancing sellar mass (arrows). **(B)** MRI scan shows the mass with a flow void (arrows). **(C)** Angiogram shows the left cavernous sinus internal carotid aneurysm (arrows).

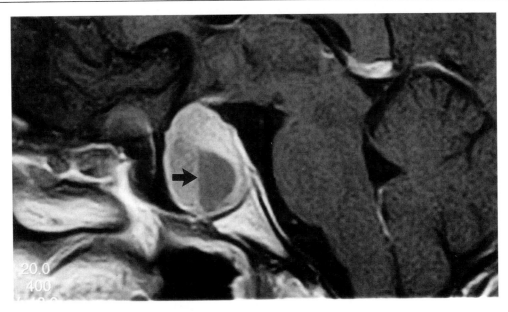

Figure 20-4 MRI studies from a 47-yr-old man with pituitary apoplexy. A fluid–fluid level is shown (arrow) in this 3.1 × 2.5 × 1.9 cm sellar mass.

of tumor regrowth. If the recurrent tumor is primarily intrasellar, we typically monitor these patients annually and perform a second transsphenoidal surgery if and when chiasmal compression occurs. This approach avoids the rare, but potentially devastating side effects of radiation therapy. However, if the recurrent tumor is inaccessible to a second transsphenoidal surgery (e.g., cavernous sinus) and progressive growth is documented, then radiation therapy is indicated. Conventional pituitary radiation therapy involves a total dose of 45–50 gy administered in 20 fractions over 4 wk. Risks of radiation therapy to the sellar region include vision loss, hypopituitarism, tumorigenesis, and neurocognitive dysfunction *(10)*. Gamma-Knife radiosurgery has the advantages of increased dose in targeted areas and single-day administration. However, with this more potent targeted therapy, there is greater potential risk of optic nerve or chiasmal damage. Gamma-Knife therapy is usually limited to patients who lack suprasellar tumor extension and tumors at least 5 mm distant from the optic chiasm.

Because of its slow rate of effectiveness, radiation therapy is usually not considered as primary therapy for the patient with a nonfunctioning pituitary tumor. Frequently, observation is in order in the asymptomatic patient with an incidentally discovered pituitary mass (Figure 7). A cautious treatment approach should also be considered in the elderly patient or patients who are not good surgical candidates. Although dopamine agonists (e.g., bromocriptine, cabergoline) and somatostatin analogs (e.g., octreotide) have proven to be excellent treatment options for patients with prolactinomas and growth hormone-secreting tumors, no effective pharmacologic therapy has been found for the nonfunctioning pituitary tumor. The overall goals in the treatment of the patient with a nonfunctioning pituitary adenoma are to restore normal vision, if impaired, and to preserve normal anterior and posterior pituitary function.

NONFUNCTIONING PITUITARY ADENOMA PRESENTING AS A PITUITARY INCIDENTALOMA

Two byproducts of the revolution in diagnostic imaging techniques over the past three decades are unintended discoveries and

uncertainty for the patient and clinician. To address the uncertainty associated with pituitary incidentalomas, clinicians need a clear understanding of the definitions, differential diagnoses, and options for assessment with respect to functional status and malignant potential.

A pituitary incidentaloma is defined as a sellar mass lesion serendipitously discovered by radiologic examination, in the absence of symptoms or clinical findings suggestive of pituitary-dependent disease. This "new" clinical entity is the result of technological advances in computed tomography (CT) and MRI. The diagnosis of an incidental pituitary mass is infrequent because approx 11% of individuals are found to have pituitary adenomas at autopsy *(11)* and the resolving power of imaging techniques increases with each new generation of scanners. With CT scanning, 8% of 373 normal subjects from three studies had focal apparent lesions >3 mm in diameter *(12–14)*. With MRI of the sella, 20% of 152 normal subjects from 2 studies showed focal hypodense lesions within the pituitary gland of ≥3 mm in diameter *(15,16)*. Only apparent microadenomas (≤10 mm) have been detected in all of the normal subject studies completed to date. In the two studies that have been published on patients with pituitary incidentalomas, 56% of patients had macroadenomas (>10 mm) *(17,18)*.

The two major categories of diagnostic possibilities include the non-functioning sellar mass and minimally hyperfunctioning pituitary tumor (Table 3). The most common finding is that of a clinically silent pituitary microadenoma. The evaluation should start with a history and physical examination directed at signs and symptoms of pituitary hyper- or hypofunction. The majority of these patients will have clinically nonfunctioning pituitary tumors that may be associated with subtle pituitary hormone or visual field deficits. Individualization of the evaluation based on the clinical circumstance is key in the assessment of the pituitary incidentaloma patient. Patient age and tumor size are two major factors that affect degree of diagnostic testing and follow-up. A panel of tests to consider in screening for pituitary tumor hyper- and hypofunction states includes: serum levels of PRL, IGF-1,

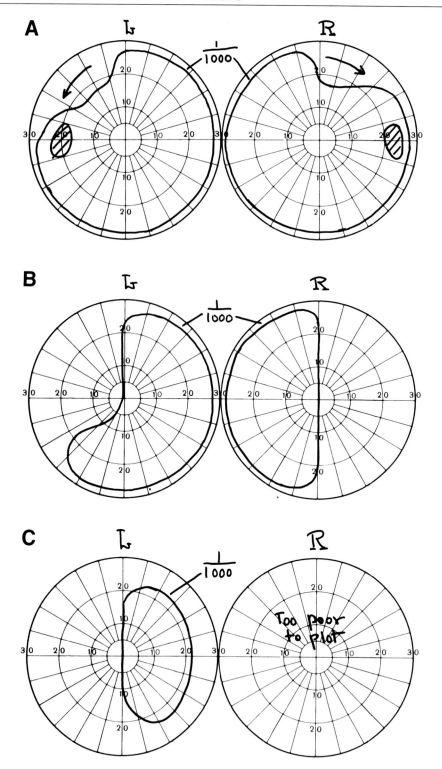

Figure 20-5 Visual fields by quantitative perimetry. The suprasellar extension of a pituitary tumor can compress the optic chiasm, and visual field defects may progress from superior bitemporal quadrantopsia (**A**) to bitemporal hemianopsia (**B**), and eventually, blindness (**C**).

Table 2
Treatment Options
for Clinically Nonfunctioning Pituitary Tumors

Transsphenoidal surgery
    To debulk large invasive tumors in patients with visual field loss
        owing to chiasmal compression
    To cure patients with tumors that do not invade the cavernous
        sinuses
Observation
    To determine biological and clinical behavior of the tumor mass
        for asymptomatic patients without visual field loss
Radiation therapy (standard or γ-knife radiosurgery)
    To treat residual pituitary tumor following surgical debulking
Pharmacologic therapy
    No effective agent is currently available

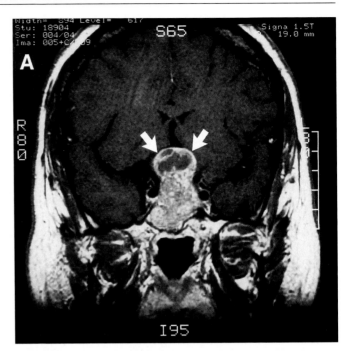

LH, FSH, pituitary-dependent sex hormone (testosterone or estradiol), thyroid-stimulating hormone (TSH), and T4, as well as 24-h urinary cortisol excretion and morning urine osmolality. Visual fields by quantitative perimetry should be performed in all patients with apparent pituitary adenomas ≥8 mm in diameter. Pituitary hypofunction is usually not seen unless the patient has a macroadenoma.

Primary pituitary malignancy is very rare (19), and the initial presentation of these patients is owing to hormone hypersecretion (usually ACTH or PRL) and symptoms associated with an invasive pituitary tumor. Therefore, the probability of a pituitary carcinoma presenting as a pituitary incidentaloma is virtually zero. Metastasis to the pituitary gland is another rare cause of an intrasellar mass (20). Between 1950 and 1996, only 52 patients were diagnosed with metastatic disease to the pituitary at the Mayo Clinic (21). In these cases, metastatic disease to the pituitary was typically found 4 yr after the diagnosis of the primary cancer. However, in 21% of the cases, the primary malignancy was diagnosed after the finding of metastatic disease to the pituitary. The discovery of metastatic disease to the pituitary was incidental in only 2 of the 52 cases. Therefore, although possible, the incidental discovery of a mass in the sella owing to metastatic disease is extremely unlikely. The optimal management approach to a patient with a pituitary incidentaloma is debated (22,23). The algorithm shown in Figure 8 is based on the following understanding about pituitary incidentalomas:

- Clinically nonfunctioning pituitary microadenomas are common and rarely result in symptoms.
- Surgical intervention should be based on evidence of hormonal hypersecretion, visual field defects, or mass effects.
- The growth rate of benign pituitary tumors may be extremely slow.
- The possibility of malignancy (primary or metastatic) in the typical intrasellar pituitary incidentaloma patient is extremely improbable.

CONCLUSION

Clinically nonfunctioning pituitary tumors are usually macroadenomas that fail to cause a clinically recognizable hormone-dependent syndrome. They are usually discovered because of local mass-effect symptoms, symptoms of hypopituitarism, or as incidentalomas when performing imaging for unrelated reasons.

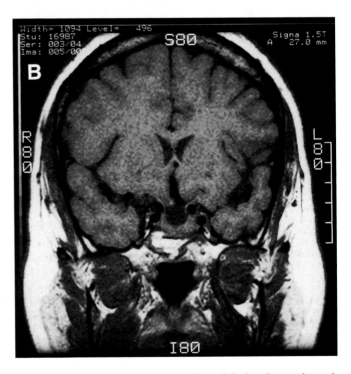

Figure 20-6 MRI scan shows a 4-cm lobulated gonadotroph adenoma preoperatively (**A**) and the sellar appearance 3 mo following transsphenoidal surgery (**B**). (Reprinted with permission from ref. 2. Copyright 1996 by Mayo Foundation for Medical Education and Research.)

Because most of these patients present with mass-effect symptoms, surgical debulking is usually indicated. An effective form of pharmacotherapy is not yet available for the clinically nonfunctioning pituitary tumor. The discovery of the incidental pituitary mass is increasing because of the technological advances in CT and MRI. In this group of patients, the most common finding

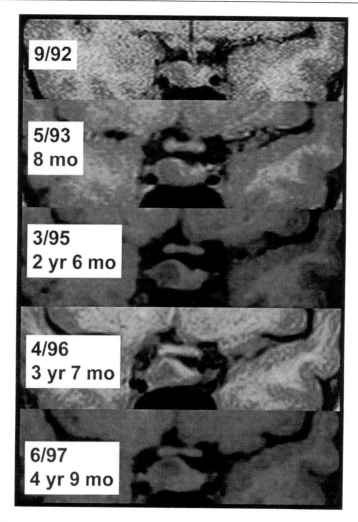

Figure 20-7 Serial MRI from a 38-yr-old woman with an incidentally discovered pituitary mass found in the investigation of headaches. The 9-mm microadenoma was shown to grow over the 5 yr of follow-up.

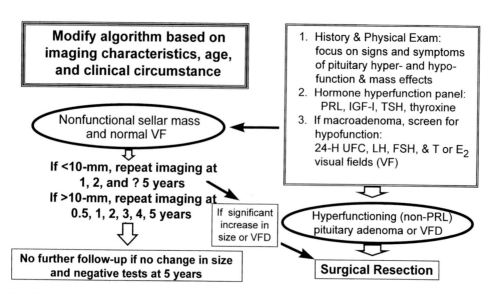

Figure 20-8 Algorithm for the evaluation and management of the pituitary incidentalomas.

Table 3
Differential Diagnosis
of the Incidentally Discovered Pituitary Mass

Nonfunctioning sellar mass
    Clinically silent benign pituitary adenoma
    Pituitary cyst
    Craniopharyngioma
    Infiltrative disease (e.g., lymphocytic hypophysitis, histiocytosis
        X, sarcoidosis, Wegener's granulomatosis)
    Hemorrhage into a pituitary tumor (apoplexy)
    Infections (e.g., bacterial, fungal, tuberculosis)
    Germline tumor (e.g., germinoma, dysgerminoma, dermoid,
        teratoma)
    Meningioma
    Gliomas
    Hemangiopericytoma
    Metastatic carcinoma
    Carotid artery aneurysm
    Vascular malformation
Hyperfunctioning mass
    Pituitary tumors with mild degrees of hypersecretion (LH, FSH,
        PRL, GH, ACTH, TSH)

is a clinically silent pituitary microadenoma. Thus, hormonal screening is indicated for subtle pituitary hyperfunction and hypofunction. Treatment decisions are based on evidence of hormonal hypersecretion, visual field defects, or mass effects.

REFERENCES

1. McCormick WF, Halmi NS. Absence of chromophobe adenomas from a large series of pituitary tumors. Arch Pathol 1971;92:231–238.
2. Young WF Jr, Scheithauer BW, Kovacs KT, Horvath E, Davis DH, Randall RV. Gonadotroph adenoma of the pituitary gland: A clinico-pathologic analysis of 100 cases. Mayo Clin Proc 1996;71:649–656.
3. Ho DM, Hsu CY, Ting LT, Chiang H. The clinicopathological characteristics of gonadotroph cell adenoma: A study of 118 cases. Hum Pathol 1997;28:905–911.
4. Girod C, Mazzuca M, Trouillas J, Tramu G, Lheritier M, Beauvillain J-C, et al. Light microscopy, fine structure and immunohistochemistry studies of 278 pituitary adenomas. In: Derome PJ, Jedynak CP, Peillon F, ed. Pituitary Adenomas: Biology, Physiopathology and Treatment. Asclepios Publishers, France, 1980, pp. 3–18.
5. Horvath E, Kovacs K, Killinger DW, Smyth S, Platts ME, Singer W: Silent corticotropic adenomas of the human pituitary gland: A histologic, immunocytologic, and ultrastructural study. Am J Pathol 1980;98:617–638.
6. Braithwaite SS, Clasen RA, D'Angelo CM. Silent corticotroph adenoma: Case report and literature review. Endocr Pract 1997;3:297–301.
7. Snyder PJ. Gonadotroph and other clinically nonfunctioning pituitary adenomas. Cancer Treat Res 1997;89:57–72.
8. Arafah BM. Reversible hypopituitarism in patients with large nonfunctioning pituitary adenomas. J Clin Endocrinol Metab 1986;62:1173–1179.
9. Katznelson L, Alexander JM, Bikkal HA, Jameson JL, Hsu DW, Klibanski A. Imbalanced follicle-stimulating hormone beta-subunit hormone biosynthesis in human pituitary adenomas. J Clin Endocrinol Metab 1992;74:1343–1351.
10. McCord MW, Buatti JM, Fennell EM, Mendenhall WM, Marcus RB Jr, Rhoton AL, et al. Radiotherapy for pituitary adenoma: Long-term outcome and sequelae. Int J Radiol Oncol Biol Physics 1997;39:437–444.
11. Molitch ME. Pituitary incidentalomas. Endocrinol Metab Clin North Am 1997;26:725–740.
12. Chambers EF, Turski PA, LaMasters D, Newton TH. Regions of low density in the contrast-enhanced pituitary gland: Normal and pathologic processes. Radiology 1982;144:109–113.
13. Wolpert SM, Molitch ME, Goldman JA, Wood JB. Size, shape, and appearance of the normal female pituitary gland. Am J Roentgenol 1984;143:377–381.
14. Peyster RG, Adler LP, Viscarello RR, Hoover Ed, Skarzynski J. CT of the normal pituitary gland. Neuroradiology 1986;28:161–165.
15. Chong BW, Kucharczyk W, Singer W, George S. Pituitary gland MR: A comparative study of healthy volunteers and patients with microadenomas. Am J Neuroradiol 1994;15:675–679.
16. Hall WA, Luciano MG, Doppman JL, Patronas NJ, Oldfield EH. Pituitary magnetic resonance imaging in normal human volunteers: Occult adenomas in the general population. Ann Intern Med 1994;120:817–820.
17. Donovan LE, Corenblum B. The natural history of the pituitary incidentaloma. Arch Intern Med 1995;155:181–183.
18. Reincke M, Allolio B, Saeger W, Menzel J, Winkelmann W. The "incidentaloma" of the pituitary gland: Is neurosurgery required? JAMA 1990;263:2772–2776.
19. Pernicone PJ, Scheithauer BW, Sebo T, Kovacs KT, Horvath E, Young WF Jr, et al. Pituitary carcinoma: A clinicopathologic study of 15 cases. Cancer 1997;79:804–812.
20. Losa M, Grasso M, Giugine E, Mortini P, Acerno S, Giovanelli M. Metastatic prostatic adenocarcinoma presenting as a pituitary mass: Shrinkage of the lesion and clinical improvement with medical treatment. Prostate 1997;32:241–245.
21. Heshmati HM, Young WF Jr, Scheithauer BW. Metastases to the pituitary gland: A survey of 52 cases. 79th Annual Meeting of the Endocrine Society, Abstract #P3-77, Minneapolis, June 11–14, 1997, p. 456.
22. Aron DC, Howlett TA. Pituitary incidentalomas. Endocrinol Metab Clin North Am 2000;29:205–221.
23. Howlett TA, Como J, Aron DC. Management of pituitary incidentalomas: a survey of British and American endocrinologists. Endocrinol Metab Clin North Am 2000;29:223–230.

21 Pituitary Tumors in Children

NALIN GUPTA, MD, PHD AND JAMES T. RUTKA, MD, PHD

INTRODUCTION

The vast majority of pituitary tumors in children are benign lesions. The challenge for the clinical team, usually the neurosurgeon, endocrinologist, and neuroradiologist, is to diagnose those tumors accurately that arise in the suprasellar and sellar region, and to direct the initial and long-term treatment of these patients (1–3).

Pituitary tumors fall into the category of midline supratentorial tumors, which includes craniopharyngiomas, optic chiasmatic and hypothalamic gliomas, germ-cell tumors, and a number of rare entities. Nonmalignant masses, such as arachnoid cysts and Rathke's cleft cysts, are also found in this area. Diagnostic confusion occurs because all of these lesions can cause overlapping clinical patterns that are often indistinguishable from each other. The symptoms and signs at presentation provide important clues, because most adenomas in children produce physiologically active hormones. Therefore, the goals of this chapter are to:

1. Describe the clinical presentation of pediatric pituitary adenomas.
2. Describe management issues that are specific to the pediatric population.
3. Illustrate characteristics of other sellar and parasellar masses that differentiate them from pituitary adenomas.

As a broad generalization, the management of verified pituitary adenomas in children follows the recommendations for the adult population. Endocrinological investigations, both static and dynamic, play a critical role in diagnosing pituitary adenoma subtypes and determining the need for endocrine replacement. Imaging studies prior to treatment, particularly magnetic resonance imaging (MRI), are absolutely crucial to narrow the diagnosis and define the anatomy. The transsphenoidal approach, safe and effective in children, is the preferred option for the majority of pituitary adenomas.

NORMAL DEVELOPMENT OF THE PITUITARY GLAND

The adenohypophysis (pars distalis, intermedialis, and tuberalis) is derived from the anterior wall of Rathke's pouch, an epithelial outgrowth of the primitive buccal cavity (the stomodeum) that forms on approximately day 24 of embryonic life. This epithelially derived tissue meets the neurohypophysis, which extends inferi-

orly as an outgrowth of the hypothalamus (Figure 1). The pars intermedia is a poorly defined collection of cells that are remnants of the posterior wall of Rathke's pouch. The cleft between the anterior and posterior wall usually regresses, but on rare occasions can expand and cause symptoms.

Fetal adenohypophysial cells are well differentiated and appear to produce all trophic hormones. Higher levels of most pituitary hormones are produced in the last two trimesters of fetal development and during the first two postnatal months (4–7). This physiological change may account for the morphological change seen by MRI during the first year of life. In neonates, the pituitary gland is bulbous with a convex superior border (8,9). After the first few postnatal months, the pituitary gradually lengthens, and the superior border becomes flat or slightly concave, which is the normal configuration during most of adolescence and adulthood (10).

Increased secretion of gonadotrophins during normal puberty, and also with central precocious puberty, will lead to an increase in pituitary size (11,12). During normal puberty, this is more prominent in girls than in boys. Accompanying this increase in height is a change in shape of the superior pituitary border from flat or concave to convex. Following puberty, the mean pituitary height decreases in both sexes.

EPIDEMIOLOGY

Because only about 2% of all pediatric brain tumors are pituitary adenomas, as a rough calculation, 30–40 new patients with adenomas reach medical attention each year in North America (13). Certainly by this measure, pituitary adenomas in children are rare entities. The pediatric subpopulations of three large institutional series of pituitary tumors (Centre Foch, the Mayo Clinic, and the University of California San Francisco) were recently analyzed and reported (14–16). The percentages of patients in the pediatric category were 2.1% (66/3200), 2.03% (36/1776) and 5.34% (119/2330) for Centre Foch (≤16 yr/old), Mayo Clinic (<18 yr/old), and UCSF (<18 yr/old), respectively.* The breakdown of adenomas by hormone subtype in each series is summarized in Table 1.

Some conclusions can be reached regarding the occurrence of adenoma subtypes by studying these three reports, which represent the largest collections of pediatric pituitary adenomas in the literature. Pituitary tumors in children under 5 yr of age are exceedingly rare. In prepubertal children (5–11 yr of age),

From: *Diagnosis and Management of Pituitary Tumors* (K. Thapar, K. Kovacs, B. W. Scheithauer, and R. V. Lloyd, eds.), ©Humana Press Inc., Totowa, NJ.

*The UCSF study includes patients from birth to 20 yr of age. To allow comparison, these figures are for those patients <18 yr of age only.

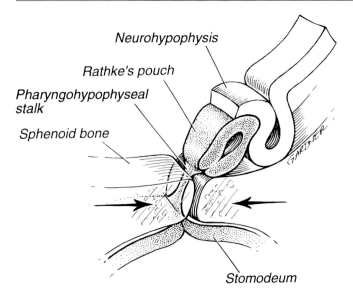

Neurohypophysis

Rathke's pouch

Pharyngohypophyseal
stalk

Sphenoid bone

Stomodeum

Figure 21-1 A schematic description of the embryological progenitors of sellar and parasellar structures. Rathke's pouch arises from an outpocketing of stomodeum (ectoderm) and gives rise to the adenohypohysis. The pharyngohypophyseal stalk, which connects the stomodeum and Rathke's pouch, is divided by the sphenoid bone as it grows together (arrows), isolating Rathke's pouch and the neurohypophysis within the sella. (From: ref. *80*. Reprinted with permission.)

corticotroph adenomas seem to predominate. Males are in the majority in this age group in the Centre Foch and Mayo Clinic series. Over all age groups, however, females are in the majority. With the onset of puberty, the number of prolactinomas rises markedly. These are more common in females and seem to account for the overall predominance of females in the Mayo Clinic and UCSF series. Prolactinomas were the most common tumors in the UCSF series (Figure 2). At the Centre Foch, corticotroph adenomas were more common than prolactinomas. Defining the upper limit of the "pediatric age group" seems critical because of a peak in the incidence of prolactinomas in the 18–20 yr age group *(15,17)*. Including this group in a series seems to result in prolactinomas being reported as the most common tumor. Compared to the adult population, the number of "nonfunctioning" or clinically silent adenomas is very low in children. In all three series, they represent <10% of the total.

CLINICAL FEATURES

The diagnostic decisions made by clinicians are dictated by the biology of the pituitary adenoma. Essentially, pituitary adenomas present with either an obvious hypersecretion syndrome or neurological deficits owing to local compressive effects. The majority of adenomas in children secrete clinically significant levels of at least one pituitary hormone. A patient presenting with the protean effects of hormonal excess should lead to an early suspicion of a hormonally active adenoma. Differences between adenoma subtypes are summarized below. Despite modern advances, vigilance is necessary, especially because the onset of symptoms precedes definitive diagnosis and treatment by years *(15)*. Clinically apparent glycoprotein-secreting adenomas (thyroid-stimulating hormone [TSH], luteinizing hormone [LH], and follicle-stimulating hormone [FSH]) are exceedingly rare in the pediatric population. Only three case reports of TSH-secreting adenomas occurring in children are reported in the literature *(18–20)*.

PROLACTINOMAS   In a Mayo Clinic study of non-ACTH-secreting tumors in children, the most common presenting symptoms for patients with prolactinomas were menstrual dysfunction (91%, females only), headache (61%), and galactorrhea (49%) *(17)*. The female-to-male ratio was 4.9:1. In males, hypogonadism, gynecomastia with galactorrhea, and delayed pubertal development were the predominant presenting symptoms. Of note, there were no prepubertal patients in this series. Other reported signs and symptoms include growth arrest, visual disturbances, and hypopituitarism. The most common hormone deficiency was for growth hormone (GH). Prolactin levels were raised for all patients with prolactinomas. Immunostaining revealed that 52% of the non-ACTH-secreting tumors stained for prolactin only, a figure far higher when compared to the adult patients from this institution. Interestingly, in the UCSF series, 21% of patients with prolactinomas were reported to have experienced pituitary apoplexy *(15)*.

Compared to corticotroph adenomas, prolactinomas tend to be macroadenomas with 15–28% reported as invading adjacent structures *(15,17)*. In the Mayo Clinic group, tumors in boys were all macroadenomas *(17)*. Macroadenomas tend to have higher prolactin levels when compared to microadenomas *(15,17)*. The lack of a clear developmental milestone, like menarche, may account for later diagnosis in boys resulting in larger tumors with higher prolactin levels at diagnosis.

CORTICOTROPH ADENOMAS   Corticotroph adenomas that secrete clinically significant levels of ACTH are one cause of the characteristic physical transformation that presents as Cushing's syndrome. The challenge for the clinician is twofold: first, making the diagnosis of hypercortisolism, and second, distinguishing whether patients have a pituitary adenoma (Cushing's disease), primary adrenal disease, or an ectopic ACTH source *(21,22)*.

Unfortunately, the findings of Cushing's syndrome are not specific and the impetus for further investigation rests with clinical suspicion *(22)*. In a recent National Institutes of Health (NIH) Clinical Center study of 59 children with Cushing's syndrome, it is telling that the average duration of symptoms prior to diagnosis was 3 yr. Although the vast majority of patients with hypercortisolism possess cushingoid features, some clinical characteristics are more common. In the NIH study, the most common presenting signs and symptoms were: weight gain (90%), growth retardation (83%), amenorrhea (78%), hirsutism (78%), and skin striae (61%) *(23)*. Other reports echo these findings *(16,21,24–26)*. Two interesting observations are present in the NIH study. First, in the Cushing's disease subgroup, Tanner stages were 3.8 and 2.5 standard deviations (sd) above values for normal subjects for breast and testes, respectively. Second, although mean height was 1.3 sd below those of normal subjects, the growth rate was a striking 3.7 sd below normal. For the clinician, early pubertal development and growth failure should trigger a vigorous search for etiology. In particular, growth failure is a serious sign that requires early treatment to prevent irreversible short stature. School performance was normal in the 20 patients for whom data were available.

Cushing's disease is the most common cause of Cushing's syndrome. Eighty-five percent of the children in the NIH study had Cushing's disease. The average age of presentation with primary adrenal disease (10 yr) or ectopic corticotrophin secretion (11 yr) was younger than those with Cushing's disease (14 yr). As with other studies, it appears that corticotroph adenomas rarely grow to large sizes. Of the 39 pituitary adenomas identified by pathology, only 2 were macroadenomas.

Table 1
Pediatric Pituitary Adenomas According to Hormonal Type in Three Institutional Series[a]

Tumor type	Centre Foch		Mayo Clinic		UCSF	
	Number	%	Number	%	Number	%
Prolactinoma	18	27.3	15	41.7	60	50.4
Cushings disease/ Nelson's syndrome	36	54.5	16	44.4	45	37.8
Gigantism/acromegaly	8	12.1	3	8.3	10	8.4
Nonfunctioning	4	6.1	2	5.6	4	3.4
Total	66	100	36	100	119	100

[a]The Centre Foch series included patients under 16 yr of age; the Mayo Clinic series included patients under 18 yr of age; and the UCSF series included patients who were <20 yr old (*n* = 136). For purposes of comparison with the other two series, the UCSF data presented in this table is from only those patients <18 yr old (*n* = 119).

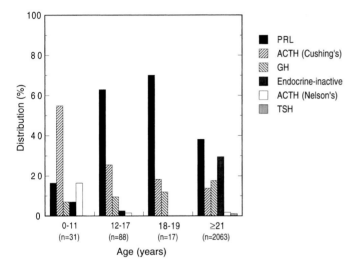

Figure 21-2   Frequency of pituitary adenomas by age as reported in the UCSF series. Age refers to age of onset of symptoms in children and to age of surgery in adults. The percentage in each age group add up to 100. The different adenoma types are listed in the same order for each age group. Note, TSH applies to adults only. (From: ref. *15*. Reprinted with permission.)

SOMATOTROPH ADENOMAS   The clinical syndrome of gigantism is associated with overproduction of GH prior to epiphyseal plate closure. As expected, the vast majority of these patients present with rapid linear growth or with acromegalic characteristics, such as soft-tissue thickening, enlargement of hands and feet, and coarse facial features. Acromegalic features can develop in children in the absence of gigantism. Somatotroph adenomas most commonly appear in adolescence. Only two case reports describe a GH-secreting pituitary adenoma in an infant or child *(27,28)*. The majority of somatotroph adenomas in the UCSF series were reported to be macroadenomas. In addition, 6 out of 11 cases were described as having invasive properties.

An interesting subset of children with gigantism have the McCune-Albright syndrome: hyperprolactinemia, polyostotic fibrous dysplasia, skin pigmentation, precocious puberty, and gigantism. The endocrinological manifestations are believed to be owing to hyperplasia of bihormonal mammosomatotrophs *(29–31)*. One case of mammosomatotroph hyperplasia is described in the absence of the McCune-Albright syndrome *(32)*. Mammosomatotrophs are reported to be more common during fetal life *(33)*.

Because electron microscopy is required to establish conclusively the presence of both GH and prolactin in the same cells, the incidence of mammosomatotrophs may be underestimated. Excessive stimulation by growth hormone releasing hormone (GHRH) also results in somatotroph hyperplasia *(32,34)*.

NONFUNCTIONING ADENOMAS   As expected, patients with nonfunctioning adenomas present with neurological deficits and are larger than secreting adenomas. In the four patients of the UCSF series, the median tumor size was 35 mm, and all presented with focal neurological deficits. Although many of these adenomas in adults are believed to produce glycoprotein or variants of normal hormones, the very small number of these tumors in children have prevented detailed immunohistochemical analysis of their origin and biology.

INVESTIGATION AND TREATMENT OF PEDIATRIC PITUITARY ADENOMAS

As a generalization, the first step in the investigation of a child suspected of harboring a pituitary lesion is to define which hormone is in excess and if there are superimposed hormone deficiencies. As is most often the case with macroadenomas, GH levels are affected first, usually followed by the gonadotropins (LH and FSH), then TSH, and finally adrenocorticotropic hormone (ACTH) *(35)*. The second step, often using dynamic endocrine tests (i.e., the dexamethasone suppression test), is to localize hormone hypersecretion to a central site (i.e., hypothalamus), a pituitary origin (i.e., adenoma), or a target organ (i.e., adrenal cortex or ectopic). The third step relies on imaging to narrow the pathological diagnosis. The final step is definitive treatment, usually surgical resection or biopsy and/or bromocriptine for prolactinomas, and radiation therapy in selected cases. The principles of investigation and dynamic endocrine testing are essentially the same for children and adults. The reader is referred to other chapters for details regarding these issues. Some points that are specific to children are outlined in this section.

ENDOCRINOLOGICAL INVESTIGATIONS   The robust circadian cortisol pattern normally does not become established until 1 yr of age *(36,37)*. This is usually not a practical concern, since pituitary adenomas rarely arise in infants. As with adults, baseline investigations, such as 24-h urinary free cortisol, 17-hydroxy-corticosteroid, and creatinine, are done in children to determine if hypercortisolemia is present. Values should be normalized to body surface area to allow comparison between patients and also for follow-up, because total glucocorticoid values increase as children grow. Plasma cortisol levels are easily available, but individual values are of little help. Several samples taken through the day are needed to provide meaningful information. The low-dose dexamethasone suppression test (30 µg/kg) is used to confirm the presence of Cushing's syndrome, whereas the high-dose test (120 µg/kg) is used to distinguish the pituitary-dependent forms of Cushing's syndrome from those with ectopic ACTH secretion (23). Although urinary cortisol levels can be used to judge suppressibility, serum cortisol measurements provide greater sensitivity (22). Using these tests as well as measurements of plasma ACTH and stimulation with ovine corticotropin-releasing hormone (CRH), the cause of Cushing's syndrome can be narrowed. It must be emphasized that admission of young children may be required for compliance with certain dynamic tests and tests requiring multiple venipunctures.

During the first two trimesters, fetal levels of prolactin are slightly higher than in adults (38). During the last trimester, fetal levels reach maternal levels (150–200 µg/L). Within 2 mo of birth, prolactin levels decrease to prepubertal levels, which are somewhat less than adult levels. During puberty, levels rise and finally stabilize at adult levels. The relative stability of basal prolactin levels usually means that dynamic tests are not required. A demonstration of elevated serum prolactin should prompt a search for a sellar lesion. Because prolactin is the only pituitary hormone whose dominant hypothalamic control is inhibitory, virtually any lesion that compresses the pituitary stalk or hypothalamus can cause moderate prolactin elevations (50–200 µg/L). High serum prolactin levels (>200 µg/L) should focus attention towards the pituitary gland. Other important causes of hyperprolactinemia in adults, such as renal failure, estrogens, or dopamine antagonists, are not as relevant in the pediatric population.

DIAGNOSTIC IMAGING Modern imaging techniques are essential for diagnosis, surgical planning, and clinical follow-up of the wide variety of tumors and cysts that occur in the sellar and suprasellar region in children (discussed in detail below). The use of MRI as a screening tool must be distinguished from its utility in patients with definite symptoms attributable to the sellar area. In general, any child with endocrinological and/or visual symptoms should have imaging of the sellar region.

The normal development of the pituitary gland should not be confused with pathological events. During the first 2 mo of life, the anterior lobe has a high signal intensity on T1-weighted images (8,39). After approx 2 mo, the anterior lobe becomes isointense with normal brain tissue. Because the posterior pituitary normally has a high signal intensity (40,41), distinguishing the posterior from the anterior pituitary during the first few months of life can be difficult (10). As mentioned above, the pituitary gland enlarged during puberty, more in females than in males, and then gradually reduced in size in the postpubertal period.

The vast majority of adenomas are hypointense with respect to the normal gland on T1-weighted images, whereas only one-half are hyperintense on T2-weighted images (Figure 3) (42,43). However, up to 40% of asymptomatic individuals will have a focal hypointensity in the pituitary gland on unenhanced T1-weighted images (44). It is reported that those adenomas that are isointense on T2-weighted images are fibrous and more difficult to remove (45). Whether this is a consistent association is unknown. As a reflection of the limited vascularity of pituitary adenomas, most show less contrast enhancement compared to the normal gland when imaged immediately after contrast injection. If imaging is

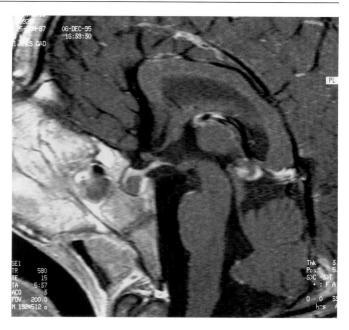

Figure 21-3 Gadolinium-enhanced, sagittal MRI of 8-yr female with syndrome of cortisol excess. The MRI shows an enlarged gland with a central area of low signal intensity. Note is also made of nonpneumatized sphenoid sinus, which must be recognized preoperatively by the neurosurgeon wishing to approach such a lesion by the transsphenoidal route.

delayed, however, an adenoma may enhance to become isointense compared to the normal gland and consequently escape detection (1). For pituitary adenomas, unenhanced MRI is reported to be equal to contrast-enhanced computerized tomography (CT), but gadolinium adds to the sensitivity and specificity of MRI (46–49). The sensitivity of gadolinium-enhanced MRI for the detection of microadenomas is estimated to be 85–90% (43).

Surgical planning often requires clarification of the following issues: degree of sphenoid sinus pneumatization, presence of septa within the sphenoid sinus (Figure 3), and the position of the carotid arteries in relation to the lateral walls of the sphenoid sinus. Coronal CT images with 3-mm slices are very useful for demonstrating bony anatomy. In addition, in certain centers and most other countries, CT scanning is more readily available than MRI.

SURGICAL TREATMENT The prevailing philosophy for treating pediatric tumors is primary surgical resection whenever possible. Adjuvent agents, such as bromocriptine, somatostatin, or focused radiation, may be considered when residual or recurrent tumor is present. The majority of pediatric pituitary tumors reported in the literature have been treated by transsphenoidal adenomectomy alone or in combination with other therapy (14–16,23). Tumor size and extension into suprasellar and parasellar structures dictate whether an additional transcranial procedure or a primary transcranial procedure is to be done. In the UCSF series, of 157 procedures for pituitary adenomas, 145 were transsphenoidal and only 10 were transcranial (15).

The standard sublabial, transseptal approach is safe and effective in children. Because the vast majority of children with pituitary tumors are older than 5 yr of age, the cranial vault and midface are already adequately developed. There have been no reports associated with abnormal midface development following a transsphenoidal procedure. The major technical consideration is the presence of an incompletely pneumatized, or "conchal," sphenoid sinus *(14,16,50)*. In this case, a high-speed drill is used to create a passage to the sella. Entering a substantial intercavernous sinus in the dura of the sellar floor may cause significant bleeding that is usually stopped by packing. Identifying macroadenomas and most microadenomas intraoperatively is usually straightforward. Failure to identify a microadenoma on preoperative imaging studies despite endocrinological evidence of the presence of a pituitary tumor may warrant further testing. Preoperative bilateral inferior petrosal sinus sampling of ACTH, pre- and post-CRH stimulation, can often lateralize a microadenoma *(22,51)*. Technically, performing catheterization of the inferior petrosal sinus is difficult in patients younger than 5 yr of age. If this technique is not available or not informative, then exploration of the gland is indicated during the procedure.

Following removal of the pituitary tumor, the sella must be reconstructed to reduce the likelihood of a CSF leak. Postoperative management is directed toward measurement of fluid balance, detection of cerebrospinal fluid (CSF) leaks, and assessment of visual function. Postoperative complications are few. Mortality has been reduced to zero in most centers. The most common sources of morbidity are transient diabetes insipidus, CSF leaks, cranial nerve palsies, and hypopituitarism. Long-term management revolves around the management of hypopituitarism, which may range from temporary postoperative hormone supplement to lifelong replacement therapy.

Failure of surgery to remove completely a pituitary tumor may be known immediately if tumor is known to be left behind, early in the postoperative period following imaging studies, or later with persistence of increased hormone levels or new clinical symptoms. In the pediatric population, even in those children older than 5 yr, radiation is generally reserved for recurrent, progressively growing tumors, which have been incompletely resected. With prolactinomas, there is the additional option of bromocriptine *(see below)* before radiotherapy must be considered.

BROMOCRIPTINE Although transsphenoidal adenomectomy is the treatment of choice for microadenomas and many macroadenomas, the availability and efficacy of bromocriptine and other dopamine agonists have resulted in medical therapy supplanting surgery in the treatment of prolactinomas *(52,53)*. In a study of five adolescents (three females and two males) with prolactin-secreting macroadenomas, Tyson et al. used bromocriptine as initial treatment in four patients *(54)*. One patient underwent surgery owing to acute visual symptoms prior to bromocriptine treatment. All five patients demonstrated clinical, radiographic, and hormonal response to therapy. Importantly, two of the older females showed resumption of normal menses. The expectation that medical therapy may allow for physiological responses of some anterior lobe hormones is tempered by the fact that bromocriptine is a lifelong medication with serious compliance issues for children. The effects of bromocriptine on neurological and endocrinological function when begun in childhood and continued over a lifetime are unknown. The efficacy of newer dopamine agonists in children is also unknown.

Replacement therapy for other hormones is guided by the specific pituitary deficiency in question. In children with prolactinomas, the most important concern is an accompanying GH deficiency, which, if untreated, will result in growth arrest. Although there is a theoretical concern of tumor regrowth caused by GH replacement *(55,56)*, in a child with short stature who is GH-deficient and on bromocriptine, replacement therapy is indicated *(57)*.

OUTCOME Treatment outcome is determined by using either early or late measures. The surgeon's operative assessment, the child's clinical status, imaging studies, and hormone levels are typically used immediately following treatment. Long-term outcome requires assessment of radiological, endocrinological, and clinical parameters. An unresolved issue at present is the length of disease free follow-up that is required to state with certainty that a cure has been achieved. Reaching conclusions based on pediatric studies in the literature is difficult owing to differences in outcome measures used, treatment protocols, and length of follow-up. In general, initial operative cure rates (surgical impression and postoperative hormone levels) are generally in the 70–100% range. Among these patients, however, recurrence rates vary widely between reported studies.

Although earlier reports characterized pituitary tumors as being more aggressive and invasive *(58–60)*, current studies suggest that initial cure rates and invasiveness are the same as the adult population *(17,61)*. Among prolactinomas, the size of the tumor and surgical success correlate with preoperative prolactin levels *(14,17)*. Macroadenomas, as expected, are less amenable to complete resection and often require bromocriptine and/or radiation. Boys, in particular, present with larger tumors and higher prolactin levels. The use of radiation and bromocriptine as adjunctive therapy results in long-term recurrence rates for macroadenomas approaching that of microadenomas *(17)*. From the Mayo Clinic, Partington et al. report an initial control rate of 100% for prolactinomas, although 33% required additional therapy *(16)*. After follow-up for a median period 79 mo, all had normal prolactin levels.

In ACTH-secreting tumors from the Mayo Clinic study, there was an 80% initial control rate as measured by serum cortisol levels, but 25% of these cases recurred within the median follow-up period of 54 mo *(16)*. In a more recent study from the same institution of only those patients with Cushing's disease, a much more cautious conclusion is reached *(62)*. Of a total of 22 patients, fully 42.2% experienced recurrence 10 yr after surgery. Of note, 58% of tumors in females recurred compared to only 10% in males. Only one tumor was a macroadenoma, and none were invasive. This study suggests that follow-up of 10 yr or longer may be needed in order to determine if the initial procedure was curative. By comparison, the UCSF group reported a 6% recurrence rate with ACTH-secreting tumors after a median follow-up of 4.1 yr *(15)*. The NIH series reported a 5% recurrence rate, but median follow-up was only 22 mo *(23)*.

It appears that GH-secreting tumors in children present with larger tumors, and in one series, the majority could not be adequately treated by surgery alone leading to additional therapy, such as radiation and/or somatostatin *(14)*. The overall results in children with GH-secreting tumors appear to be poorer than in adults *(14,63,64)*.

DIFFERENTIAL DIAGNOSIS OF PARASELLAR LESIONS

INTRODUCTION Although the presence of an obvious hypersecretion syndrome is highly suggestive of a pituitary adenoma, other sellar lesions may produce overlapping clinical symptoms and signs. Although it is impractical to order a complete battery of laboratory tests on all patients suspected of endocrine abnormalities, a detailed history and physical examination will direct subsequent investigations. All children must receive a complete neurological examination, which includes the careful listing of developmental milestones. School performance is an important indicator of behavioral and intellectual performance. If there are any doubts about the child's intellectual ability, neuropsychological testing is imperative. This is of particular importance for those children who might ultimately receive cranial irradiation. A child's growth, weight, and sexual development (particularly menarche and the menstrual cycle in females) must be documented. Neuro-ophthalmological assessment includes careful fundoscopy, measurement of visual acuity, and mapping of visual fields using Goldman or Humphreys perimetry. Bedside examination of visual pathways is inadequate to document visual deficits accurately. Even if symptoms do not exist before treatment, assessment of the visual and endocrine systems before and after treatment is useful to determine if morbidity has occurred and as a baseline for future follow-up.

In most patients, CT and/or MRI of the sellar and suprasellar region is the touchstone by which intracranial pathology is ascertained with confidence and a provisional diagnosis made. A patient presenting with a complete clinical picture of endocrine and visual dysfunction is usually imaged promptly. The dilemma rests with the investigation of children with mildly suggestive, yet very common signs, such as obesity or pubertal milestones differing from peers or siblings. The decision to investigate is dependent on the clinical suspicion and skill of the physician. Given the incidence of midline supratentorial lesions in children, the improved results associated with early treatment, and the potential for permanent effects on growth and development, physicians should err on the side of caution and obtain imaging studies early.

CRANIOPHARYNGIOMA   Clinical Features   Craniopharyngiomas account for 6–9% of all pediatric brain tumors (13,65). Their origins and treatment have been the subject of some controversy.[†] In children, approximately one-half of sellar and suprasellar tumors are craniopharyngiomas with a peak incidence between 5 and 14 yr of age (13,67–69). It should be noted that equal numbers of craniopharyngiomas are found in children and adults. Craniopharyngiomas arise from neoplastic transformation of remnants of Rathke's pouch. Histologically, these tumors consist of an external layer of columnar epithelium, a middle layer of polygonal cells, and a central epithelial matrix that often undergoes degeneration leading to cyst formation. Two pathological varieties are described: the classic adamintomatous type found both in children and adults, and the squamous papillary type found almost exclusively in adults (70–75). Although some studies report improved outcome with the squamous papillary type, a recent study showed no difference in clinical behavior between the two types (70,75,76).

In the series from The Hospital for Sick Children, the most common presenting symptoms or signs were headache (68%), short stature (54%), and hydrocephalus (48%) (68,77). Craniopharyngiomas are classified according to location as prechiasmatic, retrochiasmatic, or sellar (77). Prechiasmatic tumors tend to present with visual disturbances, whereas retrochiasmatic tumors cause obstructive hydrocephalus and raised intracranial pressure. Hypopituitarism, which manifests as growth failure in children, is common (68,78). Interestingly, among the prechiasmatic tumors, endocrinopathy is rare.

The heterogeneous composition and variable architecture of craniopharyngiomas are reflected in their appearance on CT and MRI. The findings of cysts, calcifications, and contrast enhancement of the cyst wall on CT is virtually diagnostic of craniopharyngioma. MRI, however, is the modality of choice for defining the anatomical relationships between tumor and adjacent neural structures (Figure 4). Cysts, which are present in approx 80% of tumors, often contain a highly proteinaceous and cholesterol-containing fluid (colloquially termed "machinery oil fluid") that is iso- to hyperintense on T1-weighted MRIs (79). Solid tumors with extensive calcification appear hypointense on T1- and T2-weighted MRIs. Craniopharyngiomas can be mistaken for Rathke's cleft cysts (RCCs) or epithelial cysts (80), but sufficient differences exist on MRI between these entities and pituitary adenomas for the diagnosis to be made in most instances.

Treatment   Analysis of the results of patients with craniopharyngioma in the literature is hampered by differences between studies in patient profiles, treatment protocols, follow-up intervals, and the evolution of treatment strategies. As a generalization, either radical resection with follow-up, or subtotal resection with cranial irradiation is the preferred modality of treatment. The crux of the debate hinges on which strategy is best in avoiding the morbidity and mortality associated with radical surgical resection or the long-term effects of cranial irradiation. Subtotal resection alone almost invariably leads to recurrence. Once there is recurrence, the possibility of subsequent cure is markedly reduced.

The "benign" pathology of the tumor suggests that modern neurosurgical techniques should be able to affect cures. Only Matson and Crigler, however, were able to report a zero recurrence rate following surgery (81). Despite the feeling that "total" resection was carried out, the recurrence rates in recent surgical series varied from 7 to 29% (68,82,83). In the Hospital for Sick Children series, although the recurrence rate was 29%, the functional status of the patient group was excellent (68). In Yasargil's series, an overall 7% recurrence rate was reported (83). It should be noted that in this same series, the mortality rate among the 51 children operated on for the first time was 7.8% (within the first year after operation), and 26.3% among the 19 patients who received a second procedure.

Since the first report of irradiation of craniopharyngiomas by Carpenter (84), evidence has accumulated that suggests subtotal resection or biopsy followed by irradiation is another approach that may result in few recurrences with good functional outcomes (78,85–91). The recurrence rates range from 7 to 25%, similar to the series using radical surgery only.

Given the information currently available, certain treatment guidelines can be suggested. Gross total surgical resection should only be attempted by skilled pediatric surgeons with considerable experience.[§] If gross total resection is not technically possible, subtotal resection should be followed by irradiation. Follow-up imaging and careful neuroendocrine assessment are mandatory. For young children, cranial radiation is postponed to prevent delayed complications. For intrasellar tumors, the transsphenoidal approach appears to give excellent results. In a series of patients with sellar craniopharyngiomas treated with total removal by the transsphenoidal approach (29 cases), the recurrence rate was 7% (94). The excellent results in this series are partially attributed to the diaphragma sella acting as a physical barrier preventing

---

[†]Papers from a symposium devoted entirely to the subject of craniopharyngioma were recently published as a supplement to *Pediatric Neurosurgery (66)*. The interested reader is referred to this publication for an in depth discussion of the issues introduced in this chapter.

[§]For details of surgical techniques and approaches, the reader is referred to the appropriate sources (69,77,83,92–94).

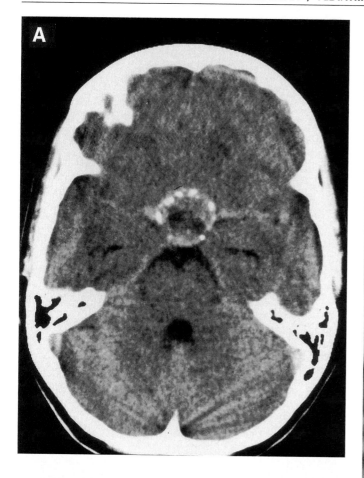

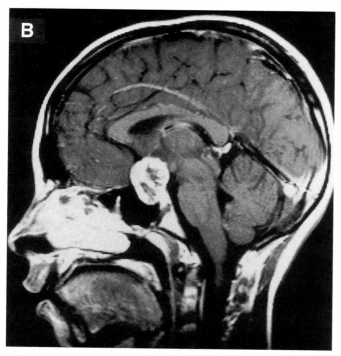

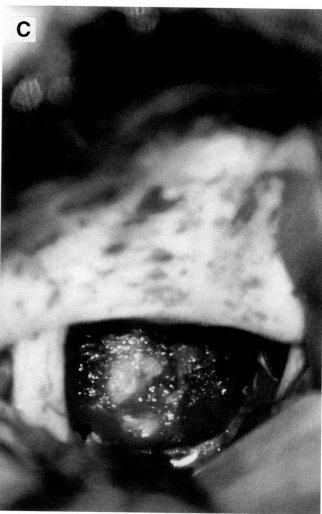

Figure 21-4 (A) Axial CT scan of 10-yr-old female presenting with unilateral visual failure. Dense calcifications are noted within the capsule of the lesion suggesting the diagnosis of craniopharyngioma. (B) Gadolinium-enhanced sagittal MRI scan of same patient demonstrating sellar and suprasellar localization of the tumor. The patient's presentation with unilateral visual failure and the information from the MRI scan suggest a prechiasmatic location of the tumor. (C) Intraoperative photograph of same patient following a right subfrontal approach. The tumor is clearly seen between the two optic nerves in the prechiasmatic space. A gross total resection of this tumor was achieved, and the patient has been well without recurrence for 5 yr.

tumor extension into the hypothalamus and adjacent vascular structures.

Intracavitary bleomycin was originally described by Takahashi et al. as a useful adjunctive therapy for primarily cystic tumors *(95)*. Currently, bleomycin is delivered into the tumor cyst through an Ommaya reservoir over 6 wk. The tumor does not appear to be eradicated, but the cyst wall frequently undergoes fibrosis *(92,96–98)*. This is useful preoperatively, because in some instances, the thickened cyst wall will retract from the surrounding brain, thereby facilitating excision *(98)*. Leakage of bleomycin into the subarachnoid space, however, can cause neurological deterioration *(99)*. Other treatment modalities, such as stereotactic radiation and intracavitary irradiation, are being assessed at the current time *(100,101)*.

OPTIC PATHWAY GLIOMAS   Clinical Features   Optic pathway gliomas account for approx 1–5% of pediatric brain tumors. Histologically, these tumors are low-grade astrocytomas with pilocytic astrocytes and Rosenthal fibers. Patients with tumors restricted to the optic nerve present with visual loss, proptosis, and optic atrophy. These are found in 15% of children with neurofibromatosis 1 (NF-1) when screened with CT *(102)*. By MRI, most optic pathway gliomas have been found to involve the chiasm and/or hypothalamus, and usually present with visual disturbance and symptoms attributable to obstructive hydrocephalus (headaches, vomiting, and decreased level of consciousness). Endocrine symptoms include growth arrest, hypothyroidism, hyperprolactinemia, and delayed puberty *(103–105)*. Some hypothalamic gliomas can cause precocious puberty, presumably owing to loss of central GHRH inhibition. Infants with hypothalamic involvement can present with the diencephalic syndrome of Russell, which consists of increased appetite, paradoxical weight loss, elevated serum GH levels, and hyperactive behavior *(106,107)*. Most patients with these tumors are <10 yr of age, which is an important distinguishing feature, since most pediatric pituitary adenomas are found in the second decade of life *(108,109)*.

The behavior of these tumors is inconsistent. Gliomas restricted to the optic nerve, although rare, can be cured with resection alone and have excellent long survival rates. Chiasmatic and hypothalamic gliomas possess similarly innocent histology, yet display more aggressive and relentless growth *(104,108,109)*. Patients with NF-1 appear to have tumors that possess more indolent characteristics *(106,110)*. Although rare, some tumors are known to involute after resection *(104)*. The intrinsic and infiltrative nature of these tumors on imaging studies provides an important clue in differentiating these tumors from pituitary adenomas and craniopharyngiomas. CT scans demonstrate a low-density suprasellar lesion that enhances following contrast administration. Similarly, T1-weighted MRIs reveal a low signal heterogeneous mass, at times cystic, involving the optic pathways, and when large, extending into the adjacent temporal lobe, frontal lobe, or hypothalamus (Figure 5). There is usually increased signal within the mass on T1-weighted images following gadolinium administration.

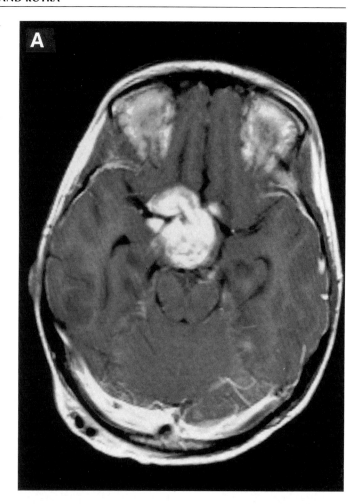

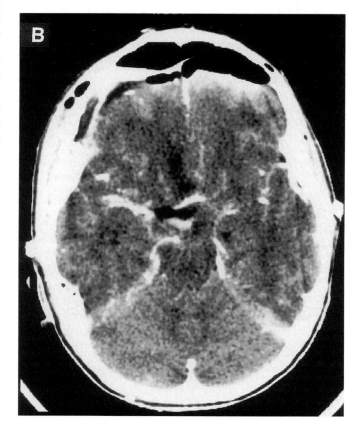

Figure 21-5   *(opposite right)* **(A)** Gadolinium-enhanced axial MRI scan of 8-yr-old male who presented with a bitemporal field defect, and signs and symptoms of raised intracranial pressure. A CSF shunt has been inserted. A large suprasellar lesion is seen occupying the region of the optic chiasm. The tumor extends into the right sylvian fissure and envelops the right middle cerebral artery. **(B)** Immediate postoperative scan of the same patient following a unilateral orbitotomy and right subfrontal approach. The tumor was found to originate from the chiasm and was radically but subtotally excised. Postoperatively, his vision has improved, and he has not developed signs of pituitary failure.

Treatment The definitive management of optic pathway gliomas is uncertain, because their proximity to critical basal neuro-anatomical structures often prevents complete resection. In these patients, the most efficacious adjunctive therapy remains unknown. Radiation therapy may be an effective means of controlling the growth of residual tumor and reducing the severity of symptoms *(108,111–114)*. The use of radiation therapy in children is a double-edged sword because of the inevitability of serious delayed complications. Clear-cut intellectual impairments occur even in children receiving low-dose craniospinal axis irradiation (1800–2400 cgy) for leukemia, *(115,116)*. In children with brain tumors, particularly those under 5 yr of age, the neuropsychological and endocrine consequences of cranial irradiation (4000–6000 cgy) are more severe *(117–124)*. It should be noted that factors, such as hydrocephalus, seizure disorders, and brain dysfunction, are independent factors that can contribute to neuropsychological impairment. Additional problems directly attributed to radiation can also occur. In the Hospital for Sick Children series, four children developed a second malignancy in the radiation field and five developed symptomatic moya-moya disease *(104)*.

Several institutions have explored the use of chemotherapy to delay radiation therapy, often with favorable results *(106,109,125–129)*. In general, the use of chemotherapy is associated with a high percentage of relapse, but this may "buy" time to allow the child to reach an age when radiation therapy is associated with fewer adverse sequelae *(130)*. The most effective chemotherapeutic agent and regimen remains unclear. In summary, the current trend favors initial surgical resection followed by chemotherapy. Tumor irradiation is reserved for children demonstrating clinically symptomatic tumor progression.

GERM-CELL TUMORS Although more common in the pineal region, approximately one-third of germ-cell tumors are found in the suprasellar area *(131,132)*. The major types of germ-cell tumors are germinomas, embryonal carcinoma, choriocarcinoma, and teratoma (immature and mature). The most common variety are germinomas, the majority of which arise in the pineal area. There is an overall male-to-female ratio of 3:1, except in the suprasellar area where the majority occur in females. Except for mature teratomas, all germ-cell tumors are malignant and possess the capacity for tissue invasion and metastasis. The classic clinical presentation of germinomas consists of diabetes insipidus, visual disturbance, and hypopituitarism, which clearly overlaps with primary pituitary lesions and other sellar masses *(133)*.

Germinomas are typically homogeneously and brightly enhancing irregular masses *(134,135)*. T1-weighted MRIs are low to isointense compared to white matter, whereas T2-weighted images are iso- to hyper-intense to white matter (Figure 6). Other germ-cell tumors can display a variety of features, such as cystic change, calcification, and/or fat. Mature teratomas can potentially have differentiated tissues derived from three germ-cell layers. This can obviously lead to a heterogeneous appearance on imaging studies. Complete imaging of the craniospinal axis is suggested to exclude spread through CSF pathways. Tumor markers, such as α-fetoprotein and human chorionic gonadotropin, obtained from serum and CSF, can assist in diagnosis and assessment of recurrence. Imaging and laboratory tests, however, do not replace an open procedure for obtaining tissue for pathological diagnosis. Because many germ-cell tumors contain mixed elements, several tissue samples should be taken to ensure a representative histological impression.

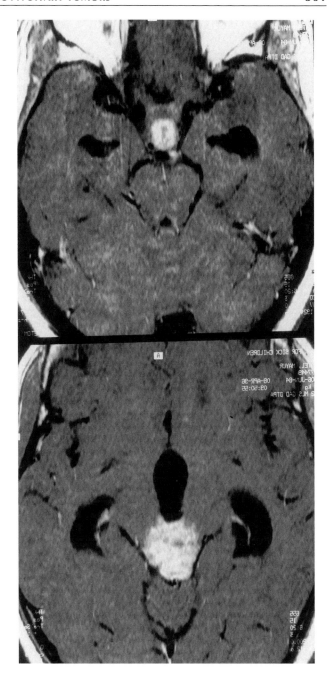

Figure 21-6 Gadolinium-enhanced axial images of a 10-yr-old male who presented with headaches, papilledema, and diabetes insipidus. The images reveal tumor deposits occurring simultaneously in the pineal and suprasellar regions highly suggestive of a germ-cell tumor. An endoscopic biopsy of the pineal region mass was performed. CSF and serum were taken for marker studies, and a ventriculo-peritoneal shunt was inserted. The α-fetoprotein in the serum and CSF was markedly elevated. The diagnosis was nongerminomatous germ-cell tumor, and the patient is receiving preirradiation chemotherapy. The suprasellar lesion could be visualized at the time of pineal tumor biopsy anterior to the mamillary bodies, and posterior to the lamina terminalis within the floor of the third ventricle.

Initial treatment is surgery followed by chemotherapy in children under 5 yr of age, with radiation for older children. The exquisite sensitivity of germinomas to external beam radiotherapy has led to excellent long-term survival rates. The 5-yr survival

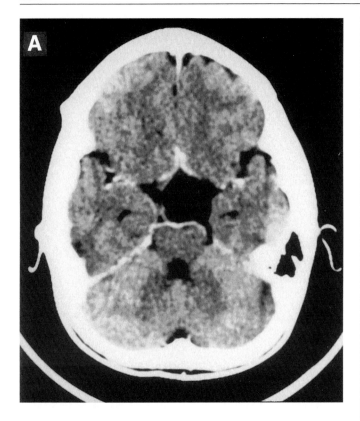
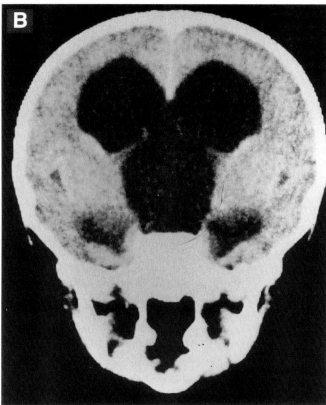

Figure 21-7 **(A)** Axial CT scan demonstrating hypodense lesion in the suprasellar region compatible with an arachnoid cyst. **(B)** Coronal CT scan in a different patient demonstrating a large arachnoid cyst, which has invaginated into the third ventricle causing marked, obstructive hydrocephalus.

rates for germinomas are in the range of 80–90% *(132,136)*. In most pediatric institutions, the trend is to delay or eliminate craniospinal irradiation. Wolden and colleagues suggest that in patients with intracranial germ-cell tumors and a negative craniospinal axis examination, prophylactic spinal irradiation can be avoided *(136)*. Other types of germ-cell tumors, unfortunately, are not nearly as radiosensitive as germinomas. In the past, a "test dose" of 2000 cgy was used as a diagnostic tool mainly, because pineal region surgery was associated with an unacceptable level of morbidity. In the current era, because most areas of the brain can now be safely approached surgically and radiation itself causes serious deleterious effects, this method of evaluation is to be avoided.

ARACHNOID CYSTS Arachnoid cysts are congenital fluid containing cavities that are lined by arachnoid cells and collagen *(137)*. The fluid within the cyst is identical to CSF. Although the cerebello-pontine angle is the most common site, approx 9% arise in the sellar and suprasellar region *(137)*. Various pathogenetic mechanisms have been proposed, including a "ball-valve" leading to one-way CSF flow *(138)*, secretion by arachnoid cells *(139)*, and anomalous duplication of the arachnoid during development *(137)*. Children with suprasellar arachnoid cysts present with hydrocephalus and increasing head size, compression of neural structures (ataxia, nystagmus, cranial nerve palsies, seizures, and developmental delay), and/or neuroendocrine dysfunction *(140)*. The "bobble-head doll" sign, a characteristic nodding of the head, occurs infrequently with suprasellar arachnoid cysts *(140)*.

Diagnosis is made following imaging studies that reveal a thin-walled cyst containing fluid isointense with CSF (Figure 7). A suprasellar arachnoid cyst can be mistaken for a third ventricular cyst on CT, but a sagittal MRI should demonstrate a membrane intervening between the cyst proper and the floor of the third ventricle. The aim of treatment is cyst decompression. From this point, two viewpoints are expressed in the literature. In some studies, craniotomy and cyst fenestration is successful and is recommended as the initial treatment, with cysto-peritoneal shunting reserved for failures *(141,142)*. Other institutions favor primary placement of a cysto-peritoneal shunt *(3,143)*. Recent advances in neuro-endoscopy allow primary cyst fenestration to be done with little or no morbidity. A ventriculo-peritoneal shunt may be inserted later if necessary. Minimally invasive techniques are likely to supplant open craniotomy in the treatment of benign developmental cysts.

RATHKE'S CLEFT CYSTS (RCCs) The pars intermedia of the adenohypophysis usually contains one or more small cysts lined with simple cuboidal or columnar epithelium, variably ciliated. These are believed to be remnants of the Rathke's pouch, hence the name Rathke's cleft cysts (RCCs). It is likely that RCCs are one end of a spectrum of epithelially derived cysts, including epidermoid cysts, dermoid cysts, and craniopharyngiomas, that are found in the sellar and suprasellar area *(80)*. RCCs, in contrast to craniopharyngiomas, lack neoplastic characteristics, but may contain areas of squamous metaplasia, which are found in craniopharyngiomas *(80,144)*. The majority of children with RCCs present with pituitary dysfunction and a visual field deficit. Imaging studies reflect the nature of the cyst contents *(145)*. If cyst contents are low in protein, the image is low-density on CT scans with low signal on T1 and mixed or high signal on T2-weighted

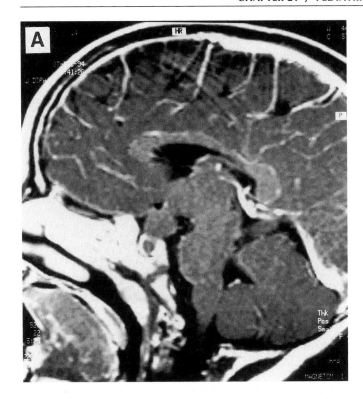

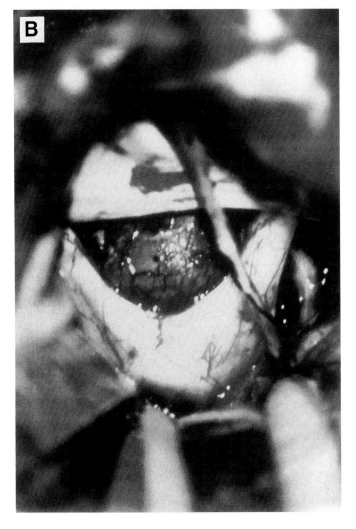

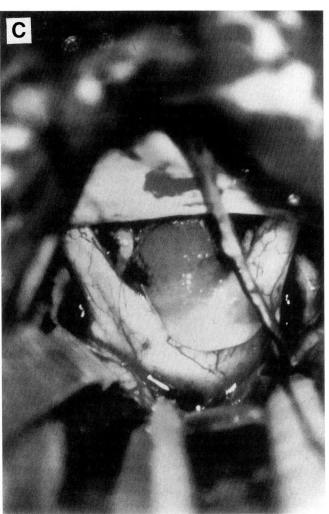

Figure 21-8 **(A)** Gadolinium-enhanced sagittal MRI scan demonstrating iso-intense lesion, which takes origin in the sellar, but extends in a bulbous fashion into the suprasellar space. Again, the nonpneumatization of the sphenoid sinus is appreciated in this 3-yr-old female who presented with diabetes insipidus. **(B)** Following a subfrontal approach, the lesion is visualized anterior to the chiasm. Note is made of the intact unilateral olfactory nerve coursing across the right optic nerve. **(C)** Following incision of the capsule, thick, gelatinous material exuded onto the chaism. The lesion was decompressed by cyst aspiration, and the capsule was removed. The diagnosis is RCC. There has been no recurrence of the lesion after 3 yr.

MR images *(146,147)* (Figure 8). CT scans in some cases demonstrate an enhancing margin corresponding to the cyst wall *(144,147)*. There is considerable imaging and clinical overlap with other cystic masses, such as pituitary adenoma, cystic craniopharyngioma, cysticercosis, arachnoid cyst, epidermoid cyst, empty sella, and mucocele. Treatment usually requires cyst wall biopsy and cyst drainage. Although this is believed to effect cure in most cases, RCCs can recur so follow-up is required.

SUMMARY

The challenge with pediatric sellar lesions is threefold. First, it rests with the internist or pediatrician to determine which signs and symptoms, among a constellation caused by tumors of the supratentorial midline, require further investigation. Second, once an intracranial mass is detected, the overall clinical and pathological assessment requires considerable expertise with laboratory investigations and imaging studies. Although surgical intervention is usually the initial treatment for the majority with these tumors, a multitude of other treatment options must be carefully weighed. Finally, attentive management of endocrine function is mandatory in the postoperative period and possibly for the duration of the child's life. Although certain tumors, such as craniopharyngiomas, large macroadenomas, and some germ-cell tumors, demonstrate aggressive characteristics that lead to a poor outcome or death, results in most cases are excellent with frequent cure or long-term remission. Future goals with respect to pituitary adenomas are the earlier detection of symptomatic tumors, development of more specific hormone antagonists, and the refinement of surgical and radiosurgical techniques.

ACKNOWLEDGMENTS

The authors thank B. W. Chong (Department of Radiology, University of Utah) for critically reviewing this chapter, and Michael J. Harrsion and Gilbert Gardner (David Grant Medical Center, Travis AFB, CA) for graciously supplying the illustration used in Figure 1.

REFERENCES

1. Chong BW, Newton TH. Hypothalamic and pituitary pathology. Radiol Clin North Am 1993;31:1147–1153.
2. Styne DM. The therapy for hypothalamic-pituitary tumors. Endocrinol Metab Clin North Am 1993;22:631–648.
3. Rutka JT, Hoffman HJ, Drake JM, Humphreys RP. Suprasellar and sellar tumors in childhood and adolescence. Neurosurg Clin North Am 1992;3:803–820.
4. Asa SL, Kovacs K, Laszlo FA, Domokos, I, Ezrin, C. Human fetal adenohypophysis. Histologic and immunocytochemical analysis. Neuroendocrinology 1986;43:308–316.
5. Fisher DA, Klein, AH. Thyroid development and disorders of thyroid function in the newborn. N Engl J Med 1981;304:702–712.
6. Kaplan SL, Grumbach MM, Aubert ML. The ontogenesis of pituitary hormones and hypothalamic factors in the human fetus: maturation of central nervous system regulation of anterior pituitary function. Recent Prog Horm Res 1976;32:161–243.
7. Thliveris JA, Currie RW. Observations on the hypothalamo-hypophyseal portal vasculature in the developing human fetus. Am J Anat 1980;157:441–444.
8. Wolpert SM, Osborne M, Anderson M, Runge VM. The bright pituitary gland-a normal MR appearance in infancy. AJNR 1988;9:1–3.
9. Tien RD, Kucharczyk J, Bessette J, Middleton, M. MR imaging of the pituitary gland in infants and children: changes in size, shape, and MR signal with growth and development. N Engl J Med 1992;158:1151–1154.
10. Elster AD, Sanders TG, Vines FS, Chen MY. Size and shape of the pituitary gland during pregnancy and post partum: measurement with MR imaging. Radiology 1991;181:531–535.
11. Sharafuddin MJ, Luisiri A, Garibaldi LR, Fulk DL, Klein JB, Gillespie, KN, et al. MR imaging diagnosis of central precocious puberty: importance of changes in the shape and size of the pituitary gland. AJR 1994;162:1167–1173.
12. Elster AD, Chen MYM, Williams DW III, Key LL. Pituitary gland: MR imaging of physiologic hypertrophy in adolescence. Radiology 1990;174:681–685.
13. Pollack IF. Brain tumors in children. N Engl J Med 1994;331:1500–1507.
14. Dyer EH, Civit T, Visot A, Delalande O, Derome P. Transsphenoidal surgery for pituitary adenomas in children. Neurosurgery 1994;34:207–212.
15. Mindermann T, Wilson CB. Pediatric pituitary adenomas. Neurosurgery 1995;36:259–268.
16. Partington MD, Davis DH, Laws ER Jr, Scheithauer BW. Pituitary adenomas in childhood and adolescence. J Neurosurg 1994;80:209–216.
17. Kane LA, Leinung MC, Scheithauer BW, Bergstralh EJ, Laws ER Jr, Groover RV, et al. Pituitary adenomas in childhood and adolescence. J Clin Endocrinol Metab 1994;79:1135–1140.
18. Nyhan WL, Green M. Hyperthyroidism in a patient with a pituitary adenoma. J Pediatr 1964;65:583–589.
19. Avramides A, Karapiperis A, Triantafyllidou E, Vayas S, Moshidou A, Vyzantiadis A. TSH-secreting pituitary macroadenoma in an 11-year-old girl. Acta Paediatr 1992;81:1058–1060.
20. Suntornlohanakul S, Vasiknanont P, Mo-Suwan L, Phuenpathom N, Chongchitnant N. TSH secreting pituitary adenoma in children: a case report. J Med Assoc Thai 1990;73:175–178.
21. Bickler SW, McMahon TJ, Campbell JR, Mandel S, Piatt JH, Harrison MW. Preoperative diagnostic evaluation of children with Cushing's syndrome. J Pediatr Surg 1994;29:671–676.
22. Trainer PJ, Grossman A. The diagnosis and differential diagnosis of Cushing's syndrome. Clin Endocrinol (Oxford) 1991;34:317–330.
23. Magiakou MA, Mastorakos G, Oldfield EH, Gomez MT, Doppman JL, Cutler GB Jr, et al. Cushing's syndrome in children and adolescents. Presentation, diagnosis, and therapy. N Engl J Med 1994;331:629–636.
24. Mindermann T, Wilson CB. Pituitary adenomas in childhood and adolescence. J Pediatr Endocrinol Metab 1995;8:79–83.
25. Weber A, Trainer PJ, Grossman AB, Afshar F, Medbak S, Perry LA, et al. Investigation, management and therapeutic outcome in 12 cases of childhood and adolescent Cushing's syndrome. Clin Endocrinol (Oxford) 1995;43:19–28.
26. Styne DM, Grumbach MM, Kaplan SL, Wilson CB, Conte FA. Treatment of Cushing's disease in childhood and adolescence by transsphenoidal microadenomectomy. N Engl J Med 1984;310:889–893.
27. Gelber SJ, Heffez DS, Donohoue PA. Pituitary gigantism caused by growth hormone excess from infancy. J Pediatr 1992;120:931–934.
28. Blumberg DL, Sklar CA, David R, Rothenberg S, Bell J. Acromegaly in an infant. Pediatrics 1989;83:998–1002.
29. Geffner ME, Nagel RA, Dietrich RB, Kaplan SA. Treatment of acromegaly with a somatostatin analog in a patient with McCune-Albright syndrome. J Pediatr 1987;111: 740–743.
30. Kovacs K, Horvath E, Thorner MO, Rogol AD. Mammosomatotroph hyperplasia associated with acromegaly and hyperprolactinemia in a patient with the McCune-Albright syndrome: a histologic, immunocytologic and ultrastructural study of the surgically-removed adenohypophysis. Virchows Arch A Pathol Anat Histopathol 1984;403:77–86.
31. Polychronakos C, Tsoukas G, Ducharme JR, Letarte J, Collu R. Gigantism and hyperprolactinemia in polyostotic fibrous dysplasia (Mc Cune-Albright syndrome). J Endocrinol Invest 1982;5:323–326.
32. Moran A, Asa SL, Kovacs K, Horvath E, Singer W, Sagman U, et al. Gigantism due to pituitary mammosomatotroph hyperplasia. N Engl J Med 1990;323:322–327.
33. Asa SL, Kovacs K, Horvath E, Losinski NE, Laszlo FA, Domokos I, et al. Human fetal adenohypophysis. Electron microscopic and ultrastructural immunocytochemical analysis. Neuroendocrinology 1988;48:423–431.
34. Sano T, Asa SL, Kovacs K. Growth hormone-releasing hormone-producing tumors: clinical, biochemical, and morphological manifestations. Endocr Rev 1988;9:357–373.
35. Aron DC, Tyrrell JB, Wilson CB. Pituitary tumors. Current concepts in diagnosis and management. West J Med 1995;162:340–352.
36. Sippell WG, Dorr HG, Bidlingmaier F, Knorr D. Plasma levels of aldosterone, corticosterone, 11-deoxycorticosterone, progesterone, 17-hydroxyprogesterone, cortisol, and cortisone during infancy and childhood. Pediatr Res 1980;14:39–46.
37. Franks RC. Diurnal variation of plasma 17-hydroxycorticosteroids in children. J Clin Endocrinol Metab 1967;27:75–78.
38. Arafah BM, Kailani S, Selman WR. Physiology and pathophysiology of prolactin secretion. In: Barrow DL, Selman WR, eds. Neuroendocrinology, Williams and Wilkins, Baltimore, 1992, pp. 95–112.

39. Cox TD, Elster AD. Normal pituitary gland: changes in shape, size, and signal intensity during the 1st year of life at MR imaging. Radiology 1991;179:721–724.

40. Kucharczyk J, Kucharczyk W, Berry I, de Groot J, Kelly W, Norman D, et al. Histochemical characterization and functional significance of the hyperintense signal on MR images of the posterior pituitary. AJR 1989;152:153–157.

41. Colombo N, Berry I, Kucharczyk J, Kucharczyk W, de Groot J, Larson T, et al. Posterior pituitary gland: appearance on MR images in normal and pathologic states. Radiology 1987;165:481–485.

42. Kucharczyk W, Davis DO, Kelly WM, Sze G, Norman D, Newton TH. Pituitary adenomas: high-resolution MR imaging at 1.5 T. Radiology 1986;161:761–765.

43. Elster AD. Modern imaging of the pituitary. Radiology 1993; 187:1–14.

44. Chong BW, Kucharczyk W, Singer W, George S. Pituitary gland MR: a comparative study of healthy volunteers and patients with microadenomas. AJNR 1994;15:675–679.

45. Snow RB, Johnson CE, Morgello S, Lavyne MH, Patterson RH Jr. Is magnetic resonance imaging useful in guiding the operative approach to large pituitary tumors? Neurosurgery 1990;26:801–803.

46. Stein AL, Levenick MN, Kletzky OA. Computed tomography versus magnetic resonance imaging for the evaluation of suspected pituitary adenomas. Obstet Gynecol 1989;73:996–999.

47. Davis PC, Hoffman JC Jr, Spencer T, Tindall GT, Braun IF. MR imaging of pituitary adenoma: CT, clinical, and surgical correlation. AJR 1987;148:797–802.

48. Newton DR, Dillon WP, Norman D, Newton TH, Wilson CB. Gd-DTPA-enhanced MR imaging of pituitary adenomas. AJNR 1989;10:949–954.

49. Stadnik T, Stevenaert A, Beckers A, Luypaert R, Buisseret T, Oxteaux M. Pituitary microadenomas: diagnosis with two-and three-dimensional MR imaging at 1.5 T before and after injection of gadolinium. Radiology 1990;176:419–428.

50. Ludecke DK, Herrmann HD, Schulte FJ. Special problems with neurosurgical treatments of hormone-secreting pituitary adenomas in children. Prog Exp Tumor Res 1987;30:362–370.

51. Oldfield EH, Chrousos GP, Schulte HM, Schaaf M, McKeever PE, Krudy AG, et al. Preoperative lateralization of ACTH-secreting pituitary microadenomas by bilateral and simultaneous inferior petrosal venous sinus sampling. N Engl J Med 1985;312: 100–103.

52. Cunnah D, Besser M. Management of prolactinomas. Clin Endocrinol (Oxford) 1991;34:231–235.

53. Molitch ME, Elton RL, Blackwell RE, Caldwell B, Chang RJ, Jaffe R, et al. Bromocriptine as primary therapy for prolactin-secreting macroadenomas: results of a prospective multicenter study. J Clin Endocrinol Metab 1985;60:698–705.

54. Tyson D, Reggiardo D, Sklar C, David R. Prolactin-secreting macroadenomas in adolescents. Response to bromocriptine therapy. Am J Dis Child 1993;147:1057–1061.

55. Arslanian SA, Becker DJ, Lee PA, Drash AL, Foley TP Jr. Growth hormone therapy and tumor recurrence. Findings in children with brain neoplasms and hypopituitarism. Am J Dis Child 1985;139: 347–350.

56. Clayton PE, Shalet SM, Gattamaneni HR, Price DA. Does growth hormone cause relapse of brain tumours? Lancet 1987;1:711–713.

57. Oberfield SE, Nino M, Riddick L, Pang S, Nagel M, Khandji A, et al. Combined bromocriptine and growth hormone (GH) treatment in GH-deficient children with macroprolactinoma in situ. J Clin Endocrinol Metab 1992;75:87–90.

58. Fraioli B, Ferrante L, Celli P. Pituitary adenomas with onset during puberty. Features and treatment. J Neurosurg 1983;59:590–595.

59. Gaini SM, Giovanelli M, Forni C, Villani R, Scuccimarra A, Carteri A, et al. Pituitary adenomas in infancy and childhood. Mod Probl Paediatr 1976;18:220–225.

60. Ortiz-Suarez H, Erickson DL. Pituitary adenomas of adolescents. J Neurosurg 1975;43:437–439.

61. Maira G, Anile C. Pituitary adenomas in childhood and adolescence. Can J Neurol Sci 1990;17:83–87.

62. Leinung MC, Kane LA, Scheithauer BW, Carpenter PC, Laws ER Jr, Zimmerman D. Long term follow-up of transsphenoidal surgery for the treatment of Cushing's disease in childhood. J Clin Endocrinol Metab 1995;80:2475–2479.

63. Ross DA, Wilson CB. Results of transsphenoidal microsurgery for growth hormone-secreting pituitary adenoma in a series of 214 patients. J Neurosurg 1988;68:854–867.

64. Tindall GT, Oyesiku NM, Watts NB, Clark RV, Christy JH, Adams DA. Transsphenoidal adenomectomy for growth hormone-secreting pituitary adenomas in acromegaly: outcome analysis and determinants of failure. J Neurosurg 1993;78:205–215.

65. Rorke LB. Introductory survey of brain tumors. In: Cheek WR, ed. Pediatric Neurosurgery. W. B. Saunders, Philadelphia, 1994, pp. 351–355.

66. Epstein FJ, Handler MH. Craniopharyngioma: the answer. Pediatr Neurosurg 1994;21(Suppl 1):S1–S132.

67. Carmel PW, Antunes JL, Chang CH. Craniopharyngiomas in children. Neurosurgery 1982;11:382–389.

68. Hoffman HJ, De Silva M, Humphreys RP, Drake JM, Smith ML, Blaser SI. Aggressive surgical management of craniopharyngiomas in children. J Neurosurg 1992;76:47–52.

69. Carmel PW. Brain tumors of disordered embryogenesis. In: Youmans JR, ed. Neurological Surgery. W. B. Saunders, Philadelphia, 1996, pp. 2761–2781.

70. Adamson TE, Wiestler OD, Kleihues P, Yasargil MG. Correlation of clinical and pathological features in surgically treated craniopharyngiomas. J Neurosurg 1990;73:12–17.

71. Banna M. Craniopharyngioma in adults. Surg Neurol 1973; 1:202–204.

72. Burger PC, Scheithauer BW, Vogel FS. Surgical Pathology of Nervous System and Its Coverings, 3rd ed. Churchhill Livingston, New York, 1991.

73. Giangaspero F, Burger PC, Osborne DR, Stein RB. Suprasellar papillary squamous epithelioma ("papillary craniopharyngioma"). Am J Surg Pathol 1984;8:57–64.

74. Petito CK, DeGirolami U, Earle KM. Craniopharyngiomas: a clinical and pathological review. Cancer 1976;37:1944–1952.

75. Weiner HL, Wisoff JH, Rosenberg ME, Kupersmith MJ, Cohen H, Zagzag D, et al. Craniopharyngiomas: a clinicopathological analysis of factors predictive of recurrence and functional outcome. Neurosurgery 1994;35:1001–1010.

76. Kahn EA, Gosch HH, Seeger JF, Hicks SP. Forty-five years experience with the craniopharyngiomas. Surg Neurol 1973;1:5–12.

77. Hoffman HJ, Kestle J. Craniopharyngiomas. In: Cheek WR, ed. Pediatric Neurosurgery. W. B. Saunders, Philadelphia, 1994, pp. 418–428.

78. Baskin DS, Wilson CB. Surgical management of craniopharyngiomas. A review of 74 cases. J Neurosurg 1986;65:22–27.

79. Pusey E, Kortman KE, Flannigan BD, Tsuruda J, Bradley WG. MR of craniopharyngiomas: tumor delineation and characterization. AJR 1987;149:383–388.

80. Harrison MJ, Morgello S, Post KD. Epithelial cystic lesions of the sellar and parasellar region: a continuum of ectodermal derivatives? J Neurosurg 1994;80:1018–1025.

81. Matson DD, Crigler JFJ. Management of craniopharyngioma in childhood. J Neurosurg 1969;30:377–399.

82. Wen DY, Seljeskog EL, Haines SJ. Microsurgical management of craniopharyngiomas. Br J Neurosurg 1992;6:467–474.

83. Yasargil MG, Curcic M, Kis M, Siegenthaler G, Teddy PJ, Roth P. Total removal of craniopharyngiomas. Approaches and long-term results in 144 patients. J Neurosurg 1990;73:3–11.

84. Carpenter RC, Chamberlin GW, Frazier CH. The treatment of hypophyseal stalk tumors by evacuation and irradiation. AJR 1937;38:162–177.

85. Regine WF, Kramer S. Pediatric craniopharyngiomas: long term results of combined treatment with surgery and radiation. Int J Radiat Oncol Biol Phys 1992;24:611–617.

86. Regine WF, Mohiuddin M, Kramer S. Long-term results of pediatric and adult craniopharyngiomas treated with combined surgery and radiation. Radiother Oncol 1993;27:13–21.

87. Danoff BF, Cowchock FS, Kramer S. Childhood craniopharyngioma: survival, local control, endocrine and neurologic function following radiotherapy. Int J Radiat Oncol Biol Phys 1983;9:171–175.

88. Wen BC, Hussey DH, Staples J, Hitchon PW, Jani SK, Vigliotti AP, et al. A comparison of the roles of surgery and radiation therapy in the management of craniopharyngiomas. Int J Radiat Oncol Biol Phys 1989;16:17–24.

89. Weiss M, Sutton L, Marcial V, Fowble B, Packer R, Zimmerman R, et al. The role of radiation therapy in the management of childhood craniopharyngioma. Int J Radiat Oncol Biol Phys 1989; 17:1313–1321.

90. Manaka S, Teramoto A, Takakura K. The efficacy of radiotherapy for craniopharyngioma. J Neurosurg 1985;62:648–656.

91. Fischer EG, Welch K, Shillito J Jr, Winston KR, Tarbell NJ. Craniopharyngiomas in children. Long-term effects of conservative surgical procedures combined with radiation therapy. J Neurosurg 1990;73:534–540.

92. Wisoff JH. Surgical management of recurrent craniopharyngiomas. Pediatr Neurosurg 1994;21(Suppl 1):108–113.

93. Maira G, Anile C, Rossi GF, Colosimo C. Surgical treatment of craniopharyngiomas: an evaluation of the transsphenoidal and pterional approaches. Neurosurgery 1995;36:715–724.

94. Laws ERJ. Transsphenoidal removal of craniopharyngioma. Pediatr Neurosurg 1994;21(Suppl 1):57–63.

95. Takahashi H, Nakazawa S, Shimura T. Evaluation of postoperative intratumoral injection of bleomycin for craniopharyngioma in children. J Neurosurg 1985;62:120–127.

96. Broggi G, Franzini A, Cajola L, Pluchino F. Cell kinetic investigations in craniopharyngioma: preliminary results and considerations. Pediatr Neurosurg 1994;21(Suppl 1):21–23.

97. Broggi G, Giorgi C, Franzini A, Servello D, Solero CL. Preliminary results of intracavitary treatment of craniopharyngioma with bleomycin. J Neurosurg Sci 1989;33:145–148.

98. Hoffman HJ. Surgical management of craniopharyngioma. Pediatr Neurosurg 1994;21(Suppl 1):44–49.

99. Haisa T, Ueki K, Yoshida S. Toxic effects of bleomycin on the hypothalamus following its administration into a cystic craniopharyngioma. Br J Neurosurg 1994;8:747–750.

100. Lunsford LD, Pollock BE, Kondziolka DS, Levine G, Flickinger JC. Stereotactic options in the management of craniopharyngioma. Pediatr Neurosurg 1994;21(Suppl 1):90–97.

101. Pollock BE, Lunsford LD, Kondziolka D, Levine G, Flickinger JC. Phosphorus-32 intracavitary irradiation of cystic craniopharyngiomas: current technique and long-term results. Int J Radiat Oncol Biol Phys 1995;33:437–446.

102. Listernick R, Charrow J, Greenwald MJ, Esterly NB. Optic gliomas in children with neurofibromatosis type 1. J Pediatr 1989; 114:788–792.

103. Cohen ME, Duffner PK. Optic pathway tumors. Neurol Clin 1991;9:467–477.

104. Hoffman HJ, Humphreys RP, Drake JM, Rutka JT, Becker LE, Jenkin D, et al. Optic pathway/hypothalamic gliomas: a dilemma in management. Pediatr Neurosurg 1993;19:186–195.

105. Johnson DL, McCullough DC. Optic nerve gliomas and other tumors involving the optic nerve and chiasm. In: Cheek WR, ed. Pediatric Neurosurgery. W. B. Saunders, Philadelphia, 1994, pp. 409–417

106. Rodriguez LA, Edwards MS, Levin VA. Management of hypothalamic gliomas in children: an analysis of 33 cases. Neurosurgery 1990;26:242–246.

107. DeSousa AL, Kalsbeck JE, Mealey J Jr, Ellis FD, Muller J. Optic chiasmatic glioma in children. Am J Ophthalmol 1979;87:376–381.

108. Pierce SM, Barnes PD, Loeffler JS, McGinn C, Tarbell NJ. Definitive radiation therapy in the management of symptomatic patients with optic glioma. Survival and long-term effects. Cancer 1990; 65:45–52.

109. Packer RJ, Sutton LN, Bilaniuk LT, Radcliffe J, Rosenstock JG, Siegel KR, et al. Treatment of chiasmatic/hypothalamic gliomas of childhood with chemotherapy: an update. Ann Neurol 1988; 23:79–85.

110. Venes JL, Latack J, Kandt RS. Postoperative regression of opticochiasmatic astrocytoma: a case for expectant therapy. Neurosurgery 1984;15:421–423.

111. Nishio S, Takeshita I, Fujiwara S, Fukui M. Optico-hypothalamic glioma: an analysis of 16 cases. Childs Nerv Syst 1993;9:334–338.

112. Kovalic JJ, Grigsby PW, Shepard MJ, Fineberg BB, Thomas PR. Radiation therapy for gliomas of the optic nerve and chiasm. Int J Radiat Oncol Biol Phys 1990;18:927–932.

113. Danoff BF, Kramer S, Thompson N. The radiotherapeutic management of optic nerve gliomas in children. Int J Radiat Oncol Biol Phys 1980;6:45–50.

114. Flickinger JC, Torres C, Deutsch M. Management of low-grade gliomas of the optic nerve and chiasm. Cancer 1988;61:635–642.

115. Rowland JH, Glidewell OJ, Sibley RF, Holland JC, Tull R, Berman A, et al. Effects of different forms of central nervous system prophylaxis on neuropsychologic function in childhood leukemia. J Clin Oncol 1984;2:1327–1335.

116. Copeland DR, Fletcher JM, Pfefferbaum-Levine B, Jaffe N, Ried H, Maor M. Neuropsychological sequelae of childhood cancer in long-term survivors. Pediatrics 1985;75:745–753.

117. Duffner PK, Cohen ME. The long-term effects of central nervous system therapy on children with brain tumors. Neurol Clin 1991; 9:479–495.

118. Duffner PK, Cohen ME. Long-term consequences of CNS treatment for childhood cancer, Part II: Clinical consequences. Pediatr Neurol 1991;7:237–242.

119. Cohen ME, Duffner PK. Long-term consequences of CNS treatment for childhood cancer, Part I: Pathologic consequences and potential for oncogenesis. Pediatr Neurol 1991;7:157–163.

120. Duffner PK, Cohen ME, Thomas P. Late effects of treatment on the intelligence of children with posterior fossa tumors. Cancer 1983;51:233–237.

121. Hirsch JF, Renier D, Czernichow P, Benveniste L, Pierre-Kahn A. Medulloblastoma in childhood. Survival and functional results. Acta Neurochir (Wien) 1979;48:1–15.

122. Raimondi AJ, Tomita T. Medulloblastoma in childhood: comparative results of partial and total resection. Childs Brain 1979;5:310–328.

123. Roman DD, Sperduto PW. Neuropsychological effects of cranial radiation: current knowledge and future directions. Int J Radiat Oncol Biol Phys 1995;31:983–998.

124. Schultheiss TE, Kun LE, Ang KK, Stephens LC. Radiation response of the central nervous system. Int J Radiat Oncol Biol Phys 1995;31:1093–1112.

125. Packer RJ, Savino PJ, Bilaniuk LT, Zimmerman RA, Schatz NJ, Rosenstock JG, et al. Chiasmatic gliomas of childhood. A reappraisal of natural history and effectiveness of cranial irradiation. Childs Brain 1983;10:393–403.

126. Moghrabi A, Friedman HS, Burger PC, Tien R, Oakes WJ. Carboplatin treatment of progressive optic pathway gliomas to delay radiotherapy. J Neurosurg 1993;79:223–227.

127. Janss AJ, Grundy R, Cnaan A, Savino PJ, Packer RJ, Zackai EH, et al. Optic pathway and hypothalamic/chiasmatic gliomas in children younger than age 5 years with a 6-year follow-up. Cancer 1995;75: 1051–1059.

128. Chamberlain MC, Grafe MR. Recurrent chiasmatic-hypothalamic glioma treated with oral etoposide. J Clin Oncol 1995;13: 2072–2076.

129. Petronio J, Edwards MS, Prados M, Freyberger S, Rabbitt J, Silver P, et al. Management of chiasmal and hypothalamic gliomas of infancy and childhood with chemotherapy. J Neurosurg 1991; 74:701–708.

130. Duffner PK, Horowitz ME, Krischer JP, Friedman HS, Burger PC, Cohen ME, et al. Postoperative chemotherapy and delayed radiation in children less than three years of age with malignant brain tumors. N Engl J Med 1993;328:1725–1731.

131. Jennings MT, Gelman R, Hochberg F. Intracranial germ-cell tumors: natural history and pathogenesis. J Neurosurg 1985;63:155–167.

132. Hoffman HJ, Otsubo H, Hendrick EB, Humphreys RP, Drake JM, Becker LE, et al. Intracranial germ-cell tumors in children. J Neurosurg 1991;74:545–551.

133. Sklar CA, Grumbach MM, Kaplan SL, Conte FA. Hormonal and metabolic abnormalities associated with central nervous system germinoma in children and adolescents and the effect of therapy: report of 10 patients. J Clin Endocrinol Metab 1981;52:9–16.

134. Fujimaki T, Matsutani M, Funada N, Kirino T, Takakura K, Nakamura O, et al. CT and MRI features of intracranial germ cell tumors. J Neurooncol 1994;19:217–226.

135. Tien RD, Barkovich AJ, Edwards MS. MR imaging of pineal 0tumors. AJR 1990;155:143–151.

136. Wolden SL, Wara WM, Larson DA, Prados MD, Edwards MS, Sneed PK. Radiation therapy for primary intracranial germ-cell tumors. Int J Radiat Oncol Biol Phys 1995;32:943–949.

137. Rengachary SS, Watanabe I. Ultrastructure and pathogenesis of intracranial arachnoid cysts. J Neuropathol Exp Neurol 1981; 40:61–83.

138. Smith RA, Smith WA. Arachnoid cysts of the middle cranial fossa. Surg Neurol 1976;5:246–252.

139. Go KG, Houthoff HJ, Blaauw EH, Havinga P, Hartsuiker J. Arachnoid cysts of the sylvian fissure. Evidence of fluid secretion. J Neurosurg 1984;60:803–813.

140. Pierre-Kahn A, Capelle L, Brauner R, Sainte-Rose C, Renier D, Rappaport R, et al. Presentation and management of suprasellar arachnoid cysts. Review of 20 cases. J Neurosurg 1990;73: 355–359.

141. Galassi E, Piazza G, Gaist G, Frank F. Arachnoid cysts of the middle cranial fossa: a clinical and radiological study of 25 cases treated surgically. Surg Neurol 1980;14:211–219.

142. Raffel C, McComb JG. To shunt or to fenestrate: which is the best surgical treatment for arachnoid cysts in pediatric patients? Neurosurgery 1988;23:338–342.

143. Ciricillo SF, Cogen PH, Harsh GR, Edwards MS. Intracranial arachnoid cysts in children. A comparison of the effects of fenestration and shunting. J Neurosurg 1991;74:230–235.

144. Voelker JL, Campbell RL, Muller J. Clinical, radiographic, and pathological features of symptomatic Rathke's cleft cysts. J Neurosurg 1991;74:535–544.

145. Kucharczyk W, Peck WW, Kelly WM, Norman D, Newton TH. Rathke cleft cysts: CT, MR imaging, and pathologic features. Radiology 1987;165:491–495.

146. Whyte AM, Sage MR, Brophy BP. Imaging of large Rathke's cleft cysts by CT and MRI: report of two cases. Neuroradiology 1993;35:258–260.

147. Oka H, Kawano N, Suwa T, Yada K, Kan S, Kameya T. Radiological study of symptomatic Rathke's cleft cysts. Neurosurgery 1994;35:632–636.

22 Invasive Pituitary Adenoma and Pituitary Carcinoma

PETER J. PERNICONE, MD AND BERND W. SCHEITHAUER, MD

GROWTH PATTERNS IN PITUITARY ADENOMA

Pituitary adenomas comprise approx 10% of all intracranial tumors. Taking their origin in the anterior lobe, most grow in a slow, expansible manner and are composed of cytologically benign cells resembling those of the normal adenohypophysis. Fully 75% are endocrinologically functional, secreting growth hormone (GH), prolactin (PRL), adrenocorticotropic hormone (ACTH), or thyroid-stimulating hormone (TSH), either alone or in various combination. The remainder are functionally "silent," producing either luteinizing hormone (LH)/follicle-stimulating hormone (FSH) and/or α-subunit, or no immunostainable hormones at all. Conventional adenoma variants and their pathobiologic characteristics are fully discussed in Chapter 7.

In terms of their size, adenomas vary markedly, ranging from microadenomas (≤10 mm) to macroadenomas (>10 mm), some measuring several centimeters (Figures 1,2). Within the gland, they may be either discrete or microinvasive of surrounding adenohypophysial tissue (Figures 1,2). A high proportion of macroadenomas are functionally "silent" and present with mass effects, including visual loss, headache, and endocrine hypofunction. Nonetheless, endocrinologically silent tumors, such as null-cell and LH/FSH adenomas, often cause mild hyperprolactinemia owing to compression of the pituitary stalk ("stalk section effect").

EXTENSION PATTERNS Extension, with or without invasion, may occur in a variety of directions with corresponding clinical signs and symptoms *(1)*. Tumors that superiorly exit the sella by superior extension through its often incomplete orifice, or by penetration of the sellar diaphragm may compress the optic chiasm, displace the hypothalamus, or even enter the third ventricle (Figures 3–8). Such growth often produces visual field defects and hypothalamic dysfunction, but may also cause hydrocephalus. Either lateral extension or invasion may result in involvement of the cavernous sinus (Figures 9,10) *(1–4)*. Since anatomic variation exists in the completeness of the dural septum comprising the lateral sellar wall *(5)*, it may be radiographically difficult to distinguish extension from invasion of the sinus (Figure 9). On occasion, such normally occurring defects are readily apparent at surgery. Adenomas entering the cavernous sinus may surround

and compress the intracavernous carotid artery as well as cranial nerves III, IV, V, and VI (Figures 9,10,11B). Only rarely do they compromise the artery, by encirclement or infiltration of its adventitia. Anterior extension may compress the olfactory or optic nerves *(6)*, whereas posterior extension can result in clival destruction or in compromise of midbrain or brainstem function. On the rare occasion, a pituitary adenoma mimics a primary clival neoplasm *(7)*. Orbital extension or invasion is quite unusual, but typically presents with exophthalmos *(8)*. Inferior extension permits a tumor access to the sphenoid sinus and, in some cases, the nasopharynx *(1,9)* (Figure 6,7,10A). In such instances, the sellar floor may undergo marked attenuation owing to pressure atrophy alone, or may demonstrate focal destruction owing to dural and osseous invasion (Figure 3C,7). Occasional patients present as a "nasal polyp" *(10)*.

INVASION Although pituitary adenomas may attain impressive size and show a variety of extension patterns, they generally maintain a cleavage plane with respect to surrounding tissues *(1–3,11–13)*. A subset of tumors does, however, demonstrate a propensity for infiltrative and destructive growth *(1–3,11–14)* (Figures 8–11). Termed "invasive adenomas," they are equipped with the biochemical means of infiltrating dura, bone, blood vessel, adventitia, and nerve sheath *(15)*. Brain invasion is rare and is generally considered a manifestation of "pituitary carcinoma" (*see* Pituitary Carcinoma below). Invasive adenomas may be difficult, if not impossible, to eradicate by surgical means alone. Although the majority are macroadenomas, small intrasellar adenomas may also demonstrate radiographically or grossly apparent invasion. For the purpose of our discussion, the definition of invasion will be that of radiographically or operatively apparent invasion of dura, bone, cavernous sinus, and so forth. It is this subset of tumors, as opposed to that showing microscopic dural invasion alone, which is thought to be clinically and prognostically relevant. Indeed, simple microscopic dural involvement alone is not considered significant in that it is an all too common finding, one directly related to tumor size. For example, Selman et al. *(13)*, in a systematic study involving random transsphenoidal sampling of paratumoral dura, found rates of microscopic invasion in microadenomas, macroadenomas, and in macroadenomas with suprasellar extension to be 69, 88, and 94%, respectively. In contrast, the overall frequency of gross, operatively apparent invasion in that series was only 40%. It is of note that the occurrence of invasion, as defined herein, can be related to a tumors functional state as well

From: *Diagnosis and Management of Pituitary Tumors* (K. Thapar, K. Kovacs, B. W. Scheithauer, and R. V. Lloyd, eds.), ©Humana Press Inc., Totowa, NJ.

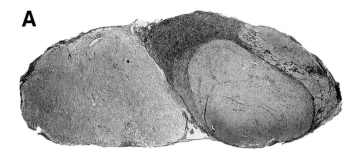

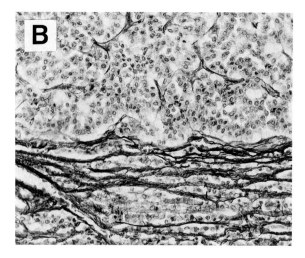

Figure 22-1 Adenoma confined to the anterior lobe showing blunt compressive growth of surrounding gland (**A**). A reticulin stain demonstrates the reticulin-poor adenoma compressing the reticulin-rich gland in which acini are compressed (**B**).

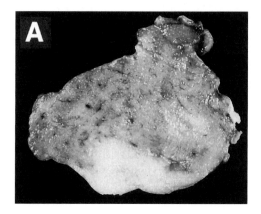

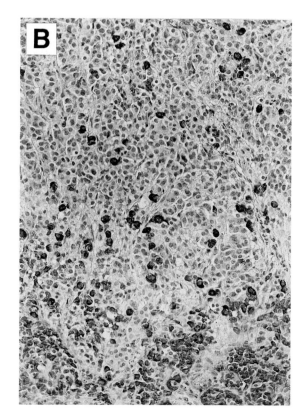

Figure 22-2 Macroadenoma in horizontal section shown overrunning and replacing the anterior lobe, but sparing posterior lobe (**A**). The tumor extended outside the sella. Invasion of individual adenoma cells into surrounding anterior lobe. Immunostain for GH (**B**).

(Table 1). Endocrinologically, functioning lesions are far more often invasive.

Compared to noninvasive adenomas, frankly invasive examples more often appear cellular, demonstrate mitotic activity, and exhibit some degree of nuclear atypia, particularly nucleolar prominence. Of morphologic parameters, cellular pleomorphism alone is perhaps least predictive of invasion or aggressive behavior.

BEHAVIOR OF SPECIFIC ADENOMA TYPES As previously noted, there is an association between the direction of extension and frequency of invasion of pituitary adenomas and their

function or immunotype (12) (Table 1). Only salient features are summarized below. Details regarding the pathology of adenoma subtypes are discussed in detail in Chapter 7.

PRL Cell Adenomas At the time of surgery, these common tumors demonstrate invasive growth in up to 52% of cases (12). Invasive macroadenomas occur most commonly in postreproductive females and in males (16), populations wherein this tumor produces high PRL levels and exhibits increased proliferative activity (17). Moreover, PRL cell adenomas show a tendency to undergo inferior extension with involvement of the sphenoid sinus

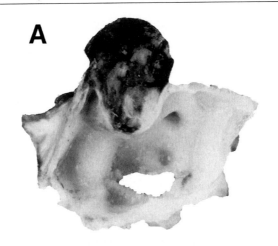

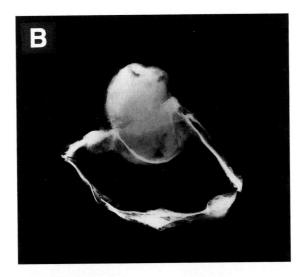

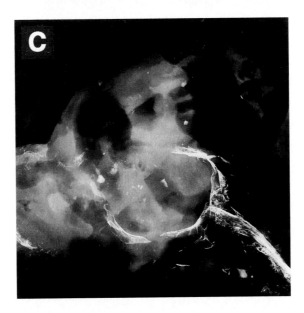

Figure 22-3 Macroadenoma with prominent suprasellar extension (**A**). A specimen X-ray demonstrates significant erosion and thinning of sellar floor (**B**). Invasive macroadenoma with irregular margins and destructive growth (specimen X-ray) (**C**). (Courtesy of P. C. Burger, Johns Hopkins Medical Center, Baltimore, MD).

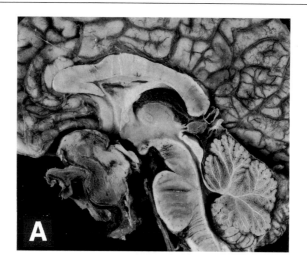

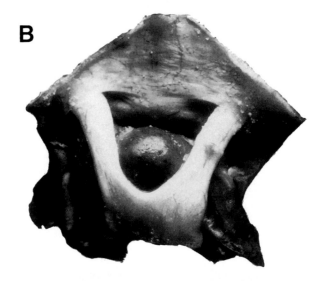

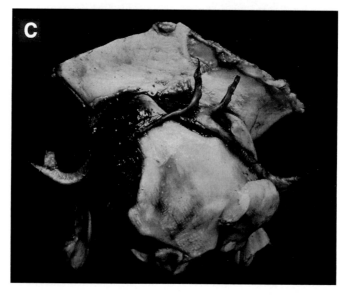

Figure 22-4   Macroadenoma with prechiasmal and superior extension (**A**). Superior view of sella and optic chiasm. Note the superior displacement of the chiasm (**B**). A larger macroadenoma causes posterior displacement and stretching of overlying optic chiasm (**C**). When protracted, demyelination of the chiasm is followed by axonal loss.

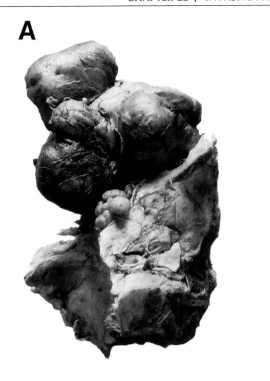

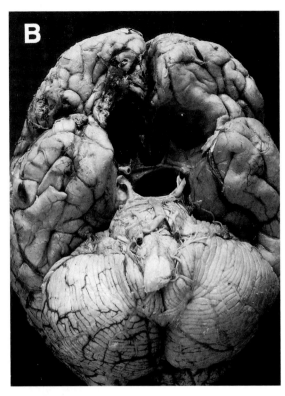

Figure 22-5 Multinodular macroadenoma with suprasellar extension (**A**). Note the severe compressive effects on surrounding brain (**B**).

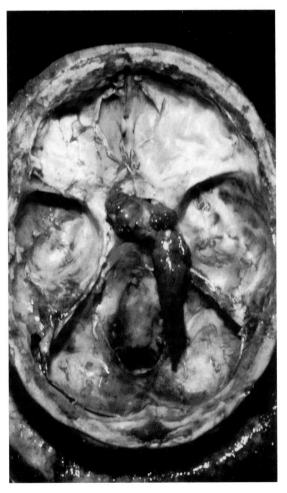

Figure 22-6 Macroadenoma with superior and posterolateral posterior fossa extension.

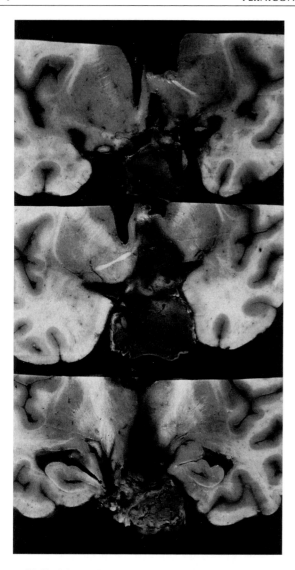

Figure 22-7 Macroadenoma with involvement of third ventricle and inferior extension into sphenoid sinus area.

and occasionally of the nasopharynx *(9,18)*. Extensive skull base destruction may also be seen. It is in such cases that conformation of tumor type is of real prognostic significance, since dopamine agonist therapy may cause tumor involution.

GH Cell Adenoma. *See* **Plurihormonal Adenoma below.**

Mixed GH Cell–PRL Cell Adenoma This, the most frequent of GH- and PRL-producing adenomas, consists of two morphologic and functional cell types. Patients typically present with acromegaly and variable hyperprolactinemia. Invasion occurs in approx 30% *(12)*.

Acidophil Stem-Cell Adenoma This far less common form of GH- and PRL-producing pituitary adenoma represents <1% of all adenomas and is composed of cells sharing ultrastructural features of somatotrophs and lactotrophs *(19)*. In addition to occasional fibrous bodies and misplaced exocytoses, these fascinating monomorphous neoplasms possess abnormal, often giant mitochondria that may be light microscopically evident as a large, cytoplasmic vacuole. The pathologist must be aware of their often subtle clinical presentation, which includes mild hyperprolactinemia, but only rarely acromegaly. Although acidophil stem-

cell adenomas may clinically be confused with PRL cell adenomas, associated PRL levels are far lower than in prolactinomas of comparable size. Ultrastructural study is required to confirm the diagnosis. Acidophil stem-cell adenomas are notorious for their aggressive behavior and their tendency to invade the sphenoid sinus, a feature seen in approx 50% of cases *(19)*.

Corticotroph Cell Adenoma In the Mayo Clinic experience, the majority (approx 85%) of corticotrophic tumors associated with Cushing's disease are intrasellar microadenomas; of these, <10% are invasive (unpublished data). In the small subgroup of macroadenomas, invasion is noted in up to approx two-thirds.

Aggressive corticotropic adenomas are encountered with particular frequency in Nelson's syndrome *(20–23)*, an iatrogenic condition wherein a patient having Cushing's disease, but an unrecognized pituitary adenoma has undergone bilateral adrenalectomy. About one-third of such patients subsequently present with an aggressive ACTH-producing macroadenoma and pigmentation at an average of 10 yr following adrenalectomy. The majority of operated Nelson's adenomas are invasive *(12)*. Furthermore, a significant proportion of pituitary carcinomas are Nelson's tumors *(see* Pituitary Carcinoma *below)*. Fortunately, with the emergence of more sensitive means of detecting pituitary microadenomas, e.g., thin-section magnetic resonance imaging (MRI) with gadolinium administration and petrosal sinus sampling, Nelson's syndrome is rapidly disappearing.

Finally, silent corticotrophic adenomas frequently exhibit aggressive behavior. Defined as clinically nonfunctioning adenomas immunoreactive for proopiomelanocortin (POMC) derivatives including ACTH, they comprise approx 5% of corticotrophic tumors. In one early series describing such tumors, 82% were invasive *(24)*. A more recent study of the two variants of silent corticotroph cell adenomas *(25)* found significant differences in the behavior of subtype I adenomas, those morphologically resembling ordinary ACTH cell adenomas, and the weakly periodic acid-Schiff (PAS)-positive and ACTH-immunoreactive, granule-sparse tumors of subtype II. These differences related to patient gender (M:F 6:1 vs 1.7:1), frequency of radiographic or gross invasion (44 vs 71%), and postoperative pituitary failure (38 vs 86%). Use of postoperative radiotherapy (44 vs 57%) did not differ. The same was true of proliferation indices, the mean being 0.6% in both. To date, the only silent corticotrophic tumor to metastasize have been of the subtype II variety *(25)* *(see* Pituitary Carcinomas below).

Gonadotrophic Cell Adenomas In both men and women, these now well-characterized adenomas typically present as macroadenomas *(26)*. Although they produce FSH and/or LH and often α-subunit as well, blood levels of LH/FSH are infrequently elevated and unassociated with endocrine effects *(26)*. In men, these include decreased libido or impotence *(27)*. Bilateral testicular enlargement owing to an FSH increase is only rarely seen. Clinical recognition of gonadotropin excess in women may be difficult, especially since elevated levels normally occur after menopause *(28)*. In the Mayo Clinic experience with 100 gonadotropic adenomas, all were macroadenomas *(26)*. Among these, gross invasion was observed in only 21% of cases, the lowest rate of any adenoma type.

TSH Cell Adenomas This rare tumor comprises no more than 1 or 2% of pituitary adenomas *(29,30)*. Although it occurs in the setting of either hypo- or hyperthyroidism, most TSH adenomas arise in a background of thyroid ablation with resultant TSH cell

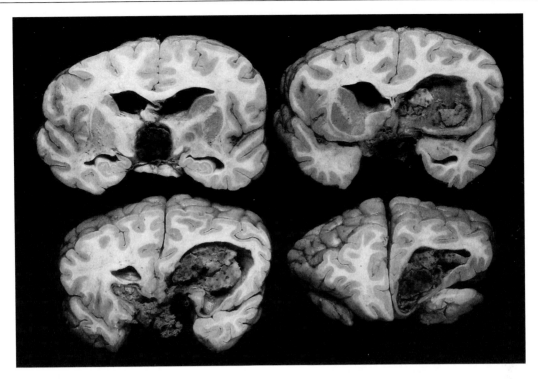

Figure 22-8 Penetration of tumors into the ventricular system is a rare finding. Its mechanism is poorly understood, but appears to be by way of third ventricular entry, thus implying brain invasion.

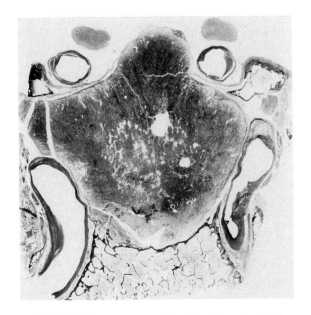

Figure 22-9 Whole-mount coronal section through sella. On occasion, a macroadenoma encroaches on the cavernous sinuses by blunt compressive growth.

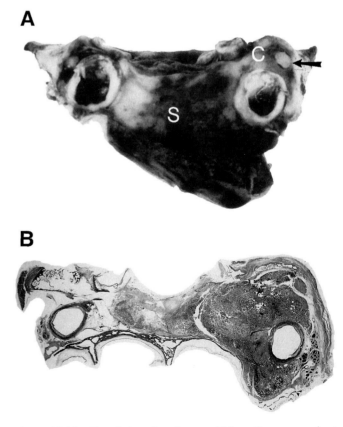

Figure 22-10 Grossly invasive adenoma. This section, a coronal cut through the cavernous (c) and sphenoid (s) sinuses, shows entrapment of a cranial nerve (arrow) and the nearby carotid artery surrounded by tumor (**A**). Whole-mount section of another invasive tumor shows massive replacement of one cavernous sinus (**B**). Such invasion precludes operative curve.

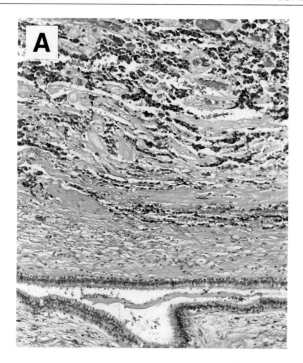

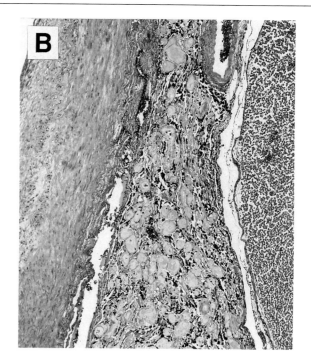

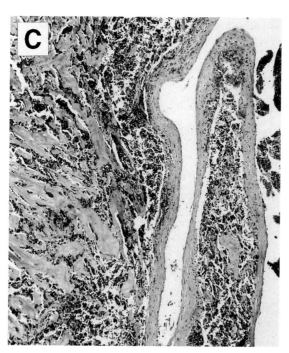

Figure 22-11   Invasive pituitary adenoma involving sphenoid sinus mucosa **(A)**, plying between cavernous nerve sinus wall and a cranial nerve **(B)**, and a dural venous sinus **(C)**.

hyperplasia. The latter may be massive and can simulate adenoma *(31)* (see Chapter ??). In one study, all were macroadenomas, and 70% were invasive *(12)*. Despite occasional nuclear pleomorphism, mitotic figures are infrequent *(32,33)*, and the MIB-1-labeling index is usually low. It has been suggested that TSH adenomas occurring in women tend to be smaller and less often invasive than in men *(30)*. TSH cell carcinomas are rare *(see below)*.

Plurihormonal Adenomas   Of this diverse group of adenomas, the majority are GH-producing *(34,35)*. In the Mayo experience, this is the most common (>90%) form of acromegaly associated adenoma. It produces the amino acid hormones GH and PRL as well as glycoprotein hormones, usually α-subunit, and/or TSH. Their cellular composition varies from monomorphous (usually densely granulated GH cell) to bi- or plurimorphous (GH and TSH cell or GH, PRL, and TSH cell). Fully 50% of plurihormonal tumors are grossly invasive *(12)*. Interestingly, one recent study found acromegaly associated tumors exhibiting growth hormone-releasing hormone production to be more often invasive *(36)*; the effect appears to be the result of autocrine stimulation. Too few

Table 1
Gross Invasion
in Pituitary Adenomas by Type[a]

GH cell	50%
PRL cell	52%
GH/PRL cell	31%
Acidophil stem cell	50%
ACTH cell (Cushing)	15%
ACTH cell (Nelson)	50%
Silent ACTH	82%
FSH/LH cell	21%
TSH cell	75%
Null cell	42%
Plurihormonal	52%
Silent subtype III	75%

[a]Modified from Scheithauer et al. *(12).*

plurihormonal adenomas of other type (PRL-ACTH, PRL-TSH, and so forth) have been reported to comment on their behavior.

Null-Cell Adenomas Whether on the oncocytic or nononcocytic end of the null-cell spectrum, this form of pituitary adenoma is unassociated with clinical or biochemical evidence of hormone secretion *(29).* Its relation to gonadotroph cell adenomas is unclear, but a recent, large comparative immunohistochemical study of ultrastructurally characterized tumors showed strong similarities *(37).* Most are large tumors at the time of diagnosis. Invasion is evident in approx 40% *(12).*

Silent Subtype III Adenomas Although originally thought to belong to the corticotroph cell line *(38),* the majority are immunonegative for POMC derivatives *(39)* apparently derived from an unknown cell type. These tumors have only recently been characterized *(39).* These uncommon tumors often masquerade as prolactinomas, particularly in young females. Histologically, their growth pattern is often diffuse. Cellular and nuclear pleomorphism may be considerable, but the MIB-1-labeling index is low. Some contain few cells positive for pituitary hormones, whereas in others, several hormones or hormone groups are represented. Their ultrastructure is distinctive showing the cells to be highly differentiated and to resemble glycoprotein hormone-producing cells. Distinctive features include nuclear spheridia and relative abundance of smooth endoplasmic reticulum. The vast majority (75%) of silent subtype III adenomas are radiographically or grossly invasive.

Ectopic Adenomas Rare pituitary adenomas are truly ectopic in location *(40).* Differentiated remnants of Rathke's pouch or of its stalk apparently give rise to most examples. Best-known among such rests is the so-called pharyngeal pituitary, a derivative of the stalk or of the pouch occurring in the midline mucosa of the nasal septum or in mucoperiosteum nearby the vomerosphenoidal junction *(40–42).* Also frequently reported are ectopic adenomas occurring in the sphenoid sinus *(18,43).* Entirely suprasellar adenomas most likely arise from anterior lobe cells residing along the supradiaphragmatic portion of the pituitary stalk (pars tuberalis). Correlating radiographic and operative data precludes confusion of ectopic adenomas with extrasellar invasion of a conventional adenoma primary in the sella.

PROLIFERATION AND MOLECULAR MARKERS OF INVASION The ability to predict a tumor's biologic behavior early in the clinical course would give surgeons, endocrinologists, and radiation oncologists an advantage in providing timely and appropriate therapy. As previously noted, cytologic features pro-

vide no particular insight into the behavior of pituitary tumors. On the other hand, mitotic activity, a subject discussed in greater detail *(see* Pituitary Carcinoma *below),* is correlated with aggressive behavior, both invasiveness and metastasis *(32).* Proliferation marker expression is also related to aggressive growth. Specifically, MIB-1, an antibody reacting in paraffin-embedded tissue with the cell-cycle-specific nuclear antigen Ki-67, has been found to be increased in invasive adenomas (Figure 12). One recent study of adenomas found MIB-1 proliferation indices >3% to be associated with invasive growth and possibly to their increased likelihood of recurrence *(33).* Only recently have investigators undertaken to identify molecular markers of invasive adenomas. Immunohistochemical expression of the p53 gene product, a nuclear phosphoprotein that arrests damaged cells in the G1 phase of the cell cycle, has been evaluated. Significant staining for p53 protein has been demonstrated in a minority of invasive adenomas, being found in up to 15% in one series *(44);* reactivity was lacking in noninvasive tumors. Loss of the normal tumor-suppressive effect of p53 protein thus appears to support tumor progression. In another study, expression of both the cytokine interleukin 6 and heat shock protein-27 (HSP-27) was significantly increased in invasive adenomas as compared to normal pituitary tissue and noninvasive tumors *(45).* Another study showed significantly reduced expression of the metastasizing suppressor gene nm-23 in invasive tumors *(46).* Finally, expression of type IV collagenase and matrix metalloproteinase-9 (MMP-9) has also been found to be greater in invasive than in noninvasive adenomas *(15).*

CYTOGENETICS AND TUMOR BEHAVIOR Studies of the cytogenetic features of pituitary adenomas have been undertaken in an effort to identify karyotypic patterns associated with aggressive behavior. In one series abnormalities were more often found in hormonally functioning tumors than in null-cell adenomas; cytogenetic changes most often involved chromosomes 1, 4, 7, and 19 *(47).* The study found no significant karyotypic differences between invasive and noninvasive tumors, despite the fact that functioning tumors are more often invasive *(12).*

PITUITARY CARCINOMA

A recent large study found that approx 0.2% of primary adenohypophyseal tumors eventually undergo either or both craniospinal/brain metastasis (Figures 13,14) or systemic spread *(48)* (Figure 15). Such rare behavior is the *sine qua non* of "pituitary carcinomas." To date, about 70 well-documented examples have been reported in the English literature *(21–25,48–103).* Brain invasion is also generally considered "malignant behavior," but is rarely documented premortem since operative procedures, particularly transphenoidal surgery, do not lend themselves to visualizing or sampling brain involvement (Figure 16). The histologic and cytologic characteristics of pituitary carcinomas vary from bland and monotonous to frankly malignant (Figures 16–18).

The vast majority of pituitary carcinomas, certainly more than the once estimated 75%, are hormone-producing and endocrine-active. PRL cell carcinomas are the most commonly subtype *(66,67,69,73,75,76,82,86,88,89,91,93,100,101).* No doubt many of what were reported as endocrinologically "nonfunctioning" carcinomas were of this type, since they antedated the characterization and measurement of this hormone. Second in frequency are ACTH-producing tumors *(21–23,50,51,53,55,57,65,77,84),* one of which was a silent subtype II tumor *(25).* Relatively few GH cell carcinomas have been reported to date *(56,63,70,79,83);* all but

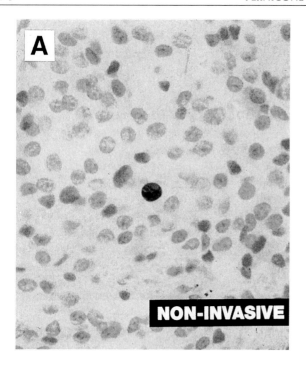

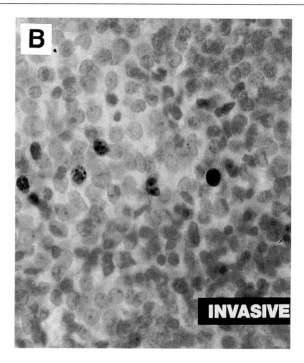

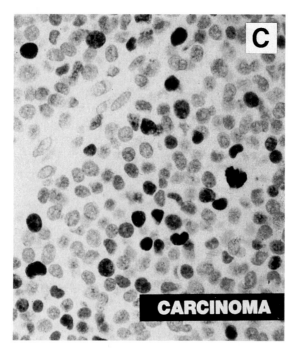

Figure 22-12   Immunostain for MIB-1 in noninvasive adenoma (**A**), invasive adenoma (**B**), and pituitary carcinoma (**C**). Note increasing MIB-1 expression.

one patient with gigantism *(103)* were acromegaly associated. Only one TSH *(92)*, one FSH/LH-producing tumor *(97)*, and three null-cell carcinomas *(48,80,85)* have also been reported. In most instances, the early clinical presentation of what will be pituitary carcinomas is that of an invasive macroadenoma with associated diplopia and headache. As expected, PRL-producing tumors present with amenorrhea/galactorrhea or impotence, corticotropic tumors with Cushing's syndrome. Several clinical and pathologic differences exist between PRL- and ACTH-producing carcinomas. In our recent series of 15 pituitary carcinomas *(48)*, the

latency period between the sellar "adenoma" presentation and the manifestation of metastasis is approximately half as long in PRL tumors (mean 4.7 yr) as compared to ACTH-producing tumors (mean 9.5). The overall latency period in pituitary carcinoma cases is surprisingly wide, ranging from a few months to as many as 18 yr *(48)*. Finally, metastases of PRL-producing tumors were less often limited to the craniospinal axis (29%) than were those of ACTH cell carcinomas (43%).

Although the question of whether pituitary carcinomas are malignant in their *in situ* or sellar phase, or whether they undergo

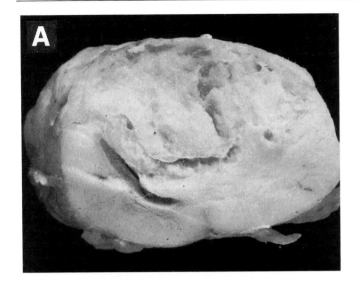

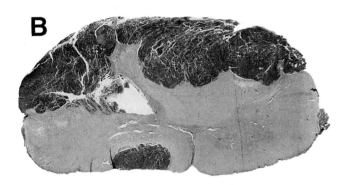

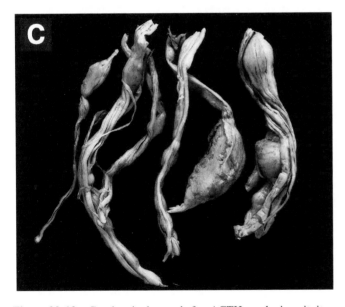

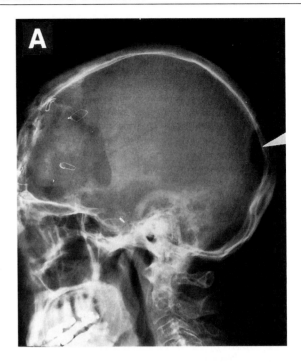

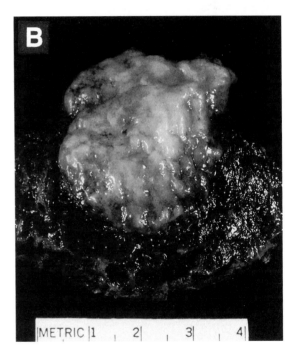

Figure 22-14 Systemic metastases in pituitary carcinoma. Common sites of involvement include bone (**A**) and liver (**B**).

Figure 22-13 Craniospinal spread of an ACTH-producing pituitary carcinoma. Extensive seeding of the spinal subarachnoid space resulted in spinal cord invasion (**A,B**) and encasement of cauda equina nerve roots (**C**).

transition from adenomas remains unsettled, the latter notion would best explain the often long intervals to and multiple recurrences that antedate metastasis. Both the relatively frequent occurrence of invasion in patently benign adenomas, and their marked

variation in cytologic appearance and even mitotic activity explain our present inability to make a diagnosis of malignancy prior to the occurrence of metastasis (Figure 17). Even ultrastructural studies, which occasionally show only a hint of specific differentiation, provide little help (Figure 18). The pathogenetic mechanisms that might underlie the transformation of an adenoma to a metastasizing tumor are unknown. Like other tumors undergoing discontinuous spread, those of the pituitary must acquire the ability to move freely through extracellular matrix and to invade blood vessels. Apparently, invasive adenomas share some, but not all of the

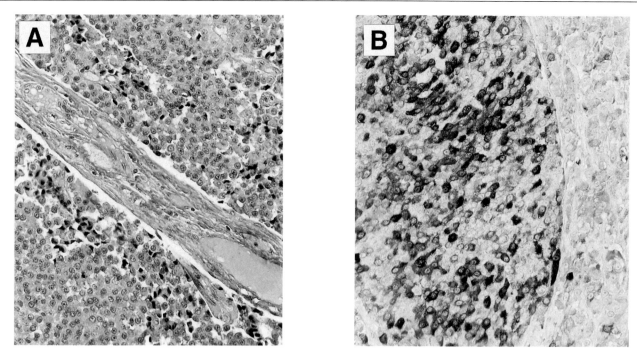

Figure 22-15 Monotonous cytologically bland ACTH carcinoma metastatic to lymph node (**A**). Immunostain for ACTH (**B**).

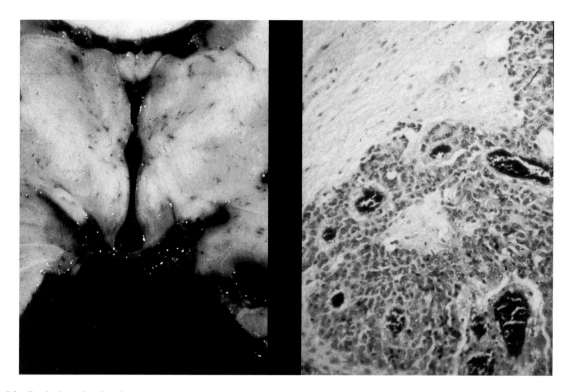

Figure 22-16 Brain invasion in pituitary carcinoma is a feature rarely documented in life.

attributes of pituitary carcinomas. Although for tumors occurring in many organ systems, routes of metastasis are well known, those of the pituitary, a gland situated in a dura-lined bony cavity at the base of the skull, are not readily apparent. At least two routes can be postulated. If, by invasion or extension, a tumor gains accesses to the cavernous sinus, its cells could embolize through the jugular veins to the right heart and on to lung, a site from which secondary systemic metastases could emanate. Alternatively, in some indi-

viduals, malignant cells could bypass the lungs and pass from the right to the left side of the heart through an incompletely closed foramen ovale. Invasion of sphenoid sinus lymphatics could give rise to cervical lymph node metastases. Based on our literature review, sites of metastases of pituitary carcinoma vary and include the brain, spinal cord, liver, lymph nodes, ovary, heart, and lung. It is of note that although one of our postulated mechanisms of systemic spread is via the lungs, pulmonary involvement is

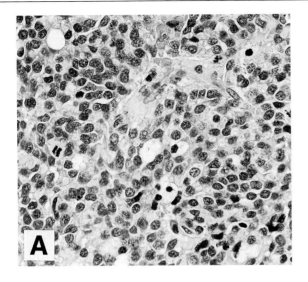
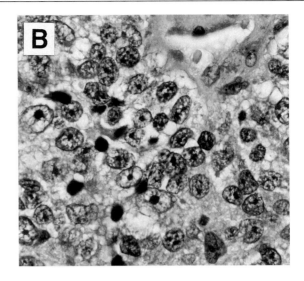
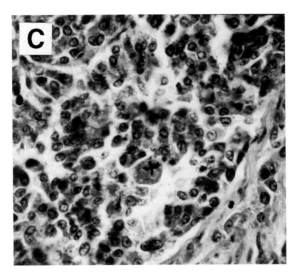

Figure 22-17 Pituitary carcinomas while variable histologic features, including monotonous cytology with only rare mitotic figures (**A**, arrow), monotonous cytology with frequent mitoses (**B**, arrows), marked cytologic atypia (**C**).

infrequently seen. Craniospinal spread is more readily understood and is no doubt by direct involvement of the leptomeninges. The question must be raised whether mechanical effects of surgical intervention promote metastases. Although nearly all patients with pituitary carcinoma have undergone at least one resection, either transsphenoidal hypophysectomy or craniotomy, 1 of our 15 patients did not undergo surgery of the primary sellar tumor prior to the development of metastatic disease *(48)*. This interesting patient with an ACTH carcinoma had only radiation, but developed osseous metastases 18 yr thereafter.

Finally, a subset of patients with ACTH-producing tumors undergo bilateral adrenalectomy alone, thus developing pituitary carcinomas in the setting of Nelson's syndrome. Protracted lack of negative feedback on the undetected adenoma presumably promotes malignant transformation. Not surprisingly, this group often has a remarkably long adenoma–carcinoma latency period, the average being 15 yr *(48)*.

Once pituitary carcinomas manifest by virtue of either systemic or craniospinal metastasis, therapeutic options are limited. Adjuncts most commonly employed are irradiation and surgical decompression. For patients with PRL-producing tumors, dopam-

ine agonists, such as bromocriptine or pergolide, offer only palliation. Initially these agents result in a decrease in serum PRL levels and retard tumor growth, but PRL cell carcinomas typically "escape" these pharmacologic effects. With regrowth, PRL levels often rise to remarkably high levels, some exceeding 20,000 ng/mL (normal; female 4–30, males 4–23). Hormone levels in cases of corticotroph carcinoma are also quite variable. One patient in our series had an ACTH level of 280,000 pg/mL (normal 23 pg/mL) and a β-endorphin of 16,000 pg/mL (normal <60 pg/mL) *(48)*.

Despite rare long-term survivors, the prognosis of patients with pituitary carcinoma is poor. In our recent study of 15 cases, only one patient survived 8 yr, this being a 62-yr-old male with a carcinoma and recurrent cerebellar metastases treated by repeated resections. Sixty-six percent of patients died within 1 yr of their presentation with metastases. Of these, the majority (75%) had systemic metastases. Exclusive of death in the postoperative period, the mean survival of the entire study population was approx 2 yr (range 0.25–8 yr), that of patients with craniospinal and systemic metastasis being 2.6 and 1.0 yr, respectively.

Since invasiveness is an indicator of malignancy in a number of tumor systems, one may question the value of separating inva-

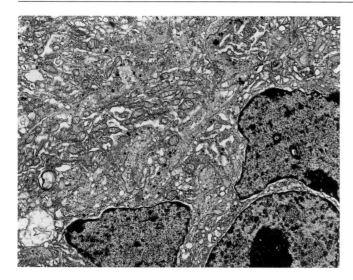

Figure 22-18 Ultrastructure of PRL carcinoma. The oncocytic lesion lacks the hallmarks of prolactin cells, i.e., abundance of rough endoplasmic reticulum and obvious misplaced exocytoses.

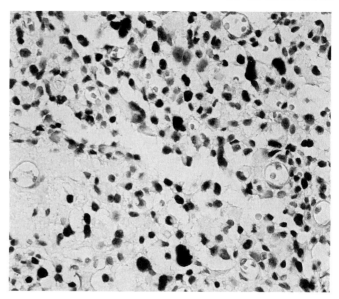

Figure 22-19 P53 immunostain in pituitary carcinoma. Note strong nuclear staining pattern.

sive pituitary adenomas from carcinomas. There are a number of compelling clinical reasons for maintaining the distinction. As a rule, invasive adenomas are locally aggressive lesions successfully managed by a combination of surgery, radiation, and pharmacologic agents. Aside from endocrinopathy, their effects as well as those of carcinomas include cranial nerve injury, nasal or sinus obstruction, hydrocephalus, and compromise of hypothalamic or brainstem function. However, patients with pituitary carcinomas also experience morbidity owing to central nervous system (CNS) or to systemic metastases. The latter often involve multiple organs. Furthermore, there are dramatic differences in survival between patients with invasive adenoma and carcinoma. As previously noted, 66% of our 15 carcinoma patients were dead of disease within 1 yr of diagnosis, fully 75% having succumbed to systemic metastases. Finally, data regarding proliferative activity and p53 gene expression in carcinomas also indicate that they represent a unique category of pituitary tumor (Figures 12,19). Comparison of mean MIB-1-labeling indices (33) and the frequency with which p53 protein immunoreactivity is seen (44) in noninvasive and invasive adenomas as well as pituitary carcinomas showed statistically significant differences between each tumor category (Figure 12). Respective values were as follows: noninvasive adenomas (1%, 0%; invasive adenomas (4.5%, 15%); pituitary carcinomas (12%, 100%). In these same study groups, a significant association between the presence of mitotic figures and tumor behavior was also noted, as evidenced by progressive increments in the proportion of cases expressing mitotic figures in the categories of noninvasive adenoma, invasive adenoma, and pituitary carcinoma (3.9, 21.4, and 66.7%, respectively). The mitotic index, however, appeared to be a less-informative parameter, being extremely low in all cases (mean = 0.016% ± 0.005 [± SEM]). Although the mean mitotic index in pituitary carcinomas (0.09% ± 0.035) was significantly higher than the mean mitotic index of either noninvasive adenomas (0.02% ± 0.002) or invasive adenomas (0.013% ± 0.005), no practical threshold value capable of distinguishing these three groups was evident (Figure 17). Thus, mitotic figures are present, they do provide some indication of the behavior and invasive potential of pituitary tumors.

Ideally, pathologists and clinicians should be able to predict which tumors will behave as carcinoma. In as much as nearly all carcinomas arise in invasive, endocrinologically active tumors, one could nearly eliminate from consideration all nonfunctioning and noninvasive adenomas. Next, we could postulate that the 15% of p53-positive invasive adenomas represent a unique, aggressive subset (see Atypical Adenoma below). If this is correct, p53 immunoreactivity of clinically invasive adenomas might be of prognostic utility. Clearly, the significance of MIB-1 labeling, p53 protein expression, and of other molecular markers in predicting behavior deserves further study.

ATYPICAL ADENOMA

("ADENOMA OF UNCERTAIN MALIGNANT POTENTIAL" [AUMP]) Recently, it has been suggested that adenohypophyseal tumors might be amenable to histopathologic grading (48). According to this scheme, macroadenomas with elevated MIB-1-labeling indices, but lacking p53 immunoreactivity would be considered "atypical adenomas" or AUMP. Such "higher-risk" patients would require careful follow-up and might be candidates for adjuvant therapy. In addition, tumors with both high proliferation indices and p53 oncoprotein expression would be placed directly into the pituitary carcinoma category. Criticisms of this approach include (1) paucity of hard data regarding the prognosis of both these tumor groups, and (2) the dependence of this approach on immunohistochemistry with its variations in method, vagueries of staining, and interpretative subjectivity. As a result, the new World Health Organization classification of adenohypophyseal tumors has placed highly proliferative, p53-immunoreactive tumors in an "atypical adenoma" category, but continues to require metastases as *the sine qua non* of pituitary carcinoma (104,105). Ideally, this approach will permit clinicians to target high-risk patients early in their course, thus preventing the occurrence of metastases. No doubt, future studies will elucidate the molecular biologic events underlying the pathobiology of aggressive pituitary neoplasms.

DIFFERENTIAL DIAGNOSIS Aside from pituitary adenomas, a variety of often invasive neoplasms may involve the sella, including meningioma, craniopharyngioma, chordoma, germ-cell tumor, nasopharyngeal carcinoma, metastatic carcinoma, sarcomas of the skull base, and even salivary gland tumors *(106)*. This spectrum of lesions is discussed in detail in Chapter 7. Attention to histologic, immunohistochemical, and ultrastructural features as well as to clinical and radiographic data invariably permits the distinction of these various neoplasms from pituitary adenoma or carcinoma.

SPECIMEN HANDLING AND DIAGNOSTIC METHODS

The management of pituitary adenomas is a team effort requiring communication among various medical specialists. As the final recipient of tumor tissue, the pathologist should be aware of relevant clinical, radiographic, and biochemical data from the onset in that it will be necessary to correlate this information with the results of intraoperative studies as well as of permanent section and immunohistochemical preparations *(104,105)*. Intraoperative tissue evaluation is best accomplished by cytologic smear or touch preparations. These simple techniques involve alcohol fixation of a smear or imprint, followed by staining with hematoxylin and eosin. These readily permit confirmation of the presence or absence of adenoma tissue as well as triaging of the specimen in case of an alternative diagnosis. Although frozen section assessment may occasionally be necessary, this method compromises immunohistochemical studies and renders tissue useless for ultrastructural examination. As a result, care must be taken to save as much unfrozen tissue as possible for ancillary studies. Smears, frozen sections, and routine histologic stains provide little information regarding the aggressive potential of a pituitary adenoma. As a rule, the best immediate indicators of invasion and aggressiveness are radiographic data and intraoperative findings. Occasionally, however, one encounters a tumor with sufficient atypia, particularly nucleolar prominence and mitotic activity, to suggest an aggressive adenoma or even a carcinoma. Since ultrastructural characterization is of necessity in identifying certain inherently aggressive adenoma variants, e.g., acidophil stem-cell and silent subtype III adenomas, a fragment of tissue should routinely be fixed in glutaraldehyde. Only a small amount of tissue—as little as 1 mm—is required.

REFERENCES

1. Jefferson G. The Invasive Adenomas of the Anterior Pituitary. CC Thomas, Springfield, IL, 1972.
2. Trumble HC. Pituitary tumors: observations on large tumours which have spread widely beyond the confines of the sella turcica. Br J Surg 1951;39:7–24.
3. Martins AN, Hayes GJ, Kempe LG. Invasive pituitary adenomas. J Neurosurg 1965;22:268–276.
4. Knosp E, Steiner E, Kitz K, Matula C. Pituitary adenomas with invasion of the cavernous sinus space: a magnetic resonance imaging classification compared with surgical findings. Neurosurgery 1993;33:610–618.
5. Dolenc VV. Anatomy of the cavernous sinus. In: Anatomy and Surgery of the Cavernous Sinus. Springer-Verlag, Vienna, 1989, pp. 3–6.
6. Arita K, Uozumi T, Yano T, Sumida M, Muttaquin Z, Hibino H, et al. MRI visualization of complete bilateral optic nerve involvement by pituitary adenoma: a case report. Neuroradiology 1993;35(7):549–550.
7. Wong K, Raisanen J, Taylor SL, McDermott MW, Wilson CB, Gutin PH. Pituitary adenoma as an unsuspected clival tumor. Am J Surg Pathol 1995;19:900–903.
8. Spiegel PH, Karcioglu ZA. Orbital invasion by pituitary adenoma. Am J Ophthalmol 1994;117:270–271.
9. Ivy SC, Luk CRC, John KC, Chou MRC, Chou FRCR, Leung S. Pituitary adenoma presenting as sinonasal tumor: pitfalls in diagnosis. Hum Pathol 1996;27:605–609.
10. Luk IS, Chan J, Chow SM, Leung S. Pituitary adenoma presenting as sinonasal tumor: pitfall in diagnosis. Hum Pathol 1996;27:605–609.
11. Scheithauer BW. Surgical pathology of the pituitary: the adenomas. Part II. Pathol Annu 1984;19(part 2):269–329.
12. Scheithauer BW, Kovacs KT, Laws ER, Randall RV. Pathology of invasive pituitary tumors with special reference to functional classification. J Neurosurg 1986;65:733–744.
13. Selman WR, Laws ER, Scheithauer BW, Carpenter SM. The occurrence of dural invasion in pituitary adenomas. J Neurosurg 1986;64:402–407.
14. Blevins LS Jr, Verity DK, Allen G. Aggressive pituitary tumors. Oncology 1998;12:1307–1312.
15. Kawamoto H, Vozumi I, Kawamoto K, Mrita K, Yano I, Hirohata T. Type IV collagenase activity and cavernous sinus invasion in human pituitary adenomas. Acta Neurochir Wien 1996;138:390–395.
16. Randall RV, Scheithauer BW, Laws ER, Abboud CF, Ebersold MJ, Kao PC. Pituitary adenomas associated with hyperprolactinemia: a clinical and immunohistochemical study of 97 patients operated on transsphenoidally. Mayo Clin Proc 1985;60:753–762.
17. Calle-Rodrique R, Giannini C, Scheithauer BW, Lloyd RV, Wollan PC, Kovacs K, Stefaneanu L, Ebright AB, Abboud C, Davis DH. Prolactinomas in males and females: a comparative clinicopathologic study. Mayo Clin Proc 1998;73:1045–1052.
18. Langford L, Batsakis JG. Pituitary gland involvement of the sinonasal tract. Ann Otol Rhinol Laryngol 1995;104:167–169.
19. Horvath E, Kovacs K, Singer W, Smyth HS, Killinger DW, Erzin C, et al. Acidophil stem cell adenoma of the human pituitary: clinicopathologic analysis of 15 cases. Cancer 1981;47:761–771.
20. Cohen KL, Noth RH, Pechinksi T. Incidence of pituitary tumors following adrenalectomy. A long-term follow-up study of patients treated for Cushing's disease. Arch Intern Med 1978;138:575–579.
21. Imai T, Funahashi H, Tanaka Y, Tobinaga J, Wada M, Mortia-Matsuyama T, et al. Adrenalectomy for treatment of Cushing syndrome: results in 122 patients and long-term follow-up studies. World J Surg 1996;20:781–786.
22. Garrao AF, Sobrinho LG, Oliveira P, Bugalho MJ, Boavida JM, Raposo JF, et al. ACTH-producing carcinoma of the pituitary with haematogenic metastases. Eur J Endocrinol 1997;137:176–180.
23. Lormeau B, Miossec P, Sibony M, Valensi P, Attali JR. Adrenocorticotropin-producing pituitary carcinoma with liver metastases. J Endocrinol Invest 1997;20:230–236.
24. Horvath E, Kovacs K. Killinger DW, Smyth HS, Platts ME, Singer W. Silent corticotropic adenomas of the human pituitary gland. Am J Pathol 1980;98:617–638.
25. Jaap AJ, Scheithauer BW, Kovacs K, Horvath E, Lloyd RV, Meyer FB, et al. Clinically silent corticotroph tumors of the pituitary. Neurosurgery (in press).
26. Young WF Jr, Scheithauer BW, Kovacs K, Horvath E, Davies DH, Randall RV. Gonadotroph adenoma of the pituitary gland: a clinicopathologic analysis of 100 cases. Mayo Clin Proc 1996;71:649–656.
27. Beckers A, Stenaert A, Mashiter K, Hennen G. Follicle-stimulating hormone-secreting pituitary adenomas. J Clin Endocrinol Metab 1985;61:525–528.
28. Daneshdoost L, Gennarelli TA, Bashey HM, Savino PJ, Sergott RC, Bosley TM, et al. Recognition of gonadotroph adenomas in women. N Engl J Med 1991324:589–594.
29. Kovacs K, Horvath E. Tumors of the pituitary gland. Atlas of Tumor Pathology, 2nd Ser, Fas 21. Armed Forces Institute of Pathology, Washington, DC, 1986, pp. 1–264.
30. Minderman T, Wilson CB. Thyrotropin-producing pituitary adenomas. J Neurosurg 1993;79:521–527.
31. Pioro EP, Scheithauer BW, Laws ER Jr, Randall RV, Kovacs K, Horvath E. Combined thyrotroph and lactotroph cell hyperplasia simulating prolactin-secreting pituitary adenoma in long-standing primarily hypothyroidism. Surg Neurol 1988;29:218–226.

32. Thapar K, Yamada Y, Scheithauer BW, Kovacs K, Yamada S, Stefaneanu L. Assessment of mitotic activity in pituitary adenomas and carcinomas. Endocr Pathol 1996;7:215–221.

33. Thapar K, Kovacs K, Scheithauer BW, Stefaneanu L, Horvath E, Murray D, et al. Proliferative activity and invasiveness among pituitary adenomas and carcinomas. An analysis using the MIB-1 antibody. Neurosurgery 1994;35:1012–1017.

34. Horvath E, Scheithauer BW, Kovacs K, Randall RV, Laws ER, Thorner MO, Tindall GT, et al. Pituitary adenomas producing growth hormone, prolactin, and one or more glycoprotein hormones: a histologic, immunohistochemical, and ultrastructural study of four surgically removed tumors. Ultrastruct Pathol 1983;5:171–183

35. Scheithauer BW, Horvath E, Kovacs K, Laws ER Jr, Randall RV, Ryan N. Plurihormonal pituitary adenomas. Semin Diagn Pathol 1986;3:69–82.

36. Thapar K, Kovacs K, Stefaneanu L, Scheithauer BW, Killinger DW, Lloyd RV, et al. Overexpression of the growth hormone-releasing hormone gene in acromegaly-associated pituitary tumors. Am J Pathol 1997;151(3):769–784.

37. Kontogeorgos G, Kovacs K, Horvath E, Scheithauer BW. Null cell adenomas, oncocytomas, and gonadotroph adenomas of the human pituitary: an immunocytochemical and ultrastructural analysis of 300 cases. Endocrinol Pathol 1993;4:20–27.

38. Horvath E, Kovacs K, Killinger DW, Smyth HS, Platts ME, Singer W. Silent corticotropic adenomas of the human pituitary gland; a histologic, immunocytologic and ultrastructural study. Am J Pathol 1980;98:617–638.

39. Horvath E, Kovacs K, Smyth HS, Killinger DW, Scheithauer BW, Randall R, et al. A novel type of pituitary adenoma: morphological features and clinical correlations. J Clin Endocrinol Metab 1988; 66:1111–1118.

40. Lloyd RV. Ectopic pituitary adenomas. In: Surgical pathology of the pituitary gland. 1993, WB Saunders Co., Philadelphia, 116–120.

41. Boyd JD. Observations on the human pharyngeal hypophysis. J Endocrinol 1956;14:66–77.

42. Melchionna RH, Moore RA. The pharyngeal pituitary gland. Am J Pathol 1938;14:763–771.

43. Slonin SM, Haykal HA, Cushing GW, Freidberg SR, Lee AK. MRI appearances of an ectopic pituitary adenoma: case report and review of the literature. Neuroradiology 1993;35:546–548.

44. Thapar K, Scheithauer BW, Kovacs K, Pernicone PJ, Laws ER. p53 expression in pituitary adenomas and carcinomas correlation with invasiveness and tumor growth fractions. Neurosurgery 1996; 38:765–771.

45. Gandour-Edwards R, Kapadia SB, Janacka IP, Martinez AJ, Barnes L. Biologic markers of invasive pituitary adenomas involving the sphenoid sinus. Mod Pathol 1996;8:160–164.

46. Irofumi T, Herman V, Weiss M, Melmed S. Purine-binding factor (nm23) gene expression in pituitary tumors: marker of adenoma invasiveness. J Clin Endocrinol Metab 1995;80:1733–1738.

47. Rock JP, Babu VR, Drumheller T, Chason J. Cytogenetic findings in pituitary adenoma: results of a pilot study. Surg Neurol 1993; 40:224–229.

48. Pernicone PJ, Scheithauer BW, Sebo TJ, Kovacs KT, Horvath E, Young WF Jr, et al. Pituitary carcinoma: a clinicopathologic study of 15 cases. Cancer 1997;79:804–812.

49. Gilmour MD. Carcinoma of the pituitary gland with abdominal metastases. J Pathol Bacteriol 1932;35:265–269.

50. Cohen H, Dible JH. Pituitary basophilism associated with basophil carcinoma of the anterior lobe of the pituitary gland. Brain 1936;59:395–407.

51. Forbes W. Carcinoma of the pituitary gland with metastases to the liver in a case of Cushing's syndrome. J Pathol Bacteriol 1947;59:137–144.

52. Feiring EH, Davidoff LM, Zimmerman HM. Primary carcinoma of the pituitary. J Neuropathol Exp Neurol 1953;12:205–222.

53. Sheldon WH, Golden A, Bondy PK. Cushing's syndrome produced by a pituitary basophil carcinoma with hepatic metastases. Am J Med 1954;17:134–142.

54. Mobert A. A case of pituitary chromophobe adenoma with metastases in the heart. Acta Pathol Microbiol Scand 1959;45:243–249.

55. Salassa RM, Kearns TP, Kernohan JW, Sprague RG, MacCarty CS. Pituitary tumors in patients with Cushing's syndrome. J Clin Endocrinol Metab 1959;19:1523–1539.

56. Newton TH, Burhenne HJ, Palubinskas AJ. Primary carcinoma of the pituitary. Am J Roent Radium Ther Nuclear Med 1962;87:110–119.

57. Scholz DA, Gastineau CF, Harrison EG. Cushing's syndrome with malignant chromophobe tumor of the pituitary and extracranial metastasis: report of a case. Mayo Clin Proc 1962;37:31–42.

58. Madonick MJ, Rubinstein LJ, Dasco MR, Ribner H. Chromophobe adenoma of pituitary gland with subarachnoid metastases. Neurology 1963;13:836–840.

59. Epstein JA, Epstein BS, Molho L, Zimmerman HM. Carcinoma of the pituitary gland with metastases to the spinal cord and roots of the cauda equina. J Neurosurg 1964;21:846–853.

60. Soltare GB, Jatlow P. Adenohypophysial carcinoma: case report. J Neurosurg 1967;26:624–632.

61. Fleischer AS, Reagan T, Ransohoff J. Primary carcinoma of the pituitary with metastasis to the brain stem: case report. J Neurosurg 1972;36:781–784.

62. D'Abrera V St E, Burke WJ, Bleasel KF, Bader L. Carcinoma of the pituitary gland. J Pathol 1973;109:335–343.

63. Ogilvy K, Jakubowski J. Intracranial dissemination of pituitary adenomas. J Neurol Neurosurg Psychiatry 1973;36:199–205.

64. Rocoy J, Carrillo R, Garcia J, Bravo G. Dissemination of pituitary adenomas: a case report. Acta Neurochirurgica 1974;31:123–130.

65. Queiroz LS, Facure NO, Facure JJ, Modesto NP, deFaria JL. Pituitary carcinoma with liver metastases and Cushing syndrome. Arch Pathol 1975;99:32–35.

66. Martin NA, Hales M, Wilson CB. Cerebellar metastasis from a prolactinoma during treatment with bromocriptine. J Neurosurg 1981;55:615–619.

67. Cohen DL, Diengdoh JV, Thomas DGT, Himsworth RL. An intracranial metastasis from a PRL secreting pituitary tumor. Clin Endocrinol 1983;18:259–264.

68. Kaiser FE, Orth DN, Mukai K, Oppenheimer JH. A pituitary parasellar tumor with extracranial metastases and high, partially suppressible levels of adrenocorticotropin and related peptides. J Clin Endocrinol Metab 1983;57:649–653.

69. U HS, Johnson C. Metastatic prolactin-secreting pituitary adenoma. Hum Pathol 1984;15:94–96.

70. Myles ST, Johns RD, Curry B. Clinicopathological conference: carcinoma of the pituitary gland with metastases to bone. Can J Neurol Sci 1984;11:310–317.

71. Papotti M, Limone P, Riva C, Gatti G, Bussolati G. Malignant evolution of an ACTH-producing pituitary tumor treated with intrasellar implantation of 90Y. Appl Pathol 1984;2:10–21.

72. Zafar MS, Mellinger RC, Chason JL. Cushing's disease due to pituitary carcinoma. Henry Ford Hosp J 1984;32:61–65.

73. Glasser RW, Finkenstedt G, Skrabal F, Twerdy K, Grunert V, Mayr U, et al. Multiple intracranial metastases from a prolactin-secreting pituitary tumor. Clin Endocrinol 1985;22:17–27.

74. Nudleman KL, Choi B, Kusske JA. Primary pituitary carcinoma: a clinical pathological study. Neurosurgery 1985;16:90–95.

75. Plangger CA, Twerdy K, Grunert V, Weiser G. Subarachnoid metastases from a prolactinoma. Neurochirurgia 1985;28:235–237.

76. Scheithauer BW, Randall RV, Laws ER, Kovacs KT, Horvath E, Whitaker MD. Prolactin cell carcinoma of the pituitary: clinicopathologic, immunohistochemical, and ultrastructural study of a case with cranial and extracranial metastases. Cancer 1985;55:598–604.

77. Casson IF, Walker BA, Hipkin LJ, Davis JC, Buxton PH, Jeffreys RV. An intrasellar pituitary tumour producing metastases in liver, bone and lymph glands and demonstration of ACTH in the metastatic deposits. Acta Endocrinologica 1986;111:300–304.

78. Gabrilove JL, Anderson PJ, Halmi NS. Pituitary proopiomelanocortin-cell carcinoma occurring in conjunction with a glioblastoma in a patient with Cushing's disease and subsequent Nelson's syndrome. Clin Endocrinol 1986;25:117–126.

79. Hashimoto N, Handa H, Nishi S. Intracranial and intraspinal dissemination from a growth hormone-secreting pituitary tumor. J Neurosurg 1986;64:140–144.

80. Kuroki M, Tanaka R, Yokoyama M, Shimbo Y, Ikuta F. Subarachnoid dissemination of a pituitary adenoma. Surg Neurol 1987;28:71–76.

81. Luzi P, Miracco C, Lio R, Malandrini A, Piovani S, Venezia SG, et al. Endocrine inactive pituitary carcinoma metastasizing to cervical lymph nodes: a case report. Hum Pathol 1987;18:90–92.

82. Muhr C, Bergstrom M, Lundberg PO, Hartman M, Bergstrom K, Pellettieri L. Malignant prolactinoma with multiple intracranial metastases studied with positron emission tomography. Neurosurgery 1988;22:374–379.

83. Mountcastle RB, Roof BS, Mayfield RK, Mordews DB, Sagel J, Biggs PJ, et al. Case report: pituitary adenocarcinoma in an acromegalic patient: response to bromocriptine and pituitary testing: a review of the literature on 36 cases of pituitary carcinoma. Am J Med Sci 1989;298:109–118.

84. Nawata H, Higuchi K, Ikuyama S, Kato K, Ibayashi H, Mimura K, et al. Corticotropin-releasing hormone and adrenocorticotropin-producing pituitary carcinoma with metastases to the liver and lung in a patient with Cushing's disease. J Clin Endocrinol Metab 1990;127:1068–1073.

85. Sakamoto T, Yasunobu I, Fushimi S, Kowada M, Saito M. Primary pituitary carcinoma with spinal cord metastasis—case report. Neurol Med Chir 1990;30:763–767.

86. Popovic EA, Vattuone JR, Siu KA, Busmanis I, Pullar MJ, Dowling J. Malignant prolactinomas. Neurosurgery 1991;29:127–130.

87. Atienza DM, Vigersky RJ, Lack EE, Carriaga M, Rusnock EJ, Tsou E, et al. Prolactin-producing pituitary carcinoma with pulmonary metastases. Cancer 1991;68:1605–1610.

88. Berezin M, Gutman I, Tadmor R, Horowitz A, Findler G. Malignant prolactinoma. Acta Endocrinol 1992;127:476–480.

89. Peterson T, MacFarlane IA, MacKenzie JM, Shaw MD. Prolactin secreting pituitary carcinoma. J Neurol Neurosurg Psychiatry 1992;55:1205–1206.

90. Tonner D, Belding P, Moore SA, Schlechte JA. Intracranial dissemination of an ACTH secreting pituitary neoplasm—a case report and review of the literature. J Endocrinol Invest 1992;15:387–391.

91. Assies J, Verhoeff NPLG, Bosch DA, Hofland LJ. Intracranial dissemination of a macroprolactinoma. Clin Endocrinol 1993;38:539–546.

92. Mixson AJ, Friedman TC, Katz DA, Fenerstein IM, Taubenberger JK, Colandrea JM, et al. Thyrotropin-secreting pituitary carcinoma. J Clin Endocrinol Metab 1993;76:529–533.

93. Walker JD, Grossman A, Anderson JV, Ur E, Trainer PJ, Benn J, et al. Malignant prolactinoma with extracranial metastases: a report of three cases. Clin Endocrinol 1993;38:411–419.

94. Cusimano MD, Ohori P, Martinez AJ, Jungreis C, Wright DC. Pituitary carcinoma. Skull Base Surg 1994;4:46–51.

95. Jamjoon A, Moss T, Coakham H, Jamjoon ZA, Anthony P. Cervical lymph node metastases from a pituitary carcinoma. Br J Neurosurg 1994;8:87–92.

96. Taylor WA, Uttley D, Wilkins PR. Multiple dural metastases from a pituitary adenoma. J Neurosurg 1994;81:624–626.

97. Beauchesne P, Trouillas J, Barra LF, Brennon J. Gonadotropic pituitary carcinoma: a case report. Neurosurgery 1995;37:810–816.

98. Frost AR, Tenner S, Tenner M, Rollhauser C, Tabbara SO. ACTH-producing pituitary carcinoma presenting as the cauda equina syndrome. Arch Pathol Lab Med 1995;119:93–96.

99. O'Brien DP, Phillips JP, Rawluk DR, Farrell MA. Intracranial metastases from pituitary adenoma. Br J Neurosurg 1995;9:211–218.

100. Saeger W, Bosse U, Pfingst E, Schierke G, Kulinna H, Atkins D, et al. Prolactin producing hypophyseal carcinoma. Case report of an extremely rare metastatic tumor. Pathologe 1995;16:354–358.

101. Bayindir C, Balak N, Gazioglu N. Prolactin-secreting carcinoma of the pituitary: clinicopathological and immunohistochemical study of a case with intracranial and intraspinal dissemination. Br J Neurosurg 1997;11:350–355.

102. Kaltsas GA, Mukherjee JJ, Plowman PN, Monson JP, Grossman AB, Besser GM. The role of cytotoxic chemotherapy in the management of aggressive and malignant pituitary tumors. 1998;83:4233–4238.

103. Rajasoorja C, Scheithauer BW, Tan, Young WF Jr. Pituitary gigantism with intracerebral metastases. The Endocrinologist 1999;9:497–501.

104. Kovacs K, Scheithauer BW, Horvath E, Lloyd RV. The world health organization classification of adenohypophysial neoplasms: a proposed five-tier scheme. Cancer 1996;78:502–510.

105. Kovacs K, Scheithauer BW, Horvath E, Lloyd RV. Tumors of the adenohypophysis. In: Solcia E, Klöppel G, Soben LH, eds. Histological Typing of Endocrine Tumors, 2nd ed. Springer-Verlag, Berlin, 2000, pp. 15–29 and 75–90.

106. Hampton TA, Scheithauer BW, Rojiani AM, Kovacs K, Horvath E, Vogt P. Salivary gland-like tumors of the sellar region. Am J Surg Pathol 1997;21:424–434.

23 Sellar Tumors Other Than Adenomas

PAUL E. McKEEVER, MD, PhD, MILA BLAIVAS, MD, PhD,
AND STEPHEN S. GEBARSKI, MD

1. EPITHELIAL ABNORMALITIES

1.1. TUMORS

1.1.1. Craniopharyngioma

Definition. Craniopharyngioma, a common epithelial neoplasm of the sellar region, is the most frequent suprasellar neoplasm in children *(1,2)*. However, neonatal or congenital tumors are very rare *(3–5)*, as are tumors in the elderly *(6)*.

Location. The majority of craniopharyngiomas are located in the suprasellar region, and about 18% are found within the sella at the time of presentation *(3,4,7–9)*. Occasionally, the neoplasm grows to giant size involving vast regions of adjacent brain *(10–12)*. Nasopharyngeal and intraventricular locations are unusual *(7,13–15)*.

Clinical Features. Presenting clinical symptoms include visual impairment, headache, hypothalamic–pituitary dysfunction, and growth retardation in children *(2,9,16–20)*. Occasionally, mental disturbances have been reported, specifically, depressive disorder in a middle-aged woman *(21)* and a case of Korsakoff psychosis *(22)*. Also reported recently was vasogenic edema *(23)*, blindness reversed by surgery *(24)*, and "acquired" Chiari-I malformation with hydromyelia that spontaneously resolved during the postoperative period *(25)*. Occasionally, patients present with chemical meningitis and abnormal cerebrospinal fluid (CSF) findings *(26–28)*.

Radiological Features. Most useful in the diagnosis of craniopharyngioma are computed tomography (CT) and magnetic resonance imaging (MRI) (Figure 1). Plain skull films and angiography are not being used as much as in the past *(17,29)*. The tumors are characterized by various amounts of soft tissue, calcium, and cysts that sometimes contain mural nodules *(20,30)*. The radiologic appearance of the neoplasm did not always correlate with the histologic features in the series of cases reported by Eldevik and coauthors *(30)*.

Macroscopic Features. Craniopharyngioma is a bosselated, usually partially cystic mass of an average 3–4 cm in size. The cyst contents vary in color from yellow to brown, resembling motor oil, and from clear to grumous and blood-stained. Calcifications are frequently found in both solid and cystic portions of the neoplasm.

Microscopic Features. The epithelial cells of the tumor are arranged in an adamantinomatous pattern in which a layer of pseudostratified columnar cells rests on basement membrane and forms palisades around loose aggregates of stellate cells. (Figure 2). The cysts are lined by columnar basal cells sitting on the basement membrane. When the latter is missing and only a thin epithelial lining is present, one has to consider an epidermoid rather than craniopharyngioma cyst. However, the validity of separation of the two was questioned in Petito and associates' paper *(5)*. Typical keratoid nodules ("wet" keratin) that may contain keratohyalin granules are frequently prominent. These keratoid nodules and/or adamantinomatous epithelium are diagnostic of craniopharyngioma on frozen sections. In the absence of the epithelium, necrotic debris with cholesterol clefts within fibrous tissue obtained from a calcified suprasellar mass, is suggestive of craniopharyngioma *(31)*.

Besides the adamantinomatous, there is a papillary craniopharyngioma that occurs more frequently in adults. It is mostly solid radiologically and is composed of well-differentiated papillary squamous epithelium (Figure 3). It lacks calcifications, keratoid nodules, and cholesterol clefts that are commonly accompanied by a foreign body giant cell reaction in adamantinomatous patterns *(20,32)*. Statistical data on the frequency of these two tumor types vary, and several papers describe the existence of combined tumors expressing the characteristics of both subtypes *(30,33,34)*. In fact, in the series of Eldevik and coauthors, only adamantinomatous and combined types were found, without a pure papillary squamous type *(30)*.

Rare tumors demonstrate sebaceous differentiation *(35)*, focal ossification *(18)*, or features of ameloblastoma and tooth bud-like structures in the "embryonal form of craniopharyngioma" *(3)*. Several cases of craniopharyngioma were reported to contain ciliated and mucin-producing cells in addition to the usual pattern, indicating a histogenetic relationship with Rathke's cleft cyst *(36,37)*. Three cases of craniopharyngioma associated with lymphocytic hypophysitis were described by Puchner and coauthors *(38)*.

Immunostaining and Ultrastructure. The epithelial cells of the neoplasm stain intensely for keratin *(39)*. In 25 craniopharyngiomas studied by Kubo and associates, the cytoplasm of the tumor cells stained positively for keratin and cytokeratin, but the staining characteristics differed from layer to layer *(40)*. The ciliated epithelium of craniopharyngioma did not stain for keratin. However, ciliated epithelium of Rathke's cleft cyst was positive for cytokeratin. Intracellular Alcian blue staining was limited to apical cells of squamous-type tumors *(41)*. Neither silver-stained

From: *Diagnosis and Management of Pituitary Tumors* (K. Thapar, K. Kovacs, B. W. Scheithauer, and R. V. Lloyd, eds.), ©Humana Press Inc., Totowa, NJ.

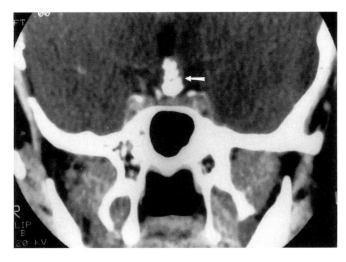

Figure 23-1   Coronal CT on a 15-yr-old boy with a craniopharyngioma. The mass extends to both intrasellar and suprasellar regions, and is densely calcified (arrow), typical for craniopharyngioma, but not seen in Rathke's cleft cysts.

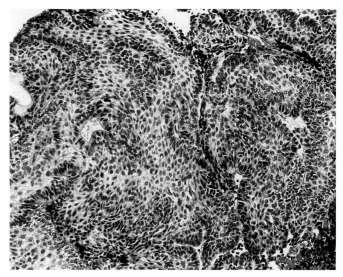

Figure 23-3   This is a hypercellular, predominantly squamous portion of craniopharyngioma.

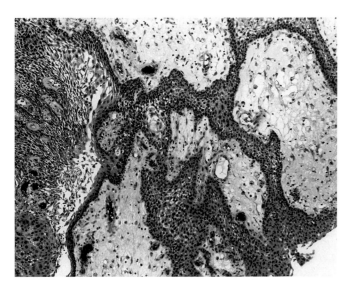

Figure 23-2   Ribbons of adamantinomatous epithelium outline loose, semicystic spaces in this craniopharyngioma.

nuclear organizer regions (AgNOR) nor proliferating cell nuclear antigen (PCNA) staining proved to be statistically significant in correlating with the tumor type and the patient's age. Szeifert and Pasztor studied staining characteristics of 13 craniopharyngiomas for pituitary hormones *(42)*. They found scattered cell groups positive for at least one hormone in 12 cases, concluding that this provided further evidence for the hypothesis of the Rathke's pouch origin of craniopharyngiomas. As a result of staining of 23 craniopharyngiomas and five normal adenohypophyses for P-glycoprotein and human chorionic gonadotropin (HCG), Tachibana and associates suggested that craniopharyngiomas produce HCG-like peptides and are unique squamous neoplasms arising in the sellar region from progenitor neuroendocrine cells *(43)*. High levels of HCG within intraparenchymal cystic fluid and CSF were suggestive of craniopharyngioma *(44)*.

Ultrastructurally, the craniopharyngioma contains numerous desmosomes, tonofilaments, and glycogen particles within the epithelial cells. Connective tissue stroma is remarkable for fenestration of capillary endothelium. "Calcifications" are a combination of calcium and phosphorus precipitations, which initially appear among the disintegrating keratinized squamous cells. Collagen and elastic fibers and cytoplasmic fibrils serve as a supportive skeleton in formations of large calcific nests *(45)*.

Differential Diagnosis.   Diagnosis of properly sampled craniopharyngioma causes no problems. One only has to identify either adamantinomatous epithelium or "wet keratin" nobs to assure the correct diagnosis. The difficulty arises when neither of them is present in the section. If gliotic parenchyma with Rosenthal fibers that frequently surrounds craniopharyngioma is sampled, pilocytic astrocytoma may be entertained as a possibility. The presence of cholesterol clefts in such tissue would be evidence of craniopharyngioma. When an epidermoid-like cyst is all that is obtained from a sellar/suprasellar lesion, craniopharyngioma may be suspected but not diagnosed.

Clinical Outcome.   Craniopharyngioma is a benign neoplasm that frequently follows an aggressive course, invading bone and compressing adjacent nervous structures. Less common is compression of the arteries *(46)*. Malignant transformation is exceedingly rare *(47)*. Overall survival in childhood craniopharyngioma is very good, especially in patients treated with surgery and radiation instead of surgery or radiation therapy alone *(48)*. There is some controversy about radical vs limited surgery. Regine and collaborators found that surgical morbidity correlated with the extent of surgery *(49)*, whereas in other series, the survival was either not influenced by the extent of surgical excision, or gross total resection was advised to lower the tumor recurrence rate *(50–53)*. Radiation treatment was strongly associated with tumor regression or absence of recurrence, particularly after subtotal resection *(30,53)*. De Vile and associates identified predictors of morbidity and tumor recurrence in correlation with modes of therapy *(54)*. They proposed a more flexible, individualized treatment approach to provide long-term tumor control with the lowest morbidity.

One more controversy surrounds the validity of their separation into solid papillary squamous and cystic adamantinomatous subtypes histologically and radiologically, and the most beneficial mode of treatment for each. Some reports support the difference between the two, whereas the others state no correlations between the survival rates and the ratio of adamantinomatous to squamous regions, the ratio of solid to cystic portion, or the age of the patients *(5,20,30,32,34,35,55–57)*. Cystic craniopharyngiomas can be treated by intratumoral injection of bleomycin *(58,59)* or by intracavitary irradiation with Yttrium-90 or Phosphorus-32 *(60–62)*. Endoscopic extirpation of three cystic craniopharyngiomas was attempted recently by Abdullah and Caemaert *(63)*. Gamma-Knife radiosurgery was successfully performed in several tumors *(64,65)*. Repeated postsurgical irradiation carries a danger of radiation-induced glioma *(66)*.

1.1.2. Nasopharyngeal Carcinoma (NPC)

Definition. NPC arises in nasopharyngeal surface epithelium and is classified into three major types: squamous cell carcinoma, nonkeratinizing carcinoma, and sinonasal undifferentiated carcinoma also known as SNUC or lymphoepithelioma.

Location. About 25% of these carcinomas invade the base of skull at the time of diagnosis *(1)*. Six major directions of tumor spread were described, with the anterior and postero-lateral directions being most common. Others include superior and supralateral extension with involvement of the sphenoid sinus, cavernous sinus, and middle cranial fossa *(2)*. NPC is a relatively rare neoplasm anywhere in the world, but is most prevalent in southern China *(3)*.

Clinical Features. Clinical symptoms are related to the localization of the original neoplasm and the directions of its spread. Early symptoms may be subtle, including epistaxis, neck pain, hearing impairment, otorrhea, rhinorrhea, and cervical lymphadenopathy *(4)*.

Radiological Features. CT was found to be the most useful radiographic technique in the diagnosis of skull base or intracranial invasion of NPC *(2)*. CT nicely demonstrates changes in both bone and soft tissue. It is sensitive enough to show subtle bone destruction. The latter allowed Miura and associates to recommend using CT in staging NPC systematically *(2)*. MRI is superior in detecting intracranial parenchymal extension.

Macroscopic Features. A typical surgical specimen consists of hemorrhagic, friable bits of soft, gray, viable, and necrotic tissue.

Microscopic Features. Keratinizing and nonkeratinizing squamous cell carcinomas have the same histological characteristics near the sella as elsewhere in the body. The cells are epithelial and cohesive. They do not extend fibrillar processes, but may elongate. Careful inspection usually reveals distinct margins between adjacent cells.

The SNUC is formed by nests, ribbons, trabeculae, or sheets of polygonal cells with moderate amount of eosinophilic cytoplasm and round to oval nuclei. Nucleoli are large, chromatin is coarse, and mitotic figures are numerous *(5)*. Vascular invasion and tumor necrosis are common. When comparing SNUC in Western and Asian patients, Lopategui and collaborators found that Asian SNUC had a broader histological spectrum *(6)*. Three morphological subtypes were identified:

1. Identical to the "Western type."
2. Histologically similar to anaplastic large-cell carcinoma of the lung.
3. Mimicking other types of NPC.

(*See* Figure 4.)

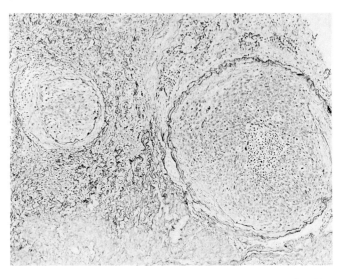

Figure 23-4 SNUC characteristically invades vessels, outlined by their perimeter of dark, wavy vascular wall reticulin. There is central necrosis in the larger intravascular tumor. Wilder's stain for reticulin.

Immunohistochemical, Cytogenetic, and Ultrastructural Features. SNUC is diffusely positive for keratin and epithelial membrane antigen and frequently also for neuron-specific enolase (NSE). It is negative for S-100 protein, HMB-45, synaptophysin, and myogenous markers *(5,7,8)*. In the series of cases reported by Lopategui et al. *(6)*, 7 of 11 tumors from Western patients stained positively for NSE, whereas only 1 of 11 Asian cases was focally reactive for NSE. Seven of 11 Asian SNUCs demonstrated positive *in situ* hybridization for Epstein-Barr virus (EBV) RNA, but all 11 Western cases were negative *(6)*. Association of NPC with EBV is well known and is frequently addressed in the literature *(6,9–12)*. This association was found to be stronger with undifferentiated and nonkeratinizing NPC than with the squamous cell NPC *(12)*. None of the 12 samples of nasopharyngeal tissue without NPC contained detectable EBV DNA in this study. However, EBV was localized by polymerase chain reaction (PCR) technique in uninvolved regions of the nasopharynx in patients with NPC *(11)*. In three well-differentiated cases of NPC without microinvasion, only a few neoplastic cells contained the EBV genome, whereas in three cases with microinvasion, the majority of the tumor cells carried the viral genome *(10)*. In all 36 cases of newly diagnosed NPC at various stages, a consistent deletion was observed at the two specific loci of the short arm of chromosome 3 *(13)*. EBV genome was also detected in 35 of these cases. In another study, all seven newly established NPC cell lines showed overexpression of c-*myc* oncogene *(14)*.

On an ultrastructural level, the undifferentiated NPC contains desmosomes and tonofilaments, in most cases, even though the absence of the latter does not preclude positive staining for keratin *(8)*.

Differential Diagnosis. Major other possible diagnoses are olfactory neuroblastoma, small-cell undifferentiated carcinoma, malignant melanoma, and rhabdomyosarcoma. Their presence of different antigenic phenotypes make the use of immunohistochemical techniques helpful in the diagnostic workup.

Two other neoplasms that occasionally infiltrate the sella from the nasopharynx are angiofibroma and adenocarcinoma resembling colonic carcinoma (ARCC) *(15–17)*. About 20% of juvenile angiofibroma cases were found to extend into the parasellar sphenoid and petrous portions of the temporal bone *(16)*. ARCC is most common in men in their 50s or 60s and is frequently associated with occupational exposure to hardwood dust *(16)*. Franquemont and collaborators *(17)* subclassified this neoplasm into papillary tubular cylinder cell type with two grades, alveolar goblet cell type, signet ring type, and a mixed pattern *(18)*. Other unusual tumors in the region of the sella are: metastatic pheochromocytoma *(19)*, adenoid cystic carcinoma *(20)*, metastatic hepatocellular carcinoma *(21)*, and two cases of metastatic lung cancer *(22,23)*.

Clinical Outcome.   The usual treatment for NPC of various types is a combination of radiotherapy, chemotherapy, and surgery. For recurrent disease after radiation, however, there is no effective treatment. An experience with an interesting novel treatment, photodynamic therapy, was recently reported by Tong and associates *(24)*. Patients with recurrent NPC were treated with an infusion of hematoporphyrin derivative followed by exposure to 630-nm wavelength light derived from a gold vapor laser. All 12 patients showed a dramatic response, demonstrated by CT and MRI, 9–12 mo after a single treatment. Intracranial and skull base involvement is a significant prognostic factor in staging NPC *(2)*. In 364 patients with newly diagnosed NPC, extensive paranasopharyngeal spread was an independent prognostic factor associated with poorer treatment outcome *(25)*. Histologic features of NPCs correlated with the prognosis: in high-grade malignant tumors, 5-yr survival occurred in 20% of cases, in intermediate malignancy, 30–40% of cases, and in low-grade malignancy, 60–72% of cases *(3)*.

1.2. CYSTS

1.2.1. Rathke's Cleft Cyst

Definition.   This cyst arises from remnants of Rathke's pouch. Rathke's pouch, also known as the craniobuccal pouch, is a midline epithelial invagination of the stomodeum that detaches and migrates dorsally. Its anterior wall thickens to form the adenohypophysis. Its posterior wall forms the intermediate lobe, which normally contains microscopic cysts that resemble miniature Rathke's cleft cysts.

Location.   Rathke's cysts occur in the intermediate lobe of the pituitary, suprasellar region, anterior sella turcica, and anterior suprasellar cistern *(1–4)*. Larger cysts extend across more than one of these locations *(4)*. Most cysts within the pituitary gland are medially situated *(5)*.

Clinical Features.   Rathke's cleft cysts often produce no symptoms, and are incidental radiographic or necropsy findings *(5,6)*. Most cysts are <2 centimeters in diameter *(1)*.

Symptomatic Rathke's cysts vary in their presentation. Of 11 symptomatic patients, 8 initially had visual problems *(7)*. Visual problems occurred in 47% of patients in another study *(8)*. Problems include reduced visual acuity, optic atrophy, visual field defects, and chiasmatic syndrome *(4,7,8)*.

In a study of 19 patients, 4 had diabetes insipidus, 3 had amenorrhea and/or galactorrhea, and 2 had panhypopituitarism. With systematic endocrinologic examination, various degrees of pituitary dysfunction were revealed *(8)*. Other abnormalities include headaches and, less commonly, epilepsy *(7,9,10)*. An unusual finding is pituitary apoplexy *(6)*. Symptomatic Rathke's cysts in identical twins suggest a hereditary predisposition *(11)*.

Numerous Rathke's cysts have been associated with pituitary adenomas *(12–17)*. In addition to symptoms described above, endocrine symptoms from the adenoma occur *(14,18)*. There are

three explanations for these occurrences, the first one being coincidental association of two common abnormalities. In a nonselected autopsy series, nearly 4% of patients had Rathke's cysts and 2% adenomas *(5)*. Thus, 8 in every 10,000 people might be expected to harbor both abnormalities.

Another explanation of some cases is a tendency for some pituitary adenomas to be cystic. Prolactinomas tend to be cystic and are among the most common adenomas reported to be associated with Rathke's cysts *(17–19)*. These cystic prolactinomas have been reported as transitional cell tumors by some authors.

Finally, a few cases present strong evidence of being true transitional tumors. These are cases with individual cells that have features of both craniobuccal epithelium and adenoma *(15,16,20)*. For example, individual cyst-lining cells have been reported to be both ciliated and contain secretory granules *(20)*.

Radiographic Features.   Rathke's cysts usually do not enlarge the sella turcica on plain X-rays *(21)*. Their cyst contents vary from homogeneous low density to slight hyperdensity relative to brain parenchyma in CT *(1)*. Contrast enhancement usually occurs in a ring near the capsule of the cyst. The variability in CT contrast enhancement among individual cysts may reflect squamous metaplasia in the wall or a peripherally displaced rim of pituitary tissue *(22,23)*. Extravasation of cyst contents may inflame nearby structures and cause enhancement *(24)*.

Cysts near the pituitary stalk may enlarge it, or shift it anteriorly or in other directions *(6,25)*. In children, a stalk to basilar artery ratio of 1 or greater should be further evaluated for cyst or other abnormality *(26)*.

The appearance of Rathke's cysts examined by MRI is variable *(22,26a)*. Although T2-weighted image hypointensity may be helpful in some cases *(6;* Figure 5), various T1- and T2-weighted image intensities occur in individual cases *(22,26a–28)*. Some of these differences in image intensities reflect the composition of the cyst contents (26a-28). In infants and children, Rathke's cleft cysts mimic cystic craniopharyngiomas *(29)*.

Specific features that suggest a Rathke's pouch cyst include a smooth contour of the lesion, absence of internal contrast enhancement, and homogenous signal intensity within the lesion *(22)*. The presence of a posterior ledge is distinctive, when present *(6)*. Rathke's cleft cyst located solely in the suprasellar region can be difficult to distinguish from craniopharyngioma. Rare skull-based cysts mimic chordoma *(27)*.

Macroscopic Features.   *In situ*, the intact cyst is round like a cranberry. A thin, gray to tan mucosa with a dull or slimy surface lines the inner wall of a thin, fibrous cyst capsule. The cyst contents vary. They may be a milky fluid or mucin, or clear and watery, light brown, waxy, or like motor oil *(26a)*.

Microscopic Features and Special Stains.   Rathke's cleft cysts are distinctive. A thin simple or pseudostratified epithelial layer of cells lies directly on fibrovascular connective tissue to form the cyst wall (Figure 6). The cuboidal to columnar epithelium often has cilia. Goblet cells with mucin are interspersed among these epithelial cells. Regions of squamous epithelium may occur.

The cyst contains an eosinophilic colloid that is positive with periodic acid schiff (PAS) and Alcian blue stains. Dead cells and lipid-filled macrophages collect in the colloid to a variable degree. Extravasation of this material may explain rare association of chronic hypophysitis with Rathke's cysts *(30)*.

Immunohistochemistry and Lectin Reactivity.   Cytokeratins are the most notable intermediate filament proteins

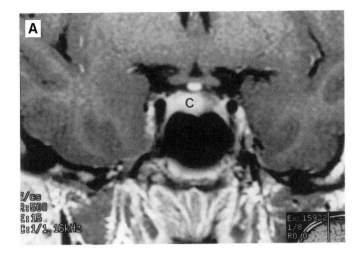
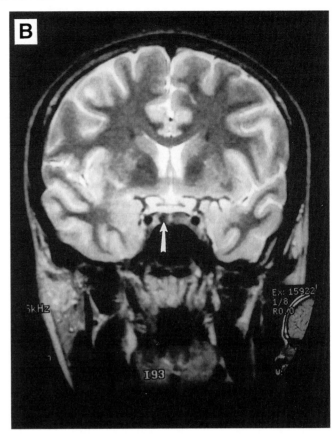

Figure 23-5 Brain MRI of a 27-yr-old woman with a Rathke's cleft cyst. **(A)** Contrast-enhanced T1-weighted coronal MRI section through the pituitary gland shows a very high-signal cyst (C) within the gland. This cyst showed the same high intensity before contrast material, typical for a Rathke's cleft cyst. It distorts the surrounding tissue, but does not invade it or show other aggressive characteristics. **(B)** Coronal T2-weighted MRI section. This cyst now shows dramatic low signal (arrow), as can be seen in Rathke's cleft cyst, choristoma, and very fresh hemorrhage. Almost no other intrasellar lesion will show such low signal on T2-weighted MRI.

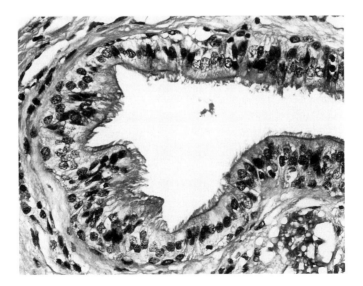

Figure 23-6 Rathke's cleft cyst is composed of ciliated columnar epithelium on a collagenous capsule. The lumen of this surgical specimen has partly collapsed. From McKeever PE, Blaivas M, Sima AAF. Neoplasms of the sellar region. In: Lloyd RV, ed. Surgical Pathology of the Pituitary Gland. Major Problems in Pathology Series. Saunders, Philadelphia, 1993, pp. 141–210.

expressed by Rathke's cyst epithelium *(18,19,31–33)*. Their cytokeratins include high-molecular-weight complex molecules *(34)*. Coexpression of glial fibrillary acidic protein (GFAP) and vimentin is focal and variable *(18,31–33,35,36)*. Similarity of their immunohistochemical profile to squamous nest of the pars tuberalis suggests a common origin *(31)*.

Other antigens expressed by Rathke's cyst epithelium include epithelial membrane antigen and secretory component *(33)*. Carcinoembryonic antigen, chromogranin, pituitary hormones, and S-100 protein are focally expressed in some cysts *(17,19,33)*.

Rathke's cyst epithelium stains with *Ulex europaeus*, peanut, and soybean agglutinins *(33,37)*. It frequently stains with *Dolichos biflorus* agglutinin and for Lewis Y, H, or A blood group antigens *(37)*.

Ultrastructural Features.
Simple or pseudostratified epithelium rests on basement membrane and connective tissue to form the wall of the cyst *(38)*. The epithelium is a mixture of ciliated and nonciliated, secretory cuboidal and columnar epithelial cells. These are mixed with goblet cells, flat cells, and basal cells *(9,39)*. The flat cells contain tonofilaments and desmosomes of squamous epithelial cells *(9)*. Some epithelial cells have a glycocalyx *(40)*. This mixture of cells resembles the mucosa in the microscopic pituitary intermediate lobe, sphenoid sinus, and in some craniopharyngiomas *(9,41,42)*.

Rathke's cysts may contain cells with secretory granules like those in pituitary cells. Follicular cysts of normal pituitary contain similar cells *(40)*.

Differential Diagnosis.
Craniopharyngioma must be distinguished from Rathke's cysts, particularly in the suprasellar region *(43*; Figure 2*)*. Although they can be cystic, craniopharyngiomas are more complex than a single, round Rathke's cyst surrounded by a thin wall. Craniopharyngiomas have solid, multicystic, or papillary regions. They are often densely calcified, unlike Rathke's cleft cysts. These regions and calcifications can be visualized best with MRI and CT, providing a major differential diagnostic feature separating them from Rathke's cysts. As a necessary part of the surgical specimen, these three-dimensional regions of a craniopharyngioma distinguish it from a Rathke's cyst. The margin of craniopharyngioma invades dorsally into brain, further distinguishing it from Rathke's cyst.

The mucocele is a cyst that resembles the Rathke's cleft cysts. Mucoceles may be multiple and bilateral *(44)*. They can arise in association with other neoplasms *(45)*. Magnetic resonance images of mucoceles are usually more hyperintense on T1- and T2-weighted images than Rathke's cleft cysts *(46)*. Most important to distinguish these two entities is location. Mucoceles are located in paranasal sinuses, the sphenoid sinus being potentially the most confusing owing to its proximity to the sella where most Rathke's cysts reside. However, this is seldom a problem since a mucocele expands the air cell and remodels its walls, whereas a Rathke's cyst will expand the sella. Differentiation of these two structures is usually straightforward with CT and MRI.

Colloid cysts histologically resemble Rathke's cysts. However, colloid cysts are located in the third ventricle, usually near the foramen of Monroe, far rostral and dorsal to Rathke's cyst territory, making differentiation rather simple with MRI or CT. In the rare confusing case, electron-dense secretory granules and oncocytic changes in some of the lining cells are reported to distinguish the Rathke's cyst in this context *(40)*. Similarly, pituitary hormone expression among the various lining cells distinguishes some Rathke's cysts *(33)*.

Choroidal epithelial cysts and fragments of choroid plexus papillomas can resemble suprasellar Rathke's cyst and can be more problematic with MRI and CT. However, fortunately these lesions almost always arise along the roof of the ventricle, where the choroid plexus is located. The rare large suprasellar Rathke's cyst will almost always be associated with the floor of the third ventricle and be central in the suprasellar cistern. With the choroid origin, they will be positive with immunostaining for prealbumin, and negative for 56/66-kilodalton cytokeratins and for epithelial membrane antigen *(35)*. Ultrastructural uniformity of a microvillous epithelial cell without a glycocalyx or mucin distinguishes choroid plexus derivatives *(40)*.

Other cysts do not resemble Rathke's cysts and should be distinctive on H&E-stained slides. Keratinous debri within epidermoid cysts generally distinguishes them from Rathke's cysts filled with mucin. CT and MRI can help differentiate these since epidermoid cysts are usually centered off midline and are loculated. Partial differences in lectin profiles of these cysts are reported *(37)*. Rare cysts display features of both Rathke's and epidermoid cysts *(47)*. The arachnoid cyst contains a thinner lining than the Rathke's cyst, and the arachnoid cyst lining cells are syncytial. CT and MRI shows the arachnoid cyst to contain fluid with attenuation and signal characteristics nearly identical to CSF.

Therapy and Clinical Outcome.
Rathke's cysts are benign. Symptomatic cysts can be excised surgically. Aspiration of cyst contents has been used as an alternative to excision. Most patients show visual and endocrinologic improvements, but patients with panhypopituitarism or diabetes insipidus did not show improvement in these abnormalities *(8)*. Collapse of the cyst and development of a scar are reported complications of cyst drainage that can cause progressive visual loss and require surgical correction *(48)*.

1.2.2. Epidermoid Cyst

Definition.
The epidermoid cyst is lined by benign keratinizing squamous epithelium on a connective tissue base, and in contrast to the dermoid cyst, contains no cutaneous adnexa within its wall.

Location.
In an autopsy series of 41 parasellar tumors, four were epidermoid cysts *(1)*. About one-third of all craniospinal epidermoid cysts occur in the parasellar region. They may be found in the midline and have been associated with defects of neural tube closure, suggesting the epithelial rest as a possible origin of the epidermoid cyst *(2)*. They may occur intra- or extradurally with erosion of underlying bone. Some of them are attached to main arteries *(3)*. Rare epidermoid tumors grow *en plaque* along the base of the skull to enter the pituitary region. These tumors are much more difficult to diagnose, and they recur more readily.

Clinical Features.
These tumors have an insidious onset, significant size when they become symptomatic, and mass effect seen in imaging studies *(4)*. A case of parasellar epidermoid cyst in a 70-yr-old woman reported by Torbiak and coworkers presented with subarachnoid hemorrhage *(5)*.

Radiographic Features.
MRI signal intensity varies with varying amount of lipids within the cyst contents, and the T1-weighted images change from high to low signal *(6)*. Mafee and coworkers compared petrous epidermoid cysts and cholesterol granuloma cysts and found that they have identical characteristics on CT. On MRI, the epidermoid cysts exhibited short T1- and long T2-characteristics. Intradural epidermoid cyst may show

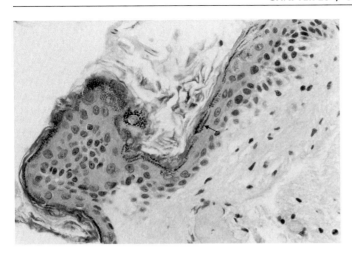

Figure 23-7 Suprasellar epidermoid cyst is lined by dark, granular keratinizing squamous epithelium on a fibrous base. Cytoplasmic dark keratin granules are conspicuous (arrow). The lumen is filled with flaky keratinous debris.

in addition curvilinear areas of higher intensity on T1-weighted images *(7)*.

Macroscopic Features. The cysts are soft, irregular or nodular, and encapsulated. They may contain areas of calcification within a pearly white, waxy substance or fluid rich in cholesterol.

Microscopic Features. Epidermoid cysts are lined by squamous epithelium covered by layers of laminated keratinous material that is exfoliating within the cyst lumen (Figure 7). These cysts are benign lesions that rarely may dedifferentiate into squamous cell carcinoma *(8,9)*.

Immunohistochemical and Ultrastructural Features. No special stains or electron microscopy is usually required for the diagnosis; however, if such a need arises in fragmented surgical material, one may use immunoperoxidase stains with cytokeratins and epithelial membrane antigen. Seven lectins applied to four epidermoid cysts had comparable binding affinities with skin, whereas the binding profile of one parasellar dermoid cyst was identical with that of keratinizing oral mucosa and of the other one with the buccal mucosa *(10)*.

Differential Diagnosis. The major differential diagnoses for epidermoid cyst in this location are dermoid cyst, Rathke's cleft cyst, and craniopharyngioma. The dermoid cyst wall is thicker and contains skin appendages within the connective tissue beneath the epidermal layer. The Rathke's cleft cyst has a distinct lining and becomes part of a differential diagnosis when that lining has undergone squamous metaplasia. The metaplastic squamous lining lacks degeneration that is typical of epidermoid cyst and that fills the latter.

Craniopharyngiomas are more difficult to differentiate when the specimen is small or fragmented since epidermoid cysts can be a component of typical craniopharyngioma *(11)*. When they are present, the most reliable features to differentiate craniopharyngioma from epidermoid cyst are palisaded adenomatous epithelium, nodules of "wet" keratin, calcifications; or thick papillae of squamous epithelium with fibrovascular cores in a papillary subtype of craniopharyngioma.

Clinical Outcome. Surgical excision of the entire cyst is curative. If a part of the cyst lining is left behind, the cyst will recur.

If the cyst wall ruptures during surgery, inflammation and gliosis of the adjacent tissue develop.

Bejarano and coworkers reported an infected epidermoid cyst of the sphenoid bone that presented on CT as a dense, sclerotic, expansile lesion *(12)*. In the review of 22 cases of craniocerebral epidermoid and 10 dermoid tumors, it was emphasized that a significant number of intradural tumors were difficult to excise because of their adherence to adjacent functionally important structures. The latter was related to higher morbidity and mortality and justified the statement that because of its extremely slow growth, complete resection should not be the goal of treatment at the risk of injury to the adjacent neurovascular structures *(4)*.

1.2.3. Dermoid Cyst

Definition. This cyst has an inner lining of skin, including cutaneous adnexa. It is "skin-like."

Location. Parasellar dermoid tumors are either intrasellar, suprasellar, or both *(1)*. A dermoid cyst occurred in the greater wing of the sphenoid bone *(2)*, but they are rare in this location. Dermoid tumors are more common in the ovaries, spinal canal, and other midline brain structures *(3)*. One patient had dermoid cysts in the pituitary and ovary *(1)*.

Clinical Features. Symptoms from parasellar dermoid cysts arise in the sensitive structures nearby. Symptoms vary depending on whether the cyst compresses hypophysis, stalk, or the visual system. Diabetes insipidus, hyperprolactinemia owing to pituitary stalk compression, and precocious puberty have been reported *(1)*. The cysts can cause visual symptoms and have been suspected of causing atypical angina pectoris by disturbing hypothalamic function *(1,4)*.

Radiographic Features. CT and MRI reveal the dermoid to be primarily cyst, rather than a solid tumor. The surrounding capsule may enhance with contrast media and be slightly thickened, but there should be no frank solid mass. MRI may demonstrate a low intensity on T1-weighted images *(1)*, but mixtures of hair and cholesterol of high-T1 signal intensity usually make the lesion bright on T1-weighted images, though a heterogeneous image is also possible *(5,6)*. MRI detects ruptured cyst contents better than CT owing to the high signal of the cyst contents on T1-weighted images *(6)*. However, CT is also usually quite effective, showing droplets of very low attenuation lipid distributed about the water-attenuation CSF.

Macroscopic Features. The cyst contains soft, greasy squamous and sebaceous debri. It is not as firm as tissue and can be easily compressed between fingers. Many dermoid cysts also contain hair, facilitating their recognition. The cyst wall is firm with gray to white collagen. Its inner lining is covered with epidermis.

Microscopic Features. Squamous epithelial debris is mixed with a variable amount of hair in the cyst contents. The cyst is a single cavity. The cyst wall consists of keratinizing, well-differentiated squamous epithelium. This epidermis overlies dermal collagen within which hair follicles and sebaceous glands are evident (Figure 8). The wall may also contain fibroadipose tissue.

Immunohistochemistry and Ultrastructure. The epithelium expresses keratin and epithelial membrane antigen, and has the ultrastructural features of epidermis. These are rarely needed for diagnosis, because its structure is so distinctive.

Differential Diagnosis. Hair follicles and sebaceous glands distinguish the dermoid cyst from an epidermoid cyst, from craniopharyngioma, and from other cystic abnormalities except ter-

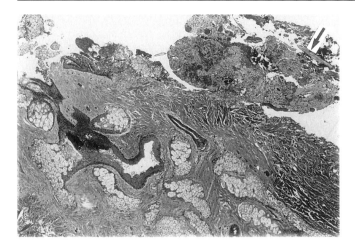

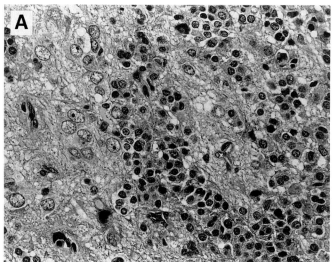

Figure 23-8   The dermoid cyst contains keratinizing squamous epithelium and cutaneous adnexa. Longitudinal profiles of hair shafts have sharp borders (arrow) and contain linear dark streaks.

atoma. The teratoma (Figure 59) may generate dermoid cysts as part of its multiple germ-cell layers of neoplastic tissue (1,3,7). Teratoma is excluded from the differential diagnosis when complete sampling fails to demonstrate additional tissue elements, like muscle, cartilage, or tissue of endodermal origin.

Clinical Outcome.   If a dermoid cyst is totally resected without spilling its contents, it is cured. Resection can be a special problem in the sellar region, where it may be difficult to separate from vital structures (1,4). Ruptured dermoid cysts can produce sterile meningitis and inflammation, histologically similar to a ruptured abscess. Squamous epithelial cells, hair, or cholesterol clefts may be evident within the inflammation (3).

2. NERVOUS SYSTEM TUMORS

2.1. NEURONAL TUMORS

2.1.1. Gangliocytoma

Definition.   Gangliocytomas or ganglioneuromas are composed of neoplastic neurons. A portion of these are sufficiently mature to be recognized on H&E-stained slides.

Location.   Gangliocytomas and related tumors occur throughout the brain and spinal cord, but are more common in cerebrum, particularly temporal lobe and the floor of the third ventricle (1–3). Most gangliocytomas that occur within the sella are mixed with pituitary adenoma (4,5; Figures 9,10).

Clinical Features.   Most cerebral gangliocytomas occur in children and young adults. Four-fifths of gangliocytoma cases occur in patients <30 yr of age (3). In contrast, gangliocytomas in the sella predominate in adults over 30 yr of age (5).

Most intrasellar gangliocytomas are associated with endocrine signs (6–12). Acromegaly is most common (5,7). Other cases show amenorrhea-galactorrhea or Cushing's syndrome (6).

It is of interest that many gangliocytomas that are not associated with pituitary adenoma also have endocrine signs (5). These gangliocytomas may produce pituitary hormone-releasing factors that stimulate overproduction by the adenohypophysis (9). Other nonadenomatous gangliocytomas are associated with hypopituitarism, diabetes mellitus, or diabetes insipidis (5,10). Hydrocephalus, somnolence, and eating disorder were associated with a third ventricular gangliocytoma (2).

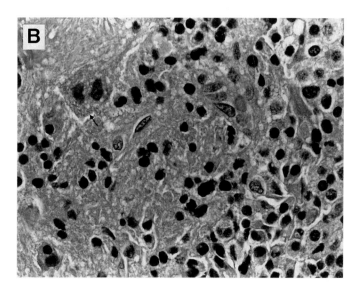

Figure 23-9   Gangliocytoma mixed with a prolactin-producing adenoma from within the sella of a young woman. **(A)** Fibrillary zones contain ganglion cells with large, round nucleoli within large, round, and oval nuclei with sparse chromatin. Zones with a higher density of smaller epithelioid cells are adenoma. **(B)** A "smudgy" binucleated neuron (arrow) is present in the gangliocytic portion of the specimen. Adenoma cells are nearby.

Radiographic Features.   Signal intensities vary on MRI since these masses may have large cysts, but the stroma is similar to gray matter on T1-weighted images. Gangliocytomas generally enhance, at least partially, with contrast media. CT may show sellar erosion or extension into sinuses (5).

Macroscopic Features.   These parasellar and sellar tumors are usually small, gray, and firm to touch. They are well demarcated from surrounding tissue. Cases in children tend to be larger and extend beyond the sella (5). Larger cerebral tumors may be macrocystic or extensively calcified.

Microscopic Features.   Irregularly oriented mature neuronal elements frequently display binucleated forms (Figure 9). The largest neurons of parasellar and sellar tumors contain prominent Nissl substance and are watermelon- to banana-shaped. They resemble large neurons in the hypothalamic nuclei. Their nuclei are large and vesicular, and they have large, round nucleoli

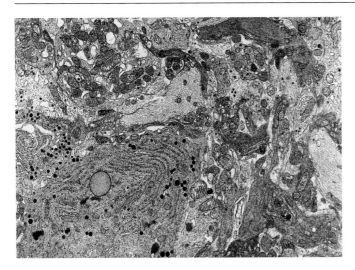

Figure 23-10 Same case as Figure 9. Electron micrograph of a portion of adenoma cell cytoplasm containing abundant RER and 250-nm secretory granules. Neurites next to adenoma cell are cell processes of the gangliocytoma. They contain a mixture of smaller clear synaptic vesicles and 80-nm dense core neurosecretory granules (X12,200, UALC stain).

(Figure 9). In gangliocytomas, the glial stroma is inconspicuous, in contrast to gangliogliomas where the glial component is neoplastic. Gangliocytomas may contain calcospherites and calcification of the vascular walls. Occasionally, neuronal precursors produce small perivascular clusters of mononuclear cells (11).

Immunohistochemistry and Special Stains. Synaptophysin and neurofilament protein stains identify the gangliocytoma cells. Synaptophysin is more sensitive, but less specific. It stains adenoma cells (5). Well-differentiated neurons can be identified with neurohistologic stains. Silver stains, such as Bielschowsky stain, identify their axons. Cresyl violet stain highlights their Nissl substance.

Ultrastructural Features. Stacks of cytoplasmic rough endoplasmic reticulum (Nissl substance), neurites, and synaptic vesicles identify gangliocytic cells (7,8; Figure 10). Individual cases show cytoplasmic inclusions like zebra bodies (12).

Gangliocytomas mixed with pituitary adenomas generally show sparse secretory granules in the adenomatous component (Figure 10). In individual cases, misplaced granule exocytosis, whorled rough endoplasmic reticulin (RER), and fibrous bodies occur (5,7,12). Some cases show transitional cells with features intermediate between adenoma and ganglion cells (7).

Differential Diagnosis. Cerebral gangliocytomas must be distinguished from normal gray matter. Evidence of neuronal neoplasia includes hypercellularity and disarray of neurons, binucleated neurons, and pleomorphism. Gangliocytomas may display heavy bands of fibrous tissue or perivascular round cells, but these are not invariably present. Serial radiographic evidence of growth over a time interval is good evidence of neoplasia.

Hypothalamic hamartomas may present a problem in the differential. These can be identified by their similarity to hypothalamic gray matter, and are more fibrillar, more organized, and less cellular than gangliocytomas. They tend not to enlarge over time. Hypothalamic hamartomas are related to the hypothalamus, floor of the third ventricle, or tuber cinereum by their location within one of these structures or attachment to it by a stalk.

In the cerebrum, ganglioglioma and giant-cell astrocytoma resemble gangliocytomas. However, these have neoplastic glial elements that distinguish them from gangliocytoma. The glial element must be evaluated. A section lightly stained for GFAP with immunoperoxidase (less than half the usual time in substrate for the peroxidase) and counterstained with hematoxylin aids this determination, lending a better view of glial nuclei. Reactive glia in a gangliocytoma show smaller, rounder, less angulated, and less crowded nuclei than neoplastic glia of giant-cell astrocytoma or ganglioglioma.

Within the sella, the main problem is recognition of gangliocytes among adenoma and adenohypophyseal cells. Gangliocytes are larger than these other cells, and their nuclei more prominent. If neuronal markers are used to confirm gangliocytes, choose markers that stain neurites like antineurofilament or Bielschowsky silver stain. Electron microscopy is most definitive in difficult cases.

Therapy and Clinical Outcome. Gangliocytomas eventually enlarge and grow over intervals of time. However, they grow extremely slowly. They are frequently controlled by surgery. Total removal is preferable, but not always possible near clinically sensitive hypothalamic structures.

2.1.2. Hypothalamic Hamartoma

Definition. Hypothalamic hamartoma is a mass of mature disorganized neural tissue that forms a tumor-like structure; however the lesion behaves more as a malformation than a neoplasm.

Location. Hypothalamic neuronal hamartomas are usually small, well-defined masses attached to the tuber cinereum, the mammillary bodies, or to the floor of the third ventricle; some are attached by a thin stalk. Rarely, they can be very large. An intrasellar neuronal hamartoma associated with growth hormone-producing pituitary adenoma containing amyloid was reported in a 63-yr-old man (1).

Clinical Features. Hamartomas may present with endocrine abnormalities, including precocious puberty, visual impairment, epilepsy, and behavioral abnormalities (2–8). Occasionally, they are associated with various developmental abnormalities, such as absent pituitary, polydactyly, Chiari I malformation, and others (5,6,9,10). A classification of the hypothalamic hamartomas into four subgroups was proposed recently (6). It was based on clinical and topographical data obtained from 42 selected cases.

Radiographic Features. MRI usually demonstrates a small, discrete, round mass of variable signal intensity, but very similar to gray matter (Figures 11,12). The lesion is characteristically stable, over long periods of time. Occasionally, the lesion demonstrates a rim of isointense signal with a hyperintense center on T2-weighted sequences (7). Contrast enhancement is usually poor, nearly identical to other gray matter.

Macroscopic Features. The small nodule has a rather smooth outer surface with a pale and smooth cut surface. Many hamartomas resemble gray matter.

Microscopic Features. Histologically, the lesion is formed by aggregates of mature neurons that vary in size and may be separated by bands of axons and glial cells (Figure 13). Binucleated ganglionic cells are extremely rare (8). Rarely, other tissues, for example, adipose tissue, are found included within (3).

Immunohistochemical and Ultrastructural Features. These features reflect glial and neuronal properties of the cells forming the lesion. Glia are GFAP positive. Neurons stain for neurofilaments and synaptophysin.

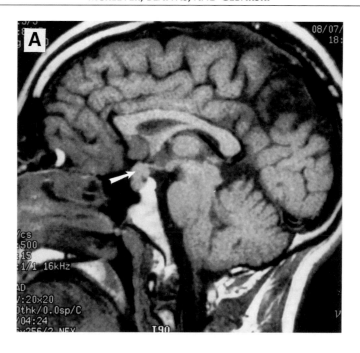

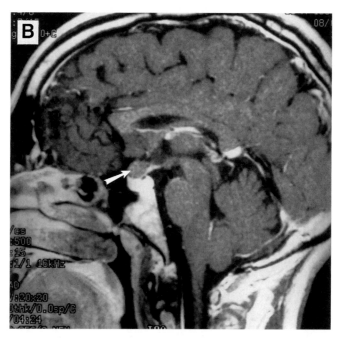

Figure 23-11 Sagittal MR images of a 39-yr-old man with a hypothalamic hamartoma. **(A)** T1-weighted MRI before contrast material. The hamartoma (arrow) extends from the tuber cinereum into the sella turcica anterior to the infundibulum. As is typical for these lesions, it has signal very similar to normal gray matter. **(B)** After iv contrast material is administered, the hamartoma (arrow) enhances to the same intensity as normal gray matter. The lush normal enhancement of the pituitary infundibulum and pituitary gland make these structures easy to separate from the hamartoma.

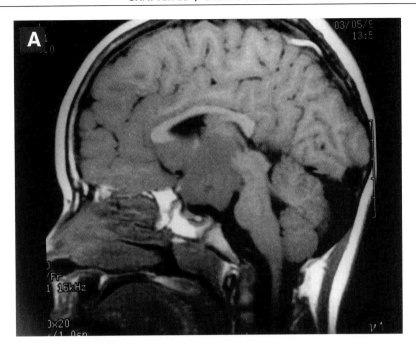

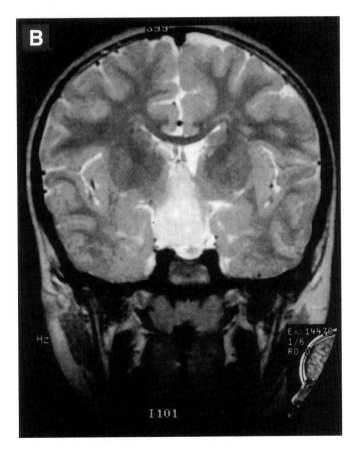

Figure 23-12 Brain MRI on a 5-yr-old boy with hypothalamic hamartoma. These hamartomas can attain very large dimensions, but always retain their nonaggressive character. (**A**) Sagittal noncontrast T1-weighted MRI shows the large gray matter intensity mass causing dramatic, but benign-appearing distortion of the sella turcica and diencephalon. (**B**) Coronal T2-weighted MRI through the hamartoma shows only slightly higher signal intensity than normal gray matter and some heterogeneity, as can be seen in these lesions. However, there is no invasion of surrounding brain, despite the large size of this lesion.

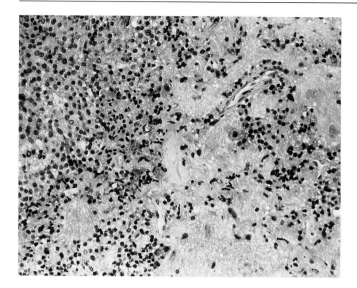

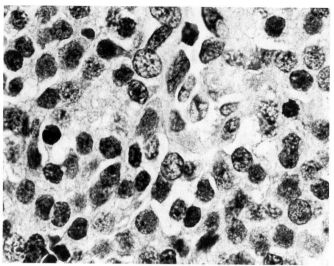

Figure 23-13 Hypercellular pituitary adenoma occupies one-half of the field, whereas the other half is a hypocellular lesion made of large, mature neurons on a fibrillary background. Small cells in between are glia along with some adenoma cells.

Figure 23-14 This olfactory neuroblastoma shows a few fibrillar cellular processes that distinguish it from small cell carcinoma and lymphoma. Round and pleomorphic nuclei crowd together. This and their high nuclear-to-cytoplasmic ratio produce a tumor that looks blue on H&E stain. This tumor invaded the ethmoid region and cribriform plate of a middle-aged man. From McKeever PE, Blaivas M, Sima AAF. Neoplasms of the sellar region. In: Lloyd RV, ed. Surgical Pathology of the Pituitary Gland. Major Problems in Pathology Series. Saunders, Philadelphia, 1993, pp. 141–210.

Asa and associates *(11)* reported a case of hamartoma accompanied by growth hormone-producing adenoma and suggested that the neurosecretory activity of the hamartoma induced the development of the adenoma. Scheithauer et al. *(2)* and Slowik et al. *(3)* suggested that secretory granules within the neuronal processes of hamartoma cells had the effect of growth hormone-releasing factor responsible for the adenoma development. In a similar case of Iwase and coworkers, some neuronal cells stained positively with S-100 and growth hormone-releasing factor *(1)*. On electron microscopy, neuronal processes with neurotubules interdigitated with adenoma cells.

Differential Diagnosis. Since the ectopic neural and glial tissue forming the hamartoma is normal in appearance, the major differential diagnosis is entrapped gray matter. Lack of normal gray matter organization is a helpful feature.

On the other hand, "the cytologic normality" helps to distinguish the hamartoma from a gangliocytoma and a ganglioglioma. The ganglioglioma contains binucleated, "smudged," or misshapen neurons, and frequently exhibits a cystic background and perivascular lymphocytic inflammation. Radiologic evidence of no enlargement for years or decades favors hamartoma.

Therapy and Clinical Outcome. Hypothalamic hamartomas are benign in their behavior. If the patient is symptomatic, surgical removal is curative. They are occasionally found incidentally postmortem or at the time of pituitary adenoma resection.

2.1.3. Olfactory Neuroblastoma

Definition. This tumor is also called esthesioneuroblastoma. It is a tumor composed of neuroblasts thought to arise from olfactory neurosensory epithelium.

Location. Olfactory neuroblastomas are usually found near the cribriform plate rostral to the sella in the superior portion of the nasal cavity among the olfactory sensory cells. Intracranial involvement is secondary to local extension from the cribriform plate, and less often by metastasis into the cranial vault *(1)*.

Olfactory neuroblastomas can occur primarily in the sellar and parasellar regions. This increases their likelihood of confusion with pituitary adenoma. Fortunately, this site of occurrence is rare *(2–4)*.

Clinical Features. Olfactory neuroblastomas occur in patients of all ages, but their peak incidences are during the second and sixth decades *(5)*. They usually cause epistaxis and nasal obstruction *(6)*. Clinical presentation reflects the extent of involvement of surrounding structures. Cranial nerve signs and symptoms occur *(2,6,7)*. An olfactory neuroblastoma has caused paraneoplastic Cushing's syndrome without invading the hypothalamus or pituitary *(8)*.

Radiographic Features. Radiographic and surgical anatomic information will frequently suggest the correct diagnosis. Tumors of mixed density are often large before discovery *(2,7,9,10)*. Tumors may grow on both sides of the cribriform plate producing a nasal mass and frontal lobe mass. Erosion of the cribriform plate, sinus walls, and other bones of the skull base occurs *(9,11)*. The bone lesions are more apparent on CT images than MRI. MRI is useful to define the soft tissue extension, especially regarding the degree of intracranial spread *(11)*. The sella may be rarely involved primarily. It is more often affected by secondary invasion from the nasal and anterior cranial fossa *(2,4)*. The mass is usually quite homogeneous, low signal on T2-weighted MRI, and usually shows lush contrast enhancement. CT shows modestly high density before contrast material is given, consistent with the lesion's high nuclear-to-cytoplasmic ratio.

Macroscopic Features. The tumor is gray and semitranslucent with many small vessels. Its consistency varies from soft to firm. Specimens may include respiratory mucosa or portions of skull invaded by tumor.

Microscopic Features. The olfactory neuroblastoma is a densely cellular neoplasm. Monotonous groups of small, round nuclei cluster between dissecting bands of fibrovascular stroma. Scant cytoplasm surrounds these nuclei that have minimal to moderate pleomorphism. The cells have fibrillary processes (Figure 14). This fibrillarity is critical to the diagnosis. It is evident on most cases stained with H&E *(12)*. Homer Wright rosettes or Flexner rosettes are often inconspicuous. When found, they are valuable diagnostic features. Mitotic indices vary substantially.

Fibrovascular stroma is highly variable. It can be very thick and resemble desmoplasia of carcinoma in some tumors, or it can be minimal *(13)*.

Immunohistochemistry and Special Stains. Olfactory neuroblastomas express neuroectodermal antigens *(10,13–18)*. Many have S-100 protein and Leu 7 reactivity, and all react with neuron-specific enolase *(13–15)*. The relatively broad specificity of these antigens includes other neoplasms like gliomas, choristomas, schwannomas, and ganglioma cell tumors. Neuronal markers like synaptophysin, neurofilament, β-tubulin, and microtubule-associated protein-2 have more restricted specificity. However, immunostaining does not detect each marker on all olfactory neuroblastomas *(13–15)*. If a panel of neuronal markers is used, at least one is usually positive *(15)*. Olfactory neuroblastomas have tyrosine hydroxylase *(10)*, occasionally express cytokeratin *(14)*, and rarely contain melanin pigment *(19)*.

Fibrillar cellular processes are an important feature of olfactory neuroblastoma cells. If crowded cells or fibrous stroma confound these features on H&E, S-100 protein or neuronal enolase stains that do not stain collagen will enhance them. More specific detection can be sought with silver stains for axons or antineurofilament stains. However, the former may crossreact with collagen, and the latter is not always positive. If reactivity is equivocal, the case should be examined ultrastructurally.

Ultrastructural Features. Electron microscopy reveals fibrillar cellular processes in olfactory neuroblastoma *(6,9,10,17,18,20–22)*. Cellular processes contain microtubles and filaments in a neuritic pattern *(22,23)*. Neurosecretory granules are variable in abundance. They average 180 nm in diameter *(9,10,21–23)*. A few tumors contain more specific structures that resemble immature olfactory vesicles *(9)*.

Differential Diagnosis. The more malignant SNUC must be distinguished from olfactory neuroblastoma. Small epithelioid cells form clusters and ribbons in the SNUC *(9,13,21,24)*, in contrast to fibrillar neuroblastoma cells. SNUC characteristically invades vessels. When present, Homer Wright rosettes with fibrillary cores or Flexner rosettes with central lumens rimmed by a distinct pink border distinguish the neuroblastoma. Neuroblastoma nuclei are more uniformly round than SNUC nuclei.

Neuronal markers plus S-100 protein are recommended to distinguish olfactory neuroblastoma from SNUC. Some neuroblastomas stain for S-100 protein, neurofilaments, or neurotubules, which SNUC lacks *(13–15)*. Synaptophysin is a sensitive marker for neuroblastoma, which can elucidate difficult cases. It can be found in virtually all olfactory neuroblastomas *(15)*.

Synaptophysin is relatively specific for neuronal cells, but will not distinguish olfactory neuroblastoma from a gangliocytoma, hypothalamic hamartoma, or ganglioneuroma. These tumors have lower cellular density than olfactory neuroblastoma, and are almost never found in the same location as olfactory neuroblastomas.

Other neoplasms that resemble olfactory neuroblastoma are lymphoma and melanoma, but these, too, only rarely show extension centered about the cribriform plate. These neoplasms lack the neuronal markers described above. Lack of fibrillar cellular processes and presence of lymphocytic markers distinguish lymphomas. Ultrastructural morphometry distinguishes them also *(25)*.

Leukocyte immunohistochemical markers like leukocyte common antigen (LCA) are recommended for difficult lymphomas *(26,27)*.

Melanomas are histochemically similar because they share S-100 reactivity and capability of melanin production with neuroblastomas *(14,19)*. Features on H&E like larger cells, nuclei, and nucleoli than neuroblastomas will identify most melanomas. Neurosecretory granules and neuronal markers revealed by ultrastucture or immunoperoxidase distinguish other neuroblastomas from melanoma.

Most pituitary adenomas have more cytoplasm and less cellular density than olfactory neuroblastoma. Aggressive adenomas and ectopic nasopharyngeal adenomas may cause confusion. Pituitary peptide hormone immunohistochemical markers are recommended to distinguish pituitary adenomas from neuroblastoma *(28)*.

Clinical Outcome. The prognosis of olfactory neuroblastoma is relatively good. Complete resection often results in a cure *(12,13)*. This outcome argues for considering these tumors as neuronal rather than embryonal neoplasms.

2.2. GLIAL TUMORS

2.2.1. Pilocytic Astrocytoma (Infundibuloma)

Definition. Pilocytic means hair-cell, referring to its long cytoplasmic processes. Pituitary astrocytomas of the sellar region originate from "pituicytes" of neurohypophysis and infundibulum and are usually pilocytic (Figure 15). Their histologic appearance is similar to that of pilocytic astrocytomas elsewhere in the brain *(1)*.

Location. Pilocytic astrocytomas of hypothalamus and optic chiasm (*see* Figures 16 and 17 in Subheading 2.2.2.), which spread to the sellar region, are much more common than pilocytic astrocytomas originating in posterior pituitary and infundibulum *(2,3,4)*. Jänisch noted a relatively higher proportion of eosinophilic astrocytomas in infancy than in later childhood *(5)*.

Clinical Features. The patients present with visual impairment, headache, occasionally dizziness, and as reported in one case, transient amnestic syndrome after spontaneous hemorrhage into the tumor *(3–6)*. Jänisch reported lateral ventricular hydrocephalus and di-encephalic emaciation or failure to thrive in infants with these neoplasms *(5)*.

Radiographic Features. CT and MRI show a globular or nodular enhancing mass that may have cystic components and infiltrate adjacent structures *(3,5,8)*. In a nonpilocytic astrocytoma in the neurohypophysis reported by Hurley and collaborators, the sellar mass with suprasellar extension was isointense on T1-weighted images, had moderate enhancement with gadolinium, and had an increased signal on proton-density-weighted and T2-weighted images *(7)*.

Macroscopic Features. Soft, vascular, pink, or gray fragments of tissue are usually recovered from surgery. They may be gelatinous and translucent.

Microscopic Features. The majority of neurohypophyseal and hypothalamic astrocytomas are pilocytic. They are characterized by a biphasic pattern of loose, microcystic regions occasionally of oligodendroglial-like cells displaying a perinuclear halo, and more compact areas with thick piloid fibers and Rosenthal fibers (Figures 15,18,19). However, Hurley and collaborators reported a pituicytoma in a 26-yr-old female that was not a pilocytic variant *(7)*. In their case, the tumor was hypercellular, with oval nuclei and prominent nucleoli, indistinct cell borders, moderate pleomorphism, and rich capillary network. There were no mitotic figures and no Rosenthal fibers.

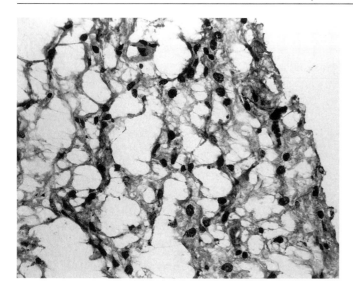

Figure 23-15 This hypocellular cystic pilocytic astrocytoma from the region of the infundibulum is composed of small astrocytic nuclei on a fibrillary background. Frozen section.

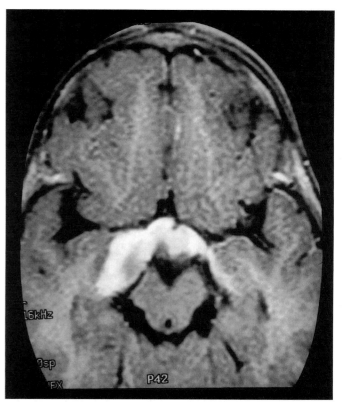

Figure 23-17 Brain MRI of a 1-yr-old girl with an optic glioma. On this axial post-iv contrast T1-weighted MRI, dramatic pathologic contrast enhancement is seen in the optic chiasm and bilateral optic tracts. Such enhancement characteristics are typical for pilocytic astrocytoma.

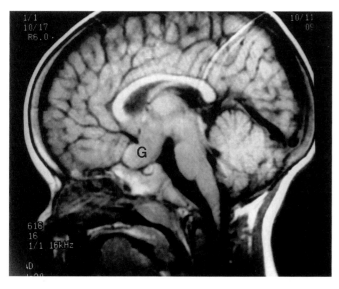

Figure 23-16 Brain MRI of a 2-yr-old girl with optic glioma. This noncontrast T1-weighted sagittal image dramatically shows extension of a large mass (G) along the path of the visual apparatus, typical for this lesion.

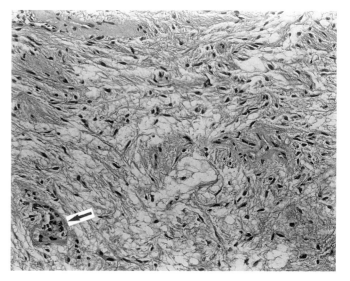

Figure 23-18 Optic nerve glioma from the chiasm of a young woman is filled with numerous fibrillar cellular processes, some aligned in parallel. Its cytologic features are those of a pilocytic astrocytoma. Cellular density is low. Some vascular walls are hypercellular (arrow).

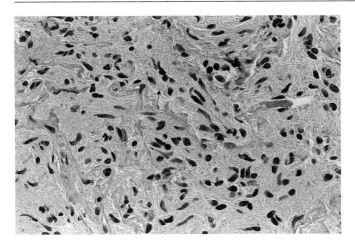

Figure 23-19 Optic nerve glioma contains light hyaline Rosenthal fibers (arrow), and dark spindled and oval nuclei speckled with fine chromatin.

Immunohistochemical, Ultrastructural, and Cytogenetic Features. The neoplastic cells usually stain positively for GFAP, vimentin, and S-100; and negatively for cytokeratin and epithelial membrane antigen (EMA). In a case of a nonpilocytic variant of astrocytoma, electron microscopy revealed two cell populations, some with electron-dense and some with lucent cytoplasm. There were intermediate filaments, broad cell junctions, and no secretory granules *(6)*.

In a study of 27 low-grade astrocytomas of childhood conducted by White and associates, hypothalamic pilocytic astrocytomas showed similar chromosomal changes to the pilocytic astrocytomas originating elsewhere in the central nervous system (CNS). These features constituted gains of chromosomes 7 and 8, and less commonly, chromosomes 4, 6, 11, 12, and 15 *(9)*.

Differential Diagnosis. In the presence of all typical histologic characteristics, the diagnosis of pilocytic astrocytoma poses no problem. When Rosenthal fibers are very scant or absent, the neoplasm can be classified as "consistent with pilocytic astrocytoma" *(9)*. Other differential diagnoses include grade II fibrillary astrocytoma, or higher-grade astrocytoma, if cell density and mitoses are prominent. Other entities under consideration in this location are granular cell tumor, ganglioglioma, hamartoma, and teratoma.

Clinical Outcome. Recent data support the previous observation that pilocytic astrocytomas rarely evolve into higher-grade astrocytomas *(9)*. Recent studies showed that attempting radical surgery in hypothalamic pilocytic astrocytomas (especially with spread to the adjacent parenchyma) carries significant risk. Treatment with chemotherapy with or without previous conservative surgery may provide a mean survival up to 10 yr *(8)*. It also allows one to delay local radiation that can be deleterious to the young developing brain *(10)*. Youth and the presence of neurofibromatosis type 1 predicted a more aggressive course in a series of 20 patients evaluated by Valdueza and coworkers *(3)*.

2.2.2. Optic Nerve Glioma

Definition. The vast majority of optic nerve gliomas are histologically benign pilocytic astrocytomas (*see* Subheading 2.2.1.), but malignant gliomas have been reported (*see* Subheading 2.2.3.). The nebulous term "optic glioma" is entrenched,

perhaps appropriately in this location where obtaining an adequate biopsy is difficult.

Location. These gliomas occur within optic nerve or optic chiasm. Tumor involving the optic chiasm may also involve the hypothalamus and third ventricle. It may not be possible to determine whether a large tumor originated in the optic pathway or in the hypothalamus.

Clinical Features. Optic nerve gliomas involve mostly young subjects *(1,2)*. Although most are histologically benign, their location compromises vision. Patients present with visual loss in one eye (optic nerve glioma) or both (chiasmatic glioma). Chiasmatic gliomas may cause hypothalamic symptoms. Orbital involvement causes proptosis *(3)*.

At least 10% of optic nerve gliomas are associated with von Recklinghausen's disease *(1,2)*. These gliomas are often multiple. Davis *(4)* reported that in approx 40% of the cases, there was bilateral involvement.

Malignant optic nerve gliomas are rare. Many of them evolve from optic gliomas associated with von Recklinghausen's disease *(5,6)*. Gliomas in adults exhibit more aggressive characteristics with rapid growth and infiltration of the temporal lobes and hypothalamus. They may display features of malignant astrocytomas.

The incidence of optic gliomas is approx 1% of all intracranial neoplasms. The incidence in pediatric materials is approx 4% since these tumors usually affect the younger population *(7)*.

Radiographic Features. Optic gliomas enlarge the nerve in which they grow. Their elongated vs round shape is governed by whether they are enclosed by the optic nerve sheath, or grow out into either the orbit or the hypothalamus (Figure 16). Like all pilocytic astrocytomas, they usually enhance well with iv contrast media *(8;* Figure 17).

Macroscopic Features. Optic nerve gliomas are gray and semitranslucent. Red vascular markings may be prominent. Consistency varies, but some are very soft and mucinous.

Microscopic Features. Optic nerve gliomas have the structure of compact pilocytic astrocytomas dissected by fibrovascular stroma, some of which may be residual trabeculae of the optic nerve. By 1993 World Health Organization (WHO) criteria, they are the lowest grade, grade I *(9)*. They extend fibrillar cellular processes of considerably higher density than their nuclei, imparting a pink tone on H&E stains (Figure 18). Cellular processes often gather in parallel bundles and may show diagnostically useful Rosenthal fibers. Protein granule degeneration may be seen in the cytoplasm. They may demonstrate microcystic regions or myxomatous changes, but they tend not to form large cysts *(10)*. Leptomeningeal invasion occurs, even from low-grade tumors. In von Recklinghausen's disease, optic gliomas tend to produce pronounced arachnoidal hyperplasia and extensive tumor infiltration of the leptomeninges *(4,5)*.

Nuclei are round to spindled with clear regions and finely stippled chromatin (Figure 19). Nuclei may be pleomorphic without changing their histologic grade from grade I *(9)*. Mitoses and nuclear crowding are uncommon, and suggest anaplastic change *(11)*. Proof of this rare event awaits evidence of widespread brain invasion or cerebrospinal metastasis. Histologic features of malignant nonpilocytic optic gliomas are described in Subheading 2.2.3.

Immunohistochemistry and Special Stains. The immunohistochemical stain for GFAP has supplanted others as the method of choice for identifying these gliomas *(12)*. Cells and their hair-like processes are highly GFAP-positive. Rosenthal fibers are only positive at their periphery, their central portion being immunoreactive for α-β-crystallin *(13,14)*. While eosinophilic granular bodies are reactive with the above reagents *(15)*, they are most easily and economically distinguished with PAS stain.

Ultrastructural Features. The neoplastic astrocytes and their cellular processes contain 7- to 8-nm intermediate filaments. Although these filaments are recognizable arranged like a bundle of hay grabbed in the hand, they are more definitively identified by a GFAP stain. Rosenthal fibers and eosinophilic granular bodies are electron-dense *(14,15)*.

Differential Diagnosis. Reactive gliosis is most likely to be confused with an optic glioma. Any irritation can produce gliosis, but craniopharyngioma is a particular menace here because of the fibrillary nature and considerable amount of gliosis it generates. Rosenthal fibers frequently accompany this gliosis. Careful radiologic interpretation and surgical sampling should preclude this problem, but the latter is compromised by the clinical sensitivity of this neuroanatomic region. An optic glioma may produce microcysts and mucinous degeneration not usually seen in gliosis, but this is not entirely reliable. This leaves the radiologist's interpretation and surgeon's *in situ* observations key to the diagnoses. In their absence, diagnostic certainty may be impossible unless epithelial tissue from craniopharyngioma is present in the specimen.

Ganglion cell tumors and hamartomas are a potential source of confusion. Since the optic nerve lacks neurons, this is only a concern with posterior growth of a chiasmatic tumor. Immunohistochemical staining with synaptophysin and neurofilament stains, followed by careful evaluation of the marked neurons for abnormal crowding, pleomorphism, and binucleated neurons is recommended. Pilocytic astrocytomas may trap hypothalamic neurons, but do not diffusely intermingle with them, a difference that can be appreciated on a GFAP stain. Hypothalamic hamartomas resemble hypothalamic gray matter and generally lack Rosenthal fibers.

Therapy and Clinical Outcome. Like pilocytic astrocytomas in other locations, optic nerve gliomas usually grow very slowly. Total excision and cure are often possible *(8)*. The clinical outcome of chiasmatic and adult forms is less favorable *(8,16–18)*. The prognosis of rare malignant optic gliomas is dismal.

2.2.3. High-Grade Glioma

Definitions. The commonly used term "high-grade glioma" refers to the grade of malignancy of a glial tumor (astrocytoma, oligodendroglioma, ependymoma, and their variants). The WHO brain tumor classification system is used here. Its grade I is the lowest grade of malignancy, and grade IV the highest. Anaplastic gliomas (grade III) and glioblastomas (grade IV) are considered to be high-grade gliomas.

High-grade gliomas around the sella are often associated with prior therapeutic radiation of a previous tumor, commonly craniopharyngioma or adenoma. Before a correlation between radiation and a second tumor is entertained, minimal criteria *(1–3)* pertain:

1. The second tumor should be located within the region irradiated.
2. The first and second tumors should be histologically different types.
3. Asymptomatic latency should be long enough to indicate that the second tumor was not present at the time of irradiation.

Location. Most spontaneous high-grade gliomas near the sella are reported arising from the optic nerve, chiasm, or tracts *(4–8)*. They are rarer than the lower-grade optic nerve glioma or pilocytic astrocytoma (Subheading 2.2.2.).

Postirradiation gliomas occur within the previous radiation field. Depending on the extent of this field, the glioma may arise in the optic chiasm, thalamus, basal ganglia, brainstem, ventral frontal or temporal lobe, or in other areas beyond the scope of this chapter *(9–12)*. Improvements in conformal radiotherapy should reduce the incidence of distant inadvertent radiotherapy-induced neoplasia.

Clinical Features. Spontaneous high-grade optic gliomas tend to occur in the adult to geriatric age groups *(6–8,13)*. Rapidly progressive unilateral or bilateral visual loss is often accompanied by periorbital discomfort or headaches *(5)*. Amaurosis may occur. With progression, hemiplegia may follow *(7)*.

Postirradiation gliomas usually occur 4–25 yr after radiation of a pituitary adenoma or craniopharyngioma *(2,3,9–11,14–21)*. The average latent interval is 10 yr. Total radiation doses range from 45 to 66 gy. One study suggests an incidence of 1% of the irradiated patient population at risk *(3)*. This 18-yr study (N. Shitara, personal communication) extrapolates to an estimated yearly incidence of over 50 gliomas/100,000 in this radiated population, or more than 15 times the baseline incidence of 2.8 gliomas/100,000 in the general population of Japan *(21a)*. Other studies estimate the relative risk of a second tumor at 9.4 times and 16 times greater than the general population *(22,23)*.

Symptoms of postradiation gliomas vary with the site of involvement, but they progress rapidly. Headache and visual or other functional deficits occur. Seizures accompany cerebral involvement.

Radiographic Features. Radiographic features are highly variable owing to locational and histopathologic differences between cases *(4,8,13)*. Generally, there is an abnormal mass that enhances with contrast media. MRI shows enhancement with gadolinium on T1-weighted images that may be brighter at the tumor periphery forming a "ring" of enhancement. The infiltrative neoplasm can enlarge as well as deform anatomic structures *(7)*. Tumor enlargement is frequently evident even within weeks of follow-up.

Macroscopic Features. Most high-grade gliomas are gray, stippled with red dots of intravascular blood, and fleshy or gelatinous *(24)*. Their margin with surrounding brain or optic nerve is indistinct. They may be cystic *(13)*.

Glioblastomas are more heterogeneous than anaplastic astrocytomas. They may contain friable, pale necrosis, brown recent hemorrhage, or yellow remote hemorrhage.

Microscopic Features. Most parasellar high-grade gliomas are astrocytic (glioblastomas and anaplastic astrocytomas). They have cells that extend fibrillar cytoplasmic processes. They are crowded with pleomorphic and hyperchromatic nuclei, some of which are spindled. Mitoses are evident. In addition to the above features, glioblastomas contain coagulation necrosis and/or proliferation of cells in vascular walls *(25; Figure 20)*.

Less common anaplastic oligodendrogliomas have rounder nuclei and less cellular processes than astrocytic gliomas *(2)*. They may contain necrosis and vascular proliferation.

The high-grade gliomas occurring after parasellar radiation are structurally similar to those in patients who have never received therapeutic radiation. However, surrounding tissue may show

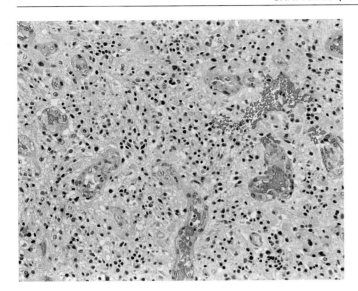

Figure 23-20   This glioblastoma occurred in the temporal lobe of an elderly man 8 yr following its irradiation. It is composed of numerous small fibrillar cells with mitoses. There is extensive proliferation of vascular wall cells.

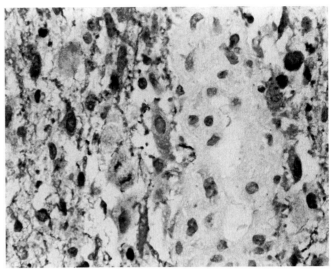

Figure 23-21   Same tumor as Figure 20 stained for GFAP. Parenchymal cells are GFAP-positive, but cells in vertical longitudinal section of vessel are negative.

evidence of prior radiation, including necrosis that particularly involves white matter, and vascular wall necrosis, hyalinization, or cavitation *(26)*.

Immunohistochemistry.   High-grade gliomas express GFAP (Figure 21). Anaplastic astrocytomas generally have the most immunoreactivity, and anaplastic oligodendrogliomas have less GFAP. Microgemistocytes in anaplastic oligodendrogliomas have globules of cytoplasmic GFAP near their round nuclei *(27)*. Glioblastomas vary widely from case to case in numbers of GFAP-positive cells, but will show at least focal GFAP immunoreactivity.

Ultrastructural Features.   Anaplastic astrocytomas and glioblastomas contain bundles of 7 nm intermediate filaments in their cytoplasm around nuclei and within cellular processes. Anaplastic oligodendrogliomas have clear, watery cytoplasm with few organelles. Scattered cells contain bundles of 7-nm intermediate filaments.

Differential Diagnosis.   Growth within the optic nerve and GFAP immunoreactivity distinguish the spontaneous malignant glioma of optic pathways from other malignancies affecting this region. Despite this, its rarity, aggressive growth, and inaccessibility have limited surgical diagnosis of this entity until recently *(4,6,7)*. It differs from the pilocytic astrocytoma of optic pathways by its hypercellularity, anaplastic nuclear features, mitoses, and when present, necrosis. Pilocytic astrocytomas have lower cellular density, more intense fibrillarity of cell processes often in bundles, distinctive Rosenthal fibers, and protein granule degeneration.

Clinical circumstances narrow the differential of postirradiation high-grade gliomas. Recurrent previously treated tumor is a consideration. Nearly all first tumors were either GFAP-negative pituitary adenomas or craniopharyngiomas. Pituitary hormone and chromogranin further identify the adenoma, whereas the craniopharyngioma is distinctively epithelial by light and electron microscopy. Second tumors, other than high-grade glioma, include sarcoma and meningioma, both of which lack GFAP found in the glioma.

Clinical Outcome.   The combination of aggressive and infiltrative neoplasm, late presentation, plus clinically sensitive and therapeutically hazardous location join to produce a dismal prognosis *(7,8)*. Malignant optic gliomas generally produce bilateral blindness followed by death within a year *(5,8)*.

Spontaneous gliomas have more therapeutic options than postirradiation gliomas. One study advocates aggressive radiation and chemotherapy treatment protocols to prolong the survival of these patients *(28)*.

2.2.4. Granular Cell Tumor (GCT)

Definition.   The GCT is usually a benign lesion of Schwann cell origin or heterogeneous cell origin with common morphologic features and immunophenotype that reflect abundant intracellular lysosomes.

Location.   The GCT arises most commonly from the head and neck region and is the most frequent intrinsic tumor of the neurohypophysis and infundibulum. Small GCTs are found incidentally in 1–6.5% of autopsies *(1,2)*. The incidence becomes even higher, up to 17%, if serial sections of hypophysis are examined *(3)*.

Clinical Features.   Incidental small aggregates of granular cells found in the neurohypophysis or lower portion of the pituitary stalk are usually clinically asymptomatic. When they enlarge and compress the pituitary, optic chiasm, or hypothalamus, headaches, visual disturbances, or hypopituitarism develop. Diabetes insipidus and hydrocephalus are less common. Symptomatic tumors occur most frequently in women in the fourth and fifth decades *(4)*. GCT is usually a single tumor; however, recently, a case of multiple (124 lesions) skin GCTs in an 11-yr-old girl was reported *(5)*. They were associated with face and skull defects, EEG and other neurologic abnormalities, diffuse hypotonia, and pulmonary stenosis.

Radiological Features   The GCT is a well-circumscribed, homogeneous, vascular, intrasellar, or suprasellar mass that enhances with contrast on CT and produces a vascular blush on angiography *(6)*. In a rare case of malignant GCT, CT showed a large, soft tissue mass in the infratemporal fossa that caused destruction

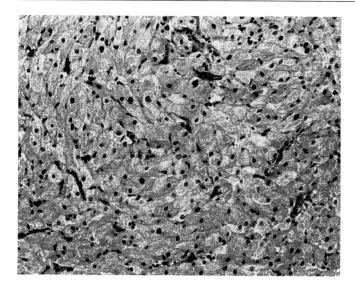

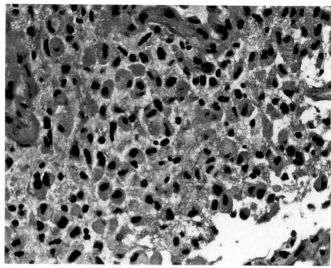

Figure 23-22   The granular cell tumor is formed by sheets of cells with distinctly granular cytoplasm and small, rounded nuclei with no mitotic figures.

Figure 23-23   This anaplastic astrocytoma arising from the temporal lobe has rounded cell bodies with granular cytoplasm and pleomorphic nuclei.

of the mandible and involved the floor of the left orbit and the cavernous sinus *(7)*.

Macroscopic Features.   To a neurosurgeon, GCT is a "tough, nonsuckable, vascular tumor" *(6)*. The surgical specimen is usually a small, firm, gray or tan, and spherical or lobulated nodule. A malignant GCT is also firm and solid *(5)*.

Microscopic Features.   The GCT is a nonencapsulated tumor nodule composed of compactly arranged large cells with granular cytoplasm (Figure 22). Luse and Kernohan recognized three distinct patterns. The first and most common in the neurohypophysis is a sharply demarcated nodule formed by irregular columns of large, irregularly polygonal cells around thin-walled vessels *(3)*. Abundant eosinophilic cytoplasm is filled with fine and coarse granules. The small, round, or oval nuclei contain small nucleoli. A second, less frequent pattern is remarkable for poor demarcation of the tumor and arrangement of the cells in irregular strands. The cells are elongated, with large nuclei, irregular in shape, coarse chromatin, and prominent nucleoli. Indistinct plasmalemmal outlines create a syncytial appearance. The third pattern was only seen in two tumors of the pituitary stalk in which large, sharply circumscribed nodules were formed by slender elongated granular cells with blurred cytoplasmic outlines and small elongated nuclei. The cells whorled around small vessels. Mitotic figures were not found in any of these patterns.

Several cases of malignant GCT have been reported *(8,9)*. A malignant GCT of the infratemporal fossa was composed of solid sheets of pleomorphic, polygonal, or fusiform cells with eccentric vesicular nuclei and occasional prominent nucleoli *(7)*. Up to four mitotic figures per high-power field were commonly seen along with tumor necrosis and perineural/intraneural invasion. Features associated with malignant behavior included necrosis, marked nuclear pleomorphism with hyperchromasia, and any mitotic activity. These tumors were also much larger in size and poorly circumscribed. The latter feature appears to be relevant only to the intracranial GCT, since even benign ones elsewhere in the body can have indistinct margins *(7)*.

Immunohistochemical and Ultrastructural Features.
Cytoplasmic granules in all GCT, intracerebral or elsewhere

in the body, stain positively with PAS. In general, the neoplastic cells react strongly with S-100 protein, NSE, vimentin, KP1(CD68), and in some cases with α-1-antitrypsin and lectins *(10–14,15)*.

In malignant GCT, α-1-antitrypsin and KP1 were negative *(7)*. Three cases of congenital GCT reported by Filie and coworkers were negative for S-100 protein and NSE, suggesting a different origin of this tumor compared to the adult GCT that is presumed to be of Schwann cell origin *(15)*. Other markers, such as keratin, desmin, smooth muscle actin, CD57, CD15, HMB45, myoglobin, and MAC387, were negative *(15–17)*.

Intracerebral GCT are rare and in most cases stain negatively with S-100 protein and vimentin; however, in some cases, S-100 and even GFAP stained positively *(13,14)*. This occasional GFAP positivity is a reflection of heterogeneity of GCT. Granular cells are encountered in a variety of neoplastic and nonneoplastic lesions in different body sites. Oligodendrogliomas, intracranial schwannomas, astrocytomas (Figure 23), and meningiomas occasionally contain foci of granular cells *(15)*. The latter were considered to be of degenerative nature. Uncommon hemispheric tumors composed predominantly or exclusively of granular cells are variably GFAP-positive and are considered to be astrocytomas with granular cell differentiation *(15,16,17a)*. A temporal lobe anaplastic astrocytoma with granular cell differentiation demonstrated positive GFAP and S-100 staining, and negative EMA *(17)*, whereas five hemispheric astrocytomas (two low-grade and three anaplastic) reported by Geddes and coauthors expressed diffuse cytoplasmic EMA staining with no true membrane staining *(15a)*. The authors concluded that "the granular change is a degenerative phenomenon that, like lipidization, can occur in tumors of different cell type *(15a)*."

Ultrastructurally, the tumor cells contain numerous membrane-bound autophagic vacuoles with myelin figures and other cellular debris. In cases of astrocytomas with granular cell differentiation, intracytoplasmic filaments were also identified *(15a,16,17a)*. In GCT of Schwann cell origin, incomplete basal lamina was present *(7)*.

Differential Diagnosis.   Because of its location and clinical presentation, GCT of sellar and adjacent regions is easily mistaken

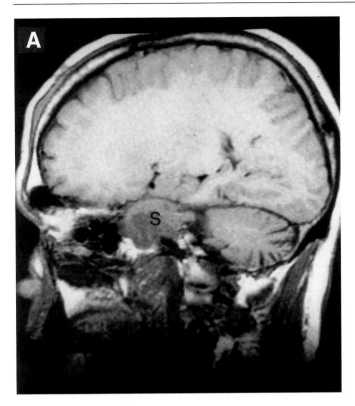
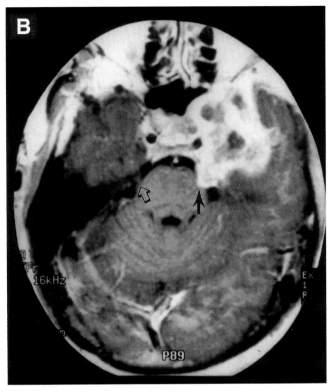

Figure 23-24 Brain MRI of a 44-yr-old man with a cavernous sinus schwannoma. Schwannomas can be difficult to differentiate from meningiomas on MRI since both can present as inhomogeneous, brightly enhancing masses centered about the cavernous sinus. However, noncontrast CT usually shows higher attenuation in meningiomas compared to schwannomas, and there is also usually a more fusiform contour of the schwannoma as it follows the involved cranial nerve. In this case, MRI shows this fusiform nature best on sagittal imaging. **(A)** Sagittal, noncontrast, T1-weighted image showing the schwannoma (S). The fusiform nature of this lesion along the path of the fifth cranial nerve is apparent. **(B)** The lesion is invasive, extending into the sella turcica and sphenoid sinus in this axial image obtained after iv contrast. There is a rather distinctive protuberance of mass (arrow) extending along the cisternal path of the fifth nerve, the nerve of origin for this neoplasm. This is typical for schwannoma, but unusual for meningioma. For comparison, look at the normal cisternal portion of the right fifth nerve (open arrow).

for adenoma, craniopharyngioma, or optic glioma. In cases of astrocytoma with granular cell differentiation, a small biopsy can be confused with an infarct, demyelinating disease, or a metastatic carcinoma *(15a)*. Adequate sample size and special stains with or without the addition of electron microscopy will aid in the diagnosis.

Clinical Outcome. GCT is usually a benign tumor, with only about 36 malignant cases reported *(7–9)*. The malignant GCT recurs locally and also metastasizes to regional lymph nodes and lungs as the most common sites *(7)*. Generally, GCT is not radiosensitive. However effective radiation treatment of one extracranial GCT was reported *(17)*.

2.2.5. Schwannoma

Definition. Most commonly a benign neoplasm, the schwannoma is formed by Schwann cells with spindled or small, rounded nuclei arranged in two distinct patterns, Antoni A and Antoni B. Their nonneoplastic counterparts surround axons in the peripheral nervous system.

Location. Intracranial schwannomas most commonly arise in the 8th cranial nerve and, less frequently, in the 5th and 7th cranial nerve *(1)*. Occasionally, they originate from the 9th and 3rd nerves *(1,2)*. Only a few sellar region schwannomas have been reported *(3–6)*. In one case, the tumor was located in the tuberculum sellae *(5)*, and in the other one, it arose from the trigeminal nerve and extended in a suprasellar direction *(6)*. Two of five

nasopharyngeal schwannomas extended into the middle cranial fossa *(7)*. An unusual case of intracerebral schwannoma with enlargement of the sella was reported by Ghatak and collaborators *(8)*.

Clinical Features One intrasellar schwannoma presented with panhypopituitarism, whereas in another endocrine dysfunction was absent *(3,4)*. A patient with intracerebral schwannoma accompanied by sellar enlargement presented with seizures followed by hemiparesis, visual disturbances, facial weakness, and other symptoms *(8)*. Progressive visual loss was also reported in a case of cystic schwannoma involving the sphenoid sinus and base of the skull *(9)*, and in nasopharyngeal schwannomas invading the ethmoid and sphenoid sinuses *(7)*.

Radiologic Features. Parasellar schwannomas often follow cranial nerves as a fusiform tumor (Figure 24). Routine skull roentgenograms of a 63-yr-old woman with intracerebral schwannoma showed erosion of the posterior clinoid processes and enlargement of the sella turcica. A radionuclide brain scan revealed an area of increased uptake in the right deep parietal area *(8)*. In a case of ethmoid sinus and nasal cavity schwannoma, on MRI there was a 3 × 4 cm mass with low signal intensity on the T1-weighted images and high signal intensity on the T2-weighted images with moderate homogeneous enhancement after Gadolinium injection *(7,10)*.

Macroscopic Features. The tumors are usually firm in consistency and yellowish-tan in color. The one in the ethmoid sinus was friable (10). The aforementioned intracerebral schwannoma presented as a solid, granular tumor with yellowish concretions on the surface lying within a large cyst (8).

Microscopic Features. The histologic appearance of schwannoma is quite standard regardless of location. Two types of cellular arrangement are recognized, of which Antoni A type usually predominates and is formed by interwoven bundles of spindled cells occasionally arranged in palisades (Verocay bodies). The Antoni B type is looser and myxoid. Small vessels usually have thick, hypocellular, hyalinized walls and sometimes are clustered together. Nuclear pleomorphism may be prominent, but in the absence of mitotic figures, it is considered to be degenerative or "ancient" change (3,5,10). These regressive changes occasionally extend to focal calcification and ossification (8).

Nasopharyngeal schwannomas invading the middle cranial fossa in the series of Hasegawa et al. were more cellular than usual and lacked an identifiable capsule (7). Benhaiem-Sigaux and coworkers reported an unusual epithelioid variant of schwannoma arising in the acoustic nerve (11). Only two other cases of intracranial epithelioid schwannoma existed in the literature prior to their paper. Histologically, besides well-recognizable features of schwannoma with Antoni A and B areas and thick hylanized vessels, there were clear, large, polygonal epithelioid cells isolated or in small cords or islets. The epithelioid component predominated over spindle-cell tumor.

A cystic schwannoma with large portions of the tumor occupied by Antoni B region involving the sphenoid sinus was reported by DiNardo and Mellis (9).

Immunohistochemical and Ultrastructural Features. Schwannomas express strong positivity for S-100 protein. In some series, they were also positive for Leu-7 and KP1 (CD68) (10,12). No difference was found in immunoreactivity for KP1 or S-100 protein in Antoni A compared to Antoni B areas. A few cases also stained positively for GFAP (12).

Epithelioid schwannoma showed strong positivity for S-100 protein in the cytoplasm of both Schwann cells and epithelioid cells. Vimentin, GFAP, Leu-7, EMA, NSE, HMB45 and cytokeratin were negative in both cell types (11).

Differential Diagnosis. Sellar schwannomas can be misinterpreted as meningioma, chordoma, or myxoma when the cystic Antoni B portion is prominent. A case of cystic schwannoma involving the sphenoid sinus was diagnosed initially as a destructive myxoma (9). Immunopositivity for S-100 protein distinguished schwannoma from myxoma microscopically.

In cases of epithelioid schwannoma, the differential diagnosis with a melanoma or carcinoma may be difficult; however, negative Fontana, PAS and anti-HMB45 staining rule out malignant melanoma, whereas absence of cytokeratin staining rules out metastatic carcinoma (11).

Clinical Outcome. In order to reverse or alleviate symptoms, complete or *en bloc* removal was achieved in the cases of sphenoid sinus cystic schwannoma, intracerebral schwannoma with enlargement of the sella turcica, sphenoid sinus and nasal cavity schwannoma, and epithelioid schwannoma (8–11). With 1-yr of follow-up, the above patients retained some minor clinical symptoms but showed no radiologic recurrence.

3. MENINGEAL TUMORS

3.1. MENINGIOMA

3.1.1. Definition. This is a tumor composed of meningeal cells from the membranes that cover the brain and spinal cord.

3.1.2. Location. Meningiomas arise in the dura and arachnoid membranes, are uncommon in choroid plexus, and are rare within CNS tissue. Their distribution at different meningeal sites is not random. Sites around the sella are frequent sites of occurrence of meningiomas (1–4). Olfactory, suprasellar, and parasellar meningioma together comprise 14% of parapituitary tumors (5). Olfactory meningiomas occur near the cribriform plate and olfactory grove, parasellar meningiomas occur in the medial sphenoid wing or the lateral portion of the sella turcica, and suprasellar meningiomas attach to the tuberculum sellae.

Suprasellar meningiomas have attracted special attention (3,4,6–8). They represent between 5 and 10% of all meningiomas (6–8). They may arise from arachnoid cells of the villous processes of the venous sinuses (9), which surround the hypophysis under the diaphragma sellae. They occur at the diaphragma sellae, tuberculum sellae, under the optic nerve, or laterally or behind the infundibulum anterior to the dorsum sellae (10,11).

3.1.3. Clinical Features. The peak incidence of suprasellar meningiomas occurs in females between 30 and 39 yr of age, and in males between 50 and 59 yr of age (4). Meningiomas are more common in women at a ratio of about 3:2 (12), and in suprasellar meningiomas, a ratio of 4:1 (3,6,8).

Most suprasellar meningiomas present with chiasmal syndrome, consisting of primary optic atrophy and bitemporal hemianopsia with a normal sella turcica and no endocrinopathy (3,6,7). Anosmia and involvement of the 3rd, 4th, 5th, and 6th nerves and mental changes are more prominent with olfactory and parasellar meningioma (1,3). Anterior clinoid meningiomas produce oculomotor problems of gradual onset (13).

Intrasellar meningiomas may present with galactorrhea and amenorrhea, suggesting a "stalk sign," a hypothalamic–pituitary dysfunction with inhibition of prolactin inhibitory factor (14). Others lack endocrine symptoms, growing larger until visual symptoms occur (15,16).

Rare meningiomas occur after radiation. Their numbers are so low and meningiomas so common that it is difficult to rule out incidental association. Twenty years after radiation for a chromophobe adenoma, one patient developed an orbital roof meningioma (17).

3.1.4. Radiographic Features. Meningiomas are, generally, quite vascular, and usually enhance with contrast media. On MRI, they generally do not displace the pituitary (18). They are often isointense with gray matter on T1-weighted MRI images (19). Globular meningiomas often show an extension of contrast enhancement along the dura called a "tail sign." This tissue often shows meningioma trailing off into reactive dural thickening. Cavernous sinus meningiomas may involve local vessels and nerves (Figure 25). Other tumors grow along the dura producing a thick, flat tumor called meningioma *en plaque*. These tend to occur along the sphenoid ridge. MRI is the modality of choice in evaluating the parenchyma of suprasellar meningiomas (20), but CT better defines bone involvement.

Accompanying hyperostosis of underlying bone is a common feature of suprasellar meningiomas (49%) and olfactory meningiomas (62%) (4). Hyperostosis and blistering are best demonstrated by CT (21). Parasellar meningiomas often invade nearby structures. In a series of 24 meningiomas of the lateral sella turcica, 14 invaded the cavernous sinus and 8 invaded the sella turcica (2).

3.1.5. Macroscopic Features. Most meningiomas are gray with prominent vascular markings. Their consistency varies from

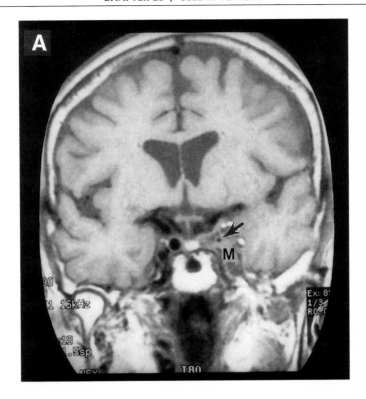

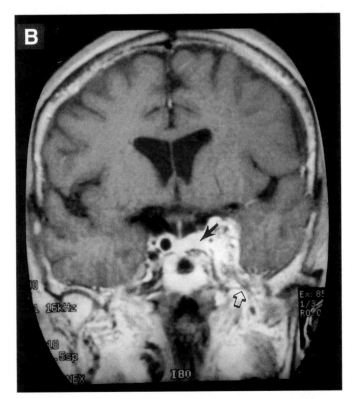

Figure 23-25 Brain MRI of a 74-yr-old woman with meningioma. **(A)** Precontrast T1-weighted imaging of a cavernous sinus meningioma (M) shows the invasive nature of the lesion, encasing and narrowing the internal carotid artery (arrow). **(B)** After iv contrast is administered, rather homogeneous pathologic contrast enhancement of the lesion is shown, including its extension into the sella turcica (arrow). There is also some extension of the lesion along the mandibular division of the fifth nerve (open arrow).

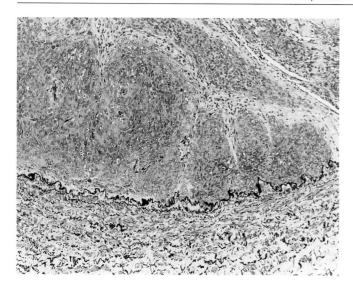

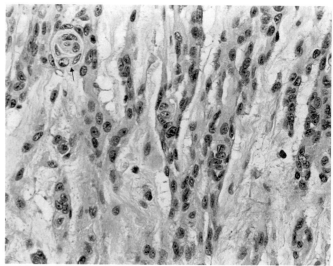

Figure 23-26 Meningothelial meningiomas resemble a syncytium. They are common in the skull base near the sella. This meningioma grew *en plaque* in the skull base, and occluded the arterial lumen while leaving the vascular wall and its dark wavy elastin (below) intact. Movat's pentachrome stain. From McKeever PE, Blaivas M, Sima AAF. Neoplasms of the sellar region. In: Lloyd RV, ed. Surgical Pathology of the Pituitary Gland. Major Problems in Pathology Series. Saunders, Philadelphia, 1993, pp. 141–210.

Figure 23-27 This chordoid meningioma from the skull base of an adult man resembles chordoma except for its small meningothelial whorls (arrow) and nuclear features.

soft to firm with increasing collagen content. Meningothelial meningiomas are softer than fibrous meningiomas. Calcifications in some tumors make them gritty on slicing. The surfaces of meningiomas are smooth or bosselated. Yellow lipid or gelatinous mucin content is not common in meningiomas near the sella *(3,6,13–16)*.

3.1.6. Microscopic Features. This tumor has many variants. Collections of cases around the sella suggest the same variety as seen elsewhere *(3,4,6–8,11,13,15)*. Among these variants, certain features provide strong evidence of meningioma *(22)*. For example, a "syncytial" pattern is distinctive (Figure 26). It is the characteristic pattern of meningothelial meningiomas and is evident focally in other types.

Cellular whorls characterize the meningioma (Figure 27). Whorls are concentric clusters of flat cells that resemble cabbage leaves or onion bulbs *(23)*. Whorls are prominent in transitional meningiomas, and focal in other types.

Psammoma bodies are concentrically laminated calcifications. They predominate in psammomatous meningioma, and occur focally in other types. They are particularly useful for diagnosis around the sella when surrounded by flat cells.

The nuclei of meningiomas vary with individual types from oval to spindled. Intranuclear cytoplasmic inclusions are common. Sharp nuclear angulations and conspicuous mitoses are not present, except in aggressive variants of WHO grade higher than grade I *(24)*. These are rare around the sella.

Studies show that the more common meningothelial, fibroblastic, and transitional variants of meningioma are well represented in and around the sella, as they are at other locations *(3,4,6–8,11,13,15)*. The meningothelial (endotheliomatous, syncytial) meningioma is the prototypic "syncytial" meningioma (Figure 26). Individual boundaries between the cells are not seen on paraffin sections. Its nuclei are typically oval, often with cytoplasmic inclusions. Whorls and psammoma bodies are generally sparse.

Meningothelial meningioma is a headache in the sella, as it were, because it resembles pituitary adenoma.

Fibroblastic (fibrous) meningiomas are composed of flat cells with spindled nuclei. Their nuclei are more hyperchromatic than in the meningothelial variant. Their stroma is collagenous, often showing conspicuously thick bundles of collagen that may calcify.

Transitional meningiomas are the easiest meningioma to identify. They contain both syncytial and fibroblastic elements. Most show whorls, psammoma bodies, and clusters of "syncytial" cells.

Psammomatous meningioma are found near the sella *(3)*. They contain mostly concentrically laminated psammoma bodies with syncytial cells filling spaces between the conspicuous psammoma bodies.

The presence of rare and new variants of meningioma in or around the sella is incompletely documented. There is ample room for scholarly reports about these. A very unusual granular suprasellar meningioma had clusters of granular cells *(25)*. These were negative for both GFAP and S-100 excluding astrocyte or Schwann cell derivation. (Granular meningioma is the most common spontaneously occurring meningeal tumor in rats *[26]*.) A suprasellar lymphoplasmacyte-rich meningioma featured nests and cords of epithelial cells with prominent cytoplasm among fibrous stroma *(27)*. Surprisingly, it expressed GFAP, a glial marker, in addition to standard epithelial membrane antigen and vimentin markers found in meningiomas.

Unique to the sellar region is occurrence of a parasellar meningioma with a pituitary adenoma *(28)*. Among seven confirmed cases that share these two tumors, four were meningotheliomatous meningiomas of the sphenoid ridge or the tuberculum sellae which occurred together with nonsecreting chromophobe adenomas *(28–31)*, two fibroblastic meningiomas with eosinophilic adenomas *(32,33)*, and one transitional meningioma with a chromophobe adenoma *(34)*. The two neoplasms were located in proximity to each other in five of these cases. No causal relationship between these two tumors has been proven.

3.1.7. Immunohistochemistry, Cytogenetics, and Special Stains. Most meningiomas contain epithelial membrane antigen, at least focally *(35)*. The high intensity of vimentin expres-

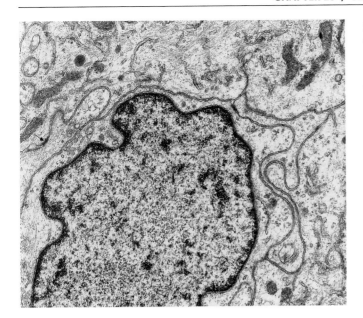

Figure 23-28 This recurrent meningothelial meningioma of the skull base has the typical ultrastructural appearance of dark, fuzzy desmosomes (arrow) "stapling" together its interdigitated cellular processes. Uranyl acetate and lead citrate; × 16,300. From McKeever PE, Blaivas M. In: Sternberg S, Antonioli D, Kempson R, Carter D, Eggleston J, Oberman HA, eds. Diagnostic Surgical Pathology, vol. 1, Raven, New York, 1989, pp. 357–359.

sion by meningiomas has stimulated its use on these tumors. This should be done only in combination with other markers, since many other tumors express vimentin. Expression of S-100 protein by meningiomas is highly variable *(36)*. Partial or complete loss of chromosome 22 is the most common cytogenetic abnormality.

Meningiomas contain a variable amount of parenchymal reticulin and fibrous tissue *(22)*. Fibrous meningiomas have the most collagen, detectable with Masson's trichrome stain.

3.1.8. Ultrastructural Features.   The ultrastructural basis of the so-called syncytial features of meningiomas are numerous tightly interdigitating cellular processed joined by desmosomes (Figure 28). These hold meningioma cells tightly together during tissue processing. The distinctive appearance of these structures and the dearth of specific histochemical and immunohistochemical markers of meningioma cells maintain electron microscopy as an important alternative for the diagnosis of difficult cases *(37)*. In the sella, this particularly helps to confirm the meningothelial type of meningioma.

3.1.9. Differential Diagnosis.   In the sella, pituitary adenoma is a major source of confusion with meningothelial meningioma. Granular cytoplasm suggests adenoma on H&E stains, but is not entirely reliable, and is complicated by the granular meningioma *(25)*. Similarly, syncytial features suggest meningioma, but whorls are more definitive, when present. Since some adenomas calcify, psammoma bodies are only distinctive when surrounded by flat meningioma cells.

Chromogranin and pituitary peptide hormone immunohistochemical stains distinguish pituitary adenomas from all meningiomas, including meningothelial types. These should be applied as a battery of stains, such as prolactin, growth hormone, adrenocorticotrophic hormone, and chromogranin, since individual adenomas are positive for only one or two of these markers. Electron

microscopy is an attractive alternative, distinguishing adenomas containing secretory granules, prominent RER and large Golgi apparatus from meningiomas with interdigitating cellular processes.

Specific types of meningioma invite other possible sources of confusion. Chordoid meningiomas resemble chordomas *(22;* Figure 27). Fibroblastic meningiomas resemble schwannomas and fibromas. Whorls confirm meningioma, when present. Ultrastructural demonstration of interdigitating cellular processes joined by desmosomes distinguishes meningiomas. Alternatively, chordomas contain mitochondrial–rough endoplasmic reticular complexes, and schwannoma cells are enveloped with basement membrane material *(22,37,38)*. Meningiomas have epithelial membrane antigen that fibromas lack and usually less S-100 protein than schwannomas.

The majority of meningiomas in and near the sella are histologically benign. They lack the mitotic activity, monotonous regions of undifferentiated cells, and necrosis of atypical meningiomas, plus anaplasia and brain invasion evident in malignant meningiomas. However, individual cases with some, but not all of these features have been reported in the pituitary *(39)*.

Hemangiopericytomas must be distinguished from meningioma. These tumors are more densely cellular than benign meningiomas. They compress their internal vessels as they grow and distort their lumens into odd shapes. They usually lack whorls, but they do have regions of pericellular basement membrane material that highlights with PAS or reticulin stains *(22)*.

3.1.10. Therapy and Clinical Outcome.   Meningiomas are benign, encapsulated tumors that can be entirely removed surgically from most intracranial locations. However, around the sella, surgical removal can be more difficult. Meningiomas that involve the tuberculum sellae are hard to approach and to dissect away from the pituitary stalk *(40)*. Meningiomas involving the inferior leaf of the diaphragma sellae require repair of the sphenoid sinus to prevent CSF leakage *(40)*. Suprasellar and optic nerve meningiomas create a serious risk of eventual blindness *(41)*.

4. MESENCHYMAL TUMORS

4.1. CHORDOMA

4.1.1. Definition.   The chordoma is a locally invasive tumor that resembles embryonic notochord. The notochord is a rod of mesoblastic tissue below the primitive groove of the embryo in the region destined to become the craniospinal axis. Chordomas may arise from remnants of notochord in the clivus or dorsum sellae called ecchordosis physaliphora.

4.1.2. Location.   Chordomas are common in and around the sella. Five percent of neoplasms in the region of the sella were chordomas in one series *(1)*. Parasellar chordomas represent at least a third of all chordomas *(2,3)*. The clivus and sphenoid regions correspond with the most cranial portion of the notochord at the spheno-occipital synchondrosis where notochordal remnants have been found in 2% of autopsies *(3,4)*. Clival chordomas often occur in younger individuals than chordomas elsewhere, but most chordomas occur in adults *(2,3)*. Chordomas can be confined within the sella *(5,6)*. This increases their likelihood of confusion with adenoma. Fortunately, totally intrasellar chordomas are rare.

4.1.3. Clinical Features.   Diplopia and visual field abnormalities are frequent symptoms. Facial paralysis and dysphagia result from tumor compression of other cranial nerves. Headaches and vomiting can occur *(2,3)*. A nasopharyngeal mass signals invasion of this region *(7)*.

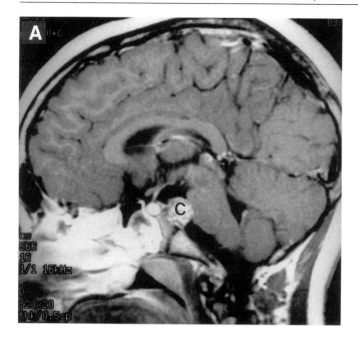
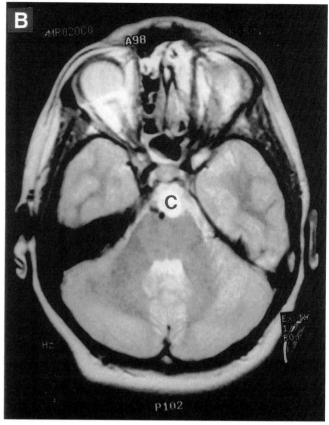

Figure 23-29 Brain MRI of an 11-yr-old girl with a chordoma. This case illustrates the ability of the chordoma to appear anywhere along the path of the notochord, which terminates at the level of the dorsum sellae and may even have rests in the meninges just above this region. **(A)** Sagittal postcontrast, T1-weighted MR image showing the chordoma (C) destroying the dorsum sellae and distorting the pons. The lush pathologic contrast enhancement is typical for this lesion. **(B)** T2-weighted axial MR image shows the very high T2 signal contained within this lesion (C), typical of this chondroid matrix neoplasm.

4.1.4. Radiographic Features. Diagnostically useful radiographic features include erosion of the tip of the clivus, and usually frank osteolytic changes *(2,8,9)*. Chordomas destroy bone of the clivus and sella, distinguishing them from many other tumors *(3,7;* Figure 29). Chordomas can compress the internal carotid artery and alter its location *(10)*. Some chordomas erode the clivus and grow into the sphenoid sinus or nasopharynx *(7)*. CT usually shows a partially "cystic" or necrotic-appearing aggressive mass with mixed, but usually, at least partially, intense contrast enhancement (Figure 30). MRI shows very distinctive, markedly high T2 signal, typical for chondroid matrix tumors (Figure 29B).

4.1.5. Macroscopic Features. Chordomas are multilobular, gelatinous, and myxoid. Clival chordomas rarely bleed spontaneously *(8,11)*. Bone erosion is evident *in situ*.

4.1.6. Microscopic Features. Cords of physaliphorous cells line up like beads on string (Figure 31). The vacuoles in these cells vary in size up to a whole-cell diameter. Many are larger than macrophage vacuoles. In contrast to perinuclear oligodendroglial vacuoles, they contain mucin and lie beside cellular nuclei. Physaliphorous cells are recognizable on fine-needle aspiration or CSF cytology specimens *(12,13)*. Immunocytochemistry and electron microscopy augment interpretation of cytologic specimens that resemble well-differentiated adenocarcinoma *(12,14,15)*.

Chordomas contain a myxoid and mucinous extracellular matrix, which stains with Alcian blue. Although it stains like mucin, this material is probably a highly glycosylated, acidic ground substance.

4.1.7. Immunohistochemistry. Chordomas express epithelial membrane antigen, two intermediate filaments (cytokeratin and vimentin), and S-100 protein (Figures 32–34) *(16–25)*. This panel of antibodies is recommended. Lack of these four markers suggests a neoplasm other than chordoma.

4.1.8. Ultrastructural Features. The large vacuoles of physaliphorous cells contain sparse, short microvilli protruding into their lumens *(26)*. Material in these large vacuoles resembles the extracellular matrix of chordomas. Dilated RER in continuity with mitochondria produces smaller cytoplasmic vacuoles *(26,27)*. Other vacuoles enclose glycogen *(28,29)*.

Chordomas contain distinctive mitochondrial–RER complexes *(28)*. Layers of RER alternate with elongated mitochondria. Bulbous ends of the mitochondria protrude from these complexes in a dumbbell configuration. The complex suggests coalescence to position mitochondrial energy close to the protein production organelles of these cells.

4.1.9. Differential Diagnosis. A typical chordoma composed of cords of vacuolated cells in a mucoid matrix is distinct from other tumors, except the chordoid meningioma *(30)*. This tumor is rare in the sellar region. Properly sampled specimens of chordoid meningioma will show meningothelial features and less immunoreactivity for S-100 protein and cytokeratin than chordoma.

Portions of a chordoma may not show the typical physaliphorous appearance, placing a premium on thorough sampling of tumors. They may be epithelioid with less matrix and resemble a pituitary

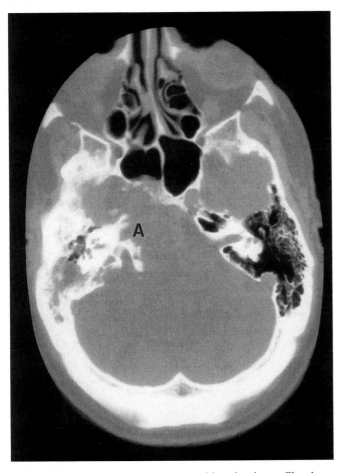

Figure 23-30   CT of a 60-yr-old man with a chordoma. Chordoma is a very aggressive lesion, easily destroying bone. It frequently originates in a parasagittal location, but usually at least approaches midline. This chordoma has destroyed not only the sella turcica, but also the apex of the temporal bone (A).

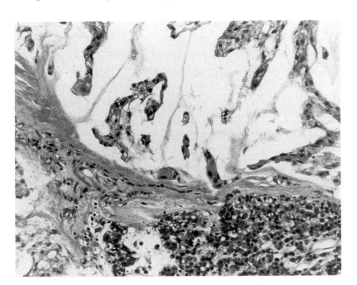

Figure 23-31   This intrasellar chordoma compresses adjacent dark adenohypophyseal cells below. Dark cords of tumor cells contrast with light myxoid material, some of which washes out during specimen processing. Courtesy of Dr. Steven C. Bauserman, Department of Pathology, University of Maryland Medical School, Baltimore, MD. From McKeever PE, Blaivas M, Sima AAF. Neoplasms of the sellar region. In: Lloyd RV, ed. Surgical Pathology of the Pituitary Gland. Major Problems in Pathology Series. Saunders, Philadelphia, 1993, pp. 141–210.

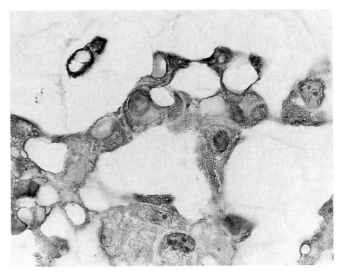

Figure 23-32   Cords of physaliphorous cells are positive for low-mol-wt cytokeratin. This important intermediate filament distinguishes chordoma from chondrosarcoma. Hematoxylin counterstain. From McKeever PE, Blaivas M, Sima AAF. Neoplasms of the sellar region. In: Lloyd RV, ed. Surgical Pathology of the Pituitary Gland. Major Problems in Pathology Series. Saunders, Philadelphia, 1993, pp. 141–210.

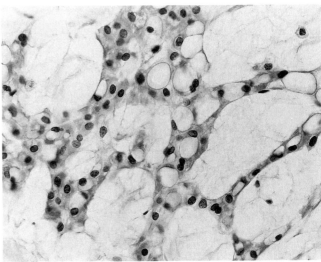

Figure 23-33   Intermediate filament expression by chordomas has a dual role. Physaliphorous cells in a section near those illustrated in Figures 32 and 34 are vimentin-positive. Hematoxylin counterstain. From McKeever PE, Blaivas M, Sima AAF. Neoplasms of the sellar region. In: Lloyd RV, ed. Surgical Pathology of the Pituitary Gland. Major Problems in Pathology Series. Saunders, Philadelphia, 1993, pp. 141–210.

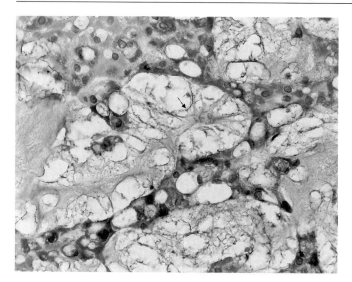

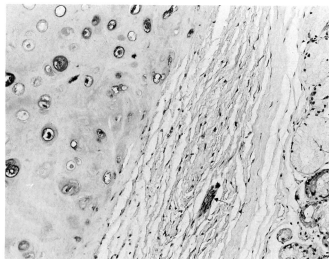

Figure 23-34   Physaliphorous cells are also positive for S-100 protein. The robust hematoxylin stain applied to this section reveals "cobwebs" (arrow) showing that much of the myxoid extracellular matrix did not wash out of this region during processing. From McKeever PE, Blaivas M, Sima AAF. Neoplasms of the sellar region. In: Lloyd RV, ed. Surgical Pathology of the Pituitary Gland. Major Problems in Pathology Series. Saunders, Philadelphia, 1993, pp. 141–210.

Figure 23-35   This tumor contains single- and double-nucleated S-100 protein-positive neoplastic cells in a chondroid matrix, seen on left. However, these cells were negative for cytokeratin and epithelial membrane antigen throughout the entire tumor. Here in the skull base it invades nasopharyngeal fibrous tissue within which is an S-100-positive nerve twig (arrow). Its biologic behavior has been that of a low-grade chondrosarcoma with relentless invasion of the skull base despite numerous resections over more than a decade. From McKeever PE, Blaivas M, Sima AAF. Neoplasms of the sellar region. In: Lloyd RV, ed. Surgical Pathology of the Pituitary Gland. Major Problems in Pathology Series. Saunders, Philadelphia, 1993, pp. 141–210.

adenoma or low-grade carcinoma, and other portions may contain spindle cells resembling a fibroblastic neoplasm *(2,3)*. Chordomas strongly express S-100 protein, vimentin, and type II procollagen reactivity, which as a group distinguish them from carcinomas *(14,16)*. Chordoma mitochondrial–RER complexes are another differential feature *(28,31)*. The possible utility of tissue polypeptide antigen and monoclonal antibody (MAb) ICR.2 in such panels remains to be determined *(32,33)*.

Chordomas lack secretory granules of pituitary adenomas that can be found ultrastructurally or immunocytochemically *(34)*. Most pituitary adenomas lack cytoplasmic vacuoles. An exception is the rare and aggressive acidophil stem-cell adenoma. Mucin in the vacuoles of chordoma cells distinguishes them from vacuoles of acidophil stem-cell adenomas. This adenoma has prolactin immunoreactivity that chordomas lack. Chordomas also lack giant mitochondria of the acidophil stem cell adenoma.

Distinguishing between chordoma and low-grade chondrosarcoma presents a particularly difficult diagnostic problem (Figure 35). This is complicated by the disputed transitional entity called a chondroid chordoma *(35,36)*. The survival of patients with chondroid chordomas is reported to be five times as long as patients with typical chordoma *(35,37)*. Seven neoplasms with structural features of chondroid chordomas have been reported. On the basis of lack of cytokeratin and epithelial membrane antigen markers of chordoma and no mixed pattern of epithelial marker reactivity, these seven tumors were interpreted as low-grade chondrosarcomas *(35)*. However, another chordoma expressed a mixture of chondromatous and chordomatous histologic features and a mixed pattern of epithelial staining *(36)*. With time, this tumor progressed toward the epithelial antigenicity of a typical chordoma, and contained monoparticulate glycogen seen in chordomas and microtubular inclusions within the endoplasmic reticulum seen in chondrosarcomas *(36)*. Transitions between conventional chordomas and malignant spindle-cell tumors have also been noted *(38)*.

4.1.10. Clinical Outcome.   Chordomas of the clivus eventually kill patients. They invade surrounding structures and compromise critical neuroanatomic structures. They may compress arteries *(10)* and rarely hemorrhage *(11)*. Nonetheless, many chordomas grow very slowly, resulting in an average survival of 4 yr. The incidence of metastases varies between reports from rare up to nearly half of the cases *(2,4)*. Studies of proliferative capacity or immunophenotyping may eventually be of prognostic value in chordomas *(35–40)*.

4.2. GIANT-CELL TUMOR OF BONE (GCTB)

4.2.1. Definition.   The GCTB is a benign, but locally aggressive neoplasm with a strong tendency to recur after surgery.

4.2.2. Location.   The GCTB is usually located within the epiphysis of long bones in the third and fourth decades of life. In the rare situation when it occurs in the skull, the most frequently affected are sphenoid and temporal bones *(1–3)*. In several cases of sellar location, it was proposed that the tumor arose from the floor of the sella in relation to the zone of endochrondral ossification of the sphenoid body and spread in lateral, caudal, and inferior directions *(1)*.

Wu and collaborators reported an unusual multicentric GCTB of sphenoid bone and sella in a 17-yr-old female *(4)*. Another very rare location was occipital bone in a 24-yr-old female who also had NF2 *(5)*. Still another rare site and age of occurrence of GCTB was reported by Curilovic in the parietal bone of a 9-yr-old female *(6)*. In a single case of GCTB associated with Turner's syndrome, it was located at the base of skull on the left middle cranial fossa floor *(7)*.

4.2.3. Clinical Features.   Most frequently, patients present with frontal headaches, visual impairment, and sometimes with field defects and oculomotor palsy. Pituitary dysfunction is rare.

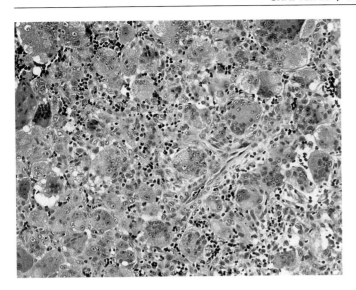

Figure 23-36 Rather evenly dispersed multinucleated giant cells are mixed with the small mononucleated cells in this giant-cell tumor of bone. From McKeever PE, Blaivas M, Sima AAF. Neoplasms of the sellar region. In: Lloyd RV, ed. Surgical Pathology of the Pituitary Gland. Major Problems in Pathology Series. Saunders, Philadelphia, 1993, pp. 141–210.

4.2.4. Radiographic Features. Early in the tumor's course, CT reveals destruction of the dorsum sellae and erosion of the sellar floor. In later stages, the tumor spreads, destroying adjacent bony structures: ethmoid, sphenoid wings, and so forth *(1)*. MRI usually shows a destructive, rather homogeneous enhancing mass that may have a few cysts, but is not dominantly cystic.

4.2.5. Macroscopic Features. A surgical specimen of GCTB is soft, friable, and hemorrhagic.

4.2.6. Microscopic Features. Histologically, the neoplasm is formed by evenly dispersed, round, benign, multinucleated giant cells on a background of sheets and clusters of small mononuclear cells (Figure 36). The nuclei of both large and small cells are rather pale, but with occasional prominent nucleoli *(3,5)*. Mitotic figures are infrequent. Recent and remote hemorrhage as well as cyst formation can be present.

4.2.7. Immunohistochemical and Ultrastructural Features. In a case of parietal skull GCTB in a 9-yr-old female, the giant cells were strongly reactive with CD68 as were normal bone osteoclasts. Mac-387 was negative. The small stromal cells were negative for both CD68 and Mac-387. The stromal cells were found to have two immunohistochemical phenotypes. One was negative for lysozyme staining in 50–80% of the cells and positive for proliferating cell nuclear antigen (PCNA) in about 30% of the nuclei. The other phenotype expressed reactivity with lysozyme, but was negative for PCNA *(6)*. In a case of GCTB infiltrating a plexiform neurofibroma reported by Opitz et al., positive Ki-67 staining and mitotic figures were moderate in numbers and restricted to the stromal cells *(5)*. Fine collagen fibers stained for collagen I, III, V, and weakly for collagen VI filled spaces between the giant and stromal cells. S-100 protein stain was negative *(5)*.

Ultrastructurally, giant cells contain numerous oval nuclei with prominent nucleoli and cytoplasmic inclusions. The plasma membrane forms microvillous protrusions. The small stromal cells are less electron-dense than giant cells, and have prominent RER in perinuclear locations and smooth plasma membranes *(5)*.

4.2.8. Differential Diagnosis. Differential diagnosis includes aneurysmal bone cyst, bone changes associated with hyperparathyroidism, chondroblastoma, osteoblastoma, chondrosarcoma, and in rare cases, germinoma since it also has a large- and small-cell population. The diagnosis of GCTB is not usually difficult owing to its characteristic histologic appearance. However, negative staining for S-100 protein distinguishes this neoplasm from chondroblastoma *(8)*. Lysozyme activity of the stromal cells in GCTB differentiates this neoplasm from chondroblastoma and osteosarcoma in which the positive cells are macrophages, whereas the stromal cells stain negatively *(6)*.

4.2.9. Clinical Outcome. GCTB is histologically benign. However, its location in the sellar region and capacity for local destruction may produce devastating results. The recommended definitive treatment is surgical excision, but whether the achieved excision should be total or subtotal remains controversial for various locations of the neoplasm *(7)*. Up to 50% of GCTB recur after curettage, and up to 10% develop distant metastases, most commonly to the lung. Thus, these tumors have to be considered potentially malignant and treated with *en bloc* excision followed by radiation therapy *(9)*. Malignant transformation of GCTB of sphenoid bone following radiotherapy has been reported *(10)*.

4.3. HEMANGIOPERICYTOMA

4.3.1. Definition. The hemangiopericytoma is a neoplasm composed of cells that resemble pericytes, myocytes, or fibroblasts. Pericytes are specialized elongated cells between vascular endothelium and tissue parenchyma.

4.3.2. Location. Hemangiopericytomas occur in the intracranial meninges. Parasellar and sellar involvement from sinonasal and orbital skull base tumors occurs *(1–6)*. Primary hemangiopericytomas of the pituitary are less common *(7–12)*. Spinal cord and systemic involvement have been associated with hemangiopericytomas around the sella *(7,13)*.

4.3.3. Clinical Features. Individual patients have presented with a variety of symptoms and signs. These include headaches, drooping of eyelids, amenorrhea, and acromegaly *(9,10,13)*. The most consistent abnormality of parasellar and suprasellar hemangiopericytomas is partial loss of visual fields *(8,10,13)*.

4.3.4. Radiographic Features. Noncontrast CT of hemangiopericytomas shows high attenuation, very similar to meningiomas. This attenuation is higher than that of surrounding brain and pituitary. Lush CT enhancement reflects the tumor's hypervascularity. The tumor margins on CT are often surprisingly distinct *(8,10,13,14)*. Reports of MRI are limited *(14)*, but usually resemble the features of an aggressive meningioma.

4.3.5. Macroscopic Features. Vascularity is prominent, coloring the lobulated translucent gray tumor with red blood. Lighter gray coloration and firmer texture results from invasion of dura, diaphragma sellae, and other collagenous structures. Macroscopic invasion of bone, pituitary, or brain is particularly common in recurrent tumors *(10,13)*.

4.3.6. Microscopic and Cytogenetic Features. The hemangiopericytoma is a "blue tumor" on routine H&E staining owing to its high cellular density (Figure 37). Vascular lumens are distorted and compressed by nearby neoplastic cells, producing lumens that resemble antlers or staghorns *(15)*. Less cellular regions of tumor often contain basement membrane material that can be highlighted with PAS or reticulin stains (Figure 38). Necrotic regions may be evident.

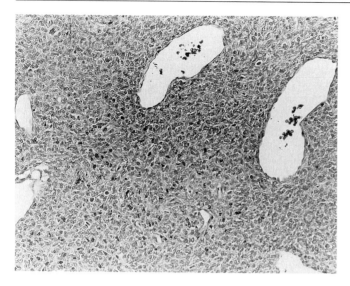

Figure 23-37 Hemangiopericytoma consists of a uniform pattern of cells with round and oval nuclei. This dense and monotonous array produces a blue tumor stained with H&E. Lucent vascular lumens are distorted by neoplastic cells into reniform shapes. From McKeever PE, Blaivas M, Sima AAF. Neoplasms of the sellar region. In: Lloyd RV, ed. Surgical Pathology of the Pituitary Gland. Major Problems in Pathology Series. Saunders, Philadelphia, 1993, pp. 141–210.

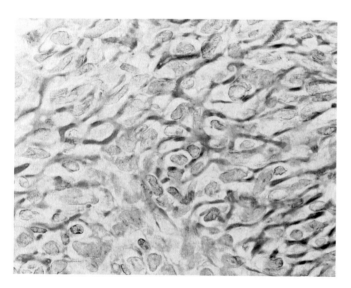

Figure 23-38 The dark "mortar" between these hemangiopericytoma cells is glycosylated pericellular collagen or reticulin. PAS stain. From McKeever PE, Blaivas M, Sima AAF. Neoplasms of the sellar region. In: Lloyd RV, ed. Surgical Pathology of the Pituitary Gland. Major Problems in Pathology Series. Saunders, Philadelphia, 1993, pp. 141–210.

Oval nuclei predominate, but some tumors have pleomorphic and hyperchromatic regions. Nucleoli are small. Mitoses are present and sometimes frequent.

Local invasion of dura, bone, pituitary, or brain occurs, and is a major problem in cases with multiple recurrences. The most common pathway for brain and pituitary invasion is along the penetrating vessels, rather than direct infiltration of parenchyma by solitary neoplastic cells.

Deletions that involve the long arm of chromosome 12 are common in hemangiopericytomas. This suggests the possibility of

a tumor suppressor gene in the 12q13-15 region *(16)*. Numerous other chromosome abnormalities occur, particularly after radiotherapy *(17)*.

4.3.7. Immunohistochemistry. Reactivity for vimentin and not for other cytoplasmic markers is typical of hemangiopericytomas. Rare hemangiopericytomas express focal muscle-specific actin and epithelial membrane antigen reactivity suggestive of pericytes, but this is not the common pattern *(1,2,4,6,18–23)*. Their basement membrane material contains type IV collagen *(2)*.

4.3.8. Ultrastructural Features. Lack of immunoreactivity for all but the relatively nonspecific vimentin and basement membrane markers invites diagnosis of hemangiopericytomas by electron microscopy. Often the neoplastic cells are surrounded by extracellular materials *(24)*. Intercellular collagens usually resemble basal lamina, but large collagen fibers are present in some cases. In other cases, the basal lamina is thick and multilaminated *(20)*.

Cells have thick cytoplasmic processes and intermediate filaments distributed diffusely throughout the cytoplasm. One-third of hemangiopericytomas show neoplastic cells differentiated like pericytes, but statistics for parasellar tumors are unknown.

4.3.9. Differential Diagnosis. In the region around the sella, meningioma, pituitary adenoma, and carcinoma must be considered. These alternatives all tend to show more eosinophilic cytoplasm than hemangiopericytomas, except for sinonasal undifferentiated carcinomas. Hyperostosis of nearby bone suggests meningioma *(25)*.

From an immunohistochemical perspective, meningioma and carcinoma express cell-surface epithelial membrane antigen. Carcinomas express cytokeratin, more variable in meningiomas and adenomas. Pituitary adenomas contain secretory granules that will be positive for at least one peptide hormone (prolactin, growth hormone, adrenocorticotropic hormone [ACTH], gonadotrophic hormone) or for chromogranin. Hemangiopericytomas are negative for all of the above immunohistochemical markers except for uncommon cytokeratin expression.

Electron microscopy distinguishes the interdigitating cellular processes of meningiomas and secretory granules of primary pituitary tumors from hemangiopericytoma cells surrounded by basal laminae *(1,23)*. When esthesioneuroblastoma is a consideration, its neurites and neurosecretory granules are distinctive.

4.3.10. Therapy and Clinical Outcome. Hemangiopericytomas recur relentlessly. Local recurrences are common, causing particular agony in tumors involving clinically sensitive structures around the sella. Control of local recurrence is never assured *(26)*, and this is complicated by the threat of distant metastasis *(7)*. Implantation of radioactive seeds have been used to augment surgery in the treatment of certain cases *(7,8,11)*.

4.4. MYXOMA

4.4.1. Definition. The myxoma is a benign tumor that originates from mesenchymal tissue *(1)*. Intracerebral myxomas are usually metastases or emboli from cardiac atrial myxomas *(2–4)*.

4.4.2. Location. The only report of a primary myxoma in the pituitary fossa was published in 1987 *(5)*. The tumor was located on the right side of the sella.

4.4.3. Clinical Features. A 38-yr-old Japanese man with primary myxoma in the pituitary fossa developed a sudden and rapid deterioration of his right-sided visual acuity. Pituitary function was not affected. A 60-yr-old woman with cerebral metastasis of an atrial myxoma presented with a 15-mo history of Jacksonian seizures *(4)*.

4.4.4. Radiographic Features. CT of a primary pituitary fossa myxoma showed an isodense mass in the right side of the pituitary fossa with suprasellar extension that was slightly and homogeneously enhanced by contrast. A metastatic atrial myxoma produced an enhancing subcortical lesion on CT.

4.4.5. Macroscopic Features. Surgical resection yielded a gray, gelatinous, semitransparent, well-circumscribed tumor within the right side of the sella *(5)*.

4.4.6. Microscopic Features. Microscopically, the tumor was composed of stellate spindled and bipolar cells with hypochromatic nuclei and a mucinous background. The cells were organized in lobules separated by connective tissue trabeculae. A cerebral metastasis of an atrial myxoma reported by Samaratunga exhibited histologic features of epithelioid hemangioendothelioma *(4)*.

4.4.7. Special Stains. The myxomatous stroma is Alcian blue-positive, hyaluronidase-digestible, and PAS-positive. The tumor cells are more intensely PAS-positive than the stroma.

4.4.8. Differential Diagnosis. Metastatic cardiac myxoma may mimic an epithelioid hemangioendothelioma. The differential diagnosis of a primary myxoma includes any lesion that has a myxomatous tissue component.

4.4.9. Clinical Outcome. Myxomas are histologically benign. However, they have the potential for local invasion of the underlying bone and, if not completely excised, they may recur *(6)*.

4.5. FIBROMA

4.5.1. Definition. This is a well-demarcated, hypocellular lesion formed by fibroblasts embedded in collagenous or hyalinized matrix.

4.5.2. Location. Few intracranial fibromas have been reported, and ones that invaded the sellar region usually originated from sphenoid bone or from the sinonasal region *(1–3)*. A case of pseudotumor of the sellar and parasellar regions with marked fibrosis was reported by Gartman and collaborators *(4)*.

4.5.3. Clinical Features. An unusual case of ossifying fibroma of sphenoid bone with coexistent mucocele presented with decreasing vision in the right eye, diplopia, headache, and galactorrhea *(2)*.

4.5.4. Radiographic Features. In the case mentioned above, both CT and MRI studies showed a large, ground-glass-appearing lesion that showed low-to-intermediate proton density and quite low signal on both T1- and T2-weighted MRI. The lesion diffusely enhanced on CT and MRI after contrast administration *(2)*. The coexistent sphenoid sinus mucocele had intermediate proton density, high T2 signal intensity, and low T1 signal intensity compared with brain. The mass itself did not enhance, but it had an intensely enhancing thin rim. In cases of psammomatoid ossifying fibromas of the sinonasal region, the radiographic studies were typical for osseous and soft tissue masses varying in appearance, with or without erosion of the adjacent bone and intracranial extension *(3)*.

4.5.5. Macroscopic Features. Fibromas are nodular, rather well-circumscribed masses; however, in the majority of the cases mentioned above, the neoplasms eroded through the bone and extended within the cranium. The density of the mass varied from hard and cartilaginous or osseous to mixed osseous and soft, depending on the amount of soft tissue mass included within *(1–3)*.

4.5.6. Microscopic Features. Pure fibromas are usually paucicellular and composed of dense eosinophilic collagenous

matrix with scattered fibroblasts. Ossifying fibromas are characterized by haphazardly arranged collagen bundles within well-vascularized stroma, spindled cells, calcific deposits, and irregular trabeculae of immature bone. The histologic appearance of aggressive psammomatoid ossifying fibromas was characterized by a cellular stroma with scattered giant cells, variable amounts of myxomatous material, and scattered small mineralized (psammomatoid) bodies *(3)*. A pseudotumor arising from sphenoid sinuses with subsequent spread to the sella demonstrated chronic inflammatory changes and dense fibrosis *(1)*.

4.5.7. Immunohistochemical and Ultrastructural Features. The cells are reactive with antivimentin antibody. Ultrastructurally, fibromas consist of fibroblasts, with an occasional admixture of myofibroblasts when the lesion is more cellular.

4.5.8. Differential Diagnosis. Two major differential diagnoses for fibromas are fibromatoses and low-grade fibrosarcoma. Fibromatoses are reactive, but potentially aggressive infiltrative lesions that are usually more collagenous and less cellular than fibromas. However, despite these features, it is sometimes difficult to differentiate between fibromatosis and a low-grade fibrosarcoma. Ossifying fibromas, on the other hand, should be differentiated from other fibro-osseous lesions.

4.5.9. Clinical Outcome. Surgical excision is the treatment of choice. For a tumor with locally aggressive behavior, such as some of the psammomatous ossifying fibromas, complete *en bloc* surgical excision is the treatment of choice and may prove curative *(3)*.

4.6. FIBROSARCOMA

4.6.1. Definition. These malignant mesenchymal neoplasms of soft tissue are composed of elongated cells that resemble fibroblasts. Sarcomas around the sella are often associated with prior therapeutic radiation of a previous tumor. Before a correlation between radiation and a second tumor is entertained, minimal criteria *(1–3)* pertain:

1. The second tumor should be located within the region irradiated.
2. The first and second tumors should be histologically different types.
3. Asymptomatic latency should be long enough to indicate that the second tumor was not present at the time of irradiation.

4.6.2. Location. Intracranial sarcomas arise in the meninges or brain. Many fibrosarcomas arise in or adjacent to the sella *(4–9)*. However, their infiltration of dura, brain, and bone confounds precise localization of many tumors *(4,8,10)*.

4.6.3. Clinical Features. Fibrosarcomas are rare tumors. The majority of fibrosarcomas arise months to years after therapeutic radiation to preceding pituitary adenomas *(4–12)*. About half of afflicted patients had received more than 30 gy to the sellar area and half in excess of 50 gy. The latent period from time of irradiation to sarcoma varies from 2.5 to more than 20 yr. Although fibrosarcoma is the most common, other types of sarcoma have followed radiotherapy *(13,14;* Figure 39).

Parasellar sarcomas are locally aggressive, affecting the optic nerves, eroding overlying brain, and compressing brainstem structures *(4,5)*. Symptoms reflect structures involved, and include headaches, partial to complete blindness, ptosis, and paralysis. Internal carotid compression, hemiparesis, and infarcts can occur *(4–9)*.

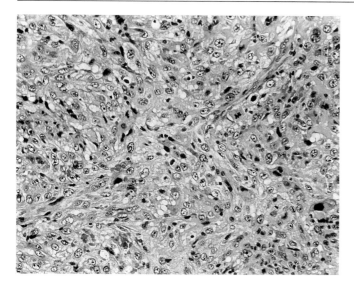

Figure 23-39 This postirradiation sarcoma with numerous mitotic spindle abnormalities is predominantly undifferentiated. It contains a few spindled cells and wisps of pink collagen. It developed in dura of the skull base in a young woman 4½ yr following therapeutic parasellar radiation.

4.6.4. Radiographic Features. Fibrosarcomas are often quite homogeneous on CT and MRI, and usually enhance with contrast media (6,7,9). CT often reveals erosion of bone (6,7). Infiltration of sphenoidal and cavernous sinuses, and of brain may be evident (4,8).

4.6.5. Macroscopic Features. Fibrosarcomas are gray tumors of variable firmness, increased by collagen and decreased by necrosis. They infiltrate and expand tissue components, making their margins obscure.

4.6.6. Microscopic Features. Fibrosarcomas are composed of elongated spindle cells with considerable pleomorphism and numerous mitoses (4,5). Their elongated nuclei are hyperchromatic and pleomorphic (15). They may show a fascicular pattern (8). Other sarcomas defy subclassification (Figure 39).

The sellar fibrosarcomas commonly show nests of pre-existing adenomas within the tumor. These adenohypophyseal or adenomatous elements seldom demonstrate malignant differentiation (16).

Spontaneously occurring fibrosarcomas of the pituitary are extremely rare (17,18). A parasellar pituitary leiomyosarcoma was reported (19). It was believed to have arisen from vascular smooth muscle cells.

4.6.7. Immunohistochemistry and Special Stains. Variable amounts of extracellular collagen are highlighted with Masson's trichrome or reticulin stains. Adenomatous elements within the sarcoma are demonstrable with pituitary hormone and chromogranin immunohistochemical stains.

4.6.8. Ultrastructural Features. Fibrosarcoma cell cytoplasm contains free ribosomes, RER, with distended cisternae, and Golgii apparatus. Glycogen may be present. Extracellular collagen fibers are evident (8,18).

4.6.9. Differential Diagnosis. Fibrous meningioma, fibroma, and hemangiopericytoma are concerns in the differential diagnosis. Meningioma and fibroma have benign nuclei and inconspicuous mitoses. Anaplastic meningioma is more difficult to distinguish. Look for rounder, meningothelial nuclei, whorls,

psammoma bodies, and epithelial membrane antigen immunoreactivity. These features may be focal and minimal in anaplastic meningioma.

Hemangiopericytomas have less angulated nuclei and more pericellular reticulum than fibrosarcoma (8,20). Distorted vascular lumens suggest hemangiopericytoma.

4.6.10. Clinical Outcome. The prognosis of fibrosarcoma in the sella is dismal. From the onset of symptoms, death occurs within months (4). In contrast to postirradiation sarcomas, primary sarcomas tend to metastasize (17).

4.7. OSTEOGENIC SARCOMA

4.7.1. Definition. Osteogenic sarcoma is a primary tumor of bone. Its malignant cells produce osteoid (1).

4.7.2. Location. Less than 9% of osteogenic sarcomas originate in the cranial bones, with the mandible being the most common site (1). Two cases of primary osteosarcoma have been reported in the sellar region. One case of suprasellar osteosarcoma developed 10 yr after radiation therapy for pituitary adenoma, and of three osteosarcomas of sphenoid bone, two were primary and one 15 yr after radiation therapy for craniopharyngioma (2–6).

4.7.3. Clinical Features. A 48-yr-old woman and a 22-yr-old man with primary osteogenic sarcoma of the sellar region presented with headache and diplopia (2,3).

4.7.4. Radiographic Features. Radiologically, osteogenic sarcoma is a rather poorly defined, osteolytic, osteoblastic, or mixed osteolytic-sclerotic neoplasm. In one of the cases of primary osteosarcoma of the sellar region, a CT scan demonstrated a homogeneous enhancing mass within the tuberculum sellae encroaching on the anterior part of the sphenoid sinus (3). The lesion often shows whorl or star-burst patterns of new bone formation.

4.7.5. Macroscopic Features. The gray or off-white nodular mass consists of firm osseous or cartilaginous regions alternating with softer fibrous portions. Small cystic or hemorrhagic regions may also be present.

4.7.6. Microscopic Features. The histologic appearance is quite variable not only from one case to another, but regionally within the same specimen. Anaplastic mesenchymal parenchyma produces osteoid and cartilage and, depending on the prevalence of each of these components, osteosarcomas are classified into three major subtypes: osteoblastic, chondroblastic, and fibroblastic.

4.7.7. Immunohistochemical and Ultrastructural Features. Immunohistochemistry and electron microscopic studies are of limited value in the diagnosis and differential diagnosis of osteosarcoma.

4.7.8. Differential Diagnosis. The major neoplasms to differentiate from osteosarcoma are chondrosarcoma, malignant fibrous histiocytoma, and uncommonly, myositis ossificans and GCTB. Each of these neoplasms exhibits distinct histologic features.

A rare case of symptomatic osteolipoma of the tuber cinereum was recently reported, whereas all previously reported cases were incidental autopsy findings (7). The neoplasm was a dumbbell-shaped bony mass identified directly behind the pituitary stalk and microscopically was composed of mature adipose tissue and compact lamellar bone with a central core of fat and bone marrow and outer fibrous tissue covering.

4.7.9. Clinical Outcome. Shinoda and coworkers emphasized the rarity and poor prognosis of primary skull osteosarcomas (8). The treatment is usually surgery with the addition of chemotherapy and, in some cases, radiotherapy *(9)*. Survival rates are similar for all three major histological subtypes of osteogenic sarcoma, i.e., osteoblastic, chondroblastic, and fibroblastic.

5. VASCULAR TUMORS

5.1. CAVERNOUS ANGIOMA (CA)

5.1.1. Definition. CA or hemangioma is a well-circumscribed hamartomatous vascular malformation composed of closely packed, thin-walled sinusoidal blood channels lined by flattened endothelium. There is no elastic lamina, muscle layer, or intervening brain parenchyma *(1–3)*.

5.1.2. Location. CA can be found anywhere in the CNS, but are most common in subcortical white matter and pons. According to some series, they are more frequent in females; however, others state that men are affected more than women *(1,2,4)*. A large percentage of Hispanic males harbor CA, and some of the cases are familial or with multiple (up to 30) CAs per patient *(2)*. Many CAs are located in middle cranial fossa, some with extension into adjacent structures *(1,5–7)*. Extracerebral CAs are rare. Most of them occur in the parasellar region and extend into the sella *(8)*. Three out of five CAs arising from the cavernous sinus extended laterally into the middle cranial fossa, medially into the sella, and anteriorly into the superior orbital feature ("endophytic" growth). The other two extended "exophytically" to the entry of the third and fourth cranial nerves *(9)*.

5.1.3. Clinical Features. A variety of clinical symptoms at presentation include seizures, focal neurologic deficit, headaches, visual disturbances, tremor, and in one case, hyperprolactinemia *(1,2,5,6)*. A remarkably large and clinically silent dumbbell-shaped pituitary CA extending to the left hypothalamus was found incidentally at the autopsy in a 72-yr-old woman with metastatic breast carcinoma *(7)*.

5.1.4. Radiographic Features. MRI is the most sensitive technique in the diagnosis of CA. Kattapong and collaborators described the following patterns: "target" lesions with central high signal surrounded by low signal (20% of cases), reticulated heterogeneous lesions (34%), hemosiderin (43%), acute blood (2%) and subacute blood (2%) *(2)*. Parasellar CAs were different by CT and MRI from intracerebral CAs: CT showed homogeneously enhanced tumor similar to a meningioma, but without calcifications or bone hyperostosis *(8)*. Characteristic MRI findings were hypodensity on T1-weighted images, and very high signal intensity on T2-weighted images along with strong homogeneous enhancement with Gadolinium *(8,9)*. Erosion of the sellar bone or ballooning of the sella without visible calcification was considered characteristic by several workers *(1,5,10)*.

5.1.5. Macroscopic Features. The CA is an aggregate of discrete vessels of various diameters combined with old and recent hemorrhage and a leather-firm rim of gliotic parenchyma.

5.1.6. Microscopic Features. CAs are composed of multiple large and small vascular channels (Figure 40). These may be filled with blood or thrombi in various stages of organization. Hemosiderin deposits, cholesterol clefts, focal hyaline thickening of the vessel walls, and calcifications are common. No intervening brain parenchyma is present in between the vessels, but the adjacent brain parenchyma is frequently gliotic.

5.1.7. Immunohistochemical Features. CAs stain positively for factor VIII, *Ulex europaeus* agglutinin I, and vimentin. Epithelial membrane antigen (EMA), cytokeratin, and carcinoembryogenic antigen stain negatively *(11)*.

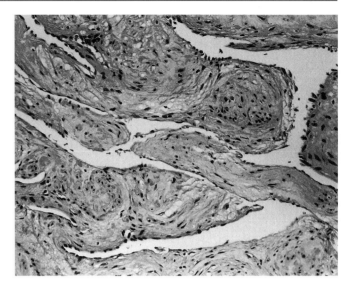

Figure 23-40 This cavernous angioma of the pituitary region is composed of thick-walled vascular channels lined by flattened cells. Thickening of the walls is owing to the proliferation of connective tissue and smooth muscle.

5.1.8. Differential Diagnosis. Diagnosis of CA usually presents no problem. The lesions to consider in the differential diagnosis are other vascular malformations and hamartomatous growths. Unlike arteriovenous malformations, the abnormal vessels in CA lack elastic laminae.

5.1.9. Clinical Outcome. CAs are thought to be hamartomatous congenital lesions that grow in size with time *(1)*. However, Kattapong and colleagues propose that the patients may not be born with MRI-identifiable CA *(2)*. The latter become visible with advancing age because of growth and/or hemorrhage. Changing size with each decade of life was interpreted as likely owing to hemorrhage and not growth. The conclusion was that CA may be more benign than previously thought.

The usual treatment for CA is surgical resection, provided the location allows radical excision without danger of massive hemorrhage *(4)*.

5.2. HEMANGIOBLASTOMA

5.2.1. Definition. The hemangioblastoma is a benign CNS tumor characterized by vacuolated stromal cells mixed with a rich capillary network. In 10–20% of cases, it is associated with von Hippel-Lindau syndrome.

5.2.2. Location. The majority of hemangioblastomas are located in the posterior fossa, with <3% being supratentorial. Of the latter, three cases of hemangioblastoma involving the pituitary gland have been reported *(1,3)*.

5.2.3. Clinical Features. Two pituitary cases were associated with von Hippel-Lindau disease *(1,2)*. The third was an obese 28-yr-old woman with no signs of a phacomatosis who presented with a 3-yr history of Chiari-Frommel syndrome *(3)*. She complained of fronto-orbital headaches, galactorrhea, and hair loss. Occasionally, obstructive hydrocephalus develops when the tumor involves the sella *(4)*.

5.2.4. Radiographic Features. On CT, hemangioblastoma presents as a sharply circumscribed isodense mass with little surrounding edema. The tumor is either solid or cystic with a mural nodule *(1,3)*. It enhances after contrast injection. Angiography

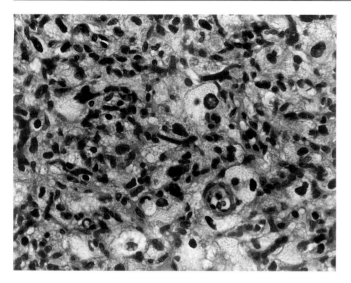

Figure 23-41 Capillary-sized vessels of the hemangioblastoma are lined by mostly uniform and small, but occasionally pleomorphic endothelial cells. Large, foamy stromal cells are prominent in between the vascular channels. From McKeever PE, Blaivas M, Sima AAF. Neoplasms of the sellar region. In: Lloyd RV, ed. Surgical Pathology of the Pituitary Gland. Major Problems in Pathology Series. Saunders, Philadelphia, 1993, pp. 141–210.

shows a highly vascular tumor with feeding vessels and persistent blush. Although formerly this was the most helpful procedure, MRI has generally replaced it in preoperative evaluation, unless therapeutic embolization is elected.

5.2.5. Macroscopic Features.   Hemangioblastomas are not encapsulated, have a red-tan or yellow color, and in about half of the cases, they are associated with cysts filled with clear fluid of high protein content.

5.2.6. Microscopic Features.   The neoplasm is highly vascularized and is composed of a mixture of dilated thin-walled capillaries lined with uniform flat endothelial cells and large, polygonal foamy cells (Figure 41). The latter vary in size and shape, and in the amount of lipid granules in their cytoplasm. The nuclei can be pleomorphic and hyperchromatic, but mitotic figures are inconspicuous. Hemangioblastomas are subclassified into three types, based on the appearance of the vascular network and the lipid content of the stromal cells: capillary, cavernous, and cellular. This subtyping bears no prognostic value.

5.2.7. Immunohistochemical, Genetic, and Ultrastructural Features.   Numerous papers address the question of the origin of the stromal cells and their role as a part of the neoplasm (5–12,13). Based on a difference between stromal and vascular cells in staining pattern for a number of markers, including NSE and factor VIII, a neuroendocrine origin was proposed (9). Endothelial origin was also suggested (14). Still another paper denied endothelial, neural, epithelial, pericytic, or neuroendocrine origin, hypothesizing a cell of origin to be an undifferentiated mesenchymal cell (12). Kepes and associates held a view that on light microscopy, the stromal cells are a heterogeneous group of cells and not a single type of cell (5). Based on positivity of all stromal cells for vimentin and α-enolase, along with most of them staining positively for NSE and aldolase C4 and the process-bearing stromal cells positive for GFAP and histiocytic markers, Ironside and coauthors concluded that the stromal cell population includes

entrapped reactive astrocytes and locally derived nonvascular cells of neuroectodermal (pial) origin (10). Only endothelial cells were positive for factor VIII-related antigen and Ulex Europaeus I lectin. The presence of a fourth type of cell within capillary hemangioblastoma, besides endothelial and stromal cells and pericytes, was suggested by Bohling and associates (15). These cells are small and granular and stain positively for erythropoietin, renin, and α-1-antitrypsin. Nemes found that spindled or stellate-shaped cells staining positively for factor XIIIa were consistently present in hemangioblastomas and were capable of transformation into vacuolated stromal cells (16). He concluded that this indicated fibrohistiocytic differentiation, which is part of the differentiation spectrum of hemangiopericytomas. The stromal cells express high levels of vascular endothelial growth factor, placental growth factor mRNA, and abundant epidermal growth factor receptor (17).

Molecular genetic analysis revealed that mutations of the von Hippel-Lindau (VHL) tumor suppressor gene occur in a significant percentage of hemangioblastomas (18). The VHL tumor suppressor gene is a suggested target for inactivation in hemangioblastomas being involved in the pathogenesis of both familial and sporadic tumors (19).

Ultrastructurally, hemangioblastomas are composed of three types of cells: endothelial, stromal, and pericytes (20). The stromal cells contain membrane-bound lipid granules. The vascular channels are lined by fenestrated endothelium. The discontinuous periendothelial cell layer is surrounded by basement membrane.

5.2.8. Differential Diagnosis.   Major differential diagnoses include pilocytic astrocytoma, particularly when the neoplasm presents as a mural nodule within a cyst, and renal cell or other clear-cell metastatic carcinoma (21–23). The latter are especially likely in patients with VHL disease. Carcinomas are EMA-positive and hemangioblastomas are NSE-positive (9,22). Pilocytic astrocytomas are more fibrillar than hemangioblastoma. This feature can be confirmed on routine paraffin or plastic sections.

5.2.9. Clinical Outcome.   Complete surgical excision is the treatment of choice. As a rule, there are no recurrences of the excised neoplasm. Radiotherapy is occasionally used for partially removed tumors. Patients with VHL must be monitored for new tumors.

5.3. GLOMUS TUMOR (GT) (GLOMANGIOMA)

5.3.1. Definition.   The GT is a rare, usually benign neoplasm arising in a glomus body. The latter is a specialized arteriovenous anastomosis serving in thermal regulation.

5.3.2. Location.   The usual sites of GT are the nail beds and pads of the fingers and toes. Extracutaneous location is uncommon; however, GT has been reported in muscle, tendon, gastrointestinal tract, mediastinum, nasal cavity, palate, trachea, and vagina (1,2). Asa and coworkers reported a glomangioma of the sellar region in 1984 (3).

5.3.3. Clinical Features.   The GT is usually a small, solitary, subcutaneous nodule that can produce significant pain (4). Cases of multiple nodules are likely to be familial, inherited via the paternal line (5). A 42-yr-old man with a sellar GT presented with headaches, followed by decreased visual activity (3).

5.3.4. Radiographic Features.   CT at the first presentation of the patient with the aforementioned sellar GT was negative for neoplasm; however, a year later, it showed a pituitary tumor with suprasellar extension (3).

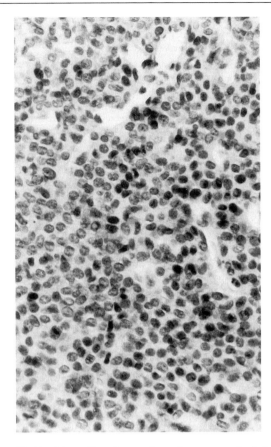

Figure 23-42 The sellar glomangioma is composed of sheets of round to oval nuclei with indistinct cytoplasm and thin vessels lined by flattened endothelium. From McKeever PE, Blaivas M, Sima AAF. Neoplasms of the sellar region. In: Lloyd RV, ed. Surgical Pathology of the Pituitary Gland. Major Problems in Pathology Series. Saunders. Philadelphia, 1993, pp. 141–210. (From Asa SL, Kovacs K, Horvath E, Ezrin C, Weiss MH. Sellar glomangioma. Ultrastruct Pathol 1994;7:49–54.).

5.3.5. Macroscopic Features. The nodule of a benign GT is well circumscribed, rather firm, and occasionally bosselated or multiple. A malignant GT in a 63-yr-old man was bluish-red, bulbous, and bled easily *(6)*.

5.3.6. Microscopic Features. The GT is formed by modified smooth muscle cells and should not be confused with the glomus jugulare tumor, which is a paraganglioma located within the mastoid bone. The sellar glomangioma of Asa and associates was composed of uniform, round, or polygonal cells with round or oval nuclei and indistinct nucleoli (Figure 42). Mitotic figures were rare, and the cell borders were poorly defined. Vascular channels lined by flat endothelium were scattered among sheets of neoplastic cells *(3)*. Depending on the proportion of vessels and smooth muscle, GT has been subclassified into conventional GT, glomangioma, and glomangiomyoma. A new subtype, epithelioid GT, was recently described by Pulitzer and coauthors *(4)*. They reported five cases of this unusual histological variant of GT. The tumors were composed of large polygonal or spindled cells with large irregularly shaped hyperchromatic nuclei and abundant eosinophilic cytoplasm. They had both epithelioid and myoid features. The epithelial regions showed cytologic atypia that was interpreted to be a manifestation of degeneration or senescence (as in

schwannomas) rather than malignancy *(4)*. The GT is usually benign. However, it can be locally infiltrative or cytologically malignant and metastasize to various organs *(6–8)*.

5.3.7. Immunohistochemical and Ultrastructural Features. Being modified smooth muscle cells, GT cells (including the ones in the "marked epithelioid" variant) are strongly immunoreactive for smooth muscle actin and occasionally desmin, and for vimentin. They are negative for S-100 and cytokeratin *(3,4,6)*. The endothelial markers, factor VIII, and CD 31 stain only the tumor endothelium. Staining for GFAP and pituitary hormones was negative in a case of sellar glomangioma *(3)*.

Ultrastructurally, the cell cytoplasm contains abundant microfilaments arranged in parallel arrays and focal densities, pinocytotic vesicles at the periphery of the cytoplasm, and well-developed basal lamina *(3,4,6)*.

5.3.8. Differential Diagnosis. Major tumors in the differential diagnosis include spindle-cell tumors, such as hemangiopericytoma, schwannoma, leiomyoma, particularly in epithelioid variants of GT, and round-cell sarcomas in cases of malignant GT *(4,6–8)*. Nuovo and collaborators found two cases of hemangiopericytoma to be positive for muscle-specific actin and vimentin, the stains that were also positive in 40 cases of GT *(9)*. According to their study, desmin was a useful marker in differentiation between the two neoplasms, since it was positive in 73% of GT and negative in hemangiopericytoma. In the other series, none of the 11 cases of hemangiopericytoma exhibited smooth muscle differentiation, whereas all of 16 GT did *(10)*. The GT rarely contains branching "stag horn" vessels commonly present in hemangiopericytoma.

Schwannomas are encapsulated and have Antoni A and B regions, hyalinized or thrombosed vessels, and stain positively with S-100, compared to the GT, which is only partially covered by a fibrous pseudocapsule, lacks Antoni A and B regions, and stains negatively with S-100. Common to both schwannoma and the epithelioid variant of GT is nuclear pleomorphism of "ancient" type *(4)*.

5.3.9. Clinical Outcome. The GT is usually a benign neoplasm that is sufficiently treated by surgical excision. This also applies to the epithelioid variant of GT that expresses marked nuclear pleomorphism *(4)*. However, malignant GT is known to recur locally and metastasize to various organs *(6)*. The sellar GT had suprasellar extension at the time of first surgery and recurred several times, despite radiation treatment *(3)*.

6. HEMATOPOIETIC NEOPLASMS

6.1. HISTIOCYTOSIS

6.1.1. Definition. The histiocytoses are a group of lesions composed of histiocytes. A plethora of named variants, some quite rare, have confounded classification systems. Recent attempts to classify these as Langerhan's cell histiocytosis have concentrated on extent of disease: solitary, multifocal, or disseminated. The most common of these to involve the parasellar region is multifocal eosinophilic granuloma or Hand-Schüller-Christian disease.

6.1.2. Location. The most common Langerhan's cell histiocytosis is called an eosinophilic granuloma. Solitary eosinophilic granuloma usually occurs within bone rather than the pituitary or hypothalamus.

Multifocal Langerhan's cell histiocytosis is called Hand-Schüller-Christian disease. About half of the time, it involves the

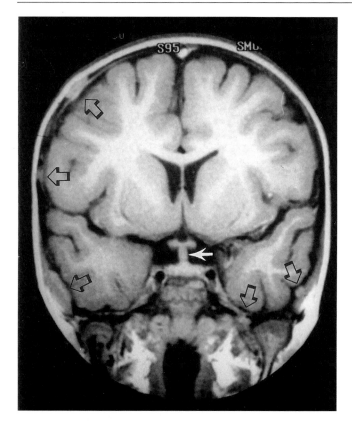

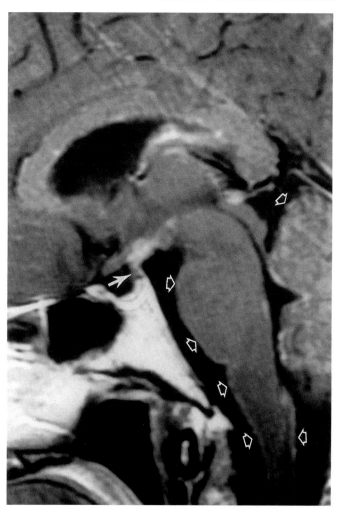

Figure 23-43 Noncontrast T1 coronal MRI of a 2-yr-old girl with Langerhans cell histiocytosis. This single image illustrates an aggressive form of Langerhans cell histiocytosis, Hand-Schüller-Christian disease. There are thickening of the infundibulum (arrow) and numerous destructive bone lesions (open arrows).

Figure 23-44 Contrast-enhanced T1 sagittal MRI of a 77-yr-old man with Langerhans cell histiocytosis. Though Langerhans cell histiocytosis is usually seen in children, it can also be seen in the older population. This image illustrates the diffuse leptomeningeal spread (open arrows) of this lesion, including the classic infundibular involvement (arrow).

hypothalamic region. Pituitary or hypothalamic involvement without bone involvement is called Gagel's granuloma *(1,2)*.

Letterer-Siwe disease is more disseminated than eosinophilic granuloma. It involves many organs, especially skin, lymphatics, and viscera.

6.1.3. Clinical Features. Histiocytosis generally strikes children and young adults, although a case that involved the pituitary of a 63-yr-old woman has been reported *(3)*. It is not very common, even among children. In a large series of parasellar tumors in children, there is only one case of histiocytosis *(4)*. The classic triad of abnormalities associated with histiocytosis is diabetes insipidus, pituitary insufficiency, and visual deterioration *(5–10)*.

Individual cases vary from the classic triad of symptoms *(11)*. Distal optic extension can produce proptosis *(12)*. Panhypopituitarism may occur without diabetes insipidus *(13)*. Other cases lack visual complaints *(2)*. Involvement of glands other than pituitary may alter the symptom complex *(14)*. Cutaneous lesions can develop *(13,15)*.

6.1.4. Radiographic Features. Thickening of the pituitary stalk is a common radiographic abnormality in parasellar histiocytosis (Figure 43) *(16–19)*. The hypothalamus may also be thickened *(18)*. In young children, the stalk will be >2.5 mm thick *(19)*. Although not specific for histiocytosis, stalk thickening plus absence of normal posterior lobe high signal intensity on T1-weighted images should arouse suspicion of this possibility *(17)*.

CT of lesions varies in intensity *(12,20,21)*. They uniformly enhance with contrast media *(12,13,20)*. Although MRI is superior to CT in evaluating the tumor parenchyma and also shows the bone lesions fairly well *(13)*, CT has particular value in evaluating bone defects often associated with histiocytosis involving the parasellar region *(17,22)*. The classic lesion fills the destroyed bone after destroying one or both tables of the skull. Abnormal soft tissue then extends out of the destroyed bone forming a "collar button" or "champagne cork" appearance.

If histiocytosis is suspected, additional lesions should be sought *(17)*. Although any part of the brain may be involved, optic and third ventricular regions are particularly susceptible *(3,12, 13,21,23–25)*. Temporal bone CT or bone scans may show additional lesions, but MRI is superior in defining the intracranial spread of disease *(17;* Figure 44).

6.1.5. Macroscopic Features. Most older lesions are firm nodules that contain collagen. They are gray to yellow, depending on their lipid content. Collagen hinders stereotactic biopsy, and

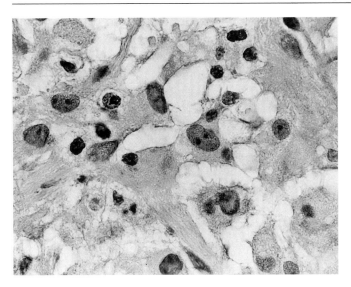

Figure 23-45 Rosai-Dorfmann disease shows large histiocytes with oval and reniform nuclei that contain leukocytes in their cytoplasm. From McKeever PE, Blaivas M, Sima AAF. Neoplasms of the sellar region. In: Lloyd RV, ed. Surgical Pathology of the Pituitary Gland. Major Problems in Pathology Series. Saunders, Philadelphia, 1993, pp. 141–210.

lesions involving the diaphragma sellae, dura, skull base, or even the brain parenchyma may be difficult to resect *(12,21)*.

New lesions of Langerhan's cell histiocytosis are less fibrotic than older lesions *(5,21)*. Other lesions are less fibrotic because they represent different variants with different constituents, including extranodal sinus histiocytosis with massive lymphadenopathy (SHML) *(12,21,23)* and xanthoma disseminatum *(26)*.

6.1.6. Microscopic Features. Cells that resemble histiocytes are the unifying structural theme of the histiocytoses. Among them, some cells will have nuclei larger than nuclei of reactive macrophages or Gitter cells. These vary from reniform nuclei to nuclei with complex folds and slits of nuclear membrane invaginations, seen well on cytologic preparations. The histiocytes contain variable amounts of lipid.

Mixed with these histiocytes are inflammatory cells, including lymphocytes, plasma cells, eosinophils, and polymorphonuclear leukocytes. Their numbers and distributions vary by case and by tissue region. Cytoplasmic leukocytes are a distinct feature of Rosai-Dorfman disease (SHML); *27*; Figure 45). Older lesions contain abundant polarizable collagen fibers. Margins of these lesions produce intense gliosis, increasing their resemblance to a glioma.

6.1.7. Immunocytochemistry. A panel of immunostains is recommended to rule out other possibilities and to subclassify the histiocytosis. This panel should include histiocytic markers like α-1-antichymotrypsin, lysozyme, and the MT1 marker. Of the numerous markers positive on individual cases, these three markers are positive on a high percentage of the histiocytoses *(28–31)*. Various histiocytoses express a T-cell marker with probable macrophage specificity *(28)*, a Hodgkin's cell marker *(32)*, and S-100 protein *(28–31)*.

S-100 protein should be included in the panel to help subclassify the histiocytosis and to test the possibility of a reactive process, more common than histiocytosis in the base of the skull. S-100 protein is present in the Langerhan's cell histio-

cyte and absent in macrophages or Gitter cells reacting to injury *(33,34)*. It is also absent in the foamy macrophages of xanthoma disseminatum *(12,26)*.

6.1.8. Ultrastructural Features. Langerhan's cell histiocytosis contains abnormal Langerhan's cells, which can be identified by their content of Birbeck granules *(25)*. These beautiful little cytoplasmic rods consist of long parallel membranes linked by cross-striations to form ultrastructural stepladders. Their rarity in some cases of Langerhan's histiocytosis diminishes the diagnostic impact of their absence. For this reason, Birbeck granules are more useful as a positive than as a negative marker.

Other constituents include variable numbers of cytoplasmic lipid and phagocytic vacuoles, mitochondria, and endoplasmic reticulum. Electron microscopy reveals the nuclear slits seen with light to be deep invaginations of the nuclear membranes with cytoplasmic penetrations.

6.1.9. Differential Diagnosis. Gliomas are a potential source of confusion. Common near the sella turcica, pilocytic astrocytomas show more fibrillar cellular processes than histiocytes, and they have distinctive Rosenthal fibers in some processes. Less common pleomorphic xanthoastrocytomas may require demonstration of their GFAP-positive cells to distinguish them from GFAP-negative histiocytosis. Other potentially confusing gliomas lack parenchymal collagen present in histiocytoses, and stainable with Masson's trichrome or silver stain for reticulin *(35)*.

Meningioma is a consideration in the differential of histiocytosis *(36)*. Some meningiomas mimick histiocytosis, particularly meningiomas with lymphoplasmacytes. Whorls and cells resembling syncytial cells characterize the meningioma. Meningothelial cells have a distinct ultrastructure of interdigitating cellular processes "stapled" together by desmosomes.

Subacute and chronic inflammation resembles histiocytosis. However, reactive and inflammatory macrophages have more uniform nuclear features than those in histiocytoses. They lack S-100 protein and Birbeck granules present in Langerhan's histiocytosis. Leukocytes do not abound in their cytoplasm like in histiocytes of SHML.

Primary lymphomas in this region have more pleomorphic lymphocytes with higher nuclear to cytoplasmic ratios than histiocytoses. These lymphoma cells show abundant mitoses and necrosis. Most are B-cell lymphomas. Histiocytic lymphomas and the immature component of malignant histiocytosis stain with monoclonal antihuman monocyte-1 (Mo1) marker *(37)*. Malignant histiocytic cells also contain ferritin *(29)*.

Presence of Birbeck granules distinguishes Langerhan's cell histiocytosis from the related disorder, extranodal sinus histiocytosis with massive lymphadenopathy (ESHML) *(3,21,25,26,37a)*. On the other hand, lymphocytes within the cytoplasm of large histiocytes is more definitive evidence of ESHML than lack of Birbeck granules. The large histiocytes of ESHML may also contain other types of blood cells *(23)*.

6.1.10. Therapy and Clinical Outcome. Individual histiocytoses respond differently to radiation and chemotherapy. Some cases respond to these *(11,15)*. Other cases are resistant *(13,38,39)*.

Chronic histiocytosis produces growth retardation in children *(40)*. About half of the patients who present with primary Langerhan's histiocytosis of the hypothalamus subsequently develop secondary lesions in other central nervous locations *(6–10,25)*.

6.2. LYMPHOMA

6.2.1. Definition.
The lymphoma is a neoplasm composed of a monoclonal proliferation of malignant lymphocytes. Compared to other malignancies, like glioblastoma and melanoma, the lymphoma is called a "small-cell tumor." However, compared with other lymphomas, the cells of parasellar lymphomas are rather large in some cases. With rare exceptions *(1)*, parasellar lymphomas are primary brain lymphomas.

6.2.2. Location.
Primary parasellar lymphomas usually involve the hypothalamus. They do this either directly or by invasion from the thalamus or basal ganglia *(2–10)*. Sinonasal lymphoma may invade the parasellar region through the destruction of bone *(11)*. Primary intrasellar lymphomas are rare.

Many primary CNS lymphomas are multicentric *(12)*. The occurrence of multiple brain masses or CSF metastases with signs of hypothalamic dysfunction raises strong suspicion of CNS lymphoma with hypothalamic involvement *(10)*.

6.2.3. Clinical Features.
Hypothalamic dysfunction determines the presenting symptoms. Diabetes insipidus is most common *(3,5)*. Other signs of hypothalamic invasion by lymphomas include hypoglycemia and weight loss *(4,6–8)*. Hypothalamic invasion interrupting neural pathways from cells producing prolactin-inhibitory factor in the hypothalamus are suggested to be important to the association of a prolactin-producing adenoma with a primary lymphoma *(2)*. A complex tumor mixed with lymphoma has been reported to contribute to diabetes mellitus in one patient *(9)*.

The incidence of primary CNS lymphomas is increasing. Part of its increase results from its occurrence among immunosuppressed individuals and those infected with human immunodeficiency virus (HIV). Another part probably reflects better immunohistochemistry and better diagnosis *(13)*. Despite all of this, in a study of pituitary lesions of patients with acquired immunodeficiency syndrome (AIDS), not 1 of 12 CNS lymphomas actually invaded the pituitary *(14)*. Dramatic regression of hypothalamic lymphomas occurs with steroid therapy *(5)*. Steroidal regression has been advocated as a diagnostic test, but it lacks specificity.

6.2.4. Radiographic Features.
MRI of suprasellar lymphomas is close to isointense on T1-weighted images and consistently hyperintense on proton density and T2-weighted images *(15)*. Cranial nerve enhancement with gadolinium may be seen *(16)*. Lymphomas usually show moderately high attenuation on CT and usually enhance homogeneously.

6.2.5. Macroscopic Features.
Lymphomas are gray or tan, and soft. Some are like a viscous liquid, almost pouring out from their surroundings. The softness and diffuse margins resemble that of high-grade gliomas. These features are hard to appreciate on many biopsies, since their deep location in clinically sensitive neuroanatomic regions has stimulated stereotactic biopsies *(17–19)*. Although adequate for straightforward cases, this approach may not provide sufficient tissue for complete analysis of other cases, including T-cell lymphomas *(20)*.

6.2.6. Microscopic Features and Special Stains.
A hypercellular infiltrate of small- to medium-sized malignant cells, which are nonfibrillar and noncohesive, suggests lymphoma. These features are highlighted on good touch preparations that show isolated, round neoplastic cells without processes (Figure 46).

Another feature often missing on stereotactic biopsies is a perivascular distribution of neoplastic cells with vascular wall invasion (Figure 47). Vascular wall invasion is well seen with a

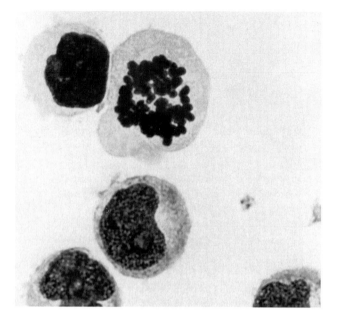

Figure 23-46 Lymphoma cells have nuclear pleomorphism, mitotic activity, and high nuclear cytoplasmic ratios. Lack of cellular processes among single, noncohesive cells rules out many other small-cell malignancies. Cytologic preparation, Wright's stain. From McKeever PE, Blaivas M, Sima AAF. Neoplasms of the sellar region. In: Lloyd RV, ed. Surgical Pathology of the Pituitary Gland. Major Problems in Pathology Series. Saunders, Philadelphia, 1993, pp. 141–210.

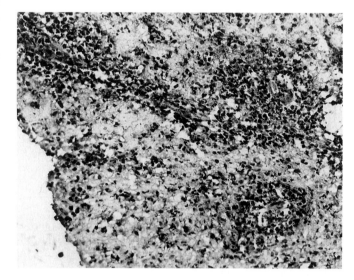

Figure 23-47 This primary CNS lymphoma infiltrated brain just above the hypothalamus. Malignant cells cluster around vessels and within their walls, and are less dense in brain tissue. This produces an ominous multifocal pattern of "dark clouds." From McKeever PE, Blaivas M, Sima AAF. Neoplasms of the sellar region. In: Lloyd RV, ed. Surgical Pathology of the Pituitary Gland. Major Problems in Pathology Series. Saunders, Philadelphia, 1993, pp. 141–210.

collagen stain like Masson's trichrome. It distinguishes vascular walls from parenchyma and simultaneously shows the neoplastic cells with standard counterstaining. Cytologic features of neoplastic cells within vascular walls and parenchyma are identical in lymphomas, in contrast to endothelial proliferations of malignant gliomas and desmoplasia of carcinomas.

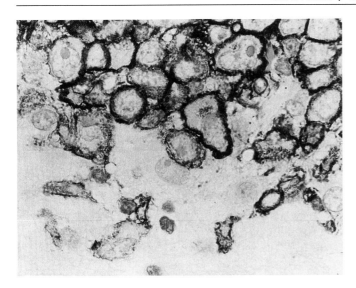

Figure 23-48 Typical staining of brain lymphoma cells with cell surface reactivity for B-cell markers like L26. The cells have large nuclei with peripheral margination of clumped chromatin, and huge nucleoli. From McKeever PE, Blaivas M, Sima AAF. Neoplasms of the sellar region. In: Lloyd RV, ed. Surgical Pathology of the Pituitary Gland. Major Problems in Pathology Series. Saunders, Philadelphia, 1993, pp. 141–210.

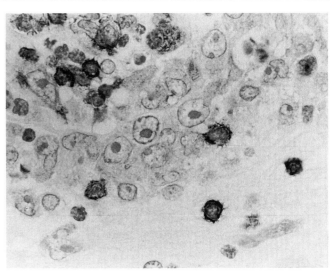

Figure 23-49 Same lymphoma as Figure 48 stained for T-cell marker UCHL-1. Lymphoma cells are negative, but smaller reactive T-cells are positive. McKeever PE, Blaivas M, Sima AAF. Neoplasms of the sellar region. In: Lloyd RV, ed. Surgical Pathology of the Pituitary Gland. Major Problems in Pathology Series. Saunders, Philadelphia, 1993, pp. 141–210.

Histiocytic lymphoma may be more common in hypothalamic lymphomas than other primary CNS locations *(2)*. Morphology of lymphomas varies from small-cell to plasmacytoid to large-cell immunoblastic *(21,22)*.

6.2.7. Immunohistochemistry. Reliable immunophenotypic markers for paraffin sections of routine formalin-fixed tissues have revolutionized the identification of B-cell lymphomas from small samples of tissue like stereotactic biopsies *(23)*. Most primary brain lymphomas, including parasellar examples, are B-cell lymphomas. Thus, they are positive for the L26 (CD20) marker of B-cells (Figure 48). Most are also positive for common leukocyte antigen (CLA; LCA) (CD45). Although neoplastic cells are usually negative for T-cell markers like A6 (CD45RO) or UCHL-1 (CD45R), there may be many reactive T-cells mixed with lymphoma cells (Figure 49).

For difficult cases, the immunostaining panel may be expanded with additional markers, such as MB1, MB2, MT2, LN-1 (CDw75), LN-2 (CD74), LN-3, and KP1 (CD68) *(21,23)*. Immunostaining for subtypes of immunoglobulin heavy and light chains is less useful for lymphomas than myelomas. However, *in situ* hybridization for light-chain mRNA has been recommended *(13)*.

6.2.8. Ultrastructural Features. Immunophenotyping has superseded electron microscopy for diagnosis of most lymphomas. Primary CNS lymphomas show round cells with little cytoplasm and no specific organelles *(24,25)*. Tumor vasculature is fenestrated *(26)*.

6.2.9. Differential Diagnosis. The lymphoma is a hypercellular small-cell malignancy. Other such tumors in the sellar region include the olfactory neuroblastoma and SNUC. Location is an important differential consideration. When the tumor arises in the hypothalamus, its more likely to be a lymphoma.

Olfactory neuroblastoma and SNUC cells lack lymphoid markers, including LCA and L26. Care should be taken to interpret immunohistochemically stained sections counterstained with hematoxylin to identify markers on neoplastic cells, since reactive lymphocytes may be present in any of these tumors. Lymphomas lack the neuronal markers present on olfactory neuroblastomas, including synaptophysin, neurofilaments, and S-100 protein *(27,28)*, and they lack epithelial markers of carcinomas, including cytokeratin and epithelial membrane antigen.

In contrast to the relatively nondescript ultrastructure of lymphomas, other small round cell tumors that might be mistaken for lymphomas have distinct features *(29)*. Olfactory neuroblastomas contain 150- to 350-nm dense core granules in cell bodies and processes. Carcinomas have epithelial features and may show intercellular junctions.

6.2.10. Clinical Outcome. In general, the prognosis of parasellar lymphoma patients is poor. CSF metastases occur, and more rarely, extraneural metastases are found *(10)*. MRI is useful in monitoring recurrence *(5)*. Intravenous chemotherapy has induced remission in a lymphoma metastasizing to the hypophysis *(1)*.

6.3. PLASMACYTOMA AND MULTIPLE MYELOMA

6.3.1. Definition. The plasmacytoma is a solitary neoplasm composed of plasma cells. If there are multiple lesions, the neoplasm is then called multiple myeloma. Parasellar plasmacytomas frequently progress to multiple myeloma *(1,2)*.

6.3.2. Location. Plasma cell neoplasms occur in the skull and soft tissues of the head, including the parasellar, hypothalamic, and intrasellar regions. Intrasellar and hypothalamic plasmacytomas are rare *(2–8)*.

Approximately 9 out of 10 extramedullary plasma cell neoplasms occur in the head and neck region *(9,10)*. Since at least three-fourths of these involve the sinonasal region, direct parasellar extension can occur. Review of previous studies may confirm the diagnosis.

6.3.3. Clinical Features. A plasmacytoma may be asymptomatic or present with diplopia and other cranial nerve signs, depending on its proximity to these sensitive structures *(3,6–8)*.

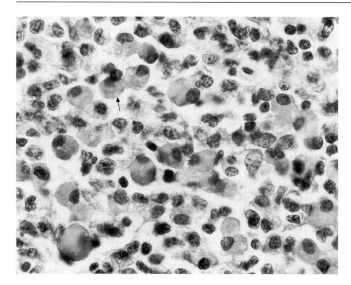

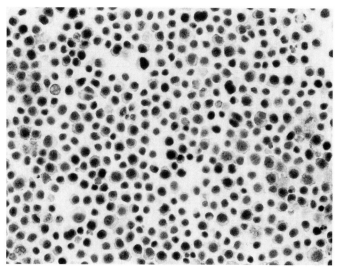

Figure 23-50   This plasmacytoma from the sphenoid bone is filled with plasma cells, some of which contain multiple light eosinophilic Russell bodies (arrow) producing a "mulberry" appearance in their cytoplasm. From McKeever PE, Blaivas M, Sima AAF. Neoplasms of the sellar region. In: Lloyd RV, ed. Surgical Pathology of the Pituitary Gland. Major Problems in Pathology Series. Saunders, Philadelphia, 1993, pp. 141–210.

Figure 23-51   Less-differentiated plasma cells in this systemic myeloma that involved the soft palate still show cells with dark cytoplasm and a perinuclear clear space. There are a few binucleated cells. From McKeever PE, Blaivas M, Sima AAF. Neoplasms of the sellar region. In: Lloyd RV, ed. Surgical Pathology of the Pituitary Gland. Major Problems in Pathology Series. Saunders, Philadelphia, 1993, pp. 141–210.

Depending on the extent of hypothalamic involvement, endocrine function may or may not be disturbed *(3,6,8)*.

Clinical features of intrasellar plasmacytomas are not very distinctive. Two intrasellar plasmacytomas were initially diagnosed as pituitary adenomas. The subsequent systemic course of the illness did not occur until 3–5 mo later, leading to the diagnosis *(1,4)*. This raises the question of whether there may be a fraction of plasmacytomas that do not progress to multiple myeloma and might elude correct diagnosis in the sella.

Multiple myeloma will have systemic manifestations *(1,2,4,8)*. A second tumor or lytic lesion should raise suspicion. Serum or urinary protein abnormalities may indicate a monoclonal gammopathy *(1,8)*.

6.3.4. Radiographic Features.   Myeloma may be isointense with brain tissue on T1-weighted images and hyperintense on T2-weighted images *(8)*. Destruction of the sella or surrounding skull bone may occur. Lytic lesions elsewhere in the skull or other bones may be evident *(1,4,7,11)*. Entirely intrasellar plasmacytomas may be radiographically indistinguishable from pituitary adenoma *(1)*.

6.3.5. Macroscopic Features.   The plasmacytoma varies from fleshy to soft and gelatinous. It is red-brown to gray. Bone lesions are lytic. The defects are often small and round with relatively distinct margins.

6.3.6. Microscopic Features.   Well-differentiated plasmacytomas resemble monotonous aggregates of mature plasma cells in abnormal locations *(2,9)*. Stained with H&E, they have round nuclei with clumped chromatin that resemble a clock face or cartwheel. Nuclei are peripherally displaced in purple cytoplasm with a prominent perinuclear clear space. Bi- or trinucleated cells may be evident. Cytoplasmic Russell bodies may occur. They are aggregated immunoglobulin that show as orange-pink, round globules (Figure 50). All ranges of immaturity may occur (Figure 51). Poorly differentiated myeloma cells may resemble plasmacytoid lymphocytes or bone marrow precursor cells.

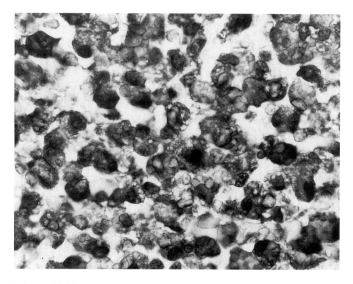

Figure 23-52   All cells contain cytoplasmic IgG in this sphenoidal plasmacytoma. They were κ light-chain positive, and negative for other immunoglobulin markers. From McKeever PE, Blaivas M, Sima AAF. Neoplasms of the sellar region. In: Lloyd RV, ed. Surgical Pathology of the Pituitary Gland. Major Problems in Pathology Series. Saunders, Philadelphia, 1993, pp. 141–210.

6.3.7. Immunohistochemistry.   Myeloma cells produce a monoclonal or highly restricted class of immunoglobulins (Figure 52). They stain for only a single light chain, either κ or λ *(12)*. They are positive for epithelial membrane antigen.

6.3.8. Ultrastructural Features.   Well-differentiated neoplastic plasma cells contain a highly developed RER. This is the material that colors the cytoplasm blue on H&E stains and produces immunoglobulin protein from mRNA. The RER cisternae often contain crystalline or amorphous aggregates of this protein, the ultrastructural equivalent of Russell bodies. There is a well-developed Golgi apparatus, corresponding to the perinuclear clear space on H&E stain *(9,13)*. Less-differentiated cells contain fewer of these cytoplasmic organelles.

6.3.9. Differential Diagnosis. A solitary intrasellar plasmacytoma bears a remarkable resemblance to a pituitary adenoma when stained with H&E *(14)*. Both neoplasms are composed of cells with high secretory capacity, producing a similar appearance. Electron microscopy has established the correct diagnosis in many reported cases *(2,4,13)*. Pituitary adenomas have large, dense secretory granules, intercellular junctions, and pericellular basal laminae that myelomas lack *(13)*. When cases progress to multiple myeloma, bone marrow biopsy or laboratory electrophoresis are definitive *(1,8)*.

Immunocytochemistry can reveal monoclonal expression of an immunoglobulin (Ig) heavy-chain subtype and κ or λ light chain *(12,13)*. This immunoreactivity differs from pituitary hormone immunoreactivity of adenoma and from histiocytes and inflammation.

Primary brain lymphomas have high nuclear to cytoplasmic ratios and infiltrate in and around vessel walls producing prominent perivascular cuffs *(15,16)*. Plasma cells have immunoreactivity for epithelial membrane antigen and frequently lack activity for leukocyte common antigen. All of these features help to differentiate myeloma from lymphomas *(17,18)*. Myelomas often lack L26, LN1, LN2, MB1, MB2 or MB3 MAb of B-cells *(19)*. Myelomas tend to have more monoclonal immunoglobulin in their cytoplasm than lymphomas. However, immunoglobulin secretion is their most characteristic feature. Therefore, when it is positive, serum protein electrophoresis is a reliable assay to distinguish multiple myeloma from lymphoma.

Chronic inflammatory process are polyclonal. Careful inspection for inflammatory cells other than plasma cells usually confirms this difference from myeloma. In more difficult cases, examination of heavy- and light-chain subclasses for neoplastic expression of monoclonality can be done *(19)*.

Plasma cells associated with monoclonal gammopathy of undetermined significance (MGUS) lack the marker against natural killer cells CD56 and have inconspicuous staining with the MB2 MAb to an intracytoplasmic B-cell antigen *(20,21)*. These are less aggressive than myelomas positive for common acute lymphoblastic leukemia antigen (CALLA) *(22)*.

6.3.10. Clinical Outcome. Parasellar plasma cell neoplasms exhibit a highly variable range of outcomes. Although individual exceptions occur, these general rules govern most cases. The majority of intrasellar plasmacytomas progress to multiple myeloma *(1,2,4,13)*. In contrast, solitary sinonasal plasmacytomas rarely progress, particularly if removed as a polyp. A plasmacytoma that involves bone is more likely to progress to multiple myeloma than one in soft tissue.

Multiple myeloma is treated with radiation and chemotherapy *(2,8,23)*. As with other radiated tumors in this region, the treatment may be complicated by optic neuropathy *(24)*.

7. GERM-CELL TUMORS

7.1. GERMINOMA AND OTHER GERM-CELL TUMORS

7.1.1. Definition. The germinoma is the most common intracranial germ-cell neoplasm. It resembles the testicular seminoma and the ovarian dysgerminoma.

Less common germ-cell tumors include endodermal sinus tumor, embryonal carcinoma, choriocarcinoma, and teratoma. Their usual presentation as mixed tumors precludes their separate discussion. All except teratoma *(see* Subheading 7.2.) are included here.

7.1.2. Location. Intracranial germ-cell tumors arise along the midline from the suprasellar cistern to the pineal gland 95% of the time *(1)*. The percentage of germ-cell tumors that arise in the suprasellar cistern varies from 18% (Japan) to 37% (United States) *(1,2)*. Most of these are germinomas *(1,2)*. Another 6–13% of germ-cell tumors involve both pineal and suprasellar regions *(1–4)*.

The group of various germ-cell tumors are slightly more common in the pineal than the suprasellar region *(1,2)*. On the other hand, the majority of germinomas arise in the suprasellar region, and the pineal gland is more involved with nongerminomatous germ-cell tumors *(1)*.

7.1.3. Clinical Features. Two-thirds of patients are diagnosed in adolescence *(1,2)*. Other cases occur in children to middle-aged adults. Males are more commonly afflicted.

Diabetes insipidus is the most common clinical manifestation of patients with suprasellar germinoma *(5–7)*. Signs of hypopituitarism are very common, including hypogonadism, hypocortisolism, hypothyroidism, growth delay, and pubertal delay *(5,6)*. Visual disturbances, headache, or vomiting occur in about half of the cases. A few patients have cranial nerve paresis, papilledema, or ataxia *(5,6)*. Anorexia nervosa has occasionally been associated with germinoma. One-third of patients with anorexia and an intracranial lesion had a germ-cell tumor in one study *(8)*.

Small series of patients with both suprasellar and pineal germinomas have been reported. In these cases, the initial symptoms have been similar to solitary suprasellar germinomas. Pineal symptoms developed subsequently *(4)*.

Germinomas with an intrasellar component do not always present with diabetes insipidus. Optic and endocrinologic symptoms may mimic pituitary adenoma *(9)*.

Rarely, germinomas are associated with clinical syndromes. In addition to a hypophyseal stalk germinoma, a Klinefelter's syndrome patient had a mediastinal teratocarcinoma *(10)*. Another patient with mental retardation and characteristic facial features of Cornelia de Lange syndrome had a suprasellar germinoma *(11)*. A third patient had multiple tumors, including a third ventricular germinoma, and a hypothalamic cystic mixed astrocytoma and oligodendroglioma *(12)*.

7.1.4. Radiographic Features. CT reveals a hyperdense soft tissue mass that enhances inhomogeneously with contrast *(6;* Figure 53). More modern studies evaluate the tumor with MRI. On T1-weighted images, germinoma signal intensity is moderately low to isointense *(6,13,14)*. On T2-weighted images, signal intensity is usually hyperintense *(6,13,14)*. Regions of different intensity are common *(13)*. Frank enhancement with MRI contrast is typical of germinoma *(13,15)*.

The majority of germinomas have a suprasellar component *(13)*. These well-marginated, round, or lobular tumors have prolonged T1 and T2 relaxation times *(15)*. They usually displace the third ventricle, but seldom the carotid artery or optic chiasm *(14,16)*. They do not calcify or erode the dorsum sellae *(6,14,17)*.

Many suprasellar germinomas have an intrasellar component *(9,13)*. The intrasellar component can be confused with pituitary

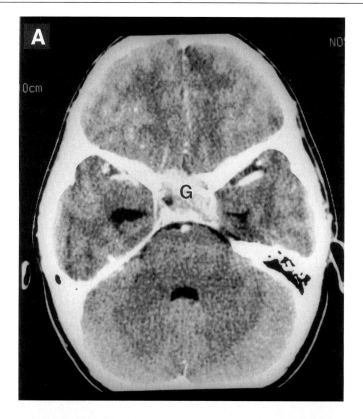

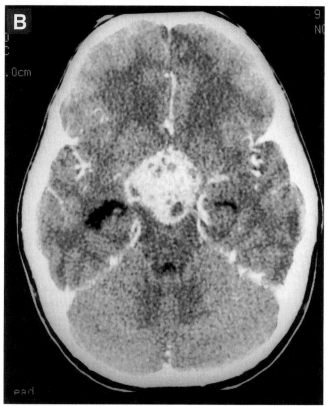

Figure 23-53   Post-iv contrast brain CT of a 9-yr-old boy with a germinoma. **(A)** This axial CT section through the sella turcica shows an inhomogeneously enhancing mass (G) entering the sella turcica and distorting the pituitary gland. **(B)** This slightly more rostral section shows the extension of the inhomogeneously enhancing mass to distort the base of the frontal lobes and the mesencephalon. The inhomogeneous texture of this lesion is typical for perisellar germinomas.

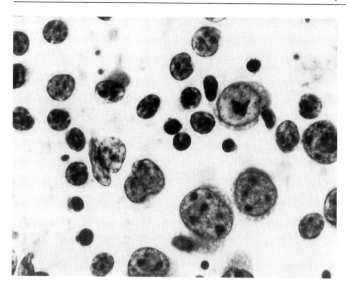

Figure 23-54 This germinoma shows typical large epithelioid cells with large nuclei and large, irregular nucleoli. These are mixed with small lymphocytes. Cytologic preparation stained with H&E. From McKeever PE, Blaivas M, Sima AAF. Neoplasms of the sellar region. In: Lloyd RV, ed. Surgical Pathology of the Pituitary Gland. Major Problems in Pathology Series. Saunders, Philadelphia, 1993, pp. 141–210.

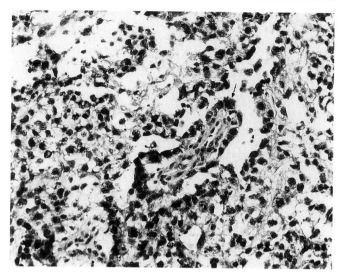

Figure 23-55 This mixed endodermal sinus tumor and germinoma contains Schiller-Duval bodies (arrow). From McKeever PE, Blaivas M, Sima AAF. Neoplasms of the sellar region. In: Lloyd RV, ed. Surgical Pathology of the Pituitary Gland. Major Problems in Pathology Series. Saunders, Philadelphia, 1993, pp. 141–210.

adenoma *(9)*. This problem is increased in germinomas, which are predominantly or exclusively intrasellar *(18,19)*. Displacement of the pituitary anteriorly suggests a germinoma; displacement superiorly suggests adenoma *(20)*. The MRI signal of intrasellar germinoma shows absence of the normal hyperintense signal of posterior pituitary on T1-weighted images *(21)*. Some germinomas expand the sella *(19)*.

7.1.5. Macroscopic Features. Germinomas are gray tumors with distinct margins up against surrounding tissue. They vary in firmness depending on their collagen content. Other germ-cell tumors may be softer or more vascular than germinoma. Teratomas are described under Subheading 7.2.

Germinoma tissue needs careful handling to preserve its histologic features. Small samples may show only the lymphocytes creating the appearance of a lymphoid proliferation or only large cells that resemble carcinoma. The lymphocytes dry out quickly under hot lamps and smear easily, producing streaks of hematoxylinophilic material obscuring cellular detail.

7.1.6. Microscopic Features. Histologic features of germinoma show two distinct cell populations. Large, neoplastic, epithelioid cells contain large, round, vesiculated nuclei with prominent pleomorphic nucleoli (Figure 54). These cells contain glycogen. Small lymphocytes comprise the second cell population.

Other germ-cell tumors include endodermal sinus tumor (yolk sac tumor), choriocarcinoma, and embryonal carcinoma. These are usually mixed with germinoma and/or each other in the sellar region. Compared with germinoma, lymphocytes are relatively sparse in pure choriocarcinoma, embryonal carcinoma, or endodermal sinus tumors. Teratomas are described separately (Subheading 7.2.).

Endodermal sinus tumors are composed of epithelial ribbons and papillae that resemble yolk sac membranes. They contain Schiller-Duvall bodies *(22)*. These are papillae with vascular cores that protrude into clear channels. Both papillae and channels are

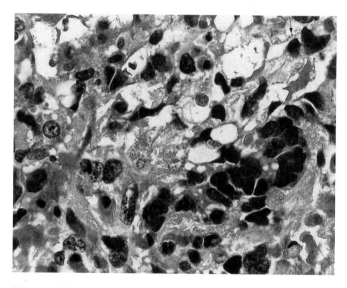

Figure 23-56 Cytoplasmic and extracellular eosinophilic globules (arrow) up to 5 μm in diameter occur in this endodermal sinus tumor portion of mixed germ-cell tumor. These are globules of AFP (Figure 58).

lined by cuboidal epithelium (Figure 55). Eosinophilic globules occur in and around the epithelium (Figure 56).

Embryonal carcinoma is composed of primitive epithelial cells with many mitoses and necrosis. These cells may form sheets or glandular conglomerates.

Choriocarcinoma is composed of huge syncytial and smaller trophoblastic cells. These are recognizable on H&E stains. The two layers of large and small trophoblastic cells line up beside each other.

7.1.7. Immunohistochemistry. Germinomas contain placental alkaline phosphate (PlAP) *(23,24)*. Membranous reactivity predominates (Figure 57). Ninety-three percent of germinomas are positive for PlAP *(2)*. In contrast, 25% of embryonal carcinomas and no choriocarcinoma are positive.

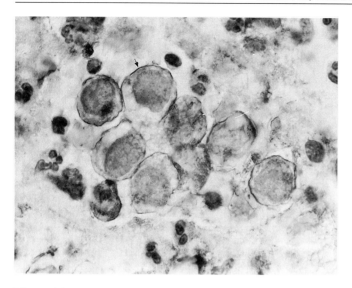

Figure 23-57   This germinoma is positive (arrow) for placental alkaline phosphatase (PlAP). From McKeever PE, Blaivas M, Sima AAF. Neoplasms of the sellar region. In: Lloyd RV, ed. Surgical Pathology of the Pituitary Gland. Major Problems in Pathology Series. Saunders, Philadelphia, 1993, pp. 141–210.

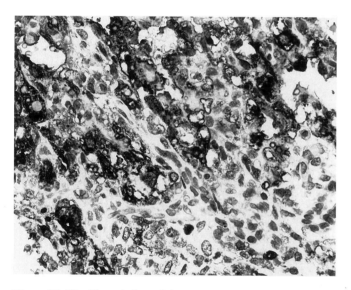

Figure 23-58   The endodermal sinus tumor component of this mixed germ-cell tumor is immunohistochemically positive for cytoplasmic AFP. Some AFP is globular, and some globules are extracellular.

Angiotensin-I-converting enzyme (ACE) is detectable in germinoma tissues as well as in plasma of affected patients (25–27). Embryonal carcinomas and teratocarcinoma are negative (25).

The majority of endodermal sinus tumors and embryonal carcinomas are positive for α-fetoprotein (AFP) (2,27–29; Figure 58). The majority of choriocarcinomas express human chorionic gonadotropin (HCG) (2,27). Germinomas do not usually stain with these markers (2,6,27).

Suprasellar germinomas are reported to lack epithelial membrane antigen (EMA), cytokeratin (CK), and vimentin markers expressed by pineal germinomas (30). This pattern is virtually identical to gonadal germinomas.

The small cells in germinomas are a polyclonal collection of T-lymphocytes, B-lymphocytes, and natural killer cells (31–34).

These antigens can be stained with A6 for T-cells and L26 for B-cells. Provocative evidence suggests these small cells are different than lymphocytes elsewhere (35). Confirmation is eagerly awaited.

7.1.8. Ultrastructural Features.   Nucleolonemae are large, complex labyrinthine or fenestrated nucleoli (36–38). These are a distinctive ultrastructural feature of germinomas. Intranuclear membranous profiles are also distinctive. Other ultrastructural features of germinomas, including tubuloreticular structures, annulate lamellae, glycogen, and distended RER, are relatively nonspecific features (36–38). The ultrastructural features of parasellar germinomas resemble those of gonadal seminomas and dysgerminomas (39).

7.1.9. Differential Diagnosis.   A major consideration in the differential diagnosis of germinoma is carcinoma. This includes embryonal carcinoma, metastatic carcinoma, and local carcinoma. Most local carcinomas like sinonasal undifferentiated carcinoma and salivary tumors invade the parasellar region secondarily. Careful attention to their anatomic origin distinguishes them.

Metastatic pulmonary carcinoma with lymphocytic infiltrates of its regions of desmoplasia resembles germinoma. Mucin production favors adenocarcinoma. PlAP can be helpful, but 7% of germinomas do not express PlAP, and a few metastatic carcinomas express PlAP (40). Ultrastructural analysis can be useful. Most helpful is the anatomical distribution. A solitary suprasellar mass is highly suggestive of germinoma. A solitary mass or multiple intracranial masses outside of the midline pituitary–pineal axis requires search to rule out an occult systemic primary.

Anatomic distribution is not helpful in distinguishing local embryonal carcinoma from germinoma. Embryonal carcinoma classically produces epithelial structures that resemble acini. Alternatively, lymphocytes are prominent in germinoma, and a pure germinoma lacks AFP.

Sampling problems may produce a specimen loaded with lymphocytes that can be confused with hypophysitis or lymphoma. A careful search for the other component, large epithelioid cells, should include immunohistochemical markers. The lymphocytes in germinomas are smaller than lymphoma cells and are polyclonal.

7.1.10. Therapy and Clinical Outcome.   Histologic diagnosis and extent of disease are critical prognostic factors in germ-cell tumors (1). Pure germinomas are highly radiosensitive even when given <45 gy (41,42). Pure germinomas properly treated have a significantly longer survival than mixed and nongerminomatous germ-cell tumors. This places a premium on checking serum or CSF for AFP and HCG, and on surgical excision of a large portion of tumor to evaluate properly the possibility of a mixed germ-cell tumor (2).

Tumor involvement of the hypothalamus, third ventricle, or spinal cord significantly decreases survival (1). Systemic metastases are less common from suprasellar than from pineal germinomas, perhaps reflecting the larger percentage of pure germinomas around the sella (1,43). Ten percent of patients who require ventriculosomatic shunts develop abdominal or pelvic metastases (1,33).

7.2. TERATOMA

7.2.1. Definition

The teratoma is a complex neoplasm composed of a variety of heterogeneous tissues, typically reflecting more than one of the three embryonal germ layers. Russell and Rubinstein separated them into mature teratomas formed by well-differentiated tissues from all three layers and immature teratomas that contain less-differentiated elements derived from one or all germinal layers (1).

7.2.2. Location. Teratomas of the sellar region are rare and usually occur in children and young adults. Two of 74 patients with parasellar tumors had malignant intrasellar teratoma *(2)*. Two of 41 patients with parasellar tumors, in an autopsy series that included patients of all ages, had teratomas *(3)*. In two unusual cases, the sellar region was secondarily occupied by a teratoma in neonates who presented with facial teratoma associated with craniopharyngeal canal *(4,5)*.

7.2.3. Clinical Features. Five children ages 5–10 yr with suprasellar teratoma had symptoms of diabetes insipidus, visual disturbance, hypopituitarism, and occasionally increased intracranial pressure *(6)*. Craniofacial teratomas in various locations can present prenatally with macrocrania and polyhydramnios, difficult delivery, or postnatally with brain herniation, hydrocephalus, respiratory distress, or feeding problems owing to a large, life-threatening mass *(7)*.

7.2.4. Radiographic Features. Teratomas are usually multilobulated masses, often large, with complex radiologic characteristics *(7*; Figure 59). In a 19-yr-old man with immature teratoma mixed with germinoma, the skull radiographs and tomography of the sella turcica demonstrated mild enlargement of the sella and irregular demineralization and thinning of the sellar floor and the dorsum sellae *(8)*. Similar findings were reported in a 33-yr-old man with an intrasellar tumor that was classified as teratoid and not a teratoma since only two germinal layer representatives were identified *(9)*. CT in both of these cases demonstrated an enhancing intrasellar mass. However, CT and MRI often show a heterogeneous mass, typical for a neoplasm of multilayer embryonic origin.

7.2.5. Macroscopic Findings. These neoplasms are bulky and irregular in consistency. They have soft regions alternating with firm ones and some cystic spaces. Specific tissues like cartilage, brain, or epithelium may be evident.

7.2.6. Microscopic Features. In the mature teratoma, tissues representing all three germinal layers are mixed together and are benign and well differentiated (Figure 60). For example, solid or cystic areas of squamous epithelium may be mixed with glandular or tubular structures lined by various types of epithelium, mature glial and neuronal tissue, and possibly cartilage separated by stretches of mesenchymal stroma. Only one of the five cases reported by Tekeuchi et al. was benign, even though it occurred in the youngest of all five patients *(6)*. The other four cases were mixed germ-cell tumors, a combination of teratoma with germinoma, choriocarcinoma, or carcinoma (*see* Subheading 7.1.). Immature elements of teratoma that are prognostically important most frequently are embryonal neural epithelial structures that resemble neuroblastoma, medulloepithelioma, or ependymoblastoma.

7.2.7. Immunohistochemical Features. Teratomas stain positively with a variety of different markers depending on their constituents. These include vimentin for mesenchymal tissues, keratin and possibly epithelial membrane antigen for epithelial tissues, and GFAP for glial tissue. If other types of germ-cell tumors are mixed within, they stain with appropriate markers, such as placental alkaline phosphatase, β-HCG, α-fetoprotein.

7.2.8. Differential Diagnosis. Teratomas are not difficult to diagnose when surgical sampling is complete and the elements of all three germinal layers are present. Inadequate sampling generates a whole list of diagnoses depending on which portion or portions of the neoplasm were biopsied, particularly in cases where the teratoma includes elements of other germ-cell tumors.

7.2.9. Clinical Outcome. Mature teratomas are amenable to complete surgical excision with a good prognosis. In a rare case when an immature teratoma can be removed in its entirety, the outcome is also good. However, half of the patients with nonremovable immature teratoma died within the first year according to Jennings and collaborators *(10)*.

8. OTHER TUMORS

8.1. PARAGANGLIOMA

8.1.1. Definition. Paraganglioma, chemodectoma, or glomus jugulare tumor (compare with Subheading 5.3.) is a neuroendocrine tumor that arises in association with sympathetic and parasympathetic ganglia.

8.1.2. Location. Paragangliomas have been reported in intrasellar and suprasellar locations *(1–3)*. The origin of paragangliomas in this location is not clear since paraganglionic cells have not been found in the pituitary gland. It seems likely, as was suggested by Ho et al. *(4)* and Steel et al. *(3)*, that they arise from small aggregates of paraganglion cells migrating along the tympanic branch of the XII cranial nerve where they were found residing occasionally, or from nearby sources of specialized neural crest cells. Paragangliomas arising in the carotid bodies, glomus jugulare, nasal region, or temporal bone may rarely extend into the cranial cavity to involve the parasellar region.

8.1.3. Clinical Features. The patients present with headaches that can be associated with nausea and vomiting *(3)*. One patient had hypopituitarism *(1)*; another developed a pheochromocytoma-like syndrome owing to a catecholamine-secreting paraganglioma arising within the pterygopalatine fossa *(5)*. Visual field examination was normal in all of these patients.

8.1.4. Radiographic Features. The mass is nearly uniformly contrast-enhancing on MRI. It may extend into adjacent structures and usually demonstrates little abnormal vascularity on angiography *(2,3)*. As with other paragangliomas, the surrounding bone can be remodeled, but seldom shows frank destruction.

8.1.5. Macroscopic Features. The tumor was soft, pinkish-white, and bled readily when sectioned in the cases of Steel and collaborators. One of them was encapsulated, but eroded through the floor of the pituitary fossa *(3)*. In another case, the tumor encased both carotid arteries and compressed left mesial temporal lobe, left cerebral peduncle, extending to the left foramen ovale. In the case of Bilbao and associates, the intrasellar mass was firm and indistinguishable from normal pituitary tissue *(1)*.

8.1.6. Microscopic Features. The neoplasm is formed by round, oval, or polyhedral cells with abundant finely granular cytoplasm and centrally placed slightly hyperchromatic nuclei. The "Zellballen" pattern is not as clear as in paragangliomas in other locations; rather, the cells are arranged in vague lobules separated by vascular connective tissue bands.

8.1.7. Immunohistochemistry and Ultrastructure. Two cell types are recognizable: more prominent chief cells and sustentacular cells. The chief cells stain positively with chromogranin, and the sustentacular cells that vary in numbers from one case to another stain for S-100 protein. Paragangliomas characteristically stain positively for catecholamines and methionine-enkephalin *(6)*. They do not stain for pituitary hormones.

The neurosecretory granules of paragangliomas as of many other endocrine tumors are better visualized in electron micrographs or toluidine blue-stained resin-embedded section than in H&E-stained paraffin sections *(7)*. They range from 150 to 300 nm

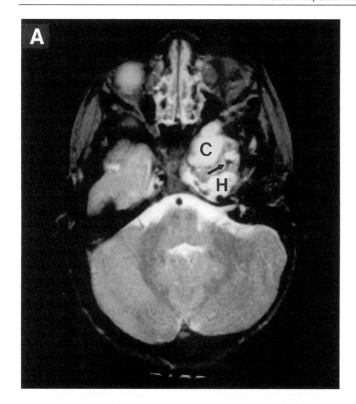

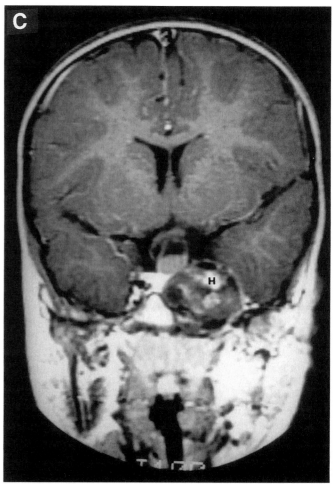

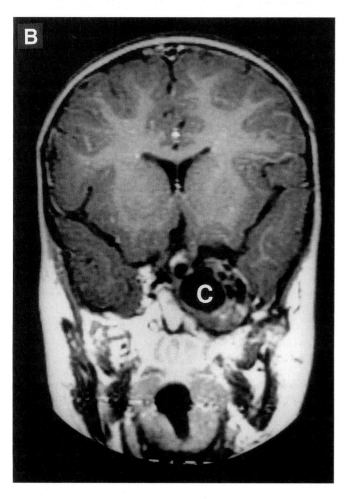

Figure 23-59 Brain MRI of a 3-yr-old girl with a teratoma. **(A)** T2-weighted axial MR image shows the typical complex signal character of a teratoma. There are cysts of two different signal intensities, with a dense isthmus of stroma between them. The anterior cyst (C) signal is similar to that of CSF, owing to its mainly serous content. The isthmus of stroma shows some pathologic contrast enhancement (panels B and C) and a few dense calcified regions, delineated as low signal on this image (arrow). The posterior more complex cyst (H) has higher signal contents on both T2- and T1-weighted imaging, consistent with cholesterol and/or hemorrhage. **(B)** Coronal T1-weighted MR section after iv contrast through the anterior cyst (C) shows the low T1 signal of the mainly water-containing cyst and some of the enhancing surrounding stroma. **(C)** Coronal T1-weighted MR section after iv contrast shows the partially enhancing stroma surrounding the high signal of the posterior cyst (H).

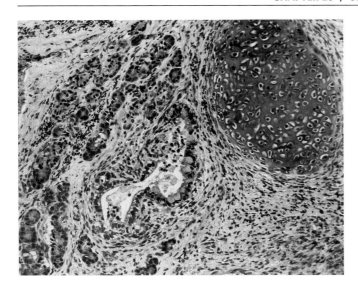

Figure 23-60 Representatives of multiple germinal layers are in one section of this mature sellar teratoma: glandular acini, gut-like epithelium, hyaline cartilage, and mesodermal stroma. From McKeever PE, Blaivas M, Sima AAF. Neoplasms of the sellar region. In: Lloyd RV, ed. Surgical Pathology of the Pituitary Gland. Major Problems in Pathology Series. Saunders. Philadelphia, 1993, pp. 141–210.

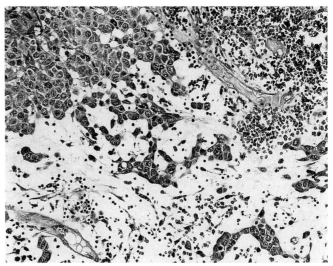

Figure 23-61 This melanoma is composed of epithelioid cells. It resembles carcinoma or chordoma. From McKeever PE, Blaivas M, Sima AAF. Neoplasms of the sellar region. In: Lloyd RV, ed. Surgical Pathology of the Pituitary Gland. Major Problems in Pathology Series. Saunders, Philadelphia, 1993, pp. 141–210.

in diameter and are membrane-bound. Glycogen, lipopigment, microfilaments and microtubles are present in many cells. Thick basement membrane surrounds clusters of tumor cells *(1)*.

8.1.8. Differential Diagnosis. Paragangliomas can be distinguished from most pituitary adenomas by their different hormone content. They rarely present a diagnostic problem as long as one is aware of their possible occurrence in the region of the pituitary gland.

8.1.9. Therapy and Clinical Outcome. For most paragangliomas of the head and neck, surgical excision is the treatment of choice. Additional radiotherapy is also recommended, particularly in cases of incomplete surgical removal. Two patients reported by Steel et al. remained stable 12 mo after treatment *(3)*.

8.2. MELANOMA

8.2.1. Definition. The melanoma is a malignant tumor composed of neoplastic melanocytes and pigmented cells found in a few tissues, but most prominently in the skin.

8.2.2. Location. Parasellar primary melanomas occur in the intrasellar, suprasellar, sinonasal, and sphenoid regions *(1–7)*. They are rare in all of these locations. The origin of intrasellar melanomas is not known, but may be melanocytes in the meninges or Rathke's pouch *(2,8)*. Metastatic melanoma is covered in another chapter.

8.2.3. Clinical Features. Common chief complaints are headaches and decreased vision. Impaired memory has been reported. Clinical signs include optic disk atrophy and signs of hypopituitarism *(2,4,8)*.

8.2.4. Radiographic Features. Melanomas are masses of heterogeneous, and often high CT density. They expand the pituitary fossa and erode the dorsum sellae *(2)*. Radiographic features vary depending on the structures involved and can include meningeal involvement *(1,3,5,9)*. MRI often shows the paramagnetic behavior of melanin. The T1 signal will be high, but the T2 signal will be low. Amelanotic melanoma does not show this paramagnetic behavior.

8.2.5. Macroscopic Features. The most characteristic feature of melanoma is its jet black color *(3)*. However, this is seen more often in better-differentiated tumors, some of which may be melanocytomas rather than malignant melanomas. Common color variants range in gray tones, the lightest of which are nonpigmented and indistinguishable from adenomas and gliomas *(2–5,8)*. Regional hemorrhage adds mixtures of red, brown, and yellow *(7)*. Soft regions of necrosis occur. Some melanomas invade locally and spread through the meninges, imparting a diffuse margin *(1,9–12)*.

8.2.6. Microscopic Features and Special Stains. Melanomas are composed of malignant epithelioid to spindled cells that contain variable amounts of small, dark brown melanin granules (Figure 61). These cytoplasmic granules are on average smaller, darker, and more uniform in size and shape than hemosiderin granules *(13)*. Melanin does not stain with Perl's stain for iron like hemosiderin. It does react with the Fontana stain. Some melanomas provide no light microscopic evidence of melanin granules.

Nuclei are pleomorphic with dark chromatin (Figure 61). Nucleoli are often, but not invariably quite large and are pleomorphic. Pyknotic nuclei and regions of coagulation necrosis occur. Mitoses are often conspicuous, but tumors vary. Individual sellar melanomas contain papillae and less mitoses *(2)*. Hemorrhage is common *(7)*.

Tumor margins may be highly infiltrative, particularly into the meninges *(14)*. Other margins are abrupt. Still other melanomas form a fibrous capsule between the melanoma and surrounding tissues.

8.2.7. Immunohistochemistry. Melanomas express S-100 protein *(1,15)*. They express the β-subunit of S-100, and sometimes α as well *(16)*.

Melanomas react with the HMB-45 antibody *(17,18*; Figure 62). HMB-45 stains an antigen in lipoid cytoplasmic vacuoles *(17)*. Its specificity is more restricted than the S-100 stain, but HMB-45 stains other pigmented tumors like melanotic schwannoma and glioma. Like many MAbs, its staining power is improved using

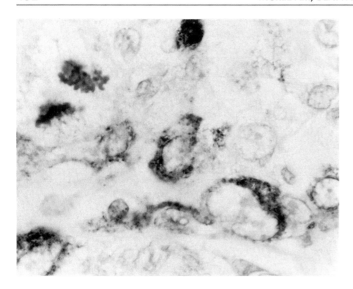

Figure 23-62 Same tumor as Figure 61 is positive for granular cytoplasmic HMB-45. From McKeever PE, Blaivas M, Sima AAF. Neoplasms of the sellar region. In: Lloyd RV, ed. Surgical Pathology of the Pituitary Gland. Major Problems in Pathology Series. Saunders, Philadelphia, 1993, pp. 141–210.

signal amplification procedures like avidin–biotin immunohistochemistry *(19)*. With proper amplification, HMB-45 will stain certain amelanotic melanomas. The antibody ME1-14 reacts with 60% of melanomas in cytologic preparations *(15)*. It targets α-chondroitin sulfate proteoglycan.

8.2.8. Ultrastructural Features. The amelanotic melanoma is the most challenging melanoma to recognize and confirm. Electron microscopy aids identification of these tumors by revealing nonpigmented premelanosomes. These cytoplasmic organelles are 100 × 400 nm ellipsoidal, membrane-bound structures. The most characteristic lamellar and spiral premelanosomes contain striated cores of parallel filaments and coils of filaments, respectively, that produce zigzag patterns *(20,21)*.

Mature melanosomes are electron-dense structures that become larger than premelanosomes. They are found in pigmented melanomas and usually do not require electron microscopy for their identification.

8.2.9. Differential Diagnosis. Pigmented melanomas provide little diagnostic challenge in the sellar region. The more indolent melanocytoma and melanotic schwannoma cause theoretical concern, but are extremely rare near the sella *(3,22)*. Both tumors have less anaplastic nuclear features, lower mitotic rates, and are less invasive than malignant melanoma.

Nonpigmented melanomas have a broader differential and are more challenging. Since melanomas are uniformly S-100-positive, lack of S-100 suggests another malignancy, such as an S-100-negative type of carcinoma or sarcoma. Since melanomas are positive for β S-100 and pituitary adenomas are not, this provides a potential distinction *(16)*. However, production of a pituitary hormone guarantees identification of the adenoma *(23)*. Olfactory neuroblastoma and primitive neuroectodermal tumors can be distinguished by their synaptophysin reactivity, which melanoma lacks *(1)*.

CK immunoreactivity suggests carcinoma or chordoma, and EMA reactivity adds meningioma to the list. Melanomas are CK- and EMA-negative, and negative for GFAP. GFAP distinguishes

gliomas from melanoma *(24)*. If any nonmelanin-producing neoplasm is in the differential, it can be excluded if the tumor is HMB-45-positive or contains premelanosomes by electron microscopic examination *(21)*.

8.2.10. Clinical Outcome. Although individual cases are highly variable, the usual prognosis is poor. Solitary, well-circumscribed tumors that can be totally removed and show minimal mitotic activity have the best prognosis *(3,25)*. Some of these solitary tumors may not be melanomas.

ACKNOWLEDGMENTS

We thank Dianna Banka and Peggy Otto for skillfully preparing the manuscript. Mark Deming provided superb light micrographs. Yinru Sieracki, Barbara Rogers, and Toby Booker provided fine electron micrographs. This work was supported in part by US HHS PHS National Institutes of Health grant 1 R01 CA68545 and P03 CA46592.

REFERENCES

1.1.1. Craniopharyngioma

1. Hoffman HJ. Craniopharyngiomas. Prog Exp Tumor Res 1987; 30:325–334.
2. Richmond I, Wilson CB. Parasellar tumors in children I. Clinical presentation, preoperative assessment, and differential diagnosis. Child's Brain 1980;7:73–84.
3. Yamada H, Haratake J, Narasaki T, Oda T. Embryonal craniopharyngioma. Case report of the morphogenesis of a craniopharyngioma. Cancer 1995;75:2971–2977.
4. Lederman GS, Recht A, Loeffler JS, Dubusson D, Kleefield J, Schnitt SJS. Craniopharyngioma in an elderly patient. Cancer 1987;60:1077–1080.
5. Petito CK, DeGirolami U, Earle KM. Craniopharyngiomas. Cancer 1976;37:1944–1952.
6. Akimura T, Kameda H, Abiko S, Aoki H, Kido T. Intrasellar craniopharyngioma. Neuroradiology 1989;31:180–183.
7. Byrne MW, Sessions DG. Nasopharyngeal craniopharyngioma. Case report and literature review. Ann Otol Rhinol Laryngol 1990;99:633–639.
8. Neetens A, Selosse P. Oculomotor anomalies in sellar and parasellar pathology. Opthalmologia 1977;175:80–104.
9. Hiramatsu K, Takahashi K, Ikeda A, Arimori S. A case of intrasellar craniopharyngioma. Tokai J Exp Clin Med 1987;12:135–140.
10. Young SC, Zimmerman RA, Nowell MA, Hackney, Grossman RI, Goldberg HI. Giant cystic craniopharyngiomas. Neuroradiology 1987;29:468–473.
11. Kuwabara S, Seo H, Ishikawa S. Huge, dense, cystic craniopharyngioma with unusual extensions. Case report. Neurol Med Chir (Tokyo) 1987;2737–2741.
12. Sener RN. Giant craniopharyngioma extending to the anterior cranial fossa and nasopharynx. Am J Roentgenology 1994;162:441–442.
13. Sharma RR, Davis CH, Lynch PG. Intraventricular craniopharyngioma. Surg Neurol 1994;42:551–552.
14. Graziani N, Donnet A, Bugha TN, Dufor H, Figarella-Branger D, Grisoli F. Ectopic basisphenoidal craniopharyngioma: case report and review of the literature. Neurosurgery 1994;34:346–349.
15. Kanungo N, Just N, Black M, Mohr G, Glikstein R, Rochon L. Nasopharyngeal craniopharyngioma in an unusual location. Am J Neuroradiol 1995;16:1372–1374.
16. Sklar CA. Craniopharyngioma: endocrine abnormalities at presentation. Pediatr Neurosurg 1994;1:18–20.
17. Lee JS, Tsai WY, Liu HM, Lin MY, Tu YK. Growth retardation as the initial manifestation of intracranial tumors: report of two cases. Acta Paediatr Sinica 1994;35:157–162.
18. Palaoglu S, Akbay A, Mocan G, Oncol B, Ozcan OE, Ozgen T, et al. Ossified adamantinomatous type craniopharyngiomas. A series of 13 patients. Acta Neurochir 1994;127:166–169.

19. Paja M, Lucas T, Garcia-Uria J, Salame F, Barcelo B, Estradada J. Hypothalamic-pituitary dysfunction in patients with craniopharyngioma. Clin Endocrinol 1995;42:467–473.

20. Crotty TB, Scheithauer BW, Young WF Jr, Davis DH, Shaw EG, Miller GM, et al. Papillary craniopharyngioma: a clinicopathological study of 48 cases. J Neurosurg 1995;83:206–214.

21. Spence SA, Taylor DG, Hirsch SR. Depressive disorder due to craniopharyngioma. J Royal Soc Med 1995;88:637–638.

22. Yarde WL, Kepes JJ, O'Boynick P. Craniopharyngioma presenting as Koraskoff psychosis. Kansas Med 1995;96:22–23.

23. Kearney D, Tay-Kearney ML, Khangure MS. Craniopharyngioma and the moustache sign. Aust Radiol 1993;34:370–371.

24. al-Wahhabi B, Choudhury AR, al-Moutaery KR, Aabed M, Faqeeh A. Giant craniopharyngioma with blindness reversed by surgery. Childs Nerv System 1993;9:292–294.

25. Lee M, Rezai AR, Wisoff JH. Acquired Chiari-I malformation and hydromyelia secondary to a giant craniopharyngioma. Pediatr Neurosurg 1995;22:251–254.

26. Patrick BS, Smith RR, Bailey TO. Aseptic meningitis due to spontaneous rupture of craniopharyngioma cyst. J Neurosurg 1974;41:387–390.

27. Okamoto H, Harada K, Uozumi T, Goishi J. Spontaneous rupture of a craniopharyngioma cyst. Surg Neurol 1985;24:507–510.

28. Satoh H, Uozumi T, Arita K, Kurisu K, Hotta T, Kiya K, et al. Spontaneous rupture of craniopharyngioma cysts. A report of five cases and review of the literature. Surg Neurol 1993;40:414–419.

29. Harwood-Nash DC. Neuroimaging of childhood craniopharyngioma. Pediatr Neurosurg 1994;1:2–10.

30. Eldevik OP, Blavias M, Gabrielsen TO, Hald JK, Chandler WF. Craniopharyngioma: radiologic and histologic findings and recurrence. AJNR 1996;17:1427–1439.

31. Burger PC, Vogel FS. Surgical Pathology of the Nervous System and Its Coverings, 2nd ed. John Wiley, New York, 1982, p. 514.

32. Giangaspero F, Burger PC, Osborne DR, Stein RB. Suprasellar papillary squamous epithelioma ("papillary craniopharyngioma"). Am J Surg Pathol 1984;8:57–64.

33. Sziefert GT, Sipos L, Horath M, Sarker MH, Major O, Salomvary B, et al. Pathological characteristics of surgically removed craniopharyngiomas: analysis of 131 cases. Acta Neurochirurgica 1993;124:139–143.

34. Miller DC. Pathology of craniopharyngiomas: clinical import of pathological findings. Pediatr Neurosurg 1994;21:11–17.

35. Tsunoda S, Sakaki T, Tsutsumi A, Eguchi T, Takeshima T, Morimoto T, et al. Clinicopathological study on craniopharyngioma with sebaceous differentiation. Noshyuo Byori 1993;10:69–74.

36. Goodrich JT, Post KD, Duffy P. Ciliated craniopharyngioma. Surg Neurol 1985;24:105–111.

37. Oka H, Kawano N, Tagishita S, Kobayashi I, Saegusa H, Fujii K. Ciliated craniopharyngioma indicates histogenetic relationship to Rathke cleft epithelium. Clin Neuropathol 1997;16:103–106.

38. Puchner MJ, Ludecke DK, Saeger W. The anterior pituitary lobe in patients with cystic craniopharyngiomas: three cases of associated lymphocytic hypophysitis. Acta Neurochir 1994;126:38–43.

39. Aza SL, Kovaks K, Bilbao JM, Penz G. Immunohistochemical localization of keratin in craniopharyngiomas and squamous cell nests of the human pituitary. Acta Neuropathol 1981;54:257–260.

40. Kubo O, Tajika Y, Uchimuno H, Muragaki Y, Shimoda M, Kiyama H, et al. Immunochemical study of craniopharyngiomas. Noshyuo Byori 1993;10:131–114.

41. Uematsu Y, Komai N, Tanaka Y, Shimizu M, Naka D, Yukawa S, et al. Cellular differentiation, secretory and proliferative activities of craniopharyngiomas. Noshuyo Byori 1994;11:43–50.

42. Szeifert GT, Pasztor E. Could craniopharyngiomas produce pituitary hormones? Neurol Res 1993;15:68–69.

43. Tachibana O, Yamashima T, Yamashita J, Takabatake Y. Immunohistochemical expression of human chorionic gonadotropin and P-glycoprotein in human pituitary glands and craniopharyngiomas. J Neurosurg 1994;80:79–84.

44. Honegger J, Mann K, Thierauf P, Zrinzo A, Fahlbusch R. Human chorionic gonadotropin immunoactivity in cystic intracranial tumours. Clin Endocrinol 1995;42:235–241.

45. Sato K, Kubota T, Yamamoto S, Ishikura A. An ultrastructural study of mineralization in craniopharyngioma. J Neuropathol Exp Neurol 1986;45:463–470.

46. Launay M, Fredy D, Merland JJ, Bories J. Narrowing and occlusion of arteries by intracranial tumors: Review of the literature and report of 25 cases. Neuroradiology 1977;14:117–126.

47. Nelson GA, Bastian FO, Schlitt M, White RL. Malignant transformation in craniopharyngioma. Neurosurgery 1988;22:427–429.

48. Hetelekidis S, Barnes PD, Tao ML, Fischer EG, Schneider L, Scott RM, et al. 20-year experience in childhood craniopharyngioma. Int J Rad Oncol Biol Phys 1993;27:189–195.

49. Regine WF, Mohiuddin M, Kramer S. Long term results of pediatric and adult craniopharyngiomas treated with combined surgery and radiation. Radiat Ther Oncol 1993;27:13–21.

50. Rajan B, Ashley S, Gorman C, Jose CC, Horwich A, Bloom HJ, et al. Craniopharyngioma—long term results following limited surgery and radiotherapy. Radiother Oncol 1993;26:1–10.

51. Tomita T, McLone DG. Radical resections of childhood craniopharyngiomas. Pediatr Neurosurg 1993;19:6–14.

52. Weiner HL, Wisoff JH, Rosenberg ME, Kupersmith MJ, Cohen H, Zagzag D, et al. Craniopharyngiomas: a clinicopathological analysis of factors predictive of recurrence and functional outcome. Neurosurgery 1994;35:1001–1010.

53. Mark RJ, Lutge WR, Shimizu KT, Tran LM, Selch MT, Parker RG. Craniopharyngioma: treatment in the CT and MR imaging era. Radiology 1995;197:195–198.

54. DeVile CJ, Grant DB, Kendall BE, Neville BG, Stanhope R, Watkins KE, et al. Management of childhood craniopharyngioma. J Neurosurg 1996;85:73–81.

55. Adamson TE, Wiestler OD, Kleihues P, Tasargil MG. Correlation of clinical and pathological features in surgically treated craniopharyngiomas. J Neurosurg 1990;73:12–17.

56. Kahn EA, Gosch HH, Seeger JF, Hicks SP. Forty-five years experience with the craniopharyngiomas. Surg Neurol 1973;1:5–12.

57. Kawano N, Oka H, Suwa T, Ito H, Yada K, Kameya T, et al. Origin of craniopharyngioma: an electron microscopic study. Noshuyo Byori 1993;10:117–123.

58. Hoffman HJ. Surgical management of craniopharyngioma. Pediatr Neurosurg 1994;21:44–49.

59. Cavalheiro S, Sparapani FV, Franco JO, da Silva MC, Braga FM. Use of bleomycin in intratumoral chemotherapy for cystic craniopharyngioma. Case report. J Neurosurg 1996;84:124–126.

60. Lange M, Kirsch CM, Steude U, Oeckler R. Intracavitary treatment of intrasellar cystic craniopharyngiomas with 90-Yttrium by transsphenoidal approach—a technical note. Acta Neurochirurgica 1995;135:206–209.

61. Pollock BE, Lunsford LD, Kondziolka D, Levine G, Flickinger JC. Phosphorus-32 intracavitary irradiation of cystic craniopharyngiomas: current technique and long-term results. Int J Radiat Oncol Biol Phys 1995;33:437–446.

62. Liu Z, Tian Z, Yu X, Li S, Huang H, Kang G, Xu Y, et al. Stereotactic intratumour irradiation with nuclide for craniopharyngiomas. Chinese Med J 1996;109:219–222.

63. Abdullah J, Caemaert J. Endoscopic management of craniopharyngiomas: a review of 3 cases. Minimally Invasive Neurosurg 1995;38:79–84.

64. Kobayashi T, Tanaka T, Kida Y. Stereotactic gamma radiosurgery of craniopharyngiomas. Pediatr Neurosurg 1994;21:69–74.

65. Yamamoto M, Ide M, Umebara Y, Hagiwara S, Jimbo M, Takakura K. Gamma knife radiosurgery for brain tumors: postirradiation volume changes compared with preradiosurgical growth fractions. Neurologia Medico-Chirurgica 1996;36:358–363.

66. Tolnay M, Kaim A, Probst A, Ulrich J. Subependymoma of the third ventricle after partial resection of a craniopharyngioma and repeated postoperative irradiation. Clin Neuropath 1995;15:63–66.

1.1.2. Nasopharyngeal Carcinoma (NPC)

1. Million RR. The myth regarding bone and cartilage involvement by cancer and the likelihood of cure by radiotherapy. Head Neck 1989;11:30–40.

2. Miura T, Hirabuki N, Hisiyama K, Hasimoto T, Kawai R, Yoshida J, Sasaki R, Matsunaga T, Kozuka T. Computed tomographic findings of nasopharyngeal carcinoma with skull base and intracranial involvement. Cancer 1990;65:29–37.

3. Hsu YC, Chen CL, Hsu MM, Lynn TC, Tu SM, Huang SC. Pathology of nasopharyngeal carcinoma. Proposal of new histologic classification correlated with prognosis. Cancer 1987;59:945–951.

4. Komoroski EM. Nasopharyngeal carcinoma: early warning signs and symptoms. Pediatric Emergency Care 1994;10:284–286.

5. Mills SE, Fechner RE. Undifferentiated neoplasms of the sinonasal region: Differential diagnosis based on clinical, light microscopic, immunohistochemical, and ultrastructural features. Semin Diagn Pathol 1989;6:316–328.

5a. McKeever PE, Blaivas M, Sima AAF. Neoplasms of the sellar region. In: Lloyd RV, ed. Surgical Pathology of the Pituitary Gland. Major Problems in Pathology Series. WB Saunders, Philadelphia, 1993, pp. 141–210.

6. Lopategui JR, Gaffey MJ, Frierson HF, Chan JKC, Mills SE, Chang KL, et al. Detection of Epstein-Barr viral RNA in sinonasal undifferentiated carcinoma from Western and Asian patients. Am J Surg Pathol 1994;18:391–398.

7. Wick MR, Stanley SJ, Swanson PE. Immunohistochemical diagnosis of sinonasal melanoma, carcinoma, and neuroblastoma with monoclonal antibodies HMB-45 and anti-synaptophysin. Arch Pathol Lab Med 1988;112:616–620.

8. Taxy JB, Hidvegi DF, Battifora H. Nasopharyngeal carcinoma: Antikeratin immunohistochemistry and electron microscopy. Am J Clin Pathol 1985;83:320–325.

9. Shanmugaratham K, Chan SH, De-The G, Goj JE, Khor TH, Simons MJ. Histopathology of nasopharyngeal carcinoma. Correlations with epidemiology, survival rates and other biological characteristics. Cancer 1979;44:1029–1044.

10. Yeung WM, Zong YS, Chiu CT, Chan KH, Sham JS, Choy DT, et al. Epstein-Barr virus carriage by nasopharyngeal carcinoma in situ. International Journal of Cancer 1993;53:746–750.

11. Lung ML, Sham JS, Lam WP, Choy DT. Analysis of Epstein-Barr virus in localized nasopharyngeal carcinoma tumors. Cancer 1993;71:1190–1192.

12. Niemhom S, Maeda S, Raksakait K, Petchclai B. Epstein-Barr virus DNA in nasopharyngeal carcinoma in Thai patients at Ramathibodi Hospital, Bangkok. Southeast Asian J Trop Med Public Health 26 Suppl 1995;1:325–328.

13. Choi PHK, Suen MWM, Huang DP, Lo K-W, Lee JCK. Nasopharyngeal carcinoma: genetic changes, Epstein-Barr virus infection, or both. Cancer 1993;72:2873–2878.

14. Lin CT, Chan WY, Chen W, Huang HM, Wu HC, Hsu MM, et al. Characterization of seven newly established nasopharyngeal carcinoma cell lines. Lab Invest 1993;68:716.

15. Austin MB, Mills SE. Neoplasms and neoplasm-like lesions involving the skull base. Ear, Nose and Throat 1986;65:25–52.

16. Ward PH, Thompson R, Calcaterra T, Kadin MR. Juvenile angiofibroma: A more rational therapeutic approach based upon clinical and experimental evidence. Laryngoscope 1974;84:2181–2194.

17. Franquemont DW, Fechner RE, Mills SE. Histologic classification of sinonasal intestinal-type adenocarcinoma. Am J Surg Pathol 1991;15:368–375.

18. Yu L, Fleckman AM, Chadha M, Sacks E, Levetan C, Vikram B. Radiation therapy of metastatic pheochromocytoma: case report and review of the literature. Am J Clin Oncol 1996;19:389–392.

19. Dickhoff P, Wallace CJ, MacRae ME, Campbell WN. Adenoid cystic carcinoma: an unusual sellar mass. Can Assoc Radiol J 1993;44:393–395.

20. Sim RS, Tan HK. A case of metastatic hepatocellular carcinoma of the sphenoid sinus. J Laryngol Otol 1994;108:503,504.

21. Izumihara A, Orita T, Tsurutani T, Kajiwara K, Matsunaga T, Hatano M. Pineal and suprasellar metastasis of lung cancer: case report and review of the literature. Comput Med Imaging Graph 1995;19:435–437.

22. Struk DW, Knapp TR, Munk PL, Poon PY. Pituitary and intradural spinal metastases: an unusual initial presentation of lung cancer. Can Assoc Radiol J 1995;46:118–121.

23. Kida A, Endo S, Iida H, Yamada Y, Sakai F, Furusaka T, et al. Clinical assessment of squamous cell carcinoma of the nasal cavity proper. Auris, Nasus, Larynx. 1995;22:172–177.

24. Tong MC, van Hasselt CA, Woo JK. Preliminary results of photodynamic therapy for recurrent nasopharyngeal carcinoma. Eur Arch Oto-Rhino-Laryngol 1996;253:189–192.

25. Chua DT, Sham JS, Kwong DL, Choy DT, Au GK, Wu PM. Prognostic value of paranasopharyngeal extension of nasopharyngeal carcinoma. Cancer 1996;78:202–210.

1.2.1. Rathke's Cleft Cyst

1. Kucharczyk W, Peck WW, Kelly WM, Norman D, Newton TH. Rathke cleft cysts: CT, MR imaging, and pathologic features. Radiology 1987;165:491–495.

2. Graziani N, Dufour H, Figarella-Branger D, Donnet A, Bouillot P, Grisoli F. Do the suprasellar neurenteric cyst, the Rathke cleft cyst and the colloid cyst constitute a same entity? Acta Neurochir (Wien) 1995;133:174–180.

3. Cavallo AV, Murphy MA, McKelvie PA, Cummins JT. An epithelial cyst of the suprasellar region. Aust N Z J Surg 1993;63:490–493.

4. Yamamoto M, Jimbo M, Ide M, Umebara Y, Hagiwara S, Kubo O. Recurrence of symptomatic Rathke's cleft cyst: a case report. Surg Neurol 1993;39:263–268.

5. Teramoto A, Hirakawa K, Sanno N, Osamura Y. Incidental pituitary lesions in 1,000 unselected autopsy specimens. Radiology 1994;193:161–164.

6. Kleinschmidt-DeMasters BK, Lillehei KO, Stears JC. The pathologic, surgical, and MR spectrum of Rathke cleft cysts. Surg Neurol 1995;44:19–27.

7. Rao GP, Blyth CP, Jeffreys RV. Ophthalmic manifestations of Rathke's cleft cysts. Am J Ophthalmol 1995;119:86–91.

8. Eguchi K, Uozumi T, Arita K, Kurisu K, Yano T, Sumida M, et al. Pituitary function in patients with Rathke's cleft cyst: significance of surgical management. Endocr J 1994;41:535–540.

9. Matsushima T, Fukui M, Fujii K, Kinoshita K, Yamakawa Y. Epithelial cells in symptomatic Rathke's cleft cysts. A light- and electron-microscopic study. Surg Neurol 1988;30:197–203.

10. Yoshida J, Kobayashi T, Kageyama N, Kanzaki M. Symptomatic Rathke's cleft cyst. Morphological study with light and electron microscopy and tissue culture. J Neurosurg 1977;47:451–458.

11. Hayashi Y, Yamashita J, Muramatsu N, Sakuda K, Nitta H. Symptomatic Rathke's cleft cysts in identical twins. Case illustration. J Neurosurg 1996;84:710.

12. Nishio S, Fujiwara S, Morioka T, Fukui M. Rathke's cleft cysts within a growth hormone producing pituitary adenoma. Br J Neurosurg 1995;9:51–55.

13. Arita K, Uozumi T, Takechi A, Hirohata T, Pant B, Kubo K, et al. A case of Cushing's disease accompanied by Rathke's cleft cyst: the usefulness of cavernous sinus sampling in the localization of microadenoma. Surg Neurol 1994;42:112–116.

14. Ikeda H, Yoshimoto T, Katakura R. A case of Rathke's cleft-cyst within a pituitary adenoma presenting with acromegaly. Do "transitional cell tumors of the pituitary gland" really exist? Acta Neuropathol 1992;83:211–215.

15. Pearl GS, Takei Y, Kurisaka M, Seyama S, Tindall GT. Cystic prolactinoma: a variant of "transitional cell tumor" of the pituitary. Am J Surg Pathol 1981;5:85–91.

16. Kepes JJ. Transitional cell tumor of the pituitary gland developing from a Rathke's cleft cyst. Cancer 1978;41:337–343.

17. Nishio S, Mizuno J, Barrow DL, Takei Y, Tindall GT. Pituitary tumors composed of adenohypophysial adenoma and Rathke's cleft cyst elements: a clinicopathological study. Neurosurgery 1987;21:371–377.

18. Ikeda H, Niizuma H, Fujiwara S, Suzuki J, Sasano N. A case of prolactinoma in close association with Rathke's cleft cyst. No Shinkei Geka 1987;15:999–1003.

19. Miyagi A, Iwasaki M, Shibuya T, Kido G, Kushi H, Miyagami H, et al. Pituitary adenoma combined with Rathke's cleft cyst. Case report. Neurol Med Chir (Tokyo) 1993;33:643–650.

20. Nakasu S, Nakasu Y, Kyoshima K, Watanabe K, Handa J, Okabe H. Pituitary adenoma with multiple ciliated cysts: transitional cell tumor? Surg Neurol 1989;31:41–48.

21. Oka H, Kawano N, Suwa T, Yada K, Kan S, Kameya T. Radiological study of symptomatic Rathke's cleft cysts. Neurosurgery 1994;35:632–637.

22. Naylor MF, Scheithauer BW, Forbes GS, Tomlinson FH, Young WF. Rathke cleft cyst: CT, MR, and pathology of 23 cases. J Comput Assist Tomogr 1995;19:853–859; Erratum 20:171.

23. Okamoto S, Handa H, Yamashita J, Ishikawa M, Nagasawa S. Computed tomography of intra- and suprasellar epithelial cysts (symptomatic Rathke cleft cysts). Am J Neuroradiol 1985;6:515–519.

24. McKeever PE, Blaivas M. The brain, spinal cord, and meninges. In: Sternberg SS, Antonioli DA, Carter D, Mills SE, Oberman HA, eds. Diagnostic Surgical Pathology. Raven, New York, 1994, pp. 409–492.

25. Sumida M, Uozumi T, Yamanaka M, Mukada K, Arita K, Kurisu K, et al. Displacement of the normal pituitary gland by sellar and juxtasellar tumors: surgical-MRI correlation and use in differential diagnosis. Neuroradiology 1994;36:372–375.

26. Seidel FG, Towbin R, Kaufman RA. Normal pituitary stalk size in children: CT study. Am J Roentgenol 1985;145:1297–1302.

26a. Sumida M, Uozumi T, Mukada K, Arita K, Kurisu K, Eguchi K. Rathke cleft cysts: correlation of enhanced MR and surgical findings. AJNR Am J Neuroradiol 1994;15:525–532.

27. Meyer JR, Quint DJ, McKeever PE, Boland M, Ross DA. Giant Rathke cleft cyst. AJRN Am J Neuroradiol 1994;15:533–536.

28. Skjodt K, Loft Edal A, Nepper-Rasmussen HJ, Skjdt K. Rathke's cleft cyst. Two cases with uncommon MR signals. Acta Radiol 1996;37:596–598.

29. Christophe C, Flamant-Durand J, Hanquinet S, Heinrichs C, Raftopoulos C, Sariban E, et al. MRI in seven cases of Rathke's cleft cyst in infants and children. Pediatr Radiol 1993;23:79–82.

30. Wearne MJ, Barber PC, Johnson AP. Symptomatic Rathke's cleft cyst with hypophysitis. Br J Neurosurg 1995;9:799–803.

31. Marin F, Boya J, Lopez-Caronell AL, Borregon A. Immunohistochemical localization of intermediate filament and S-100 proteins in several non-endocrine cells of the human pituitary gland. Arch Histol Cytol 1989;52:241–248.

32. Kasper M, Karsten U. Coexpression of cytokeratin and vimentin in Rathke's cysts of the human pituitary gland. Cell Tissue Res 1988;253:419–424.

33. Lach B, Scheithauer BW, Gregor A, Wick MR. Colloid cyst of the third ventricle. A comparative immunohistochemical study of neuraxis cysts and choroid plexus epithelium. J Neurosurgery 1993;78:101–111.

34. Uematsu Y, Komai N, Hirano A, Shimizu M, Tanaka Y, Naka D, et al. Cytokeratin immunohistochemical study of epithelial cysts in the central nervous system: with special reference to origins of colloid cyst of the third ventricle and Rathke's cleft cyst in the sella. Noshuyo Byori 1993;10:43–52.

35. Inoue T, Matsushima T, Fukui M, Iwaki T, Takeshita I, Kuromatsu C. Immunohistochemical study of intracranial cysts. Neurosurgery 1988;23:576–581.

36. Ikeda H, Yoshimoto T, Suzuki J. Immunohistochemical study of Rathke's cleft cyst. Acta Neuropathol 1988;77:33–38.

37. Niikawa S, Yamada H, Sakai N, Ando T, Zhang W, Hara A, et al. Distribution of cellular carbohydrate moieties in human dysontogenetic brain tumors, especially in craniopharyngioma and epidermoid/dermoid. Acta Neuropathol (Berl) 1992;85:71–78.

38. Miyagami M, Tsubokawa T. Histological and ultrastructural findings of benign intracranial cysts. Noshuyo Byori 1993;10:151–160.

39. Diengdoh JV, Scott T. Electron-microscopical study of a Rathke's cleft cyst. Acta Neuropathol (Berl) 1983;60:14–18.

40. Lach B, Scheithauer BW. Colloid cyst of the third ventricle. A comparative ultrastructural study of neuraxis cysts and choroid plexus epithelium. Ultrastruct Pathol 1992;16:331–349.

41. Hirano A, Hirano M. Benign cystic lesions in the central nervous system. Light and electron microscopic observations of cyst walls. Child's Nerv Syst 1988;4:325–333.

42. Cinti S, Sbarbati A, Balercia G, Cigolini M. An ultrastructural study on muciparous microcysts of the human adenohypophysis. Acta Anat 1985;121:94–98.

43. Barrow DL, Spector RH, Takei Y, Tindall GT. Symptomatic Rathke's cleft cysts located entirely in the suprasellar region: review of diagnosis, management, and pathogenesis. Neurosurgery 1985;16:766–772.

44. Schaeffer BT, Som PM, Sacher M, Lanzieri CF, Solodnik P, Lawson W, et al. Coexistence of a nasal mucoepidermoid carcinoma and sphenoid mucoceles: CT diagnosis and treatment implications. J Comput Assist Tomogr 1985;9:803–805.

45. Alleva MD, Werber JL, Kimmelman CP. Pathologic quiz case 2. Fibromyxoma of the ethmoidal sinus with secondary sphenoidal sinus mucocele. Arch Otolaryngol Head Neck Surg 1989;115:878–879.

46. Karnaze MG, Sartor K, Winthrop JD, Gado MH, Hodges FJ. Suprasellar lesions: Evaluation with MR imaging? Radiology 1986;161:77–82.

47. Verkijk A, Bots GT. An intrasellar cyst with both Rathke's cleft and epidermoid characteristics. Acta Neurochir 1980;51:203–207.

48. Fischer EG, DeGirolami U, Suojanen JN. Reversible visual deficit following debulking of a Rathke's cleft cyst: a tethered chiasm? J Neurosurg 1994;81:459–462.

1.2.2. Epidermoid Cyst

1. Lana-Peixoto MA, Pittella JE, Arouca EM. Primary intracranial tumors: Analysis of a series of consecutive autopsies and biopsies. Arq Neuropsiquiatr 1981;39:13–24.

2. Sadeh M, Goldhammer Y, Schacked I, Tadmar R, Godel V. Basal encephalocele associated with suprasellar epidermoid cyst. Arch Neurol 1983;39:250–252.

3. Launay M, Fredy D, Merland JJ, Bories J. Narrowing and occlusion of arteries by intracranial tumors: Review of the literature and report of 25 cases. Neuroradiology 1977;14:117–126.

4. Gormley WB, Tomecek FJ, Qureshi N, Malik GM. Craniocerebral epidermoid and dermoid tumours: a review of 32 cases. Acta Neurochir 1994;128:115–121.

5. Torbiak CW, Mazagri R, Tchang SP, Clein LJ. Parasellar epidermoid cyst presenting with subarachnoid hemorrhage. Can Assoc Radiol J 1995;46:392–394.

6. Horowitz BL, Chari MV, James R, Bryan RN. MR of intracranial epidermoid tumors: correlation of in vivo imaging with in vitro ^{13}C spectroscopy. Am J Neuroradiol 1990;11:299–302.

7. Mafee MF, Kumar A, Heffner DK. Epidermoid cyst (cholesteatoma) and cholesterol granuloma of the temporal bone and epidermoid cysts affecting the brain. Neuroimaging Clin North Am 1994;4:561–578.

8. Salyer D, Carter D. Squamous carcinoma arising in the pituitary gland. Cancer 1973;31:713–718.

9. Lewis AJ, Cooper PW, Kassel EE, Schwartz ML. Squamous cell carcinoma arising in suprasellar epidermoid cysts. J Neurosurg 1983;59:538–541.

10. Nakasu S, Matsumura K, Nioka H, Handa J. Lectin histochemistry of dermoid and epidermoid cysts of the central nervous system. Noshuyo Byori 1993;10:11–17.

11. Petito CK, DeGirolami U, Earle KM. Craniopharyngiomas. Cancer 1976;37:1944–1952.

12. Bejarano PA, Broderick DF, Gado MH. Infected epidermoid cyst of the sphenoid bone. Am J Neurol 1993;14:771–773.

1.2.3. Dermoid Cyst

1. Klonoff DC, Kahn DG, Rosenzweig W, Wilson CB. Hyperprolactinemia in a patient with a pituitary and an ovarian dermoid tumor: Case report. Neurosurgery 1990;26:335–339.

2. Mortada A. Dermoid cysts of great wing of sphenoid bone. Br J Ophthalmol 1970;2:131–133.

3. McKeever PE, Blaivas M. The brain, spinal cord, and meninges. In: Sternberg SS, Antonioli DA, Carter D, Mills SE, Oberman HA, eds. Diagnostic Surgical Pathology, 2nd ed. Raven, New York, 1994, pp. 409–492.

4. Hashimoto T, Kubota S, Shimizu T, Beppu T. A case of suprasellar tumor associated with so-called atypical angina pectoris. No Shinkei Geka (Neurol Surg) 1976;4:979–984.

5. Graham DV, Tampieri D, Villemure JG. Intramedullary dermoid tumor diagnosed with the assistance of magnetic resonance imaging. Neurosurgery 1988;23:765–767.

6. Smith AS, Benson JE, Blasner SI, Mizushima A, Tarr RW, Bellon EM. Diagnosis of ruptured intracranial dermoid cyst: value of MR over CT. AJNR Am J Neuroradiol 1991;12:175–180.

7. Hirano A, Hirano M. Benign cystic lesions in the central nervous system. Light and electron microscopic observations of cyst walls. Child's Nerv Cyst 1988;4:325–333.

2.1.1. Gangliocytoma

1. Scheithauer BW, Kovacs K, Randall RV, Horvath E, Okazaki H, Laws ER. Hypothalamic neuronal hamartoma and adenohypophyseal neuronal choristoma: their association with growth hormone adenoma of the pituitary gland. J Neuropathol Exp Neurol 1983;42:644–648.

2. Beal MF, Kleinman GM, Ojemann RG, Hochberg FH. Gangliocytoma of third ventricle: hyperphagia, somnolence, and dementia. Neurology 1981;31:1224–1228.

3. Russel DS, Rubinstein LJ. Pathology of Tumours of the Nervous System. Williams and Wilkins, London, 1989.

4. Burchield KJ, Shaw COM, Kelly WA. A mixed functional microadenoma and ganglioneuroma of the pituitary fossa. Case Report. J Neurosurg 1983;58:416–420.

5. Towfighi J, Salam MM, McLendon RE, Powers S, Page RB. Ganglion cell-containing tumors of the pituitary gland. Arch Pathol Lab Med 1996;120:369–377.

6. Li JY, Racadot O, Kujas M, Kouadri M, Peillon F, Racadot J. Immunocytochemistry of four mixed pituitary adenomas and intrasellar gangliocytomas associated with different clinical syndromes: acromegaly, amenorrhea-galactorrhea, Cushing's disease and isolated tumoral syndrome. Acta Neuropathol (Berl) 1989;77:320–328.

7. Horvath E, Kovacs K, Scheithauer BW, Lloyd RV, Smyth HS. Pituitary adenoma with neuronal choristoma (PANCH): composite lesion or lineage infidelity? Ultrastruct Pathol 1994;18:565–574.

8. Saeger W, Puchner MJ, Ludecke DK. Combined sellar gangliocytoma and pituitary adenoma in acromegaly or Cushing's disease. A report of 3 cases. Virchows Arch 1994;425:93–99.

9. Asa SL, Scheithauer BW, Bilbao JM, Horvath E, Ryan N, Kovacs K, et al. A case of hypothalamic acromegaly: A clinicopathologic study of six patients with hypothalamic gangliocytomas producing growth hormone-releasing factor. J Clin Endocrinol Metab 1984;58:796–803.

10. Shuangshoti S, Samranvej P. Hypothalamic and pancreatic lesions with diabetes mellitus. J Neurol Neurosurg Psychiatry 1975;38:1003–1007.

11. Zulch KJ. Biologie und Pathologie der Hirngeschwulste. In: Olivecrona H, Tonnis W, eds. Handuch der Neurochirugie, vol. 3. Springer Verlag, Berlin, 1956, p. 381.

12. Kamel OW, Horoupian DS, Silverberg GD. Mixed gangliocytoma-adenoma: a distinct neuroendocrine tumor of the pituitary fossa. Hum Pathol 1989;20:1198–203.

2.1.2. Hypothalamic Hamartoma

1. Iwase T, Nishizawa S, Baba S, Hinokuma K, Sugimura H, Nakamura SI, et al. Intrasellar neuronal choristoma associated with growth hormone-producing pituitary adenoma containing amyloid deposits. Hum Pathol 1995;62:925–928.

2. Scheithauer BW, Kovacs K, Randall RV, Horvath E, Okazaki H, Laws ER. Hypothalamic neuronal hamartoma and adenohypophyseal neuronal choristoma: their association with growth hormone adenoma of the pituitary gland. J Neuropathol Exp Neurol 1983;42:644–648.

3. Slowik F, Fazekas I, Balint K, Gazso L, Pasztor E, Czirjak D, Lapis K. Intrasellar hamartoma associated with pituitary adenoma. Acta Neuropathol 1990;80:328–333.

4. Colaco MP, Desai MP, Choksi CS, Shah KN, Mehta RU. Hypothalamic hamartomas and precocious puberty. Indian J Pediatr 1993;60:445–450.

5. Cheng K, Sawamura Y, Yamauchi T, Abe H. Asymptomatic large hypothalamic hamartoma associated with polydactyly in an adult. Neurosurgery 1993;32:458–460.

6. Valdueza JM, Cristante L, Dammann O, Bentele K, Vortmeyer A, Saeger W, et al. Hypothalamic hamartomas: with special reference to gelastic epilepsy and surgery. Neurosurgery 1994;34:949–958.

7. Turjman F, Xavier JL, Froment JC, Tran-Minh VA, David L, Lapras C. Late MR follow-up of hypothalamic hamartomas. Child's Nervous System 1996;12:63–68.

8. Hamilton RL. Precocious puberty. (Case of the month). Brain Pathol 1997;7:711,712.

9. Hall JG, Pallister PD, Clarren SK, Beckwith JB, Wiglesworth FW, Fraser FL, et al. Congenital hypothalamic hamartoblastoma, hypopituitarism, imperforate anus, and postaxial polydactyly—a new syndrome? 1. Clinical causal and pathogenic considerations. Am J Med Genet 1980;7:47–74.

10. Nurbai MA, Tomlinson BE, Lorigan-Forsythe B. Infantile hypothalamic hamartoma with multiple congenital abnormalities. Neuropathol Appl Neurobiol 1985;11:61–70.

11. Asa SL, Bilbao JM, Kovacs K, Linfoot JA. Hypothalmic neuronal hamartoma associated with pituitary growth hormone cell adenoma and acromegaly. Acta Neuropathol 1980;52:231–234.

2.1.3. Olfactory Neuroblastoma

1. Rodas RA, Erkman-Balis B, Cahill DW. Late intracranial metastasis from esthesioneuroblastoma: case report and review of the literature. Neurosurgery 1986;19:622–627.

2. Burke DP, Gabrielsen TO, Knake JE, Seeger JF, Oberman HA. Radiology of olfactory neuroblastoma. Radiology 1980;137:367–372.

3. Jakumeit HD. Neuroblastoma of the olfactory nerve. Acta Neurochir 1971;25:99–108.

4. Sarwar M. Primary sellar-parasellar esthesioneuroblastoma. AJR 1979;133:140,141.

5. Elkon D, Hightower SI, Lim ML, Cantrell RN, Constable WC. Esthesioneuroblastoma. Cancer 1979;44:1087–1094.

6. Schochet SS Jr, Peters B, O'Neal J, McCormick WF. Intracranial esthesioneuroblastoma. A light and electron microscopic study. Acta Neuropathol (Berl) 1975;31:181–118.

7. Rosengren JE, Jing BS, Wallace S, Danziger J. Radiographic features of olfactory neuroblastoma. Am J Roentgenology 1979;132:945–948.

8. Reznik M, Melon J, Lambricht M, Kaschten B, Beckers A. Neuroendocrine tumor of the nasal cavity (esthesioneuroblastoma). Apropos of a case with paraneoplastic Cushing's syndrome. Ann Pathol 1987;7:137–142.

9. Ng KH, Poon WS, Poon CYF, South JR. Intracranial olfactory neuroblastoma mimicking carcinoma: report of two cases. Histopathology 1988;12:393–403.

10. Takahashi H, Wakabayashi K, Ikuta F, Tanimura K. Esthesioneuroblastoma: a nasal catecholamine-producing tumor of neural crest origin. Demonstration of tyrosine hydroxylase-immunoreactive tumor cells. Acta Neuropathol (Berl) 1988;75:522–527.

11. Levine PA, Paling MR, Black WC, Cantrell RW. MRI vs high resolution CT scanning: Evaluation of the anterior skull base. Otolaryngol Head Neck Surg 1987;96:260–267.

12. Mills SE, Firerson HF Jr. Olfactory neuroblastoma. A clinicopathologic study of 21 cases. Am J Surg Pathol 1985;9:317–327.

13. Mills SE, Fechner RE. "Undifferentiated" neoplasms of the sinonasal region: Differential diagnosis based on clinical, light microscopic, immunohistochemical, and ultrastructural features. Semin Diagn Pathol 1989;6:316–328.

14. Taxy JB, Bharani NK, Mills SE, Frierson HF, Gould VE. The spectrum of olfactory neural tumors. A light-microscopic immunohistochemical and ultrastructural analysis. Am J Surg Path 1986;10:687–695.

15. Frierson HF Jr, Ross GW, Mills SE, Frankfurter A. Olfactory neuroblastoma. Additional immunohistochemical characterization. Am J Clin Pathol 1990;94:547–553.

16. Perentes E, Rubinstein LJ. Immunohistochemical recognition of human neuroepithelial tumors by anti-Leu 7 (HNK-1) monoclonal antibody. Acta Neuropathol (Berl) 1986;69:227–233.

17. Durham JC, Olfactory neuroblastoma. Ear Nose Throat J 1989; 68:185,186.

18. Miyaguchi M, Kitaouku S, Sakai S, Uda H. Clinical and histopathological studies of olfactory neuroblastoma. Auris Nasus Larynx 1989;16:157–163.

19. Curtis JL, Rubinstein LJ. Pigmented olfactory neuroblastoma. A new example of melanotic neuroepithelial neoplasm. Cancer 1982;49:2136–2143.

20. Takahashi H, Ohara S, Yamada M, Ikuta F, Tanimura K, Honda Y. Esthesioneuroepithelioma: a tumor of true olfactory epithelium origin. An ultrastructural and immunohistochemical study. Acta Neuropathol (Berl) 1987;75:147–155.

21. Ferris CA, Schnadig VJ, Quinn FB, Des Jardins L. Olfactory neuroblastoma. Cytodiagnostic features in a case with ultrastructural and immunohistochemical correlation. Acta Cytol 1988;32:381–385.

22. Chaudhru AP, Haar JG, Koul A, Nickerson PA. Olfactory neuroblastoma (esthesioneuroblastoma): a light and ultrastructural study of two cases. Cancer 1979;44:554–579.

23. Spalke G, Mennel HD, Martin G. Histogenesis of olfactory neuroblastoma. I. Electron microscopy of typical human case. Pathol Res Pract 1985;180:516–520.

24. Frierson HF, Mills SE, Fechner RE, Taxy JB, Levine PA. Sinonasal undifferentiated carcinoma: An aggressive neoplasm derived from Schneiderian epithelium and distinct from olfactory neuroblastoma. Am J Surg Pathol 1986;10:771–779.

25. Payne CM, Smith WL, Grogan TM, Nagle RB, Paplanus SH, Palmer T. Ultrastructural morphometry distinguishes Burkitt's-like lymphomas from neuroendocrine neoplasms: Useful criteria applied to the evaluation of a poorly differentiated neuroendocrine neoplasm of the nasal cavity masquerading as Burkitt's-like lymphoma. Mod Pathol 1989;8:35–45.

26. Warnke RA, Gatter KC, Falini B, Hildreth P, Woolston RE, Pulford K, et al. Diagnosis of human lymphoma with monoclonal antileukocyte antibodies. N Engl J Med 1983;309:1275–1281.

27. Kurtin PJ, Pinkus GS. Leukocyte common antigen—a diagnostic discriminant between hematopoietic and non-hematopoietic neoplasms in paraffin sections using monoclonal antibodies: Correlation with immunologic studies and ultrastructural localization. Hum Pathol 1985;16:353–365.

28. McKeever PE, Lloyd RV. Tumors of the pituitary gland region. In: Garcia JH, Budka H, McKeever PE, Sarnat HB, Sima AAF, eds. Neuropathology: The Diagnostic Approach. Mosby-Yearbook, Philadelphia, 1997, pp. 219–222.

2.2.1. Pilocytic Astrocytoma (Infundibuloma)

1. Russell DS, Rubinstein LJ. Pathology of tumours of the nervous system Baltimore, Williams & Wilkins 1988, pp. 377–378.

2. Scothorne CM. Glioma of the posterior lobe of the pituitary gland. J Pathol Bacteriol 1955;69:109–112.

3. Valdueza JM, Lohmann F, Dammann O, Hagel C, Eckert B, Freckmann N. Analysis of 20 primarily surgically treated chiasmatic hypothalamic/pilocytic astrocytomas. Acta Neurochir 1994;126:44–50.

4. Tekkok IH, Tahta K, Saglam S. Optic nerve glioma presenting as a huge intrasellar mass. Case report. J Neurosurg Sci 1994;38:137–140.

5. Jänisch W. Brain tumors in infancy. J Neuropathol Exp Neurol 1995;55s–56s.

6. Sorenson EJ, Silbert PL, Benarroch EE, Jack CR, Parisi JE. Transient amnestic syndrome after spontaneous hemorrhage into a hypothalamic pilocytic astrocytoma. J Neurol Neurosurg Psych 1995;58:761–763.

7. Hurley TR, D'Angelo CM, Clasen RA, Wilkinson SB, Passavoy RD. Magnetic resonance imaging and pathological analysis of a pituicytoma: case report. Neurosurgery 1994;35:314–317.

8. Sutton LN, Molloy PT, Sernyak H, Goldwein J, Phillips PL, Rorke LB, et al. Long-term outcome of hypothalamic/chiasmatic astrocytomas in children treated with conservative surgery. J Neurosurg 1995;83:583–589.

9. White FV, Anthony DC, Yunis EJ, Tarbell NJ, Scott RM, Schofield DE. Nonrandom chromosomal gains in pilocytic astrocytomas of childhood. Hum Pathol 1995;26:979–986.

10. Nishio S, Morioka T, Takeshita I, Shono T, Inamura T, Fujiwara S, et al. Chemotherapy for progressive pilocytic astrocytomas in the chiasmo-hypothalamic regions. Clin Neurol Neurosurg 1995;97: 300–306.

2.2.2. Optic Nerve Glioma

1. Reese AB. Tumors of the Eye and Adnexa. Atlas of Tumor Pathology Fascicle 38, Armed Forces Institute of Pathology, Washington DC, 1956, pp. 31–42.

2. Russel DS, Rubinstein LJ. Pathology of Tumours of the Nervous System. Williams and Wilkins, London, 1989.

3. Rush JA, Younge BR, Campbell RJ, MacCarty CS. Optic glioma. Long-term follow-up of 85 histopathologically verified cases. Ophthalmology 1982;89:1213–1219.

4. Davis FA. Primary tumors of the optic nerve (a phenomenon of Recklinghausen's disease) a clinical and pathological study with a report of five cases and review of the literature. Arch Ophthalmol 1940;23:735–821.

5. Borit A, Richardson EP. The biological and clinical behavior of pilocytic astrocytoma of the optic pathway. Brain 1982;105:161–187.

6. Rubinstein LJ. Tumeurs et hamartomes dans la neurofibromatose central. In: Michaux L, Feld M, eds. Les Phakomatoses Cerebrales. SPEI Editeurs, Paris, 1963, p. 427.

7. Matson D. Neurosurgery of Infancy and Childhood. Thomas, Springfield IL, 1969, pp. 523–536.

8. Alvord EC, Lofton S. Gliomas of the optic nerve or chiasm. Outcome by patients age, tumor site, and treatment. J Neurosurg 1988;68:85–98.

9. Kleihues P, Burger PC, Scheithauer BW. Histologic Classification of Tumours of the Central Nervous System. Springer-Verlag, New York, 1993.

10. Verhoeff FH. Tumors of the optic nerve. In: Penfield W, ed. Cytology and Cellular Pathology of the Nervous System, vol. 3. Hoeber, New York, 1932, p. 1027.

11. Dirks PB, Jay V, Becker LE, et al. Development of anaplastic changes in low-grade astrocytomas of childhood. Neurosurgery 1994;34:68–78.

12. Cáccamo DV, Rubinstein LJ. Tumors: Applications of immunocytochemical methods. In: Garcia JH, Budka H, McKeever PE, Sarnat HB, Sima AAF, eds. Neuropathology: The Diagnostic Approach. Mosby-Yearbook, Philadelphia, 1997, pp. 193–218.

13. Clark GB, Henry JM, McKeever PE. Cerebral pilocytic astrocytoma. Cancer 1985;56:1128–1133.

14. Lach B, Sikorska M, Rippstein P, Gregor A, Staines W, Davie TR. Immunoelectron microscopy of Rosenthal fibers. Acta Neuropathol (Berl) 1991;81:503–509.

15. Murayama S, Bouldin TW, Suzuki K. Immunocytochemical and ultrastructural studies of eosinophilic granular bodies in astrocytic tumors. Acta Neuropathol (Berl) 1992;83:408–414.

16. Horwich A, Bloom HJG. Optic gliomas: radiation therapy and prognosis. Int J Radiol Oncol Biol Phys 1985;11:1067–1079.

17. Hoyt WF, Mechel LG, Lessell S, Schatz NJ, Suckling RD. Malignant optic glioma of adulthood. Brain 1973;96:121–132.

18. Spoor TL, Kernnerdell JS, Martinez AJ, Zorub D. Malignant gliomas of the optic nerve pathways. Am J Ophthalmol 1980;89:284–292.

2.2.3. High-Grade Glioma

1. McKeever PE, Blaivas M, Sima AAF. Neoplasms of the sellar region. In: Lloyd RV, ed. Surgical Pathology of the Pituitary Gland, vol. 27, Livolsi VA, ed. Major Problems in Pathology. WB Saunders, Philadelphia, 1993, pp. 141–210.

2. Huang CI, Chiou WH, Ho DM. Oligodendroglioma occurring after radiation therapy for pituitary adenoma. J Neurol Neurosurg Psychiatry 1987;50:1619–1624.

3. Kitanaka C, Shitara N, Nakagomi T, Nakamura H, Genka S, Nakagawa K, et al. Postradiation astrocytoma: Report of two cases. J Neurosurg 1989;70:469–474.

4. Millar WS, Tartaglino LM, Sergott RC, Friedman DP, Flanders AE. MR of malignant optic glioma of adulthood. AJNR Am J Neuroradiol 1995;16:1673–1676.

5. Spoor TC, Kennerdell JS, Martinez AJ, Zorub D. Malignant gliomas of the optic nerve pathways. Am J Ophthalmol 1980;89:284–292.

6. Harper CG, Stewart-Wynne EG. Malignant optic glioma in adults. Arch Neurol 1978;35:731–735.

7. Manor RS, Israeli J, Sandbank U. Malignant optic glioma in a 70 year old patient. Arch Ophthalmol 1976;94:1142–1144.

8. Taphoorn MJ, de Vries-Knoppert WA, Ponssen H, Wolbers JG. Malignant optic glioma in adults. Case report. J Neurosurg 1989;70:277–279.

9. Ushio Y, Arita N, Yoshimine T, Nagatani M, Mogami H. Glioblastoma after radiotherapy for craniopharyngioma: Case report. Neurosurgery 1987;21:33–38.

10. Hufnagel TJ, Kim JH, Lesser R, Miller JM, Abrahams JJ, Piepmeier J, et al. Malignant glioma of the optic chiasm eight years after radiotherapy for prolactinoma. Arch Opthalmol 1988;106:1701–1705.

11. Zampieri P, Zorat PL, Mingrino S, Soattin GB. Radiation-associated cerebral gliomas. A report of two cases and review of the literature. J Neurosurg Sci 1989;33:271–279.

12. Shimizu H, Fujiwara K, Kobayashi S, Kitahara M. A case of paraventricular anaplastic astrocytoma following radiation therapy for craniopharyngioma. No Shinkei Geka 1994;22:357–362.

13. Barbaro NM, Rosenblum ML, Maitland CG, Hoyt WF, Davis RL, Maroon JC. Malignant optic glioma presenting radiologically as a "cystic" suprasellar mass: Case report and review of the literature. Neurosurgery 1982;11:787–789.

14. Marus G, Levin CV, Rutherfoord GS. Malignant glioma following radiotherapy for unrelated primary tumors. Cancer 1986;58:886–894.

15. Suda Y, Mineura K, Kowada M, Ohishi H. Malignant astrocytoma following radiotherapy in pituitary adenoma: Case report. No Shinkei Geka 1989;17:783–788.

16. Komaki S, Komaki R, Choi H, Correa-Paz F. Radiation and drug induced intracranial neoplasm with angiographic demonstration. Neurol Med Chir (Tokyo) 1977;17:55–62.

17. Sogg RL, Donaldson SS, Yorke CH. Malignant astrocytoma following radiotherapy of a craniopharyngioma. J Neurosurg 1978;48:622–627.

18. Gutjahr P, Dieterich E, Risiko. Risk of a second malignant neoplasm after successful treatment of a malignant tumor in children. Dtsch Med Wochenschr 1979;104:969–972.

19. Piatt JH, Bluie JM, Schold SC, Burger PC. Glioblastoma multiforme after radiotherapy for acromegaly. Neurosurgery 1983;13:85–89.

20. Liwnicz BH, Berger TS, Liwnicz RG, Aron BS. Radiation-associated gliomas: A report of four cases and analysis of post-radiation tumors of the central nervous system. Neurosurgery 1985;17:436–445.

21. Maat-Schiemann MLC, Bots GTAM, Thomeer RTWM, Vielvoye GJ. Malignant astrocytoma following radiotherapy for craniopharyngioma. Br J Radiol 1985;48:480–482.

21a. Committee of Authors. National Epidemiologic Study, July, 1982.

22. Brada M, Rajan B, Ross G, Traish D, Ashley S, Ford D. Long-term tumor control and toxicity following conservative surgery and radiotherapy in the treatment of pituitary adenoma. Br J Cancer 1993;67(Supple XX):27.

23. Tsang RW, Laperriere NJ, Simpson WJ, Brierley J, Panzarella T, Smyth HS. Glioma arising after radiation therapy for pituitary adenoma. A report of four patients and estimation of risk. Cancer 1993;72:2227–2233;73:492.

24. Tamura M, Misumi S, Kurosaki S, Shibasaki T, Ohye C. Anaplastic astrocytoma 14 years after radiotherapy for pituitary adenoma. No Shinkei Geka 1992;20:493–497.

25. McKeever PE, Blaivas M, Nelson JS. The diagnosis of brain and spinal tumors by conventional light microscopic methods. In: Garcia JH, Budka H, McKeever PE, Sarnat HB, Sima AAF, eds. Neuropathology: The Diagnostic Approach. Mosby-Yearbook, Philadelphia, 1997, pp. 31–96.

26. McLaughlin PW, Schea R, McKeever PE, Boothman DA. Radiobiological effects and changes in gene expression in the central nervous system in response to ionizing radiation. In: Levin AJ, Schmidek HH, eds. Molecular Genetics of Nervous System Tumors. Wiley-Liss, New York, 1993, pp. 163–177.

27. Burger PC, Scheithauer BW. Tumors of the central nervous system. In: Rosai J, Sobin LH, ed and assoc ed. Atlas of Tumor Pathology, fasc 10, 3rd ser. Armed Forces Institute of Pathology, Washington, DC, 1994.

28. Albers GW, Hoyt WF, Forno LS, Shratter LA. Treatment response in malignant optic glioma of adulthood. Neurology 1988;38:1071–1074.

2.2.4. Granular Cell Tumor (GCT)

1. Kovacs K, Horvath E. Tumors of the pituitary gland. Armed Forces Institute of Pathology, Washington DC, 1986.

2. McCormick WF, Hamlmi BS. Absence of chromophobe adenomas from a large series of pituitary tumors. Arch Pathol 1971;92:231–238.

3. Luse SA, Kernohan JW. Granular cell tumors of the stalk and posterior lobe of the pituitary gland. Cancer 1955;8:616–622.

4. Vaquero J, Leunda G, Gabezudo JM, Salazar AR, Miguel de J. Granular pituicytomas of the pituitary stalk. Acta Neurochir 1981;59:209–215.

5. Bakos L. Multiple cutaneous granular cell tumors with systemic defects: a distinct entity? Int J Dermatol 1993;32:432–435.

6. Becker DH, Wilson CB. Symptomatic parasellar granular cell tumor. Neurosurgery 1981;8:173–180.

7. Simsir A, Osborne BM, Greenbaum E. Malignant granular cell tumor: A case report and review of the recent literature. Hum Pathol 1996;27:853–858.

8. Thunold S, Von Eyben FE, Maehle B. Malignant granular cell tumor of the neck: Immunohistochemical and ultrastructural studies of a case. Histopathology 1989;14:655–662.

9. O'Donovah DG, Kell P. Malignant granular cell tumor with intraperitoneal dissemination. Histopathology 1989;14:417–428.

10. Lloyd RV, Warner TF. Immunohistochemistry of neuron-specific enolase. In: DeLellis RA, ed. Advances in Immunohistochemistry. Masson, New York, 1984, pp. 127–140.

11. Nathrath WBJ, Remberger K. Immunohistochemical study of granular cell tumors. Demonstration of neuron specific enolase, S100 protein, laminin and alpha-1-antichymotrypsin. Virchows Arch (Pathol Anat) 1986;408:421–434.

12. Liwnicz BH, Liwnicz RG, Huff JS, McBride BH, Tew JM. Giant granular cell tumor of the suprasellar area: Immunohistochemical and electron microscopic studies. Neurosurgery 1984;15:246–251.

13. Gambini C, Ruelle A, Palladino M, Boccardo M. Intracerebral granular cell tumor. Case report. Pathologica 1990;82:83–88.

14. Dickson DW, Suzuki KI, Kanner R, Weitz S, Horoupian DS. Cerebral granular cell tumor: Immunohistochemical and electron microscopic study. J Neuropathol Exp Neurol 1986;45:304–314.

15. Filie AC, Lage JM, Azumi N. Immunoreactivity of S100 protein, α-1-antitrypsin, and CD68 in adult and congenital granular cell tumors. Mod Pathol 1996;9:888–892.

15a. Geddes JF, Thom M, Robinson SFD, Revesz T. Granular cell tumor change in astrocytic tumors. Am J Surg Pathol 1996;20:55–63.

16. Nakamura T, Hirato J, Hotchi M, Kyoshima K, Nakamura Y. Astrocytoma with granular cell tumor-like changes. Report of a case with histochemical and ultrastructural characterization of granular cells. Acta Pathol Jpn 1990;40:206–211.

17. Rosenthal SA, Livolsi VA, Turrisi AT. Adjuvant radiotherapy for recurrent granular cell tumor. Cancer 1990;65:897–900.

17a. Melaragno MJ, Prayson RA, Murphy MA, Hassenbusch SJ, Estes ML. Anaplastic astrocytoma with granular cell differentiation: Case report and review of the literature. Hum Pathol 1993;24:805–808.

2.2.5. Schwannomas

1. Ho K-L. Schwannoma of the trochlear nerve. J Neurosurg 1981;55:132–134.

2. Lennda G, Vaquero J, Cabezudo J, Garcia-Uria J, Bravo G. Schwannoma of the oculomotor nerve. Report of four cases. J Neurosurg 1982;57:563–565.

3. Wilberger JE Jr. Primary intrasellar schwannoma. Case report. Surg Neurol 1989;32:156–158.

4. Perone TP, Robinson B, Holmes SM. Intrasellar schwannoma: Case report. Neurosurgery 1984;14:71–73.

5. Goebel HH, Shimokawa K, Schaake TH, Kremp A. Schwannoma of the sellar region. Acta Neurochir 1979;48:191–197.

6. Chadduk WN. Unusual lesions involving the sella turcica. S Med J 1973;66:948–955.

7. Hasegawa SL, Mentzel T, Fletcher CDM. Schwannomas of the sinonasal tract and nasopharynx. Mod Pathol 1997;10:777–784.

8. Ghatak NR, Norwood CW, Davis CH. Intracerebral schwannoma. Surg Neurol 1975;3:45–47.

9. DiNardo LJ, Mellis MG. Cystic schwannoma of the sphenoid sinus and skull base. Ear, Nose Throat J 1993;72:816–818.

10. Cotton RT, Goodman ML. A 12-year-old boy with progressive nasal obstruction. N Engl J Med 1995;332:1285–1291.

11. Benhaiem-Sigaux N, Ricolfi F, Keravel Y, Poirier J. Epithelioid schwannoma of the acoustic nerve. Clin Neuropathol 1996;15:231–233.

12. Kurtin PJ, Bonin DM. Immunohistochemical demonstration of the lysosome-associated glycoprotein CD68 (KP-1) in granular cell tumors and schwannomas. Hum Pathol 1994;25:1172–1184.

3.1. Meningioma

1. Ugrumov VM, Ignatyeva GE, Olushin VE, Tigliev GS, Polenov AL. Parasellar meningiomas: diagnosis and possibility of surgical treatment according to the place of original growth. Acta Neurochir 1979;Suppl 28:373–374.

2. Bonnal J, Brotchi J, Born J. Meningiomas of the lateral portion of the sella turcica. Acta Neurochirurgica 1979;28(Suppl):385,386.

3. Solero CL, Giombini S, Morello G. Suprasellar and olfactory meningiomas. Report on a series of 153 personal cases. Acta Neurochir 1983;67:181–194.

4. Synom L. Olfactory grove and suprasellar meningiomas. In: Krayenbuhl H, ed. Advances and Technical Standards in Neurosurgery, vol. 4. Springer Verlag, New York, 1977, pp. 67–91.

5. Banna M, Baker HL, House OW. Pituitary and parapituitary tumours on computed tomography. Br J Radiol 1980;53;1123–43.

6. Ehlers N, Malmros R. The suprasellar meningioma. A review of the literature and presentation of a series of 31 cases. Acta Ophthalmol Suppl 1973;121:1–73.

7. Ley A, Gabas E. Meningiomas of the tuberculum sellae. Acta Neurochir Suppl 1979;28:402–404.

8. Krenkel W, Frowein RA. Suprasellar meningiomas. Acta Neurochir 1974;31:280.

9. Russel DS, Rubinstein LJ. Pathology of Tumours of the Nervous System. Williams and Wilkins, London, 1989.

10. Busch E, Mahneke A. A case of meningioma from the diaphragm of the sella turcica. Zbl Neurochir 1954;14:25–28.

11. Demailly PW, Guiat G. Meningiomes du diaphragme sellaire. Bull Soc D'Ophthalm 1970;2:191–193.

12. Kepes JJ. Meningiomas. Biology, Pathology and Differential Diagnosis. Masson, New York, 1982, pp. 64–149.

13. Papo I, Villani R, Giovanelli M, Scarpelli M, Salvolini V, Pasquini U, et al. Angioblastic parasellar extradural tumours. Acta Neurochirurgica, Suppl 1979;28:438–444.

14. Shah RP, Leavens ME, Samaan NA. Galactorrhea, amenorrhea, and hyperprolactinemia as manifestations of parasellar meningioma. Arch Int Med 1980;140:1608–1612.

15. Grisoli F, Vincentelli F, Raybaud C, Harter M., Guibout M, Baldini M. Intrasellar meningioma. Surg Neurol 1983;20:36–41.

16. Hardy J, Roberst F. Un meningiome de la sella turcique variete sous diaphragmatique (exerese par voie transphenoidale) Neurochirurgie 1969;15:535–544.

17. Meyrignac C, N'Guyen JP, Blatrix C, Degos JDD. Meningiome post radique. Complication tardive de l irradiation de la sella turcique. La Nouv Presse Med 1981;10:3246–3247.

18. Sumida M, Uozumi T, Yamanaka M, Mukada K, Arita K, Kurisu K, et al. Displacement of the normal pituitary gland by sellar and juxtasellar tumours: surgical MRI correlation and use in differential diagnosis. Neuroradiol 1994;36:372–375.

19. Johnsen DE, Woodruff WW, Allen IS, Cera PJ, Funkhouser GR, Coleman LL. MR imaging of the sellar and juxtasellar regions. Radiographics 1991;11:727–758.

20. Hershey BL. Suprasellar masses: diagnosis and differential diagnosis. Semin Ultrasound Comput Tomogr Magn Reson 1993;14:215–231.

21. Dietemann JL, Cromero C, Tajahmady T, Baumgartner J, Gangi A, Kastler B, et al. CT and MRI of suprasellar lesions. J Neuroradiol 1992;19:1–22.

22. McKeever PE, Blaivas M, Nelson JS. The diagnosis of brain and spinal tumors by conventional light microscopic methods. In: Garcia JH, Budka H, McKeever PE, Sarnat HB, Sima AAF, eds. Neuropathology: The Diagnostic Approach. Mosby-Yearbook, Philadelphia, 1997, pp. 31–96.

23. McKeever PE, Brissie NT. Scanning electron microscopy of neoplasms removed at surgery: Surface topography and comparison of meningioma, colloid cyst, ependymoma, pituitary adenoma, schwannoma and astrocytoma. J Neuropathol Exp Neurol 1977;36:875–896.

24. Kleihues P, Burger PC, Scheithauer BW. Histologic Classification of Tumours of the Central Nervous System. Springer-Verlag, New York, 1993.

25. Friede RL, Yasargil MG. Suprasellar neoplasm with a granular cell component. J Neuropathol Exp Neurol 1977;36:769–782.

26. Mitsumori K, Maronpot RR, Boorman GA. Spontaneous tumors of the meninges in rats. Vet Pathol 1987;24:50–58.

27. Wanschitz J, Schmidbauer M, Maier H, Rossler K, Vorkapic P, Budka H. Suprasellar meningioma with expression of glial fibrillary acidic protein: a peculiar variant. Acta Neuropathol (Berl) 1995;90:539–544.

28. Yamada K, Hatayama T, Ohta M, Sakoda K, Uozumi T. Coincidental pituitary adenoma and parasellar meningioma. Case report. Neurosurgery 1986;19:267–270.

29. O'Connell JEA. Intracranial meningioma associated with other tumors involving the central nervous system. Br J Surg 1961;48:373–383.

30. Kitamura K, Nakamura N, Terao H, Hayakawa I, Kamano S, Ishijima T, et al. Primary brain tumors. Brain Nerve 1965;17:109–117.

31. Probst A. Combined occurrence of Cushing syndrome, hypophyseal adenoma and suprasellar meningioma. Case report. Zentralbl Neurochirurg 1971;32:75–82.

32. Bunick EM, Mills LC, Rose LI. Association of acromegaly and meningiomas. JAMA 1978;240:1267–1268.

33. Hyoda A, Nose T, Maki Y, Enomoto T. Pituitary adenoma and meningioma in the same patient. Neurochir (Stuttg) 1982;25:66–67.

34. Brennan TG Jr, Rao CVGK, Robinson W, Itani A. Case report: Tandem lesions. Chromophobe adenoma and meningioma. J Comput Assisted Tomogr 1977;1:517–520.

35. Sautner D, Saeger W, Ludecke DK. Tumors of the sellar region mimicking pituitary adenomas. Exp Clin Endocrinol 1993;101:283–289.

36. Meis JM, Ordonez NG, Bruner JM. Meningiomas: An immunohistochemical study of 50 cases. Arch Pathol Lab Med 1986;110:934–937.

37. Mrak RE. Ultrastructural diagnosis of tumors of the nervous system. In: Garcia JH, Budka H, McKeever PE, Sarnat HB, Sima AAF, eds. Neuropathology: The Diagnostic Approach. Mosby-Yearbook, Philadelphia, 1997, pp. 97–192.

38. McKeever PE, Lloyd RV. Tumors of the pituitary gland region. In: Garcia JH, Budka H, McKeever PE, Sarnat HB, Sima AAF, eds. Neuropathology: The Diagnostic Approach. Mosby-Yearbook, Philadelphia, 1997, pp. 219–262.

39. Thomas HG, Dolman CL, Berry K. Malignant meningioma: Clinical and pathological features. J Neurosurg 1981;55:929–934.

40. Kinjo T, al-Mefty O, Ciric I. Diaphragma sellae meningiomas. Neurosurgery 1995;36:1082–1092.

41. Jallu A, Kanaan I, Rahm B, Siqueria E. Suprasellar meningioma and blindness: a unique experience in Saudi Arabia. Surg Neurol 1996;45:320–323.

4.1. Chordoma

1. Lana-Peixoto MA, Pittella JE, Arouca EM. Primary intracranial tumors: Analysis of a series of consecutive autopsies and biopsies. Arquivos de Neuroi-Psiquiatria 1981;39:13–24.

2. Volpe R, Mazabraud A. A clinicopathologic review of 25 cases of chordoma. Am J Surg Pathol 1983;7:161–170.

3. Austin MB, Mills SE. Neoplasms and neoplasm-like lesions involving the skull base. Ear Nose Throat J 1986;65:25–52.

4. McKeever PE, Blaivas M, Sima AAF. Neoplasms of the sellar region. In: Lloyd RV, ed. Surgical Pathology of the Pituitary Gland. Major Problems in Pathology Series. Saunders, Philadelphia, 1993, pp. 141–210.

5. Mathews W, Wilson CB. Ectopic intrasellar chordoma: Case report. J Neurosurg 1974;40:260.

6. Belza J. Double midline intracranial tumors of vestigial origin: Contiguous intrasellar chordoma and suprasellar craniopharyngioma: Case report. J Neurosurg 1966;25:199.

7. Perzin KH, Pushparaj N. Nonepithelial tumors of the nasal cavity, paranasal sinuses, and nasopharynx. Cancer 1986;57:784–796.

8. Franquemont DW, Katsetos CD, Ross GW. Fatal acute pontocerebellar hemorrhage due to an unsuspected spheno-occipital chordoma. Arch Pathol Lab Med 1989;113:1075–1078.

9. Kendall BE. Cranial chordomas. Br J Radiol 1977;50:687–698.

10. Launay M, Fredy D, Merland JJ, Bories J. Narrowing and occlusion of arteries by intracranial tumors: Review of the literature and report of 25 cases. Neuroradiology 1977;14:117–126.

11. Koga N, Kadota Y, Hatashita S, Hosaka Y, Sugamura J, Sakakibara T, et al. A case of clivus chordoma showing hemorrhage in the posterior fossa. No Shinkei Geka 1988;16:1417–1421.

12. Kontozoglou T, Qizilbash AH, Sianos J, Stead R. Chordoma: Cytologic and immunocytochemical study of four cases. Diagn Cytopathol 1986;2:55–61.

13. Marigil MA, Pardo-Mindan FJ, Joly M. Diagnosis of chordoma by cytologic examination of cerebrospinal fluid. Am J Clin Pathol 1983;80:402,403.

14. Apaja-Sarkkinen M, Vaananen K, Curran S, Siponen P, Autio-Harmainen H. Carcinomatous features of cervical chordoma in a fine needle aspirate. Acta Cytologica 1987;31:769–773.

15. Finley JL, Silverman JF, Dabbs DJ, West RL, Dickens A, Felman PS, et al. Chordoma: diagnosis by fine-needle aspiration biopsy with histologic, immunocytochemical, and ultrastructural confirmation. Diagn Cytopathol 1986;2:330–337.

16. Bouropoulou V, Bosse A, Roessner A, et al. Immunohistochemical investigation of chordomas: Histogenetic and differential diagnostic aspects. Current Topics Pathol 1989;80:183–203.

17. Coindre JM, Rivel J, Trojani M, DeMascarel I, DeMascarel A. Immunohistological study in chordomas. J Pathol 1986;150:61–63.

18. Meis JM, Giraldo AA. Chordoma: an immunohistochemical study of 20 cases. Arch Pathol Lab Med 1988;112:553–556.

19. Miettinen M, Lehto V-P, Dahl D, Virtanen I. Differential diagnosis of chordoma, chondroid, and ependymal tumors as aided by anti-intermediate filament antibodies. Am J Pathol 1983;112:160–169.

20. Nakajima T, Kameya T, Watanabe S, et al. An immunoperoxidase study of S-100 protein distribution in normal and neoplastic tissues. Am J Surg Pathol 1982;6:715–727.

21. Nakamura Y, Becker LE, Marks A. S-100 protein in human chordoma and human and rabbit notochord. Arch Pathol Lab Med 1983;107:118–120.

22. Okajima K, Honda I, Kitagawa T. Immunohistochemical distribution of S-100 protein in tumors and tumor-like lesions of bone and cartilage. Cancer 1988;61:792–799.

23. Rutherfoord GS, Davies AG. Chordomas—ultrastructure and immunohistochemistry: a report based on the examination of six cases. Histopathology 1987;11:775–787.

24. Salisbury JR, Isaacson PG. Demonstration of cytokeratins and an epithelial membrane antigen in chordomas and human fetal blood. Am J Surg Pathol 1985;9:791–797.

25. Schmitt FC, Bacchi CE. S-100 protein: Is it useful as a tumor marker in diagnostic immunocytochemistry? Histopathology 1989;15:281–288.

26. Kay S, Schatzki PF. Ultrastructural observations of a chordoma arising in the clivus. Hum Pathol 1972;3:403–413.

27. Pardo-Mindan FJ, Guillen FJ, Villas C, Vazquez JJ. A comparative ultrastructural study of chondrosarcoma, chordoid sarcoma, and chordoma. Cancer 1981;47:2611–2619.

28. Erlandson RA, Tandler B, Lieberman PH, Higinbotham NL. Ultrastructure of human chordoma. Cancer Res 1968;28:2115–2125.

29. Ho KL. Ecchordosis physaliphora and chordoma: a comparative ultrastructural study. Clin Neuropathol 1985;4:77–86.

30. McKeever PE, Blaivas M, Nelson JS. The diagnosis of brain and spinal tumors by conventional light microscopic methods. In: Garcia JH, Budka H, McKeever PE, Sarnat HB, Sima AAF, eds. Neuropathology: The Diagnostic Approach. Mosby-Yearbook, Philadelphia, 1997, pp. 31–96.

31. Mrak RE. Ultrastructural diagnosis of tumors of the nervous system. In: Garcia JH, Budka H, McKeever PE, Sarnat HB, Sima AAF, eds. Neuropathology: The Diagnostic Approach. Mosby-Yearbook, Philadelphia, 1997, pp. 97–192.

32. Burger PC, Makek M, Kleihues P. Tissue polypeptide antigen staining of the chordoma and notochordal remnants. Acta Neuropathol (Berl) 1986;70:269–272.

33. Imrie SF, Sloane JP, Ormerod MG, Styles J, Dean CJ. Detailed investigation of the diagnostic value of tumour histopathology of ICR.2, a new monoclonal antibody to epithelial membrane antigen. Histopathology 1990;16:573–581.

34. McKeever PE, Lloyd RV. Tumors of the pituitary gland region. In: Garcia JH, Budka H, McKeever PE, Sarnat HB, Sima AAF, eds. Neuropathology: The Diagnostic Approach. Mosby-Yearbook, Philadelphia, 1997, pp. 219–262.

35. Brooks JJ, LiVolsi VA, Trojanowski JQ. Does chondroid chordoma exist? Acta Neuropathol 1987;72:229–235.

36. Mierau GW, Weeks DA. Chondroid chordoma. Ultra Pathol 1987;11:731–737.

37. Ohshima T, Sakamoto M, Takasugi S, Matsumoto K, Asano N, Kouyama Y. Three cases of intracranial chordoma. Typical chordoma and chondroid chordoma. No Shinkei Geka 1984;12:591–598.

38. Hruban RH, Traganos F, Reuter VE, Huvos AG. Chordomas with malignant spindle cell components. A DNA flow cytometric and immunohistochemical study with histogenetic implications. Am J Pathol 1990;137:436–447.

39. Cho KG, De Armond SJ, Barnwell S, Edwards MSB, Hoshino T. Proliferative characteristics of intracranial and spinal tumors of developmental origin. Cancer 1988;62:740–748.

40. Spaar F-W, Spaar U, Markakis E. DNA in chordomas of the clivus Blumenbachi. Neurosurg Rev 1990;13:219–229.

4.2. Giant Cell Tumor of Bone (GCTB)

1. Viale GL. Giant cell tumours of the sellar region. Acta Neurochir 1977;38:259–268.

2. Jacas R, Bermejo A. Giant cell tumors of the sellar region Acta Neurochirurgica 1979;(Suppl)28:416–417.

3. Wolfe JT, Scheithauer BW, Dahlin DC. Giant cell tumor of the sphenoid bone. Review of 10 cases. J Neurosurg 1983;59:322–327.

4. Wu KK, Ross PM, Mitchell DC, Sprague HH. Evolution of a case of multicentric giant cell tumor over a 23-year period. Clin Orthop Rel Res 1986;213:279–288.

5. Opitz H, Petersen D, Heiss E, Duffner F, Meyermann R. Giant cell tumor of the occipital bone in a case of von Recklinghausen neurofibromatosis. Clin Neuropathol 1996;15:226–230.

6. Curilovic A, Eich GF, Stallmach T. Giant cell tumor in a skull of a 9-year-old child: immunohistochemistry to confirm a diagnosis rare for age and site. Pediatr Pathol Lab Med 1995;15:769–779.

7. Rock JP, Mahmood A, Cramer HB. Giant cell tumor of skull base. Am J Otol 1994;15:268–272.

8. Monda L, Wick MR. S-100 protein immunostaining in the differential diagnosis of chondroblastoma. Hum Pathol 1985;16:287–293.

9. Bertoni F, Unni KK, Beabout JW, Ebersold MJ. Giant cell tumors of the skull. Cancer 1992;70:1124–1132.

10. Martins AN, Dean DF. Giant cell tumor of sphenoid bone: Malignant transformation following radiotherapy. Surg Neurol 1984;2:105–107.

4.3. Hemangiopericytoma

1. Eichhorn JH, Dickersin GR, Bhan AK, Goodman ML. Sinonasal hemangiopericytoma. A reassessment with electron microscopy, immunohistochemistry, and long-term follow-up. Am J Surg Pathol 1990;14:856–66.
2. D'Amore ES, Manivel JC, Sung JH. Soft-tissue and meningeal hemangiopericytomas: an immunohistochemical and ultrastructural study. Hum Pathol 1990;21:414–423.
3. Davidson GS, Hope J. Meningeal tumors of childhood. Cancer 1989;63:1205–1210.
4. Iwaki T, Fukui M, Takeshita I, Tsuneyoshi M, Tateishi J. Hemangiopericytoma of the meninges: a clinicopathologic and immunohistochemical study. Clin Neuropathol 1988;7:93–99.
5. Austin MB, Mills SE. Neoplasms and neoplasm-like lesions involving the skull base. Ear Nose Throat J 1986;65:57–73.
6. Winek RR, Scheithauer BW, Wick MR. Meningioma, meningeal hemangiopericytoma (angioblastic meningioma), peripheral hemangiopericytoma, and acoustic schwannoma. A comparative immunohistochemical study. Am J Surg Pathol 1989;13:251–261.
7. Kumar PP, Good RR, Skultety FM, Masih AS, McComb RD. Spinal metastases from pituitary hemangiopericytic meningioma. Am J Clin Oncol 1987;10:422–428.
8. Kumar PP, Good RR, Cox TA, Leibrock LG, Skultety FM. Reversal of visual impairment after interstitial irradiation of pituitary tumor. Neurosurgery 1986;18:82–84.
9. Nikonov AA, Matsko DE. Pituitary hemangiopericytoma. Arkhiv Patholagii 1985;47:79–83.
10. Mangiardi JR, Flamm ES, Cravioto H, Fisher B. Hemangiopericytoma of the pituitary fossa: case report. Neurosurgery 1983;13:58–62.
11. Kumar PP, Good RR, Leibrock LG, Mawk JR, Yonkers AJ, Ogren FP. High activity iodine 125 endocurietherapy for recurrent skull base tumors. Cancer 1988;61:1518–1527.
12. Orf G. "Angioreticuloma" of the sella turcica. Acta Neurochir (Wien) 1970;23:63–78.
13. Yokota M, Tani E, Maeda Y, Morimura T, Kakudo K, Uematsu K. Acromegaly associated with suprasellar and pulmonary hemangiopericytomas. Case report. J Neurosurg 1985;62:767–771.
14. Takahashi S, Higano S, Ishii K, Matsumoto K, Shimanuki Y, Ishibashi T, et al. CT and MR image findings of sphenoidal masses. Nippon Igaku Hoshasen Gakkai Zasshi 1994;54:751–760.
15. McKeever PE, Blaivas M, Nelson JS. The diagnosis of brain and spinal tumors by conventional light microscopic methods. In: Garcia JH, Budka H, McKeever PE, Sarnat HB, Sima AAF, eds. Neuropathology: The Diagnostic Approach. Mosby-Yearbook, Philadelphia, 1997, pp. 31–96.
16. Mandahl N, Örndal C, Heim S, Willén H, Rydholm A, Bauer HCF, et al. Aberrations of chromosome segment 12q13-15 characterize a subgroup of hemangiopericytomas. Cancer 1993;71:3009–3013.
17. Gollin SM, Janecka IP. Cytogenetics of cranial base tumors. J Neurooncol 1994;20:241–254.
18. Theunissen PH, Debets-Te Baerts M, Blaauw G. Histogenesis of intracranial haemangiopericytoma and haemangioblastoma. An immunohistochemical study. Acta Neuropathol 1990;80:68–71.
19. Schurch W, Skalli O, Lagace R, Seemayer TA, Gabbiani G. Intermediate filament proteins and actin isoforms as markers for soft-tissue tumor differentiation and origin. III. Hemangiopericytomas and glomus tumors. Am J Pathol 1990;136:771–786.
20. Dardick I, Hammar SP, Scheithauer BW. Ultrastructural spectrum of hemangiopericytoma: a comparative study of fetal, adult, and neoplastic pericytes. Ultrastruct Pathol 1989;15:111–154.
21. Moss TH. Immunohistochemical characteristics of haemangiopericytic meningiomas: comparison with typical meningiomas, haemangioblastomas and haemangiopericytomas from extracranial sites. Neuropathol Appl Neurobiol 1987;13:467–480.
22. Miettinen M. Antibody specific to muscle actins in the diagnosis and classification of soft tissue tumors. Am J Pathol 1988;130:205–215.
23. Nakamura M, Inoue HK, Ono N, Kunimine H, Tamada J. Analysis of hemangiopericytic meningiomas by immunohistochemistry, electron microscopy and cell culture. J Neuropathol Exp Neurol 1987;46:57–71.
24. Mrak RE. Ultrastructural diagnosis of tumors of the nervous system. In: Garcia JH, Budka H, McKeever PE, Sarnat HB, Sima AAF, eds. Neuropathology: The Diagnostic Approach. Mosby-Yearbook, Philadelphia, 1997, pp. 97–192.
25. Dietemann JL, Cromero C, Tajahmady T, Baumgartner J, Gangi A, Kastler B, et al. CT and MRI of suprasellar lesions. J Neuroradiol 1992;19:1–22.
26. Rice CD, Kersten RC, Mrak RE. An orbital hemangiopericytoma recurrent after 33 years. Arch Opthalmol 1989;107:552–556.

4.4. Myxoma

1. Stout AP. Myxoma: The tumor of primitive mesenchyme. Ann Surg 1948;127:706–719.
2. Branch CL, Laster DW, Kelly DL. Left atrial myxoma with cerebral emboli. Neurosurgery 1985;16:675–680.
3. Budzilovich G, Aleksic S, Greco A, Fernandez J, Harris J, Finegold M. Malignant cardiac myxoma with cerebral metastases. Surg Neurol 1979;11:461–469.
4. Samaratunga H, Searle J, Cominos D, Le Fevre I. Cerebral metastasis of an atrial myxoma mimicking an epithelioid hemangioendothelioma. Am J Surg Path 1994;18:107–111.
5. Nagatoni M, Mori M, Takomoto N, Arita N, Ushio Y, Hayakawa T, et al. Primary myxoma in the pituitary fossa: Case report. Neurosurgery 1987;20:329–331.
6. Ghosh BC, Huvos AG, Gerold FP, Miller TR. Myxoma of the jaw bones. Cancer 1973;31:237–240.

4.5. Fibroma

1. Frank E, Derauz J-P, de Tribolet N. Chondromyxoid fibroma of the petrous-sphenoid junction. Surg Neurol 1987;27:182–186.
2. Sterling KM, Stollman A, Sacher M, Som PM. Ossifying fibroma of sphenoid bone with coexistent mucocele: CT and MRI. J Comput Assisted Tomogr 1993;17:492–494.
3. Wenig BM, Vinh TN, Smirniotopoulos JG, Fowler CB, Houston GD, Heffner DK. Aggressive psammomatoid ossifying fibromas of the sinonasal region: a clinicopathologic study of a distinct group of fibro-osseous lesions. Cancer 1995;76:1155–1165.
4. Gartman JJ, Powers SK, Fortune M. Pseudotumor of the sellar and parasellar areas. Neurosurgery 1989;24:896–901.

4.6 Fibrosarcoma

1. McKeever PE, Blaivas M, Sima AAF. Neoplasms of the sellar region. In: Lloyd RV, ed. Surgical Pathology of the Pituitary Gland, vol. 27, Livolsi VA, ed. Major Problems in Pathology. WB Saunders, Philadelphia, 1993, pp. 141–210.
2. Huang CI, Chiou WH, Ho DM. Oligodendroglioma occurring after radiation therapy for pituitary adenoma. J Neurol Neurosurg Psychiatry 1987;50:1619–1624.
3. Kitanaka C, Shitara N, Nakagomi T, Nakamura H, Genka S, Nakagawa K, et al. Postradiation astrocytoma: Report of two cases. J Neurosurg 1989;70:469–474.
4. Shi T, Farrell MA, Kaufman JCE. Fibrosarcoma complicating irradiated pituitary adenoma. Surg Neurol 1984;22:277–283.
5. Powell HC, Marshall LF, Ignelzi RJ. Post-irradiation pituitary sarcoma. Acta Neuropath (Berl) 1977;39:165–167.
6. Martin WH, Cail WS, Morris JL, Constable WC. Fibrosarcoma after high energy radiation therapy for pituitary adenoma. AJR 1980;135:1087–1090.
7. Martin WH, Cail WS, Morris JL, Constable WC. Fibrosarcoma after high energy radiation therapy for pituitary adenoma. Am J Neuroradiol 1980;1:469–472.
8. Sato K, Hayashi M, Komai T, Kubota T, Kawano H, Handa Y. Clinical and histological study of pituitary fibrosarcoma following radiotherapy for pituitary adenoma. Case report. Neurol Med Chir (Toyko) 1990;30:888–892.

9. Nagatani M, Ikeda T, Otsuki H, Mizuta T, Mori S, Ushio Y, et al. Sellar fibrosarcoma following radiotherapy for prolactinoma. No Shinkei Geka 1984;12(3 Suppl):339–346.

10. Coppeto JR, Roberts M. Fibrosarcoma after proton-beam pituitary ablation. Arch Neurol 1979;36:380,381.

11. Terry RD, Hyams VJ, Davidoff LM. Combined non-metastasizing fibrosarcoma and chromophobe tumor of the pituitary. Cancer 1959;12:791–798.

12. Walzp TA, Brownell B. Sarcoma: A possible late result of effective radiation therapy for pituitary adenoma. Report on two cases. J Neurosurgery 1966;24:901–907.

13. Amendola BE, Amendola MA, McClatchey KD, Miller CH. Radiation associated sarcoma; a review of 23 patients with post-radiation sarcoma over a 50-year period. Am J Clin Oncol 1989;12:411–415.

14. Amine ARC, Sugar O. Suprasellar osteogenic sarcoma following radiation for pituitary adenoma. J Neurosurg 1976;44:88–91.

15. Schrantz JL, Araoz CA. Radiation induced meningeal fibrosarcoma. Arch Pathol 1972;93:26–31.

16. Pieterse S, Dinning TAR, Blumbergs PC. Post-irradiation sarcomatous transformation of a pituitary adenoma: a combined pituitary tumor. J Neurosurg 1982;56:283–286.

17. Willis RA. Pathological study of tumors of the pituitary region. Med J Aust 1938;1:281–291.

18. Mena H, Garcia JH. Primary brain sarcomas: light and electron microscopic features. Cancer 1978;42:1298–307.

19. Anderson WR, Cameron JD, Tsai SH. Primary intracranial leiomyosarcoma. Case report with ultrastructural study. J Neurosurg 1980;53:401–405.

20. Dardick I, Hammar SP, Scheithauer BW. Ultrastructural spectrum of hemangiopericytoma: a comparative study of fetal, adult, and neoplastic pericytes. Ultrastruct Pathol 1989;15:111–54.

4.7. Osteogenic Sarcoma

1. Dahlin DL, Uuni KK. Bone Tumors, 4th ed, Charles C. Thomas, Springfield IL, 1986, p. V271.

2. Kleinsasser O, Albrecht H. Zur Kenntnis der Osteosarcome des Stirn-und Keilbeines Arch Ohren Heilk 1957;170:595–603.

3. Reichenthal E, Cohen ML, Manor R, Marshak G, Matz S, Shalit MN. Primary osteogenic sarcoma of the sellar region. Case report J Neurosurg 1981;55:299–302.

4. Lee YY, Van Tassel P, Raymond AK, Edeiken J. Craniofacial osteosarcomas: Plain film, CT and MR findings in 46 cases. AJR 1988;150:1397–1402.

5. Tanaka S, Nishio S, Morioka T, Fukui M, Kitamura K, Hikita K. Radiation-induced osteosarcoma of the sphenoid bone. Neurosurgery 1989;25:640–643.

6. Amine ARC, Sugar O. Suprasellar osteogenic sarcoma following radiation for pituitary adenoma. Case report. J Neurosurg 1976;44:88–91.

7. Mackenzie IRA, Girvin JP, Lee D. Symptomatic osteolipoma of the tuber cinereum. Clin Neuropathol 1996;15:60–62.

8. Shinoda J, Kimura T, Funakoshi T, Iwata H, Tange K, Kasai C, Miyata Y. Primary osteosarcoma of the skull—a case report and review of the literature. J Neuro-Oncol 1993;17:81–88.

9. Salvati M, Ciappetta P, Capoccia G, Capone R, Raco A. Osteosarcoma of the skull. Report of a post-Paget and post-radiation case in an elderly woman. Neurosurg Rev 1994;17:73–76.

5.1. Cavernous Angioma (CA)

1. Voigt K, Yasargil MG. Cerebral cavernous hemangiomas or cavernomas. Neurochirurgia 1976;19:59–68.

2. Kattapong VJ, Hart BL, Davis LE. Familial cerebral cavernous angiomas: clinical and radiologic studies. Neurology 1995;45:492–497.

3. Challa VR, Moody DM, Brown WR. Vascular malformations of the central nervous system. J Neuropathol Exp Neurol 1995;54:609–621.

4. Acciarri N, Padovani R, Giulioni M, Gaist G, Acciarri R. Intracranial and orbital cavernous angiomas: a review of 74 surgical cases. Brit J Neurosurg 1993;7:529–539.

5. Kawai K, Fukui M, Tanaka A, Kuramoto S, Kitamura K. Extracerebral cavernous hemangioma of the middle fossa. Surg Neurol 1978;9:19–25.

6. Shimabukuro H, Shinoda S, Yamada N, Iwasa H, Masuzawa T, Sato F. Parasellar cavernous hemangioma presenting with hyperprolactinemia. Case report Neurol Med Chir (Tokyo) 1984;24:212–216.

7. Sansone ME, Liwnicz BH, Mandybur TI. Giant pituitary cavernous hemangioma. Case Report J Neurosurg 1980;53:124–126.

8. Shen WC, Lee SK. CT and MRI of parasellar cavernous hemangioma in two cases. J Formos Med Assoc 1992;91:S165–S169.

9. Lombardi D, Giovanelli M, de Tribolet N. Sellar and parasellar extra-axial cavernous hemangiomas. Acta Neurochirurgica 1994;130:47–54.

10. Moore T, Ganti SR, Mawad ME, Hilal SK. CT and angiography of primary extradural juxtasellar tumors. AJNR 1985;145:491–496.

11. Gray MH, Rosenberg AE, Dickersin GR, Bhan AK. Cytokeratin expression in epithelioid vascular neoplasms. Hum Pathol 1990;21:212–217.

5.2. Hemangioblastoma

1. Rho YM. Von Hippel-Lindau's disease: A report of five cases. Can Med Assoc J 1969;101:135–142.

2. Dan NG, Smith DE. Pituitary hemangioblastoma in a patient with von Hippel-Lindau disease. Case report. J Neurosurg 1975;42:232–235.

3. Grisoli F, Gambarelli D, Raybaud C, Guibout M, Leclercq T. Suprasellar hemangioblastoma. Surg Neurol 1984;22:257–262.

4. Kupersmith MJ, Berenstein A. Visual disturbances in von Hippel-Lindau disease. Ann Ophthalmol 1981;Feb:195–197.

5. Kepes JJ, Rengachary SS, Lee SH. Astrocytes in hemangioblastomas of the central nervous system and their relationship to stromal cells. Acta Neuropathol (Berlin) 1979;47:99–104.

6. Tanimura A, Nakamura V, Hachisuka H, Tanimura Y, Fukumura A. Hemangioblastoma of the central nervous system: Nature of the stromal cells as studied by the immunoperoxidase technique. Hum Pathol 1984;15:866–869.

7. Kochi N, Tani E, Kaba K, Natsume S. Immunohistochemical study of fibronectin in hemangioblastomas and hemangiopericytomas. Acta Neuropathol (Berlin) 1984;64:229–233.

8. Kamitani H, Masauzawa H, Sato J, Kanazawa I. Capillary hemangioblastoma: Histogenesis of stromal cells. Acta Neuropathol (Berlin) 1987;73:370–378.

9. Feldenzer JA, McKeever PE. Selective localization of γ-enolase in stromal cells of cerebral hemangioblastomas. Acta Neuropathol (Berlin) 1987;72:281–285.

10. Ironside JW, Stephenson TJ, Royds JA, Mills PM, Taylor CB, Rider CC, et al. Stromal cells in cerebellar hemangioblastomas: An immunohistochemical study. Histopathology 1988;12:29–40.

11. Grant JW, Gallagher PJ, Hedinger C. Hemangioblastoma. An immunohistochemical study of ten cases. Acta Neuropathol (Berlin) 1988;76:82–86.

12. Frank TS, Trojanowski JQ, Roberts SA, Brooks JJ. A detailed immunohistochemical analysis of cerebellar hemangioblastoma: An undifferentiated mesenchymal tumor. Mod Pathol 1989;2:638–651.

13. Kawamura J, Garcia JH, Kamiyo Y. Cerebellar hemangiomas: Histogenesis of stromal cells. Cancer 1987;31:1528–1540.

14. Ho K-L. Ultrastructure of cerebellar capillary hemangioblastoma. I. Weibel-Palade bodies and stromal cell histiogenesis. J Neuropathol Exp Neurol 1984;43:592–608.

15. Bohling T, Haltia M, Rosenlof K, Fyhrquist F. Erythropoietin in capillary hemangioblastoma. An immunochemical study. Acta Neuropathol (Berlin) 1987;74:324–328.

16. Nemes Z. Fibrohistiocytic differentiation in capillary hemangioblastoma. Hum Pathol 1992;23:805–810.

17. Bohling T, Hatva E, Kujala M, Claesson-Welsh L, Alitalo K, Haltia M. Expression of growth factors and growth factor receptors in capillary hemangioma. J Neuropathol Exp Neurol 1996;5:522–527.

18. Oberstrass J, Reifenberger G, Reifenberger J, Wechsler W, Collins P. Mutation of the von Hippel-Lindau tumour suppressor gene in capillary haemangioblastomas of the central nervous system. J Pathol 1996;179:151–156.

19. Tse J, Wong JH, Lo K-W, Poon W-S, Huang D, Ng J-K. Molecular genetic analysis of the von Hippel-Lindau disease tumor suppressor gene in familial and sporadic cerebral hemangioblastomas. Am J Clin Pathol 1997;107:459–466.

20. Chaudhry AP, Moutes M, Cohn GA. Ultrastructure of cerebellar hemangioblastoma. Cancer 1978;42:1834–1838.

21. Clelland CA, Treips CS. Histological differentiation of metastatic renal carcinoma in the cerebellum from cerebellar hemangioblastoma in von Hippel-Lindau's disease. J Neurol Neurosurg Psychiatry 1989;52:162–166.

22. Mills SE, Ross GW, Perentes E, Nakagawa Y, Scheithauer BW. Cerebellar hemangioblastoma: Immunohistochemical distinction from metastatic renal cell carcinoma. Surg Pathol 1990;3:121–132.

23. Crocker J, Carey MP, Allcock R. Hemangioblastoma and renal clear cell carcinoma distinguished by means of the AgNOR method. Am J Clin Pathol 1990;93:555–557.

5.3. Glomus Tumor (GT) Glomangioma

1. Enzinger FM, Weiss SW. Soft Tissue Tumors, 3rd ed. St. Louis, Mosby, 1995. pp. 704–713.

2. Kim YI, Kim JH, Suh JS, Ham EK, Suh KP. Glomus tumor of the trachea. Report of a case with ultrastructural observation. Cancer 1989;64:881–886.

3. Asa SL, Kovacs K, Horvath E, Ezrin C, Weiss MH. Sellar gliomangioma. Ultrastruct Pathol 1984;7:49–54.

4. Pulitzer DR, Martin PC, Reed RJ. Epithelioid glomus tumor. Hum Pathol 1995;26:1022–1027.

5. Mey van der AGL, Maaswinkel-Mooy PD, Cornelisse CJ, Schmidt PH, Kamp van de JJP. Genomic imprinting in hereditary glomus tumors: Evidence for new genetic theory. Lancet 1989;8675:1292–1294.

6. Brathwaite CD, Poppiti R Jr. Malignant glomus tumor: A case report of widespread metastases in a patient with multiple glomus body hamartomas. Am J Surg Pathol 1996;20:233–238.

7. Harvey JS, Walker F. Solid glomus tumor of the pterygoid fossa: A lesion mimicking an epithelial neoplasm of low-grade malignancy. Hum Pathol 1987;18:965–966.

8. Gould EW, Manivel JC, Albores-Saavedra J, Monforte H. Locally infiltrative glomus tumors and glomangiosarcomas. Cancer 1990;65:310–318.

9. Nuovo MA, Grimes MM, Knowles DM. Glomus tumors: A clinicopathologic and immunohistochemical analysis of forty cases. Surg Pathol 1990;3:31–45.

10. Porter PL, Bigler SA, McNutt M, Gown AM. The immunophenotype of hemangiopericytomas and glomus tumors, with special reference to muscle protein expression: An immunohistochemical study and review of the literature. Mod Pathol 1991;4:46–42.

6.1. Histiocytosis

1. Russel DS, Rubinstein LJ. Pathology of Tumours of the Nervous System. Williams and Wilkins, London, 1989.

2. Scholz M, Firsching R, Feiden W, Breining H, Brechtelsbauer D, Harders A. Gagel's granuloma (localized Langerhans cell histiocytosis) in the pituitary stalk. Clin Neurol Neurosurg 1995;97:164–166.

3. Hou-Jensen K, Rawlinson DG, Hendrickson M. Proliferating histiocytic lesion (Histiocytosis-X?). Cancer 1973;32:809–821.

4. Richmond I, Wilson CB. Parasellar tumors in children. I. Clinical presentation, preoperative assessment, and differential diagnosis. Child's Brain 1980;7:73–84.

5. MacCumber MW, Hoffman PN, Wand GS, Epstein JI, Beschorner WE, Green R. Opthalmic involvement in aggressive histiocytosis X. Opthalmology 1990;97:22–27.

6. Rimoin DL. Hereditary forms of growth hormone deficiency and resistance. Birth Defects 1976;12:15–29.

7. Hirata Y, Sakamoto N, Yoshimoto Y, Kato Y, Matsukura S. Diabetes insipidus and galactorrhea caused by histiocytosis X. Endocrinol Jpn 1975;22:311–318.

8. Schneider J, Guthert H. Histiozytosis X of the hypothalamus. Zentralb Allg Pathol 1975;119:49–55.

9. Gates RB, Friesen H, Samaan NA. Inappropriate lactation and amenorrhea: Pathological and diagnostic considerations. Acta Endocrinol 1973;72:101–114.

10. Lampert IA, Catovsky D, Bergier N. Malignant histiocytosis: A clinicopathological study of 12 cases. Br J Haematol 1978;40:65–77.

11. Ma JT, Ho FC, Wang C, Lam KS, Yeung RT. Primary hypothyroidism and essential hypernatremia in a patient with histiocytosis X. Aust N Z J Med 1985;15:72–74.

12. Asai A, Matsutani M, Kohno T, Fujimaki T, Tanaka H, Kawaguchi K, et al. Leptomeningeal and orbital benign lymphophagocytic histiocytes. J Neurosurg 1988;69:610–612.

13. Tabarin A, Corcuff JB, Dautheribes M, Merlio JP, Cochet C, Maire JP, et al. Histiocytosis X of the hypothalamus. J Endocrinol Invest 1991;14:139–145.

14. Gaines P, Chan JC, Cockram CS. Histiocytosis X involving the thyroid and hypothalamus. Postgrad Med J 1991;67:680–682.

15. Catalina PF, Rodrìguez Garcìa M, de la Torre C, Pàramo C, Garcìa-Mayor RV. Diabetes insipidus for five years preceding the diagnosis of hypothalamic Langerhans cell histiocytosis. J Endocrinol Invest 1995;18:663–666.

16. Peyster RG, Hoover ED. CT of the abnormal pituitary stalk. AJNR Am J Neuroradiol 1984;5:49–52.

17. Tien RD, Newton TH, McDermott MW, Dillon WP, Kucharczyk J. Thickened pituitary stalk on MR images in patients with diabetes insipidus and Langerhans cell histiocytosis. AJNR Am J Neuroradiol 1990;11:703–708.

18. Maghnie M, Arico M, Villa A, Genovese E, Beluffi G, Severi F. MR of the hypothalamic-pituitary axis in Langerhans cell histiocytosis. AJNR Am J Neuroradiol 1992;13:1365–1371.

19. Schmitt S, Wichmann W, Martin E, Zachmann M, Schoenle EJ. Pituitary stalk thickening with diabetes insipidus preceding typical manifestations of Langerhans cell histiocytosis in children. Eur J Pediatr 1993;152:399–401.

20. O'Sullivan RM, Sheehan M, Poskitt KJ, Graeb DA, Chu AC, Joplin GF. Langerhans cell histiocytosis of hypothalamus and optic chiasm: CT and MR studies. J Comput Assisted Tomogr 1991;15:52–55.

21. Lopez P, Estes ML. Immunohistochemical characterization of the histiocytes in sinus histiocytosis with massive lymphadenopathy: Analysis of an extranodal case. Hum Pathol 1989;20:711–715.

22. Broadbent V, Dunger DB, Yeomans E, Kendall B. Anterior pituitary function and computed tomography/magnetic resonance imaging in patients with Langerhans cell histiocytosis and diabetes insipidus. Med Pediatr Oncol 1993;21:649–654.

23. Mir R, Aftalion B, Kahn LB. Sinus histiocytosis with massive lymphadenopathy and unusual extranodal manifestations. Arch Pathol Lab Med 1985;109:867–870.

24. Moscinski LC, Kleinschmidt-DeMasters BK. Primary eosinophilic granuloma of frontal lobe. Cancer 1985;9:284–288.

25. Eriksen B, Janinis J, Variakojis D, Winter J, Russel E, Marder R, et al. Primary histiocytosis X of the parieto-occipital lobe. Hum Pathol 1988;19:611–614.

26. Knobler RM, Neumann RA, Gebhart W, Radaskiewicz TH, Ferenic P, Widhalm K. Xanthoma disseminatum with progressive involvement of the central nervous and hepatobiliary systems. J Am Acad Dermatol 1990;23:341–346.

27. McKeever PE, Blaivas M. The brain, spinal cord, and meninges. In: Sternberg SS, Antonioli DA, Carter D, Mills SE, Oberman HA, eds. Diagnostic Surgical Pathology, Raven, New York, 1994, pp. 409–492.

28. Kahn HJ, Thorner PS. Monoclonal antibody MT1: A marker for Langerhans cell histiocytosis. Pediatr Pathol 1990;10:375–384.

29. Ya-You JI, Yan-Fang L, Bo-Yun W, De-Yun Y. An immunocytochemical study on the distribution of ferritin and other markers in 36 cases of malignant histiocytosis. Cancer 1989;64:1281–1289.

30. Salisbury JR, Hall PA, Williams HC, Mangi MH, Mufti GJ. Multicentric reticulohistiocytosis. Detailed immunophenotyping confirms macrophage origin. Am J Surg Pathol 1990;14:687–693.

31. Eisen RN, Buckley PJ, Rosai J. Immunophenotypic characterization of sinus histiocytosis with massive lymphadenopathy. Semin Diagn Pathol 1990;7:74–82.

32. Andreesen R, Brugger W, Sohr GW, Kross KJ. Human macrophages can express the Hodgkin's cell-associated antigen Ki-1 (CD30). Am J Pathol 1989;134:187–192.

33. Rabkin MS, Kjeldsberg CR, Wittwer CT, Marty J. A comparison study of two methods of peanut agglutinin staining with S-100 immunostaining in 29 cases of histiocytosis X (Langerhans' cell histiocytosis). Arch Pathol Lab Med 1990;114:511–515.

34. Ornvold K, Ralfkiaer E, Carstensen H. Immunohistochemical study of the abnormal cells in Langerhans cell histiocytosis (histiocytosis X). Virchows Arch 1990;416:403–410.

35. McKeever PE, Balentine JD. Histochemistry of the nervous system, In: Spicer SS, ed. Histochemistry in Pathologic Diagnosis, vol. 22, Schwartz MK, ed. Clinical and Biochemical Analysis, Marcel-Dekker, New York, 1987, pp. 871–957.

36. Carey MP, Case CP. Sinus histiocytosis with massive lymphadenopathy presenting as a meningioma. Neuropathol Appl Neurobiol 1987;13:391–398.

37. Sacchi S, Artusi T, Selleri L, Temperani P, Zucchini P, Vecchi A, et al. Sinus histiocytosis with massive lymphadenopathy: immunological, cytogenetic and molecular studies. Blut 1990;60:339–344.

37a. Nemes Z, Thomazy V. Diagnostic significance of histiocyte-related markers in malignant histiocytosis and true histiocytic lymphoma. Cancer 1988;62:1970–1980.

38. DiMaggio LA, Lippes HA, Lee RV. Histiocytosis X and pregnancy. Obstet Gynecol 1995;85:806–809.

39. Faivre J, Pecker J, Ferrand B. Posterior fossa syndrome terminating the course of histiocytosis X. Study of lesions of the central nervous system. Association with polyvinylpyrrolidone thesaurismosis. Semaine des Hôpetaux 1975;51:2229–2237.

40. Calzada LD, Chaussain JL, Job JC. Growth retardation in histiocytosis X. Evaluation of anterior pituitary function. Semaine des Hôpitaux 1978;54:1251–1256.

6.2. Lymphoma

1. Jonkhoff AR, Huijgens PC, Schreuder WO, Teule GJ, Heimans JJ. Hypophyseal non-Hodgkin's lymphoma presenting with clinical panhypopituitarism successfully treated with chemotherapy. J Neurooncol 1993;17:155,156.

2. Roggli VL, Suzuki M, Armstrong D, McGavran MH. Pituitary microadenoma and primary lymphoma of brain associated with hypothalamic invasion. Am J Clin Pathol 1979;71:724–727.

3. Patrick AW, Campbell IW, Ashworth B, Gordon A. Primary cerebral lymphoma presenting with cranial diabetes insipidus. Postgrad Med J 1989;65:771,772.

4. Peters FT, Keuning JJ, deRooy HA. Primary cerebral malignant lymphoma with endocrine defect. Case report and review of the literature. Neth J Med 1986;29:406–410.

5. Hirata K, Izaki A, Tsutsumi K, Kaminogo M, Baba H, Shibata S, et al. A case of primary hypothalamic malignant lymphoma with diabetes insipidus. No Shinkei Geka 1989;17:461–466.

6. Ashworth B. Cerebral histiocytic lymphoma presenting with loss of weight. Neurology 1982;32:894–896.

7. Anonymous. Case records of the Massachusetts General Hospital. Weekly clinicopathological exercises. Case 31-1982. A 50-year-old woman with an acute neurologic disorder and changing CT-scan findings. N Engl J Med 1982;307:359–368.

8. Hadfield MG, Vennart GP, Rosenblum WI. Hypoglycemia: Invasion of the hypothalamus by lymphosarcoma. Metastasis to blood glucose regulating centers. Arch Pathol 1972;94:317–321.

9. Shuangshoti S, Samranvej P. Hypothalamic and pancreatic lesions with diabetes mellitus. J Neurol Neurosurg Psychiatry 1975;38:1003–1007.

10. Kunze P, Hoppe W, Riedel C, Doge H. Primary malignant lymphoma of the central nervous system. Primares malignes Lymphom des Zentralnervensystems. Psychiatr Neurol Med Psychol (Leipz) 1980;32:373–381.

11. Mills SE, Fechner RE. "Undifferentiated" neoplasms of the sinonasal region: Differential diagnosis based on clinical, light microscopic, immunohistochemical, and ultrastructural features. Semin Diagn Pathol 1989;6:316–328.

12. McKeever PE, Blaivas M, Nelson JS. The diagnosis of brain and spinal tumors by conventional light microscopic methods. In: Garcia JH, Budka H, McKeever PE, Sarnat HB, Sima AAF, eds. Neuropathology: The Diagnostic Approach. Mosby-Yearbook, Philadelphia, 1997.

13. McKeever PE. Insights about brain tumors gained through immunohistochemistry and in situ hybridization of nuclear and phenotypic markers. J Histochem Cytochem 1998; 46:585–594.

14. Sano T, Kovacs K, Scheithauer BW, Rosenblum MK, Petito CK, Greco CM. Pituitary pathology in acquired immunodeficiency syndrome. Arch Pathol Lab Med 1989;113:1066–1070.

15. Karnaze MG, Sartor K, Winthrop JD, Gado MH, Hodges FJ. Suprasellar lesions: Evaluation with MR imaging? Radiology 1986;161:77–82.

16. Marx AS, Blake P, Ross M, Atlas S, Brown D. Gadolinium enhancement of the cisternal portion of the oculomotor nerve: Clinical and pathological significance. Neuroradiology 1991;33:S151.

17. Feiden W, Bise K, Steude U. Diagnosis of primary cerebral lymphoma with particular reference to CT-guided stereotactic biopsy. Virchows Arch 1990;417:21–28.

18. Hitchcock E, Morris CS. Immunocytochemical techniques in stereotactic biopsy. Stereotact Funct Neurosurg 1989;53:21–28.

19. Nakamine H, Yokote H, Itakura T, Hayashi S, Komai N, Takano Y, et al. Non-Hodgkin's lymphoma involving the brain. Diagnostic usefulness of stereotactic needle biopsy in combination with paraffin-section immunohistochemistry. Acta Neuropathol (Berlin) 1989;78:462–461.

20. Namiki TS, Nichols P, Young T, Martin SE, Chandrasoma P. Stereotaxic biopsy diagnosis of central nervous system lymphoma. Am J Clin Pathol 1988;90:40–45.

21. Murphy JK, O'Brien CJ, Ironside JW. Morphologic and immunophenotypic characterization of primary brain lymphomas using paraffin-embedded tissue. Histopathology 1989;15:449–460.

22. Nakhleh RE, Manivel JC, Hurd D, Sung JH. Central nervous system lymphomas: Immunohistochemical and clinicopathologic study of 26 autopsy cases. Arch Pathol Lab Med 1989;113:1050–1056.

23. Davey FR, Elghetany MT, Kurec AS. Immunophenotyping of hematologic neoplasms in paraffin-embedded tissue sections. Am J Clin Pathol 1990;(Suppl) S17–S26.

24. Slowik F, Jellinger K. Membranous changes in primary malignant CNS lymphomas. Acta Neuropathol 1989;79:86–93.

25. Johnson PC. Ultrastructural study of two central nervous system lymphomas. Acta Neuropathol Suppl (Berlin) 1975;6:155–160.

26. Shibata S. Sites of origin of primary intracerebral malignant lymphoma. Neurosurg 1989;25:14–19.

27. Taxy JB, Bharani NK, Mills SE, et al. The spectrum of olfactory neural tumors. A light-microscopic immunohistochemical and ultrastructural analysis. Am J Surg Pathol 1986;10:687–695.

28. Ross GW, Mills SE, Frankfurter A, et al. Immunohistochemical characterization of human olfactory neuroblastomas with multiple markers. J Neuropathol Exp Neurol 1988;47:3479 (abstract).

29. Min KW. Usefulness of electron microscopy in the diagnosis of "small" round cell tumors of the sinonasal region. Ultrastruct Pathol 1995;19:347–363.

6.3. Plasmacytoma and Multiple Myeloma

1. Bitterman P, Ariza A, Black RA, Allen WE, Lee SH. Multiple myeloma mimicking pituitary adenoma. Computerized Radiol 1986;10:201–205.

2. Ariel-Sanchez J, Rahman S, Strauss RA, Kaye GI. Multiple myeloma masquerading as a pituitary tumor. Arch Pathol 1976;101:55–56.

3. Goriachkina GP. Solitary plasmacytoma of the hypothalamus. Arkh Patol 1979;41:53–57.

4. Poon M-C, Prchal JT, Murad TM, Galbraith JG. Multiple myeloma masquerading as chromophobe adenoma. Cancer 1979;43:1513–1516.

5. Harrison LB, Schnall S, Cardinale FS, Farber LR. Multiple myeloma presenting as a pituitary tumor. Int J Radiat Oncol Biol Phys 1987;13:653–654.

6. Evans PJ, Jones MK, Hall R, Scanlon MR. Pituitary function with a solitary intrasellar plasmacytoma. Postgrad Med J 1985;61:513,514.

7. Losa M, Terreni MR, Tresoldi M, Marcatti M, Campi A, Triulzi F, et al. Solitary plasmacytoma of the sphenoid sinus involving the pituitary fossa: A case report and review of the literature. Surg Neurol 1992;37:388–393.

8. Kanoh T, Okuda T, Hayashi M, Yumoto Y. Multiple myeloma presenting as parasellar syndrome and cranial nerve palsies. Rinsho Ketsueki 1996;37:260–264.

9. Mills SE, Fechner RE. Undifferentiated neoplasms of the sinonasal region: Differential diagnosis based on clinical, light microscopic, immunohistochemical, and ultrastructural features. Semin Diagn Pathol 1989;6:316–328.

10. Fu Y-S, Perzin KH. Nonepithelial tumors of the nasal cavity, paranasal sinuses and nasopharynx. A clinicopathologic study. IX. Plasmacytomas. Cancer 1978;42:2399–2406.

11. Takahashi S, Higano S, Ishii K, Matsumoto K, Shimanuki Y, Ishibashi T, et al. CT and MR imaging findings of sphenoidal masses. Nippon Igaku Hoshasen Gakkai Zasshi 1994;54:751–760.

12. Sautner D, Saeger W, Ludecke DK. Tumors of the sellar region mimicking pituitary adenomas. Exp Clin Endocrinol 1993;101:283–289.

13. Urbanski SF, Bilbao JM, Horvath E, Kovacs K, So W, Ward JV. Intrasellar solitary plasmacytoma terminating in multiple myeloma: A report of a case including electron microscopical study. Surg Neurol 1980;14:223–236.

14. Estopinan V, Riobo P, Fernandez G, Varela C. Intrasellar plasmacytoma simulating a pituitary adenoma. Letter. Med Clin (Barc) 1987;89:128.

15. Murphy JK, O'Brien CJ, Ironside JW. Morphologic and immunophenotypic characterization of primary brain lymphomas using paraffin-embedded tissue. Histopathology 1989;15:449–460.

16. Roggli VL, Suzuki M, Armstrong D, McGavran, MH. Pituitary microadenoma and primary lymphoma of brain associated with hypothalamic invasion. Am J Clin Pathol 1979;71:724–727.

17. Kurtin PJ, Pinkus GS. Leukocyte common antigen—a diagnostic discriminant between hematopoietic and nonhematopoietic neoplasms in paraffin sections using monoclonal antibodies: Correlation with immunologic studies and ultrastructural localization. Hum Pathol 1985;16:353–365.

18. Pinkus GS, Kurtin PJ. Epithelial membrane antigen—a diagnostic discriminant in surgical pathology: Immunohistochemical profile in epithelial, mesenchymal, and hematopoietic neoplasms using paraffin sections and monoclonal antibodies. Hum Pathol 1985;16:929–940.

19. Davey FR, Elghetany MT, Kurec AS. Immunophenotyping of hematologic neoplasms in paraffin-embedded tissue sections. Am J Clin Pathol 1990;(Suppl) S17–S26.

20. Van Camp B, Durie BGM, Spier C, De Waele M, Van Riet I, Vela E, et al. Plasma cells in multiple myeloma express a natural killer cell-associated antigen: CD56 (NKH-1; Leu-19). Blood 1990;76:377–382.

21. Dehou MF, Schots R, Lacor P, Arras N, Verhavert P, Kloppel G, Van Camp B. Diagnostic and prognostic value of the MB2 monoclonal antibody in paraffin-embedded bone marrow sections of patients with multiple myeloma and monoclonal gammopathy of undetermined significance. Am J Clin Pathol 1990;94:287–291.

22. Kurabayashi H, Kubota K, Murakami H, Tamura J, Sawamura M, Nogiwa E, et al. Ultrastructure of myeloma cells in patients with common acute lymphoblastic leukemia antigen (CALLA)-positive myeloma. Cancer Res 1988;48:6234–6237.

23. Jacquet G, Vuillier J, Viennet A, Godard J, Steimle R. Solitary plasmacytoma simulating pituitary adenoma. Neurochirurgie 1991;37:67–71.

24. Guy J, Mancuso A, Beck R, Moster ML, Sedwick LA, Quisling RG, et al. Radiation-induced optic neuropathy: A magnetic resonance imaging study. J Neurosurg 1991;74:426–432.

7.1. Germinoma and Other Germ-Cell Tumors

1. Jennings MT, Gelman R, Hochberg F. Intracranial germ-cell tumors: Natural history and pathogenesis. J Neurosurg 1985;63:155–167.

2. Inoue HK, Haganuma H, Ono N. Pathobiology of intracranial germ-cell tumors: Immunochemical, immunohistochemical, and electron microscopic investigations. J Neuro Oncol 1987;5:105–115.

3. Fetell MR, Stein BM. Neuroendocrine aspects of pineal tumors. Neurol Clin 1986;4:877–905.

4. Sugiyama K, Uozumi T, Kiya K, Mukada K, Arita K, Kurisu K, et al. Intracranial germ cell tumor with synchronous lesions in the pineal and suprasellar regions: Report of six cases and review of the literature. Surg Neurol 1992;38:114–120.

5. Buchfelder M, Fahlbusch R, Walther M, Mann K. Endocrine disturbances in suprasellar germinomas. Acta Endocrinol (Copenh) 1989;120:337–342.

6. Legido A, Packer RJ, Sutton LN, D'Angio G, Rorke LB, Bruce DA, et al. Suprasellar germinomas in childhood. Cancer 1989;63:340–344.

7. Nishio S, Inamura T, Takeshita I, Fukui M, Kamikaseda K. Germ cell tumor in the hypothalamo-neurohypophysial region: Clinical features and treatment. Neurosurg Rev 1993;16:221–227.

8. Chipkevitch E. Brain tumors and anorexia nervosa syndrome. Brain Dev 1994;16:175–182.

9. Kidooka M, Okada T, Nakejima M, Handa J. Intra- and suprasellar germinoma mimicking a pituitary adenoma—case report. Neurol Med Chir (Tokyo) 1995;35:96–99.

10. Konig R, Schonberger W, Grimm W. Mediastinal teratocarcinoma and hypophyseal stalk germinoma in a patient with Klinefelter syndrome. Klin Padiatr 1990;202:53–56.

11. Sugita K, Izumi T, Yamaguchi K, Fukuyama Y, Sato A, Kajita A. Cornelia de Lange syndrome associated with a suprasellar germinoma. Brain Dev 1986;8:541–546.

12. Shuangshoti S. Combined occurrence of third ventricular germinoma and hypothalamic mixed glioma. J Surg Oncol 1986;31:148–152.

13. Sumida M, Uozumi T, Kiya K, Mukada K, Arita K, Kurisu K, et al. MRI of intracranial germ cell tumors. Neuroradiology 1995;37:32–37.

14. Karnaze MG, Sartor K, Winthrop JD, Gado MH, Hodges FJ. Suprasellar lesions: Evaluation with MR imaging? Radiology 1986;161:77–82.

15. Kollias SS, Barkovich AJ, Edwards MS. Magnetic resonance analysis of suprasellar tumors of childhood. Pediatr Neurosurg 1992;17:284–303.

16. Richmond I, Wilson CB. Parasellar tumors in children. I. Clinical presentation, preoperative assessment, and differential diagnosis. Child's Brain 1980;7:73–84.

17. Karnaze MG, Sartor K, Winthrop JD, Gado MH, Hodges FJ. Suprasellar lesions: Evaluation with MR imaging. Radiology 1986;161:77–82.

18. Shen DY, Guay AT, Silverman ML, Hybels RL, Freidberg SR. Primary intrasellar germinoma in a woman presenting with secondary amenorrhea and hyperprolactemia. 1984;15:417–420.

19. Baskin DS, Wilson CB. Transsphenoidal surgery of intrasellar germinomas. Report of two cases. J Neurosurg 1983;59:1063–1066.

20. Sumida M, Uozumi T, Yamanaka M, Mukada K, Arita K, Kurisu K, et al. Displacement of the normal pituitary gland by sellar and juxtasellar tumors: Surgical-MRI correlation and use in differential diagnosis. Neuroradiology 1994;36:372–375.

21. Fujisawa I, Asato R, Okumura R, Nakano Y, Shibata T, Hamanaka D, et al. Magnetic resonance imaging of neurohypophyseal germinomas. Cancer 1991;68:1009–1014.

22. McKeever PE, Blaivas M, Sima AAF. Neoplasms of the sellar region. In: Lloyd RV, ed. Surgical Pathology of the Pituitary Gland. Major Problems in Pathology Series. Saunders, Philadelphia, 1993, pp. 141–210.

23. Ono N, Inoue HK, Naganuma H, Kunimine H, Zama A, Tamura M. Diagnosis of germinal neoplasm in the thalamus and basal ganglia. Surg Neurol 1986;26:24–28.

24. Koide O, Iwai S, Kanno T, Kanda S. Isoenzymes of alkaline phosphatase in germinoma cells. Am J Clin Pathol 1988;89:611–616.

25. Saint-Andre JP, Alhenc-Gelas F, Rohmer V, Chretien MF, Bigorgne JC, Corvol P. Angiotensin-I-converting enzyme in germinomas. Hum Pathol 1988;19:208–213.

26. Rohmer V, Saint-Andre JP, Alhenc-Gelas F, Corval P, Vigorgne JC. Angiotensin I-converting enzyme in a suprasellar germinoma. Am J Clin Pathol 1987;87:281–284.

27. Yamagami T, Handa H, Yamashita J, Okumura T, Paine J, Haebara H, et al. An immunohistochemical study of intracranial germ cell tumours. Acta Neurochir 1987;86:33–41.

28. Harms D, Janig U. Germ cell tumours of childhood. Report of 170 cases including 59 pure and partial yolk-sac tumours. Virchows Arch 1986;409:223–239.

29. Ulbright TM, Roth LM, Brodhecker CA. Yolk sac differentiation in germ cell tumors. Am J Surg Pathol 1986;10:151–164.

30. Nakagawa Y, Perentes E, Ross GW, Ross AN, Rubinstein LJ. Immunohistochemical differences between intracranial germinomas and their gonadal equivalents. An immunoperoxidase study of germ cell tumours with epithelial membrane antigen, cytokeratin, and vimentin. J Pathol 1988;156:67–72.

31. Vaquero J, Coca S, Magallon R, Ponton P, Martinez R. Immunohistochemical study of natural killer cells in tumor-infiltrating lymphocytes of primary intracranial germinomas. J Neurosurg 1990;72:616–618.

32. Sawamura Y, Hamou MF, Kuppner MC, de Tribolet N. Immunohistochemical and in vitro functional analysis of pineal-germinoma infiltrating lymphocytes: Report of a case. Neurosurgery 1989;25:454–457.

33. Paine JT, Handa H, Yamasaki T, Yamashita J. Suprasellar germinoma with shunt metastasis: Report of a case with an immunohistochemical characterization of the lymphocyte subpopulations. Surg Neurol 1986;25:55–61.

34. Saito T, Tanaka R, Kouno M, Washiyama K, Abe S, Kumanishi T. Tumor-infiltrating lymphocytes and histocompatibility antigens in primary intracranial germinomas. J Neurosurg 1989;70:81–85.

35. Nitta T, Hishii M, Sato K, Okumura K. Immunohistochemical characterization of small, lymphoid-like cell populations within germinomas: immunologic and molecular approaches to diagnosis. Cancer Lett 1995;90:183–189.

36. Koide O, Iwai S, Matsumura H. Intranuclear membranous profiles in germinoma cells—a variant of nuclear pockets and intranuclear annulate lamellae. Acta Pathol Jpn 1985;35:605–619.

37. Hassoun J, Gambarelli D, Pellissier JF, Henin D, Toga M. Germinomas of the brain. Light and electron microscopic study. A report of seven cases. Acta Neuropathol Suppl (Berl) 1981;7:105–108.

38. Matsumura H, Setoguti T, Mori K, Ross ER, Koto A. Endothelial tubuloreticular structures in intracranial germinomas. Acta Pathol Jpn 1984;34:1–9.

39. Tabuchi K, Yamada O, Nishimoto A. The ultrastructure of pinealomas. Acta Neuropathol (Berlin) 1973;24:117–127.

40. Wick MR, Swanson PE, Manivel JC. Placental-like alkaline phosphatase reactivity in human tumors: An immunohistochemical study of 520 cases. Hum Pathol 1987;18:946–954.

41. Jennings MT, Gelman R, Hochberg F. Intracranial germ-cell tumors: Natural history and pathogenesis. J Neurosurg 1985;63:155–67.

42. Ono N, Kakegawa T, Zama A, Nakamura M, Inoue HK, Tamura M, et al. Factors affecting functional prognosis in survivors of primary central nervous system germinal tumors. Surg Neurol 1994;41:9–15.

43. Delahunt B. Suprasellar germinoma with probable extracranial metastases. Pathology 1982;14:215–218.

7.2. Teratoma

1. Russell DS, Rubinstein LJ. Pathology of Tumours of the Nervous System, 5th ed. Williams & Wilkins, Baltimore, 1989, p. 681.

2. Richmond I, Wilson CB. Parasellar tumors in children I. Clinical presentation, preoperative assessment, and differential diagnosis. Child's Brain 1980;7:73–84.

3. Lana-Peixoto MA, Pittella JE, Arouca EM. Primary intracranial tumors: Analysis of a series of consecutive autopsies and biopsies. Arquivos de Neuroi-Psiquiatria 1981;39:13–24.

4. Wilson JW, Gehweiler JA. Teratoma of the face associated with a patent canal extending into the cranial cavity (Rathke's pouch) in a three-week old child. J Pediatr Surg 1970;5:349–359.

5. Senae MO, Segall HD. CT diagnosis of an atypical nasopharyngeal teratoma in a newborn. AJNR 1987;8:710–712.

6. Tekeuchi J, Morik, Moritake K, Tani F, Waga S, Handa H. Teratomas in the suprasellar region: Report of five cases. Surg Neurol 1975;3:247–255.

7. Smirniotopoulous JG, Chiechi MV. Teratomas, dermoids, and epidermoids of the head and neck. Radiographics 1995;15(6):1437–1455.

8. Page RB, Plourde PV, Coldwell D, Heald JI, Weinstein J. Intrasellar mixed germ-cell tumor. Case report. J Neurosurg 1983;58:766–770.

9. Merchut MP, Biller J, Ghobrial M, Fine M. Adult intrasellar teratoid tumor. J Clin Neuro-Opthalmol 1986;6:175–180.

10. Jennings MT, Gelman R, Hochberg F. Intracranial germ-cell tumors: Natural history and pathogenesis. J Neurosurg 1985;63:155–167.

8.1. Paraganglioma

1. Bilbao JM, Horvath E, Kovacs K, Singer W, Hudson AR. Intrasellar paraganglioma associated with hypopituitarism. Arch Pathol Lab Med 1978;102:95–98.

2. Flint EW, Claassen D, Pang D, Hirsch WL. Intrasellar and suprasellar paraganglioma: CT and MR findings. Am J Neuroradiol 1993;14:1191–1193.

3. Steel TR, Dailey AT, Born D, Berger MS, Mayberg MR. Paragangliomas of the sellar region: Report of two cases. Neurosurgery 1993;32:844–847.

4. Ho KC, Meyer G, Garancis J, Hanna J. Chemodectoma involving the cavernous sinus and semilunar ganglion. Hum Pathol 1982;13:942–943.

5. Walker PJ, Fagan PA. Catecholamine-secreting paraganglioma of the pterygopalatine fossa: Case report. Am J Otol 1993;14:306–308.

6. Lloyd RV, Sisson JC, Shapiro B, Verhofstad AAJ. Immunohistochemical localization of epinephrine, norepinephrine, catecholamine-synthesizing enzymes, and chromogranin in neuroendocrine cells and tumors. Am J Pathol 1986;125:45–54.

7. Silverstein AM, Quint DJ, McKeever PE. Intradural paraganglioma of the thoracic spine. Am J Neuroradiol 1990;11:614–616.

8.2. Melanoma

1. Wick MR, Stanley SJ, Swanson PE. Immunohistochemical diagnosis of sinonasal melanoma, carcinoma, and neuroblastoma with monoclonal antibodies HMB-45 and anti-synaptophysin. Arch Pathol Lab Med 1988;112:616–20.

2. Scholtz CL, Siu K. Melanoma of pituitary. Case report. J Neurosurg 1976;45:101–103.

3. Kasumova SIU, Inauri GA. Melanotic tumor of the hypophysis. Vopr-Onkol 1980;26:64–66.

4. Roos B. Isolated melanoma of the pituitary. Fortschr Hals Nasen Ohrenheilkd 1965;12:193–198.

5. Shinbor T, Vyama E, Eto K, Kohrogi H, Araki S. An autopsy cases of malignant melanoma possibly originating in the sphenoid sinus. Rinsho-Shinkeigaku 1988;28:636–642.

6. Delank KW, Ballantyne AJ. Tumors of the nasal cavity occurring after hypophysectomy. Neurochirurgia (Stuttg) 1993;36:203–206.

7. Chappell PM, Kelly WM, Ercius M. Primary sellar melanoma simulating hemorrhagic pituitary adenoma: MR and pathologic findings. AJNR Am J Neuroradiol 1990;11:1054–1056.

8. Neilson JM, Moffat AD. Hypopituitarism caused by a melanoma of the pituitary gland. J Clin Pathol 1963;16:144–149.

9. Moseley RP, Davies AG, Bourne SP, Popham C, Carrel S, Monro P, et al. Neoplastic meningitis in malignant melanoma: Diagnosis with monoclonal antibodies. J Neurol Neurosurg Psychiatry 1989;52:881–886.

10. Wick MR, Stanley SJ, Swanson PE. Immunohistochemical diagnosis of sinonasal melanoma, carcinoma, and neuroblastoma with monoclonal antibodies HMB-45 and anti-synaptophysin. Arch Pathol Lab Med 1988;112:616–620.

11. Christensen E. Two cases of primary intracranial melanoma. Acta Chir Scand 1941;85:90–98.

12. Gibson JB, Burrows D, Weir WP. Primary melanoma of the meninges. J Pathol Bacteriol 1957;74:419–438.

13. McKeever PE, Blaivas M, Nelson JS. The diagnosis of brain and spinal tumors by conventional light microscopic methods. In: Garcia JH, Budka H, McKeever PE, Sarnat HB, Sima AAF, eds. Neuropathology: The Diagnostic Approach. Mosby-Yearbook, Philadelphia, 1997, pp. 31–96.

14. Moseley RP, Davies AG, Bourne SP, Popham C, Carrel S, Monro P, et al. Neoplastic meningitis in malignant melanoma: Diagnosis with monoclonal antibodies. J Neurol Neurosurg Psychiatry 1989;52:881–886.

15. Shoup SA, Johnson WW, Siegler HF, Tello JW, Schlom J, Bigner DD, et al. A panel of antibodies useful in the cytologic diagnosis of metastatic melanoma. Acta Cytol 1990;34:385–392.

16. Hayashi K, Hoshida Y, Horie Y, Takahashi K, Taguchi K, Sonobe H, et al. Immunohistochemical study on the distribution of alpha and beta subunits of S-100 protein in brain tumors. Acta Neuropathol (Berlin) 1991;81:657–663.

17. Duray PH, Ernstoff MS, Titus-Ernstoff L. Immunohistochemical phenotyping of malignant melanoma: A procedure whose time has come in pathologic practice. Pathol Annu 1990;25 (pt 2):351–377.

18. Smoller BR, Hsu A, Krueger J. HMB-45 monoclonal antibody recognizes an inducible and reversible melanocyte cytoplasmic protein. J Cutan Pathol 1991;18:315–322.

19. McKeever PE. Insights about brain tumors gained through immunohistochemistry and in situ hybridization of nuclear and phenotypic markers. J Histochem Cytohem 1998; 46:585–594.

20. Erlandson RA. Diagnostic Transmission Electron Microscopy of Human Tumors: The Interpretation of Submicroscopic Structures in Human Neoplastic Cells. Masson, New York, 1983, pp 71–79.

21. Mrak RE. Ultrastructural diagnosis of tumors of the nervous system. In: Garcia JH, Budka H, McKeever PE, Sarnat HB, Sima AAF, eds. Neuropathology: The Diagnostic Approach. Mosby-Yearbook, Philadelphia, 1997, pp. 97–192.

22. Burger PC, Scheithauer BW. Tumors of the central nervous system. In: Rosai J, Sobin LH, ed and assoc ed. Atlas of Tumor Pathology, fasc 10, 3rd ser. Armed Forces Institute of Pathology, Washington, DC, 1994, pp. 1–452.

23. McKeever PE, Spicer SS. Pituitary histochemistry. In: Spicer SS, ed. Histochemistry in Pathologic Diagnosis, vol. 22, Schwartz MK, ed. Clinical and Biochemical Analysis, Marcel-Dekker, New York, 1987, pp 603–645.

24. Cáccamo DV, Rubinstein LJ. Tumors: Applications of immunocytochemical methods. In: Garcia JH, Budka H, McKeever PE, Sarnat HB, Sima AAF, eds. Neuropathology: The Diagnostic Approach. Mosby-Yearbook, Philadelphia, 1997, pp. 193–218.

25. Moffat FL, Ketcham AS. Metastatic proclivities and patterns among APUD cell neoplasms. Semin Surg Oncol 1993;9:443–452.

24 Tumor-like Lesions of the Sellar Region

WOLFGANG SAEGER, MD

PITUITARY HYPERPLASIA

For a long time, the existence of pituitary hyperplasia which is defined as an increase in cell number was the object of controversial discussion. The main difficulty is the definition of the normal percentages of cells in the regular pituitary. The second problem is the nonuniform distribution of the different cell types. Therefore, for an exact identification of hyperplasia, the whole anterior pituitary has to be studied, serial sections should be cut, and morphometry performed. Using those methods, Trouillas et al. *(1)* found a density of adrenocorticotropic (ACTH) cells between 2.5 and 60% in the different zones. These problems refer mostly to diffuse hyperplasia (Table 1).

The difficulty in nodular hyperplasia is the differentiation from microadenoma. Whereas nodular hyperplasia shows a small focus, which is composed of nearly exclusively one cell type in a preserved area of a slightly coarsened basic structure, the microadenoma presents a widely monomorphous composition of cells in a destroyed basic structure. For identification of basic structure, special stains for reticulin fibers can be helpful. Hyperplasia can be found in 6.0% of unselected postmortem pituitaries from patients without known pituitary dysfunction (Table 2) *(2)*. Most (81%) are nodular, and some (13%) appear to be of diffuse type. ACTH cell hyperplasia is most frequent (73% of hyperplasia in postmortem pituitaries) followed by prolactin cell hyperplasia (16%) and oncocytic hyperplasia (5%), 3.8% of all pituitaries harbor strongly increased hyperplastic ACTH cells in the posterior gland (so-called basophil invasion). Pituitary hyperplasia (Table 3) is less commonly diagnosed in surgical specimens in postmortem material, because in surgical specimens, only parts of the pituitary are included and the remaining parts may contain hyperplasia. In our surgical specimens, slight hyperplasia of follicle-stimulating hormone/luteinizing hormone (FSH/LH) cells are most frequent (57%) followed by ACTH hyperplasias (35%) *(2)*.

GH CELL HYPERPLASIA Growth hormone (GH) cell hyperplasia is found in association with tumors producing growth hormone-releasing hormone (GHRH) *(3–5)*. The hyperplasia is characterized by enlarged acini, distorted pattern, and strongly increased numbers of GH cells. The electron microscope reveals a well-developed rough endoplasmic reticulum, large Golgi areas, and a dense granulation with large secretory granules in those cells

(6). GH cell hyperplasia without this rare association is uncommon (Tables 2 and 3) and mostly not interpretable. A very rare case of a child with acromegalic gigantism owing to diffuse hyperplasia of mammosomatotrophs without GHRH-producing tumor was described *(7)*.

PROLACTIN CELL HYPERPLASIA Hyperplasia of prolactin cells is a frequent finding in postmortem pituitaries (Table 2) *(2)* and is often coincidental with adenomas of the same, but also of other types *(8)*. They can also develop in cases with lesions or distortions of the pituitary stalk by defects in the transport of pituitary-inhibiting factors, which lead to a reduced inhibition of the prolactin cells and result in a hyperstimulatory hyperplasia of prolactin cells. In our material, this was found (Table 3) in some pituitaries harboring adenomas (Figure 1) or craniopharyngiomas with suprasellar growth. They were also often found adjacent to active prolactin-secreting adenomas in surgical specimens *(9)*, whereas in other series *(10)*, these hyperplasia were not as frequent. Prolactin cell hyperplasia can mimic a prolactin cell adenoma clinically *(11,12)*. In one of these cases, a transition of hyperplasia into an adenoma was demonstrable *(12)*.

Transgenic female mice overexpressing galanin in the pituitary develop prolactin cell hyperplasia and hyperprolactinemia *(13)*. Whereas prolactin cell hyperplasia develops in rodents after treatment with estrogens, there is no evidence for the occurrence of hyperplasia after estrogen medication in humans. During pregnancy and lactation the number of prolactin cells increases greatly, resulting in a weight increase of the pituitary by 100%. Since the GH cell number decreases under these circumstances, it was assumed that GH cells can transform into mammosomatotrophs and into prolactin cells, or that the progenitor cell develops mostly into prolactin cells and less into GH cells *(14)*.

The hyperplastic prolactin cells in pregnancy show a well-developed rough endoplasmic reticulum (Figure 2), decreased granulation, and increased elongated cytoplasma *(15)* referred to as pregnancy cells.

ACTH CELL HYPERPLASIA ACTH cell hyperplasia may be diffuse (25%), nodular (15%), or dispersed (60%) *(2)* (Table 2). Nodular and dispersed types present a coarsened basic structure with increased size of acini (Figures 3 and 4). The single ACTH cells may be of normal size or slightly increased in size. By ultrastructural examination, the ACTH cells are ovoid to angular, and face the capillaries. The relatively electron-opaque cytoplasm contains a well-developed Golgi complex, moderately demonstrable rough endoplasmic reticulum, and usually numerous spherical or oval secretory granules measuring 200–400 nm. Type I

From: *Diagnosis and Management of Pituitary Tumors* (K. Thapar, K. Kovacs, B. W. Scheithauer, and R. V. Lloyd, eds.), ©Humana Press Inc., Totowa, NJ.

Table 1
Types of Hyperplasia

Term	Definition
Diffuse hyperplasia	Diffusely increased number of one pituitary cell type
Nodular hyperplasia	Small nodule composed nearly exclusively of one pituitary cell type; alveolar basic structure may be distorted
Dispersed hyperplasia	Several nodules of one cell type
Absolute hyperplasia	Increased number of one cell type without decrease of other cell types
Relative hyperplasia	Increased number of one cell type and simultaneous decrease of other cell types
Primary hyperplasia	Development without regulatory disturbance
Secondary hyperplasia	Development from regulatory hyperstimulation

cytokeratin filaments are present in the paranuclear region, where lysosomal vacuoles are also demonstrable, the so-called enigmatic bodies (15). Crooke's cells with typical hyaline changes and paranuclear vacuoles are developed only in those patients who are hypercortisolemic (16). Therefore, some conclusions can be drawn from the presence of Crooke's cells. If they can be found, a hypercortisolism must exist. If they are lacking, a significant hypercortisolism can be excluded (17). Most ACTH cell hyperplasia found in surgical or postmortem specimens do not correlate to any dysfunction, but in cases with arterial hypertension, they appear to be more frequent (18). Adjacent to clinically nonactive ACTH cell adenomas, they developed in about 10% of cases, but also in other adenoma types, ACTH cell hyperplasia can be found in up to 15% of cases (Table 2). In the para-adenomous pituitary with active ACTH adenomas in Cushing's disease, they have been found in up to 50% of cases (10) (Figure 4). Since transformations of those hyperplasia into adenomas are demonstrable in a number of cases (19,20), we can conclude that ACTH cell hyperplasia in Cushing's disease may be an early stage of an ACTH cell adenoma. That does not mean that adenomas usually arise as a downstream consequence of excess trophic influences from the hypothalamus. They may also arise as a result of an intrinsic pituitary defect (16). Patients with CRH-producing tumors can develop endocrine active hyperplasia inducing Cushing's disease (21,22). These tumors can be located in various organs (23,24). They stimulate the ACTH cell system chronically and induce hyperplasia. Corticotropin-releasing hormone- (CRH) producing gangliocytomas in the sellar region are very rare (25,26). ACTH cell hyperplasia can transform into ACTH cell adenomas in rare cases as reported previously (2). ACTH cell hyperplasia as the cause of pituitary Cushing's disease is very rare (27–30) and can be diagnosed only in those cases in which an ACTH cell adenoma cannot be demonstrated. Since those adenomas can be extremely small, its demonstration may be very difficult, time-consuming, and expensive. An apparently unique case, an ACTH cell hyperplasia with Cushing's disease adjacent to a Crooke's cell adenoma, was previously described (31). Since the latter presumably cannot be the source of hyperfunction, the hyperplasia had to have been hyperfunctional.

In cases with primarily untreated Addison's disease, the ACTH cells develop diffuse and nodular hyperplasia, and increase in size forming so-called Crooke-Russel's cells, which show decreased numbers of enigmatic bodies and of secretory granules and enlarged euchromatic nuclei. Such ACTH cell hyperplasia may transform into tumorlets, and also into ACTH cell microadenomas (32).

In the intermedia zone of autopsy pituitaries ACTH cell hyperplasia occur in 29% of men and in 14% of women (33). The corticotrophs of the neurohypophysis, the so-called basophil invasion, are increased in number in 13% of postmortem pituitaries (17). In most cases, they are coincidental with adenohypophyseal hyperplasia of the corticotrophs. Two-thirds of these patients suffered from arterial hypertension (17). Irrespectively of hypertension, the degree of migration of ACTH cells increases with patient age and is more common in men than in women (34).

TSH CELL HYPERPLASIA Thyroid-stimulating hormone (TSH) cell hyperplasia is mainly diffuse and less frequent nodular or dispersed. The TSH cells are mostly enlarged. The immunoreactivity for TSH may be strongly indicative of a high storage of TSH or may be weakly suggestive of a minimal storage of the hormone. TSH cell hyperplasia can be accompanied by prolactin cell hyperplasia and lead to an increase in size and weight of the pituitary (35). Stimulated TSH cells are enlarged and characterized by a vacuolated slightly PAS-positive cytoplasm, which may also harbor large strongly PAS-positive globules. They are called thyroidectomy cells. In the electron microscope (15), the rough endoplasmic reticulum is strongly increased and dilated as being responsible for light microscopical vacuolation. The Golgi complexes are also enlarged. The secretory granules vary in size and number. Hyperplasia is induced by chronic hyperstimulation owing to hypothyroidism (36) or TSH-stimulating drugs and hormones (37).

In long-standing primary hypothyroidism, diffuse and nodular TSH cell hyperplasia was found in 69 and 25% of pituitaries, in 12% of glands in the intermediate stages between nodular hyperplasia and the development of microadenoma, and in 8% thyrotropic adenomas demonstrable (36).

GONADOTROPH CELL HYPERPLASIA The frequency of hyperplasia of gonadotroph cells is controversial in the literature. Whereas Lloyd (38) did not find it in surgically resected pituitaries, our material reveals a slight, but significant diffuse hyperplasia of FSH and /or LH cells in many patients with metastasizing cancers of the breast or prostate who were palliatively treated by total hypophysectomy (39). Hyperplastic gonadotroph cells are mostly also hyperstimulated showing a slight increase in size, densely arranged vacuoles, and variably diminished granules in the cytoplasm. These cells have been called castration cells or gonadectomy cells. Electron microscopically (15,39), the vacuoles are formed by strongly dilated rough endoplasmic reticulum. The Golgi apparatus is enlarged, and the number of secretory granules decreased.

The cause of gonadotroph hyperplasia is a chronic hypogonadism, which may be primary or secondary from gonadectomy. Chronic therapy with gonadotropins stimulating drugs (37) may also lead to gonadotroph cell hyperplasia. Transition of gonadotroph cells hyperplasia into an adenoma has not been observed to date.

INFLAMMATORY LESIONS

Pituitary inflammation is comprised of a number of inflammatory processes that are totally different in their etiology, pathogenesis, and structure. All can enlarge the pituitary or form local

Table 2
Types of Hyperplasias in Postmortem Pituitaries[a]

Cell type	Diffuse hyperplasia	Nodular hyperplasia	Dispersed hyperplasia	Total	Coincidental with adenoma of same cell type	Coincidental with adenoma of other cell type
GH cell	1			1		
Prolactin cell	2	13	1	16	5	2
ACTH cell	18	11	43	72	10	11
TSH cell	2			2		
FSH/LH cell			1	1		
Null cell		2		2	1	
Oncocyte	1	3	1	5		
Total	24	29	46	99		

[a]Author's unpublished data.

Table 3
Types of Hyperplasia in Surgical Specimens[a]

Cell type	Without adenoma	With adenoma of same cell type	With adenoma of other cell type	With other tumor
GH cell	2	1	0	0
Prolactin cell	5	1	4	1 Craniopharyngioma
ACTH cell	28	2	1	2 Carcinoids of bronchus
TSH cell	0	0	0	0
FSH/LH cell	46	0	0	0
Total	81	4	5	3

[a]Author's unpublished data.

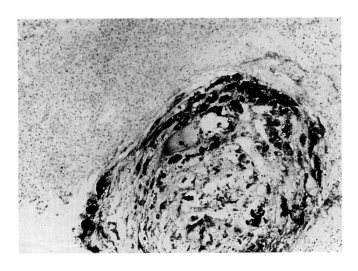

Figure 24-1 Prolactin cell hyperplasia adjacent to a densely granulated GH cell adenoma (above and left). Antiprolactin, hematoxylin, ×110.

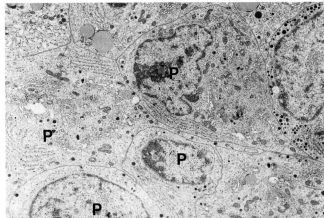

Figure 24-2 Prolactin cell hyperplasia adjacent to a sparsely granulated GH cell adenoma: prolactin cells (P) with sparse secretory granules and slightly increased rough endoplasmic reticulum. Uranyl–acetate–lead citrate, ×6100.

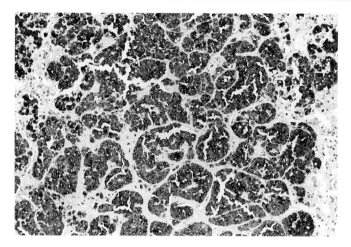

Figure 24-3 ACTH cell hyperplasia in postmortem pituitary without known endocrinopathy. Anti-ACTH hematoxylin, ×125.

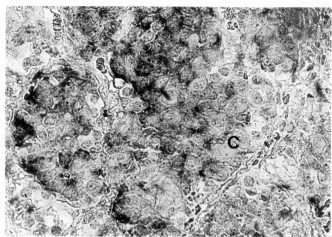

Figure 24-4 Nodular ACTH cell hyperplasia intermingled with Crooke's cells (C) adjacent to an ACTH cell adenoma in Cushing's disease. ISH for POMC mRNA-digoxigenin, ×450.

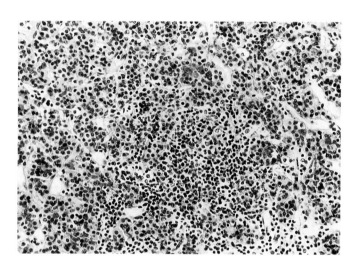

Figure 24-5 Lymphocytic hypophysitis: infiltration with lymphocytes in the connective tissue and partly in the acini of the anterior lobe. PAS-reaction hematoxylin, ×225.

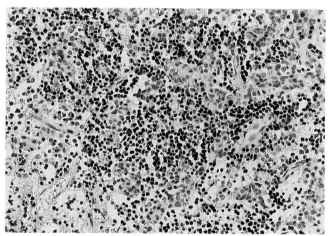

Figure 24-6 Lymphocytic hypophysitis: dense inflammation with T-lymphocytes in the anterior lobe. Anti-CD 43-hematoxylin, ×225.

tumor-like lesions involving surrounding tissues. Three types of inflammation are autochthonous pituitary diseases: lymphocytic hypophysitis, the granulomatous hypophysitis, the xanthomatous hypophysitis and secondary hypophysitis.

LYMPHOCYTIC HYPOPHYSITIS The interstitial tissue of the adenohypophysis is more or less densely infiltrated by lymphocytes (Figures 5 and 6). The more lymphocytes that are present, the more parenchymal acini are involved by the inflammation. Necrosis of hormone-producing cells correlates with the severity of the process.

The lympocytes are mostly accompanied by plasmacytes. They are mainly T-lymphocytes expressing T-markers by immunohistology (40) (Figure 6). Often the intermediate zone is densely infiltrated, and the posterior lobe may also be involved (41). The pituitary is often strongly diffusely enlarged showing suprasellar expression so that some patients have been operated on with the clinical diagnosis of the pituitary tumor. In the differential diagnosis, focal accumulations of lymphocytes mostly in the intermedi-

ate zone have to be considered in cases that are suspicious for hypophysitis (Figure 7). Those foci are found in about 7% of all postmortem pituitaries (40) and do not have any biological significance. The etiology of lymphocytic hypophysitis is apparently autoimmunopathic, since many of the patients suffer from other immunopathies (thyroiditis, autoimmune gastritis) (41), or it develops during pregnancy or after delivery (42).

Whereas case reports from former decades comprised nearly exclusively females, there is an increasing number of men with lymphocytic hypophysitis presenting mostly with symptoms of a pituitary tumor (40,43,44) or of hypopituitarism (40,41).

IDIOPATHIC GRANULOMATOUS HYPOPHYSITIS We differentiate the idiopathic granulomatous hypophysitis (40,45–47) from the granulomatous hypophysitis secondary to a generalized granulomatosis in Boeck's disease or tuberculosis. The granulomas are composed of epithelioid cells, multinucleated giant cells, and some follicular stellate cells (Figure 8). They are accompanied by lymphocytes, mainly of T-type, and by fibrosis of mostly

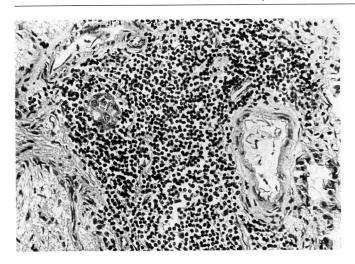

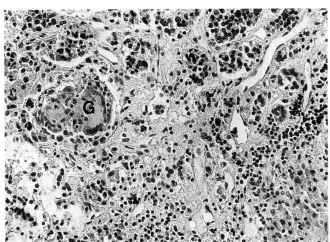

Figure 24-7 Focal accumulation of lymphocytes in the intermediate lobe in normal postmortem pituitary. Hematoxylin-eosin, ×270.

Figure 24-8 Granulomatous hypophysitis: granuloma with giant cells (G), fibrosis of stroma and lymphocytic infiltrates. Hematoxylin-eosin, ×270.

low extension. The granulomatous inflammation destroys the pituitary acini. The giant cells can contain needle-shaped anisotropic cytoplasmic inclusions positive for prolactin, but most cases are free of demonstrable inclusions *(40,45)*.

Granulomatous hypophysitis enlarges the pituitary and gives the impression of tumorous growth. The etiology is unknown. The diagnosis can be made with certainty only in those patients who are definitively free of a generalized granulomatosis *(40)*. Otherwise the possibility of a secondary involvement of the pituitary cannot be excluded.

XANTHOMATOUS HYPOPHYSITIS   Xanthomatous hypophysitis is characterized by infiltration of the anterior lobe by foamy histiocytes, granulation tissue, and cellular debris *(48,49)*. The histiocytes express CD68 *(48)* and in one study *(49)* also S100-Protein and CD1a. The etiology of this inflammation is unknown.

SECONDARY HYPOPHYSITIS   In the neighborhood of craniopharyngiomas, the anterior pituitary can show granulation tissue, fibroses, and inflammatory lymphocytic infiltrates of B- and T-type *(40,50)*. The composition of hormone-producing cells is regular. The basic structure is focally loosened. This inflammation is strongly localized and does not extend to the whole gland. It can be found in about 10% of surgically removed craniopharyngiomas *(50)*, but the incidence is probably higher. Most specimens of craniopharyngioma contain no surrounding tissue or only a very small rim besides the tumor, so that the real incidence remains obscure. The authors *(50)* call it secondary hypophysitis, because it develops only adjacent to tumorous lesion. This inflammation itself does not clinically appear as a tumor, but can simulate a greater tumor mass, since it is represented by the tumor itself.

SARCOIDOSIS   Sarcoidosis as a multisystemic granulomatous tissue disease affecting many organs. Clinical signs of involvement of the central nervous system are found in about 5% of all patients with sarcoidosis. Symptoms of a hypothalamic–pituitary disease are present in <1% *(51,52)*.

Neurosarcoidosis affects mainly the leptomeninges of the brain base and posterior fossa, but also the parenchyma of the infundibulum and the floor of the third ventricle as well as the optic nerves. Fifty percent of cases with neurosarcoidosis involve the hypo-

thalamus leading to hypothalamic dysfunctions in less than each second cases *(51)*. Adenohypophysial dysfunction and diabetes insipidus are somewhat uncommon in these patients. The sarcoidosis appears to develop downward from the hypothalamus to the infundibulum, the pituitary stalk, and the neurohypophysis. The anterior pituitary is least affected, but in some cases it may be extensively involved.

Microscopically the characteristic features are noncaseating granulomas with multinucleated giant cells, which may contain Schaumann bodies. They are surrounded by lymphocytes and fibroses. With increasing duration of the disease, granulomas and infiltration diminish, whereas fibrosis and calcifications increase *(51)*.

The definitive diagnosis of sarcoidosis requires biopsy, but histology of the pituitary cannot differentiate between idiopathic granulomatous hypophysitis and involvement by generalized sarcoidosis.

LANGERHANS' HISTIOCYTOSIS   The etiology of Langerhans' histiocytosis, also called histiocytosis X, comprising the eosinopilic granuloma, Hand-Schüller-Christian disease, and Abt-Letterer-Sive disease, was unclear for many decades. Nowadays it is thought to be a proliferation of the mononuclear phagocytic system.

About 25% of patients with Langerhans' histiocytosis present with involvement of the nervous system *(51)*. Lesions are found in the hypothalamus and the pituitary stalk, but not in the anterior pituitary.

Clinically, the lesions appear as mostly suprasellar tumors, but also can present as slight enlargement of the pituitary gland with bowing of the diaphragma *(53)*. Microscopically, histiocytes with foamy cytoplasm, nonvacuolated histiocytes, eosinophilic granulocytes, multinucleated giant cells, lymphocytes, plasmacytes, and glial cells in a predominantly perivascular arrangement are found.

Capillaries are increased showing enlarged plump endothelial cells. The typical histiocytes called Langerhans' cells contain folded nuclei. Ultrastructurally, Birbeck granules may be present. They are composed of short double membranes. Langerhans' histiocytes are immunoreactive for S-100-protein. Patients suffer most often from diabetes insipidus and less frequently from hypo-

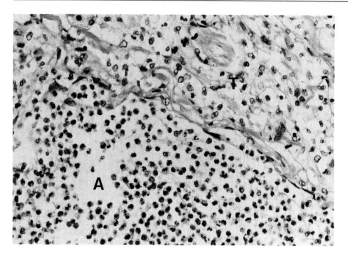

Figure 24-9 Septic abscess in the anterior lobe: focal necrosis and densely arranged granulocytes (A) surrounded by granulation tissue (T). Hematoxylin-eosin, ×270.

thalamic dysfunctions, including obesity, hypogonadism, and growth retardation.

INFECTIONS

ABSCESS Pituitary abscesses develop from sepsis, as a result of septic embolism, or as secondary extension from an adjacent suppurative process (meningitis, sinusitis, thrombophlebitis of the cavernous sinus). Microabscesses in the neurohypophysis are not rare autopsy findings in septic patients, representing a clinically insignificant preterminal complication *(51)*. β-Hemolytic streptococcus, pneumococcus, and listeria have been identified as etiologic agents. Pituitary abscesses simulate pituitary tumors or meningitis. In chronic abscesses, hypopituitarism may develop.

Abscesses can originate in cysts *(54)*, craniopharyngioma *(50)*, or adenomas *(55)*. In these cases, necroses in the lesions and its bacterial infection are the basis of abscess development. Microscopically, the typical structures of an abscess are found: the necrosis is densely infiltrated by granulocytes and surrounded by granulation tissue, which extends into the pituitary parenchyma (Figure 9).

OTHER BACTERIAL GRANULOMATOSES In the tertiary stage of syphilis, gumma formation can be found in the sella region *(56)*, but nowadays this is extremely rare, whereas in decades before antibiotic therapy, it was somewhat common. Gummas with central necroses, surrounding granulation tissue, giant cells, and accompanying lymphocytes are present as active signs of inflammation. They can transform into scars with fibrous defects of the pituitary *(57)*. Both lobes can be involved. In cases with lesions of the neurohypophysis, diabetes insipidus was found *(56)*. In those cases, the syphilitic nature of the process may remain obscure.

Actinomycosis principally caused by *Actinomyces israeli* is a common saprophyte in the tonsils and mouth, but may become pathogenic. It develops in damaged or hypoxic tissues and forms fistulas filled with pus. Microscopically, actinomyces is identified by radiated colonies of granules and filaments being PAS- and Gram-positive *(58)*. Fistulas can extend from the mouth or tonsils to the meninges and the sella, and mimic a space-occupying lesion *(57)*.

TUBERCULOMA Pituitary tuberculomas appearing as isolated manifestations of the disease are rare. Clinically, they can mimic pituitary adenomas *(59–62)*. Microscopically they show a typical granulomatous inflammatory process with giant cells of Langhans' type, epithelioid histiocytes, fibroses in the periphery, and caseation necroses in the center. Acid-fast bacilli were rarely found. The adenohypophysis can be destroyed locally.

Hypophysial tuberculomas are secondary to hematogenous dissemination mostly from the lung. The differential diagnosis includes idiopathic granulomatous hypophysitis and generalized Boeck's disease. In doubtful cases regarding the diagnosis is of tuberculosis, modern methods of molecular biology (restriction enzyme analyses) should be used *(63)*.

FUNGAL AND PARASITIC INFECTIONS With the increasing spread of acquired immunodeficiency syndrome (AIDS), fungal and parasitic infections are being found *(64–66)* (Table 4) with increasing frequency in the pituitary that have not been observed before AIDS was established. Large abscesses or tumor-like lesions are very rare in AIDS. A large pituitary necrosis owing to toxoplasmosis followed by panhypopituitarism was published as a case report *(67)*.

PARASITOSES Parasitoses in the sella or pituitary appear very rarely, but can look clinically like a tumor, so clinicians and pathologists should be aware of the possibility of parasitosis in the sellar region. More often *(68)*, the basal cisterns and the subarachnoidal space or the meninges are involved in cerebral parasitoses. Therefore, theoretically an amoebiasis can develop an abscess with throphozoites or granulomas in the suprasellar region. Cysticercosis can show calcified cysts and fibroses in the basal cisterns. Strongyloidiasis may present larvae, necroses, and abscesses in the subarachnoidals space. Aspergillus, blastomyces, or chromoblastomycosis can show abscesses in the meninges. Histoplasmosis leads to necroses and granulomas in the meninges. Nocardiosis produces abscesses and rarely granulomas in the meninges. Zygomycosis can involve the sphenoid sinus and the sellar bone with inflammatory reactions around blood vessels and extensive necroses *(69)*.

Pathologists should try to identify the parasites within the lesions using special stainings (methenamine silver, PAS, Giemsa, immunostainings for some organisms). Infectious organisms usually reach the sellar region by the hematogenous route, mostly by the arterial system or more rarely the valveless venous plexus *(68)*.

MUCOCELES Increased pressure within the sphenoidal sinus owing to a blocking of the ostium secondary to inflammation, trauma, or tumor results in a mucocele. It is defined as a propulsion through a defect in the bony wall of the sinus into the intracranial area. The cavity contains thickened mucus. The wall is composed of flattened respiratory epithelium, fibrous tissue, and surrounding compressed tissue (brain, bone, pituitary) *(70,71)*. The bone reacts with increased trabecula formation and fibroses of its marrow. The propulsion into the sellar region can clinically mimic a cystic tumour *(72)*. Morphological identification of a mucocele should not be very difficult.

Clinically, sphenoid mucoceles usually develop over a long period with nonspecific headaches and late onset of visual loss, but with very rare exceptions, unlike in pituitary adenomas, a typical bitemporal hemianopsia or pituitary insufficiency is not present *(73)*.

CYSTIC LESIONS

Various cystic lesions can be present in the sellar region (Table 5). Because their proliferative activity is different, exact morphological identification is necessary.

Table 4
Pathology of the Pituitary in AIDS

Authors	Number of autopsies with AIDS	Infections with					
		Necroses %	Cytomegaly virus %	Cryptococcus %	Toxoplasma %	Pneumocystis carinii %	Mycobacterium tuberculosis %
Ferreiro and Vinters (64)	88	11%	3%	1%			
Groll et al. (65)	109	8%	6%	2%	1%		
Klatt et al. (66)	565		1%	2%	0.4%	0.4%	0.2%

Table 5
Cystic Lesions of the Sellar Region (75,76,77,78)

Type	Location	Histological features	Immunostaining
Rathke's cleft cyst	Intrasellar between anterior and posterior pituitary; suprasellar	Predominantly columnar epithelial lining with variable degrees of ciliation and goblet cells	Cytokeratin, vimentin, GFAP (74,79,80)
Epidermoid cyst	Parasellar; suprasellar	Lined by squamous epithelium with a linear keratohyaline granule layer, flattened linear sheaves of keratin	Keratins of low molecular weight in the basal cell layer, of high molecular weight in the spinocellular layer
Dermoid cyst	Suprasellar; parasellar	Lined by keratinized squamous epithelium; skin adnexa demonstrable in the cyst wall	Like epidermoid cyst
Arachnoidal cyst	Suprasellar	Lined by flattened arachnoid cells and collagen; rarely chronic inflammatory cells	Fibronectin, laminin, collagen type 4, procollagen type 3 (81,82,83), neural cell adhesion molecule (84)
Empty sella	Intrasellar	Lined by collagenous connective tissue; flattened arachnoid cells may be present	Like arachnoidal cyst
Craniopharyngioma	Suprasellar; intrasellar	Adamantinomatous or squamous epithelium with an irregular keratohyalin granule layer partially invading surrounding parenchyma, granulation tissue	Keratins of high molecular weight mainly in the squamous prickle cells; keratins of low molecular weight mainly in the peripherally palisading cells; occasionally, estrogen-receptor (78); leukemia inhibitory factor (85)
Cystic pituitary adenoma	Intrasellar; suprasellar; parasellar	Strands of adenoma cells, granulation tissue, necroses, edema, siderin deposits	Pituitary hormones, neuron-specific enolase, synaptophysin

RATHKE'S CLEFT CYSTS   Although Rathke's pouch closes in early embryonic life, its apical extremity persists until postnatal life, forming a cleft between the anterior and the posterior pituitary. It is lined by cuboidal or columnar epithelium, but ciliated cells and goblet cells may also be present (Table 5). They express cytokeratin (74).

These pouch remnants can develop cysts of different sizes and be localized partially or entirely in the suprasellar region. The wall of the cysts contains fibrovascular connective tissue and a single layer of cuboidal or columnar epithelium, or may have ciliated cells with microvilli or goblet cells with mucin (75) (Figure 10). Squamous cells with tonofilaments can also be developed. Cytokeratins, vimentin, and glial fibrillary acidic protein (GFAP) are often coexpressed (79,80). The cavity contains a serous fluid or, rarely, a mucoid substance (86). It can be combined with lymphocytic adenohypophysitis (87) or clinically appear as a noncystic hypothalamic mass (87).

ARACHNOID CYSTS   Arachnoid cysts are localized in the sylvian fissure or in the cerebello-pontine angle. The suprasellar region (88) and the clivus are rare (<3%) localizations of this type of cyst (89) (Table 5). They can be regarded as a developmental

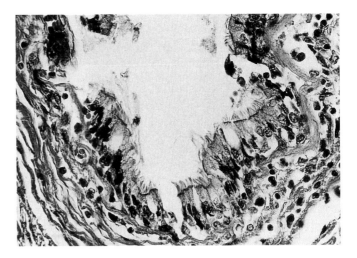

Figure 24-10   Rathke's cyst in the intermediate lobe with ciliated columnar cells. Hematoxylin-eosin, ×340.

abnormality of the arachnoid. The cyst wall is lined by a vascular collagenous membrane and flattened syncytial arachnoid cells. Immunohistological , they express fibronectin, laminin, collagen type IV, and procollagen type III *(81–83)*. Arachnoid cells are interrupted by discrete groups of similar cells on the inner side of the membrane. Electron microscopic studies show *(89)* that the cysts are formed by splittings of the arachnoid membrane, which are compensated for by thick layers of collagen. The cysts are totally separated from the inner layer of the dura mater *(90)*. They are filled with colorless fluid, which can be rich in protein and xanthochrome. The surrounding collagen may show iron pigment-containing macrophages and rare chronic inflammatory cells. Very rarely arachnoidal cysts can be localized in the sella and clinically give the impression of an empty sella *(91)*. The cysts may be clinically silent and be discovered as incidental findings or may present as space-occupying lesions *(78)*.

EMPTY SELLA SYNDROME   A reduction in the volume of the contents of the sella leads to the empty sella syndrome, which may be primary or secondary. The primary type is characterized by a rudimentary development or a total aplasia of the diaphragma sellae. Through this widely open connection, the pressure of the cerebrospinal fluid compresses the pituitary gland to the sphenoid bone. The hypophysial fossa is enlarged and mostly filled with cerebrospinal fluid, whereas the pituitary gland is compressed and flattened at the bottom of the hypophysial fossa. Evident structural alterations of the compressed pituitary parenchyma were not found. Immunohistological studies revealed all pituitary cell types *(92)*. Maldevelopments of the diaphragma are not rare. Autopsy studies demonstrated a fully developed diaphragma in 42% of adults, a medium-sized diaphragma (not more than 3 mm) with a broad peripheral ring in 38%, and a very small ring in 20% *(93)*. Although the diaphragm is nearly lacking in these 20% of adults, autopsy studies have shown that a primary empty sella developed only in 5% of adults *(94)*.

A secondary empty sella syndrome can develop after surgical hypophysectomy, infarction, and necroses of the pituitary or its adenomas *(95)* if the pituitary is resected or shrunken and the remaining "empty" sella filled with cerebrospinal fluid.

Clinically the empty sella syndrome has to be differentiated from cysts and cystic tumors (Table 5). Fifteen percent of the patients show a mild hyperprolactinemia *(96)*. The development of hypopituitarism appears to be related to the degree of sellar enlargement *(97)*. In children and adolescents, an empty sella was demonstrated in 8.8% of patients with isolated GH deficiency, in 34.9% of patients with multiple deficiency, in 5.9% of patients with hypogonadotropic hypogonadism, and in 40.0% of patients with an idiopathic delayed puberty *(97)*. On the other hand, an empty sella can also be found in cases with hyperpituitarism owing to coexisting hypersecreting pituitary adenomas *(73,98)*.

OTHER CYSTIC LESIONS   For craniopharyngeomas *see* Chapter 23, for cystic adenomas *see* Chapter 7, for epidermoid/dermoid cyst *see* Chapter 23.

VASCULAR LESIONS

Suprasellar or intrasellar aneurysms of the carotid arteries or suprasellar aneurysms of the anterior and posterior communicating arteries can clinically resemble expanding pituitary tumors (Figure 11). Owing to compression of adjacent structures, visual defects can develop in cases with suprasellar aneurysms *(99)*. The sellar bone may be asymmetrically destroyed *(73)*. Aneurysms can deeply indent the third ventricle and produce abnormalities of

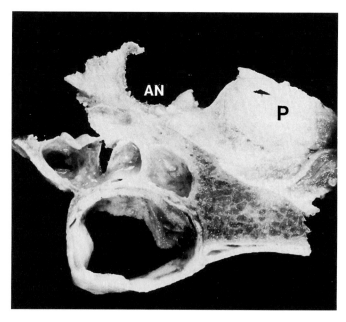

Figure 24-11   Aneurysm of the carotid artery (AN) beside the pituitary (P).

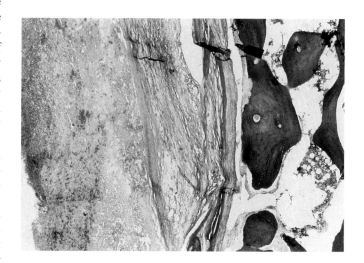

Figure 24-12   Aneuryms of the carotid artery (right) with granulation tissue adjacent to sellar bone (left). van Gieson, ×100.

pituitary function either by compressing its stalk or vasculature *(51)*. Intrasellar aneuryms may induce a hypopituitarism *(73)*.

Histologically, typical degenerative sclerotic changes of the arterial wall are usually found, but also chronic inflammatory alterations may be present (Figure 12).

Aneurysms may be demonstrable in conjunction with pituitary adenomas *(73,100)*, but causal correlations do not appear to exist. Complications of aneurysms can be bleeding into the sella or chiasmatic cisterns, and the development of arteriovenous fistulas in the cavernous sinus *(101)*.

MISCELLANEOUS

CHORISTOMA, HAMARTOMA, GANGLIOCYTOMA, AND GANGLIOGLIOMA   A choristoma is defined as a tumor-like proliferation or growth of heterotopic tissue *(102)*. Hamartomas are defined as tumor-like masses comprising an excess of tissues, which are normal to the site of occurrence. Gangliocytomas are composed of mature tumorous neuronal elements. The former term "ganglioneuroma" was used for the same entity (103). A ganglioglioma has to be diagnosed if the tumor contains tumorous neuronal and glial elements (103). Pituitary choristomas are mostly very small tumors arising in the neurohypophysis, probably from its pituicytes (104). For small foci of these cells, the term "tumorettes" also is used. These tumorettes are found in 1–2% of unselected autopsy material (104). They are localized in the posterior lobe or the lower part of the pituitary stalk. Larger tumors of these kind are uncommon. They correspond to granular cell tumors or granular cell myoblastomas, which develop in other organs from Schwann cells. They show a sharp demarcation and loose to more dense arrangements of relatively large cells with excentric nuclei and granular PAS-positive cytoplasm. They can be immunostained for S100 protein, NSE, and Leu-7 (77). The term "neuronal choristoma" or "neuronal hamartomas" (77) was used for tumors that are composed of mature neurons and occasional glial constituents. Since these glial components are thought to be not tumorous, but reactive astrocytes only (25,26), the terms "neuronal choristoma" and "neuronal hamartoma" should be replaced by "gangliocytoma". The genuine hamartoma of the sellar region is a congenital tumerous mass arising in the hypothalamus and containing neuronal, glial, and occasionally ependymal cell elements. Variations include lipoma, osteolipoma, and tuberous sclerosis (105), but these three tumors have to be designated as teratomas owing to the content of noncerebral tissues.

Sixty-five percent of sellar gangliocytomas are associated with a pituitary adenoma (25). Seventy-four percent of patients with these tumors suffer from hormonal oversecretion from the pituitary, mostly from acromegaly.

Gangliocytomas are localized mostly in the sella and are radiologically indistinguishable from ordinary pituitary adenomas. If gangliocytomas are combined with pituitary adenomas, the gangliocytomas often are found as a spherical mass sitting centrally on the adenoma. Histologically gangliocytomas are characterized by ganglionic cells of variable size and shape. The nuclei are large and the nucleoli prominent. Binucleate cells are often present. The cytoplasm is variably broad, acidophilic, and partly elongated. With silver staining, an extensive network of nerve axons becomes apparent (106).

Immunohistochemistry reveals expression of neuronal markers as synaptophysin, neuron-specific enolase (NSE), or neurofilament protein. GHRH is demonstrable in cases with acromegaly and some of the very rare cases with inactive gangliocytomas. CRH is demonstrable in most of the rare gangliocytomas associated with Cushing's disease (Figure 13) and in very few gangliocytomas with acromegaly. Somatotropin release-inhibiting hormone (SRIH) is present in about two-thirds of gangliocytomas (25).

Single cases have been positive for glucagon, vasoactive intestinal polypeptide (VIP), bombesin, and gastrin (25). In some tumors, glial cells expressing S100 protein or GFAP have been demonstrable (25,26). They represent reactive cells and are found not to be tumorous (26). Therefore, the term "ganglioglioma" is not justified for these tumors.

Electron microscopic studies show (Figure 14) well-developed microvesicles, sparse, small- to medium-sized and partly oval secretory granules, sparse rough endoplasmic reticulum, numerous mitochondria, and winding cellular membranes are found (26).

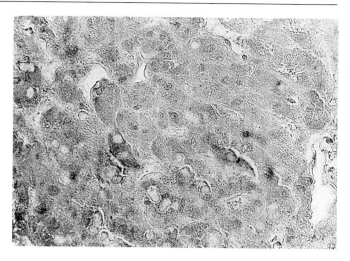

Figure 24-13 Intrasellar CRH-gangliocytoma adjacent to ACTH cell adenoma in Cushing's disease: differently intense immunostaining for CRH. Anti-CRH, ×440.

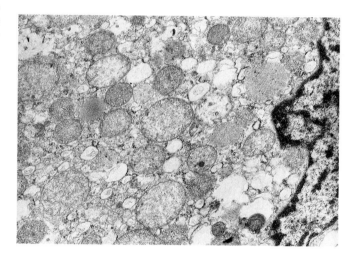

Figure 24-14 Intrasellar CRH-gangliocytoma: slightly lobated nucleus, large mitochondria, many synaptic vesicles. Uranyl-acetate-lead citrate, ×12,400.

In cases of combined gangliocytomas and adenomas, both tumors are very closely associated and often intermingled with one another. In Cushing's disease, sellar gangliocytomas are accompanied by ACTH cell hyperplasia in about half of these very rare cases, whereas the other half shows ACTH cell adenomas (26; Figure 15). The hyperplasia of these cases may represent an early stage of adenoma.

FIBROUS DYSPLASIA Fibrous dysplasia is a benign monostotic or polyostotic benign proliferation of fibrous tissue and bone, and frequently involves the craniofacial bones. Because it produces widely variable radiographic images, it can look like a real tumor in the sellar region. The monostotic form is usually diagnosed before 30 yr of age in about 75% of patients. The gnathic lesions often lead to obvious deformities, but are otherwise asymptomatic (107).

Genetic studies revealed clonal structural aberrations, suggesting that fibrous dysplasia is a neoplastic lesion developing as the result of somatic mutations (108). Patients with polyostotic fibrous

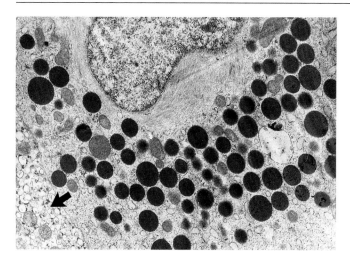

Figure 24-15   Densely granulated ACTH cell adenoma beside CRH gangliocytoma (arrow) (same tumor as Figure 14). Uranyl–acetate– lead citrate, ×12,400.

dysplasia often have macular pigmented skin lesions, a precocious puberty, and rarely multiple fibromyxomatous soft tissue tumors comprising the McCune-Albright syndrome. This can be combined with acromegaly owing to GH-secreting pituitary tumors *(109)*.

Morphologically we find fibrous tissue, mineralized bone, cysts with amber or bloody fluid, and cartilage nodules. The bony trabeculae are irregularly shaped. The fibrous stroma can be highly cellular with little collagen or sparsely cellular with much collagen or myxomatous *(107)*. Multinucleated giant cells of osteoclastic type may be present. At the periphery, the fibroosseous tissue infiltrates between the trabeculae of the normal bone.

The differential diagnosis comprehends well-differentiated osteosarcomas and fibrosarcomas. Recurrences following curretages or surgical resections are common. Malignant transformations into sarcomas are very rare *(107)*.

REFERENCES

1. Trouillas J, Guigard MP, Fonlupt P, Souchier C, Girod C. Mapping of corticotropic cells in the normal human pituitary. J Histochem Cytochem 1996;44:473–479.
2. Saeger W. Latent hyperplasias and adenomas in post-mortem pituitaries. Endocr Pathol 1995;6:379–380.
3. Garcia-Luna PP, Leal-Cerro A, Montero C, Scheithauer BW, Campanario A, Dieguez C, et al. A rare cause of acromegaly: ectopic production of growth-hormone releasing factor by a bronchial carcinoid tumor. Surg Neurol 1987;27:563–568.
4. Scheithauer BW, Carpenter PC, Bloch B, Brazeau P. Ectopic secretion of a growth hormone-releasing factor: report of a case of acromegaly with bronchial carcinoid tumor. Am J Med 1984;76:605–616.
5. Ezzat S, Asa SL, Stefaneanu L, Whittom R, Smyth H, Horvath E, et al. Somatotroph hyperplasia without pituitary adenoma associated with a long standing growth hormone-releasing hormone-producing bronchial carcinoid. J Clin Endocrinol Metab 1994;78:555–560.
6. Thorner MO, Perryman RL, Cronin MJ, Rogol AD, Draznin M, Johanson A, et al. Somatotroph hyperplasia: successful treatment of acromegaly by removal of a pancreatic islet tumor secreting a growth hormone-releasing factor. J Clin Invest 1982;70:965–977.
7. Moran A, Asa SL, Kovacs K, Horvath E, Singer W, Sagman U, et al. Gigantism due to pituitary mammosomatotroph hyperplasia. New Engl J Med 1990;323:322–327.
8. Kovacs K, Ryan N, Horvath E, Ezrin C, Penz G. Prolactin cells of the human pituitary gland in old age. J Gerontol 1977;32:534–540.
9. Landolt AM, Minder H. Immunohistochemical examination of the paraadenomatous "normal" pituitary. An evaluation of prolactin cell hyperplasia. Virchows Arch A Pathol Anat Histopath 1984;403:181–193.
10. Saeger W, Lüdecke DK. Pituitary hyperplasia. Definition, light and electron microscopical structures and significance in surgical specimens. Virchows Arch A Pathol Anat Histopath 1983;399:277–287.
11. Jay V, Kovacs K, Horvath E, Lloyd RV, Smyth HS. Idiopathic prolactin cell hyperplasia of the pituitary mimicking prolactin cell adenoma: a morphological study including immunocytochemistry, electron microscopy and *in situ* hybridization. Acta Neuropath (Wien) 1991;82:147–151.
12. Peillon F, Dupuy M, Li JY, Kujas M, Vincens M, Mowszowicz I, et al. Pituitary enlargement with suprasellar extension in functional hyperprolactinemia due to lactotroph hyperplasia: a pseudotumoral disease. J Clin Endocrinol Metab 1996;73:1008–1015.
13. Cai A, Hayes JD, Patel N, Hyde JF. Targeted overexpression of galanin in lactotrophs of transgenic mice induces hyperprolactinemia and pituitary hyperplasia. Endocrinology 1999;140:4955–4964.
14. Stefaneanu L, Kovacs K, Lloyd RV, Scheithauer BW, Young-WFJ, Sano T, et al. Pituitary lactotrophs and somatotrophs in pregnancy: a correlative in situ hybridization and immunocytochemical study. Virchows Arch B Cell Pathol Incl Mol Pathol 1992;62:291–296.
15. Horvath E, Kovacs K. Fine structural cytology of the adenohypophysis in rat and man. J Electron Microsc Tech. 1988;8:401–432.
16. Thapar K, Kovacs K, Laws ER, Jr. The classification and molecular biology of pituitary adenomas. In: Symon L, editor. Advances and technical standards in neurosurgery. Springer, Wien, New York, 1995, pp. 3–53.
17. Saeger W, Geisler F, Lüdecke DK. Pituitary pathology in Cushing's disease. Pathol Res Pract 1988;183:592–595.
18. Saeger W, Schröder H. ACTH-Zellhyperplasien der Adeno- und der Neurohypophyse und ihre Beziehungen zur arteriellen Hypertonie. Pathologe 1985;6:141–148.
19. Saeger W. Zur Ultrastruktur der hyperplastischen und adenomatösen ACTH-Zellen beim Cushing-Syndrom hypothalamisch-hypophysärer Genese. Virchows Archiv Path Anat 1974;362:73–88.
20. Caselitz J, Saeger W. The ultrastructure of the pituitary gland under chronic stimulation of the ACTH-cells in human pathology and animal experiments. Endokrinologie 1979;74:163–176.
21. Carey RM, Varma SK, Drake CR, Thorner MO, Kovacs K, Rivier J, et al. Ectopic secretion of corticotropin-releasing factor as a cause of Cushing's syndrome. New Engl J Med 1984;311:13–20.
22. Schteingart DE, Lloyd RV, Akil H, Chandler WF, Ibarra-Perez G, Rosen SC, et al. Cushing's syndrome secondary to ectopic corticotropin-releasing hormone-adrenocorticotropin secretion. J Clin Endocrinol Metab 1986;63:770–775.
23. Asa SL, Kovacs K, Vale W, Petrusz P, Vecsei P. Immunohistologic localization of corticotropin-releasing hormone in human tumors. Am J Clin Pathol 1987;87:327–333.
24. Saeger W, Reincke M, Scholz GH, Lüdecke DK. Ektop ACTH-oder CRH-bildende Tumoren mit Cushing-Syndrom. Zbl Allg Path Pathol Anat 1993;139:157–163.
25. Puchner MJA, Lüdecke DK, Saeger W, Riedel M, Asa SL. Gangliocytomas of the sellar region—a review. Exp Clin Endocrinol Diabetes 1995;103:129–149.
26. Saeger W, Puchner MJA, Lüdecke DK. Combined sellar gangliocytoma and pituitary adenoma in acromegaly or Cushing's disease. A report of 3 cases. Virchows Archiv Path Anat 1994;425:93–99.
27. Young WF, Jr., Scheithauer BW, Gharib H, Laws ER, Jr., Carpenter PC. Cushing's syndrome due to primary multinodular corticotrope hyperplasia. Mayo Clin Proc 1988;63:256–262.
28. Salgado LR, Mendonca BB, Goldman J, Semer M, Knoepfelmacher M, Tsanaclis AM, et al. Failure of partial hypophysectomy as definitive treatment in Cushing's disease owing to nodular corticotrope hyperplasia: Report of four cases. Endocr Pathol 1995;6:57–66.

29. McKeever PE, Koppelman MCS, Metcalf D, Quindlen E, Kornblith PL, Strott CA, et al. Refractory Cushing's disease caused by multinodular ACTH-cell hyperplasia. J Neuropathol Exp Neurol 1982;41:490–499.

30. Schnall AM, Kovacs K, Brodkey JS, Pearson OH. Pituitary Cushing's disease without adenoma. Acta Endocr (Kbh.) 1980; 94:297–303.

31. Horvath E, Kovacs K. The adenohypophysis. In: Kovacs K, Asa SL, eds. Functional Endocrine Pathology. Oxford, Blackwell Scientific Publ., 1991, pp. 245–282.

32. Scheithauer BW, Kovacs K, Randall RJ. The pituitary in untreated Addison's disease. Arch Pathol Lab Med 1983;197:484–487.

33. Horvath E, Kovacs K, Lloyd RV. Pars intermedia of the human pituitary revisited: Morphologic aspects and frequency of hyperplasia of POMC-peptide immunoreactive cells. Endocr Pathol 1999;10:55–64.

34. Lloyd RV, D'Amato CJ, Thiny MT, Jin L, Hicks SP, Chandler WF. Corticotroph (basophil) invasion of the pars nervosa in the human pituitary: localization of proopiomelanocortin peptides, galanin and peptidylglycine alpha-amidating monooxygenase-like immunoreactivities. Endocr Pathol 1993;4:86–94.

35. Khalil A, Kovacs K, Sima AAF, Burrow GN, Horvath E. Pituitary thyrotroph hyperplasia mimicking prolactin-secreting adenoma. J Endocrinol Invest 1984;7:399–404.

36. Scheithauer BW, Kovacs K, Randall RV, Ryan N. Pituitary gland in hypothyroidism. Histologic and immunocytologic study. Arch Pathol Lab Med 1985;109:499–504.

37. Saeger W. Effect of drugs on pituitary ultrastructure. Microsc Res Techn 1992;20:162–176.

38. Lloyd RV. Non-neoplastic pituitary lesions, including hyperplasia. In: Lloyd RV, editor. Surgical Pathology of the Pituitary Gland, 27th ed. W.B. Saunders Company, Philadelphia, 1993, pp. 25–33.

39. Saeger W, Schmidt W, Lüdecke DK. Metastases in the pituitary gland. Morphological studies of postmortem and surgical series. In: Georgii A, editor. Verhandlungen der Deutschen Krebsgesellschaft, Vol. 4. G. Fischer, Stuttgart, 1983, pp. 857.

40. Sautner D, Saeger W, Lüdecke DK, Jansen V, Puchner MJA. Hypophysitis in surgical and autoptical specimens. Acta Neuropath (Wien) 1995;90:637–644.

41. Thodou E, Asa SL, Kontogeorgos G, Kovacs K, Horvath E, Ezzat S. Clinical case seminar: Lymphocytic hypophysitis: Clinicopathological findings. J Clin Endocrinol Metab. 1995;80:2302–2311.

42. Feigenbaum SL, Downey DE, Wilson CB, Jaffe RB. Transsphenoidal pituitary resection for preoperative diagnosis of prolactin-secreting pituitary adenoma in women: Long term follow-up. J Clin Endocrinol Metab 1996;81:1711–1719.

43. Riedl M, Czech T, Slootweg J, Czernin S, Hainfellner JA, Schima W, et al. Lymphocytic hypophysitis presenting as a pituitary tumor in a 63-year-old man. Endocr Pathol 1995;6:159–166.

44. Lee JH, Laws ER, Jr., Guthrie BL, Dina TS, Nochomovitz LE. Lymphocytic hypophysitis: occurrence in two men. Neurosurgery 1994;34:159–163.

45. Püschel W, Wernert N, Hinkeldey KKM, Brittner-Flemmer V, Remberger K. Granulomatöse Hypophysitis. Bericht über drei Fälle und Literaturübersicht. Pathologe 1992;13:100–103.

46. Scanarini M, D'Avella D, Rotilio A, Kitromilis N, Mingrino S. Giant-cell granulomatous hypophysitis: a distinct clinicopathological entity. J Neurosurg 1989;71:681–686.

47. Yoshioka M, Yamakawa N, Saito H, Yoneda M, Nakayama T, Kuroki M, et al. Granulomatous hypophysitis with meningitis and hypopituitarism. Intern Med 1992;31:1147–1150.

48. Folkerth RD, Price DL, Schwartz M, Black PM, Degirolami U. Xanthomatous hypophysitis. Am J Surg Pathol 1998;22:736–741.

49. Deodhare SS, Bilbao JM, Kovacs K, Horvath E, Nomikos P, Buchfelder M, et al. Xanthomatous hypophysitis: A novel entity of obscure etiology. Endocr Pathol 1999;10:237–241.

50. Puchner MJA, Lüdecke DK, Saeger W. The anterior pituitary lobe in patients with cystic craniopharyngiomas: three cases of associated lymphocytic hypophysitis. Acta Neurochir (Wien) 1994;126: 38–43.

51. Scheithauer BW. The hypothalamus and neurohypophysis. In: Kovacs K, Asa SL, eds. Functional Endocrine Pathology. Blackwell Scientific Publ., Oxford, 1991, pp. 170–245.

52. Stern BJ, Krumholz A, Johns C, Scott P, Nissim J. Sarcoidosis and its neurological manifestations. Arch Neurol (Chic.) 1985;42:909–917.

53. Nishio S, Mizuno J, Barrow DL, Takei Y, Tindall GT. Isolated histiocytosis X of the pituitary gland: case report. Neurosurgery 1987;21:718–721.

54. Domingue JN, Wilson CB. Pituitary abscesses: report of seven cases and review of the literature. J Neurosurg 1977;46:601–608.

55. Bjerre P, Riishede J, Lindholm J. Pituitary abscess. Acta Neurochir (Wien) 1983;68:187–193.

56. Jones GM. Diabetes insipidus. Clinical observations in forty-two cases. Arch Intern Med 1944;74:81–93.

57. Fassbender HG. Pathologische Anatomie der endokrinen Drüsen. In: Kaufmann E, Staemmler M, ed. Lehrbuch der speziellen pathologischen Anatomie. Walter de Gruyter, Berlin, 1956, pp. 1427–1587.

58. Brown JR. Human actinomycosis: a study of 181 subjects. Hum Pathol 1973;4:319–330.

59. Brooks MH, Dumlao J, Bronsky D, Waldstein SS. Hypophysial tuberculoma with hypopituitarism. Am J Med 1973;54:777–781.

60. Delsedime M, Aguggia M, Cantello R, Chiado-Cuttin I, Nicola G, Torta R, et al. Isolated hypophyseal tuberculoma: case report. Clin Neuropathol 1988;7:311–313.

61. Esposito V, Fraioli B, Ferrante L, Palma L. Intrasellar tuberculoma. Neurosurgery 1987;21:721–723.

62. Pereira J, Vaz R, Carvalho D, Cruz C. Thickening of the pituitary stalk: A finding suggestive of intrasellar tuberculoma? Case report. Neurosurgery 1995;36:1013–1015.

63. Matthews R. Application of molecular biology to the diagnosis and typing of bacterial and fungal pathogens. In: Rapley R, Walker MR, eds. Molecular diagnostics. Blackwell Scientific Publ., Oxford, 1993, pp. 396–402.

64. Ferreiro J, Vinters HV. Pathology of the pituitary gland in patients with the acquired immune deficiency syndrome (AIDS). Pathology 1988;20:211–215.

65. Groll A, Schneider M, Althoff PH, Falkenbach A, Helm EB, Keul HG, et al. Morphologie und klinische Bedeutung pathologischer Veränderungen an Nebennieren und Hypophyse bei AIDS. Dtsch med Wschr 1990;115:483–488.

66. Klatt EC, Nichols L, Noguchi TT. Evolving trends revealed by autopsies of patients with the acquired immunodeficiency syndrome. 565 autopsies in adults with the acquired immunodeficiency syndrome, Los Angeles, CA, 1992–1993. Arch Pathol Lab Med 1994;118:884–890.

67. Milligan SA, Katz MS, Craven PC, Strandberg DA, Russell IJ, Becker RA. Toxoplasmosis presenting as panhypopituitarism in a patient with the acquired immune deficiency syndrome. Am J Med 1984;77:760–763.

68. Scaravilli F. Parasitic and fungal infections. In: Adams JH, Duchen LW, eds. Greenfields neuropathology. 5th ed. Arnold, London, 1992, pp. 400–446.

69. Ellis CJK, Daniel SE, Kennedy PG, Oppenheimer SM, Scaravilli F. Rhinoorbital zygomycosis. J Neurol Neurosurg Psychiat 1985;48: 455–458.

70. Berendes J. Über eine Mucocele der Keilbeinhöhle. Arch Ohrenheilk 1939;146:189–193.

71. Hyams VJ, Batsakis JG, Michaels L. Tumors of the respiratory tract and ear. Armed Forces Institute of Pathology, Washington, 1988.

72. Abla AA, Maroon JC, Wilberger JE, Kennerdell JS, Deeb ZL. Intrasellar mucocele simulating pituitary adenoma: Case report. Neurosurgery 1986;18:197–199.

73. Post K, McCormick PC, Bello JA. Differential diagnosis of pituitary tumors. Endocrinol Metab Clin N Amer 1987;16:609–645.

74. Asa SL, Kovacs K, Bilbao JM, Penz G. Immunohistochemical localization of keratin in craniopharyngiomas and squamous cell nests of the human pituitary. Acta Neuropath (Wien) 1981;54:257–260.

75. Harrison MJ, Morgello S, Post KD. Epithelial cystic lesions of the sellar and parasellar region: A continuum of ectodermal derivatives? J Neurosurg 1994;80:1018–1025.

76. Asa SL. Tumors of the pituitary gland. Armed Forces Institute of Pathology, Washington, D.C., 1998.

77. McKeever PE, Blaivas M, Sima AAF. Neoplasms of the sellar region. In: Lloyd RV, ed. Surgical Pathology of the Pituitary Gland. W.B. Saunders Company, Philadelphia, PA, 1993, pp. 141–210.

78. Thapar K, Kovacs K. Neoplasms of the sellar region. In: Bigner DD, McLendon RE, Bruner JM, Tamariz AS, eds. Russell and Rubinstein's pathology of tumors of the nervous system, Vol. 2, Part II, Pathologic Anatomy, 6th ed. Arnold, London, 1998:561–680.

79. Kasper M, Karsten U. Coexpression of cytokeratin and vimentin in Rathke's cysts of the human pituitary gland. Cell Tissue Res 1988;253:419–424.

80. Marin F, Boya J, Lopez-Carbonell A, Borregon A. Immunohistochemical localization of intermediate filament and S-100 proteins in several non-endocrine cells of the human pituitary gland. Arch Histol Cytol 1989;52:241–248.

81. Inoue T, Matsushima T, Fukui M, Iwaki T, Takeshita I, Kuromatsu C. Immunohistochemical study of intracranial cysts. Neurosurgery 1988;23:576–581.

82. Rutka JT, Giblin J, Dougherty DV, McCulloch JR, de Armond SJ, Rosenblum ML. An ultrastructural and immunocytochemical analysis of leptomeningeal and meningioma cultures. J Neuropathol Exp Neurol 1986;45:285–303.

83. Ikeda H, Yoshimoto T, Suzuki H. Immunohistochemical study of Rathke's cleft cyst. Acta Neuropath (Wien) 1988;77:33–38.

84. Bruner JM, Tien RD, Enterline DS. Tumors of meninges and related tissues. In: Bigner DD, McLendon RE, Bruner JM, Tamariz AS, eds. Russell and Rubinstein's pathology of tumors of the nervous system, Vol. 2, Part II, Pathologic Anatomy. 6th ed. Arnold, London, 1998, pp. 67–140.

85. Tran A, Kovacs K, Stefaneanu L, Kontogeorgos G, Scheithauer BW, Melmed S. Expression of leukemia inhibitory factor in craniopharyngioma. Endocr Pathol 1999;10:103–108.

86. Turpin G, Kujas M, van Effenterre R, Requeda E, Heshmati HM, Racadot J, et al. Les cystes mucigènes de l'hypophyse. Trois observations. Presse Med 1984;13:1319–1321.

87. Nishioka H, Ito H, Miki T, Wada J, Sano T. Lymphocytic adenohypophysitis associated with Rathke's cleft cyst. Endocr Pathol 1995;6:337–343.

88. Wenzel M, Salcman M, Kristt DA, Gellad FE, Kapcala LP. Pituitary hyposecretion and hypersecretion produced by a Rathke's cleft cyst presenting as a noncystic hypothalamic mass. Neurosurgery 1989;24:424–428.

89. Rengachary SS, Watanabe I. Ultrastructure and pathogenesis of intracranial arachnoid cysts. J Neuropathol Exp Neurol 1982;40:61–83.

90. Harding BN. Malformations of the nervous system. In: Adams JH, Duchen LW, editors. Greenfield's neuropathology, 5th ed. Arnold, London, 1992, pp. 521–638.

91. Guiot G, Olson D, Hertzog E. Kystes arachnoidiens intra-sellaires. Neuro-Chirurgie (Paris) 1971;17:539–548.

92. Bergeron C, Kovacs K, Bilbao JM. Primary "empty sella." A histologic and immunocytologic study. Arch Intern Med 1979; 139:248–249.

93. Busch W. Die Morphologie der Sella turcica und ihre Beziehung zur Hypophyse. Virchows Archiv Path Anat 1951;320:437–458.

94. Bergland RM, Ray BS, Torack RM. Anatomical variations in the pituitary gland and adjacent structures in 225 human autopsy cases. J Neurosurg 1968;28:93–99.

95. Ahmed M, Rifai A, Al Jurf M, Akhtar M, Woodhouse NJY. Classical pituitary apoplexy presentation and follow-up of 13 patients. Horm Res 1989;31:125–132.

96. Vance ML. Medical progress—Hypopituitarism. New Engl J Med 1994;330:1651–1662.

97. Cacciari E, Zucchini S, Ambrosetto P, Tani G, Carla G, Cicognani A, et al. Empty sella in children and adolescents with possible hypothalamic-pituitary disorders. J Clin Endocrinol Metab 1994; 78:767–771.

98. Domingue JN, Wing SD, Wilson CB. Coexisting pituitary adenomas and partially empty sellas. J Neurosurg 1978;48:23–28.

99. Raymond LA, Tew J. Large suprasellar aneurysms imitating pituitary tumour. Neurol Neurosurg Psychiatr 1978;41:83–87.

100. Lippman HH, Onofrio BM, Baker HL. Intrasellar aneurysm and pituitary adenoma: Report of a case. Mayo Clin Proc 1971;46: 532–535.

101. Chakeres DW, Curtin A, Ford G. Magnetic resonance imaging of pituitary and parasellar abnormalities. Radiol Clin North Am 1989;27:265–281.

102. Zülch KJ. Other malformative tumors and tumor-like lesions. In: Anonymous Brain Tumors. Their Biology and Pathology, 3rd ed. Springer, Berlin, 1986, pp. 426–450.

103. Takahashi H, Wakabayashi K, Kawai K, Ikuta F, Tanaka R, Takeda N, et al. Neuroendocrine markers in central nervous system neuronal tumors (gangliocytomas and ganglioglioma). Acta Neuropath (Berlin) 1989;77:237–243.

104. Kovacs K, Horvath E. Tumors of the pituitary gland. Armed Forces Institute of Pathology, Washington, DC, 1986.

105. Treip CS. The hypothalamus and pituitary gland. In: Adams JH, Duchen LW, editors. Greenfield's neuropathology, 5th ed. Arnold, London, 1992, pp. 1046–1082.

106. Zülch KJ. Tumors of neuroepithelial tissue. In: Anonymous Brain Tumors. Their Biology and Pathology, 3rd ed. Springer, Berlin, 1986, pp. 210–343.

107. Fechner RE, Mills SE. Tumors of the bones and joints. Washington, DC, Armed Forces Institute of Pathology, 1992.

108. Mertens F, Albert A, Heim S, Lindholm J, Brosjo O, Mitelman F, et al. Clonal structural chromosome aberrations in fibrous dysplasia. Gene Chromosome Cancer 1996;11:271–272.

109. Chanson P, Dib A, Visot A, Derome PJ. McCune-Albright syndrome and acromegaly: clinical studies and responses to treatment in five cases. Eur J Endocrinol 1994;131:229–234.

25 Pituitary Tumors

Future Perspectives

GREGORY M. MILLER, PhD, XUN ZHANG, PhD, AND ANNE KLIBANSKI, MD

During the past decade, research developments have broadened our understanding and raised new questions regarding the pathogenesis and therapy of pituitary tumors. X-chromosome inactivation studies have established that most pituitary adenomas are clonal in origin, indicating that somatic mutations are responsible for tumor formation *(1)*. Pituitary tumor research in the future will likely lead to the identification of genes underlying neoplastic transformation, and offer novel strategies for medical therapies to limit tumor progression and eliminate the clinical manifestations of hormone excess. Advances in our understanding of hormone regulation have identified abnormalities in hormone biosynthesis and secretion in human pituitary tumors. However, aberrant hormonal regulation may be uncoupled from neoplastic cell proliferation in some pituitary tumor types. The identification of hypothalamic and growth factor receptor expression patterns in neoplastic pituitary tissue is only the first step in determining the role of these receptors in mediating both hormone secretion and tumor growth. Basic research investigating receptor structure/function and intracellular signaling pathways has translated into successful medical management for many patients with prolactinomas and somatotroph adenomas, and current investigations are the basis of future strategies for the treatment of both secretory and nonsecretory pituitary adenoma subtypes. Recent research findings that may lead to new investigative and therapeutic strategies for pituitary tumors will be reviewed.

PITUITARY TUMOR PATHOGENESIS

Although X-chromosome inactivation studies have shown that pituitary tumors arise owing to somatic mutations, the identification of specific causal genetic rearrangements, deletions, or mutations has been elusive in the vast majority of tumors. The only mutations consistently found in pituitary adenomas are in a growth-promoting oncogene, *gsp*, present almost exclusively in a significant minority of somatotroph tumors *(2)*. These activating mutations are single amino acid substitutions that result in stabilization of guanine nucleotide stimulatory protein (G_s) α into its active state resulting in constitutive activation of adenylyl cyclase *(3)*. An important question is whether a specific underlying somatic mutation leading to the formation of a somatotroph tumor would

impact on tumor hormonal or biologic characteristics. One possibility is that the identification of such a mutation in a tumor sample may be a predictive factor in tumor size, recurrence, or level of hormone hypersecretion. To date, no study has demonstrated this. The majority of acromegalic patients have tumors that do not have *gsp* mutations, and these patients are not clinically distinguishable from those patients who have tumors with *gsp* mutations. It therefore seems more likely that different underlying mutations will lead to a somatotroph tumor of a common phenotype.

Studies have now demonstrated that mutations in oncogenes that are common in aggressive or malignant human tumors are extremely rare in pituitary adenomas. The few reported findings of mutated oncogenes have been associated with pituitary metastatic transformations and not with pituitary adenomas. Mutations in the p53 tumor suppresser gene have been shown to be present in up to 50% of all human cancers. Although mutations in p53 are an early event in some tumors, such as in astrocytic gliomas, or a late event, occurring during the malignant progression from adenoma to carcinoma, no mutations in p53 have been found in any pituitary adenomas *(4,5)*. Point mutations in the H-*ras* gene have been identified in pituitary metastases, but not in primary pituitary carcinomas or pituitary adenomas *(6)*. Protein kinase C (PKC) plays an important role in signal transduction, and is associated with the regulation of hormone release, mitogenesis, and tumor proliferation. A point mutation in the PKC α-isoform has been found in an invasive subpopulation of pituitary tumors, but not in pituitary adenomas *(7)*. Allelic deletions on chromosome 11 have been identified in 18% of pituitary tumors *(8)*. This finding raises the possibility that inactivation of a gene on chromosome 11 may be an important initiating event in the development of a pituitary adenoma. Recently, a putative tumor suppressor gene, *MEN1*, was identified on chromosome 11q13 *(9,10)*. Mutation of this gene has been associated with hereditary multiple endocrine neoplasia type I syndrome, characterized by the development of tumors of the pancreas, the parathyroid, and the anterior pituitary *(11)*. However, numerous studies have shown that somatic mutations of *MEN1* are rare in sporadic pituitary tumors, suggesting that it does not play a prominent role in the pathogenesis of such tumors *(12–14)*. Meanwhile, the high frequency of allelic loss on chromosome 11q13 in sporadic pituitary tumors suggests that there may be another gene in this region involved in pituitary tumorigenesis. Allelic losses in other chromosomes have been described, but occur at much lower frequency. In addition, no evidence of amplifica-

From: *Diagnosis and Management of Pituitary Tumors* (K. Thapar, K. Kovacs, B. W. Scheithauer, and R. V. Lloyd, eds.), ©Humana Press Inc., Totowa, NJ.

tion or rearrangement in 10 recognized cellular oncogenes has been found (8). Overexpression of c-myc has been reported in a cross-section of pituitary adenoma phenotypes (15). However, none of these mutations in and of themselves are sufficient to explain pituitary tumor pathogenesis. Therefore, somatic mutations in genes potentially important to neoplastic transformation remain to be identified for the majority of pituitary adenoma phenotypes. The observation that mutations common in many cancers are not found in pituitary adenomas may reflect the differences between factors that govern neoplastic initiation and progression in adenomas vs those factors involved in the multistep, multihit process of malignant transformation.

Where then might somatic mutations in pituitary adenomas occur? Mutations could occur anywhere along the signaling pathway, from a cell-surface receptor to a nuclear transcription factor. Mutations in regulatory proteins for hormone production and secretion or growth signaling pathways may play an important role in pituitary tumorigenesis, but it is also possible that an adenoma phenotype may be the result of a receptor mutation. A somatic mutation in a cell-surface receptor could potentially lead to a constitutive activation or a loss of function. An activating mutation in a stimulatory G-protein-linked receptor, or loss of function in an inhibitory G-protein linked receptor could have cellular effects similar to gsp mutations. Recently, somatic mutations have been identified in the VI transmembrane domain of the G-protein-linked thyrotropin receptor in hyperfunctioning autonomous thyroid adenomas (16,17). These mutations were found to be single amino acid substitutions that result in constitutively high cAMP levels within the adenoma and when transiently transfected into COS cells. This finding strongly implicates the VI transmembrane domain as a hot spot for constitutively activating mutations in G-protein-linked receptors. To date, however, no mutations in any G-protein-linked receptors have been identified in any pituitary adenomas. In addition to gsp, somatic mutations in other G-proteins may play a role in neoplastic transformation. For example, mutations in the α-subunit of Gq result in enhanced phospholipase C production in transiently transfected NIH-3T3, COS-7, and HEK-293 cell lines (18,19). Further, the NIH-3T3 cells expressing a mutant Gq were transformed, as illustrated by their capacity to form foci in soft agar (19).

Another class of membrane receptors activate tyrosine or serine/threonine kinases following ligand binding and dimerization. Mutations in these receptors could result in constitutive activation of kinases or truncated receptor proteins that lack intracellular signaling domains, creating dominant negative phenotypes, which would block signaling. A constitutively activating mutation in a receptor tyrosine kinase has been found in the c-kit proto-oncogene in the human mast cell leukemia cell line, HMC-1 (20). Point mutations in the c-kit proto-oncogene result in constitutive phosphorylation and activation of this receptor in the absence of ligand, and have been associated with neoplastic growth of mast cells (21). Conversely, genetic alteration in the intracellular kinase domain of a receptor kinase can produce receptors that act as dominant negatives. In a recent study, kinase-deficient activin type II receptor mutants, which lack the intracellular domain of the receptor, were unable to phosphorylate type I receptors and acted as dominant negatives when transfected into COS cells (22). Together, these findings raise the as yet unproven possibility that a somatic mutation in a receptor tyrosine or serine/threonine kinase could promote pituitary neoplastic transformation.

Activin is a member of transforming growth factor-β (TGF-β) cytokine family, which, functioning through its specific membrane serine kinase receptors, inhibits proliferation in a variety of cells (23). Originally identified in ovarian fluid and found to regulate pituitary follicle-stimulating hormone (FSH) production in a classic endocrine fashion, it is also expressed locally in pituitary (23,24). It has been shown that activin induces growth arrest in several pituitary cell lines, such as mouse corticotroph AtT20 (25) and rat somatotroph GH_3 (26). However, activin fails to inhibit cell proliferation in most clinically nonfunctioning human pituitary tumors investigated, suggesting a defect in the signaling pathway in these tumors (27). Despite the fact that no somatic mutation in activin/TGF-β type I and II receptor genes was found in 64 human pituitary adenomas (28), it has been reported that human pituitary tumors specifically express several truncated activin type I receptors, that lack various C-terminal kinase subdomains (29). These truncated type I receptors can form complexes with the type II receptor but fail to mediate signal controlling gene transcription and cell proliferation (30). Therefore, the tumor-specific expression of these truncated activin receptors in human pituitary adenomas may contribute to uncontrolled cell growth and pituitary tumorigenesis.

Somatic mutations in pituitary tumors that may be involved in neoplastic transformation may occur further along the intracellular signaling pathway, in the cellular machinery involved in transcriptional regulation or cell-cycle regulation, or in a genetic rearrangement resulting in overexpression of a growth-promoting factor or underexpression of a tumor suppressor factor. For example, overexpression of the cAMP-responsive transcription factor CREB, an intermediate in the proliferative response to cAMP, has been reported in all of 15 GH-secreting tumors studied, suggesting a role for CREB-induced genes in somatotroph transformation (31). Also, it has been shown that activin-mediated inhibition of cell growth is accompanied by altered activities of cell cycle factors. For example, activin up-regulates the mitotic inhibitor p21[Waf1/Cip1] and suppresses cyclin D2, a cell cycle-dependent kinase, resulting in hypophosphorylation and activation of the tumor suppressor Rb protein (32–34). Mitotic inhibitors such as p21[Waf1/Cip1] and p27[Kip1] prevent progression of G1 to S phase in the cell cycle by binding to the cyclin/cyclin-dependent kinase complexes and inhibiting their activities. Interestingly, p27[Kip1] knockout mice develop ACTH-secreting tumors (35–37). However, no mutation in p27[Kip1] gene and deletion of p27[Kip1] locus has been found in human pituitary tumors, although decreased p27[Kip1] protein levels have been observed in some pituitary tumors (38–40). Therefore, other mechanisms for p27[Kip1] inactivation at the posttranslational level may be involved in a subset of pituitary adenomas. In another report, parathyroid adenomas have been shown to overexpress cyclin D1, a cell-cycle-dependent kinase protein (41). This overexpression is the result of a chromosomal inversion in which the cyclin D1 gene, CCND1, comes under the control of the parathyroid hormone promoter. Cyclin D1 is also overexpressed in human esophageal tumors and the HCE7 human esophageal carcinoma cell line (42). The expression of an antisense cyclin D1 in this cell line produces a marked inhibition of cell proliferation and a loss of tumorigenicity when transplanted into nude mice, suggesting a direct role of this protein in tumorigenesis (43). It is anticipated that future studies will reveal which if any of these potential mechanisms will be shown to play a causal role in pituitary tumor development.

Recently, a novel gene named pituitary tumor-transforming gene *(PTTG)* was isolated from rat pituitary tumor cell lines *(44)* and subsequently cloned from the human *(45)*. When overexpressed in NIH3T3 cells, it causes malignant cell transformation and stimulates production of basic fibroblast growth factor (bFGF), an important angiogenic factor and growth regulator of human pituitary tumors *(44,45)*. It also has been found to inhibit sister-chromatid separation, therefore contributing to aneuploid and genetic instability *(46)*. *PTTG* is highly expressed in all human malignant tumor cell lines examined, while its expression in normal tissues is very restricted *(45,47)*. Also, increased expression of human *PTTG* is reported in most pituitary adenomas investigated, suggesting its involvement in pituitary tumorigenesis *(48,49)*. It will be important to investigate its tumor-specific expression and precise function in cell proliferation in order to understand further the molecular events governing the formation of human pituitary tumors.

TRANSITIONAL RESEARCH: FUTURE DIRECTIONS

DEVELOPING NEW PHARMACEUTICAL THERAPIES

One line of research has been directed toward characterizing cell-surface receptors in pituitary tumors, and determining whether biosynthetic defects, overexpression, or tumor-specific expression can be found. The identification of receptors expressed in pituitary adenomas may have direct clinical application to treatments for patients with pituitary adenomas by providing the basis of future drug development. The use of the somatostatin analog, Octreotide, has been an important adjunctive medical therapy for patients with somatotroph tumors. Five somatostatin receptor subtype (SSTR) genes have recently been cloned and characterized. Messenger RNA analysis in pituitary adenomas has demonstrated that SSTR2 and SSTR5, both of which have high affinity for Octreotide, are present in virtually all GH-secreting adenomas as well as in other pituitary tumor phenotypes *(50–52)*. One unanswered question is whether tumors differ in the amount of SSTR subtype gene expression, functional SSTR protein translated, or cell-surface density, and whether these characteristics determine octreotide efficacy. Possibly a mutation in an SSTR is present in those patients who are not responsive to Octreotide.

In contrast to secretory tumors, such as prolactinomas, in which suppression of hormone secretion by bromocriptine is typically accompanied by a decrease in adenoma size, octreotide treatment may have a pronounced effect on growth hormone secretion in somatotroph adenomas with little or no effect on tumor mass. The dissociation between the regulation of hormone secretion and antiproliferative actions has previously been shown using a hypothalamic-releasing hormone agonist. For example, GnRH analogs were initially thought to be an ineffective treatment for gonadotropin-secreting tumors, because such tumors typically fail to show gonadotropin desensitization with chronic GnRH analog administration. However, GnRH antagonist administration in patients with such tumors has been shown to result in decreased hormone secretion without an effect on tumor size. In this case, levels of hormone secretion are minimal compared to tumor mass, and suppression of hormone levels is likely unrelated to underlying proliferative factors. The presence of a variety of SSTR subtypes in all pituitary tumor phenotypes, along with the demonstrated antiproliferative actions of somatostatin in numerous experimental systems, suggests that a future drug therapy for the treatment of patients with pituitary adenomas may include novel somatostatin analogs with

altered affinities for specific SSTRs, resulting in an agonist with strong antiproliferative actions.

In addition to the development of more effective peptide analogs, future therapies may be directed at alleviating the clinical manifestations of pituitary tumors with the use of specific hormone antagonists. One exciting prospect is the development of a selective growth hormone antagonist. Growth hormone uses two different sites to bind two identical growth hormone receptor molecules. The receptor complex is activated following sequential dimerization. A successful antagonist may be a mutant growth hormone analog that would allow the initial binding event, but not the second binding event, thereby preventing dimerization and activation of the receptor. Such an antagonist may be of great value in managing the clinical symptoms of acromegaly. It is unknown, however, what effect a growth hormone antagonist has in vivo and what effect it may have on tumor proliferation.

There are currently no pharmaceutical treatments for many pituitary adenoma subtypes, including corticotroph adenomas. In one recent study, however, two ACTH-secreting macroadenomas were cultured and treated with antisense POMC oligonucleotides. Significant reductions in POMC mRNA levels in the cells and ACTH levels secreted into culture media were observed following treatment *(53)*. This study raises the interesting possibility that the use of specific DNA sequences as pharmaceutical agents may be a new avenue of drug treatment for pituitary tumor patients.

TUMOR LOCALIZATION AND DETECTION
In vivo imaging using MRI, CT, and PET has been utilized in the diagnosis and localization of pituitary microadenomas and in determining the extent of parasellar invasion of macroadenomas. These radiological techniques provide morphological detail suitable for tumor localization, but cannot distinguish tumor hormone phenotype. Radionuclide-labeled analogs have been used for the in vivo visualization of dopamine D2 receptor- and somatostatin receptor-positive tumors. With regard to somatostatin receptors, 123I-labeled Tyr3-octreotide has been used to identify somatostatin receptor-positive GH-secreting pituitary adenomas. Furthermore, there appears to be a correlation between ^{123}I-labeled Tyr3-octreotide uptake and the presence of a therapeutic response to octreotide *(54)*. This finding suggests that pituitary scintigraphy may have prognostic value in determining the efficacy of drugs, such as octreotide, as an adjunctive medical therapy for patients with pituitary tumors. The use of other radiopharmaceuticals for the detection of pituitary tumors and the visualization of specific receptors may be applicable to the screening of potential ligands as drug treatments for individual patients. The assessment of morphological detail provided by MRI, CT, and PET, along with the ability to visualize receptors using pituitary scintigraphy will likely become more sophisticated and result in the ability to resolve images at a cellular level.

GENE THERAPY FOR PITUITARY TUMORS?
The identification of genes responsible for cellular transformation and tumor proliferation may be critical to the development of future therapies for many patients with pituitary tumors. An intriguing question is whether future medical treatments for pituitary adenoma patients can be based on targeting therapeutic intervention to a tumor-specific genetic defect. A molecular genetic therapy for the treatment of pituitary adenoma patients may involve gene therapy to destroy adenomous cells specifically or alter the neoplastic phenotype of the tumor cells such that normal cellular functions are restored. If a somatic mutation causes a clonal expansion of the

tumor, gene therapy may be implemented so that the mutant allele responsible for promoting tumorigenesis is corrected.

The major difficulties revolve around how to express transgenes permanently in human cells and the practicality of using this approach for such patients. The potential widespread applications of gene therapy will ensure the development of novel methodologies for delivering transgenes to cells. In addition to the issues of gene delivery are issues of target specificity. In the coming years, methodology developed to target gene expression to specific body organs may be applicable to targeting genetic alterations to pituitary adenomas. It may be important to consider that the pituitary may have a unique location for future gene therapy applications directed at producing transgene products that would act on neoplastic tissue. The hypothalamic–pituitary portal system is a venous blood supply that allows minute quantities of hypothalamic secretions to act on pituitary cell-surface receptors prior to diffusion into the general circulation. Gene therapy for pituitary adenomas may involve targeting transgenes to hypothalamic neurons that project to the median eminence. Proteins from transduced genes could be secreted into the portal vasculature and delivered to the pituitary. Therefore, a mechanism to deliver concentrated protein product to the adenoma tissue while leaving other body tissues to receive only diffused transgene products already exists. Whether such an approach is feasible, practical, and therapeutically sound will remain important future questions.

ACKNOWLEDGMENTS

This work was supported by NIH grants R01DK40947 and DK09281. We would like to thank Joseph M. Alexander for his helpful suggestions.

REFERENCES

1. Alexander JM, Biller BM. K, Bikkal H, Zervas NT, Arnold A, Klibanski A. Clinically nonfunctioning pituitary tumors are monoclonal in origin. J Clin Invest 1990;86:336–340.
2. Landis CA, Masters SB, Spada A, Pace AM, Bourne HR, Vallar L. GTPase inhibiting mutations activate the alpha chain of Gs and stimulate adenylyl cyclase in human pituitary tumours. Nature 1989;340:692–696.
3. Spada A, Arosio M, Bassetti M, Vallar L, Clementi E, Bazzoni N. Mutations in the alpha subunit of the stimulatory regulatory protein of adenylyl cyclase (Gs) in human GH-secreting pituitary adenomas. Pathol Res Pract 1991;187:567–570.
4. Herman V, Drazin NZ, Gonsky R, Melmed S. Molecular screening of pituitary adenomas for gene mutations and rearrangements. J Clin Endocrinol Metab 1993;77:50–55.
5. Levy A, Hall L, Yeudall WA, Lightman SL. p53 gene mutations in pituitary adenomas: rare events. Clin Endocrinol 1994;41:809–814.
6. Karga HJ, Alexander JM, Hedley-Whyte ET, Klibanski A, Jameson JL. Ras mutations in human pituitary tumors. J Clin Endocrinol Metab 1992;74:914–919.
7. Alvaro V, Levy L, Dubray C, Roche A, Peillon F, Querat B, et al. Invasive human pituitary tumors express a point-mutated alpha-protein kinase-C. J Clin Endocrinol Metab 1993;77:1125–1129.
8. Boggild MD, Jenkinson S, Pistorello M, Boscaro M, Scanarini M, McTernan P, et al. Molecular genetic studies of sporadic pituitary tumors. J Clin Endocrinol 1994;78:387–392.
9. Bystrom C, Larsson C, Blomberg C, Sandelin K, Falkmer E. Localization of the MEN-1 gene to a small region within chromosome 11q13 by deletion mapping in tumors. Proc Natl Acad Sci USA 1990;87:1968–1972.
10. Chandrasekharappa SC, Guru SC, Manickam P, Olufemi SE, Collins FS, Liotta LA, Crabtree JS, et al. Positional cloning of the gene for multiple endocrine neoplasia-type I. Science 1997;276:404–407.

11. Marx SJ. Familial multiple endocrine neoplasia type I. Mutation of a tumor suppressor gene. Trend Endocrinol Metab 1989;1:76–82.
12. Zhaung Z, Ezzat SZ, Vortmeyer AO, Weil R, Oldfield EH, Park WS, Pack S, et al. Mutations of the MEN1 tumor suppressor gene in pituitary tumors. Cancer Res 1997;57:5446–5451.
13. Prezant TR, Levine J, Melmed S. Molecular characterization of the men1 tumor suppressor gene in sporadic pituitary tumors. J Clin Endocrinol Metab 1998;83:1388–1391.
14. Schmidt MC, Henke RT, Stangl AP, Meyer-Puttlitz B, Stoffel-Wagner B, Schramm J, von Deimling A. Analysis of the MEN1 gene in sporadic pituitary adenomas. J Pathol 1999;188:168–173.
15. Woloschak M, Roberts JL, Post K. c-myc, c-fos, and c-myb gene expression in human pituitary adenomas. J Clin Endocrinol Metab 1994;79:253–257.
16. Parma J, Duprez L, Van Sande J, Cochaux P, Gervy C, Mockel J, et al. Somatic mutations in the thyrotropin receptor gene cause hyperfunctioning thyroid adenomas. Nature 1993;365:649–651.
17. Porcellini A, Ciullo I, Pannain S, Fenzi G, Avvedimento E. Somatic mutations in the VI transmembrane segment of the thyrotropin receptor constitutively activate cAMP signalling in thyroid hyperfunctioning adenomas. Oncogene 1995;11:1089–1093.
18. Conklin BR, Chabre O, Wong YH, Federman AD, Bourne HR. Recombinant Gq alpha. Mutational activation and coupling to receptors and phospholipase C. J Biol Chem 1992;267:31–34.
19. De Vivo M, Chen J, Codina J, Iyengar R. Enhanced phospholipase C stimulation and transformation in NIH-3T3 cells expressing Q209LGq-alpha-subunits. J Biol Chem 1992;267:18,263–18,266.
20. Furitsu T, Tsujimura T, Tono T, Ikeda H, Kitayama H, Koshimizu U, et al. Identification of mutations in the coding sequence of the proto-oncogene c-kit in a human mast cell leukemia cell line causing ligand-independent activation of c-kit product. J Clin Invest 1993;92:1736–1744.
21. Tsujimura T, Furitsu T, Morimoto M, Kanayama Y, Nomura S, Matsuzawa Y, et al. Substitution of an aspartic acid results in constitutive activation of c-kit receptor tyrosine kinase in a rat tumor mast cell line RBL-2H3. Internatl Arch All Immunol 1995;106:377–385.
22. Tsuchida K, Vaughan JM, Wiater E, Gaddy-Kurten D, Vale WW. Inactivation of activin-dependent transcription by kinase-deficient activin receptors. Endocrinology 1995;136:5493–5503.
23. Mathews LS. Activin receptor and cellular signaling by the receptor serine kinase family. Endocr Rev 1994;15:310–325.
24. Alexander JM, Swearingen B, Tindall GT, Klibanski A. Human pituitary adenomas express endogenous inhibin subunit and follistatin messenger ribonucleic acids. J Clin Endocrinol Metab 1995;80:147–152.
25. Bliezikjian LM, Blount AL, Campen CA, Gonzalez-Manchon C, Vale W. Activin-A inhibits proopiomelanocortin messenger RNA accumulation and adrenocorticotropin secretion of AtT20 cells. Mol Endocrinol 1991;5:1389–1395.
26. Billestrup N, Gonzalez-Manchon C, Potter E, Vale W. Inhibition of somatotroph growth and growth hormone biosynthesis by activin in vitro. Mol Endocrinol 1990;4:356–362.
27. Danila DC, Inder WJ, Zhang X, Alexander JM, Swearingen B, Hedley-Whyte E. T, Klibanski A. Activin effects on neoplastic proliferation of human pituitary tumors. J Clin Endocrinol Metab 2000;85:1009–1915.
28. D'Abronzo FH, Swearingen B, Klibanski A, Alexander JM. Mutational analysis of activin/transforming growth factor-b type I and type II receptor kinases in human pituitary tumors. J Clin Endocrinol Metab 1999;84:1716–1721.
29. Alexander JM, Bikkal HA, Zervas NT, Laws ER Jr, Klibanski A. Tumor-specific expression and alternate splicing of messenger ribonucleic acid encoding activin/transforming growth factor-β receptors in human pituitary adenomas. J. Clin. Endocrinol. Metab. 1996;81:783–790.
30. Zhou Y, Sun H, Danila DC, Johnson SR, Sigai DP, Zhang X, Klibanski A. Truncated activin type I receptor Alk4 isoforms are dominant negative receptors inhibiting activin signaling. Submitted, 2000.

31. Bertherat J, Chanson P, Montminy M. The cyclic adenosine 3', 5'-monophosphate-responsive factor CREB is constitutively activated in human somatotroph adenomas. Mol Endocrinol 1995;9:777–783.

32. Sehy DW, Shao LE, Yu AL, Tsai WM, Yu J. Activin A-induced differentiation in K562 cells is associated with a transient hypophosphorylation of Rb protein and the concomitant block of cell cycle at G1 phase. J Cell Biochem 1992;50:255–265.

33. Zauberman A, Oren M, Zipori D. Involvement of p21$^{WAF1/Cip1}$, CDK4 and Rb in activin A mediated signaling leading to hepatoma cell growth inhibition. Oncogene 1997;15:1705–1711.

34. Yamato K, Koseki T, Ohguchi M, Kizaki M, Ikeda T, Nishihara T. Activin A induction of cell-cycle arrest involves modulation of cyclinD2 and p21$^{CIP1/WAF1}$ in plasmacytic cells. Mol Endocrinol 1997;11:1044–1052.

35. Nakayama K, Ishida N, Shirane N, Inomata A, Inoue T, Shishido N, Horii I, et al. Mice lacking p27^{Kip1} display increased body size, multiple organ hyperplasia, retinal dysplasia, and pituitary tumors. Cell 1996;85:707–720.

36. Kiyokawa H, Kineman RD, Manova-odorova KO, Soares VC, Hoffman ES, Ono M, Khanam D, et al. Enhanced growth of mice lacking the cyclin-dependent kinase inhibitor function of p27^{Kip1}. Cell 1996;85:721–732.

37. Fero ML, Rivkin M, Tasch M, Porter P, Caroe CE, Firpo E, Polyak K, Tsai LH, Broudy V, Perlmutter RM, Kaushansky K, Roberts JM. A syndrome of multiorgan hyperplasia with features of gigantism, tumorigenesis, and female sterility in p27^{Kip1}-deficient mice. Cell 1996;85:733–744.

38. Tanaka C, Yoshimoto K, Yang P, Kimura T, Yamada S, Moritani M, Sano T, et al. Infrequent mutations of P27^{Kip1} gene and trisomy 12 in a subset of human pituitary adenomas. J Clin Endocrinol Metab 1997;82:3141–3147.

39. Dahia PL, Aguiar RC, Honegger J, Fahlbush R, Jordan S, Lowe DG, Lu X, et al. Mutation and expression analysis of the p27/Kip1 gene in corticotropin-secreting tumors. Oncogene 1998;16:69–76.

40. Bamberger CM, Fehn M, Bamberger AM, Ludecke DK, Beil FU, Saeger W, Schulte HM. Reduced expression levels of the cell-cycle inhibitor p27Kip1 in human pituitary adenomas. Eur J Endocrinol 1999;140:250–255.

41. Motokura T, Bloom T, Kim HG, Juppner H, Ruderman JV, Kronenberg HM, et al. A novel cyclin encoded by a bc11-linked candidate oncogene. Nature 1991;350:462–463.

42. Jiang W, Zhang YJ, Kahn SM, Hollstein MC, Santella RM, Lu SH, et al. Altered expression of the cyclin D1 and retinoblastoma genes in human esophageal cancer. Proc Natl Acad Sci USA 1993;90:9026–9030.

43. Zhou P, Jiang W, Zhang YJ, Kahn SM, Schieren I, Santella RM, et al. Antisense to cyclin D1 inhibits growth and reverses the transformed phenotype of human esophageal cancer cells. Oncogene 1995;11:571–580.

44. Pei L, Melmed S. Isolation and characterization of a pituitary tumor-specific transforming gene (PTTG). Mol Endocrinol 1997;11:433–441.

45. Zhang X, Horwitz GA, Prezant TR, Valentini A, Nakashima M, Bronstein MD, Melmed S. Structure, expression, and function of human pituitary tumor-transforming gene (PTTG). Mol Endocrinol 1999;13:156–166.

46. Zou H, McGarry TJ, Bernal T, Kirschner MW. Identification of a vertebrate sister-chromatid separation inhibitor involved in transformation and tumorigenesis. Science 1999;285:418–422.

47. Dominquez A, Ramos-Morales F, Ramero F, Rios RM, Dreyfus F, Tortolero M, Pintor-Toro JA. *hpttg*, a human homologue of rat *pttg*, is overexpressed in hematopoietic neoplasms. Evidence for a transcriptional activation function of hPTTG. Oncogene 1998;17:2187–2193.

48. Zhang X, Horwitz GA, Heaney AP, Nakashima M, Prezant TR, Bronstein MD, Melmed S. Pituitary tumor transforming gene (PTTG) expression in pituitary adenomas. J Clin Endocrinol Metab 1999;84:761–767.

49. Saez C, Japon MA, Ramos-Morales F, Ramero F, Segura DI, Tortolero M, Pintor-Toro JA. *hpttg* is over-expressed in pituitary adenomas and primary epithelial neoplasias. Oncogene 1999;18:5473–5476.

50. Greenman Y, Melmed S. Heterogeneous expression of two somatostatin receptor subtypes in pituitary tumors. J Clin Endocrinol Metab 1994;78:398–403.

51. Greenman Y, Melmed S. Expression of three somatostatin receptor subtypes in pituitary adenomas: Evidence for preferential SSTR5 expression in the mammosomatotroph lineage. J Clin Endocrinol Metab 1994;79:724–729.

52. Miller GM, Alexander JM, Bikkal HA, Katznelson L, Zervas NT, Klibanski A. Somatostatin receptor subtype gene expression in pituitary adenomas. J Clin Endocrinol Metab 1995;80:1386–1392.

53. Woloschak M, Post K, Roberts JL. Effects of antisense DNA on POMC mRNA and ACTH levels in cultured human corticotroph adenoma cells. J Endocrinol Invest 1994;17:817–819.

54. Ur E, Mather SJ, Bomanji J, Ellison D, Britton K, Grossman AB, et al. Pituitary imaging using a labelled somatostatin analogue in acromegaly. Clin Endocrinol 1992;36:147–150.

INDEX

ABC peroxidase method, 94
Abscesses, 190, 454
Acetylcholine, 52
Acidophil stem-cell adenomas, 124, 125–126 *fig.*
 invasive growth, 374
Acquired immunodeficiency syndrome (AIDS), 454, 455 *table*
Acromegaly, 1–3, 167–168
 anterior pituitary function tests, 300
 bones and joints in, 296–297
 bromocriptine for, 191, 253–254
 cardiovascular system in, 297
 central nervous sytem in, 297–298
 clinical aspects, 296–298
 combination treatment for, 306
 DA therapy for, 305
 diagnosis, 300–302
 L-DOPA and, 8
 dopamine agonists for, 253–257
 ectopic GHRH secretion in, 299–300
 ectopic GH secretion in, 300
 endocrine organs in, 298
 familial, 300
 follow-up in, 306–307
 gastrointestinal system in, 297
 genitourinary system in, 297
 GHBP and, 301
 GH concentrations and, 300
 GH excretion and, 301
 GH paradoxical responses and, 301–302
 GH-receptor antagonists for, 257, 306
 GHRH test, 302
 GH secretion and, 296
 GH urinary excretion of, 301
 hyperprolactinemia in, 302–303
 IGF-1 and, 301
 IGF-BP3 and, 301
 immune system in, 298
 irradiation in, 304
 malignancies and, 299
 McCune-Albright syndrome and, 300
 medical therapy, 305–307

Acromegaly (*cont.*),
 MEN 1 and, 300
 metabolic changes in, 299
 multihormonal adenomas and, 302–303
 neurological examination, 300
 neuromuscular system in, 297–298
 octreotide and, 304, 305–306
 ophthalmological examination, 300
 oral glucose test for, 300
 peripheral nervous sytem in, 297–298
 physiognomy in, 296
 pituitary insufficiency and, 303
 pituitary tumors and, 5
 prevalence, 295
 pulmonary system in, 297
 radiation therapy of, 270–271
 radiological examination, 300
 scintigraphic methods, 302
 somatostatin analogs and, 305–306
 stereotactic radiosurgery in, 304
 surgery for, 271, 303–304
 treatment of, 8, 255–257, 303–307
ACTH, *see* Adrenocorticotrophic hormone (ACTH)
Actinomycosis, 454
Activin, 462
Adenohypophysial tumors, 9
Adenohypophysis, 41
 cells, 97–107
 follicles in, 110 *fig.*
 salivary gland remnants, 107, 111 *fig.*
 squamous metaplasia of, 106, 111 *fig.*
 vasculature, 107
Adenoma of uncertain malignant potential (AUMP), 382
Adrenocorticotrophic hormone (ACTH), 6, 7, 42, 49–50
 actions, 49–50
 cell adenomas
  incidence of, 62, 63 *table,* 65
 cell hyperplasia, 449–450
 cells, 99, 101–103
 Cushing's disease and, 326
 in Cushing's syndrome, 320–322
 feedback control, 49
 HT control, 49
 hypersecretion of, 168
 loss of, 166

From: *Diagnosis and Management of Pituitary Tumors* (K. Thapar, K. Kovacs, B. W. Scheithauer, and R. V. Lloyd, eds.), © Humana Press Inc., Totowa, NJ

Adrenocorticotrophic hormone (ACTH)-producing adenomas, 124, 127–129

Adrenocorticotrophic hormone (ACTH)-producing tumors, 377, 378, 381

Adrenocorticotrophic hormone (ACTH)-secreting tumors
    ISH study of, 156–157

Age
    in pediatric pituitary tumors, 353–354
    pituitary adenomas and, 61, 63–65
    visual outcomes and, 192–193

cAMP response element binding protein (CREB), 72

Aneurysms, of the carotid artery, 456

Angiography, 201

Anterior cerebral arteries, 36, 38

Anterior chiasmal syndrome, 180–181, 182 *fig.*

Anterior choroidal artery, 36

Anterior communicating artery, 36

Apoplexy, pituitary, 188–190, 195, 205–207

Arachnoid cysts, 392, 455–456
    pediatric, 362

Argentaffin methods, 93

Arginine-vasopressin/SV40 large T-antigen
    mice transgenic for, 86

Argyrophil preparations, 93

Arteries
    aneurysms of, 456
    carotid, 20, 25, 26
    cerebral, 36, 38
    choroidal, 36
    communicating, 36
    of inferior cavernous sinus, 26
    McConnell's capsular, 26
    meningohypophyseal, 26
    ophthalmic, 36
    posterior cerebral, 36
    surgical injury to, 235
    thalamoperforating, 36
    of third ventricle, 37

Atrophy, optic, 192

Atypical adenomas, 382–383

Autopsy, tumors found at, 5–6, 63–65

B

Babinski, M.J., 3

Basophilia, 104 *fig.,* 112–113

Beadles, C.F., 3

Béclère, A., 3

Benda, C., 3

Binasal hemianopia, 181

Bitemporal hemianopia, 180, 186 *fig.*

Bleomycin
    with pediatric craniopharyngiomas, 360

Boyce, R., 3

Brainstem
    surgical injury to, 236

Bromocriptine, 190–191, 221, 222, 239
    for acromegaly, 253–254
    for clinically nonfunctioning adenomas, 258–259
    for Cushing's disease, 258
    for hyperprolactinemia, 248
    long-term considerations, 250
    macroadenomas and, 249 *table*

Bromocriptine, 190–191, 221, 222, 239 (*cont.*)
    microadenomas and, 250
    octreotide with, 257, 306
    oral alternatives, 251, 286
    in pediatric pituitary tumors, 357
    pharmacology, 247–248
    pregnancy and, 240, 251–252, 289–291
    for prolactinomas, 248–250, 269–270, 285–286
    psychosis and, 251
    resistance to, 251, 286
    side effects, 250–251, 285–286

C

Cabergoline, 222, 252–253, 286

Calcitonin
    tumorigenesis and, 83

Carcinoma
    pituitary, 8–9, 377–382
        invasive tumors cf., 381–382

Carotid arteries, 20, 25, 26
    aneurysms of, 456
    internal, 35

Castration cells, 108 *fig.*

Cavernous angiomas (CAs), 417

Cavernous sinus, 25–26, 28–29
    imaging of, 205, 206 *fig.*
    surgical injury, 235

Cell proliferation markers, 9

Cerebral arteries, 36, 38

Cerebrospinal fluid (CSF)
    leaks, 357
    rhinorrhea, 235

Chemotherapy, *see* Medical therapy

Chiari-Frommel syndrome, 6

Chiasm, *see* Anterior chiasmal syndrome; Optic chiasm

Children
    arachnoid cysts in, 362
    corticotroph adenomas in, 354
    cortisol pattern in, 355–356
    craniopharyngiomas in, 207
    Cushing's disease in, 354
    Cushing's syndrome in, 354, 356
    germ-cell tumors in, *see* Germ-cell tumors, pediatric
    gigantism in, 355
    McCune-Albright syndrome in, 355
    nonfunctioning adenomas in, 355
    optic pathway gliomas in, *see* Optic pathway gliomas, pediatric
    pituitary tumors in, 65, 353–364
    prolactin in, 356
    prolactinomas in, 354
    Rathke's cleft cysts (RCCs) in, *see* Rathke's cleft cysts (RCCs), pediatric
    somatotroph adenomas in, 355
    surgery
        visual outcomes, 194

Chondrosarcomas
    chordomas *vs.,* 412

Chordomas
    clinical features, 409
    clinical outcome, 412
    definition, 409
    differential diagnosis, 410, 412

Chordomas (*cont.*)
  immunohistochemistry, 410
  location, 409
  macroscopic features, 410
  microscopic features, 410
  radiographic features, 410
  ultrastructural features, 410
Choristomas, 456
Choroidal artery, 36
Choroidal epithelial cysts, 392
Choroid plexus papillomas, 392
Circadian rhythms, *see also* Endocrine rhythms; Infradian rhythms
  in growth hormone (GH), 52–53
  prolactin (PRL), 54
  in thyrotropin-stimulating hormone (TSH), 49
Clinically nonfunctioning adenomas, 62, 63 *table,* 347
  bromocriptine for, 258–259
  in children, 355
  hormonal evaluation, 344
  imaging, 344, 345–347 *fig.,* 350 *fig.*
  as incidentalomas, 347, 349
  medical therapy, 258, 347
  presentation, 343–344
  radiation therapy, 273–274, 347
  surgery, 273–274
  treatment, 344, 347, 349 *table*
  visual abnormalities and, 344, 348 *fig.*
Clinically nonfunctioning tumors
  surgical results, 244
Colloid cysts, 392
Colney Hatch Lunatic Asylum, 3
Communicating arteries, 36
Comparative genomic hybridization (CGH), 160
Computed tomography (CT) scanning, 169, *see also* Imaging;
        Magnetic resonance imaging (MRI)
  of craniopharyngiomas, 207–208
  of cystic lesions, 211
  of diabetes insipidus, 214
  of germ-cell tumors, 208
  of gliomas, 210
  of granular cell myoblastomas, 210–211
  of hypothalamic hamartomas, 211–212, 213 *fig.*
  of meningiomas, 208–210
  of pituitary abscesses, 214
  of pituitary adenomas, 204–207
  of pituitary gland, 201–203
  of pituitary hyperplasias, 211
  of primary sellar melanoma, 211
  of vascular and ischemic lesions, 214–215
  vs. magnetic resonance imaging (MRI), 201
Corticotroph adenomas, 124, 127–129
  in children, 354
  invasive growth, 374
  silent, 135, 139 *fig.,* 141 *fig.*
  surgical results, 242–243
Corticotroph cells, 99, 101–103
Corticotroph hyperplasia, 146
Corticotropin-releasing hormone (CRH), 71
  simulation test for Cushing's disease, 320–321
Cortisol, 168, 170
  in children, 355–356
  Cushing's disease and, 326

Craniopharyngiomas, 185, 187, 189 *table,* 194
  clinical features, 387
  clinical outcome, 388–389
  definition, 387
  differential diagnosis, 388
  epidermoid cysts *vs.,* 393
  imaging of, 207–208
  immunostaining, 387–388
  location, 387
  macroscopic features, 387
  microscopic features, 387
  pediatric
    bleomycin with, 360
    clinical features, 358
    imaging, 358, 359 *fig.*
    irradiation of, 358
    recurrence, 358
    surgery, 358, 360
    treatment, 358, 360
  radiological features, 387
  ultrastructure, 388
Crooke's hyalinization, 102–103, 103 *fig.,* 129
CT scanning, *see* Computed tomography (CT) scanning
Cushing, Harvey, 4, 5, 6
Cushing's disease, 5, 65, 170, 205 *fig.,* 227–228, 242
  ACTH secretion and, 326
  bilateral adrenalectomy for, 327
  bromocriptine for, 258
  in children, 354
  clinical features, 317–318
  complications, 324
  cortisol production and, 326
  CRH simulation test for, 320
  cyproheptadine for, 258
  dexamethasone and, 320
  etiology, 317
  etomidate for, 326
  follow-up, 323–324
  interstitial radiation for, 326
  IPSS for, 321–322
  irradiation in, 325–326
  ketoconazole for, 257–258, 326
  medical therapy, 326
  metyrapone for, 258, 320–321, 326
  mitotane (*o,p'DDD*) for, 258, 326
  octreotide for, 258
  pathogenesis, 317
  pituitary imaging and, 321
  postoperative evaluation, 323–324
  radiation therapy, 272, 325–326
  recurrence, 324–325
  residual disease, 324
  RU 486 for, 326
  sodium valproate for, 258
  surgery, 272, 322–325
  surgical outcomes, 324
  trilostane for, 326
  venous sampling, 321–322
Cushing's syndrome, 65, 71, 168–169
  ACTH dependency in, 320
  biochemical tests, 320–321
  in children, 354, 356

Cushing's syndrome (*cont.*)
    diagnosis, 319–21
    differential diagnosis, 320–321, 323 *table*
    pseudo-Cushing states, 319–320
    RU 486 for, 326
Cyclic AMP, 72
Cyclin-dependent kinase (CDK) inhibitors, 66, 74–75
Cyproheptadine, 258
Cystic lesions, 454–456
    imaging, 211

D

D_2 binding, 221, 223
Del Castillo syndrome, 6
Dermoid cysts, 393–394
Desmopressin acetate (dDAVP), 170–171
Dexamethasone
    Cushing's disease and, 320
Diabetes, 240
Diabetes insipidus (DI), 167, 170
    imaging of, 214
Diaphragma sellae, 16, 20
Diaphragma sella meningiomas, 187, 194
Diethylstilbestrol (DES), 81
Diplopia, 184–185
L-DOPA, 8
Dopamine (DA), 42, 49, 53, 142–143, 237
Dopamine (DA) agonists, 252–253
Dopamine (DA) agonist therapy, 170
    for acromegaly, 253–257, 305
    for prolactinomas, 221–222, 269–270, 284–285, 286, 287–288,
        288–289
Dopamine receptor studies, 219, 220–221
Double immunostaining, 94
Drug therapy, *see* Medical therapy
Dwarfism
    GH-deficient, 203–204
Dynamic MRI, 204, 205 *fig.*

E

Ectopic adenomas
    invasion by, 377
Electron microscopy, 95–96
Empty sella syndrome, 190, 193–194, 195, 456
Endocrine hypothalamus (HT)
    anatomy, 43–44
Endocrine rhythms, 43
Epidemiology
    of pediatric pituitary adenomas, 353–354
    of pituitary adenomas, 57–66
Epidermoid cysts, 392–393
Estrogen
    tumorigenesis and, 81–83
Estrogen receptor (ER), 81
Estrogen replacement, 171
Etomidate
    for Cushing's disease, 326
Euthyroidism, 338
Extra-ocular muscle (EOM) palsy, 189
Extra-ocular muscle paresis, 192

F

Fertility
    prolactinomas and, 239–240, 289
Fibroblast growth factor (FGF), 75
Fibroblast growth factor-2 (FGF-2), 75–76
Fibroblast growth factor-4 (FGF-4) (hst), 76
Fibromas, 415
Fibrosarcomas, 415–416
Fibrous dysplasia, 457–458
F-fluorodeoxyglucose, 219, 220, 223
Follicle-stimulating hormone (FSH), 6–7, 42, 48
    cell adenomas, 62
Foramen of Monro, 30
Forbes-Albright syndrome, 6
Foster Kennedy syndrome, 185
Fröhlich, A., 2–3
Frozen section, 113–115, 116 *fig.*
Fungal infections, 454

G

Gadolinium-enhanced MRI, 356
Galactorrhea, 8, 281
Gallstones
    octreotide and, 257, 306
Gamma-Knife radiosurgery, 4, 274, 304, 325–326, 347
Gangliocytomas, 9, 394–395, 457
    hypothalamic, 9
Gangliogliomas, 457
Gender
    in pediatric pituitary tumors, 354
    in pituitary adenomas, 61–62, 63–65, 132–33
Gene expression, 9
Germ-cell tumors
    imaging of, 208
    pediatric
        clinical features of, 361
        irradiation of, 362
        treatment of, 361–362
Germinomas
    clinical features, 425
    clinical outcome, 428
    definition, 425
    differential diagnosis, 428
    immunohistochemistry, 427–428
    location, 425
    macroscopic features, 427
    microscopic features, 427
    radiographic features, 425–427
    therapy, 428
    ultrastructural features, 428
Giant-cell tumor of bone (GCTB), 412–413
Gigantism, 2, 298–299
    in children, 355
Gliomas
    classification, 402
    high-grade, 402–403
    imaging of, 210
    optic nerve, *see* Optic nerve gliomas
    optic pathway, *see* Optic pathway gliomas
Glomus tumor (GT), 418–419
Glucocorticoid replacement, 170

Glycoprotein hormones/SV40 large T-antigen
α-subunit, mice transgenic for, 86
Glycoprotein α-subunit (α-TSH), 334
Goiter, 333
Gonadal steroid replacement, 171
Gonadectomy, 84
Gonadotroph adenomas, 131–133, 134 *fig.*, 136 *fig.*
invasion by, 374
ISH analysis of, 157–158
octreotide for, 259
Gonadotroph cells, 100 *fig.*, 106, 107 *fig.*
Gonadotroph hyperplasia, 148, 450
Gonadotrop hormones
action, 47
chemical structure, 46
receptors, 47
secretion, 47
Gonadotropin-releasing hormone (GnRH), 47–48
analogs, 463
antagonists and, 259
neurons, 47
pulse generator activity, 47–48
receptors, 47
secretion, 47–48
Gonadotropin-releasing hormone receptor (GnRH-R) gene/SV40
large T-antigen
mice transgenic for, 86
Gonadotropins, 6–7
secretion, 48
G-proteins, 65, 72
Gramegna, A., 3
Granular cell myoblastoma
imaging of, 210–211
Granular cell tumors (GCTs), 403–405
Granulomatoses, 454
Growth hormone binding protein (GHBP)
acromegaly and, 301
Growth hormone (GH), 6, 42, 50–53
actions, 50
adenomas, 115, 117
endocrinologic remission, 240–241
recurrence, 242
surgical results, 240–242
antagonists, 463
cell adenomas
incidence of, 62, 63, 65
PRL cell adenomas and, 374
cells, 97–99
hyperplasia, 449
circadian rhythm, 52–53
deficiency, 171
dwarfism and, 203–204
excessive production, 167–168
feedback mechanisms, 295
GH₃ cell line, 83–84
HT control, 50–51
metabolic factors, 295
octreotide and, 254–255
paradoxical responses, 301–302
receptor, 295
receptor antagonists
acromegaly and, 257

Growth hormone (GH) (*cont.*)
secretion, 52–53
ectopic, in acromegaly, 300
physiology, 295–296
tumors
bromocriptine and, 191
ISH study of, 156
somatostatin analog treatment of, 222
urinary excretion, 301
Growth hormone (GH)F-1 gene, 75
Growth hormone-releasing hormones (GHRH), 51–52, 66, 71, 75
ectopic expression of, 84–85
neural control, 51–52
secretion
ectopic, in acromegaly, 299–300
test
in acromegaly, 302
Growth hormone-releasing peptides (GHRPs), 51
gsp oncogene, 461
Guanosine triphosphate, 65, 72

H

Hamartomas, 456–457
clinical features, 395
clinical outcome, 398
definition, 395
differential diagnosis, 398
gangliocytomas *vs.*, 395
imaging of, 211–212, 213 *fig.*
immunohistochemical features, 395
location, 395
macroscopic features, 395
microscopic features, 395
radiographic features, 395
therapy, 398
ultrastructural features, 398
Hand-Schüller-Christian disease, 419–420
Hardy, Jules, 4–5, 225
Hemangioblastomas, 417–418
Hemangiopericytomas, 413–414
Hematoxylin and eosin (H&E) stain, 92–93
Hemianopia
binasal, 181
bitemporal, 180, 186 *fig.*
homonymous, 181
monocular, 181, 183 *fig.*
Hemifield slide phenomena, 184, 186 *fig.*
Hemolytic plaque assay, 9
Hereditary hypertrophic osteoarthropathy, 1
Histiocytosis, 419–421
Histochemistry, 91–93
Homonymous hemianopia, 181
Hormone replacement therapy in pediatric pituitary tumors, 357
Hormone secretion, 9, 41–42
rhythms of, 43
Horsley, V., 4
H-*ras* gene, 461
Hst gene, 76
Human β-actin/HPV oncogene type 16 E6/E7 ORFs
mice transgenic for, 87
Human β-thyrotropin (hTSH)/SV40T antigen
mice transgenic for, 86

Hutchinson, W., 2
Hybridization, 155
   in situ, see In situ hybridization
Hypercortisolism, 168, 242–243, 319, 325
Hyperplasia, 145–148, 449–450
   ACTH cell, 449–450
   corticotroph, 146
   GH cell, 449
   gonadotroph, 148, 450
   imaging, 211
   lactotroph, 145–146, 239
   pituitary, 145–148, 449–450
   PRL cell, 449
   somatotroph, 145, 146 *fig.,* 147 *fig.*
   thyrotroph, 146–148
   TSH cell, 450
   types of, 450 *table,* 451 *table*
Hyperprolactinemia, *see also* Prolactinomas
   in acromegaly, 302–303
   bromocriptine for, 248
   causes, 167
   ectopic, 283
   eutopic, 282–283
   with medium-large adenomas, 222–223
   pathologic, 282
   physiologic, 281–282
Hyperprolactinemic endocrine syndrome, 280–281
Hyperthyroidism, 147 *fig.,* 168, 333, 338–339
Hypertrophic pulmonary osteoarthropathy, 1
Hypogonadism, 166, 167, 169
Hyponatremia, 171
Hypophysis
   blood supply of, 44–45
Hypophysitis
   idiopathic granulomatous, 452–453
   Langerhans,' 453–454
   lymphocytic, 190, 452
   secondary, 453
   xanthomatous, 453
Hypopituitarism, 325, 334
   following radiation therapy, 275
   iatrogenic, 236
Hypothalamic hamartomas, *see* Hamartomas
Hypothalamoadenohypophysial systems, 41–42, 46–54
Hypothalamohypophysial system, 41–43
Hypothalamoneurohypophysial system, 41, 42, 45–46
Hypothalamus (HT)
   anatomy of, 43–44
   role in pituitary adenomas, 66, 71
   surgical injury to, 235
Hypothyroidism, 146–147
   pituitary tumor and, 339–340

I

Idiopathic granulomatous hypophysitis, 452–453
Imaging, 463, *see also* Computed tomography (CT) scanning;
      Magnetic resonance imaging (MRI)
   cavernous angiomas (CAs), 417
   chordomas, 410
   clinically nonfunctioning adenomas, 344, 345–347 *fig.*
   craniopharyngiomas, 387
      pediatric, 358, 359 *fig.*

Imaging (*cont.*)
   dermoid cysts, 393
   epidermoid cysts, 392–393
   fibromas, 415
   fibrosarcomas, 416
   gangliocytomas, 394
   germinomas, 425–427
   giant-cell tumor of bone (GCTB), 413
   granular cell tumors (GCTs), 403–404
   hamartomas, 395–397
   hemangioblastomas, 417–418
   hemangiopericytomas, 413
   of high-grade gliomas, 402
   Langerhans cell histiocytosis, 420
   lymphomas, 422
   melanomas, 211
   meningiomas, 208–210, 406, 407 *fig.*
   myxomas, 414–415
   nasopharyngeal carcinoma, 389
   olfactory neuroblastomas, 398
   optic nerve gliomas, 401
   osteogenic sarcomas, 416
   pilocytic astrocytomas, 399
   pituitary tumors, 201–215
      pediatric, 356
   Rathke's cleft cyst (RCC), 390
   of schwannomas, 405
   teratomas, *fig.,* 429
Immunocytochemistry
   controls in, 94–95
Immunoelectron microscopy, 9, 95–96
Immunohistochemistry, 7–8, 93–95
   chordomas, 410
   germinomas, 427–428
   hamartomas, 395
   lymphomas, 423
   meningiomas, 408–409
   optic nerve gliomas, 401–402
   pituitary tumors, 93–95, 113
   Rathke's cleft cysts (RCCs), 390–391
Inferior petrosal sinus sampling (IPSS), 321–322
Inflammatory lesions, 450–454
Infradian rhythms, 43
Infundibulum, 29, 43–44
In situ hybridization, 96, 97
   analyses of pituitary tumors, 156–158
   controls in, 155–156
   signal detection in, 155
   tissue preparation and processing, 155
Insulin-like growth factors (IGFs), 50
   IGF-1, 50, 296
      acromegaly and, 301
   IGF-BP, 296
   IGF-BP3
      acromegaly and, 301
Intercavernous venous connections, 25, 27
Internal carotid artery, 35
Interstitial radiation, 326
Intrasellar arachnoid cysts, 187, 194
Invasion, 369–370
   acidophil stem-cell adenomas, 374
   corticotroph cell adenomas, 374

Invasion (*cont.*)
cytogenetics and, 377
ectopic adenomas, 377
GH cell–PRL cell adenomas, 374
gonadotrophic cell adenomas, 374
molecular markers, 377
null-cell adenomas, 377
plurihormonal adenomas, 376–377
by PRL cell adenomas, 370, 374
proliferation marker expression, 377
silent subtype III adenomas, 377
TSH cell adenomas, 374, 376
Ionizing radiation
tumorigenesis and, 83–84
Irradiation
in acromegaly, 304
in Cushing's disease, 325–326
of pediatric craniopharyngiomas, 358
of pediatric germ-cell tumors, 362

J

Junctional scotoma of Traquair, 181

K

Kernohan and Sayre's atlas, 6
Ketoconazole, 257–258, 326
Kovacs and Horvath's atlas, 8

L

Lactotroph adenomas, 100 *fig.*, 120–121, 122 *fig.*, 143, 145 *fig.*
hyperplasia of, 145–146, 239
Lamina terminalis, 30, 38
Langerhans cell histiocytosis
clinical features, 420
clinical outcome, 421
definition, 419
differential diagnosis, 421
imaging of, 212–213
immunocytochemistry, 421
location, 419–420
macroscopic features, 420–421
microscopic features, 421
radiographic features, 420
therapy, 421
ultrastructural features, 421
Langerhans hypophysitis, 453–454
Lanreotide, 256
Letterer-Siwe disease, 420
Loss of heterozygosity (LOH), 66, 73–74
Luteinizing hormone (LH), 6, 41–42, 48
Lymphocytic adenohypophysitis
imaging of, 213–214
Lymphocytic hypophysitis, 190, 452
Lymphomas
clinical features, 422
clinical outcome, 423
definition, 422
differential diagnosis, 423
immunohistochemistry, 423
location, 422
macroscopic features, 422
microscopic features, 422

Lymphomas (*cont.*)
radiographic features, 422
staining, 422–423
ultrastructural features, 423

M

Macroadenomas
bromocriptine and, 249 *table*
cabergoline and, 253
classification, 226
definition, 112
imaging, 204–205, 206 *fig.*
surgery, 233–234, 322
Macroprolactinomas, 239
DA-agonist therapy for, 288–289
pregnancy and, 290–291
surgery for, 289
therapy for, 288–289
Magnetic resonance imaging (MRI), 169, *see also* Computed tomography (CT) scanning; Imaging
of craniopharyngiomas, 207–208
CT *vs.*, 201
of cystic lesions, 211
of diabetes insipidus, 214
dynamic, 204, 205 *fig.*
gadolinium-enhanced, 356
of germ-cell tumors, 208
of gliomas, 210
of granular cell myoblastomas, 210–211
of hypothalamic hamartomas, 211–212, 213 *fig.*
of lymphocytic adenohypophysitis, 213–214
of meningiomas, 208–210
of pituitary abscesses, 214
of pituitary adenomas, 204–207
of pituitary gland, 201–203
of pituitary hyperplasia, 211
of pituitary metastases, 208–210
of primary sellar melanomas, 211
of thyrotroph microadenomas, 334
of vascular and ischemic lesions, 215
Mamillary bodies, 29
Mamillary region, 44
Mammosomatotroph adenomas, 121, 124, 125 *fig.*, 355
MAO-B enzyme, 219, 223
Marie, Pierre, 1–2
Marie-Bamberger's disease, 1
McCune-Albright syndrome
acromegaly and, 300
in children, 355
Medial posterior choroidal arteries, 36
Medical therapy, 142–145, 170–172, *see also names of specific tumors*
future, 463
for pediatric optic pathway gliomas, 361
Melanomas, 431–432
imaging, 211
MEN 1, *see* Multiple endocrine neoplasia type 1 (MEN 1)
Meningiomas
clinical features, 406
definition, 406
differential diagnosis, 409
imaging of, 208–210

Meningiomas (*cont.*)
  immunohistochemistry, 408–409
  location, 406
  macroscopic features, 406, 408
  microscopic features, 408
  radiographic features, 406, 407 *fig*
  therapy, 409
  ultrastructural features, 409
Meningohypophyseal trunk, 26
C-L-methionine, 219, 220, 222–223
Metyrapone, 258, 320–321, 326
Microadenomas
  bromocriptine and, 250
  classification, 226
  definition, 107, 112
  imaging, 204
  pituitary hyperplasia *vs.,* 449
  surgery, 234, 322–323
Microprolactinomas, 239
  DA-agonist therapy for, 287–288
  postoperative persistent disease, 288
  pregnancy and, 290
  surgery for, 288
  therapy for, 287–288
Microwave fixation, 94
Milk secretion, 7
Mitotane (*o,p'*DDD), 258, 326
Monocular hemianopia, 181
Mucoceles, 454
Multiple endocrine neoplasia type 1 (MEN 1)
  acromegaly and, 300
  gene, 66, 74
  suppressor gene, 461
  syndrome, 76
Multiple myelomas, 423–425
Myxomas, 414–415

N

Nasopharyngeal carcinoma (NPC), 389–390
Nelson's syndrome, 243
  corticotrophic adenomas in, 374
  presentation, 327
  radiation therapy for, 273
  surgery for, 327
  treatment, 327
Neurohormones, 42
Neuro-ophthalmology, 173–195
Neurosecretion, 41–43
Neurosurgery, 169–170, *see also* Surgery
Nonfunctioning adenomas, *see* Clinically nonfunctioning adenomas
Nonparetic diplopia, 184
Northern blot hybridization, 155
Nuclear oncogenes, 73
Nucoceles, 392
Null-cell adenomas, 63 *table,* 65, 133–134, 136–137 *fig.*
  invasion by, 377
  ISH analysis of, 157–158
  oncocytic variant, 133–34, 138 *fig.*
Null cells, 106, 108 *fig.*

O

Octreotide, 143, 170, 463
  acromegaly and, 255–256, 304, 305–306
  adverse effects, 256–257
  beneficial effects, 306
  bromocriptine and, 306
  bromocriptine with, 257
  for Cushing's disease, 258
  gallstones and, 257, 306
  gastrointestinal effects, 256–257
  GH levels and, 254–255
  for gonadotroph adenomas, 259
  pharmacology of, 254–255
  pregnancy and, 255
  resistance, 305–306
  side effects, 306
  sleep apnea and, 256
  with thyrotroph adenomas, 338
  thyrotropin-secreting adenomas and, 259–260
  visual function and, 191
Olfactory neuroblastomas, 398–399
Oncogenes
  nuclear, 73
  ras, 72–73
Onococytic adenomas
  ISH analysis of, 157–158
Ophthalmic artery, 36
Ophthalmoplegia, 195
Optic atrophy, 181, 184, 192
Optic chiasm, 29, 34–35
  anatomy, 174–175
  axons in, 175
  embryology of, 173–174
  pathophysiology, 177
  vascular supply, 176–177
Optic nerve
  axons in, 175
  incipient compression, 184
  intracranial
    vascular supply of, 176–177
  pathophysiology of, 177
Optic nerve gliomas
  clinical features, 401
  clinical outcome, 402
  definition, 401
  differential diagnosis, 402
  immunohistochemistry, 401–402
  location, 401
  macroscopic features, 401
  microscopic features, 401
  radiographic features, 401
  staining, 401–402
  therapy, 402
  ultrastructural features, 402
Optic pathway gliomas, pediatric
  chemotherapy for, 361
  clinical features, 360
  radiation therapy for, 361
  treatment, 361
Optic tracts
  axons in, 176
Osteoarthropathy, 1

Osteogenic sarcomas, 416–417
Oxytocin (OT)
    chemical structure, 45
    physiological action, 46
    receptors, 45, 46

P

Pachydermoperistosis, 1
Paragangliomas, 429, 431
Parasellar lesions
    differential diagnosis of, 357–363
Parasellar tumors
    symptoms, 177–179
Parasitic infections, 454
Parasitoses, 454
Paretic diplopia, 184–185
Pars distalis, 41
Pars intermedia, 41
Pars tuberalis, 41
Paul, F.T., 4
PCR, *see* Polymerase chain reaction (PCR)
Pediatric pituitary tumors, 353–364
    age and, 353–354
    bromocriptine in, 357
    endocrinological investigations, 355–356
    epidemiology, 353–354
    gender and, 354
    hormone replacement therapy in, 357
    imaging in, 356
    petrosal sinus in, 357
    sphenoid sinus in, 357
    surgical treatment in, 356–357
    treatment outcome, 357
Pegvisomant, 306
Pergolide, 222, 252, 286
Periodic acid-Schiff (PAS) stain, 92 *fig.,* 93
Peroxidase-antiperoxidase (PAP) method, 93, 94
Petrosal sinus
    in pediatric pituitary tumors, 357
p53 gene, 74
Pharmaceutical therapy, *see* Medical therapy
Pilocytic astrocytomas, 399–401
p18^{Ink4c} gene, 87
Pit-1 gene, 75
Pit-1/SV40 large T-antigen
    mice transgenic for, 87
Pituitary abscesses, 190
    imaging of, 214
Pituitary adenomas, 107–113, *see also* Pituitary tumors
    age and, 61, 63–65
    aggressiveness, 113, 140
    anatomic diagnosis, 227
    apoplexy of, 139–140, 142 *fig.*
    CGH hybridization, 160
    clonal analysis, 158
    clonality of, 71–72
    cytogenetic analyses, 160
    diagnosis, 91
        roentgenograms in, 3
    dynamic studies of, 204
    ectopic, 207

Pituitary adenomas (*cont.*)
    endocrine diagnosis, 226–227
    endocrine effects, 166–167
    extension patterns, 369
    gender and, 61–62, 63–65, 132–33
    growth patterns in, 369–377
    hemorrhage of, 205–207
    hypothalamic role in, 66, 71
    imaging, 4, 204–207
    immunohistochemical classification, 113
    incidence, 57–61
    infarction of, 205–207
    intraoperative methods, 113–115
        frozen section, 113–115, 116 *fig.*
        permanent sections, 113–115
        smear preparations, 113–115, 116 *fig.*
    invasion by, 369–370
    management, 169–172
    manifestations, 165
    medical therapy, 142–145
    medical treatment of, 8
    molecular analysis, 160
    MRI *vs.* CT, 204–207
    neural metaplasia in, 138–139, 141 *fig.*
    pathogenesis of, 65–66
    pathology
        classifications, 112–113
        electron microscopy, 95–96
        genetic methods, 97
        histochemical techniques, 91–93
        host animal transplants, 97
        immunohistochemical techniques, 93–95
        molecular biologic methods, 97
        optic methods, 97
        reverse hemolytic plaque assay (RHPA), 96
        in situ hybridization technique, 96, 97
    PCR analysis, 159
    plasmacytomas *vs.,* 425
    presentation of, 225–226
    prevalence, 57–61
    prognosis, 172
    radiation therapy, 3–4, 142, 171–172, 195
    radiologic classification, 226
    radiology, 4
    silent, 134–135, 138, 140 *fig.,* 141 *fig.*
    size, 107, 112
    specimen handling, 383
    SSCP analysis, 159–160
    subclinical, 5–6, 63
    surgery, 4–5, 140, 142
    time trends, 61
    treatment effects, 140, 142–145
    treatment objectives, 227
    types of
        incidence of, 62–63
    WHO classification, 113, 115 *table*
    women and, 61
Pituitary apoplexy, 188–190, 195, 227
Pituitary carcinomas, 8–9, 377–382
Pituitary gland
    anatomy, 20, 25, 28–29
    congenital anomalies, 203–204

Pituitary gland (*cont.*)
  development of, 353
  function of
    history, 1
  hypoplasia of, 203
  imaging, 207
  metastasis to, 211
  normal
    imaging of, 201–203
  postsurgical appearance, 207
  pregnancy and, 203
  transcription factors in, 161
Pituitary hyperplasia, *see* Hyperplasia
Pituitary incidentalomas, 347, 349, 350–351 *table*
Pituitary infections, 454
Pituitary oncocytoma, 133–34, 138 *fig.*
Pituitary tumors, *see also* Pituitary adenomas
  acromegaly and, 5
  found at autopsy, 5–6, 63–65
  in children, 65, 353–364
  diagnosis, 165–169
  experimental models, 81–88
  extra-ocular muscle (EOM) palsy in, 189
  future perspectives, 461–464
  gene therapy, 463–464
  imaging of, 201–215
  ISH analyses of, 156–158
  management of
    visual outcomes, 190–195
  molecular biological methods, 155–161
  mutations, 461–463
  neuro-ophthalmologic evaluation, 173–195
  pathogenesis, 461–463
  prevalence, 165
  recurrences, 223
  size of, 63
  surgical removal, 233–234
  symptoms, 177–179
  targeted oncogenesis and, 85–87
  transgenic models and, 84–87
Pituitary tumor-transforming gene (PTTG), 65–66, 73, 463
$p27^{Kip\ 1}$ gene, 87, 462
Plasmacytomas, 423–425
Plurihormonal adenomas, 130–131, 132 *fig.*
  invasion by, 376–377
Polymerase chain reaction (PCR), 9
 analysis of pituitary adenomas, 159
Polyoma early region/polyoma large T-antigen
  mice transgenic for, 87
Polytomography, 201
Positron emission tomography (PET)
  in prolactinomas, 220–221
  in sellar tumors, 219–224
Posterior cerebral arteries, 36
Posterior choroidal arteries
  medial, 36
Posterior communicating artery, 36
Pregnancy
  bromocriptine and, 240, 251–252, 289–291
  macroprolactinomas and, 290–291
  microprolactinomas and, 290
  octreotide and, 255

Pregnancy (*cont.*)
  pituitary adenomas in
    visual dysfunction and, 187–188, 194–195
    pituitary gland and, 203
    prolactinomas and, 239–240, 289–291
Primary cell melanoma
  imaging of, 211
Progesterone replacement, 171
Prolactinomas, 8, *see also* Macroprolactinomas;
    Microprolactinomas
  alternative medical therapy for, 286
  alternative tumor ablative therapy for, 286
  bromocriptine for, 247–252, 285–285
  cabergoline for, 252–253, 286
  in children, 354
  clinical features, 280–281
  cystic, 238
  DA therapIES, 269–270
  DA therapies, 221–222
  diagnosis
    approach to, 283–284
    differential, 281–283
    laboratory evaluation, 283
    radiologic evaluation, 283
  dopaminergic therapy for, 237
  fertility and, 239–240, 289
  incidence of, 62, 63, 65
    in children, 65
  mass effects, 281
  medical therapy, 247–253, 285–285
  pathology of, 279–280
  pergolide for, 252, 286
  PET in, 220–221
  postoperative recurrence, 239
  pregnancy and, 239–240, 289–291
  prolactin-provocative tests, 283
  quinagolide for, 252, 286
  radiation therapy, 269–270, 287–289
  serum prolactin test, 283
  surgery, 269, 286
  surgical indicators, 238
  therapeutic objectives, 284–285
  "unsuspected," 281
Prolactin (PRL), 6, 7, 42, 53, 222, *see also*
    Hyperprolactinemia
  action, 53
  in children, 356
  circadian rhythm, 54
  feedback control, 54
  HT control, 53–54
  hypersecretion of, 167
  secretion, 53, 54
Prolactin (PRL) cell adenomas
  invasive growth, 370, 374
Prolactin (PRL) cell carcinomas, 377, 378, 381
Prolactin (PRL) cell hyperplasia, 449
Prolactin (PRL) cells, 99
Prolactin (PRL)-producing adenomas, 120–121, 144 *fig.*
Prolactin (PRL)-secreting tumors
  ISH study of, 156

Pro-opiomelanocortin (POMC) messenger RNA expression (POMC mRNA), 156–157
Protein kinase C (PKC), 72, 461
Psammoma bodies, 408
p53 suppressor gene, 461
Purine binding factor (nm23) gene, 66

Q

Quinagolide, 222, 252, 286

R

C-raclopride, 219, 220–221
Radiation therapy, 142, 171–172, 195
    of acromegaly, 270–271
    with clinically nonfunctioning adenomas, 347
    complications following, 275
    for Cushing's disease, 272
    Cushing's disease and, 325–326
    hypopituitarism following, 275
    for Nelson's syndrome, 273
    for nonfunctioning adenomas, 273–274
    for pediatric optic pathway gliomas, 361
    of pituitary adenomas, 3–4
    for prolactinomas, 287–289
    of prolactinomas, 269–270
    of thyrotroph adenomas, 336–338
Radiography, 201
Radioimmunoassays, 7
Ras oncogenes, 72–73
Rathke's cleft cysts (RCCs), 187, 194, 213 fig., 455
    clinical features, 390
    clinical outcome, 392
    definition, 390
    differential diagnosis, 392
    epidermoid cysts vs., 393
    immunohistochemistry, 390–391
    location, 390
    macroscopic features, 390
    microscopic features, 390
    pediatric, 362–363
    radiographic features, 390
    remnants, 106, 111 fig.
    stains, 390
    therapy, 392
    ultrastructural features, 392
Restriction fragment-length polymorphism (RFLP), 158
Reticulin stain, 93, 117 fig.
Retinoblastoma (Rb) gene, 66, 74, 87
Reverse hemolytic plaque assay (RHPA), 96
Rhinorrhea
    cerebrospinal fluid (CSF), 235
mRNA, 9, 65–66, 155–157

S

Salivary gland remnants, 107, 111 fig.
Sandostatin-LAR, 256
Sarcoidosis, 453
Sarcomas, see also Chondrosarcomas; Fibrosarcomas
    osteogenic, 416–417
Schwannomas, 405–406
Scintigraphy, 463
    in acromegaly, 302

See-saw nystagmus, 185
Sellar region
    anatomy, 13–26, 174
    surgery in, 232–234
Silent adenomas, 134–135, 138, 140 fig., 141 fig., 377
Silver techniques, in histochemistry, 93
Single-strand confirmation polymorphism (SSCP), 159–160
    of pituitary adenomas, 159–160
Sinonasal undifferentiated carcinoma (SNUC), 389–390
Sinuses
    basilar, 25
    cavernous, 25–26, 28–29
    petrosal, 357
    sphenoid, 15–16, 357
    venous, 25
Sinus histiocytosis with massive lymphadenopathy (SHML), 421
Sleep apnea
    octreotide and, 256
Sodium valproate, 258
Somatostatin (SMS), 8, 49, 51, 75
    analogs, 143–145, 171, 222, 305–306
    thyrotropin-secreting adenomas and, 259
Somatotroph adenomas, 117–119, see also Acromegaly; Gigantism
    in children, 355
    densely granulated, 117–118
    sparsely granulated, 118–119
Somatotroph hyperplasia, 145, 146 fig., 147 fig.
Somatotroph-lactotroph adenomas, 121, 123–124
Southern blot hybridization, 155
Sphenoid bone
    anatomy, 13–15
Sphenoidotomy, 232–233
Sphenoid sinus
    anatomy, 15–16
    in pediatric pituitary tumors, 357
    surgical approaches, 231–232
Squamous metaplasia
    of adenohypophysial cells, 106
SSCP, see Single-strand confirmation polymorphism (SSCP)
Stellate cells, 106, 109 fig.
Stereotactic radiosurgery (SRS), 274–275
    in acromegaly, 304
Suppressor genes, 73–74
    inactivation of, 66, 87
Suprachiasmatic nucleus, 43
Suprachiasmatic zone, 43
Suprasellar region
    anatomy, 26–40
    arteries, 35–36, 37–38
    neural relationships, 26
    venous relationships, 36, 39–40
Surgery, 140, 142, 169–170
    for acromegaly, 271, 303–304
    approaches
        choosing, 228–231
        transsphenoidal, 231–236
    arterial damage from, 235
    brainstem injury from, 236
    cavernous sinus injury from, 235
    complications, 234–236
    contraindications for, 228
    CSF rhinorrhea from, 235

Surgery, 140, 142, 169–170 (*cont.*)
    for Cushing's disease, 272, 322–325
    extracranial approaches, 237
    history, 225
    HT injury from, 235
    hypopituitarism from, 236
    indications for, 227–228
    of macroadenomas, 322
    of macroprolactinomas, 289
    of microadenomas, 322–323
    of microprolactinomas, 288
    nasal complications, 236
    for Nelson's syndrome, 327
    for nonfunctioning adenomas, 273–274
    for pediatric craniopharyngiomas, 358, 360
    for pediatric pituitary tumors, 356–357
    postoperative care, 234
    preoperative evaluation, 228
    for prolactinomas, 269, 286
    pterional approach, 236–237
    reoperation, 236
    results
        clinically nonfunctioning tumors, 244
        corticotroph adenomas, 242–243
        GH-secreting PIT adenomas, 240–244
        prolactin-producing PIT tumors, 239–240
        thyrotroph adenomas, 243–244
    skull base approaches, 237
    of thyrotroph adenomas, 336
    transcranial approaches, 236–237
    transsphenoidal, 169, 231–236
        visual outcomes, 192, 193
    visual outcomes, 191–192, 235
Syndrome of inappropriate antidiuretic secretion (SIADH), 167

T

Teratomas, 428–429, 430 *fig.*
Testosterone replacement, 171
Thalamoperforating arteries, 36
Third ventricle, 26
    anterior wall, 30
    arteries of, 37
    floor, 26, 29–30
    neural relationships, 26
    posterior wall, 30
    venous system and, 36
Thryrotropin, 7
Thyroidectomy, 84
Thyroid hormone replacement, 171
Thyrotroph adenomas, 129–130
    DA therapy with, 338
    endocrine testing, 334–335
    incidence, 333
    medical therapy, 338
    microadenomas, 334
    morphological studies, 335–336
    octreotide and, 259–260
    octreotide with, 338
    presentation, 333–334
    radiotherapy of, 336–338
    somatostatin and, 259
    surgery, 336
    surgical results, 243–244
    in vitro studies, 335

Thyrotroph cells, 103, 105–106
Thyrotroph hyperplasia, 146–148
Thyrotropin, 42, 48–49
    circadian rhythm, 49
    HT control, 48–49
Thyrotropin-releasing hormone (TRH), 48–49, 75
    TSH and, 334
Thyrotropin-stimulating hormone (TSH), 42, 48–49
    adenomas, 129–130
        incidence of, 62, 63 *table,* 65
        invasion by, 374. 376
    cell hyperplasia, 450
    cells, 103, 105–106
    loss of production, 166
    secretion, 333–339
    somatostatin and, 222, 259
    TRH test, 334
Transcranial surgery
    visual outcomes, 192, 194
Transcription factors, in pituitary gland, 161
Transforming growth factor-α (TGF-α), 76
Transgenic models, 9
    mice, 84–87
Transnasal resection
    visual outcomes of, 194
Trichrome stains, 93
Trilostane, 326
Trimethylaniline
    tumorigenesis and, 83
Tuber cinereum, 29
Tuberculomas, 454
Tuberculum sella meningiomas, 187, 194
Tumorigenesis, 65–66
    calcitonin and, 83
    estrogen and, 81–83
    experimental models, 81–88
    gonadectomy and, 84
    ionizing radiation and, 83–84
    suppressor genes and, 87
    thyroidectomy and, 84
    transgenic models and, 84–87
    trimethylaniline, 81–83

V

Vascular lesions, 456
Vasoactive-intestinal peptide (VIP), 53
Vasopressin (VP)
    chemical structure, 45
    physiological action, 46
    receptors, 45–46
Venous sampling, 321–322
Venous sinuses, 25
Venous system, 36, 39–40
Visual field syndrome, 179–181, 192
Visual hallucinations, 185
Visual outcomes
    age and, 192–193
    bromocriptine and, 190–191
    craniopharyngomias, 194
    duration of symptoms and, 192
    empty sella syndrome, 195
    in management of tumors, 190–195
    meningiomas, 194
    pituitary apoplexy and, 195

Visual outcomes (*cont.*)
    pregnancy and, 194–195
    prognostic factors, 192
    Rathke's cleft cysts (RCCs), 194
    reoperation and, 193
    after surgery, 191–92, 193–194
        pediatric, 194
        transcranial, 192, 194
        transnasal resection, 194
        transsphenoidal, 192, 193, 235
    tumor size and type, 193

Visual symptoms, 165–166, 177–184
Von Recklinghausen's disease, 401

W

Wilbrand's knee, 175–176, 180–181
World Health Organization
    brain tumor classification, 402
    classification of pituitary adenomas, 113, 115 *table*

X

Xanthomatous hypophysitis, 453